HEALTH ASSESSMENT

Health Assessment

LOIS MALASANOS, R.N., Ph.D.

Professor and Dean, College of Nursing, University of Florida,
Gainesville, Florida

VIOLET BARKAUSKAS, R.N., C.N.M., M.P.H., Ph.D.

Associate Professor, School of Nursing, University of Michigan,
Ann Arbor, Michigan

MURIEL MOSS, R.N., M.A.

Public Health Nurse, South Central District Health Department,
Twin Falls, Idaho; formerly Assistant Professor, Department of
Public Health Nursing, College of Nursing,
University of Illinois at the Medical Center,
Chicago, Illinois

KATHRYN STOLTENBERG-ALLEN, R.N., M.S.N.

Coordinator of Hospice Planning, Lutheran Hospital,
Moline, Illinois; formerly Assistant Professor, Department of
Public Health Nursing, College of Nursing,
University of Illinois at the Medical Center,
Chicago, Illinois

SECOND EDITION

With **934** illustrations and **5** color plates

The C. V. Mosby Company

ST. LOUIS • TORONTO • LONDON   1981

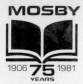

MOSBY

1906 **75** 1981
YEARS

A TRADITION OF PUBLISHING EXCELLENCE

SECOND EDITION

Copyright © 1981 by The C. V. Mosby Company

All rights reserved. No part of this book may be reproduced in any manner without written permission of the publisher.

Previous edition copyrighted 1977

Printed in the United States of America

The C. V. Mosby Company
11830 Westline Industrial Drive, St. Louis, Missouri 63141

Library of Congress Cataloging in Publication Data

Main entry under title:

Health assessment.

    Bibliography: p.
    Includes index.
    1. Nursing. 2. Medical history taking. 3. Physical diagnosis. I. Malasanos, Lois, 1928-   [DNLM:
1. Medical history taking. 2. Physical examination.
WB 205 H434]
RT48.H4   1981   616.07'5   80-27518
ISBN 0-8016-3073-8

GW/VH/VH 9 8 7 6 5   03/C/320

To our families and friends—
who encouraged and sustained us, and

To our students—
who persisted in their efforts to find knowledge
enabling them to provide better health care to their clients

Preface

This text is designed for students and beginning practitioners who are learning skills that will enable them to assess the health status of the client by obtaining a health history and performing a physical examination. Clinical skills are best acquired when learning experiences are organized and the learner is provided with opportunities to gain knowledge and to practice with experienced preceptors in settings that enhance learning (for example, a laboratory where learners can practice their new skills with each other or a clinical setting where the clients have been informed of the learner's purpose and have agreed to participate). Therefore, this text is intended for use in conjunction with structured learning experiences enabling the learner to acquire the theory and skills of health assessment.

Health assessment skills are useful to the practitioner in any clinical setting. However, this text is especially aimed at helping the student or practitioner who is preparing for a role in primary care, where the health maintenance of the client is a priority. The focus is on wellness, and the parameters of normal health are incorporated into the process of obtaining a health history and performing a physical examination. The discussion of selected problems is also included in the text as a way of demonstrating differences or deviations from the parameters of normal health. Within the framework of health maintenance, emphasis is placed on the early detection of changes in the health status of the client for the purpose of preventing a more serious problem or disability. This is compatible with the plan to assist the learner in defining the parameters of wellness and subtle or gross deviations that occur in illness.

The consumer of health care is referred to as the *client* in this text because the term implies the ability of a person, whether well or sick, to contract for health care as a responsible participant with the providers of health care. The label *patient* has been avoided because it has traditionally been used to describe someone who is ill and therefore more likely to be a dependent receiver of care. Health care providers can no longer expect consumers of care to accept health advice or treatment plans unless they have been included in the decision making process. Thus, the use of the term *client* is more appropriate in today's health care milieu.

This text is intended as a guide to assist the learner in conceptualizing the assessment of the whole person, taking into account the parameters of good health practices and the factors that impinge on health. The assessment that incorporates these components provides a basis for the development of an optimal plan for health care and health teaching that is reasonable in terms of the individual client's life situation.

To further intensify and update this commitment to the *whole person* and to instill, through the health assessment process, the individual's participation in his own health maintenance, this revision includes the Life Health Monitoring Plan (by Breslow and Somers), a preventive health care plan for the entire life of the individual. Presented in the form of goals and activities for the health care provider, the Life Health Monitoring Plan offers a definition of health care organized around the ten periods of a person's life.

The chapters on the components of the assessment, including the history, physical examination, and aspects of daily health care—nutrition and sleep—and the developmental assessment are organized in the beginning portion of the text so that the practitioner can gain an appreciation of the whole person and some aspects of individual life-styles before proceeding to the more specific assessment of the body systems.

A discussion of the purposes and techniques of interviewing precedes the chapter on the health history in order that the learner may become more sensitive to the process of obtaining information within the framework of a beginning or continuing relationship with the client. As communication is the basis for obtaining this information, the possession of keen communication skills means the difference between haphazard and effective information gathering. Therefore, within the chapter on interviews, renewed emphasis is placed on respect for empathy with the client.

Finally, the learner is encouraged to consider specific ways of organizing the assessment and of recording the data obtained. There is little value in obtaining information that is lost to the practitioner or other members of the health team at a future time when it may be of critical importance as part of an overall data base from which problems are identified and actions planned.

Because technology constantly affects the practice of health care, it is important to assess the relationship. Therefore a section on computer-assisted histories has been included, not as a replacement for written and oral health histories, but as a viable "other" approach to obtaining necessary client health histories. It is also necessary to realize that technology affects not only the practice of health care but also the health care itself. Out of this realization has grown the field of occupational medicine. The potential threat of technology to individual health prompted the inclusion of a new table, "Health Hazards of the Workplace," and a dictionary of industrial chemicals in an appendix for the benefit of the practitioner.

Stress, another manifestation of technology on individual health, is also a consideration in the assessment of health care and must be recognized as a factor in dealing with the whole person. In an attempt to assess life stresses and their relationship to the individual's susceptibility to physical and psychological problems, two tools, the Recent Life Change Questionnaire (Rahe) and the Life Experiences Survey (Sarason, Johnson, and Siegel) are included in Chapter 4, "Developmental Assessment."

New to this edition are several additions to the assessment of specific body systems. The chapter on the respiratory system includes a comprehensive new table, "Assessment Findings Frequently Associated with Common Lung Conditions." Two new sections, one dealing with murmurs and the other with hypertension, are included in the chapter on cardiovascular assessment.

The section concerning examination of joints has been expanded. "Health Assessment of the Prenatal Client" is a totally new chapter and throughout this edition new illustrations aid in the depiction of the health assessment process for the learning practitioner. Color plates have been added to further approach reality through illustration.

For the techniques utilized to assess the health of the client, we have described the standard as well as newer techniques of history taking and the use of inspection, both direct and with instruments (for example, the otoscope and ophthalmoscope), palpation, percussion, and auscultation. In addition, we have made an effort to expand on the techniques and to describe the instruments. For example, the client's history not only includes the chief complaint, present illness, review of systems, and so on, but also focuses on the daily patterns of activity and sleep and on the developmental stage or level of the individual. In those sections where the use of examination techniques (including instrumentation) pertains, those techniques and instruments are described; for example, the techniques of percussion are discussed in the chapter on the respiratory tract examination, a description of the ophthalmoscope is found in the chapter on the eye examination, a description on the otoscope accompanies the chapter on the ear examination, and material on the stethoscope accompanies the chapter on the cardiovascular examination. Thus, a discussion of the various techniques utilized in health assessment is presented with the system relevant to that technique.

Many people have contributed to the development of this text. Without their support and assistance it would not have been possible. Carrie Schopf, M.D., was our reviewer, supporter, and teacher for the first edition. Those who have provided support, review, and suggestion for the second edition are: Lawrence Allen, M.D., Robert Milas, M.D., Mary E. Milas, R.N., M.S.N., Nancy Lee, R.N., M.S.N., and Joyce Roberts, R.N., C.N.M., Ph.D. Patricia Urbanus, R.N., M.S.N., our photographer, has been consistently interested and creative in helping us despite the enormous demands made on her time. Our thanks is also extended to Scott Thorn Barrows, William R. Schwarz, Robert Parshall, Christo Popoff, and Marion Howard for their outstanding artwork. In addition, the authors would like to express their appreciation to those colleagues, students, and practitioners who have suggested changes that are included in the revision.

Lois Malasanos
Violet Barkauskas
Muriel Moss
Kathryn Stoltenberg-Allen

Contents

1   **Introduction,** 1

2   **The interview,** 25

3   **The health history,** 35

4   **Developmental assessment,** 58

5   **Nutritional assessment,** 91
Savitri Kamath, Ph.D., R.D.

6   **Assessment of sleep-wakefulness patterns,** 113

7   **General assessment, including vital signs,** 128

8   **Assessment of mental status,** 161

9   **Assessment of the skin, hair, and nails,** 180

10   **Assessment of the ears, nose, and throat,** 205

11   **Assessment of the eyes,** 223

12   **Assessment of the head, face, and neck,** 246

13   **Assessment of the lymphatic system,** 256

14   **Assessment of the breasts,** 275

15   **Assessment of the respiratory system,** 289

16   **Cardiovascular assessment: the heart and the neck vessels,** 321

17   **Assessment of the abdomen,** 348

18   **Assessment of the anus and rectosigmoid region,** 376

19   **Assessment of the male genitalia and assessment of the inguinal area for hernias,** 385

20   Assessment of the female genitalia and procedures for smears and cultures, 397

21   Health assessment of the prenatal client, 418

22   Musculoskeletal assessment, 443

23   Neurological assessment, 518

24   Assessment of the pediatric client, 559
Muriel Moss, R.N., M.A.
Joanna Schleutermann, R.N., M.P.H.

25   Assessment of the aging client, 623

26   Integration of the physical assessment, 632

27   Clinical laboratory procedures, 646

Appendix A   Health hazards of the workplace, 671

B   Table of normal values, 684

Glossary, 702

Color plates *following p. 212*

1   Some common dermatoses and cutaneous manifestations of systemic disorders

2   Ear

3   Nose

4   Mouth

5   Eyes

HEALTH ASSESSMENT

1 Introduction

RECOGNITION OF THE NEED FOR HEALTH ASSESSMENT AND UNIVERSAL HEALTH CARE

As long ago as the beginning of the Civil War an article was published recommending periodic health examinations in the interest of the early detection of disease (Dobell, 1861). This concept was adopted by the American Medical Association in 1922 in the form of a resolution advocating periodic health assessment. In 1925 the procedure was formalized in a manual published by this organization.

In 1956 the declaration that health care is a basic human right was made at a White House Conference on Aging. The general public has expressed with increasing frequency the expectation that preventive health care constitutes a fundamental part of this care. Leavell and Clark have defined preventive health care in three categories: primary, secondary, and tertiary prevention. Primary prevention involves those aspects of health care that are aimed at avoiding the contraction of a disease. Secondary prevention is aimed at stopping or attenuating the process of disease, and tertiary prevention deals with rehabilitative processes. The objective of tertiary prevention is the restoration of optimal function to a person after the disease process has been arrested.

Each level of prevention is based on a thorough assessment of the client's health status. Preventive health care can be planned only from a complete data base of both the client and his family.

Government leaders emphasize the need for provision of adequate and accessible health care for all Americans regardless of their ability to pay and regardless of where they live. The two words that frequently appear in discussions relevant to this issue are equity and access.

The need to establish facilities for health care in the communities where people live is receiving more attention among legislators. The negative aspects of asking the client to travel long distances for preventive care are increasingly clear. In many cases the distance to the physician or hospital is the major determinant of whether a client seeks care. The famous anecdote among the people of Watts makes the point well. In this community in the early 1970s the cost of a taxi to the hospital was ten dollars. These people often had to be quite sick before they sought medical help. When they did go to the hospital, they referred to themselves as being "ten dollars sick."

One way in which the government of the United States has recognized the universal need for comprehensive health care has been through the encouragement of health maintenance organizations. These institutions are designed to provide preventive health care that is community based.

On the other side of the coin, physicians control health care in the United States as a result of both legislative action and tradition. Although the number of physicians has increased to 170 per 100,000 population, a number greater than at any other time in the history of this country, there are wide gaps between the consumer, the health care demands, and the capabilities of the available physicians to meet them. The major deficit is in the number of primary care physicians prepared to provide the degree of preventive health care known to be needed. Several British writers have taken the position that it is the primary care practitioner who can give preventive care most effectively.

The process of specialization in medical practice makes it increasingly more difficult for physicians to obtain salient family and community information. At this time the majority of preventive care is performed in physicians' offices and in emergency rooms.

Care essentially involves providing prescriptions and treatment for symptomatic clients.

Thus, most health care treatment in this country is oriented toward dealing with crisis situations. Health maintenance efforts are directed toward large industrial groups, antenatal women, well babies, school children, and military groups but remains on the whole a matter of individual responsibility.

ADVANTAGES OF ASSESSMENT

The value of periodic health examinations has been attested to in several studies. As early as 1921 the Metropolitan Life Insurance Company reported a 28% reduction in mortality as a result of early disease detection incurred through periodic health examinations. Studies related to disability reported in the 1960s showed a savings in employee disability payments that amounted to four times more than the cost of the examinations; the studies also showed that as much as 13% of the disease that produces disability in executives could be detected in the periodic health examination before the disability was incurred. Although later studies have failed to substantiate the wide margins suggested in these early studies, there is little doubt that the general public would benefit not only from the early detection of disease but also from the provision of a constantly updated baseline of relevant data. This information would benefit the individual by allowing a comparison of parameters obtained during a well visit with those observed during a suspected illness; this comparison would potentially afford a more accurate diagnosis. Furthermore, significant epidemiological data obtained during these examinations would be a secondary gain.

INCREASING ACCESSIBILITY TO ASSESSMENT

The health examination is frequently the mechanism of entry into the health care system. Since accessibility has been shown to be an important factor in determining whether a client will seek health care, alternate modes of providing health care to greater numbers of people have been explored.

Recent studies have indicated that although periodic health examinations have proved beneficial, they may not necessarily need to be performed by a physician. Controlled studies comparing physicians' and nurses' problem lists after they have examined the same client show no appreciable differences. The examinations are certainly less costly to the client when they are done by health care workers other than physicians. At least one author has suggested that as many as three-fourths of the clients who visit a primary care physician for health care could be

safely monitored by an allied health professional and at a considerable financial saving. It is reasonably clear that making health services available to the entire population in an effective manner will include both medical and nurse practitioners.

That there is a need to develop a core of individuals skilled in assessing the health status of persons seeking such care has been attested to by the Russians' use of Feldsher and by the utilization of public health nurses, nurse practitioners, and physicians' assistants in the United States. These nonphysician practitioners have helped to make preventive care an actuality by increasing accessibility to the system, both through increasing the number of people able to give this care and by providing care in communities that had previously been underserved. The provision of these services is evidence of sensitivity to the public's need and an effort to make health care more convenient.

These groups of health care workers have entered into situations involving varying degrees of responsibility for patient care. In all cases they are involved in the assessment of health status; there are some differences in expectations of their abilities to identify normal versus abnormal traits. In many cases standardized treatment schedules or protocols allow these individuals to render treatment and follow-up care. This can be a workable reality in those cases where the medical community has achieved consensus as to appropriate care for specific problems.

OBJECTIVES AND TYPES OF ASSESSMENT

The purposes of health assessment include surveillance of health status, the identification of latent or occult disease, screening for a specific type of disease (called *case finding*), and follow-up care.

The public has been educated and often required to seek certain health examinations, such as well baby, preschool, premarital, precollege, prenatal, preemployment, and preinsurance examinations. Both men and women in their middle years have been educated to their increased vulnerability to disease and thus seek care at this time.

Many words have developed to describe the act of health assessment. Some of these are *physical examination, health appraisal, check-up,* and *screening examination.* These types of assessment generally include a history, a physical examination, and a routine battery of clinical laboratory tests. Such appraisals are often thought of as isolated incidents. The *periodic health examination,* on the other hand, is regarded as occurring at regular intervals. A return or follow-up visit is one that is scheduled to assess the progress or abatement of diagnosed dysfunction.

Examinations performed for the purpose of case

finding are directed at significant diseases for which there is a recognized treatment. Furthermore, definitive tests or examinations should be recognized as being specific to the condition and the population tested. In addition, there should be an early symptomatic or latent stage of the disease, so that intervention will prevent progress of the disease.

INCREASING CLIENT PARTICIPATION IN HEALTH CARE

The health assessment should accurately define the health and sick care needs for the individual at that specific point in time.

The information obtained in the interview and physical examination is used to formulate the exchanges of responsibility in defining the contract. The client should be apprised of the services available that will be useful in dealing with his problems.

The findings of the health assessment are shared with the client in a clearly understandable manner. In many cases this may mean educating him to the anatomy and physiology of his diseased tissues so that he can fully understand the meaning and level of his dysfunction.

Only with a clear definition of his problem is the client capable of assuming active involvement in decision making for his own care.

The World Health Organization (WHO) has defined health education as the active mechanism of facilitating an optimal state of social, emotional, and physical functioning that should be available to all people. Patient education is implicit in preventive care.

Primary prevention may be facilitated through teaching the client the general tenets of a healthful life-style. Some of the topics that may be explained are the optimal nutritional habits, sleep-activity patterns, exercise regimens, and recreational patterns. The client may also be warned against such potentially dangerous health patterns as smoking and diets typified by high sugar content.

The adolescent may particularly benefit by educational efforts concerning alcohol, drugs, and sexuality.

Genetic counseling may be considered one form of primary prevention, the need for which may become apparent during the course of the health assessment.

Several authors contend that individuals should be educated to the most common problems experienced by the general public in their particular geographical locale in order to take care of themselves more effectively. Moreover, the public needs sufficient information to make responsible use of the health services available to them.

In many situations clients may be taught to monitor their own disease process. More common examples are the hypertensive client who checks his own blood pressure and the diabetic client who tests for the presence of sugar and acetone in his urine. Many assessment techniques may be easily taught to clients, particularly those involving inspection and palpation.

Another form of increasing the participation of the client in the management of his health problems is one of teaching him the untoward side effects that commonly occur with medications that are prescribed for him and the steps he should take in the event these side effects happen to him.

An exploration with the client should be planned that will allow the practitioner to understand the attitudes and feelings of the client toward the health care system. Questions may be formulated that will reveal the nature of the client's earlier experiences with physicians, nurses, and allied personnel and health care agencies. This discussion may also bring out an appreciation of the kind of problems the client feels would warrant a visit to a health care agency. This information may be utilized in planning the mechanisms that will help the individual to continue in the system.

Several studies have been done that contribute to the knowledge of the client's attitudes and values toward health care. Some of the findings are useful. The client imparts to the health professional a faith in the fact that technical competence is a given, that the professional's educational preparation has guaranteed this aspect. The client further expects that all the equipment necessary for his examination is available and in working order and that all the tests necessary to explore his problems will be ordered, performed, and interpreted correctly. The health professional is expected by the client to show a genuine interest in his general welfare, that the client is worth the time required to evaluate and intervene in the disease processes the professional may find. The client frequently correlates the competence of the health professional with the amount of time the professional is willing to spend with the client, the professional's demonstrated willingness to allow the client to fully discuss his problems, and the degree to which the professional answers questions lucidly and honestly. The client is not loath to visit several health professionals if the opinion of specialists is needed in reaching a diagnosis. He is, however, better satisfied if the health professional he visits actively intervenes in his disease process.

The prospect of an individual seeking health care in relation to a specific illness corresponds directly with his perception of (1) the dangers of the disease (disability, death), (2) his own susceptibility to the disease, and (3) the possibility that the illness can be cured by the intervention of health professionals.

The levels of income and education are positively correlated with those populations who seek health care. Furthermore, those with education regarding hygiene are more prone to ensure their well-being by attaining health surveillance. They are also more likely to secure verification of symptoms that they feel may connote disease.

The aged, the poorly educated, and the socio-economically disadvantaged are less likely to feel that health care is meeting their needs. It has been shown that women, poorly educated individuals, and elderly individuals are less likely to demonstrate compliance in health care. Thus, these groups are less likely to seek a health examination, to follow the therapeutic regimen established for them, and to return for further help.

Studies have shown that women with family responsibilities only are less likely to seek health care than those with family responsibilities who have career commitments as well.

Conditions for which health care is needed and for which case finding may be necessary include self-destructive behavior leading to early death, sickness, and debility. Such conditions may be drug dependency, alcoholism, venereal disease, and obesity. Because of the stigma attached to many of these states, the affected individuals may not seek health care. Frequently, inadequate services are available for those who do. The individual feels devalued in his own estimation and is hesitant to reveal what he considers a weakness, an aberration, over which he feels he "should" have control. It has been shown that return visits of such individuals are increased by encouraging them to assume responsibility for planning.

FREQUENCY OF ASSESSMENT

There is considerable controversy surrounding the issue of how often the periodic health examination should be performed on the ostensibly healthy client. Early recommendations suggested that the health examination should be done each year. More recent evaluation of the findings of examinations by age groups suggests that younger individuals need not be assessed as frequently as older people. One recommendation is that persons under 35 years of age be assessed every 4 to 5 years, that persons 35 to 45 years of age be assessed every 2 to 3 years, and that only persons over 45 years of age undergo a thorough health assessment every year.

LIFETIME HEALTH MONITORING PLAN (LHMP)

An emphasis on preventive health care has led to the development of a proposal for a Lifetime Health Monitoring Program (LHMP) by Breslow and Somers. This plan for preventive health care provides a definition of health care for the entire life of the individual and is organized around ten periods in the person's life. The goals for health care and the criteria for the health care provider activities and patient participation are defined for each age group. The divisions adopted include the pregnancy/perinatal period, infancy (the first year), preschool child, school-aged child, adolescence, adult entry, young adult years, middle adult years, older adult years, and old age. A summary of these recommendations follows.

Table 1-1. Recommendation for the frequency of health assessment

Client's age	Frequency of health assessment
<35	Every 4 to 5 years
35 to 45	Every 2 to 3 years
>45	Every year

A. Pregnancy-perinatal age group
1. Goals
a. To improve the quality of life of this and future generations by improving the outcome of every pregnancy
b. To make available a single standard of optimal care—including specialized care where needed—for every obstetric patient regardless of her economical and social standing
c. To ensure the mother the best chance of a healthy, full-term pregnancy and rapid recovery after a normal delivery
d. To identify and categorize high- and low-risk patients and their newborns
e. To facilitate the live birth of a normal baby, free of congenital or developmental damage
f. To help both mother and father achieve the knowledge and capacity to provide for the physical, emotional, and social needs of the baby

2. Recommended assessment periods for the normal pregnant female
a. First visit—early in the first trimester (ideally, about 2 to 4 weeks after the first missed period)
b. During initial 28 to 32 weeks of gestation—every 2 to 4 weeks
c. 28 to 32 to 36 weeks of gestation—every 2 weeks
d. 36 weeks of gestation to delivery—weekly

Ideally, counseling is initiated prior to the pregnancy and in early childhood the need for a program for exercising and maintaining normal weight should be emphasized. For the female who is assessed to be obese in the childbearing years, a program of weight reduction should be accomplished prior to pregnancy. If it is determined by history that the individual smokes, the smoker is counseled to quit prior to conception. Birth control pills are generally discontinued 2 to 3 months prior to attempts to conceive.

Recommended professional services for the pregnancy/perinatal age group*

Education and counseling
Anatomic, physiologic, and psychological changes
Nutrition
Exercise
Cigarette, alcohol, and drug use
Unnecessary X-rays
Exposure to infection
Signs and symptoms of abnormalities
Travel, clothing, employment
Labor and delivery
Infant care and parenthood preparation
Contraception
Abortion, adoption

Medical evaluation
Comprehensive history and physical
Dental examination
Weight†
Blood pressure†
Urinalysis (sugar, albumin, bacteriuria)†
Hematocrit/hemoglobin‡

Medical evaluation—cont'd
Blood sugar§
Urine culture and colony count§
Blood grouping, Rh determination, Rh antibody,‡ irregular antibody screen‡
VDRL
Rubella, toxoplasmosis, cytomegalic inclusion virus, herpes simplex titer (if available as single test; otherwise, rubella and, possibly, toxoplasmosis)
Pap smear
Tuberculin test§
Abdominal exam*
Fetal heart tones*
Pelvic exam (near term)

High-risk patients
Amniocentesis
Gonorrhea culture

*From Somers, A. R.: Lifetime health monitoring: preventive care for the child in utero, Patient Care 13(3):162-178, 1979. Copyright © 1979, Patient Care Publications, Inc., Darien, Conn.
†Repeat every visit
‡Repeat in third trimester
§Not recommended for all patients by all physicians

B. Infancy (birth to age 1 year)
  1. Goals
    a. To enter the child in an ongoing system of primary health care
    b. To establish immunity against specified infectious disease
    c. To detect and prevent certain other diseases and problems, including precursors of adult diseases before irreparable damage occurs
    d. To facilitate emotional, intellectual, and physical growth and development to the infant's optimal potential
    e. To provide a basis for a lifetime of emotional stability, especially through a loving relationship with mother, father, and other family members

  2. Four to six visits for preventive health care are recommended in the first year of life. Somers recommends a visit with a nurse at 10 days of age and visits with a physician at 6 weeks, 4½ months, and 9 months.

Overall goals for children in the growing period included (1) facilitating the child's optimal physical, mental, emotional, and social growth and development; (2) establishing and maintaining a healthy, effective parent/child relationship (this goal is expanded as the child grows to include other family members as well as peers and others outside his home); and (3) establishing healthy behavioral patterns for nutrition, exercise, study, and recreation, as a basis for a healthy life-style.

Recommended preventive procedures for the first year of life*

Before discharge		After discharge	
Condition	**Procedure**	**Condition**	**Procedure**
Growth retardation	Height and weight, at birth and at discharge	Diphtheria	Immunization
	Physical examination	Pertussis	
		Tetanus	
Congenital abnormalities	Eye examination	Poliomyelitis	
Strabismus	Observation/counseling	Phenylketonuria	Blood test
Parenting disorders	Silver nitrate eye drops	Hypothyroidism	Blood test
Neonatal gonococcal ophthalmia		Tuberculosis	Skin test
		Anemia	Hematocrit/hemoglobin
Hemorrhagic disease of the newborn	Vitamin K	Growth disorders	Height, weight, head circumference
Phenylketonuria	Blood test	Nutritional problems	History and parent counseling
Hypothyroidism	Blood test		
Accidental injury or death	Parent counseling	Congenital disorders	Physical examination
Inadequate preparation for infant care	History and parent counseling	Strabismus	Eye examination
		Developmental disorders	Observation
Parent failure to bring baby for immunizations and well-baby checks	Parent counseling	Hearing defects	Observation/noisemaker test
		Accidental death or injury	Parent Counseling
		Inadequate preparation for infant care	History and parent counseling
		Acquiring a life-style that may adversely affect health and longevity	History and parent counseling
		Dental caries	Fluoride and parent counseling

*From Somers, A. R.: Lifetime health monitoring: preventive care, Patient Care 13(3):162-178, 1979. Copyright © 1979, Patient Care Publications, Inc., Darien, Conn.

C. Preschool child (ages 1 to 5)
  1. Goals
    a. To facilitate the child's optimal physical, emotional, and social growth and development
    b. To begin the child's process of socialization through happy and effective relations with parents and other family members and gradually to introduce the child to school and other aspects of the life outside the home
    c. To identify possible precursors of adult disease such as obesity or high blood pressure
  2. Generally two visits are recommended for preventive care in the second year of life. After this, the visits are spaced at every 12 or 18 months until age 5

Recommended preventive procedures for the preschool child*

The following chart summarizes the recommendations for preventive health care for the child age 1-5.

Condition	Procedure	When
Developmental abnormalities	History, observation	Each visit
Problems with parent/child relationship	History, observation, counseling	Each visit
Discipline or behavior problems	History, observation, counseling	Each visit
Nutritional problems	History, counseling, height and weight measurement	Each visit
Accidental death or injury	Counseling	Each visit
Poisoning	Counseling about syrup of ipecac	Age 15-18 months
Dental caries	Examination, counseling	Each visit
	Fluoride supplementation	Throughout tooth development years
Growth abnormalities	Height and weight	Each visit
	Head circumference	Age 15-18 months
Eye defects, strabismus	Examination	Age 15-18 months and age 24 months or each visit†
Visual acuity	Examination	Each visit, age 3 and older
Hypertension	Blood pressure determination	Each visit, age 3 and older
Hearing defects	Audiometry	Each visit, age 3 and older
Measles, mumps, rubella	Immunization	Age 15 months
Diphtheria, tetanus, pertussis	Immunization	Age 18-24 months and age 5
Poliomyelitis	Immunization	Age 18-24 months and age 5
Tuberculosis	Skin test	Every 1-2 years or only at age 5†
Anemia	Hematocrit or hemoglobin‡	Age 15-18 months, if not done at 9-12 months, and age 5
Bacteriuria	Urinalysis‡	Each visit, age 2 and older, or only age 5†
	Urine culture (girls)‡	Age 5

*From Somers, A. R.: Lifetime health monitoring: preventive care age 1 through adolescence, Patient Care 13(8):201-216, 1979. Copyright © 1979, Patient Care Publications, Inc., Darien, Conn.
†Authorities disagree over the frequency of this procedure.
‡Some authorities question whether this procedure should be included.

D. School-aged child (ages 6 to 11)
  1. Goals
    a. To facilitate the child's optimal physical, mental, emotional, and social growth and development, including a positive self-image
    b. To establish and maintain a healthy, effective parent/child relationship
    c. To establish healthy behavioral patterns for nutrition, exercise, study, and recreation as a foundation for a healthy lifestyle
  2. While some recommend only one visit for this age span, others believe that the child should receive preventive care every 1 to 2 years.

Recommended preventive procedures for the school-age child

The following chart summarizes the recommendations for preventive health care for the child age 6-11.

Condition	Procedure	When
Developmental abnormalities	History, observation	Each visit
Problems with parent/child relationship	History, observation, counseling	Each visit
Nutritional problems	History, counseling, height and weight	Each visit
Accidental death or injury	Counseling	Each visit
Dental caries	Counseling	Each visit
Growth	Height and weight	Each visit
Vision	Examination	Each visit
Hearing defects	Examination	Each visit
Hypertension	Blood pressure determination	Each visit
Scoliosis	Examination	Each visit, starting at age 8-9
Tuberculosis	Skin test†	Every 2 years
Enlarged thyroid	Examination	Each visit
Bacteriuria	Urinalysis† Urine culture (girls)†	Each visit
Smoking, drug abuse, lack of sex education	Counseling	Each visit

*From Somers, A. R.: Lifetime health monitoring: preventive care age 1 through adolescence, Patient Care 13(8):201-216, 1979. Copyright © 1979, Patient Care Publications, Inc., Darien, Conn.
†There is disagreement whether this procedure should be included.

E. Adolescence (ages 12 to 17)
1. Goals
a. To continue optimal physical, mental, emotional, and social growth and development
b. To reinforce healthy behavior patterns and discourage negative ones in physical fitness, nutrition, exercise, study, work, recreation, sex, individual relations, driving, smoking, alcohol, and drugs as a foundation for a healthy life-style
2. Recommendations for the timing of preventive care in this age span range from one visit at age 14 to 15 to a yearly session.

Recommended preventive procedures for the adolescent*

The following chart summarizes the recommendations for preventive health care for the child age 12-17.

Condition	Procedure	When
Accidental death or injury	Counseling	Each visit
Family problems	History, counseling	Each visit
School problems	History, counseling	Each visit
Negative behavior patterns	History, counseling	Each visit
Unwanted pregnancy	History, counseling	Each visit
Growth abnormalities	Height and weight	Each visit
Developmental abnormalities	Observation	Each visit
Nutritional abnormalities	History, height and weight, counseling	Each visit
Vision	Examination	Each visit
Hypertension	Blood pressure determination	Each visit
Acne	Observation	Each visit
Scoliosis	Examination	Each visit to age 15
Tetanus/diphtheria	Immunization booster	Age 15, or 10 years since previous booster
Bacteriuria	Urinalysis†	Each visit
	Urine culture (girls)†	Each visit
Tuberculosis	Skin test	Age 15 or every 2 years‡
Cervical cancer	Pap smear	Every 2 years for girls who are sexually active or who were exposed to DES in utero
Dental caries and periodontal disease	Counseling	Each visit

*From Somers, A. R.: Lifetime health monitoring: preventive care age 1 through adolescence, Patient Care 13(8):201-216, 1979. Copyright © 1979, Patient Care Publications, Inc., Darien, Conn.
†There is disagreement whether this procedure should be included.
‡There is disagreement over the frequency of this procedure.

F. Entering adulthood (ages 18 to 24)
1. Goals
a. To facilitate transition from dependent adolescent to mature independent adult with maximum physical, mental, and emotional resources
b. To achieve useful employment and maximum capacity for a healthy marriage, parenthood, and social relations
2. It is recommended that the 18- to 24-year-old adult undergo health appraisal once. After the initial health assessment the patient is asked to return every 1 to 2 years.

Recommended preventive procedures for the adult age 18-24

The following chart summarizes the recommendations for preventive health care for the patient entering adulthood. The column on the left lists the condition to be prevented or detected, the column in the middle lists the procedure to be used, and the column on the right lists how frequently the procedure should be repeated between ages 18-24.

Condition	Procedure	Frequency
Smoking	History and counseling	At least once
Unwanted pregnancy	Counseling	At least once
Problem drinking, alcoholism	History and counseling	At least once
Drug abuse	History and counseling	At least once
Accidents	History and counseling	At least once
Obesity	History and weight; counseling	Every 2-4 years
Lack of exercise	History and counseling	At least once
Hypertension	Blood pressure measurement	Every 2 years
Breast cancer	Breast exam; counseling about self-examination	Every 1-2 years
Refractive errors	Eye screen†	Once
Tetanus-diphtheria	Booster	Once if 10 years since last one
Cervical cancer	Pap smear	Every 2-3 years
Diabetes	Urinalysis†	Once
Proteinuria	Urinalysis†	Once
Bacteriuria	Urinalysis†	Once
Birth defects	Rubella titer	Once in unimmunized women
Tuberculosis	Skin test	Once
Anemia	Hematocrit or hemoglobin†	Once
Syphilis	Blood test†	Once
High cholesterol and/or triglyceride levels	Serum cholesterol,† serum triglyceride†	Once
Dental caries and periodontal disease	Dental exam and cleaning	Every 1-2 years

*From Somers, A. R.: Lifetime health monitoring: a whole life plan for well patient care, Patient Care 13(11):83-153, 1979. Copyright © 1979, Patient Care Publications, Inc., Darien, Conn.
†There is debate on whether this procedure should be included.

G. Young adult (ages 25 to 39)
 1. Goals—see goals of entering adulthood.
 2. The individual in this age group should receive preventive health care every 1 to 2 years.

Recommended preventive procedures for adults of age 25-39*

The following chart summarizes the recommendations for preventive health care for the young adult. The column on the left lists the condition to be prevented or detected, the column in the middle lists the procedure to be used, and the column on the right lists how frequently the procedure should be repeated between ages 25-39.

Condition	Procedure	Frequency
Smoking	History and counseling	Every 2 years
Obesity or poor eating habits	History and counseling	Every 2 years
	Weight	Every 2-4 years
Lack of exercise	History and counseling	Every 2 years
Accidental injury or death	History and counseling	Every 2 years
Problem drinking, alcoholism	History and counseling	Every 2-4 years
Drug abuse	History and counseling	Every 2-4 years
Unwanted pregnancy	History and counseling	Every 2 years
Hypertension	Blood pressure measurement	Every 2 years
Breast cancer	Breast examination; counseling about self-examination	Every 1-2 years
Tetanus and diphtheria	Immunization	Every 10 years
Cervical cancer	Pap smear	Every 2-3 years
Tuberculosis	Skin test	
Diabetes	Urinalysis†	Every 4 years
Bacteriuria	Urinalysis†	Every 4 years
Proteinuria	Urinalysis†	Every 4 years
Coronary artery disease	Serum cholesterol determination†	Every 4 years
Vision defects	Examination†	Every 4 years
Anemia	Hematocrit or hemoglobin†	Every 4 years
Syphilis	Blood test†	Every 4 years
Dental caries and periodontal disease	Dental examination and cleaning	Every 1-2 years

*From Somers, A. R.: Lifetime health monitoring: a whole life plan for well patient care, Patient Care 13(11):83-153, 1979. Copyright © 1979, Patient Care Publications, Inc., Darien, Conn.
†There is debate on whether this procedure should be included.

H. Middle adult (ages 40 to 59)
   1. Goals: to prolong the period of maximum physical energy and optimum mental and social activity, including adjusting to menopause.

2. Preventive health care is recommended every 2 years for those 40 to 50 years of age. However, it is recommended that individuals receive health care every year after age 50.

Recommended preventive procedures for the middle adult years (age 40-59)*

The following chart summarizes the recommendations for preventive health care for those 40 to 59 years of age. The left-hand column lists the condition to be detected or prevented, the middle column indicates the recommended screening procedure, and the right-hand column indicates how frequently to repeat the procedure.

Condition	Procedure	Frequency
Smoking	History and counseling	At least once
Problem drinking, alcoholism	History and counseling	At least once
Accidents	History and counseling	At least once
Problems related to job, family, menopause, retirement planning, etc.	History and counseling	At least once
Lack of exercise	History and counseling	At least once
Colonic cancer	History, test of stool for occult blood*	Every 2 years (annually after age 50)
Obesity	Height and weight	Every 4-5 years
Hearing problems	Screening†	Every 4-5 years
Visual impairment	Screening†	Every 4-5 years
Hypertension	Blood pressure determination	Every 2 years
Breast cancer	Physician examination	Every 1-2 years (annually after age 50)
	Counseling about self-examination	Every 1-2 years (annually after age 50)
	Mammography†	Every 1-2 years after age 50
Cervical cancer	Pap smear	Every 2 years
Anemia	Hematocrit/hemoglobin†	Every 4-5 years
Syphilis	Blood test†	Once
Tuberculosis	Skin test†	Once
Diabetes	Urinalysis†	Every 4-5 years
Renal disease	Urinalysis†	Every 4-5 years
Bacteriuria	Urinalysis†	Every 4-5 years
Tetanus/diphtheria	Immunization	Every 10 years
Dental caries/periodontal disease	Dental examination and cleaning	Every 1-2 years
High cholesterol and triglyceride levels	Serum cholesterol,† serum triglyceride†	Every 4-5 years

*From Somers, A. R.: Lifetime health monitoring: a whole life plan for well patient care, Patient Care 13(11):83-153, 1979. Copyright © 1979, Patient Care Publications, Inc., Darien, Conn.
†There is debate on whether this procedure should be included.

I. Older adult (ages 60 to 74)
  1. Goals
     a. To prolong the period of optimum physical, mental, and social activity
     b. To minimize handicapping and discomfort from the onset of chronic conditions
     c. To prepare, in advance, for retirement years
  2. Preventive health care is recommended annually.

Recommended preventive procedures for the older adult years, age 60-74*

The following chart summarizes the recommendations for preventive health care for those 60 to 74 years of age. The left-hand column lists the condition to be detected, the middle column indicates the recommended screening procedure, and the right-hand column indicates how frequently to repeat the procedure.

Condition	Procedure	Frequency
Accidental injury or death, particularly from falls	History and counseling	Every 2 years
Lack of preparation for retirement	History and counseling	Every 2 years
Nutritional problems	History and counseling	Every 2 years
	Height and weight	Every 2-4 years
Colonic cancer	History	Annually
	Test of stool for occult blood*	Annually
Hearing defects	Screening†	Every 2 years
Visual impairment	Screening†	Every 2 years
Hypertension	Blood pressure determination	Every 2 years
Breast cancer	Physician examination	Annually
	Counseling about self-examination	Annually
	Mammography†	Every 1-2 years
Cervical cancer	Pap smear	Every 2 years
Anemia	Hematocrit/hemoglobin†	Every 4-5 years
Syphilis	Blood test†	Once in this age group
Tuberculosis	Skin test†	Once in this age group
Diabetes	Urinalysis†	Every 4-5 years
Bacteriuria	Urinalysis†	
Renal disease	Urinalysis	
Tetanus/diphtheria	Immunization	Every 10 years
Dental caries and periodontal disease	Dental examination and cleaning	Every 1-2 years
Poor fitting dentures	Dental examination	Every 2-3 years

*From Somers, A. R.: Lifetime health monitoring: a whole life plan for well patient care, Patient Care 13(11):83-153, 1979. Copyright © 1979, Patient Care Publications, Inc., Darien, Conn.
†There is debate on whether this procedure should be included.

J. Old age (75 and older)
  1. Goals
     a. To prolong the period of effective activity and ability to live independently and avoid institutionalization as far as possible
     b. To minimize inactivity and discomfort from chronic conditions in terminal illness
     c. To assure as little physical and mental distress as possible
     d. To provide emotional support to patient and family.
  2. Preventive health care is recommended annually.

Recommended preventive procedures for the patient over age 75*

The following chart summarizes the recommendations for preventive health care for those over age 75. The left-hand column lists the condition to be detected or prevented, the middle column indicates the recommended screening procedure, and the right-hand column indicates how frequently to repeat the procedure.

Condition	Procedure	Frequency
Accidental injury or death, particularly from falls	History and counseling	Annually
Loss of mental acuity	History and observation	Annually
Nutritional problems	History and counseling	Annually
	Height and weight	Annually
Colonic cancer	History	Annually
	Test of stool for occult blood†	Annually
Hearing defects	Screening	Annually
Hypertension	Blood pressure determination	Annually
Breast cancer	Physician examination	Annually
	Counseling about self-examination	Annually
	Mammography†	Every 1-2 years
Cervical cancer	Pap smear	Every 2 years
Tetanus/diphtheria	Immunization	Every 10 years
Dental caries and periodontal disease	Dental examination and cleaning	Every 1-2 years
Poor fitting dentures	Dental examination	Every 2-3 years

*From Somers, A. R.: Lifetime health monitoring: a whole life plan for well patient care, Patient Care 13(11):83-153, 1979. Copyright © 1979, Patient Care Publications, Inc., Darien, Conn.
†There is debate on whether this procedure should be included.

In 1980 new guidelines were developed by the American Cancer Society for individuals *without signs or symptoms of cancer*. These recommendations would result in fewer annual examinations. The following specific recommendations were published:

1. Annual health assessment only for men and women past 40 and every 3 years for individuals between 20 and 40
2. A Pap test every 3 years for women following two negative tests a year apart
3. Proctosigmoidoscopic examinations every 3 to 5 years after age 50 following two negative examinations a year apart
4. Annual test for occult blood after age 50
5. Breast manual examination (a) by health professional every 3 years prior to age 40 and then annually; (b) self-performed each month after age 20
6. Breast mammography examination baseline check between ages 35 to 40 and annually after age 50

Annual lung and sputum examinations in the effort to detect lung cancer are *not recommended*. It should be borne in mind that those individuals who are members of high-risk groups may need more frequent examinations.

ASSESSMENT TECHNIQUES

The history and review of systems that are obtained by interviewing the individual to be examined provide subjective information. The information obtained is the verbalized perceptions and interpretations of the client. Although the major emphasis of this volume is health assessment, there are certain physiological functions and perceptions that are considered to be integral to examination of the client; these are the skills that contribute to the art of physical diagnosis. These are the processes through which objective data are obtained. The four major procedures of physical diagnosis are inspection, palpation, percussion, and auscultation. These procedures are described here and are further developed in chapters dealing with their application for specific organs and systems.

Inspection

Inspection (L. *inspectio*, the act of beholding) is the act of concentrating attention to the thorough and unhurried visualization of the client. Inspection also involves listening to any sounds emanating from the client as well as being attuned to any odors that may be present.

Lighting must be adequate. Daylight or artificial light is suitable. The specific cues to which the ex-

aminer alerts himself are discussed in Chapter 7 on general assessment.

Palpation

By palpation (L. *palpatio*, the act of touching), the examiner's hands may be used to augment the data gathered through inspection. The skilled examiner will use the most sensitive parts of the hand for each type of palpation. The pads of the fingers are thought to be most effective in those tasks requiring discrimination through touch. Vibration is detected most effectively with the palmar surface of the metacarpal phalangeal joints. Rough measures of temperature are best determined with the dorsum of the hand. The position and consistency of a structure may best be determined by employing the grasping fingers. The examiner may utilize touch to seek out and determine the extent of tenderness and tremor or spasm of muscle tissues or to elicit crepitus in bones and joints. Individual structures within body cavities, particularly the abdomen, may be palpated for position, size, shape, consistency, and mobility. The examining hand may be used to detect masses. Palpation may also serve to evaluate abnormal collections of fluid. Both light and deep palpation may be used in the examination. Light palpation is always performed first. In the case of superficial masses the fingers are moved in a circular motion in the region suspected of containing a mass. The skin and hair are examined for moisture and texture through the use of touch.

Percussion

Percussion (L. *percussio*, the act of striking) involves a cause-and-effect relationship. This summary term includes the act of striking or otherwise producing the impact of one object against another—this is the cause. The result of this rapping is the production of a shock wave that in some cases results in vibration. The vibration may produce sound waves that may reach the ear to be interpreted as sound. In the process of physical diagnosis, percussion means the striking or tapping of a body surface such as the back or the abdomen while listening with the unassisted ear or with the stethoscope.

Auenbrugger, the originator of the technique, described what has been termed *immediate percussion*. Immediate percussion means the striking of a finger or hand directly against the body. The term *mediate percussion* is used to describe the refinement in technique that was developed some time in the 19th century. Instruments called the *pleximeter* and *plexor* were devised. The plexor was a small rubber hammer, much like the reflex hammers used today. This plexor was used to strike a blow against the pleximeter, a small, flat, solid object, often made of ivory, that was held firmly in place against the client's body.

Mediate percussion using the middle finger of one hand as the plexor that strikes against the middle finger (pleximeter) of the other hand is the method in use in current clinical practice.

The passive hand is placed gently against the body surface while the distal portion of the middle finger is placed firmly against the skin. The middle finger is dealt a blow at or immediately distal to the distal interphalangeal joint with the middle finger of the other hand. The blow must be delivered crisply, sharply, and with the plexor perpendicular to the pleximeter.

The speed and force of a blow by the plexor are made possible by wrist action. The hand is flexed back on the forearm and brought forward with a clean, snapping motion that allows a fast strike and rapid removal of the plexor (Fig. 1-1) in order not to dampen the vibration. Fingernails of the plexor finger should be cut sufficiently short to avoid cutting the skin of the pleximeter. Fatty tissue overlying the tissue to be percussed may dampen the blow. In order to overcome this, it has been suggested that more force can be brought to bear on the body surface by striking the lateral aspect of the thumb. Rapid pronation of the forearm is used to provide the quick, striking movement.

The vibration produced through percussion involves only the tissue closely adjacent to the pleximeter (approximately 3 to 5 cm). Percussion over

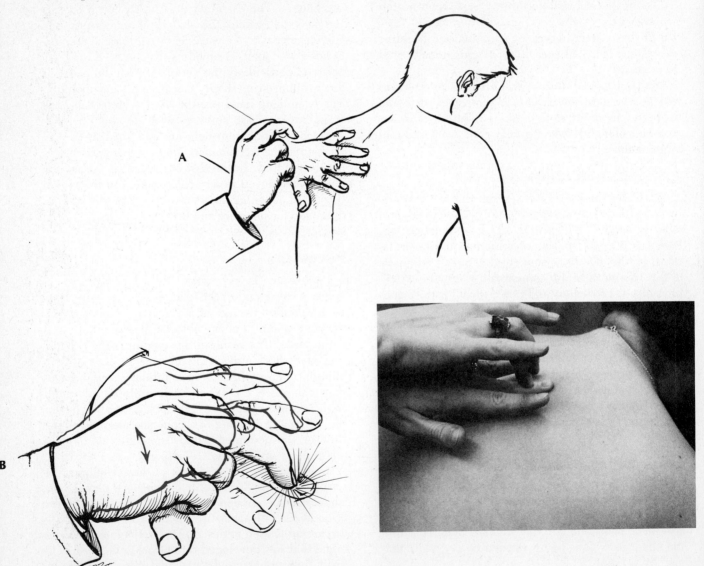

Fig. 1-1. Percussion. **A,** Positioning of the hands. **B,** Hand movement. **C,** Percussion of the posterior thorax.

bones is affected by lateral transmission of vibration.

The change from resonance to dullness is more easily perceived than the dull-to-resonant transition. Thus, the examiner organizes his percussion protocol to progress from more resonant regions to lesser ones.

Fist percussion is, as the name implies, striking with the hand in a fisted position. The blow is delivered with the lateral aspect of the hand. The purpose of this type of percussion is to elicit sensation by the vibration of the tissue. The most common applications are to stimulate pain or tenderness caused by hepatitis, cholecystitis, or kidney disease.

The sound waves that result from percussion are evaluated with reference to intensity, pitch, quality, and duration.

Sound is produced by vibrating structures. The vibrations generate a series of compression waves in the medium that is capable of sound transmission. Solids, liquids, and gases that are sufficiently elastic to convert energy to motion may transmit sound. The compression waves initiate vibrations of the tympanic membrane, which moves in and out with the frequency of the sound waves. The mechanical energy of the compression waves is transduced into neural signals by receptor structures of the middle ear. These neural signals are transmitted to the temporal cortex and perceived as sound.

Intensity, loudness. The physical property of sound called intensity produces the effect of loudness in the human auditory apparatus. As a sound wave travels through a point in the air, the air molecules are compressed and then expanded in the wake of the compression wave. The difference between maximum pressure and minimum pressure is the amplitude of the sound wave. The greater the displacement of air, the more movement during vibration of the tympanic membrane and the louder the perception of sound. Loudness is a psychological variable as well. The individual listener may be attentive to or selectively unaware of the many sounds in his environment. Furthermore, various alterations in the conduction apparatus of the ear or the sensory neural components of audition may produce alteration in the perception of sound.

Pitch, frequency. The frequency of sound is a physical property that corresponds to the number of vibrations of the sound source per second. Pitch is related to the frequency of sound.

The waveform of a sound of single frequency is sinusoidal, with perfectly matched hills (peaks) and valleys (troughs). The distance from 1 peak to the next is 1 cycle. The recording of frequency is in cycles per second (cps), or hertz (Hz). The human ear is capable of detecting sounds in the frequency range of 15 to 30 cps, to 20,000 cps. With advancing age, the human ear becomes progressively less sensitive to the higher sound frequencies. The sounds of speech and music (250 to 2,048 cps) are most frequently lost. However, most sounds of importance in physical diagnosis are in the frequency range below 1,000 cps and more particularly in the range of 40 to 500 cps. Thus, the ability to hear sounds that are important to health assessment is not compromised by aging.

Quality, harmonics. *Harmonic*, or *overtone*, refers to the physical property of sound that causes the psychological effect called quality or *timbre*. A sound of single frequency produces a pure tone. The lowest frequency at which a piano wire vibrates is called the *fundamental*. Most objects vibrate at more than one frequency. The piano wire may vibrate as a single unit or in halves or thirds that oscillate at their own frequency. These frequencies will be whole-number multiples of the single frequency. The fundamental and the multiples of the single frequency are the harmonics. Sound quality is produced by the sum of the harmonics present and their intensities. The quality is recorded in descriptive terms such as *humming*, *buzzing*, or *roaring*. The fundamental is the first harmonic. A musical sound is one wherein the mix of intensity and pitch is pleasing to the ear, whereas *noise* is the term given an unpleasant sensation. Most sounds heard in the course of the physical examination are perceived as noise.

Table 1-2. Sounds produced by percussion

Record of finding	Intensity	Pitch	Duration	Quality	Anatomical region where sounds may be encountered
Tympany	Loud	High	Moderate	Drumlike	Air in closed structure vibrates in concert with tissue surrounding it; the gastric air bubble; air in intestine
Hyperresonance	Very loud	Very low	Long	Booming	Air-filled lungs, as in emphysema
Resonance	Moderate to loud	Low	Long	Hollow	Normal lung
Dullness	Soft to moderate	High	Moderate	Thudlike	Liver
Flatness	Soft	High	Short	Flat	Muscle

An axiom of the physical examination is that, like the drum, the more air tissue contains (the less dense the tissue), the deeper, louder, and longer the sound will be. The corollary is that the more compact the tissue, the higher, fainter, and shorter the sound will be. The sounds elicited in percussion are recorded in relation to the density of the tissue being vibrated. The least dense tissues produce tympany, whereas successively more dense tissue results in hyperresonance, resonance, impaired resonance, dullness, and flatness.

The percussion hammer (see Fig. 23-47) is also used to strike a blow to tendons that serves to stretch the tendon such that a deep tendon reflex is elicited. This will be described in greater detail in the neurological examination.

Auscultation

Auscultation (L. *auscultate,* to listen to) is the process of listening for the sounds produced by the human body. The sounds of particular importance are those produced by (1) the thoracic or abdominal viscera and (2) the movement of blood in the cardiovascular system. *Direct,* or *immediate, auscultation* is accomplished by the unassisted ear, that is, without any amplifying device. This form of auscultation often involves the application of the ear directly to a body surface where the sound is most prominent. The use of a sound augmentation device such as a stethoscope in the detection of body sounds is called *mediate auscultation.*

Hippocrates described chest sounds in his writings, and Harvey mentioned heart sounds in the early 1600s. Direct, or immediate, auscultation was practiced until 1816, when Laennec devised the first stethoscope, which consisted of a series of rolled up papers held in place with gummed paper. Laennec continued to improve the device and ultimately utilized a wooden tubing with an earpiece. Later, flexible ear trumpets were modified for use in auscultation. This monaural form of mediate auscultation was succeeded by a binaural instrument in the middle of the 19th century.

The three types of stethoscopes that enjoy clinical popularity today are the acoustical, magnetic, and electronic stethoscopes.

The *acoustical stethoscope* (Fig. 1-2) is essentially a closed cylinder, which serves to inhibit the dissipation of the compression waves produced by the sound source in the column. The diaphragm of the acoustical stethoscope screens out low-frequency sounds and is therefore most effective in assessing high-frequency sounds. The diaphragm is applied firmly to the skin so that it moves synchronously with the body wall. The bell-type head is most effective in detecting low-frequency sounds. Care is taken not to flatten the skin by pressing the bell too firmly, since the vibrations of the surface tissues in response to visceral vibration are the source of sound; stretching these tissues inhibits vibration, actually converting the tissue to a diaphragm. The bell chestpiece should be wide enough to span an intercostal space in an adult and deep enough so that it will not fill with tissue.

Several sizes of earpieces are supplied with better stethoscopes. The examiner should determine which size fits the external meatus most snugly. The earpieces should occlude the meatus, thus blocking extraneous sound. However, the earpieces should not be painful to the examiner. Earpieces that are too small will enter the ear canal, causing pain. The binaurals (metal tubing) are angled somewhat toward the nose of the wearer in order to project the sound onto the tympanic membrane. The direction of the angle may be adjusted by the tension spring. The tubing should not be longer than 12 to 14 inches in order to minimize sound distortion. It is more likely that with longer tubing the sound will be diminished. An internal bore of ⅛ inch has been suggested for best sound transmission. The purpose of the stethoscope is to exclude environmental sound; the system does not magnify sound.

The Harvey stethoscope, a variation of the acoustical type, has three heads: a bell for low frequencies, a corrugated diaphragm for midrange, and a flat diaphragm for high frequencies. This stethoscope also has separate tubes leading to each head.

The *magnetic stethoscope* (Fig. 1-3) has a single head that is a diaphragm. Magnetic attraction is established between an iron disk on the interior surface of the diaphragm and a permanent magnet installed behind it in the head. A strong spring keeps the diaphragm bowed outward when not compressed against a body surface. Application of the diaphragm with the appropriate amount of pressure allows activation of the air column. A dial allows the user to adjust for high-, low-, and full-frequency sounds.

The *electronic stethoscope* (Fig. 1-4) functions as a result of vibration of a diaphragm or microphone occurring as a result of the body surface vibrations. These vibrations are transduced into electrical pulses, which are amplified and converted back to sound at a low speaker.

The use of the stethoscope is described in Chapter 15, "Assessment of the Respiratory System," and in Chapter 16, "Cardiovascular Assessment: the Heart and the Neck Vessels."

THE OPHTHALMOSCOPE

The ophthalmoscope was first used by Von Helmholtz in 1850. It provides a method of illuminating

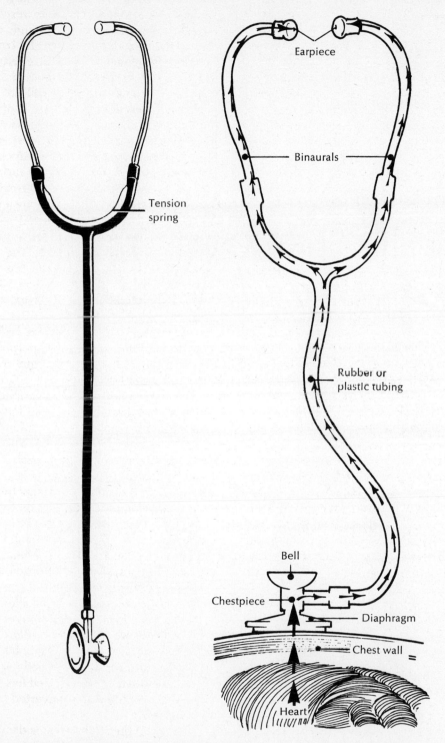

Fig. 1-2. Acoustical stethoscope. (Adapted from Patient Care, March 15, 1974. © Copyright 1974, Miller and Fink Corp., Darien, Conn. All rights reserved.)

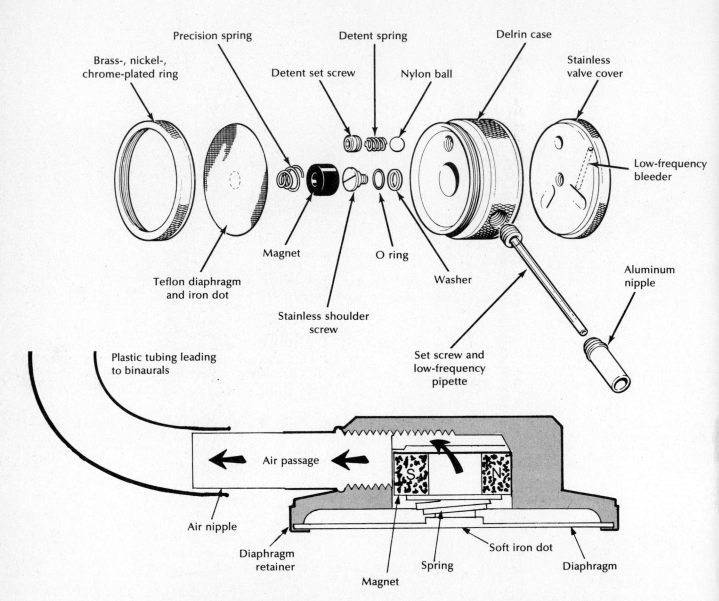

Brass-, nickel-, chrome-plated ring

Precision spring

Detent set screw

Detent spring

Nylon ball

Delrin case

Stainless valve cover

Low-frequency bleeder

Teflon diaphragm and iron dot

Magnet

Stainless shoulder screw

O ring

Washer

Set screw and low-frequency pipette

Aluminum nipple

Plastic tubing leading to binaurals

Air passage

Air nipple

Diaphragm retainer

Magnet

Spring

Soft iron dot

Diaphragm

Fig. 1-3. Magnetic stethoscope. (From Patient Care, March 15, 1974. © Copyright 1974, Miller and Fink Corp., Darien, Conn. All rights reserved.)

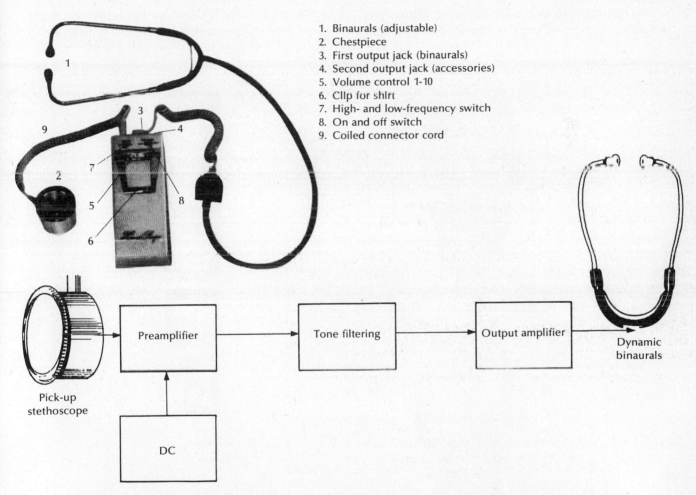

1. Binaurals (adjustable)
2. Chestpiece
3. First output jack (binaurals)
4. Second output jack (accessories)
5. Volume control 1-10
6. Clip for shirt
7. High- and low-frequency switch
8. On and off switch
9. Coiled connector cord

Fig. 1-4. Electronic stethoscope. (From Patient Care, March 15, 1974. © Copyright 1974, Miller and Fink Corp., Darien, Conn. All rights reserved.)

the interior structures of the eye and of viewing these structures as a result of an arrangement of mirrors and lenses.

The instrument and its assembly. The head of an ophthalmoscope and the five apperatures that may be available are shown in Fig. 1-5. The ophthalmoscope head is seated in the handle by fitting the male adapter end of the handle into the female receptacle of the ophthalmoscope head. The head is pushed in the direction of the handle while turning in a clockwise direction until the stop is felt.

The ophthalmoscope is turned on by depressing the button on the rheostat and turning the rheostat clockwise to the appropriate intensity of light. The instrument is turned off after use to prevent shortening the useful life of the bulb and the battery life in battery-operated ophthalmoscopes. The beginner may become familiar with the apertures by projecting them onto a piece of paper. The aperture may be changed by moving the aperture selection lever.

The structure being examined is brought into focus by rotating the lens selector dial until the image becomes clear. The instrument may be held and focused with one hand. On the front of the ophthalmoscope head is an illuminated aperture displaying the number of the lens in position before the viewing aper-

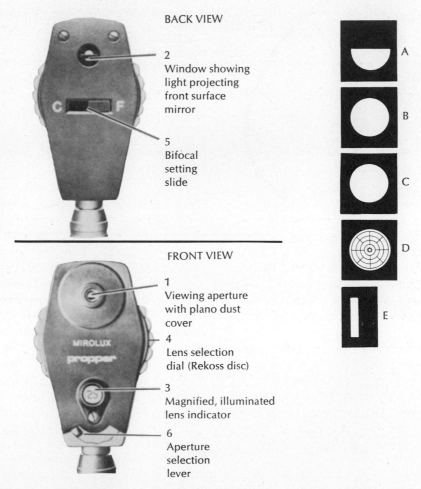

Fig. 1-5. The head and five apertures of an ophthalmoscope. **A,** Hemispot is used for small pupil examinations and to aid in eliminating the corneal light reflex. **B,** Full spot is provided in two different sizes. The small one is used for undilated pupils or to eliminate the corneal reflex in examination of the macula. The large one is used for dilated pupils. The large beam is the one most frequently used because it provides a wide field for the general fundus examination. **C,** Redfree filter is a green beam used for examining the optic disc for pallor and the retina for hemorrhages. Hemorrhages appear black with the red free filter while melanin deposits appear gray. **D,** Fixation star and polar coordinates (grid) is used to determine the fixation pattern and for relating the characteristics, size, and location of fundal lesions. **E,** Slit is used for examining the anterior segment of the eye and for determining the elevation or depression of fundal lesions.

ture. The value of the lens is indicated in diopters. Black numbers are for positive values; red figures are for negative values.

When the lens selector is rotated clockwise beginning with zero (0) the positive numbers (+1, +2, +3, +4, +5, +6, +8, +10, +12, +15, +20, +40) appear, and when the selector is rotated counterclockwise from zero (0) the negative numbers (−1, −2, −3, −4, −5, −6, −8, −10, −15, −20, −25) are seen.

The lens system can compensate for hyperopia or myopia. However, there is no correction for astigmatism.

Examination with the ophthalmoscope. The examination with the ophthalmoscope is best accomplished in a semidarkened or darkened room. It is recommended that neither the examiner nor the client wear glasses during the examination. However, if the examiner is highly astigmatic or myopic, glasses should be worn. The lens selector is moved to the dioptric value that corrects the spherical refractive error of the examiner (for most normal individuals this setting is usually 0).

In order to examine the right eye the examiner sits or stands to the patient's right side. The ophthalmoscope is held in the right hand with the viewing aperture as close as possible to the examiner's right eye. The right index finger is placed on the lens selection dial to be prepared to change lenses as necessary.

The examiner's head is placed about 1½ ft (45 cm) in front of and about 15 degrees temporal (to the right of the line of vision of the right eye). The client is instructed to look straight ahead at some fixed point at eye level. The light beam is then directed into the client's pupil. The examiner selects a strong lens with a high positive number (6 to 8 for an examiner with normal vision).

The fundus will be viewed as a red disc (the red reflex). While keeping the red reflex in view, the examiner moves slowly toward the client. The presence of cataracts or other opacities of the cornea or lens may partially or totally occlude the red reflex. Lens correction is made while moving; a strong negative lens is appropriate for viewing structures of the fundus.

The optic disc may be viewed when the examiner is approximately 3 to 5 cm from the eye. A helpful measure in sighting the optic disc is to focus on a vessel and follow it in a nasal direction to the disc. The appropriate lens is brought into the viewing aperture to provide clear definition of the structures of the fundus. The normal retina is magnified approximately 15 times. These structures are described in Chapter 11, "Assessment of the eyes." The optic disc is examined for clarity of outline and elevation. The blood vessels are followed from the disc to the periph-

ery while the examiner appraises size and structural integrity. The client is then asked to look up so that the superior retina can be examined and down so that the inferior retina can be examined. The examiner looks toward the nose for examination of the nasal retina and laterally for examination of the temporal retina. The peripheral retina may be difficult to examine if the pupils are not dilated.

Examination of the left eye is made in a manner similar to that of the right eye but by standing on the left side of the client and by using the left eye and holding the ophthalmoscope in the left hand.

It is possible to determine the degree of elevation of the retinal disc using the ophthalmoscope. The examiner first focuses on a nonedematous area close to the retinal disc. The dioptric number is read in the lens indicator aperture. Then the crescent of the optic disc is brought into clear focus and the dioptric reading is again noted. The difference between the two dioptric values divided by three is equal to the elevation in millimeters.

THE OTOSCOPE

The otoscope provides a source of illumination for examination of the external auditory canal and the tympanic membrane. The power source for the otoscope is the same as that for the ophthalmoscope. The otoscope head is seated in the same manner as the ophthalmoscope head. The speculum chosen by the examiner should be the largest one that will comfortably fit the external meatus of the client.

Examination with the otoscope. The otoscope is held in the dominant hand. The client is asked to tip his head to the side opposite from the ear being examined. The superior posterior auricle is grasped between thumb and index finger and in the adult pulled upward, backward, and slightly away from the body. This helps to straighten the external auditory canal, which is angled downward and in slightly forward in the adult. For infants, the posterior inferior auricle is grasped and pulled downward and slightly away from the body to accommodate for the external auditory canal, which is angled upward and forward. The remainder of the fingers are rested against the head to achieve pressure restraint or to move with head, should the client move with the speculum in place. Prior to insertion of the otoscope the external ear is carefully inspected for the presence of a foreign body that could be removed. Cerumen may occlude the ear. When cerumen is wet, it is viscous, sticky, and a shade of orange-yellow or, with aging, dark brown or even black when it has been in the canal a long time. Cerumen may occlude the external meatus such that the otoscope may not be passed. A cerumen spoon may be used to remove this excess.

The otoscope is advanced carefully and slowly. The inner two-thirds of the external meatus is thin and quite sensitive to pressure. Pain may be caused by too large a speculum or by sharply angling the speculum over the thin tissue covering the bone. The speculum is advanced until the tympanic membrane can be seen. It is necessary to vary the angle of the speculum in order to visualize the entire tympanic membrane. This examination is more fully explained in Chapter 10.

Suggested equipment for health assessment

Sphygmomanometer
Stethoscope
Ophthalmoscope
Otoscope
Percussion hammer
Tuning fork
Cotton balls
Cotton-tipped applicators
Tongue blades
Ruler
Tape measure—metal or nonstretchable plastic
Safety pins
Vaginal speculum
Examination gloves

BIBLIOGRAPHY

Andreopoulos, S., editor: Primary care; where medicine fails, New York, 1974, John Wiley & Sons, Inc.

Breslow, L., and Somers, A. R.: The lifetime health monitoring program: a practical approach to preventive medicine, N. Engl. J. Med. **296**:601, 1977.

Collen, M. F.: Periodic health examinations, Primary Care **3**:197, 1976.

Garfield, S. R., Collen, M. F., Richart, P. H., and others: Evaluation of new ambulatory medical care delivery system, N. Engl. J. Med. **294**:426, 1976.

Hart, C. R.: Screening in general practice, Edinburgh, 1975, Churchill Livingstone.

Javits, J.: National health care policy for the future, J. Politics Policy Law **1**:5, 1976.

Leavell, H. R., and Clark, E. G.: Preventive medicine for the doctor in his community, ed. 3, New York, 1965, McGraw-Hill Book Co.

Mushkin, S. J., editor: Consumer incentives for health care, New York, 1974, Prodist.

Rappaport, M. D., and Sprague, H. B.: The effects of tubing bore on stethoscope efficiency, Am. Heart J. **42**:605, 1951.

Somers, A. R.: Lifetime health monitoring: preventive care for the child in utero, Patient Care **13**(3):162, 1979.

Somers, A. R.: Lifetime health monitoring: preventive care: age 1 through adolescence, Patient Care **13**(8):201, 1979.

Somers, A. R.: Lifetime health monitoring: a whole-life plan for well patient care, Patient Care **13**(11):83, 1979.

Spitzer, W. O., and others: The Burlington randomized trial of the nurse practitioner, N. Engl. J. Med. **290**:251, 1974.

2 The interview

The major purpose of the interview conducted prior to the physical examination is to obtain a health history and to elicit symptoms and the time course of their development. The goal of an effective interview is a complete and accurate data base. However, although assessment may be the main emphasis of a given exchange, the primary care practitioner must bring to bear skillful communication techniques in order to establish the rapport necessary for a full sharing of the client's relevant life experiences. A climate of trust must be established that will allow a full expression of the client's needs. Furthermore, an analysis of the reactions of the client during the interview will allow the examiner to predict the ability and willingness of the client to comprehend and carry out the directions given him as part of the therapeutic plan.

The communication skills and sensitivity of the practitioner during the interview process may well be the most important examiner skills making up the assessment armamentarium. To this end, the practitioner must develop a flexible framework for obtaining the information or behavior needed in the assessment that will also facilitate the interaction necessary for a therapeutic relationship.

The most effective place to learn how to interview is at the bedside and in the clinic while dealing with actual clients. Initial interviews should be supervised by a skilled professional who will provide approbation or suggestions for modification immediately after leaving the client.

The use of a written record of the interview, called a process recording, may be helpful in identifying communication problems. However, a tape recording of a verbal interchange between the client and the practitioner may serve the same ends.

Particularly at the first interview, the client should be allowed to talk freely, to ramble on in his description of his health condition. One frequently observed error is the monopoly of the interview by the practi-

tioner. Frequently clients report that they did not mention symptoms because they did not have an opportunity or were not encouraged to do so. When one of the participants does most of the talking during the interview, in essence delivers a monologue, the other may be silent for long periods or repeat certain phrases again and again. Thus, "uh huh" or "okay" said repeatedly by one person in the interview is characteristic of stifled communication. The practitioner should bear in mind that the perception of what is being said in conversation is often decreased when one is listening to a long presentation. The most effective communication exists when the client takes an active role in the interview.

THE CONTRACT

The interview is a verbal and nonverbal exchange that provides for the beginning and development of a relationship. Initially, the participants are strangers, each presenting his own style of relating and adapting. Defining the terms of the relationship early in the interview obviates unnecessary stressors and provides goals for the participants. Common symbols—those that are consensually validated between examiner and client, that is, have the same meaning to both participants—must be achieved, since the quality of the communication will determine the value of the relationship. Unlike many others, the association between health professional and client has a mutual concern, the well-being of the client. This commonality of interest will facilitate progress toward the sharing of information, ideas, and emotions. A mutually understandable language, as well as an understanding of the significance of body language, such as gestures and facial expressions, and somatic language (signs of autonomic nervous system reactions) will increase the exchange of information between the client and the practitioner and enrich the data obtained.

Facial expressions are the most widely used nonverbal communication and the message most frequently observed by the client. Eye contact is frequently used. Human beings invite communication with another person by looking directly at him. Generally speaking, this kind of open stare is regarded positively; the person who looks another in the eye while talking is considered open and honest. However, should the person being gazed upon decline the invitation, he generally does so by averting eye contact, most often looking downward. While a short gaze may be interpreted as accessibility and interest on the part of examiner, it is important to avoid long periods of looking directly at the client because this may be interpreted as an invitation to deeper relationship by the client.

The contract, or basic operating agreement between the client and the practitioner, should include:

1. Time and place that the interview and subsequent examinations will occur
2. Duration of time involved in the present and future examinations
3. Number of sessions required
4. Expectations for participation by the client in the assessment process
5. Confidentiality of shared information and findings—responsibilities of each member
6. Rules regarding the presence of other professionals or of the client's relatives or other advocates
7. Cost to the client where applicable
8. Therapeutic goals subsequent to the assessment process

The advantage of the contract to the practitioner is that the client is relieved of misconceptions, fears, or fantasies he may have had concerning what might happen during the interview and examination. Thus, the contract establishes norms and role behavior. A social system with definable, interdependent parts, so that a change in one part effects changes in other parts, has been identified. The practitioner and the client have expectations of each other. Abrogation of responsibility threatens the relationship.

The expectation that there will be shared decision making in the management of his health care should be made very clear to the client. To this end, the client is encouraged to learn more about himself in order to identify health needs and to recognize that he has an option in determining if and how his health needs may be met.

In traditional health care relationships there is an inequity in that the health professionals is in the authority role whereas the client is, at least to some degree, dependent. The client has initiated the interview by seeking help for his problems. In his efforts to obtain aid from the professional, the client must determine the kind of information and behavior expected. The professional is obligated to analyze the client's communication pattern in order to explain to the client what is needed for the professional to give the help that is needed. The interaction provides a kind of negotiation for the terms on which the relationship can continue, that is, a contract defining the roles of the participants. The verbal and nonverbal dialogue that occurs in the first few minutes of this social exchange may well determine not only the reliability and amount of information the client will furnish to the interviewer but also the character of the relationship that follows.

SETTING

To promote the most effective attention to communication and therefore to build rapport, the practitioner should carefully construct the interview environment to avoid interruption, distraction, or discomfort. Although geographical privacy may not be a luxury that can be obtained in large clinics or in multiple bed units in the hospital, psychological protection may be provided. Some of the assurances important to the client are that (1) the client is not being heard by other clients or personnel not concerned in his care, (2) the practitioner is giving his highest level of attention to the client, and (3) the information the client is sharing will be regarded as confidential.

In the more ideal setting, the privacy of the client's thoughts and his comfort can be guaranteed by conducting the interview in a private room where optimum temperature and lighting can be controlled.

The physical position of the practitioner as related to the client can have implications in the control process. For a mutual sharing of the control of the interview or to suggest that the client has some option for control, the chairs or other furniture should be arranged so that a face-to-face alignment is possible. The commonly used position of standing over the client (looking down at) suggests that the practitioner has assumed leadership for the interchange.

Excessively long interviews are tiring to the client. There may be a need to schedule more than one session to complete the data base, particularly if the health history is complex or the client is critically ill or debilitated.

COMMUNICATION PROCESS

Anxiety is an anticipated element in an initial interview for both the health professional and the client. Some of the indications of acute anxiety that may be observed include a furrowed brow, squinting, dilated pupils, tensed facial muscles, distended neck vessels, tensed facial muscles, distended neck vessels, rapid talk, a dry mouth, frequent hand gestures, a tense posture, an increased heart rate and blood pressure, sweaty palms and axillae, and a sweaty pubic area. Shuffling of feet may indicate a desire by the client to escape the interview. The client's anxieties may be associated with the symptoms of his illness, with the practitioner's reaction to him, with fees, or with expectations of future appointments. The practitioner is concerned with the client's response to the interview, with his (the practitioner's) ability to get appropriate information, and with his ability to synthesize the data provided so that the problems can be correctly defined. The practitioner is further concerned that problem management is appropriate and that referral is properly instituted. Clues that interview items are anxiety producing are long pauses, nervous laughter, dry coughing, and sighing.

To facilitate the development of rapport, the health professional must use his communication skills to project to the client that he is interested and concerned with providing the support needed by the client. The practitioner might convey support by assuring the client, "I'll do all I can to find out what is making you feel this way." To demonstrate interest and the willingness to listen, the practitioner must also be aware of the message conveyed nonverbally.

The practitioner must deal with both the information needed and given by the client and with the process of the interview. This process is the developing relationship and will include not only what is said but those elements that are implied by words and gesture, that is, the manner in which data are supplied and withheld as well as the client's efforts to control the interview.

Particular attention is given the remarks made as the client is entering the room or as he is leaving, since these comments frequently have special significance. The client may reveal his chief complaint at these times and avoid mentioning it during the formal interview.

The amount of structure that is brought to bear in the interview is dependent on the level of organization of ego functioning exhibited by the client. In general, the client with the lesser degree of organization needs more structure in the interview in order to increase the amount of data obtained in a given period of time and to decrease anxiety.

The communication process involves feedback in that each message sent involves a response. This response affects the next message sent and its reaction. The skilled practitioner readily settles in the communication mode that is most effective for the individual client. This is particularly important in the choice of the type of questions used to obtain the health history.

A common communication error that occurs in this society is that of thinking of the next remark, thereby not fully perceiving what is being said. This is a particular hazard for the student who is not yet fully comfortable with the interview pattern. Such an individual may perceive little of valuable data being given him by the client since he must concentrate on the format of questioning as well as on how best to word the next query.

Types of questions

Open-ended questions or suggestions. Although the interview is aimed at getting more or less specific answers concerning the events surrounding the client's signs and symptoms, each point should be developed by the client in his own words. An open-ended question or suggestion is one aimed at eliciting a response that is more than one or two words in length. This type of question is effective in stimulating descriptive or comparative responses. Observation of the client as he describes a symptom may give valuable information concerning his attitudes and beliefs. In addition, it allows the client to provide information when he is ready to disclose it, he is not forced to divulge information when sharing it may trouble him. This free description may also provide clues to the alertness, or level of mental abilities, of the client and to the organization of his ego functioning, revealed through the organization of his thoughts and through his vocabulary. Furthermore, rapport is strengthened through the demonstration that the practitioner wants to invest time in hearing the thoughts of the client.

Examples of open-ended questions or suggestions are "How have you been feeling lately?" and "Tell me about your problem."

The disadvantage of this type of question is that it may result in responses that are not relevant to a specific point being assessed. The client may use the opportunity provided by an open-ended question to digress in order to avoid discussing relevant data because it is distressing to him. Although this technique might yield important information, there are times when the examiner needs data quickly and must sacrifice to get it. This is particularly true in emergency care. When the drug overdose victim rouses, the only piece of data of importance may be elicited by a closed question ("What did you take?")

Closed questions. The closed question is a type of inquiry that requires no more than a one- or two-word answer. This might be agreement or disagreement. The response may be a yes or no and may be answered nonverbally by a nod of the head. This is the kind of question most appropriate for eliciting age, sex, marital status, and other forced-choice responses.

Examples of closed questions are "What did you eat for dinner last night?" and "What medication did you take?"

The educationally impoverished or those who lack culturally enriching experiences are often more comfortable with this type of question because they know what is expected. The open-ended question may pose anxiety to the client with poor articulation, since he may be afraid that the display of his lack of verbal skill will disadvantage him with the practitioner. On the other hand, the closed question by its nature limits the amount of information that is obtained in the health history and may convey to the client that the practitioner is too busy or disinterested to listen to him. It has been observed that practitioners use more closed questions in initial interviews and when the process is stressful, as well as when time constraints are marked.

Biased or leading questions. Questions that carry a suggestion of the kind of information that should be included in the response are called *leading* or *biased*. The client is presented with an expectation by the practitioner. This kind of question may seriously limit the value of the health history. For example, the question "You haven't ever had venereal disease, have you?" implies that the possibility that the client *has had* venereal disease would be outside the limits of reality for the practitioner. The client who has experienced the disease may not say so to avoid disappointing the questioner.

The presence of emotionally charged words in a given question may make the question a biased one. For example, there is one in the question, "You haven't been masturbating, have you?" Since the Judeo-Christian ethic defines masturbating as "bad," bias has been inflicted. In this case the practitioner has suggested that the answer should be no. The client may well avoid all matters dealing with sexuality in order to avoid the possible loss of the approval of the practitioner.

The practitioner must balance the goals of efficiency and effectiveness in the interviews. In obtaining a historical data base, the practitioner asks the client many questions, the object of which is to obtain thorough, relevant information. However, a comprehensive interview is a very time-consuming activity and practitioners often attempt to save time by asking closed questions. More information is gained by open-ended questions that may supply much relevant as well as extraneous data. Therefore, the interviewer needs to consider the relative importance of the interview questions in the gathering of the data base so that he can obtain the most useful information within a reasonable time.

Use of silence

Periods of silence during the interview are helpful in making observations, such as is the client comfortable? Angry? Confused? Silence provides an opportunity to assess the level of anxiety in both the practitioner and the client. Also, the client is provided with sufficient time to carefully organize his thoughts for a coherent explanation in response to questions. The rapid presentation of questions may not allow time for sufficient thought or reflection by the client. Silence is also useful as an indicator of the amount of anxiety the client is experiencing. Silence may indicate absorbing thought, boredom, deep affection, or grief.

Methods for assuring understanding

The practitioner must use validation maneuvers to determine if both participants understand what has been said. A clear understanding of what the client is trying to say is essential to the establishment of an accurate data base. The health history should not contain assumptions of what the client meant but a clear accounting of exactly what he said. There are many techniques that provide for encouragement of the client to expand on a description or to clarify the explanation that has been given. A workable example might be "Tell me more about it."

Use of a common language. The practitioner must carefully plan questions and give particular care in selecting the vocabulary to be used in order that the client perceive the question in the same sense that it is intended by the practitioner. The practitioner is aided in processing the language and behavior of the client for what is usual or "normal" by having an understanding of cultural and ethnic differences. Medical terminology or jargon should not be used excessively. When medical diagnoses are employed, the meaning should be explained to the client when the words are first used.

Frequently, the professional uses these terms to avoid communication altogether or to terminate conversations with clients. Should the client use a medical diagnosis, the practitioner should ascertain that the client's understanding of the word matches his own. For example, many lay people believe that *neoplasm* is synonymous with *cancer*.

Planning the questions. The client is asked one question at a time. In order for the client to give the information needed for the health history, the questions must be phrased in such a way that the client knows what kind of answers are expected. When the client's response is not appropriate, a re-ordering of the question or a more explicit choice of vocabulary may be indicated. It may be helpful to emphasize the key words in the question. In designing questions, one should avoid the use of ambiguous terms, medical language, or words with more than one meaning.

Use of an example. Comparison with a common experience, that is, a concrete happening, may help to clarify an abstract concept or hazy terminology. The practitioner may use an example as part of the questioning process when the meaning is not clear. For example, the practitioner may ask the client, "Was it as large as a cherry?"

Restatement. Restatement is the formulation of what the client has said in words that are more specific; it provides an opportunity for validation of the practitioner's conception. The client is cued that he is expected to give attention to the thought by phrases such as "Do you mean . . . ," "In other words . . . ," or "If I understand you correctly. . . ."

Reflection or echoing. Reflection, or echoing, means repeating a phrase or a sentence the client has just said. The suggestion to the client that the practitioner is still involved in that part of the communication may focus further attention or rumination on that thought. The strategy is aimed toward further elaboration in the form of the recall of facts or feeling states that surrounded the circumstance. The technique should allow clarification or expansion of the information just given by the client. Examples are "You say your mother is an alcoholic?" and "Painful?"

Encapsulation or summary. Encapsulation, or summary, is a technique that allows for the condensation of facts into a well-ordered review. It is particularly useful following a rambling, detailed description. The summary further signals the client that this particular segment of the interview is terminating and suggests to him that he should give further input immediately, since closure is imminent.

Confrontation. Telling the client something about himself is known as confrontation. This may be a helpful technique to use when inconsistencies are noticed, for example, "When you tell me how painful your arm is, I notice that you are smiling. Why is this?" Confrontation may also be of use in helping the client to discuss his emotions, for example, "You say you are not uncomfortable, but you are frowning and your muscles appear very tense."

Interpretation. The examiner may arrive at a conclusion from the data the client has given. Sharing the interpretation with the client allows the individual to confirm, deny, or offer an interpretation of his own. Making an interpretation involves the risk of being wrong, and the examiner should be prepared to deal with this eventuality. The interpretation may also constitute an act of empathy or confrontation.

Interviewer: Since your mother and brother died in the same week, you must have felt very depressed.

Client: Yes, I was somewhat upset, but I had lived with my grandmother since my brother was born and really was not as close as you might expect.

Filling in omitted data

Clinical impressions reached by the practitioner must be regarded as fluid in the sense that in further conversation with the client new information may be provided. The client may withhold information if he fears that sensitive information may be shared indiscriminately or if he has not been able to trust the practitioner. Furthermore, he may regard certain facts as unimportant or irrelevant to the focus of the interview. There are many instances when the client is so eager to comply with questions that he gives a hurried accounting and leaves out significant data. In ordering the data the practitioner may note that information is missing or that there are inconsistencies. Further interviews may be scheduled. The client may simply need to be given a summary of his previous conversation in order for him to detect the areas where he needs to interject information. These gaps may be filled by direct questioning. Another method of asking for the missing facts may be to suggest to the client that the practitioner is confused and needs to be told again a particular sequence of events. A remark such as the following would invite this input: "Now, tell me again all that you remember from the time you first vomited until you came here."

In addition, the possibility of past evaluation and treatment of symptoms should be investigated. The important facts are those obtained by asking when, where, and by whom. Were laboratory or other diagnostic tests performed? Are results available? What diagnosis was made? Was a treatment instituted? Was the treatment helpful?

Obtaining data from people other than the client

The client who is critically ill, confused, or intellectually impaired may be unable to give the information necessary to an adequate history. A close relative or a person who knows the client well may be able to provide the information necessary to understand the presence or nature of problems of the individual being examined. If an ineffective attempt has been made to obtain the history from the client, it may be psychologically prudent to ask permission to go over the details again with the second person. Such comments as "I want to be sure that I have what has happened to you correctly in my mind," or "I'd like to go over this one more time to make sure I've got the facts right and in the correct order," may help to gain the client's permission to interview relatives or friends. The parents may be the only reliable source of information for the young child.

Nonverbal communication—kinesis

Nonverbal communication is that which takes place in the form of behavior patterns that are expressive in the use of (1) body movements, (2) space or territoriality, (3) voice tone, (4) time, and (5) appearance. The behaviors can convey emotional or feeling state messages or can be used to impart instruction or direction.

COMMUNICATION THROUGH BODY MOVEMENT

Some of the gestures to be observed are movements of the body, limbs, hands, or feet; facial expressions, particularly smiling and frowning; and eye behavior such as blinking, the direction of gaze, and the length of time of gaze. Posture is particularly expressive.

Extension of large muscles is associated with relaxation, whereas contraction of large muscles is associated with anxiety and fear. The individual who sits stretched out and gestures away from the body gives an aura of assurance.

Kinesis is the communication provided through body movement. The posture or movement of the client's body may provide valuable clues to his health status. The messages given by the client through his body language may provide additional and sometimes more reliable information than his words, since many persons employ less conscious control over this aspect of behavior. Thus, by his actions the client may convey thoughts that he cannot or refuses to commit to words. Interpretation of the full meaning of the gestures and action of the client must be performed against a comparison of their sociocultural meanings. For instance, the downcast eyes of the Muhammadan woman could be interpreted as the usual or normal response to the practitioner, whereas in the United States one might become alert to other indications of fear, withdrawal or depression, or lack of attentiveness. The use of eye contact assumes a good deal of meaning among Greek and Indian cultures, whereas torso messages are common in Africa.

Posture. A closed body posture is one in which the limbs are held in defensive positions, that is, close to the body, flexed, muscles tense. The arms may be held very close to the body as though hugging oneself. The position is most often interpreted as distrustful. An open body posture is one that is more relaxed, that is, limbs extended, arms hanging loosely at sides.

Facial expression. Clenched teeth (strongly contracted masseter and temporal muscles) and contracted pupils provide a message of tension and may represent an effort to avoid saying something unpleasant to the listener. This expression is generally interpreted as one of anger.

An individual who smiles constantly may be using this expression as a mask to cover feelings of fear or depression. On the other hand, this may simply be the trademark of an individual with a strong desire to please.

The person who covers his mouth with his hands may be expressing a desire to avoid talking.

Oculesics. Oculesics is the communication that occurs through glances and eye movements. The practitioner may detect signals of disagreement, aversion, or disgust in the client through subtle eye movements. Dilation of the pupils of the eyes generally accompanies pleasurable experiences, whereas offensive or unpleasant circumstances generally result in contracted pupils.

Touch. The act of touching is one of the most intimate forms of nonverbal communication. Cultural traditions prescribe the ritual of touch or define the taboos. Touch is regulated by social-distancing techniques and is apparent in all living groups. Touch has special meaning among health professionals. Many professionals conceive of themselves reaching out in support of their clients. Touch, when used judiciously, conveys a message of closeness, encouragement, and caring and plays a prominent part in the health practitioner–client interaction.

Although in American culture a pat on the back, the handshake, a gentle squeeze of the hand, or a slap on the cheek may be well understood, the practitioner must bear in mind that this community of understanding does not exist for many touching processes. The physical contact of palpation may be misperceived as it is translated from stimulus received to perception. Touch as a form of communication precedes speech in the individual's life. Manners and mores involving touch are given to the developing child through the actions of his significant others. In America there is a taboo against touching without permission to do so. So, we talk about the reassuring pat of the hand and the warm handshake and define who is permitted to do these acts. There is often confusion when the client opts to touch the health professional.

EFFECT OF SPACE OR TERRITORIALITY ON COMMUNICATION

A good deal of symbolism has been attributed to one's position in a group. Definition of a cultural group's concern or rejection is provided by distancing. The distance between the practitioner and the client may determine the relationships developed.

The size of space allowed the client may be related to status or to the differential importance accorded him.

Hall has coined the word "proxemics" to describe the use of space by people in the United States as zones that he calls intimate, personal, social, and public.

Intimate distance. Intimate distance is the distance used for physical lovemaking and intense verbal exchange and is defined as a distance of zero to 18 inches. This is the distance from which most of the clinical examination is performed. Body contact is expected during the physical examination and the practitioner must use the intimate space of the client and must be concerned with sensory overload. Thus, sensation may frequently be distorted. The presence of another body at this close distance intrudes on the senses and is sometimes overwhelming to the client.

At this close distance the odors of each body are prominent in the senses. The examiner is aware of diagnostic body odors and of the patient's general hygiene. The examiner should also be aware of his own body smells; the use of pungent toiletries is often offensive to the client. Even the heat extruded by the bodies of participants may be a part of the interchange.

This close phase is also the distance used by the client for touch and intimate skin manipulation. This may be pleasurable and reassuring or threatening to the client. Muscular tension is heightened as though in preparation for movement.

Visual detail is sharpened. The eyes are pulled inward in accommodation, and the individual may appear to squint. Vocalization may be involuntary at the near point but become low and more frequent as the periphery of this zone is approached.

Since it would appear that it is a natural instinct to maintain and protect the space immediately around us, the intrusion on the client's intimate zone should be carefully planned. The client may be carefully assessing the practitioner's use of space. His perceptions may be largely determined by what he assesses of the practitioner in the visual domain.

Frequently the use of social measures that allow the acceptance of a shortened distance for communications may be helpful; these include introductions, an explanation of the roles of the practitioner and the client, and an explanation of the benefits to be achieved by allowing the closer contact. The client should have each procedure communicated to him before its actualization with the full knowledge that he has the option to refuse. The practitioner should use simple sentences and a carefully chosen, nonthreatening vocabulary.

The hospital room or clinic office visit seriously threatens the control of space by the client. He is told where and how he must cooperate in order that his body may be invaded by tactile, visual, auditory, and olfactory probing. The culture may permit this invasion of privacy by physicians and nurses since they are given special status by the professional roles. The endowment of the role with technical skill, authority, and confidentiality protects the client from the shame that has been cultivated in him for exposure of the body to a stranger. It has been shown that when more evidence is given of the roles of health professionals and these roles are well understood, it is easier for the client to submit to the encroachment of privacy. To this end, the professional uniform of white coat, and so on, is effective, as is the health professional's careful adherence to the behaviors recognized to be part of that role.

The client needs time to adjust to the levels of the space provided for the physical examination. The interview allows a reordering of the perimeters defining the client's space bubble. The client should be allowed as much decision making as possible. He should be allowed to order the disposition of his personal belongings. Questions regarding the use of space should be seriously attended.

Personal distance. Personal distance limits physical contact and is defined as a distance of 1½ to 4 feet. Although holding and grasping are possible at the near point, touching is the form of physical contact most frequently used. Visual perception is less distorted, and there is a three-dimensional impression of the person involved. As the distance between participants lengthens, the gaze may encompass the entire face rather than a single part of it, such as the eye or the chin. Vocal volume is moderate, and body odors and heat are less intruding.

This is the ideal distance for viewing nonverbal behaviors and is the distance most frequently utilized for the interview. Trust is best developed from this distance.

Social distance. Social distance provides protection from others without one's having to declare or demand it and is defined as a distance of 4 to 12 feet. The visual image includes more of the total person, and the fine detail of the body is lost. Eye contact becomes more important. Body heat and odor are lost. Vocalization is louder and loses its aura of privacy because it can be overheard. Interaction becomes more ritualized or formal. The threat of domination is less from this distance. This distance allows a limited view of the physical aspects of the client, and his revelation of attitudes and feelings in general is censored from this distance.

VOCALICS

Vocalics is the information that is transmitted through the delivery of speech. The individual who screeches "I'm not afraid of the operation!" reveals that he is terrified.

CHRONEMICS

Chronemics is the term used to describe the information that is transmitted through the use of time. The health practitioner is generally perceived by the client to be the one of superior status in the health care visit. Thus, the client deems it appropriate to wait past the appointment time. On the other hand, the client may be revealing some of his opposing feelings by a pattern of lateness in meeting appointments.

Similarly, the person with perceived superior status is allowed to talk longer. Interruption of the practitioner by the client with an unrelated thought while the practitioner is explaining treatment requirements may signal that the client holds the advice at low value.

EFFECT OF APPEARANCE ON COMMUNICATION

Both clothing and cosmetics may be used to create an impression. In general, adults aim to reflect the current mode of "handsome" or "beautiful" and, in most cases, "young." Furthermore, financial status may be revealed by the cut of the garments or the label of the manufacturer.

Persons in the health professions, as well as the bulk of American society, are more generous and outgoing in their feelings toward the physically attractive individual. This is true of practitioners working with all age levels. The practitioner must frequently work through attitudes and emotions in order to touch the diseased individual without visible indications of restraint or repugnance, such as tensed musculature, frowns, or touching only with the fingertips.

Supportive remarks and actions should be a part of the interview process. Although it is not credible to attest to supportiveness, the practitioner should try to convey interest and understanding of the client's problem as well as the desire to help the client meet and work through problems.

Gestures that say "I like you; you're acceptable" include smiling and moving closer. The basic projec-

tion is pleasant, and the words that are chosen say nice things.

Clients have been shown to be more cooperative when they feel accepted and respected by the health care worker. Verbal or nonverbal messages expressing unfriendliness, tension, or punishment markedly inhibit the client's motivation for interaction with the interviewer.

Effective communication is best accomplished in a climate of warmth, empathy, and genuineness. The conveyance of a feeling of positive attitude toward the client may be initiated with a hospitable greeting while devoting full attention to him. Clients most frequently interpreted warmth from the behavior of health care personnel that included direct attention and appropriate eye contact by the examiner. Thus, it is important to read or write in the chart minimally while with the client. Other behaviors that have been shown to convey warmth include a relaxed posture while leaning slightly forward in an open arm position as well as appropriate smiling and nodding. Positive regard may be demonstrated by complimenting aspects of health care that the client is practicing appropriately.

The examiner should guard against communicating haste to the client because the client may believe the examiner has low regard for the interview. Some behaviors that convey impatience are frequent checking of the time, walking to the door, or standing with the hand on the door knob.

Sincerity or genuineness on the examiner's part may be conveyed by assuring that there is congruence between the remarks made to the client and the nonverbal cues accompanying the messages. Body language that does not correspond with what is being said may be confusing or frightening to the client. The facial and body movements should correspond with what is said. The interviewer may have to spend some time learning to be aware of his own facial, body, and voice behaviors in order to effectively use them in communicating with clients. While the practitioner may be frowning because of a worry unrelated to the interview, the client in process of revealing sensitive information may conclude that the information is unacceptable to the interviewer.

Body movements that may convey that the client is uncomfortable include avoidance of eye contact, stiff posture, nervous or inappropriate laughter, and tapping the foot against the floor. The examiner would do well to ask the client about his feelings when these behaviors are observed.

EMPATHY

Role taking has been suggested to be synonymous with empathy. More simply, it is voluntarily putting oneself in another person's place in one's imagination. The four phases of empathic experience include:

1. Identification—investing oneself in thinking about the person and what is happening to him
2. Incorporation—being aware and receptive of the person, rather than projecting one's own feelings and thoughts
3. Reverberation—an interaction between the feelings and experiences of the client and the examiner
4. Detachment—return to one's own identity

The insight that is a result of the experience is helpful in understanding and meeting the needs of the client. Empathy has been described by some as active listening; it is understanding and acceptance of the client's feelings. Empathic responses may be verbal, for example, "That must have made you feel very frightened" or "That must have been very painful to you." Understanding and acceptance may also be conveyed nonverbally, for example, a hand placed on the client's shoulder. Empathy is thought to be necessary to the therapeutic relationship.

HEALTH HISTORY INTERVIEW

The first step in health assessment is the interview in which the information of the health history is obtained. This is a structured interview aimed at the collection of specific information. This type of interview may present some difficulty for the individual who has been accustomed to less structured methods, that is, more nondirective techniques. While the client may give a good deal of the history—at least the description of the problem for which help is sought—without the benefit of direct questioning, the complete information of the health history may not be obtained. In that case the practitioner must ask direct questions that will provide the necessary information. In an emergency situation, the examiner may be forced to use only closed questions.

Encouraging a complete description of the symptom

The descriptions by the client of the changes he has perceived in the structure of his body or its functions are called symptoms. The interview should provide the most accurate and constructive picture of the symptom that can be obtained, since this is the base from which the client's problems can be defined.

The practitioner carefully avoids devaluing the client's symptoms by such remarks as, "You have nothing to be nervous about," or, "That's nothing; now, last week we had a really bad case."

There are eight criteria that can be used to provide this delineation: anatomical location, quality of the symptom, quantity of the symptom, time sequence of the symptom, geographical or environmental locale in which the symptom occurs, precipitating conditions that cause the symptom to be more severe, circumstances that alleviate the symptom, and other symptoms that occur in conjunction with the symptom.

Guideline	Interview items to elicit symptom description
1. Anatomical location Radiation of the symptom	"Tell me where it hurts." "Show me where it hurts."
2. Quality or character	"What does it feel like?" "Can you compare this to something you have felt in the past?"
3. Quantity	"How bad [intense] is the pain?" "How much does the pain immobilize you?" "What effect does the pain have on normal daily activities?"
4. Time sequence	"When did you first notice the pain? "How long does it last?" How often have you had it since that time?"
5. Geographical or environmental factors	"Where were you when the pain occurred?"
6. Precipitating conditions	"Do you find that the pain occurs at a certain time of day?" "Does heat or cold seem to affect the pain?" "What causes the pain?"
Conditions making the symptom more severe	"Have you noticed anything that makes the pain worse?
7. Alleviating condition	"What seems to help you when you have the pain?"
8. Concomitant symptoms	"Have you noticed any other changes that are present when you have the pain?"

To clarify the use of these guidelines in the interview setting, consider a client who comes for treatment with a chief complaint of pain (see above column).

The accuracy of the diagnostic process is dependent on exploring the ramification of these eight areas for data collection.

BIBLIOGRAPHY

Argyle, M.: The psychology of interpersonal behavior, Balitmore, 1967, Penguin Books.

Bernstein, L., Bernstein, R. S., and Dana, R. H.: Interviewing: a guide for health professionals, New York, 1974, Appleton-Century Crofts.

Bernstein, L., and Dana, R. S.: Interviewing and the health professions, New York, 1970, Appleton-Century-Crofts.

Bird, B.: Talking with patients, ed. 3, Philadelphia, 1973, J. B. Lippincott Co.

DiMatteo, M. R.: A social-psychological analysis of physician-patient rapport toward a science of the art of medicine, J. Soc. Issues **35:**12, 1979.

Ehmann, V. E.: Empathy: its origin, characteristics and process, Perspect. Psychiatr. Care **9:**72, 1971.

Engel, G. L., and Morgan, W. L., Jr.: Interviewing the patient, Philadelphia, 1973, W. B. Saunders Co.

Enelow, A. J., and Swisher, S. N.: Interviewing and patient care, New York, 1979, Oxford University Press.

Fast, J.: Body language, New York, 1970, M. Evans & Co., Inc.

Friedman, H. S.: Nonverbal communication between patients and medical practitioners, J. Soc. Issues. **35:**82, 1979.

Froehlich, R. E., and Bishop, F. M.: Clinical interviewing skills: a programmed manual for data gathering, evaluation and patient management, ed. 3, St. Louis, 1977, The C. V. Mosby Co.

Gill, M., Newman, R., and Redlich, F.: The initial interview in psychiatric practice, New York, 1954, International Universities Press.

Gordon, R.: Interviewing; strategy, techniques and tactics, Homewood, Ill., 1969, Dorsey Press.

Hall, E.: The silent language, Greenwich, Conn., 1959, Fawcett.

Hall, E.: The hidden dimension, Garden City, N.Y., 1969, Doubleday & Co., Inc.

MacKinnon, R. A., and Michels, R.: The psychiatric interview in clinical practice, Philadelphia, 1971, W. B. Saunders Co.

Morgan, W. L., Jr., and Engel, G. L.: The clinical approach to the patient, Philadelphia, 1969, W. B. Saunders Co.

Richardson, S., Dohrenwend, B. S., and Klein, D.: Interviewing, its forms and functions, New York, 1965, Basic Books, Inc., Publishers.

Sullivan, H.: The psychiatric interview, New York, 1954, W. W. Norton & Co., Inc.

Ware, J. E., Jr., Davies, A. A., and Steward, A. L.: The measurement and meaning of patient satisfaction, Health Med. Care Serv. Rev. **1:**1, 1978.

3 The health history

The health history is an extremely important part of the health assessment. Its performance is the primary vehicle by which rapport is established between the practitioner and the client. The information derived from the history-taking interview assists the practitioner in assessing and diagnosing the client's health problems and in obtaining knowledge of the client's problems and needs within the context of that particular client's life. The health history not only records the problems of the client but also describes the client as a whole and in relation to his social and physical environment. Thus, it records not only weaknesses and abnormalities but also the strengths that will support therapy and care.

Other important components of the history data base are the perceptions of the client regarding his health, his illness, and his past experiences with health delivery systems. These perceptions must be known if future care is to be relevant and, consequently, effective.

In practice, the taking of the health history is implemented in two phases: (1) the client interview phase, which elicits the information, and (2) the recording of data. The information as presented in this chapter is organized according to a systematic method for recording the history. The client interview may or may not proceed in the same sequence. Each portion of the health history discussed contains descriptions of processes for both eliciting and summarizing data. Examples of two recorded health histories are included at the end of this chapter.

Certain principles of the history-taking procedure should be emphasized. The importance of privacy seems obvious, but this principle is too often violated in actual practice. Another apparent principle is the maintenance of eye contact (Fig. 3-1), but what does one do about recording? The practitioner must immediately note specific information, such as dates, age, and so on, or it may be forgotten. Also, the client expects the practitioner to consider his information important enough to have it recorded. It is a temptation to attempt to complete the recorded history during the interview, but it is not possible to do this and simultaneously observe the client and his responses.

FORMAT

The health history, as described in this chapter, is an extremely complete one. In many actual client care situations, it may not be possible, or even appropriate, to obtain the complete history. For clients receiving continuous care, the history can be obtained in portions during several encounters.

For clients requiring episodic care, decisions regarding the data essential for immediate therapy guide the content of the history.

However, the beginning historian should practice obtaining the complete health history in order to develop skill in interviewing and in recording data and to establish priorities for focused interviews. During this practice process the learner will develop an appreciation for the client management implications of each portion of the health history.

The format used in this text for the complete health history is as follows:

A. Biographical information
B. Chief complaint or client's request for care
C. Present illness or present health status
D. Past history
E. Family history
F. Review of systems
    1. Physical
    2. Sociological
    3. Psychological
G. Developmental data
H. Nutritional data

Biographical information

At the beginning of any health record, there should be a place to record commonly used and sometimes

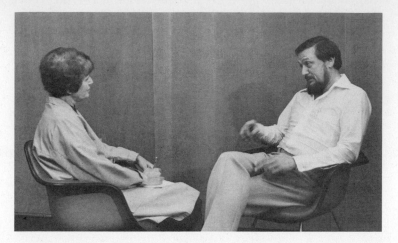

Fig. 3-1. Interview.

critically important biographical information. This information should be obtained early during the client's first visit or admission; otherwise, it may be omitted, only to be needed in an emergency or at a time when the client is unavailable or unable to respond.

The following information is to be recorded in the introductory and biographical section of the health history:

A. Full name
B. Address and telephone numbers
  1. Client's permanent
  2. Contact of client
C. Birthdate
D. Sex
E. Race
F. Religion
G. Marital status
H. Social Security number
I. Occupation
  1. Usual
  2. Present
J. Birthplace
K. Source of referral
L. Usual source of health care
M. Source and reliability of information
N. Date of interview

First, the client's name is recorded. Persons in an ethnically homogenous geographical area often have similar names. Precise identification, using first, middle, and last names, assists in assuring accurate information retrieval and coordination.

Next, the client's full mailing address and telephone number are recorded. Also recorded are the name, address, and telephone number of one of the client's friends or relatives, someone with whom he is in frequent contact and who would be willing and able to relay a message to the client in an emergency or if the client could not be located.

Birthplace, sex, race, marital status, and religion information are self-explanatory. Many health problems and needs are age, sex, race, or social situation related. This information might be correlated with problems discovered later in the history.

There are justifiable reasons for the notation of the client's Social Security number, including the precise identification of each client and a potential access to a large pool of health-related information. Potential violations of confidentiality are a disadvantage.

A significant difference may exist between the client's current and usual occupations. The nature of the difference may be indicative of the severity of the client's health problems and the level of disability resulting from them. In addition, knowledge of past occupations might provide clues to past or present environmental hazards contributing to the present illness. A mine worker with a respiratory system complaint is an example.

Knowledge of the client's birthplace provides geographical implications for the origin of problems and cultural implications for therapy and health maintenance.

If the current caregiver is not the usual and primary source of the client's care, the name and address of the individual or institution so identified should be recorded. In addition, the practitioner should record the reason for the client's entering a new health care system. The client may be in crisis, he may be dissatisfied with past care, or he may be "shopping." If the past source of care possesses significant data about the client's health and if the client intends to continue in the current health care system, the client should be asked to sign a permission for the transfer of information. Later in the health history, the practitioner will have the opportunity to record, in some detail, past patterns of health care.

Next, the practitioner makes a statement about the source of the information to follow. In most cases the source is the client, but this cannot be assumed unless the informant is specifically identified. If the information is given by someone other than the client, the degree of the informant's contact with the client should be described. For example, in the case of a child, the practitioner would utilize the history given by a grandmother who resides with the child differently from one given by a grandmother who visits the child once a week.

Along with the statement of the informant, an evaluation of his reliability is made. For example, one of the following may be stated: "inconsistent," "unclear about recent events," "evasive," or "cooperative and reliable." These statements serve as simple criteria by which the remainder of the information in the history is judged by other health care providers and may indicate a need to retake or supplement the history at a future date or to consult with other informants to determine the accuracy of the data.

The history is dated. In a situation where the client's condition changes rapidly, events can be correlated only if their temporal relationships are known.

Chief complaint or client's request for care

The chief complaint (CC) statement is a short statement, in the client's own words and recorded in quotation marks, that indicates the client's purpose for requesting health care at this time. In the case of a client who is ill, the CC statement is of the acute or chronic problem (or problems) that is the client's priority for treatment. The CC statement, whenever relevant, includes a notation of the problem's duration. The duration, as stated by the client, may not be the actual duration of the symptoms. However, it is an indication of the time during which the complaint has become intolerable enough to motivate the client to seek help.

In the case of a well client, the CC statement may be a statement of the client's request for a health examination for health screening, health promotion, or disease case-finding purposes.

The CC statement is not a diagnostic statement. Actually, it is very hazardous to state a chief complaint in diagnostic terms. For example, a client who has frequent asthmatic attacks appears for treatment with respiratory system complaints and states that he is having an "asthmatic attack." This may or may not be the case. In this early portion of the history, client and interviewer bias must be avoided; otherwise the interview and the problem solving may be set in one, and potentially a wrong, direction.

The following are examples of adequately stated chief complaints:

"Chest pain for 3 days."
"Swollen ankles for 2 weeks."
"Fever and headache for 24 hours."
"Pap smear needed. Last Pap 9/8/73."
"Physical examination needed for camp."

The following are examples of inadequately stated chief complaints:

"Thinks she might be pregnant."
"Sick."
"Nausea and vomiting."
"Hypertension."

The CC statement may seem superfluous, especially since the next section on the present illness describes the symptoms in detail. However, this is one of the few places in the recorded history of a client's encounter with the health care system where he has the opportunity to have recorded, in his own words, his needs. Too often the practitioner loses sight of the client's priorities for care. The consistent recording of a chief complaint or reason for the visit will assist in keeping the system responsive to the client's perceived needs.

In some instances the client may present several complaints. No more than three should be stated in this portion of the history and the client's stated priorities should be noted first. There is the opportunity to discuss all problems in the present illness portion of the health history.

Present illness or present health status

The present illness (PI) section describes the information relevant to the chief complaint. In the case of a client with a health problem, this portion of the health history challenges the interviewing, clinical knowledge, and written communication skills of the practitioner. The practitioner needs to learn the minute details of the chief complaint and its associated phenomena. Information must be comprehensive, it must be recorded concisely and comprehensively, and it must provide the practitioner with enough information to initiate additional assessment and the intervention measures.

The interviewing and recording for the present illness portion of the health history is especially difficult for beginning practitioners because the processes require both skill in interviewing and history taking and clinical knowledge. Outlining the progression of the present illness prior to writing the narrative discussion is sometimes helpful. Although the student learning health assessment has probably not yet learned client care management, the student may find the referral to clinical management references for the system(s) discussed with the patient will often alert him to the most valuable pieces of data and highlight important omissions, which can be incorporated in future interviews.

In the case of a well client, the interviewer usually describes the client's usual health and briefly summarizes his health maintenance needs and activities.

The following are the components of the PI section:

I. Introduction
   A. Client's summary
   B. Usual health
II. Investigation of symptoms: chronological story
   A. Onset
   B. Date
   C. Manner (gradual or sudden)
   D. Duration
   E. Precipitating factors
   F. Course since onset
      1. Incidence (frequency)
      2. Manner
      3. Duration (longest, shortest, and average times)
      4. Patterns of remissions and exacerbations
   G. Location
   H. Quality
   I. Quantity
   J. Setting
   K. Associated phenomena
   L. Alleviating or aggrevating factors
III. Negative information
IV. Relevant family information
V. Disability assessment

Introduction. The introduction to the PI section should be succinct; its major purpose is to provide the reader with a general orientation to the client.

The introduction indicates which admission or visit this particular one is for this client to the institution or service. Next, there is a short summary of the client's biographical data. Age, race, marital status, employment status, and occupation are the items of information usually recorded. If the client is being hospitalized and has been hospitalized in the past, the client's total number of hospitalizations and the number of hospitalizations for complaints related to the current illness are noted.

The practitioner next describes the client's usual health and records any significant past diagnoses or past or current health problems that might have caused the client to enjoy anything other than good health.

Investigation of symptoms: chronological story. The practitioner usually initiates the PI description by asking the client: "Tell me about it [the problem mentioned in the CC statement]," or "How did it start and what has happened since it started?" The client will usually respond to this inquiry with a long but usually diagnostically incomplete discourse about his health problems and needs. The practitioner exer-

cises skill in determining when to interrupt the client and more specifically direct his responses by asking additional, clarifying questions and when to allow the client to continue the narration of those events significant to him.

The practitioner needs a mental or actual list of the areas of symptom investigation as an aid in attaining comprehensive information. Regardless of the nature of a problem, each of the areas of investigation is relevant, and any health problem analysis would be incomplete without the description of all areas.

The practitioner also attempts to determine the chronological sequence of the client's problem. The client is apt to best remember his most recent episode of illness and in the case of a prolonged illness will need direction in tracing the problem back to its first symptomatic event. Once this first event is identified, it is investigated in detail and its date, manner of onset, duration, and precipitating factors are described in the recording.

Each symptom's course since onset is described. Frequency in a specific time interval is determined. Clients may state vaguely that they have a symptom "all the time." This may mean once a month to one client or ten times a day to another. To obtain specific information, the practitioner might ask, "How many times a day (or a week, or a month) does it occur?" Although the practitioner avoids suggesting answers with his questions, occasionally it may be necessary to pursue frequency with leading questions, for example, "Does it occur more often than five times a day?"

The practitioner determines the usual manner of onset for the illness episodes. Any change in onset is specifically mentioned. In the case of many episodes, the longest, shortest, and average durations of the episodes are noted. If there have been only several episodes, the length of each is identified.

In prolonged illnesses, the patterns of remission and exacerbation are described according to their duration and frequency. The practitioner needs to be watchful for environmental or other clues that might be precipitating factors for the illness events.

In recording, there are several suggested methods that can be used in assisting readers to easily identify temporal relationships. The practitioner describes the initial event first and then the subsequent events. The chronological story may be indexed in the left-hand column of the history sheet, using the reference base *prior to admission* (PTA). For example, the index might be listed as follows: "6 years PTA," "3 years PTA," "6 months PTA," "1 day PTA," and so on, with the corresponding narrative alongside of and below the temporal index heading.

A method of demonstrating the progression of ill-

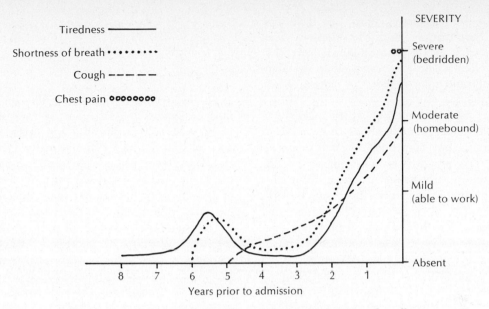

Fig. 3-2. Use of a graph to illustrate symptomatic progress of an illness.

ness is accomplished by the use of a diagram illustrating the disease process (Fig. 3-2). A diagram is especially helpful in the case of multisymptomatic illnesses.

As the chronological story evolves, the other areas of symptom investigation are integrated into the text of the narrative. Whenever appropriate, the sign's or symptom's location, quality, quantity, setting, associated phenomena, and alleviating and aggravating factors are described, especially whenever there is a change in any of them.

LOCATION. The exact site of the sign or symptom is determined. Subjective events, such as pain, pose some problem. Having a client point to the exact point of pain and trace its radiation with his finger assists in location. In recording location, one uses body hemispheres and landmarks.

QUALITY. Quality refers to the unique properties of the complaint. Signs, such as discharge, are described according to their color, texture, composition, appearance, and odor. Sound and temperature may be descriptive attributes of other phenomena.

Subjective events, such as pain, challenge the creativity of the practitioner. The quality of pain is frequently characterized as dull, aching, sharp, nagging, throbbing, stabbing, or squeezing.

Whenever appropriate, the client's descriptions are used with quotation marks.

QUANTITY. Quantity refers to the size, extent, number, or amount, for example, of the pain, rash, discharge, or lesion. With objective signs, the practitioner can use commonly understood measures, such as centimeters, cups, or tablespoons. In describing subjective events, pain, for example, one should note that evaluations such as "a little" or "a lot" have different meanings among persons. The quality of such phenomena can be more accurately understood by describing the client's response to the symptom. For example, does he have to stop and sit or does he continue on with what he is doing?

SETTING. Whenever something occurs, the client is somewhere and is either with someone or alone. Physically or psychologically the setting may have an effect on the client, and knowledge of this information may provide the practitioner with clues of the cause of the problem and implications for treatment.

ASSOCIATED PHENOMENA. Associated phenomena are those symptoms that occur with the chief complaint. They may be related to the chief complaint or may be a part of a totally different syndrome. Often the client will spontaneously identify these events. In addition, the practitioner may ask if there is anything else occurring with the chief complaint or ask about the presence or absence of certain specific events. A complete review of the implicated problem system or systems is indicated. Positive responses are recorded with a complete description of all reported symptoms. Negative responses are recorded in the negative information section.

ALLEVIATING OR AGGRAVATING FACTORS. When an illness occurs, a person often accommodates to it or treats himself. He may decrease activity, eat more or less, wait, or actively medicate and treat himself. The practitioner should nonpunitively probe into the client's actions in response to the problem and into the effect of these actions. If there has been professional intervention, the nature, source, and effect of each intervention are recorded. The client, through treatment or through accommodation, may have discovered something that alleviates the symptom. The client is asked what makes his problem better. The nature of the client's solution may provide valuable therapeutic data and may reflect the nature of his adaptation to illness.

The client is asked about that which makes the chief complaint worse. Usually clients have noticed aggravating factors but may need assistance in recalling them. The practitioner may ask about the effect of movement, positioning, or eating, for example. Again, valuable therapeutic data may be obtained.

Negative information. In analyzing a problem, one may find negative information as significant as positive information in determining the diagnosis.

Each system implicated in the PI section is thoroughly reviewed. All of the client's positive replies are recorded in the text of the chronological story. All of the negative information is recorded in this separate category of the PI section.

Relevant family history. The client is queried about any problem similar to the chief complaint in his blood relatives. Positive replies are recorded, identifying specifically the relative and his problem. A negative reply is recorded generally, for example, "None of the client's blood relatives has diabetes."

Disability assessment. The practitioner determines the extent to which the symptoms identified in the PI section have affected the client's total life. Not only are the physiological effects determined, but also the sociological, psychological, and financial impacts of the problem.

Past history

The purpose of the past history (PH) section of the health history is to identify all major past health problems of the client.

The following indicates the information to be obtained and recorded in the PH section of the health history:

- A. Past illnesses
    1. Childhood illnesses
    2. Injuries
    3. Hospitalizations
    4. Operations
    5. Other major illnesses
- B. Allergies
    1. Environmental
    2. Ingestion
    3. Drug
    4. Other
- C. Immunizations
- D. Habits
    1. Alcohol
    2. Tobacco
    3. Drugs
    4. Coffee, tea
- E. Medications taken regularly
    1. By practitioner prescription
    2. By self-prescription

The recording of childhood illnesses is probably more relevant to and more easily obtained for a child's history than for an adult's history. However, all adults should be asked minimally if they have had rheumatic fever. Whenever there is a positive reply, the age of the client at occurrence, the fact or absence of a medical diagnosis, and the sequelae of the disease are determined.

The client is asked to recall accidents and disabling injuries, regardless of whether he was hospitalized for them or was treated on an outpatient basis. The precipitating event, the extent of injury, the fact or absence of medical care, the names of the practitioner and institution, and sequelae are determined and recorded. The practitioner investigates for patterns of injuries or for the presence of consistent environmental hazards.

Descriptions of hospitalizations include all the times the client was admitted to an inpatient unit. Dates of stay, the primary practitioner, the name and address of the hospital, the admitting complaint, the discharge diagnosis, and the follow-up care and sequelae should all be recorded.

Obstetrical hospitalizations are recorded in the review of systems portion of the health history under the review of the female genital system.

Operations are recorded together, under this specific category. The history should include as complete a description of the nature of the repair or removal as is possible. However, clients are generally and unnecessarily unaware of the nature of their operations. Past records may need to be consulted for accurate and complete information.

Clients may have had major, acute illnesses or chronic illnesses that have not required hospitalization. The course of treatment, the person making the diagnosis, the the follow-up care and sequelae are noted.

Information under the categories of hospitalizations, operations, and other major illnesses may, in some cases, be redundant. Information is not recorded more than once, but the presence of a past problem is stated, and the reader is referred to the section where the original notation was made.

The practitioner specifically asks about allergies to food, environmental factors, animals, and drugs. (The practitioner should particularly ask about past administrations and reactions are noted in the record.) If the client has an allergy, specific information is obtained about the causative factor, the reaction, the diagnosis of causative factor, the therapy, and the sequelae. Caution must be exercised in assessing drug allergies. A drug reaction may not always be an allergic response; it may be an interaction with a concurrently administered drug, a misdose, or a side effect.

Habits that may have relevance to the health of an individual are excessive alcohol, coffee, or tea ingestion; smoking; and the addictive use of legal or illegal mood-altering substances. In the case of habits, the number of cigarettes, ounces, tablets, and so on, per day are noted along with the duration of the habit.

If therapy is to be logically planned by informed practitioners, it is critical that all medications that are currently being used by the client are known and recorded. Clients usually admit to vague patterns, such as "a white pill once a day for water," but forget to tell the practitioner about the aspirin or antacid they take several times a day unless they are specifically asked about nonprescription items. Here, the health practitioner has the opportunity to educate clients about the names, doses, and uses of their medications and about the necessity of knowing such information.

Family history

The purpose of the family history (FH) section is to learn about the general health of the client's blood relatives, spouse, and children and to identify any illnesses of environmental, genetic, or familial nature that might have implications for the client's current or future health problems and needs.

The practitioner inquires about the health of the client's family members, including maternal and paternal grandparents, parents, siblings, aunts, uncles, spouse, and children. Information is obtained about the current health status, presence of disease, and current age or age at death of each family member. If a member is deceased, the cause of death is recorded.

If the nature of the client's established or possible illnesses have known or suspected familial tendencies, the client is again questioned about similar problems of family members.

Inquires about the presence of the following diseases are made because of their genetic, familial, or environmental tendencies: epilepsy, diabetes, hemotological disorders (such as hemophilia, sickle cell anemia, thalassemia, hemolytic jaundice, and severe anemia), Huntington's chorea, cancer, hypertension, arteriosclerosis, gout, obesity, allergic disorders, coronary artery disease, tuberculosis, and kidney disease. The interviewer may inquire about additional diseases because of the client's family history, occupation, socioeconomic status, ethnic origins, or environment.

The information in the FH section may be outlined in the record or put in the form of a family tree chart. Fig. 3-3 is an example of such a chart.

Review of systems

The review of systems (ROS) portion of the history includes a collection of data about the past and present health of each of the client's systems. This review of the client's physical, sociological, and psychological health status may identify problems not uncovered previously in the history and provides an opportunity to indicate client strengths as well as liabilities.

Generally, the ROS portion of the history is organized from cephalad to caudad, from physical to

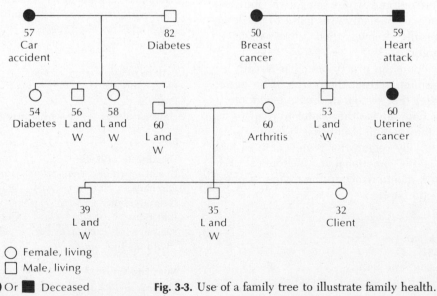

Fig. 3-3. Use of a family tree to illustrate family health.

psychosocial. Clients are instructed that they will be asked a number of questions. Both beginning and experienced interviewers normally need a checklist or written reminder of the questions usually asked each client.

PHYSICAL SYSTEMS

In the review of physical systems section, the practitioner asks about symptoms or asks a specific question and then pauses, allowing the client to think and respond. If the client responds positively, the examiner analyzes the symptoms according to the characteristics of symptoms discussed in the PI section of the history. The practitioner asks questions quickly enough to be efficient, yet slowly enough to allow the client time to think. Questions generally emphasize the presence of past or current common anatomical of functional problems of the system and the health functioning and maintenance of the system.

Obviously, the signs and symptoms need to be creatively translated into questions and terms that can be understood by the client. For example, questions concerning a symptom such as intermittent claudication would need to be presented in lay, descriptive terms.

The presence or absence of all signs or symptoms regarding which inquiry has been made is stated in the record. The general term "negative" for a total system is meaningless; the reader, if he is not the recorder, does not know which questions were asked and consequently does not know the context of "negative"; if the reader is also the recorder, he probably will not, after time, remember which specific questions were asked. An exception might exist in a health care system where the review of physical systems section is routinized and where "negative" indicates an inquiry into and a negative response to predetermined, universally known, and always-reviewed items of exploration.

In the PI section the practitioner has already reviewed the problem system thoroughly. The practitioner can, under that system in the review of physical systems section, advise the reader to refer to the PI section for information about that system.

Systems and body regions for review and exploration of health status, functional and anatomical problems, and health maintenance in the review of physical systems section are:

General

Usual state of health
Episodes of chills
Episodes of weakness or malaise
Fatigue
Fever

Recent and significant gain or loss of weight (if present, amount, time interval, and possible causes are recorded)
Sweats
Usual, maximum, and minimum weight

Skin

Usual state of health	Masses
Previously diagnosed and treated disease	Odors
	Petechiae
Color changes	Pruritus
Dryness	Temperature changes
Ecchymoses	Texture changes
Lesions	Care habits

Hair

Usual state of health	Use of dyes
Alopecia or hair loss	
Texture changes	

Nails

Usual state of health
Changes in appearance
Texture changes

Head and face

Usual state of health	Syncope
Dizziness	Unusual or frequent headache
Injuries	
Pain	

Eyes

Usual state of health
Visual acuity, without and with corrective lenses, if applicable
Cataracts
Changes in visual fields or vision
Diplopia
Excessive tearing
Glaucoma
Date of last ophthamologic examination
Visual disturbances, such as rainbows around lights, flashing lights, or blind spots
Infections
Pain
Pattern of eye examinations
Photophobia
Pruritus
Unusual discharge or sensations

Ears

Usual state of health	Tinnitus/buzzing/ringing
Use of prosthetic devices	Otalgia
Discharge	Vertigo (subjective or objective)
Hearing ability	
Infections	Care habits, especially ear cleaning
Presence of excessive environmental noise	

Nose and sinuses

Usual state of health	Pain in infraorbital or sinus areas
Olfactory ability	

Discharge (seasonal associations)
Epistaxis
Frequency of colds
Obstruction
Postnasal drip
Sinus infection
Sneezing (frequent or prolonged)

Mouth and throat

Usual state of health
Use of prosthetic devices
Abscesses
Bleeding or swelling of gums
Change in taste
Dryness
Excessive salivation
Hoarseness
Lesions
Odors
Sore throats
Voice changes
Pattern of dental care
Pattern of dental hygiene

Neck and nodes

Usual state of health
Masses
Node enlargement
Pain with movement or palpation
Swelling
Tenderness

Breasts

Usual state of health
Discharge
Masses
Pain
Tenderness
Self-examination pattern

Respiratory and cardiovascular systems

Usual state of health
Past diagnosis of respiratory or cardiovascular system disease
Cough
Cyanosis
Dyspnea (if present, amount of exertion precipitating it is recorded)
Edema
Hemoptysis
High blood pressure
Orthopnea (number of pillows needed to sleep comfortably is recorded)
Pain (exact location and radiation, effect of respiration are recorded)
Palpitations
Sputum
Stridor
Wheezing
Paroxysmal nocturnal dyspnea
Date of last roentgenogram or electrocardiogram

Gastrointestinal system

Usual state of health
Appetite
Bowel habits
Previously diagnosed problems
Abdominal pain
Ascites
Change in stool color
Hematemesis
Hemorrhoids
Hernia
Indigestion
Infections
Jaundice
Nausea
Pyrosis

Constipation
Diarrhea
Dyschezia
Dysphagia
Flatulence
Food idiosyncrasies
Rectal bleeding
Rectal discomfort
Recent changes in habits
Thirst
Vomiting
Previous roentgenograms

Urinary system

Usual state of health
Past diagnosed problems
Usual patterns of urination
Anuria
Change in stream
Dysuria
Enuresis
Flank pain
Frequency
Hematuria
Hesitancy of stream
Incontinence
Nocturia
Oliguria
Polyuria
Pyuria
Retention
Stress incontinence
Suprapubic pain
Urgency
Urine color change
Urine odor change

Genital system

Male

Usual state of health
Lesions
Impotence
Masses
Pain
Prostate problems
Swelling

Female

Usual state of health
Diagnosed problems
Lesions
Pruritus
Vaginal discharge
Frequency of Pap smear
Menstrual history
  Age at menarche
Frequency of menses
Duration of flow
Amount of flow
Date of last menstrual period (LMP)
Dysmenorrhea
Menorrhagia
Metorrhagia
Polymenorrhea
Amenorrhea
Dyspareunia
Obstetrical history (for each pregnancy)
Prenatal course
Complications of pregnancy
Duration of pregnancy
Description of labor
Date of delivery
Type of delivery (vaginal, cesarean section)
Condition, sex, and weight of baby
Postpartum course
Place of prenatal care and hospitalization

Both sexes

Ability to perform and enjoy satisfactory sexual intercourse
Infertility
Sterility
Venereal disease

Extremities and musculoskeletal system

Usual state of health
Past diagnosis of disease
Extremities
  Coldness
  Deformities
  Discoloration
  Edema
  Intermittent claudication
Muscles
  Cramping
  Pain
  Weakness
Bones and joints
  Stiffness
  Swelling
  Redness

Pain	Heat
Thrombophlebitis	Limitation of movement
	Fractures
	Back pain

Central nervous system

Usual state of health	Motor
Past diagnosis of disease	Ataxia
Anxiety	Imbalance
General behavior change	Paralysis
Loss of consciousness	Paresis
Mood change	Tic
Nervousness	Tremor
Seizures	Spasm
Speech	Sensory
Aphasia	Pain
Dysarthria	Paresthesia (hyperesthe-
Cognitive ability	sia, anesthesia)
Changes in memory	
Disorientation	
Hallucinations	

Endocrine system

History of physical growth and development
Adult changes in size of head, hands, or feet
Diagnosis of diabetes or thyroid disease
Presence of secondary sex characteristics
Dryness of skin or hair
Exophthalmos
Goiter
Hair distribution
Hormone therapy
Hypoglycemia
Intolerance to heat or cold
Polydipsia
Polyuria
Polyphagia
Postural hypotension
Weakness

Hematopoietic system

Past diagnosis of disease	Blood type
Anemia	Bruising
Bleeding tendencies	Exposure to radiation
Blood transfusion	Lymphadenopathy

SOCIOLOGICAL SYSTEM

The practitioner cannot effectively diagnose a disorder or treat a client by knowing the client's physical status only. The client is a unique and whole person. In order for therapy to be effective, the problem must be assessed and treated within the context of that person. The practitioner should, in some organized way, gather information about the sociological status of the client, as well as his psychological, developmental, and nutritional status.

The following is a suggested organization of sociological data:

A. Relationships with family and significant others
  1. Client's position in the family
  2. Persons with whom client lives
  3. Persons with whom client relates
  4. Recent family crises or changes
B. Environment
  1. Home
  2. Community
  3. Work
  4. Recent changes in environment
C. Occupational history
  1. Jobs held
  2. Satisfaction with present and past employment
  3. Current place of employment
D. Economic status and resources
  1. Source of income
  2. Perception of adequacy or inadequacy of income
  3. Effect of illness on economic status
E. Educational level
  1. Highest degree or grade attained
  2. Judgment of intellect relative to age
F. Daily profile
  1. Rest-activity patterns
  2. Social activities
  3. Special weekend activities
  4. Recent changes in daily activities
G. Patterns of health care
  1. Private and public primary care agencies
  2. Dental care
  3. Preventive care
  4. Emergency care

This outline is recommended for gathering the sociological data of the majority of adult clients; obviously, adaptations will need to be made for some individuals. Many clients may be unaccustomed to extensive questioning about nonphysical matters during the taking of a health history. The practitioner may need to explain the use of such data by stating to the client, for example, "In order to treat you most effectively, it is important that I know something about you as a person."

First, the practitioner asks about the client's role or roles in the family and household. A member may have a societally assigned role, relating to birth, for example, that of son, father, or grandfather, as well as a circumstantially defined role, for example, that of provider, "black sheep," child, and so on. Both should be identified.

Next, the practitioner inquires about the people with whom the client lives and relates on a regular basis. Information can be used to hypothesize, for example, the effect on the family of a long illness of the provider, Also, the practitioner could identify strengths in the presence of strong family or friend relationships. The client should also be asked about the closeness and compatibility of the relationships.

Sometimes unsatisfactory social relationships produce stress, which can be a factor in the exacerbation or causation of illness.

It has been epidemiologically demonstrated that there is a higher than expected incidence of morbidity in those who have undergone recent important life crises or changes. Each client should be asked if any recent event has had a significant impact on his life. Resultant positive data might provide clues of causation or implications for prevention of illness.

Physical as well as psychological environments can have a profound effect on the health status and potential of an individual. The practitioner asks about the client's satisfaction with the appearance and general comfort of his house, his community, and his work situation. The practitioner might ask if the client considers his environment healthy or unhealthy. The pursuit of "why" in the case of negative responses will provide the practitioner some insight into the client's value system, possible information regarding significant health hazards and clues to the etiology of the present illness as well as a validation of the negative response. Again, the practitioner asks about recent change or loss. Positive responses are recorded.

Occupational history information can be used to identify past environmental hazards, to determine the fit between personal ability and productivity, and to plan rehabilitation. The practitioner asks about jobs held, satisfaction with those jobs, and the place of current employment.

The practitioner does not, in many cases, need to know the exact annual income; however, he should know the source of income and the client's assessment of its adequacy. Clients whose resources are too insufficient to enable them to follow therapy must be identified early, and appropriate referral for financial assistance made. In the case of probable prolonged illness, financial reserves are discussed and recorded. If the client is covered by any health insurance, the type of insurance, the name of the insurer, and the policy number are recorded.

The educational level of the client is determined. The highest degree or grade completed is recorded. The practitioner may also wish to make a judgment regarding intellectual ability relative to age. Interviewing up to this point in the history has provided the opportunity for extensive observation of the client's understanding, response, and judgment.

Knowledge of the client's daily pattern helps the practitioner know the client as a person, with habits that encourage or impede health. The practitioner asks the client to describe a typical 24-hour day and to indicate weekend differences. Work, activity, sleep, rest, and recreational pursuits are specifically identified in the recording.

Part of the client's past social interaction has been with the health care system, and past responses may be predictive of future patterns. The client is asked about the health agencies that he has used in the past for acute, preventive, and maintenance health care. It can be determined whether the client is a health facility "shopper" or whether care has had continuity.

PSYCHOLOGICAL SYSTEM

The following is an outline of the information obtained and recorded in the psychological assessment of the client:

A. Cognitive abilities
   1. Comprehension
   2. Learning patterns
   3. Memory
B. Responses to illness and health
   1. Reaction to illness
   2. Coping patterns
   3. Value of health
C. Response to care
   1. Perceptions of the caregivers
   2. Compliance
D. Cultural implications for care
   1. Patterns of therapy
   2. Patterns of illness response

In the assessment of cognitive abilities, the practitioner determines the comprehension ability of the client. Usually this assessment is accomplished more indirectly than directly. Prior to this point in the history-taking process, the client has demonstrated his ability to respond to some rather complex questions. The recording is the judgment summary of the practitioner regarding the client's general comprehension ability.

Since education should be an essential component of all therapy, it is useful to determine the client's health-learning patterns. Some clients need personal instructions; others learn best through reading or group discussion. Knowledge of the client's preference can enable efficient use of provider effort and also involve the client in decision making concerning the process of his therapy.

A discussion of the client's behavior in past illnesses and in health will probably be predictive of future responses. The practitioner asks: "What does health mean to you, and what do you do to keep yourself healthy?" "How do you feel, and what do you do when you become slightly ill? When you become very ill?" "Who do you go to for help if you are ill?" Most clients will be able to answer these questions easily. A summary of the client's responses is recorded concisely. Information can alert the practitioner about strengths, weaknesses, and possible problems in therapy.

Skill may be required in learning the client's real responses to care, since he is often placed in a position of subjugation by the health care system. The practitioner might ask the client how comfortable he feels in asking questions of his health care providers and if he has considered himself a partner in care with them. Answers may be recorded verbatim or summarized.

The practitioner asks about the client's amount of compliance to past courses of therapy. If compliance has been minimal, reasons should be determined for noncompliance. Problems resulting from lack of understanding and financial constraints are more easily solved than problems relating to distrust, indifference, or denial.

If the client is of a cultural group different from that of the practitioner and the majority of the care providers, it would be useful to ask the client what he expects of care and therapy, what general things are done in his culture for persons with needs similar to his. If the chief complaint is of an illness, the practitioner asks about the feelings and responses of the client and his significant others to the fact of the illness. Responses may guide the care provider into more efficient and fewer unacceptable routes of intervention.

Developmental data

A detailed description of the developmental assessment is presented in Chapter 4, "Developmental Assessment."

The recording of this data minimally includes a summary of the client's development to date and a statement of current developmental functioning.

Nutritional data

A detailed description of nutritional assessment is presented in Chapter 5, "Nutritional Assessment."

The recording of data minimally includes a description of an average day's food intake, an assessment of adequacy, inadequacy, or excess of the components of the Basic Four food groups and the presence of any past nutritional problems.

COMPUTER-ASSISTED HISTORIES

Computer science is becoming an important and permanent component of health care technology, and the computer can be used to assist in obtaining the client health history. Studies have demonstrated that the use of the computer in history taking can save practitioner time, can yield a reliable, comprehensive, and readable printout, and is acceptable to clients. In personnel-deficient situations, where time allocated to history taking has been inadequate, the computer-assisted history can be superior to verbal histories.

Computer systems for history taking can be either practitioner-interactive or client-interactive. The client-interactive systems are more commonly utilized because they are more likely to save practitioner time. A number of client-interactive, computerized, history-taking systems are available. Wakefield and Yarnell (1975) describe a number of both computer-assisted and other self-administered histories that would be very helpful to those considering the use of client self-administered, data collection techniques.

Self-administered histories involve the client's either completing a paper-and-pencil questionnaire or interacting with a computer. In the paper-and-pencil questionnaire situation, the client's responses are computerized in a variety of ways and the practitioner receives a printout of responses. In the client-interactive systems, the client responds to inquiries from a computer terminal. Clients have been generally favorable to computer-assisted interviews, and printouts using such systems have been complete, accurate, and legible.

In any client self-administered system, practitioner time is needed to review the history with the client, but usually this review requires only a relatively small amount of time. The amount of time spent by the client in the history-taking process is not shortened by the computer-assisted methods, however. Client age, number of client's problems, and time required by the client to complete the instructional portion of the computer program are positively correlated with overall time needed to give a computer history, and the number of client's years of formal education is negatively correlated with overall time.

The computer-assisted history is more appropriate to the ambulatory client than to the hospitalized client. The ambulatory client can be scheduled for a computer interview, or he can complete a form for computerization with the printout to be available to the practitioner for an appointment in several days. For hospitalized clients, information is generally immediately needed, and patient access to terminals becomes problematical. Also, often the hospitalized patient is too ill to complete a questionnaire or to use a computer terminal.

Practitioner-based computer systems for history taking involve either the practitioner's direct interaction with a computer, which is programmed for questions relating to the history and into which answers are placed, or the practitioner's completion of a form that is computer-processed at a later time.

The computer-interactive systems require a terminal for each practitioner, a situation that may not be cost-effective in ambulatory care situations. The use of the questionnaire for computerization has been used more extensively. The advantage of this latter method is that a legible printout is produced, an improvement over most handwritten documents.

The computer-assisted history can be as effective as the verbal history and may be more effective because remembering items for review is not a problem. Any question that can be asked verbally can be programmed into a computer system, and computer technology allows for additional branching questions if certain significant responses are given. Prior to additional assessment and to therapy it is imperative that any client self-administered history be discussed, reviewed, and verified by the practitioner to determine the validity of significant responses: the client may have misunderstood instructions or there may have been mechanical errors reflected in the information.

As computers become more prevalent in health care systems, the use of computer-assisted histories is likely to increase. However, there will always exist situations in which the computer history is not feasible and a verbal history is necessary. Therefore, skill in history taking is, and will continue to be, an important ability of the health care practitioner.

WRITTEN RECORD OF THE HEALTH HISTORY

The written record is the permanent, legal, and working documentation of what was seen, heard, and felt during the examination. It will serve as the baseline by which subsequent changes will be evaluated and therapy advised. It is very often utilized by a reader who does not have access to the recorder and is consequently subject to interpretation.

It is important that the record be as objective, concise, and specific as possible. The history is not the place for the recorder to bias the reader with opinions of diagnoses. Other portions of a client's record allow for the recorder to elaborate on hypotheses and plans.

The record should be specific enough for the reader to clearly determine what was asked and examined, and the result of the interview and examination. An entry such as "Eyes—negative" or "Eyes—normal" does not supply information regarding procedures done, areas of the eyes examined, or the condition of the eyes. The range of "normal" is wide. Change in condition, even within the range of "normal," may be significant for an individual client.

The record, however, should be concise. Regional entries should be easily located and read. An extremely verbose and disorganized record may be less effective than an incomplete one because its appearance may frustrate the busy reader, who simply will not read it.

Two examples of recorded health histories are presented. One is an example of a history taken from an ill client who is being admitted to a hospital. The other is an example of a history taken from a well client. An example of a recorded physical examination is included in Chapter 26, "Integration of the Physical Assessment."

EXAMPLE OF A RECORDED HEALTH HISTORY: Ill client

Client: John Donald Doe
Address: 9037 N. Sheridan St.
       St. Louis, Mo. 63125
Telephone: 735-1946
Contact: Mrs. Clara Doe (mother)
Address: Same address as above; client will move in with mother after discharge from hospital
Telephone: Same telephone number as above
Birthdate: March 3, 1945   **Sex:** Male   **Race:** White
Religion: Presbyterian (inactive)   **Marital status:** Separated
Social Security number: 097-32-7259
Usual occupation: Offset printer
Present occupation: None; on disability for 1 year
Birthplace: New York, N.Y.
Source of referral: Self
Usual source of health care: Dr. Ryan
                    1346 W. North Ave.
                    St. Louis, Missouri 63122
Source and reliability of information: Client; attempted to be cooperative; however, was frequently vague about the nature and
    time of events
Date of interview: Jan. 9, 1975

Continued.

EXAMPLE OF A RECORDED HEALTH HISTORY: Ill client—cont'd

CHIEF COMPLAINT
"Pain in the left side of stomach for 2 days."

PRESENT ILLNESS

Usual health
This is the fifth Healer's Hospital admission for this 29-year-old white, separated, unemployed male who has been drinking an average of 2 to 3 fifths of hard liquor daily. Total past admissions number 8; none of these has been for abdominal complaints. Client is presently on disability income due to a diagnosis of tuberculosis (11/73). Also has a history of drug abuse and gastric ulcer.

Chronological story

14 years PTA*	Began drinking heavily and regularly.
7 years PTA	Diagnosed as having a gastric ulcer by Dr. Ryan. Treated by him on an outpatient basis with Maalox and Valium prn. Had x-rays at that time. Has complained of slight to moderate gastric discomfort and food intolerance intermittently since then. Unable to relate the specific frequency or specific characteristics of episodes of illness. States that they are usually accompanied by "hangovers." Generally experiences left upper quadrant (LUQ) discomfort, feelings of hunger, nausea, and vomiting of mucous material 6 to 8 hours after drinking heavily. Drinks heavily 3 to 4 days a week and states symptoms occur approximately 2 times a week. Appetite generally has been good. Meal patterns are erratic. Takes Valium for sleep each night. Drinks 2 to 3 8-oz bottles of Maalox per week. No pattern of follow-up care with Dr. Ryan. Symptoms relieved somewhat with Maalox. Bowel movements have been regular, formed, and brown.
1 day PTA	Had not been drinking the night before. Awoke at approximately 7:00 AM and took several alcoholic drinks (amount approximately 1 cup). An hour after an attempt to drink orange juice experienced nausea and vomiting.
	At 10:00 AM walked to his mothers home (2 blocks). On arriving, experienced a sharp, continuous, nonradiating pain in his upper left abdominal area. Indicates LUQ. The intensity required him to lie down. Position changes provided no relief. A whole bottle of Maalox did not affect the pain, which built in intensity over the next 2 hours. After 2 hours the pain remained constant but was more nagging than sharp. Tried to take some soup and orange juice but immediately vomited it. At 2:00 PM vomited again, and this time there were red streaks in the vomitus, which was a green, thick material. (Exact amount of vomitus or blood streaks unknown.)
	Throughout the remainder of the afternoon and early evening, took 5 mg Valium for a total of 4 times. Obtained no relief; pain remained nagging and continuous. Was able to walk with no increase in discomfort but felt most comfortable lying down.
	At bedtime took a sleeping pill but states it did not really help him sleep. Spent a fitful night, and the pain persisted with increased intensity. States he took his temperature at midnight and had a fever of 102° F.
Date of admission	Rose at 9:00 AM and was driven to Dr. Ryan's office but found it closed. Then came directly to Healer's outpatient clinic, where he was seen and admitted.

Negative information
Denies unusual weakness, chills, or fever prior to the onset of symptoms. Denies injury to the abdomen, unusual activity or exercise, pain in other locations, diarrhea, constipation, change in stools, jaundice, ascites, flatulence, hemorrhoids, rectal bleeding, or dysphagia.

Relevant family history
The only significant family history (hx) for a serious, persistent gastrointestinal disorder was a maternal uncle who was a heavy drinker and who died of stomach cancer at age 40.

Disability assessment
Client states that he has not felt really well in the past 7 years. Has not spent a great deal of time in bed but has not worked regularly and has been either drinking or "hung over" most of the time. Was diagnosed as having tuberculosis, 11/73, and was placed on a disability income plan at that time. This insurance will cover medical expenses.

PAST HISTORY

Childhood illnesses
Exact illnesses or dates unknown. Assumes he had all childhood illnesses, for example, measles, mumps, chickenpox; denies hx of rheumatic fever.

*PTA = prior to admission.

EXAMPLE OF A RECORDED HEALTH HISTORY: Ill client—cont'd

Injuries
Client unable to provide exact dates for any of the following:
1. Age 9 (1954). Hit in the eye by rock. States has had a permanent decrease in vision in that eye. No medical care.
2. Age 14 (1959). In an automobile accident. Was hospitalized in Lakewide Hospital, Chicago, for 1 week. Physician unknown. Discharged from hospital with no follow-up required.
3. Age 15 or 16 (1960 or 1961). Fractured right ankle while playing football. Cast applied at Johnson Hospital, Chicago, and was followed in their orthopedic clinic. Apparently healed.
4. Age 18 (1963). Head injury from blow with blunt object, which was thrown. Was unconscious for approxiatemly 30 minutes. Head sutured in emergency room (ER) of Healer's Hospital, St. Louis. No follow-up except for removal of sutures. No sequelae.
5. Age 21 (1966). Stab wound in left shoulder; was attacked and robbed. Sutured in ER of Lakewise Hospital, Chicago. No follow-up except for removal of sutures. No sequelae.

Hospitalizations
1. Age 10 (1955). Hernia repair at Lakeside Hospital, Chicago. Dates and events of hospitalization unclear.
2. Age 14 (1959). Automobile accident. See item 2 under Injuries.
3. Age 20 (1965). Pneumonia. Under the care of Dr. Warner at St. Peter's Hospital, Chicago. Hospitalized for 2 weeks during December. No follow-up.
4. Age 23 (1968). Surgery for priapism at Lakeside Hospital. Under the care of Dr. Meyer. Follow-up for 1 year after surgery because was unable to obtain an erection. No other complications or current disability.
5. Age 24 (1969). Drug overdose. Under the care of Dr. Ryan, Healer's Hospital, St. Louis. Hospitalized for 2 weeks; was to start methadone maintenance, did not. Dates of stay not known.
6. Age 26 (1971). Drug overdose. Under the care of Dr. Ryan, Healer's Hospital. In the hospital for 1 week. Discharged against medical advice.
7. Age 28 (1973). Drug overdose. Under the care of Dr. Ryan. Hospitalized at Healer's Hospital for 2 weeks (1/73). Discharged on methadone maintenance.
8. Age 28 (1973). Hemorrhoidectomy. Under the care of Dr. Ryan and Dr. Jones, Healer's Hospital. Hospitalized 1 week. No complications; 1 follow-up visit.

Operations
See Hospitalizations for details.
1. Age 10 (1955). Hernia repair.
2. Age 23 (1968). Correction of priapism.
3. Age 28 (1973). Hemorrhoidectomy.

Other major illnesses
1. Age 23 (1968). Diagnosed as having a gastric ulcer by Dr. Ryan after an outpatient evaluation including x-rays. See Present illness section for follow-up and sequelae.
2. Age 28 (1973). Tuberculosis diagnosed and treated by staff of the St. Louis Health Department as an outpatient. Medications for 1 year. Off medications for the past 3 months. Followed with yearly x-rays and evaluation.

Allergies
None known. Denies allergies to penicillin, other drugs, foods, or environmental components; has had at least 3 courses of penicillin.

Immunizations
Unknown.

Habits
Cigarettes—smokes 1 pack a day. Habit regular since age 12.
Hard drugs—all types, including heroin. 1969-1973 had a "$90.00 a day habit."
Alcohol—started to drink heavily at age 16. Drinking decreased during period of drug addiction. Has been drinking 2 to 3 fifths of hard liquor a day for the past 2 years.
Coffee—drinks 6 to 7 cups a day.

Medications
Maalox—for ulcer prn with varied dosage since 1968. Prescribed by Dr. Ryan. Client states he uses 2 to 3 8-oz bottles a week.
Valium—10 mg prn for ulcer and nervousness since 1968. Client states he uses at least 1 to 2 tablets a day.
Methadone—40 mg daily for 6 months, 1973. Given through drug abuse program.

Continued.

EXAMPLE OF A RECORDED HEALTH HISTORY: Ill client—cont'd

Medications—cont'd

Streptomycin—IM daily, dose? For TB, 11/73 to 9/74.

INH—tid for TB, 11/73 to 9/74.

Salve—namely unknown, a nonprescription drug; topically every day for scaling skin on soles of feet; since approximately 8/74.

Magnesium citrate—for constipation approximately once (×1) monthly or less frequently; prescribed by self. Uses 1 tbsp prn.

Sleeping pill—prn. Name and dose unknown. Prescribed by Dr. Ryan; 1 every night.

FAMILY HISTORY

Maternal and paternal grandparents deceased. Ages at death and causes of death unknown. Denies family hx of diabetes, blood disorders, arteriosclerosis, gout, obesity, coronary artery disease, tuberculosis, cancer, hypertension, epilepsy, kidney disease, or allergic disorders. Uncertain about health history of aunts and uncles.

Mother—age 52; alive and well.

Father—deceased, age 50, 1960; cause unknown.

Siblings—no maternal miscarriages.

1. ♀ Age 27; alive and well.
2. ♂ Age 20; deceased 1973; drug overdose.
3. ♀ Age 21; alive and well.
4. ♂ Age 18; deceased 1970; gunshot wound.
5. ♀ Age 19; alive and well.

Children

1. ♂ Age 10; alive and well.
2. ♂ Age 7; alive and well.

Wife—age 31; obese, otherwise well.

REVIEW OF PHYSICAL SYSTEMS

General

Chronically ill, white male adult; usual wt about 176 lb. Reports approximately 10-lb wt loss over the past 3- to 4-month period. Feels this is due to not eating when drinking heavily. States he has felt a generalized fatigue and malaise for over 1 year, since onset of TB, but denies requiring daily naps or extra sleep. States he cannot exercise due to fatigue. Denies chills (other than those associated with present illness), sweats, and seizures.

Skin, hair, and nails

Denies lesions, color changes, ecchymoses, petechiae, texture changes, unusual odors, or infections. Pruritus; soles of feet dry and scaling for 6 months; condition stable (using nonprescription salve, name unknown). States he has had small cracks at corners of mouth for 1 month. Denies cold sores. States hair breaks off and falls out but denies patchy alopecia. Denies brittle, cracking, or peeling nails. States bites nails. Has 1 birthmark on upper back but is not aware of any change in size or color.

Head and face

Denies pain, headache, dizziness, or vertigo. Hx of injury with blow to forehead. Reports frequent losses of consciousness after drinking; duration unknown, probably 1 to 8 hours.

Eyes

Has worn corrective lenses since 1955, age 10. States rt eye 20/20, lt eye 20/50. Hx of 1 eye injury, age 9. States visual acuity decreased after injury. Denies pain, infection, watery or itching eyes, diplopia, blurred vision, glaucoma, cataracts, decreased peripheral vision. Last ophthalmological examination 2 years ago.

Ears

Denies hearing loss. Denies discharge, pain, irritation, or ringing in ears. States he was "cut in a fight" on rt auricle. Cleans ears with a toothpick.

Nose and sinuses

Denies sinus pain, postnasal drip, discharge, epistaxis, soreness, excessive sneezing, or obstructed breathing. Denies injuries. States he has approximately 2 colds a year. Olfaction not good; attributes this to smoking.

Oral cavity

Complains of frequent dryness in mouth and cracking of lips and tongue. No false teeth. Gums bleed frequently. Denies hoarseness, pain, odor, frequent sore throats, voice change. Dental care infrequent. Brushes teeth "occasionally."

EXAMPLE OF A RECORDED HEALTH HISTORY: Ill client—cont'd

Neck
Denies pain, stiffness, or limitation of range of motion. Denies masses.

Nodes
Denies enlarged or tender nodes in neck, axillary, or inguinal area.

Breasts
Denies surgery, pain, masses, or discharge.

Chest and respiratory system
Denies pain, wheezing, asthma, or bronchitis. Hx of pneumonia, age 20 (see Hospitalizations). Denies shortness of breath or dyspnea. Sleeps on 2 pillows but is not dependent on them for breathing. Hx of TB, 1973-1974. Last chest x-ray on present admission, negative. States he had 1 episode of hemoptysis, 1968, associated with his ulcer. Details of this unclear. States he has "smoker's cough" (dry cough in the morning) but denies sputum.

Cardiovascular system
Denies chest pain, coronary artery disease, rheumatic fever, or heart murmur. Denies hypertension, palpitations, cyanosis, or diagnosis of cardiac disorder. States he has occasional slight edema in rt ankle.

Gastrointestinal system
See PI. Also see Hospitalizations re hemorrhoidectomy. Appetite good. Denies dysphagia, belching, or hematemesis. Hx of ulcer (see PI) and hernia repair (see Hospitalizations). Denies melena, clay-colored stools, or diarrhea. Takes laxative, citric magnesium, approximately ×1 monthly or less for constipation. Denies jaundice. Reports decreased appetite with alcohol intake but denies specific intolerence to any food.

Genitourinary system
Denies bladder or kidney infections, urgency, frequency, hesitancy, painful micturation, incontinence, nocturia, or polyuria, hx of VD. Denies testicular pain. Hx of surgery for priapism with inability to have erection for 1 year following (p) surgery. No dysfunction at present. States sex life is "fair." Alcohol decreases "urge." Fertile; states he has fathered 7 children.

Extremities
Hx of fractured rt ankle, age 15 or 16. Reports swelling of ankle without pain. Denies varicose veins, thrombophlebitis, joint pain, stiffness, swelling, gout, arthritis, limitation of movement, or color changes.

Back
Denies pain, stiffness, limitation of movement, or disc disease.

Central nervous system
Reports loss of consciousness (1963) following blow to head; duration approximately 30 minute. Denies clumsiness of movement, weakness, paralysis, tremor, neuralgia, or paresthesia. States he is a "nervous" person but denies hx of nervous breakdown. Hx of drug and alcohol abuse. States he will periodically (every 2 to 3 weeks) have spontaneous jerky movement of legs during rest. There are 4 to 5 movements in each episode. This has never occurred while legs were bearing weight. Denies disorientation or memory disorders. Denies seizures or epilepsy. "Passes out" frequently after heavy alcohol ingestion and sleeps for 5 to 6 hours. Wakes with headache and nausea.

Hematopoietic system
Denies bleeding, bruising, blood transfusion, or exposure to x-rays or toxic agents.

Endocrine system
Denies diabetes, thyroid disease, or intolerance to heat or cold. Growth has been within normal range.

REVIEW OF SOCIOLOGICAL SYSTEM

Family relationships
Has been separated from wife for 6 to 7 months and is in the process of being divorced. States his marital problems do not interfere with seeing his children. Plans to move to his mother's home when discharged from hospital. States relationships with his family are good.

Occupational history
Offset printer since 1971. Presently unemployed. Was advised not to work for 6 months when tuberculosis was diagnosed and has not been "able to get back to work." States he liked that occupation but expresses no urgency to return to work.

Continued.

EXAMPLE OF A RECORDED HEALTH HISTORY: Ill client—cont'd

Economic status

On disability income, because of tuberculosis and need to rest. States he does not have trouble making ends meet on present income.

Daily profile

Lives alone in a room. States he spends time during the day at home or with friends, drinking. Has no special hobbies or activities to occupy time. Has habit of heavy daily drinking. States "I just hang around all day." Does do some spur-of-the-moment traveling. Weekdays are no different than weekends. States he dropped out of college because of disinterest. Meal patterns are erratic; sleeps 8 to 10 hours every day, usually 1 AM until 9 to 11 AM.

Educational level

States he is "smart enough." Dropped out of college after 2 years because of disinterest. States he has no aspiration except to "get by in life."

Patterns of health care

Has maintained relationship with same physician for episodic care for the last 10 years. Does return for periodic examinations and follow-up when symptoms "scare him."

Environmental data

Birthplace—New York, N.Y. No travel outside of USA; no armed forces duty.

Home—plans to move to his mother's home. Will share the 5-bedroom residence with his mother and 2 siblings. Neighborhood is residential; describes it as "beautiful."

REVIEW OF PSYCHOLOGICAL SYSTEM

Cognitive abilities

Oriented to present events. Has fairly adequate vocabulary. Has a fair to poor memory. Cannot recall details of some important events. No history of psychiatric treatment.

Response to illness

States he "quit" drinking when he entered the hospital and plans to abstain in the future. Verbalizes that his health problems are his own fault and that he will die soon if he does not resolve them. States illness does not bother him except when "it gets out of control." Definition of health entails being able to play baseball again.

Response to care

States he has sometimes not followed medical advice, because of fear or because drug or alcohol did not allow him to think "straight." "People have been nice to me." States all care has been "OK."

Cultural implications

Inactive Presbyterian at present but is concerned about conflict with religious beliefs and life-style. Fourth-generation American.

DEVELOPMENTAL DATA

Adult male who has had problems with interpersonal relationships in his marriage. Has demonstrated drug and alcohol abuse since entering adulthood. Does not express concern regarding his inability to work; has abandoned his college attendance. Immediate plans for the future involve moving in with his mother and trying to stop drinking. Speaks of his children as playmates; expresses few fathering needs or activities.

NUTRITIONAL DATA

States he does not eat when drinking heavily and must build his tolerance to food by taking liquids such as soup or juices after drinking. States he does eat 3 complete meals daily when not drinking. Includes foods from the four basic food groups.

EXAMPLE OF A RECORDED HEALTH HISTORY: Well client

Client: Mary Rose Doe
Address: 1056 N. East St.
St. Louis, Mo. 60347
Telephone: 278-9274
Contact: Mrs. Elsa Smith (mother)
Address: 3496 Oak St.
St. Louis, Mo. 63047
Telephone: 926-8711
Birthdate: Feb. 6, 1945   **Sex:** Female   **Race:** Black
Religion: Methodist (active)   **Marital status:** Married
Social Security number: 396-47-8911
Usual occupation: Grade school teacher
Present occupation: Same—Greenwich School
Birthplace: St. Louis, Mo.
Source of referral: Self
Usual source of health care: St. Louis Health Maintenance Organization
4693 C. Division St.
St. Louis, Mo. 63044
Source and reliability of information: Client; cooperative, apparently reliable
Date of interview: Dec. 12, 1975.

REASON FOR VISIT

Annual physical examination; last exam, 1/74.

PRESENT HEALTH STATUS

Usual health
This is the third St. Louis Health Maintenance Organization (HMO) visit for this 30 year old black, married female school teacher who has been in good health for all of her life. Client has been hospitalized twice for the purposes of normal childbirth only. Has no major chronic diseases.

Summary
Client is presently well and requests a physical examination for health maintenance and screening purposes. Is concerned about a strong family history of hypertension and believes that monitoring of her blood pressure status is important.

Also requests a Pap smear and evaluation for continuance of oral contraceptives. Has been taking Ortho-Novum 1+50 since the birth of her last child in 1969. Client enrolled in the health plan a year ago.

PAST HISTORY

Childhood illnesses
Had rubella, chickenpox—not diagnosed by a physician. Has not had rheumatic fever.

Injuries
None.

Hospitalizations
See obstetrical data in Review of physical systems.
1. Age 20 (1965). Childbirth.
2. Age 24 (1969). Childbirth.

Operations
None.

Major illnesses
None.

Allergies
None known. Denies allergy to penicillin, other drugs, foods, or environmental components. Has had a course of penicillin (10 d, oral).

Immunizations
Had full series of diphtheria-pertussis-tetanus (DPT) when a preschooler. Had oral polio when an adolescent.

Continued.

EXAMPLE OF A RECORDED HEALTH HISTORY: Well client—cont'd

Habits
Cigarettes—smoked 15 cigarettes a day for 5 years (age 20-25).
Hard drugs—none.
Alcohol—drinks 3 to 4 mixed drinks during a weekend.
Coffee, tea—drinks approximately 10 cups of coffee a day. Drinks tea rarely.

Medications
Ortho-Novum 1+50 oral contraceptive since 1969.
Aspirin (ASA) for headache—takes approximately ×10 gr twice a month.
Milk of magnesia for constipation—takes 1 tablespoon about once a month.
One-a-Day multiple vitamins—takes 1 a day.

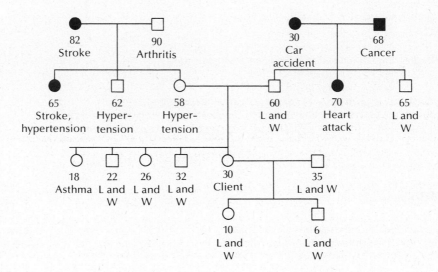

FAMILY HISTORY

Denies family history of diabetes, blood disorder, gout, obesity, tuberculosis, epilepsy, kidney disease, or gastrointestinal disease.

REVIEW OF PHYSICAL SYSTEMS

General
Usually well. Usual-minimum-maximum weight: 135-125-160 lb. No increase or decrease in weight. Denies fatigue, malaise, chills, sweats, fever, seizures, or fainting.

Skin, hair, and nails
Denies lesions, color change, ecchymoses, masses, petechiae, texture changes, pruritus, sweating, or unusual odors. No alopecia or brittle hair. Denies brittle, cracking, or peeling nails. No birthmarks. Washes hair once a week; does not use dyes.

Head and face
Denies pain, dizziness, vertigo, or history of injury or loss of consciousness.

Eyes
Has worn corrective lenses since age 7; currently wears contact lenses all day. Denies recent change in visual acuity, pain, infection, watery or itching eyes, diplopia, blurred vision, glaucoma, cataracts, or decreased peripheral vision. Last ophthalmoscopic examination 2 years ago.

Ears
Denies hearing loss, discharge, pain, irritation, or ringing in the ears. Cleans ears with cotton-tipped applicator.

Nose and sinuses
States she has sinus pain, congestion, and subsequent nasal discharge several times each winter. Takes Contact prn (approximately 1 q 12 hours × 3d) for each episode of rhinitis; gets relief. Denies epistaxis, soreness, excessive sneezing, obstructed breathing, or injuries. States olfaction is good.

EXAMPLE OF A RECORDED HEALTH HISTORY: Well client—cont'd

Oral cavity
Visits a dentist every 6 months for cleaning and examination. Brushes teeth twice a day. Denies toothache, lesions, soreness, bleeding of gums, coated tongue, disturbance of taste, hoarseness, or frequent sore throat.

Neck
Denies pain, stiffness, limitation of movement, or masses.

Nodes
Denies enlarged or tender nodes in neck, axillary, or inguinal area.

Breasts
Denies masses, pain, tenderness, or discharge. Examines breasts monthly, right after menses.

Chest and respiratory system
Denies pain, wheezing, shortness of breath, dyspnea, hemoptysis, or cough. Denies hx of asthma, pneumonia, or bronchitis. Has yearly chest x-ray, required for work in the schools.

Cardiovascular system
Denies precordial pain, palpitations, cyanosis, edema, or intermittent claudication. Frequently bicycles in summer and downhill skis in winter. Walks 2 miles a day. Denies diagnosis of heart murmur, hypertension, coronary artery disease, or rheumatic fever.

Gastrointestinal system
Denies history of gastrointestinal disease. Appetite good. Bowels active daily, stools are always brown. Denies pain, constipation, diarrhea, flatulence, vomiting, hemorrhoids, hernias, jaundice, pyrosis, or bleeding. Has never had GI x-rays.

Genitourinary system
Denies hx of bladder or kidney infections, hematuria, urgency, frequency, dysuria, incontinence, nocturia, polyuria, or VD. Menses—onset 13 years; frequency, every 26 to 30 days; duration, 5 days; flow, heavy for 3 days, light for 2 days; last menstrual period (LMP), 12/1/75. Denies dysmenorrhea, menorrhagia, metrorrhagic discharge, or pruritus. Last Pap smear, 12/74.

Obstetrical history
1. Sept. 12, 1965. Girl, 6 lb, 8 oz. Vaginal delivery at St. Francis Hospital, St. Louis. Prenatal, intrapartum, and postpartum course normal for mother and baby.
2. Oct. 9, 1969. Boy, 7 lb 2 oz. Vaginal delivery at St. Francis Hospital, St. Louis. Prenatal, intrapartum, and postpartum course normal for mother and baby.

Sexual history
Age at first intercourse was 17 years. Enjoys intercourse with husband—no dyspareunia and able to achieve satisfactory orgasm most of the time. Using oral birth control medication. Not sure yet if she will have another child. Will consider sterilization when family is complete.

Extremities
No past problems. Denies deformities, varicose veins, thrombophlebitis, joint pain, stiffness, swelling, gout, arthritis, limitation of movement, color changes, or temperature changes.

Back
No past problems. Denies pain, stiffness, or limitation of movement; no history of disc disease.

Central nervous system
No past problems. Denies loss of consciousness, clumsiness of movement, difficulty with balance, weakness, paralysis, tremor, neuralgia, paresthesia, history of emotional disorders, drug or alcohol dependency, disorientation, memory lapses, or seizures. Speech articulate.

Hematopoietic system
No past problems. Denies excessive bleeding and bruising, blood transfusions, or excessive exposure to x-rays or toxic agents. Blood type A, Rh positive.

Endocrine system
Denies history of diabetes or thyroid disease, polyuria, polydipsia, polydysplasia, intolerance to heat or cold, or hirsutism.

Continued.

EXAMPLE OF A RECORDED HEALTH HISTORY: Well client—cont'd

REVIEW OF SOCIOLOGICAL SYSTEM

Family relationships
Lives in own home with husband and 2 children. Husband is a school teacher also; couple shares finances, childrearing, and housekeeping responsibilities. Client's parents live ½ mile away, and relationships are described as "good." Couple has several close friends; also, siblings are in frequent contact. No recent family crisis or change.

Occupational history
Has been a grade school teacher for 5 years. Holds BS and MA degrees and feels secure that she can retain her job as long as she wants it. Enjoys children and states job is very satisfying.

Economic status
Client and husband achieve a combined gross income of over $30,000 a year. Feels this is very adequate. Has hospitalization insurance.

Daily profile
During the week, works 8 AM to 3 PM. Returns home around 3:30 and works until 5 PM on school work. Then cooks dinner and interacts with family. Has meetings 1 or 2 evenings a week. Weekends, client and husband usually have 1 evening out with friends, to movie or concert. Family attends church each Sunday. Client is involved with photography as a hobby. Sleeps 7 to 8 hours every night (approximately 11 PM to 7 AM).

Educational level
Highest degree attained is the master's degree. Obtains most of health knowledge by reading.

Patterns of health care
Has always had a primary care provider. Cared for by Dr. Richard Smith, a family practitioner until first pregnancy. Then seen regularly by Dr. Janice Lawson, for obstetrical and gynecological care. Family enrolled in HMO a year ago; all family members are being seen here. Dental care regular and at the HMO.

Environmental data
Birthplace—Greenwood, Miss. Grew up in Trenton, N.J.

Home—family lives in their own 8-room home in a residential St. Louis neighborhood. Client describes home as comfortable. Has lived there for 10 years.

Community—community is middle income, integrated, consisting primarily of young professional families.

Work—teaches fourth grade in a community grade school. States that the work situation is fairly good. School is in good condition, and classes are small. A recent stress is a new assistant principal with whom client does not get along. May consider transfer to another school.

REVIEW OF PSYCHOLOGICAL SYSTEM

Cognitive abilities
Oriented to time, place, and person (×3). Is articulate, asks questions, has a good memory. Able to understand directions.

Response to illness
States she has never been seriously ill, so does not know what personal response would be. Feels she is "too busy" to be ill for any length of time. Uses the resources of HMO for preventive and therapeutic needs of self and family.

Response to care
States she enjoys encounters with health care providers. States she usually follows through on the advice that is given. Feels that the services of the HMO are adequate to meet her family care needs and she has been very satisfied with the care to date.

Cultural implications
Client states she and her family are involved in a racially integrated community. She grew up in a predominantly black northern community. Cannot identify any way in which her black culture would especially affect her response to illness or therapy in the case of illness. Active Methodist; believes that religious concerns would influence her response to illness and treatment.

DEVELOPMENTAL DATA
Adult female; wife, mother, and career teacher.

EXAMPLE OF A RECORDED HEALTH HISTORY: Well client—cont'd

NUTRITIONAL DATA

Diet adequate; high in fats and carbohydrates. Has no food intolerances.

Usual breakfast—toast with butter, fried egg, orange juice, and coffee with cream.

Usual lunch—eats with school children; consists of meat, 1 vegetable, 1 carbohydrate, dessert, and beverage.

Dinner—meat (beef, chicken, or pork), salad, 1 vegetable, potato or bread, dessert, and coffee with cream.

Snacks—may have cheese and crackers, or peanuts in the evening.

BIBLIOGRAPHY

Berg, R. L.: Health status indexes, Chicago, 1973, Hospital Research and Educational Trust.

Bernstein, L., Bernstein, R. S., and Dana, R. H.: Interviewing; a guide for health professionals, ed. 2, New York, 1974, Appleton-Century-Crofts.

Bird, B.: Talking with patients, ed. 2, Philadelphia, 1973, J. B. Lippincott Co.

Blum, L. H.: Reading between the lines; doctor-patient communication, New York, 1972, International Universities Press, Inc.

Bowder, C. L., and Burnstein, A. G.: Psychosocial basis of medical practice, Baltimore, 1974, The Williams & Wilkins Co.

Froelich, R. E., and Bishop, F. M.: Clinical interviewing skills: a programmed manual for data gathering, evaluation and patient management, ed. 3, St. Louis, 1972, The C. V. Mosby Co.

Mitchell, P. H.: Concepts basic to nursing, New York, 1973, McGraw-Hill Book Co.

Small, I. F., editor: Introduction to the clinical history, Flushing, N.Y., 1971, Medical Examination Publishing Co.

Tumulty, P. A.: The effective clinician, Philadelphia, 1973, W. B. Saunders Co.

Wakefield, J. S., and Yarnell, S. R.: The history data base, ed. 3, Seattle, 1975, Medical Computer Services Assoc.

4 Developmental assessment

In performing the health assessment of a client, there is naturally much emphasis placed on the physical aspects of that assessment. The beginning practitioner is often preoccupied with assimilating new skills, handling new tools and techniques, and remembering lists of questions and components of the history and physical examination. From the onset of the learning process, however, it is important to emphasize a focus on the whole personhood of each client and to gain familiarity with a holistic frame of reference in regard to clients. This involves taking into account the life developmental process of that individual, the series of stages of maturity by which the individual progresses toward a higher level of functioning. This necessitates taking time to discuss and discover the client's world—his interaction and growth within himself, with significant others, and with society at large.

Discussing developmental stages, phases, and crises with clients can provide both practitioner and client with a sharper and deeper perspective of the client's life situation and its relationship to health or illness. An openness to discussing the life tasks of individuals can help them appreciate the appropriateness and normalcy of their feelings and behaviors, or it may assist those who seemed blocked in their ability to accomplish their tasks.

It may also help clients to review their past, to compare it to the present, to look at progressive stages and intervals, and to plan for the future, as is appropriate and necessary. Perhaps most importantly, it may serve to help a person appreciate both his similarities to others and his own unique individuality and to gain assurance in his efforts to be most fully and healthily himself.

That growth and development are continuous throughout the life cycle is a premise basic to this approach. In order to perform a developmental assessment, one must give some thought to what constitutes "growth" and "development." There are numerous components to this broad, diversified, universal, and yet infinitely unique process. These include the physical, emotional, psychological, social, and educational facets of growth. Human development in these and other areas ranges from changes that are slow, subtle, and often elusive to those that occur with almost incredible rapidity. Whatever the rate of changes, one perceives and understands them more fully in the perspective that comes with the passage of time. Gesell, Ilg, and Ames (1956) define growth as "the patterning process whereby the mutual fitness of organism and environment is brought to progressive realization" (p. 25). Growth combines integration and differentiation in all of its aspects—physical, emotional, and social. Change is a central concept; life has the remarkable property of changing with time while maintaining a core of individuality. The problem or challenge of development is "to bring opposites into effectual control and counterpoise . . . in such a manner that the individual achieves integration, choice and direction" (Gesell and others, 1956, p. 19).

During each phase or stage of human development certain aspects are ascendent or salient, yet the phases are not totally distinct or mutually exclusive.

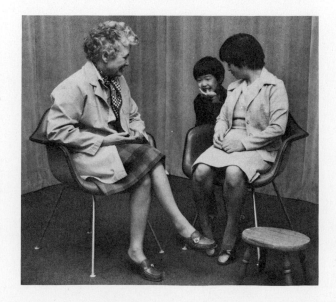

For example, "Childhood does not end nor adulthood begin around adolescence. Rather, the adult is anticipated in the child and the child persists in the adult" (Katchdourian, p. 51). Stages of development may be defined in different ways. Some are defined by physical changes, others by internal psychological events, still others by external behavior, activities, or life situations.

Erikson suggests eight developmental stages of the ego and identifies for each stage a central task and a threat to the accomplishment of that task. (These will be integrated into the discussion of the various developmental stages.) These central tasks may also be thought of as developmental "crises," although not in the sense of an acute emergency situation, which that word often describes, but rather "as a term designating a necessary turning point, a crucial moment, when development must move one way or another, marshaling resources of growth, recovery, and further differentiation" (Erikson, 1968, p. 16). It is "a period of increased vulnerability and heightened potential" (Erikson, 1976, p. 6). He describes a life "cycle" as the "tendency of individual life to 'round itself out' as a coherent experience and to form a link in the chain of generations from which it receives and to which it contributes both strength and fateful discord" (1975, p. 5).

There is a cyclic aspect to the various developmental stages. For example, young children tend to grow in spurts, then level off for a period, and adolescents tend to have cycles of untoward activity and then inner reflection. Adults also may experience periods of outward and inward involvement. Gesell, Ilg, and Ames suggest that "growth gains are consolidated during recurring periods of relative equilibrium. There is a tendency for stages of increased equilibrium to be followed by stages of lessened equilibrium when the organism makes new inner or outer thrusts into the inner or outer unknown" (1956, p. 20).

The developmental aspects of infancy and childhood have received much attention and study for several decades, and there is an abundance of literature on these phases, though much still remains to be learned and understood. Of more recent vintage are the studies and theories advanced on adolescence and old age. And latest to surface in the literature on human development is material on that age span between youth and old age, namely, middle adulthood. Similarly, there are numerous tools and tests devised to assess early childhood stages, but few to assess school-aged children and adults. Several of the infancy and early childhood assessment tools will be described; with adolescents and adults much developmental assessment is accomplished simply by talking with the client in an accepting, unrushed manner.

(Two tools that assist with adult assessment are briefly described.) Nonthreatening questions about thoughts and feelings, work, family, and other activities and an attitude of active listening will encourage clients to share significant discussion about themselves. The practitioner should not expect to learn everything about a client's developmental accomplishments in one or even in several interviews. It is a personal story that takes time and trust to be told. Furthermore, developmental assessment for a client of any age is a continuous, ongoing process. Life is more like a moving picture than a still photograph; it is changing and dynamic and should be regularly reassessed.

The approach used in this chapter will be to organize developmental assessment around seven major life stages: infancy, early childhood, childhood, adolescence, young adulthood, middle adulthood, and late adulthood. Activities characteristic of each stage, including the developmental tasks, will be described. The length of the chronological divisions will increase with age: that is, for infants, monthly changes are described; for adolescents, annual changes; and for adults, decades.

A notation on the clinician's impression of a client's developmental tasks and accomplishments can be placed in the health history after the psychological system review. See examples on pp. 52 and 56.

CONCEPTUAL FRAMEWORK OF DEVELOPMENTAL ASSESSMENT

The assessment of a child's development is carried out formally or informally by the practitioner during each examination. The opportunity to observe the development of many children enhances the ability to define the parameters of normal development, and the experienced examiner often responds to subtle behavioral cues with an intuitive hunch that all is not well with the child. However, it is usually difficult to verify this initial impression and make a determination of the presence or absence of a developmental deficit while examining a child in a busy clinical setting. The practitioner may need to plan additional time in order to focus attention on the assessment of the child's development or may need to seek the assistance of experts in child development.

The information obtained from the developmental assessment has many uses. It will aid the practitioner in providing assistance to the parents when they have questions about their child's behavior. Most parents will be interested in learning that their child is developing normally, and with anticipatory guidance they can gain a greater appreciation of ways to support the normal development of their child. The developmental assessment also provides information that can be useful at a future time. For instance, the child who has been developing in a normal fashion and then demonstrates a developmental lag presents a different problem than the child who has been consistently slower in development. Finally, the developmental assessment is helpful in screening for some of the more obvious deficits in development that deserve further investigation.

It is most important to keep in mind that the developmental assessment is not a test of the child's intelligence and does not allow the practitioner to make a diagnosis. It does allow the practitioner to collect data that indicate whether the development of the individual child is within the normal range.

Although there are many theories of development that can provide a framework for observing and assessing the development of children, the discussion in this chapter is limited. However, it is reasonable to expect that each practitioner with an interest in children will be challenged to increase understanding of the behavior presented by children of different ages.

The discussion in this section includes a conceptual framework for organizing the developmental assessment; approaches to the developmental assessment of the child, which can be incorporated into the plan for the health history and examination; and a brief discussion of selected screening tests that can be helpful to the practitioner.

A systematic appraisal of the child's development can be organized in different ways. Although each behavior of the child is part of an indivisible whole, it is clinically useful to separate behaviors into several categories whether the assessment is carried out as a part of the health examination or as a more formal procedure. Different categories of behavior are used, but many of the screening tests commonly focus on three categories: fine and gross motor development, language and communication, and personal-social behavior. These categories are especially useful in the assessment of the infant and preschool child, when observable changes occur most rapidly. When the development of the older child is being assessed, it is important to include questions about the child's adjustment to school and the grade level achieved and about his relationships with peers, siblings, and significant adults.

The stages of motor development have been documented and are well known, as is the relationship of motor skills to neuromotor organization. The practitioner will find information about the expected norms for achieving specific motor skills in most standard textbooks of pediatrics or child development. What is not usually discussed in regard to developing motor abilities is the way the child uses these skills. Is the child active and using his skills in a variety of ways? Or is the child quiet, showing little apparent interest or pleasure in walking, running, and climbing? Information as to the amount of activity may lead to questions about the environment. Does it offer too much stimulation or too little? Differences in the use of skills may also be related to organic problems, which are sometimes demonstrated by the hyperactive, impulse-ridden child.

The normal age range for the sequential development of language and communication skills is also well documented, as well as the relationship of speech development to intellectual functioning. The assessment of the child's language and communication skills should provide information about the size of the child's vocabulary, his understanding of language, his clarity of articulation, and his use of phrases and sentences. The speech of the young child is easily disturbed when there are physical problems or problems with the people in the environment. Speech disturbances may be transitory, may indicate an impairment of the hearing or speech apparatus, or may indicate the presence of a mental disability. Although a delay in speech development may be a temporary problem, it is a concern that deserves further investigation even when the child is very young.

The appraisal of the personal-social behavior of the child provides information about the child's developing awareness of himself as a person, his ability to interact with people, and his adaptive behaviors. These abilities can also be described as the intellectual, emotional, and social skills of the child. Erik Erikson's "conceptual itinerary" of the psychosocial stages of life provides a plan, or a guided overview, of the changes and adaptive behaviors of the child in each of the sequential stages of childhood.

Approaches to assessment

The practitioner with limited time would be well served to find ways to incorporate aspects of the developmental assessment into the routine health examination of every child. A good deal of information can be gained by including questions about the child's development in the history. Also, since it is traditional to include observations of the child's behavior as part of the general inspection of the physical examination, it is relatively easy to pay special attention to particular aspects of behavior in order to obtain data about the child's level of functioning. However, it is also well to keep in mind that the behavior demonstrated may not be typical because of the stress from the unfamiliar environment or the particular problems of the illness that the child is experiencing.

A modification of the "Schedule for Preventive Health Care" developed by the American Academy of Pediatrics and published in the second edition of *Standards of Child Health Care* is included in Chapter 21, "The Assessment of the Pediatric Client." It includes suggestions and recommendations for the examination of the child during each visit for health care during the first 6 years of life. Items from the Denver Developmental Screening Test that are appropriate for the chronological age of the child at the time of each visit have been incorporated. This schedule offers an example of a plan for the continuing appraisal of specific developmental milestones at the time the child is seen for health care.

Because there are limited opportunities to observe the child's behavior in the clinical setting, the history becomes the major tool for obtaining information about the child's development. First, the history allows the practitioner to obtain data about the factors that will increase the chances of the child's being at risk for problems that may interfere with his development. Una Haynes outlines many of the factors that contribute to the "at risk" status of the child. This information can be elicited from the past history of the child in the prenatal, natal, and postnatal period of life; from the family history; from the sociological assessment; from the developmental data; and from the history of illnesses and injuries. The history that reveals problems such as prematurity, precipitate delivery, or hyperbilirubinemia in the first 48 hours of life will alert the practitioner that the child is at greater risk than most children for developmental problems. However, this information should not bias the practitioner's perception of the child's development but should encourage a sense of "benign suspicion," a term used by Sally Provence (1968a) to describe the attitude of the examiner.

The pediatric history as outlined in Chapter 21 includes a developmental history that provides information about the age at which the child achieved certain developmental milestones. This information can be used to determine whether the early development was within average or normal limits. The history of the present health or present illness should include a description of the child's current level of functioning. The practitioner can review the achievements expected of the child at a specific chronological age as outlined in many texts on child development. Table 4-1 provides such an outline. Questions about these expected achievements will provide information about the child's current level of development; this information can then be included in the description of the child's present health.

Provence (1968a) mentions two questions that are helpful for the examiner to keep in mind when making judgments about the development of a child: (1) What has the child achieved in the various sectors of development that one can observe, describe, or measure? (2) How does the child make use of the skills and functions available to him? The first question requires the practitioner to find out about the developmental progress of the infant or child from helplessness at birth to his current level of development. The second question requires the practitioner to find out about the adaptation the child is making to his life. The second question is usually more difficult to answer, because it is not based on standardized developmental schedules. However, information about the child's adaptation can be obtained by asking the parent to describe the child. This description can be broadened by asking whether the child is quiet or active, happy or sad, and mischievous or very good.

Ronald Illingworth (1975) stresses that purely objective tests result in obtaining information about scorable items in the area of sensorimotor skills and that it is of great importance to also determine the child's alertness, responsiveness, and interest in surroundings, which cannot be scored. Arnold Gessell (1947) calls these latter behaviors "insurance factors." If the child demonstrates these behaviors but has delays in some of the sensorimotor behaviors, an opinion should be reserved and the child followed over a longer period of time before a judgment is made about the developmental skills of the child.

If there are questions or concerns about a child's development that are identified as the result of the routine appraisal, it would be well to set aside time so that a complete developmental assessment could be done that would include a careful review of the history of the developmental milestones and an appraisal of the child's current level of function. It would be appropriate to use one of the more structured screening tests.

DEVELOPMENTAL SCREENING TESTS

There are several screening tests that the practitioner may find useful in assessing the development of an infant or young child. Most of them require some training in order for the validity of the test to be ensured.

The clinical assessment of gestational age helps the practitioner to determine that the newborn's gestational age is accurate and to anticipate problems that are related to the infant's maturity or immaturity. Several tools designed for use during the first few days of life assess the physical and neuromuscular maturity of the infant. Included in each of the two major categories are selected items that can be scored and the total score obtained allows the practitioner

Text continued on p. 66.

Table 4-1. Child development from 1 month to 5 years*

1 MONTH

Motor

1. Moro reflex present.
2. Vigorous sucking reflex present.
3. Lying prone (face down): lifts head briefly so chin is off table.
4. Lying prone: makes crawling movements with legs.
5. Held in sitting position: back is rounded, head held up momentarily only.
6. Hands tightly fisted.
7. Reflex grasp of object with palm.

Language

8. Startled by sound; quieted by voice.
9. Small throaty noises or vocalizations.

Personal-social-adaptive

10. Ringing bell produces decrease of activity.
11. May follow dangling object with eyes to midline.
12. Lying on back: will briefly look at examiner or change his activity.
13. Reacts with generalized body movements when tissue paper is placed on face.

2 MONTHS

Motor

1. Kicks vigorously.
2. Energetic arm movements.
3. Vigorous head turning.
4. Held in ventral suspension (prone): no head droop.
5. Lying prone: lifts head so face makes an approximate 45° angle with table.
6. Held in sitting position: head erect but bobs.
7. Hand goes to mouth.
8. Hands often open (not clenched).

Language

9. Is cooing.
10. Vocalizes single vowel sounds, such as: ah-eh-uh.

Personal-social-adaptive

11. Head and eyes search for sound.
12. Listens to bell ringing.
13. Follows dangling object past midline.
14. Alert expression.
15. Follows moving person with eyes.
16. Smiles back when talked to.

3 MONTHS

Motor

1. Lying prone: lifts head to 90° angle.
2. Lifts head when lying on back (supine).
3. Moro reflex begins to disappear.
4. Grasp reflex nearly gone.
5. Rolls side to back (3-4 months).

Language

6. Chuckling, squealing, grunting, especially when talked to.
7. Listens to music.
8. Vocalizes with two different syllables, such as: a-a, la-la (not distinct), oo-oo.

Personal-social-adaptive

9. Reaches for but misses objects.
10. Holds toy with active grasp when put into hand.
11. Sucks and inspects fingers.
12. Pulls at clothes.
13. Follows object (toy) side to side (and 180°).
14. Looks predominately at examiner.
15. Glances at toy when put into hand.
16. Recognizes mother and bottle.
17. Smiles spontaneously.

4 MONTHS

Motor

1. Sits when well supported.
2. No head lag when pulled to sitting position.
3. Turns head at sound of voice.
4. Lifts head (in supine position) in effort to sit.
5. Lifts head and chest when prone, using hands and forearms.
6. Held erect: pushes feet against table.

Language

7. Laughs aloud (4-5 months).
8. Uses sounds, such as: m-p-b.
9. Repeats series of same sounds.

Personal-social-adaptive

10. Grasps rattle.
11. Plays with own fingers.
12. Reaches for object in front of him with both hands.
13. Transfers object from hand to hand.
14. Pulls dress over face.
15. Smiles spontaneously at people.
16. Regards raisin (or pellet).

5 MONTHS

Motor

1. Moro reflex gone.
2. Rolls side to side.
3. Rolls back to front.
4. Full head control when pulled to or held in sitting position.
5. Briefly supports most of his weight on his legs.
6. Scratches on table top.

Language

7. Squeals with high voice.
8. Recognizes familiar voices.
9. Coos and/or stops crying on hearing music.

Personal-social-adaptive

10. Grasps dangling object.
11. Reaches for toy with both hands.
12. Smiles at mirror image.
13. Turns head deliberately to bell.
14. Obviously enjoys being played with.

6 MONTHS

Motor

1. Supine: lifts head spontaneously.
2. Bounces on feet when held standing.

*Reprinted by permission of Walter M. Block, M. D., Child Evaluation Clinic of Cedar Rapids, Iowa © Copyright 1972.

Table 4-1. Child development from 1 month to 5 years—cont'd

---

6 MONTHS—cont'd

Motor—cont'd

3. Sits briefly (tripod fashion).
4. Rolls front to back (6-7 months).
5. Grasps foot and plays with toes.
6. Grasps cube with palm.

Language

7. Vocalizes at mirror image.
8. Makes four or more different sounds.
9. Localizes source of sound (bell, voice).
10. Vague, formless babble (especially with family members).

Personal-social-adaptive

11. Holds one cube in each hand.
12. Puts cube into mouth.
13. Resecures dropped cube.
14. Transfers cube from hand to hand.
15. Conscious of strange sights and persons.
16. Consistent regard of object or person (6-7 months).
17. Uses raking movement to secure raisin or pellet.
18. Resists having toy taken away from him.
19. Stretches out arms to be taken up (6-8 months).

8 MONTHS

Motor

1. Sits alone (6-8 months).
2. Early stepping movements.
3. Tries to crawl.
4. Stands few seconds, holding on to object.
5. Leans forward to get an object.

Language

6. Two-syllable babble, such as: a-la, ba-ba, oo-goo, a-ma, mama, dada (8-10 months).
7. Listens to conversation (8-10 months).
8. "Shouts" for attention (8-10 months).

Personal-social-adaptive

9. Works to get toy out of reach.
10. Scoops pellet.
11. Rings bell purposely (8-10 months).
12. Drinks from cup.
13. Plays peek-a-boo.
14. Looks for dropped object.
15. Bites and chews toys.
16. Pats mirror image.
17. Bangs spoon on table.
18. Manipulates paper or string.
19. Secures ring by pulling on the string.
20. Feeds self crackers.

10 MONTHS

Motor

1. Gets self into sitting position.
2. Sits steadily (long time).
3. Pulls self to standing position (on bed railing).
4. Crawls on hands and knees.
5. Walks when held or around furniture.
6. Turns around when left on floor.

Language

7. Imitates speech sounds.
8. Shakes head for "no."
9. Waves "bye-bye."
10. Responds to name.
11. Vocalizes in varied jargon-patterns (10-12 months).

Personal-social-adaptive

12. Plays "pat-a-cake."
13. Picks up pellet with finger and thumb.
14. Bangs toys together.
15. Extends toy to a person.
16. Holds own bottle.
17. Removes cube from cup.
18. Drops one cube to get another.
19. Uses handle to lift cup.
20. Initially shy with strangers.

1 YEAR

Motor

1. Walks with one hand held.
2. Stands alone (or with support).
3. Secures small object with good pincer grasp.
4. Pivots in sitting position.
5. Grasps two cubes in one hand.

Language

6. Uses "mama" or "dada" with specific meaning.
7. "Talks" to toys and people, using fairly long verbal patterns.
8. Has vocabulary of two words besides "mama" and "dada."
9. Babbles to self when alone.
10. Obeys simple requests, such as: "Give me the cup."
11. Reacts to music.

Personal-social-adaptive

12. Cooperates with dressing.
13. Plays with cup, spoon, saucer.
14. Points with index finger.
15. Pokes finger (into stethoscope) to explore.
16. Releases toy into your hand.
17. Tries to take cube out of box.
18. Unwraps a cube.
19. Holds cup to drink.
20. Holds crayon.
21. Tries to imitate scribble.
22. Imitates beating two cubes together.
23. Gives affection.

15 MONTHS

Motor

1. Stands alone.
2. Creeps upstairs.
3. Kneels on floor or chair.
4. Gets off floor and walks alone with good balance.
5. Bends over to pick up toy without holding on to furniture.

Table 4-1. Child development from 1 month to 5 years—cont'd

15 MONTHS—cont'd

Language

6. May speak four to six words (15-18 months).
7. Uses jargon.
8. Indicates wants by vocalizing.
9. Knows own name.
10. Enjoys rhymes or jingles.

Personal-social-adaptive

11. Tilts cup to drink.
12. Uses spoon but spills.
13. Builds tower of two cubes.
14. Drops cubes into cup.
15. Helps turn page in book, pats picture.
16. Shows or offers toy.
17. Helps pull off clothes.
18. Puts pellet into bottle without demonstration.
19. Opens lid of box.
20. Likes to push wheeled toys.

18 MONTHS

Motor

1. Runs (stiffly).
2. Walks upstairs—one hand held.
3. Walks backwards.
4. Climbs into chair.
5. Hurls ball.

Language

6. May say six to 10 words (18-21 months).
7. Points to at least one body part.
8. Can say "hello" and "thank you."
9. Carries out two directions (one at a time), for instance: "Get ball from table."—"Give ball to mother."
10. Identifies two objects by pointing (or picking up) such as: cup, spoon, dog, car, chair.

Personal-social-adaptive

11. Turns pages.
12. Builds tower of three to four cubes.
13. Puts 10 cubes into cup.
14. Carries or hugs a doll.
15. Takes off shoes and socks.
16. Pulls string toy.
17. Scribbles spontaneously.
18. Dumps raisin from bottle after demonstration.
19. Uses spoon with little spilling.

21 MONTHS

Motor

1. Runs well.
2. Walks downstairs—one hand held.
3. Walks upstairs alone or holding on to rail.
4. Kicks large ball (when demonstrated).

Language

5. May speak 15-20 words (21-24 months).
6. May combine two to three words.
7. Asks for food, drink.
8. Echoes two or more words.
9. Takes three directions (one at a time), for instance: "Take ball from table." "Give ball to Mommy."—"Put ball on floor."
10. Points to three or more body parts.

Personal-social-adaptive

11. Builds tower of five to six cubes.
12. Folds paper once when shown.
13. Helps with simple household tasks (21-24 months).
14. Removes some clothing purposefully (besides hat or socks).
15. Pulls person to show something.

2 YEARS

Motor

1. Runs without falling.
2. Walks up and down stairs.
3. Kicks large ball (without demonstration).
4. Throws ball overhand.
5. Claps hands.
6. Opens door.
7. Turns pages in book, singly.

Language

8. Says simple phrases.
9. Says at least one sentence or phrase of four or more syllables.
10. Can repeat four to five syllables.
11. May reproduce about 5-6 consonant sounds. (Typically: m-p-b-h-w).
12. Points to four parts of body on command.
13. Asks for things at table by name.
14. Refers to self by name.
15. May use personal pronouns, such as: I-me-you (2-2½ years).

Personal-social-adaptive

16. Builds five to seven cube tower.
17. May cut with scissors.
18. Spontaneously dumps raisin from bottle (without demonstration).
19. Throws ball into box.
20. Imitates drawing vertical line from demonstration.
21. Parallel play predominant.

2½ YEARS

Motor

1. Jumps in place with both feet.
2. Tries standing on one foot (may not be successful).
3. Holds crayon by fingers.
4. Imitates walking on tiptoe.

Language

5. Refers to self by pronoun (rather than name).
6. Names common objects when asked (key, penny, shoe, box, book).
7. Repeats two digits (one of three trials).
8. Answers simple questions, such as: "What is this?"—"What does the kitty say?"

Personal-social-adaptive

9. Builds tower of eight cubes.
10. Pushes toy with good steering.
11. Helps put things away.
12. Can carry breakable objects.
13. Puts on clothing.
14. Washes and dries hands.
15. Eats with fork.

Table 4-1. Child development from 1 month to 5 years—cont'd

2½ YEARS—cont'd

Personal-social-adaptive—cont'd

16. Imitates drawing a horizontal line from demonstration.
17. May imitate drawing a circle from demonstration.

3 YEARS

Motor

1. Stands on one foot for at least one second.
2. Jumps from bottom stair.
3. Alternates feet going upstairs.
4. Pours from a pitcher.
5. Can undo two buttons.
6. Pedals a tricycle.

Language

7. Repeats six syllables, for instance: "I have a little dog."
8. Names three or more objects in a picture.
9. Gives sex. ("Are you a boy or a girl?")
10. Gives full name.
11. Repeats three digits (one of three trials).
12. Knows a few rhymes.
13. Gives appropriate answers to: "What: swims-flies-shoots-boils-bites-melts?"
14. Uses plurals.
15. Knows at least one color.
16. Can reply to questions in at least three word sentences.
17. May have vocabulary of 750 to 1,000 words (3-3½ years).

Personal-social-adaptive

18. Understands taking turns.
19. Copies a circle (from model, without demonstration).
20. Builds three-block pyramid (⊞).
21. Dresses with supervision.
22. Puts 10 pellets into bottle in 30 seconds.
23. Separates easily from mother.
24. Feeds self well.
25. Plays interactive games, such as "tag."

4 YEARS

Motor

1. Stands on one foot for at least five seconds (two of three trials).
2. Hops at least twice on one foot.
3. Can walk heel-to-toe for four or more steps (with heel one inch or less in front of toe).
4. Can button coat or dress; may lace shoes.

Language

5. Repeats ten-word sentences without errors.
6. Counts three objects, pointing correctly.
7. Repeats three to four digits (4-5 years).
8. Comprehends: "What do you do if: you are hungry, sleepy, cold?"

4 YEARS—cont'd

Language—cont'd

9. Spontaneous sentences, four to five words long.
10. Likes to ask questions.
11. Understands prepositions, such as: on-under-behind, etc. ("Put the block *on* the table.")
12. Can point to three out of four colors (red, blue, green, yellow).
13. Speech is now an effective communication tool.

Personal-social-adaptive

14. Copies cross (+) without demonstration.
15. Imitates oblique cross (×).
16. Draws a man with four parts.
17. Cooperates with other children in play.
18. Dresses and undresses self (mostly without supervision).
19. Brushes teeth, washes face.
20. Compares lines: "Which is longer?"
21. Folds paper two to three times.
22. Can select heavier from lighter object.
23. Cares for self at toilet.

5 YEARS

Motor

1. Balances on one foot for eight to ten seconds.
2. Skips, using feet alternately.
3. May be able to tie a knot.
4. Catches bounced ball with hands (not arms) in two of three trials.

Language

5. Knows age (How old are you?")
6. Performs three tasks (with one command), for instance: "Put pen on table—close door—bring me the ball."
7. Knows four colors.
8. Defines use for: fork-horse-key-pencil, etc.
9. Identifies by name: nickel-dime-penny.
10. Asks meaning of words.
11. Asks many "why" questions.
12. Relatively few speech errors remain—90% of consonant sounds are made correctly.
13. Counts number of fingers correctly.
14. Counts by rote to 10.
15. Comments on pictures (descriptions and interpretations).

Personal-social-adaptive

16. Copies a square.
17. Copies oblique cross (×) without demonstration.
18. May print a few letters (5-5½ years).
19. Draws man with at least six identifiable parts.
20. Builds a six-block pyramid from demonstration.
21. Transports things in a wagon.
22. Plays with coloring set, construction toys, puzzles.
23. Participates well in group play.

to make a determination of gestational age. One such tool was designed by Dubowitz and coworkers (1970). A chart to estimate gestational age was developed by Brazie and Lubchenko and can be found in *Current Pediatric Diagnosis and Treatment* (Kempe, Silver, and O'Brien, 1978). Skill in administering these examinations requires practice with the supervision of an experienced clinician.

The Neonatal Behavioral Assessment Scale developed by Dr. T. Berry Brazelton and associates is designed to assess the infant's interactive behavior during the neonatal period. "It is an attempt to score the infant's available responses to his environment, and so, indirectly his effect on the environment" (Brazelton, 1973, p. 4). The test includes 27 behavioral items and repeated assessments are suggested rather than just one assessment. There are findings that suggest that this tool can be useful in predicting developmental outcomes. It can be used to discriminate between the abnormal baby and the normal baby. It is also very useful in helping parents understand their infant's behavior when parents are included in the testing process. Training in the proper administration of the test is required.*

There are few tools designed to assess infant temperament beyond the first month of life. Therefore, the tool developed by William B. Carey and Sean C. McDevitt is useful. They developed the Carey Infant Temperament Questionnaire for detecting the temperament of infants between 4 and 8 months of age. The questionnaire consists of 95 questions relating to behaviors seen during feeding, sleep, elimination, and other activities, and the parent is asked to respond according to a scale from "almost never" to "almost always." Determination of the infant's temperament or behavior is important in understanding how he interacts with his environment. The identification of the infant's temperament profile makes it possible to individualize the help offered to parents in handling and caring for their infant. The questionnaire is available from Dr. Carey.†

The Denver Developmental Screening Test (DDST) developed by W. K. Frankenburg and J. B. Dodds is a tool for the detection of developmental delays during infancy and the preschool years up to 6 years of age. It is not an IQ test but the results help in the estimation of the child's current developmental level. It is a valuable tool in determining the

child's developmental needs and provides a basis for planning anticipatory guidance. Items were selected from 12 developmental and preschool intelligence tests on the basis of (1) ease of administration and interpretation and (2) a relatively short time from the point at which a few children could perform an item to the point at which most children could perform the item. The items are organized to give an overall developmental profile with emphasis on gross motor, language, fine motor-adaptive, and personal-social skills. Both professionals and paraprofessionals can learn to administer the DDST with training. Self-instructional units are available so that each individual can learn to use a standardized method of test administration. An instructional unit is also available with a manual, workbook, and film for class instruction, and a proficiency evaluation. Requests for information about the availability of materials for training should be addressed to LADOCA.*

The Denver Articulation Screening Examination was developed by Amelia F. Drumwright, a speech pathologist, with the purpose of devising a screening test of articulation skill that would "1.) reliably detect disorders in preschool children aged 2½ to 6 years and 2.) be useful and acceptable to speech pathologists, yet readily understandable to other child workers (doctors, nurses, teachers and subprofessionals)" (Drumwright and others, 1973). The examination requires the child to repeat 22 words that represent 30 speech sounds. The examiner evaluates sound production and makes an overall judgment about the intelligibility of the child's speech. The norms are presented for children between the ages of 2½ and 6 years. The manuals, test materials, and information about training should be requested from LADOCA.

DEVELOPMENTAL STAGES
Infancy

During the brief period of infancy, from birth to 18 months, the infant develops from a dependent, helpless newborn into a person who walks, talks, and relates to different people in terms of their importance in his life. He begins interacting with his environment from the moment of birth. A rudimentary ego identity, sense of self, evolves as he gradually learns to see himself as separate from his environment and gains feelings of faith and optimism as the core problem "trust vs mistrust" (Erikson, 1968) is initially resolved. He develops intellectual and motor skills that enable him to move from almost total helplessness at birth to being an aggressive explorer at 18 months of age.

---

*A list of trained examiners who can provide training can be obtained by writing to the principal investigator, Dr. T. Berry Brazelton. There are also training films available for use with the published manual. These can be obtained by writing to Educational Development Corporation, 8 Mifflin Place, Cambridge, Mass. 02138.

†William B. Carey, M.D., 319 W. Front St., Media, Pa. 19063.

*LADOCA Project and Publishing Co.,
East 51st Ave. and Lincoln St.,
Denver, Co. 80216

The velocity of growth during the first few months and years of life is greater than at any other time but proceeds at a decelerating rate. The newborn infant, on the average, weighs 7 to 7½ pounds at birth and will lose up to 10% of that weight during the first few days of life. The birth is usually regained by the tenth day and the infant will then continue to gain steadily. He will double his birth weight during the first 4 months and then triple it by 1 year. During the second year the average weight gain is 6 to 7 pounds. The average length of the newborn is 20 inches, which will increase by 50% during the first year but will not double until 4 years of age.

Marked changes occur in the body contour during infancy. The head grows at a fairly rapid rate during the first year and the head circumference is greater than the chest circumference. Then the growth of the head slows and the chest circumference becomes greater during the second year. The thickness of the subcutaneous fat increases during the first year and reaches a peak around 9 months and then actually decreases during the second year. The plump infant becomes leaner. At birth the extremities are shorter than the trunk, with sitting height representing about 70% of body length. The extremities grow more rapidly than the trunk and at 1 year the sitting height will represent about 60% to 65% of body length. The teeth begin to erupt in the fifth or sixth month and he will have approximately six teeth by 1 year.

There are many physiological changes that occur but one of the most striking is the continued maturation and increased function of the nervous system. Myelination continues at a rapid rate during the first months of life but is not complete until several years after birth. The functional development of various body structures probably corresponds to the order of myelination and occurs in a cephalocaudal direction. Thus, the development of head control precedes sitting, standing, or walking (see Table 4-1).

There is a critical period of personality develop-ment when the child develops a "sense of trust." Successful growth during this period means that the child comes to trust the people in his environment and himself. According to Erikson (1963), a sense of trust develops when there is a mutual regulation of the baby's pattern of accepting things and the mother's way of giving them that changes as the baby develops. He says "that the family brings up a baby by being brought up by him" (p. 69). The social modality of the baby's development during the first 6 months is "to get," meaning to receive and accept. This implies a passiveness on the part of the infant that is not altogether correct. The infant influences people in his environment from the moment of birth. His first reflexive behaviors of looking, rooting, sucking, and crying elicit responses in the mother or other care-taking adults that cause them to act in ways that will meet the infant's needs. Maternal bonding is influenced by these behaviors. The social modality of the infant during the second half of the first year is "taking and holding on," which begins with the eruption of teeth and the ability to sit upright and voluntarily reach out. Erikson describes the infant as experiencing a feeling of "paradise lost" at this time because he not only is beginning to be more aware of himself as a separate person but of his mother as a separate person who can disappear. He becomes more demanding of her. The infant is also faced with the frustrations that result when his pleasure in biting or grasping and holding onto things is met with interference. There are displays of helpless rage when his strong desires are thwarted. When his behavior is understood and he continues to receive loving attention, his trust in himself and others can be maintained and strengthened.

Piaget has defined this period of cognitive development as the sensorimotor period, "the period of mental development which begins with the capacity for a few reflexes, and ends when language and other symbolic ways of representing the world first ap-

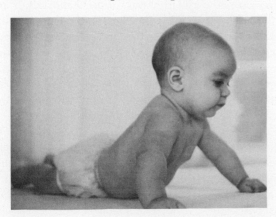

He can raise his chest off the table at 3 months of age.

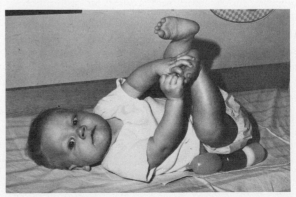

Learning is focused on body actions the first 7 to 9 months of age.

pear" (Beard, 1969, p. 33). The infant is egocentric and sensorimotor learning is related to "self." During the first 7 to 9 months of life the infant's learning is focused on body actions. Then as he gains the concept of object permanence, that things and people exist even when he cannot see them, he begins to learn about objects and people in his environment—their characteristics and relationships in space. Through a sequence of mental and physical actions and the gradual development of memory the child acquires the concept of object permanence and the awareness of himself as an object separate from his environment. It is the beginning of the child's construction of reality.

The newborn makes many rapid adjustments necessary to sustain life outside the uterus that are actually a continuum of the development during fetal life. When parasitic existence is terminated at birth, respirations are initiated and changes in the circulatory system occur, the digestive system begins to assimilate the food obtained from an external source, body wastes are excreted, and the maintenance of body heat becomes dependent on the infant's own resources. Behavior includes many reflex actions that reflect the immaturity of the nervous system but also assist in adaptation with the new environment. Some of these reflexes are discussed in Chapter 21, "The Assessment of the Pediatric Client."

The first 3 months of life can be called a period of adjustment. The newborn reflexes become more regularized during the first month and the infant learns how to search and suck and let needs be known. Sleeping and feeding patterns become more regular. The tonic neck reflex becomes more prominent at the end of the first month. During the second and third months new behaviors appear that are not reflexes. The infant begins to follow objects with his eyes, allowing exploration of the environment and coordination of movements of hand and mouth, such as sucking the thumb at will. The grasp reflex gradually lessens as more purposeful movements begin. The infant begins to prolong interesting events that occur more or less by accident. The little wails that precede crying may be continued for their own sake. And who can forget the loud, repeated, joyful squeals of the 2- to 3-month-old baby? The infant begins to smile in response to stimuli in the environment and to produce vocal sounds. Most responses are generalized and frequently involve movements of the whole body. The infant during this period has social responses but does not discriminate and any person who can satisfy his needs will be accepted.

By 3 months of age the baby becomes more discriminating. He begins to differentiate mother from others and produces special types of smiles and crying for her, which is the beginning of attachment behavior and the development of awareness of the self as separate from her. Between ages 3 and 6 months he begins to repeat actions that are interesting as well as prolong those that occur accidentally, for instance, repeatedly hitting at toys suspended in the crib to produce movement. He begins to imitate facial movements and sounds. He will look for a displaced object but will not conduct a true search. The infantile reflexes are replaced by purposeful movements, especially those seen in the development of eye-hand coordination. He begins to reach for and grasp objects with a raking motion. The tonic neck reflex and Moro reflex disappear during the fifth or sixth month. At 3 months the infant can, while in the prone position, raise head and chest from the surface with arms extended; at 4 months he can hold his head steadily while being supported in the sitting position; and at 6 months he will begin to sit without support.

The period between 6 and 12 months of life is dominated by the social modality of "taking and holding on" as described by Erikson. It is also described by Bowlby (1969) as being a period of active attachment behavior. The infant at 8 to 9 months of age has a beginning concept of object permanence and becomes fearful that the mother (object) will disappear. He actively initiates contact with her and seeks to maintain that contact. There is true searching for a vanished object, although he may expect to find it in several inappropriate places. His behavior becomes more complex and aggressive. He coordinates earlier repetitive actions into behaviors with a purposeful aim. He now explores objects more fully by rubbing, banging, and chewing them and rapidly discovers correct procedures for manipulating them. Motor development is dramatic as coordination increases. He develops the pincer grasp using the thumb and forefinger, learns to stand, and begins to walk holding onto furniture. He does more vocalizing and begins using pseudowords at about 10 to 12 months of age.

Between 12 and 18 months the infant becomes a toddler. He assumes an upright position and previously acquired motor skills are improved and expanded. Attachment behavior continues to be intense and he needs his mother close by in order to explore new places or to cope with threatening situations. Strangers will be treated with caution. However, he thoroughly enjoys his new abilities and is enthusiastically persistent and uninhibited in his attempts to manipulate things in his environment. He continues repetitive play with objects and enjoys putting things in and taking them out of a box as the experimentation with objects and object permanence continues. During the last months of this period cognitive de-

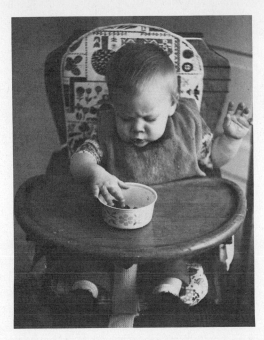

She does not use a spoon at 9 months of age

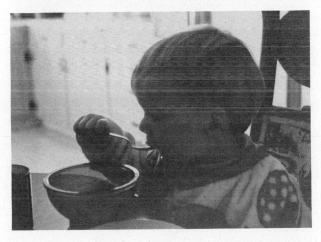

The beginning of competency at 2 years of age.

velopment is such that the infant begins to replace the earlier sensorimotor mental images that are nonverbal and have a highly personal meaning with mental symbols that are the beginning of language and he acquires approximately 20 words besides "mama" and "dada."

Early childhood

The infant moves into the early childhood years well equipped to continue learning about himself and his world. His ability to see himself as separate from his environment, his sense of trust and hope, and his developing intellectual and motor skills allow "autonomy" to blossom. Ego growth is rapid during the second and third years of life as the child

continues his exploration and learning about the objects in his environment and gains increasing mastery of his impulses and body functions. He gains a sense of autonomy, a feeling of independence as a separate person.

The ages between 3 and 6 are marked by social, emotional, and intellectual development. The child is developing a sense of himself as a social person in relation to other people. He is also learning about the physical world. As the child identifies with the parents he loves, he is motivated to be what they want him to be as well as to be like them. A conscience, or superego, develops as he begins to internalize the standards of his society as interpreted by his parents. He also becomes involved in the romance with the parent of the opposite sex and learns and accepts a sex role identity. The child's thinking remains egocentric throughout this period. He cannot take the other person's point of view and does not seek to clarify or validate his own point of view. The child learns to use symbols in representational thought and begins to think about objects, people, and actions that are not present.

This period of development is not defined by chronological age because there is overlapping with the infant years and the school years. The core problems described by Erikson are "autonomy vs shame" during the toddler years from 1 to 3 and "initiative vs guilt" during the preschool years between 3 and 6. Cognitive development during this entire period from about 18 months to 7 years is described as "preoperational" by Piaget and it is during these years that the child begins to acquire mental symbols and develop representational thought.

Growth continues at a decelerating rate. At 2 years the child will have added about 75% of his birth length to his height and at 4 years he will have doubled his birth length. Weight increments continue at a decelerating rate between 2 and 4 years of age, followed by a very gradual acceleration between 4 and 6 years. As the rate of growth in height and weight becomes slower, it also becomes less consistent month by month.

The changes in the child's physical appearance are dramatic. The toddler, as he begins to walk, looks top-heavy with his short legs and his potbelly. Fat pads obliterate the arch of the foot and most young children appear to be flat-footed until 3 or 4 years of age. There is also a tendency for the legs to bow inward and for lordosis to be apparent. The posture and body proportions change. The chest becomes larger in proportion to the head and the abdomen after 2 years of age, the extremities continue to grow faster than the trunk, and the jaw and lower face grow more rapidly than the cranium. The subcutane-

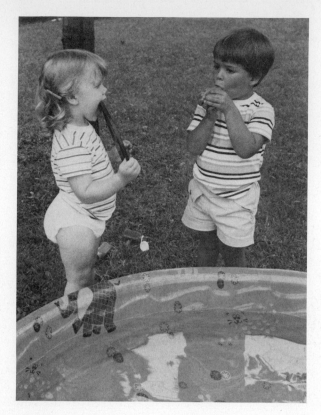

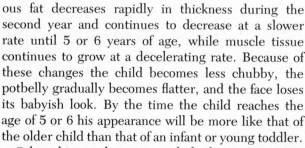

Differences in body contour and posture at 1 year of age and 3 years of age.

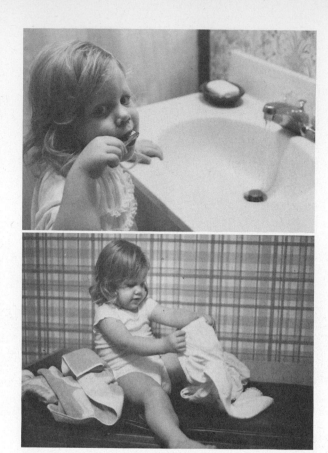

The 3½-year-old takes more responsibility for daily care.

ous fat decreases rapidly in thickness during the second year and continues to decrease at a slower rate until 5 or 6 years of age, while muscle tissue continues to grow at a decelerating rate. Because of these changes the child becomes less chubby, the potbelly gradually becomes flatter, and the face loses its babyish look. By the time the child reaches the age of 5 or 6 his appearance will be more like that of the older child than that of an infant or young toddler.

Other changes that occur include the improvement in visual acuity. The infant and young child are far-sighted and visual acuity at 2 years of age is estimated to be 20/40, compared to 20/20 between 4 and 5 years of age. The brain will reach 75% of its adult weight by 3 years and approximately 90% by 7 years. The skin changes after the first year and becomes tougher with less water content. The eruption of the primary teeth continues and the child will have the full complement of 20 primary teeth early during the third year when the second molars erupt.

During the second and third years of life, when neuromuscular coordination and intellectual development make it possible for him to actively explore and experiment, the toddler strives to establish a sense of autonomy. He is motivated to assert himself and is uninhibited in the pursuit of his own goals. He has no

limiting controls within himself and forges ahead. However, his wish to assert himself can bring him into conflict with his parents when he is confronted with the restrictions that are necessary to help him adapt to society's standards and control his primitive impulses. This is frustrating to him and tantrums are common. It can also be fear-provoking because he needs and wants his parent's love and approval. Despite his omnipotent behavior he is very dependent and wants to please. Therefore, he needs an environment that allows him to make free choices within limits that protect him from making choices that result in disappointing or disastrous consequences. Because he is not always certain of where his impulses will take him, he needs the reassurance that there are limits that protect him. The child gradually accepts limitations as he learns that he is safer and more comfortable when he pays attention to his mother instead of proceeding according to his own wishes. Attachment behaviors continue and, although he becomes increasingly able to play alone for longer periods of time, he will periodically seek his mother or go to her if threatened in any way. The young child who is faced with a new situation will venture forward with much more assurance if his mother is present. He also needs to turn to her for

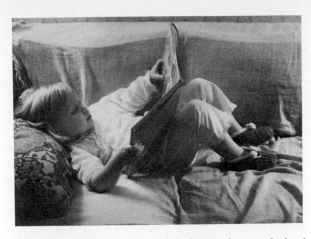

She has learned that she can lie on the couch to read a book like her mother does (3½ years).

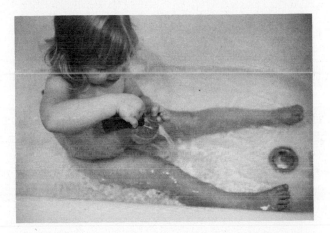

The 3½-year-old enjoys creative water play.

comfort when things get too difficult. The child during these years is sensitive to changes in the environment because his thinking is organized in a global way. His perceptions are such that, if there is one alteration, the "whole" is changed and becomes strange to him. Therefore, a consistent routine for daily activities is helpful to him. He can anticipate what will happen, learn the behaviors that are expected of him, and gain a feeling of controlling the situation and performing well. Rituals also become important at this age and reach a peak around age 2½. This is most evident at bedtime when the child is dealing with separation. If everything is done the same way each night he is reassured that his world will not change while he sleeps.

Play during these toddler years begins with exploration and discovery but, as the child gains ability to form mental images, his play becomes imaginative and imitative. He incorporates pieces of reality by imitating. He may imitate an animal or his mother's actions. The toddler appears to enjoy the company of other children but does not play with them—he plays beside them. He often treats them as if they were objects and feels free to poke, bite, or push them because he has no inner sense that this is hurtful. His egocentrism is such that if he feels no pain it must be all right. His pleasure in learning about things by touching, feeling, and manipulating is also seen in his early attempts to feed himself, brush his teeth, or drink from a cup. He is naturally messy. However, he is inclined to imitate and copy the behavior of his parents and by 3 years of age will become fairly competent.

Between 3 and 6 years of age the young child becomes more socially responsive and able to give love and affection. The development of initiative is characterized by the wish "to become," a wish to find out what kind of person he can and will be. During the earlier years he achieved a sense of himself as a separate person, a person with some power to influence his environment and control his own impulses and his body. These accomplishments make it possible for him to approach his new tasks with wonderful feelings of confidence and with lots of energy. The social modality is "to make" in the sense of "being on the make" (Erikson, 1963, p. 90). The child becomes intrusive in his desire to attack new situations (and bodies). Erikson says the child at this age intrudes into everyone's space with his locomotion and into everyone's ears with his aggressive talking. The child is noisy, active, and on the move, and thrusts himself into each situation as if driven by his curiosity and imagination. His love and admiration for his parents intensify and his identification with them increases. Sexual identification was begun at an earlier age when the child learned that he was a boy or a girl but during these preschool years it is heightened. It becomes evident as the child begins to model himself to be like the parent of the same sex and becomes acutely aware of sexual differences. His interest in the parent of the opposite sex becomes romantic, which results in conflict as he learns that he cannot displace the parent of the same sex whom he also loves. His feelings of intense love and the wish to be rid of one parent can cause anxiety and fear because the child believes that his wishes are as real as the actual deed. His task is to inhibit his sexual feelings and learn his sexual role and his role in the family. This process allows him to internalize the parents' standards and ideals and gradually develop a sense of moral responsibility. An infantile conscience develops, which makes it possible for him to resist temptation even though his parents are not present. He begins to feel guilt for misbehavior and at approximately 5 years of age he will even feel guilt for wishing to misbehave. This early conscience will be modified throughout the years of childhood as his intellectual abilities increase and his ability to identify rea-

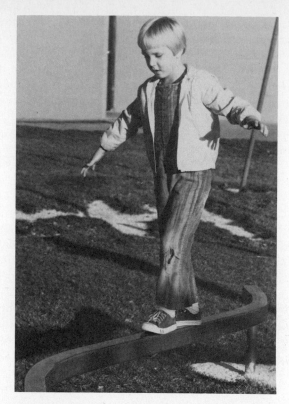

The 6-year-old has good neuromuscular coordination.

sons for moral action becomes more mature. Play during the preschool years becomes more social and imaginative. The social play of children at this age is complex as they learn to interact with each other while developing concepts, imagination, neuromuscular coordination, and language. Erikson describes this as the play age when the child is offered a micro-reality in which he uses toys to work out problems and anticipate future roles (Erikson, 1977, p. 99). Through imaginative and creative play the child tries out the roles of different people and also alleviates some of the guilt that occurs as the result of his developing conscience. In play he can be what he wants to be and gain mastery of his fears and alleviate guilt. He can feel strong and adequate instead of little and vulnerable. He can build the biggest castle or paint a beautiful picture. Through play he incorporates the behaviors of his role models, especially his parents, into his own standards of behavior, which helps him understand that he cannot replace his parent but can someday grow up and be a parent himself.

The young child's thinking during these years between 2 and 7 is limited by his egocentrism. He can see only one point of view—his own. He cannot make comparisons mentally so the logic of his own point of view cannot be challenged and he believes that everyone perceives things the same way that he does. He feels no need to justify his own conclusions and

takes little notice of how other people think. When communicating with other people he makes little attempt to relate to what the other person is saying or thinking and, if the listener is not familiar with the incident that he is talking about, his account will make no sense at all.

Cognitive development is reflected in the child's development of language. Early in the second year of life the child acquires personal, nonverbal, mental images of objects and events. His first words and gestures are also invested with unique personal meanings. His vocabulary increases rapidly during these years, which signals the appearance of thought with internal language and signs that allow him to think about objects and people not present and to anticipate future events. However, language does not immediately take the place of action thinking and the young child cannot think through a series of actions. He must actually perform them. His thinking is also characterized by "centering," which means that only one attribute of an object or event stands out in the child's perception. For instance, he can sort objects by color or by form but not by both.

Middle childhood

During the middle years of childhood, from 6 to 10 years, the child moves from the close ties to his family and home to the larger world of his peers, his school, and his neighborhood. The family romance is less intense and he is able to go out into the world. It is during this period of latency that the child is free from his earlier concentration on his sexuality and his strong basic drives. He can now direct his energy toward learning the skills and competencies of the mind and body that lead to practical achievements and accomplishments in his culture. There is tremendous intellectual growth during this lull before the storm of adolescence and the child is introduced to learning experiences that help him master the fundamental technology of his culture.

PHYSICAL GROWTH AND DEVELOPMENT

Growth during the middle years of childhood is relatively slow and smooth. The characteristic body type has emerged during the preschool years and is confirmed during the middle years; the short child remains short and the tall child remains tall. The increments in weight are less regular than seen in the young infant and child and may remain stationary for weeks at a time. The approximate annual increase in weight is about 5 to 7 pounds. The average annual increase in height is approximately 2 to 3 inches each year. Boys on the average are taller and heavier than girls until the adolescent growth spurt, which occurs earlier in girls. Although the growth spurt will be dis-

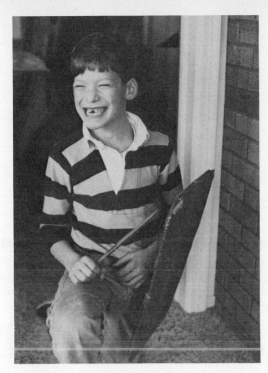

Play is creative and fun at 7 years.

cussed in relation to the child from 10 to 14 years of age, it is important to recognize that some elementary school–aged children will already have begun the growth spurt as early as age 8 or 9.

The physical changes that occur make school-aged children more agile and graceful. They become slimmer, with longer legs and a lower center of gravity than the younger child. They are stronger and better coordinated and are able to fit into the adult physical environment more easily. There is only a slight increase in the size of the cranium as nearly 90% of the growth of the brain is accomplished by age 7. The lower parts of the face continue to grow, giving the child a more mature appearance and making room for the larger teeth to erupt. The first permanent teeth to erupt at 6 to 6½ years of age are usually the mandibular central incisors. The eruption of the large permanent teeth contributes to the so-called ugly duckling appearance of the school-aged child.

The eyeball continues to grow until 10 or 12 years of age. Visual acuity is usually 20/20 between 4 and 5 years of age but depth perception is not very accurate until 6 to 7 years of age. Hearing is well established at a much earlier age. Lymphoid tissue increases steadily until puberty and then decreases. This accounts for the abundance of lymphoid tissues such as adenoids and tonsils. The skeleton continues to ossify, with cartilage being replaced by bone. The child has acquired the basic neuromuscular mechanisms by age 6 or 7 and will spend the school years in refining his

skills, resulting in an increase in motor skill and coordination. Thus, the school-aged child engages in repetition practice in all areas of neuromuscular activities from the fine motor skills of writing to the large motor skills used in baseball, bike riding, and swimming, depending on individual interests.

PSYCHOSOCIAL AND COGNITIVE DEVELOPMENT

By 6 years of age the child's personality has become structured. Through mastery of the earlier developmental crisis he has achieved a concept of self as separate from his environment, acquired a sense of trust, developed autonomy with some power over his own impulses and environment, incorporated standards of his culture as interpreted by his parents, and sublimated the desire "to make" people. According to psychoanalytical theory he has an ego, id, superego, and ego ideal. He is now ready to deal with the next core problem described by Erikson—industry vs inferiority.

During this period Erikson says the child becomes a worker. He is required to develop intellectual skills, physical skills, and social skills that contribute to his adequacy. The child is sent to school and play is transformed into work, games into competition and cooperation, and the freedom of imagination into the duty to perform (Erikson, 1977, pp. 103-104). The child's attainments in interpersonal and social development are important. The child is now able to see a higher organization of behavior in which he can and does participate. He wants to operate in socially accepted ways of thinking and behaving. He can take another person's point of view and compare it with his own. He can compare what he hears and sees with what he knows and make judgments about their reality. Also, he is able to reason and can act according to rules, which allows him to benefit from school experiences and to participate in organized play.

As the child moves into the larger world of school and peers. He will continue to need his parents' demands for conformity are placed on him by people outside the family, such as teachers, scout leaders, and peers. He will continue to need his parents' support and the approval of his teachers and other important adults, but he also needs to find his place in a group of peers. He is ready to be involved in the private world of children where adults are not always welcome. This becomes more apparent toward the end of latency when the child withdraws more into the privacy of his peer group, which is an important socializing agent. Feelings of group solidarity and belongingness are promoted by secret languages and codes as well as a common culture. Together children explore ideas and values as well as their environment.

The cognitive development of the school-aged child

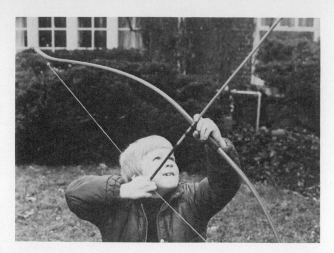

The 8-year-old concentrates on achieving a skill.

according to Piaget is characterized by the ability to begin to do mentally what he would have had to do with real action at an earlier age. "Piaget illustrated this by presenting 5-, 6-, and 7-year-old children with 6 sticks in a row and asking them to take the same number from a pile on the table. The younger children solved the problem by placing the sticks beneath the sample and matching the sticks one by one. The older children merely picked up 6 sticks and held them on their hands. The older children had counted the sticks mentally" (Elkind, 1974, p. 23). The school-aged child also sees the multiple characteristics of objects rather than centering on only one aspect. For instance, in one study Piaget placed 20 white and seven brown wooden beads in a box and asked individual 5-, 6-, and 7-year-old children if there were more white beads or more wooden beads. The young children could only respond that there were more white beads than brown beads. The older children could determine that there were more wooden beads than white beads because all of the beads were wooden (Elkind, 1974, p. 28). The older children were able to see the whole without losing sight of the uniqueness of the individual parts.

Piaget also found that it is during these years that the child masters the concept of conservation. The child begins to differentiate between the appearances of things and how they really are. Piaget's classic test is to give the child two jars of equal size containing equal amounts of liquid. The contents of one jar are then poured into two smaller containers of equal size and the child is asked whether the amount of liquid poured into the 2 smaller jars is still the same as that remaining in the other container. The younger children cannot comprehend that the liquid has been conserved when placed in smaller containers. The older children can because they can now make mental comparisons rather than actually manipulating ob-

jects, can see the whole as well as the parts, and have mastered the concept of conservation. They are ready for the cognitive task of mastering classes, relationships, and quantities.

However, this new ability to reason and to carry out mental operations in solving problems is limited in a very important respect. They can reason about concrete things but not about verbal propositions. They cannot differentiate between their own assumptions and the facts. In other words, they treat their own hypotheses as if they were facts and reject facts that do not agree with that position. Elkind has defined this as "cognitive conceit" (1974, p. 80). For instance, when the child learns that parents are not always right, there are two prevalent assumptions. One of these is that the adults are not too bright and the other is that the child knows more than the adult. Elkind points out that this behavior is often demonstrated in a spirit of fun or teasing as though the children are aware that they are using a convenient fiction.

"Cognitive conceit" is also useful in understanding the moral behavior of latency age children. Children of this age have internalized rules and know what is right and wrong. However, they continue throughout latency to break the rules they see as being made by adults. The child takes the rules as a challenge to his intellectual superiority and attempts to break them without being caught. School-aged children continue to operate with this kind of external conscience until the end of childhood when they start to formulate their own rules that will internally regulate their behavior.

Children experience success during this stage of industry as they participate in the many productive activities. They experience a sense of accomplishment that leads to the feelings of adequacy and worth vs the feelings of inferiority that come with repeated failure. School-aged children's great desire to win at games and willingness to work to achieve a variety of skills demonstrate their need to be adequate in their own eyes as well as in the eyes of others.

Preadolescence and adolescence
PREADOLESCENCE

The precise parameters of age and developmental levels begin to blend and overlap with the late childhood years. From that point on, a range of years, rather than a precise number, describes each developmental level. Some consider the "late childhood" and "early teen" years as a separate and important category known as "preadolescence." It may be helpful to think in terms of this group as youngsters from ages 9 to 12 in the fifth to eighth grades with tasks, characteristics, and behaviors that differ-

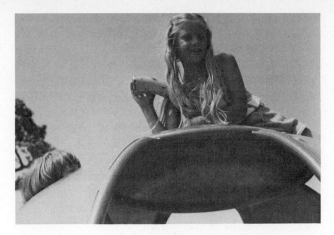

The 10-year-old enjoys her physical skills.

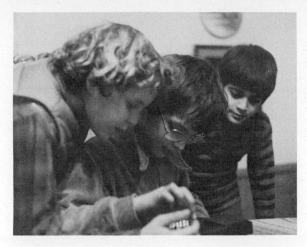

Preadolescence—establishing peer relationships.

entiate them from children and also from adolescents. Youngsters in this group are at an in-between age; they are no longer cuddly children, nor are they quite yet into the dramatic changes that mark the adolescent's world. It might be said that the tasks of preadolescence have to do with preparation for those adolescent changes that lie only a few years ahead. It is a continuation of the change in primary affiliation with the adult society and the codes of parents to an affiliation with those of their peers. Some of the patterns of the child's personality begin to loosen up and alter in some disorganization preparatory to further growth.

Preadolescents characteristically have great physical restlessness. Running is more natural than walking. Sitting still, even through a meal, may seem nearly impossible. Signs of earlier childhood problems, such as nervous habits or antics or bedwetting, may reappear temporarily before they are discarded. Muscular strength, skill, and agility are very important. In their quiet moments, which may be rather rare, preadolescents may have imaginative daydreams or may sit and stare blankly into space with apparently little on their minds. Although they may well have fears, worries, or concerns, they are not very interested in talking about them; but they may instead symbolically protect themselves from these problems by possessing toy guns, knives, or flashlights.

These years are often very trying times for parents as the parent-child bonds seem to be loosening and breaking. Although preadolescents do love and feel loyalty toward their parents, they may quite frequently treat them with surprising suspicion, distrust, and irritability. They are easily offended and respond to seemingly minor incidents with the ready accusation that adults do not understand them and, furthermore, treat them wrongly. At the same time, they

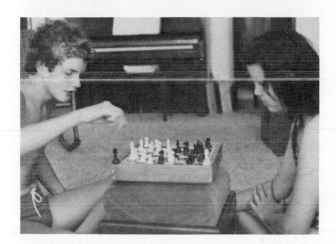

Adolescence—competition and creative conflict.

are seemingly unaware of the effect of any of their own inconsiderateness or the feelings of others and are more or less surprised when it is pointed out to them that their behavior has caused some hurt. Other adults in the neighborhood may receive more admiration than the parents receive. Parental recommendations regarding use of language and matters of appearance and cleanliness are often met with a response of indignation and frequent conflict. They are increasingly sensitive about having a parent see their bodies and about public display of affection.

At this stage, boys and girls have little to do with each other socially, although girls may move through this phase more quickly than boys. Clique and gang formation is a prominent characteristic as they establish strong identification with their peer groups. Often their pals and their peer codes do not meet with parental approval, which serves to make them all the more desirable to the preadolescent.

These changes of preadolescence are not easy for the parents, but neither are they easy for the preadolescent. There are often conflicting and painful choices, but the preadolescent must experience these in order to move on in the establishment of an individual identity.

ADOLESCENCE

The terms adolescence and adult are both derived from the Latin word *adolescere* meaning "to grow up." Both stages of life are, indeed, times of growth; however, the outward manifestations of growth during adolescence are the most dramatic. The age boundaries of adolescence are variable, although generally the teenage years (13 to 19) are used.

Adolescence is eminently a period of rapid and intense physical growth accompanied by profound changes that affect the entire organism. A physiological revolution occurs within and great concern develops over what the adolescent appears to be in the eyes of others compared with what he feels himself to be. According to Erikson (1963, 1968) the task of adolescence is the development of "ego identity" and the danger of the stage is "role confusion." The social world broadens in adolescence and the individual develops a growing sensitivity to the perceived judgments of others; he looks at himself in comparison to others.

The word conflict is often associated with the words teenager and adolescent, and it is truly a stage of conflict and turmoil, as well as one of high growth potential in the physical, sexual, and social areas. The adolescent must learn to cope with increasingly intense impulses, now vested in a maturing genital apparatus, an altering body formation, and a powerful muscle system. There is an increased craving for and intake of food, increased muscular energy and strength, and spurts of physical growth.

Breast development is often the earliest visible sign of puberty in girls, beginning normally between the ages of 8 and 13 and ending between 13 and 18. Girls' pubic hair appears at about age 11, axillary hair about a year later, and the adult pattern of hair distribution is established by about age 14. Most girls begin to menstruate at age 12 to 13, but may normally start as early as 9 or as late as 18; the early cycles tend to be irregular and are often anovulatory.

In boys, testicular enlargement is usually the first pubescent change, starting between 10 and 13 and ending between 13 and 17. The voice begins to deepen at 13 to 14. The growth of pubic hair occurs between ages 12 and 16; the growth of the beard and chest hair is usually somewhat later, around age 16. The first ejaculation usually occurs at 11 to 13 years, but the sperm are immature.

The ages 10 to 12 mark a spurt in height in girls, and by 14 to 15 their height growth is nearly com-plete. Boys of 12 to 13 have their rapid growth spurt. For some, this is preceded at about age 11 by a "stocky" or "chubby" period, which begins to decline as the spurt in height begins. By age 16, their height growth is nearly complete.

By the fourteenth year, the body of a girl is more often that of a young woman than that of a child, and for boys that year may mark a transition from boyhood to young manhood.

The behavioral traits of the adolescent years can also be described. The patterns of behavior during adolescence tend to fluctuate between outer- and inner-directedness as though the learnings of one phase need to be tested or reflected upon in the next. The adolescent needs periods for readjustment between the changing organism and the expanding environment. Growth is not a uniform, steady process but may show elements of "grown-up" helpfulness or childish lapses. It is an emotional period; the emotions should be considered symptoms of many forces —fears, struggles, and creative construction. Emotional growth requires creative struggle.

Gesell, Ilg, and Ames (1956) studied the behavioral traits of 10- to 16-year-olds. Their observations are summarized here, though the reader should be cautioned against expecting any set of behaviors during any given year. The sequence and flow of experiences are more important than the exact year during which they occur.

The 10-year-old is casual and easy-going. He gets along well with parents, siblings (unless they are 1 to 3 years younger than he), and friends. Although the attention span is rather short, there is a zest for learning. There is a delight in physical activity and a sense of fairness and sportsmanship. The 10-year-old may have explosive bursts of anger and may strike out violently, but these episodes tend to be brief and grudges are not harbored. In the area of conscience, he tends to be more aware of what is wrong than of what is right. He tends to be liberal in judgment. The shoulder shrug is a characteristic movement. "It is a golden age of developmental equipoise" (Gesell and others, 1956, p. 37).

The 11-year-old is sensitive and self-assertive, curious and talkative. He likes to be in motion, loves to argue, and may attempt to mimic and also to criticize parents. The emotional life has variable moods and peaks of intensity, which reflect the relative immaturity of the new emotional developments. In school he is an enthusiastic learner and shows increased concentration. Among friends, he may tend to stir up relationships, moving from hostilities to reconciliations. He senses increased self-reliance and claims the right to make some decisions on his own.

The 12-year-old is more balanced, more reasonable, and discrete. He relies less on forthright challenges to realize selfhood and tries to win the approval of others. A group of 12-year-olds is a high-spirited one and it has a pervasive role in shaping the attitudes of its members. He is beginning to insist that he is a child no longer. He shows some increased ability to do independent work, though preference for the group is evident. Emotional behavior is coming under increased control, there are signs of insight into self and others, and there is a blend of tolerance, humor, and enthusiasm.

The 13-year-old is more withdrawn and inner-directed. This is a reflective period—one that may be marked by spells of silence and musing. This new teenager may indulge in numerous private worries in phases of self-absorption. This is an indication of developing inner awareness, a time of releasing and reviewing inner feelings, tensions, and attitudes. Rage tends to be expressed more in words than in physical action as in the past. The 13-year-old is very sensitive to criticism and is more keenly aware of the emotional state of others. Siblings who are 2 to 5 years younger may be a source of great irritation and the parents may be found faulty, especially in problem areas the teenager is trying to resolve.

The 14-year-old is more expansive and less withdrawn. He seems to enjoy a sense of self-assurance and is anxious to be popular with peers. It is the age of interminable phone conversations, particularly for girls. There is a growing ability to consider two sides of an issue and a development in the use of language. Certain interests acquired may become life-long ones.

The 15-year-old is enigmatic and complex, yet desires to be understood by himself and others. He may appear apathetic, while he is actually preoccupied with inner-feeling states. He may appear resistant, irritable, and suspicious and may nurture feelings of revenge and violence. It is an age of increasing self-perception, a rising spirit of independence, and a loyalty to groups outside the home. Relationships in the home may deteriorate. The adolescent wants to "cut loose"; he is bored by the familiar and eager for new experiences.

The 16-year-old is often accorded more status and seen as a "pre-adult." He may have achieved some of that sought-after sense of independence, is more self-possessed, and is beginning to think more about the future in terms of a career and family.

These processes and fluctuations continue to some degree for several years in the direction of greater maturation. The task of finding an acceptable work role career, one that is personally as well as potentially economically adequate, assumes a more central position during the later high school and college years. Sheehy describes the ages of 18 to 20 as a time of "pulling up roots" (1974). College, military service, and short-term trips all provide ways of leaving the family base; peers become substitutes for family for periods of time, although rebounds to the family occur from time to time. "The tasks of this passage are to locate ourselves in a peer group role, a sex role, an anticipated occupation, an ideology or world view. As a result, we gather the impetus to leave home physically and the identity to begin leaving home emotionally" (Sheehy, 1974, p. 39). She notes that a stormy progression through this phase probably facilitates the normal progression of the adult life cycle.

Friedenberg (1959) notes the difficulty of adolescent passage in our Western society and emphasizes the importance of conflict to the individual and to society:

This process (of establishing a clear, and stable self-identification) may be frustrated and emptied of meaning in a society which, like our own, is hostile to clarity and vividness. Our culture impedes the clear definition of any faithful self-image. . . . We do not break images . . . we blur and soften them. The resulting pliability gives life in our society its familiar plastic texture. It also makes adolescence more difficult, more dangerous and more troublesome to the adolescent and to society itself. And it makes adolescence rarer. Fewer youngsters really dare to go through with it; they merely undergo puberty and simulate maturity (p. 17). . . .

The promise of maturity must be fulfilled by those who are strong enough to grow into it at their own rate as full bargaining members. Must there be conflict between the adolescent and society? The point is that adolescence is conflict—protracted conflict—between the individual and society (p. 32). . . .

Adolescent conflict is the instrument by which an individual learns the complex, subtle and precious difference between himself and his environment . . . and leads, as a high synthesis to the youth's own adulthood and to critical participation in society as an adult (p. 34).

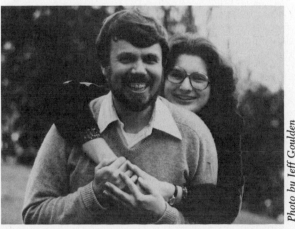

Photo by Jeff Goulden

Young adults—choosing a life-style.

Young adulthood

During the decade of ages 20 to 30, the major task is to achieve relative independence from parental figures and a sense of emotional, social, and economic responsibility for one's own life. Stevenson (1977) suggests the following developmental tasks:

1. Advancing self-development and the enactment of appropriate roles and positions in society
2. Initiating the development of a personal style of life
3. Adjusting to a heterosexual marital relationship or to another companionship style
4. Developing parenting behaviors for biological offspring, or in the broader framework of social parenting
5. Integrating personal values with career development and socioeconomic constraints

Erikson (1963), focusing more narrowly on marriage, describes the task of young adulthood as the development of affiliation or intimacy expressed as mutuality with a loved partner of the opposite sex with whom one is willing and able to regulate the cycles of work, procreation, and recreation. This involves the capacity to commit oneself "to concrete affiliations and partnerships and to develop the ethical strength to abide by such commitments, even though they may call for significant sacrifices and compromises" (p. 263). The danger of this stage is isolation or an avoidance of those persons and settings that promote and provide intimacy. A young adult whose identity work is not well underway may settle for sets of stereotyped interpersonal relationships that lead to a deep sense of isolation. This false "intimacy" bypasses the accomplishment of improved understanding of one's own inner resources and those of others.

Young adults may move out of the parental home or establish a more equal role with their parents if they stay in it. They begin to establish a style of single living, a marriage relationship, or another companionship style and adapt to the changes and compromises in expectations that their choice requires. Parenting tasks may be initiated by bearing children, adopting, becoming a foster parent, or reaching out in other ways, such as coaching children's teams or participating in child development–oriented organizations. It should also be noted that with divorce and remarriage, a frequent occurrence in American society, step-parenting and single parenting are fairly common situations. As children develop, parenting roles also develop in a reciprocal manner.

The young adult also chooses an area of study, a career, or a vocation and may begin to consider how one's belief about self and mankind affect that choice. Usually leisure time activities are selected and some

young adults include participation in local community and organizational activities in addition to career and family development. Sheehy suggests that the focus of the 20s shifts from the interior struggles of late adolescence ("Who am I?" "What is truth?") to a preoccupation with working out external situations ("Where do I go?" "How can I get there?" "How do I put my dreams into effect?"). The tasks revolve around erecting the test structure around the chosen life-style. Becoming caught up in the expectations of others is a pervasive theme, and the impulse to do what one should struggles with the impulses to be experimental and to explore alternative options.

Maturational crises of the 20s occur around these central themes: (1) attempts to increase independence from parents and parental dominance; (2) the choice of a post–secondary education course—school, a job, or the military; and (3) moving into the job or career world and establishing skills.

Middle adulthood

The middle years of adulthood may be thought of as an intermediate stage of life when growth is strongest in the areas of social and emotional development. By this time, individuals have generally chosen a lifestyle, a family or single pattern of living, and an occupation and are involved in implementing those choices. The span of time considered to cover the middle years is variable; some consider ages 40 to 65 and others, ages 30 to 70 as "middle age." However the boundaries are marked, it is probably the longest stage of an individual's life. The boundaries of this stage of life must be considered tentative and flexible. In this text the framework of 30 to 70 years of age, as described by Stevenson (1977), is used. Stevenson uses the term middlescence to describe this age span and further subdivides it into two categories: (1) the core middle years, or middlescence I, ages 30 to 50, and (2) the new middle years, or middlescence II, ages 50 to 70. The developmental tasks that she assigns to those subcategories of the middle years are presented in the boxed material on p. 79.

During the ages between 30 and 50, major goals and activities are in the areas of self-development, assistance to both the younger and older generations, and organizational endeavors. Individuals feel a need to come to terms with their own and with society's value orientations, and with the similarities and discrepancies therein. One's own value orientation may undergo a major change or numerous minor changes during these years when patterns are beginning to seem quite set but may not seem comfortably so. Individuals move into various roles and stations in a variety of settings; in the family, at work, in religious organizations, and in community and civic affairs. In Western society, much of the implementation of the goals of major institutions, including business, industry, government, education, religion, and charitable agencies, is performed by the middle-aged population. Work is a major activity and motivating force. For some the work itself is rewarding and gratifying; for others, the only rewards are the paycheck and the fringe benefits.

Much time during these years goes into promoting the growth of significant others, including one's children, parents, spouse, and friends. Erikson's seventh stage of life, generativity vs stagnation, addresses this issue of producing either another generation or something that may be passed on to the next generation. For some this means parenthood, for others this means generativity through creative acts of expression of altruism. Failure to advance to this stage or de-

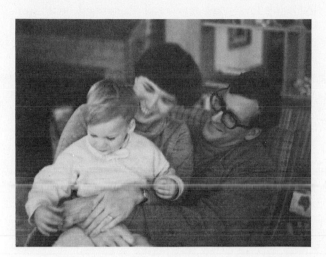

Middle adulthood—the development of a family.

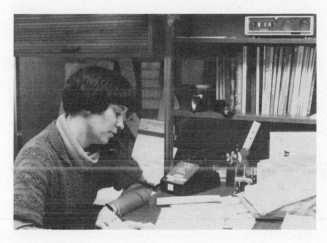

Middle adulthood—the development of a career.

Developmental tasks

**Developmental tasks of middlescence I,
the core of the middle years (30-50)***

1. Developing socioeconomic consolidation
2. Evaluating one's occupation or career in light of a personal value system
3. Helping younger persons (eg., biologic offspring) to become integrated human beings
4. Enhancing or redeveloping intimacy with spouse or most significant other
5. Developing a few deep friendships
6. Helping aging persons (eg., parents or in-laws) progress through the later years of life
7. Assuming responsible positions in occupational, social and civic activities, organizations, and communities
8. Maintaining and improving the home or other forms of property
9. Using leisure time in satisfying and creative ways
10. Adjusting to biologic or personal system changes that occur

**Developmental tasks of middlescence II,
the new middle years (50-70)**

1. Maintaining flexible views in occupational, civic, political, religious and social positions
2. Keeping current on relevant scientific, political, and cultural changes
3. Developing mutually supportive (interdependent) relationships with grown offspring and other members of the younger generation
4. Reevaluating and enhancing the relationship with spouse or most significant other or adjusting to their loss
5. Helping aged parents or other relatives progress through the last stage of life
6. Deriving satisfaction from increased availability of leisure time
7. Preparing for retirement and planning another career when feasible
8. Adapting self and behavior to signals of accelerated aging processes

*From Stevenson, J. S.: Issues and crises during middlescence, New York, 1977, Appleton-Century-Crofts.

velop this task can result, according to Erikson, in a stagnation of self or narcissistic self-indulgence. It should be noted that much of the economic effort and gain of the employed middleaged population goes toward the support of the younger and older generations. It is important that, while providing these various forms of support and assistance, the middle-aged avoid a need to completely control these other age groups.

As leisure time increases in the society, the activities that fill that larger portion are worthy of thoughtful consideration. People may choose to develop skills and talents that will serve them well in the present and in the future event of retirement. Part of self-knowledge and self-acceptance is an acknowledgement of the changes at the physical, emotional, and intellectual levels that accompany the aging process. The physical alterations may be the most difficult to accept in a culture where the signs of youthfulness are most highly acclaimed. It is most helpful to find some balance between accepting the inevitable changes in appearance while striving to maintain a high level of health with positive approaches toward exercise, diet, and the socioemotional environment. The changes of added years can also be appreciated in terms of emotional and intellectual benefits that can accrue.

During the decades of the 30s and 40s there are several maturational crises that do occur and various situational crises that can occur. Maturational crises are developmental transitions; they are stresses that occur periodically in the life cycle; situational crises are events that occur with less frequency and predictability, and for only certain individuals. Some of the predictable maturational crises in the core middle years occur in the early 30s and again in the early to mid-40s and have to do with the direction one's life seems to be taking. "Why am I doing this and not something else?" "Why am I with this person and not someone else?" "Why this career or talent or role and not another?" "Have I defined myself too narrowly?" are some of the common questions. Much soul-searching about priorities occurs and may lead to changes in residence, job, career, or spouse, or to a reevaluation and acceptance of things as they are. Individuals may approach the 30s realizing that they have expended both time and energy in doing the things their family and society indicated they "should" do. They may begin to feel too restricted by the career and personal choices made earlier and to realize that other aspects of themselves are struggling to surface and find expression. New choices and alternatives, as well as the old ones, are reconsidered and commitments may be altered or deepened. This may involve an uprooting of the life

that seemed to be so well grounded and striking out after a new vision. A job or career change may be sought, single people may renew the search for a partner, married people may feel discontent leading to a serious review of the marriage and perhaps to separation or divorce. Childless couples reconsider having children, while those who have spent a number of years raising young children may move toward involvement outside the home.

Once these struggles are decided in some way, the following few years may be characterized by a more settled situation during which people put down roots, invest in property, and work earnestly on climbing some particular career or social ladder. Much time and energy are involved in work and childrearing; satisfaction with a marriage may change.

For many individuals, the mid-30s mark a significant milestone. An awareness of life being at its halfway mark emerges. Time's passage may be felt as never before. There may be a diminishing acceptance of stereotyped roles and acknowledgement that few answers are absolute. Sheehy (1974) refers to the years of 35 to 45 as the "Deadline Decade," a time of reevaluating choices, purposes, and the expenditure of resources. It is a period of uncertainty and opportunity, a chance to restructure a narrower, earlier identity. Individuals may stumble on new aspects of themselves if they give themselves the permission to do so.

Davitz and Davitz (1976) have focused on the decade of 40 to 50 and found some similarities as well as a number of differences in the way men and women handle those years. There seems to be a generally increased awareness of one's own mortality as age-group acquaintances begin to develop illnesses and to die, often as a result of a heart attack. People in their 40s become aware, perhaps for the first time, that younger people view them as being in an older age group. Identity questions surface again, as they do with some frequency throughout the adult years, and individuals wonder: "What have I done?" "What have I become?" "Am I doing what is most fulfilling, rewarding, and satisfying for me?" "Who am I now?" Occasionally, they wonder what things might be like if they could begin again, but there is also the realization that although one might still make changes, one cannot go back to the beginning.

Parenting may be difficult, especially if the children are adolescents and working out identity problems of their own. Some parenting behaviors may be resented, although the parents may believe they are merely trying to prevent a repeat of their own mistakes. Parents may be attempting to relive their own lives through their maturing children and this is often understandably met with resentment from offspring who are seeking to lead their own lives. Concerns about aging parents also become more prominent.

During the early 40s, men may be enjoying success and promotions at work or may harbor a concern that this is the last chance to make it. Some experience tension from a fear of being passed by and are very sensitive to any indications that peers or superiors are losing confidence. While much energy goes into work or much frustration is experienced there, a sense of boredom with marriage and family life may emerge. Fears regarding sexual drive and loss of potency and masculinity may be experienced. Frustrations may be acted out at home, which tends to be the safest setting, producing more strain on the marriage and family relationship. Extramarital affairs are not uncommon. The emotions are fluctuating, moving from anger to affection and warmth and reflecting some of the internal conflicts about identity at work and at home. These conflicts occur in a context of responsibilities from which the person usually feels he or she cannot escape.

During the mid-40s, the attitude toward work may change from one of total involvement to one of lesser interest with a growing interest in developing a sport or hobby. The meaningfulness of activities is a frequent theme, as daily routines at work and home are rethought and belief in religion, politics, and relationships are reevaluated. This situation offers potential for psychological growth and a reintegration and stabilization of identity. Toward the second half of the 40s, some of the conflicts may be resolved. The stress on the marriage may promote a change in the relationship with a greater acceptance of interdependency or it may lead to a divorce and, possibly, to remarriage. Greater sexual maturity can provide an enhanced capacity to give and receive pleasure. Work may become more acceptable and viewed more in terms of its responsibilities than in terms of power. During these years aspects of the personality and talents that have been latent may begin to emerge. Physical changes are moderate; weight may increase and recovery time after exertion may be longer.

In our Western society, a woman approaches the age of 40 with a complex mixture of feelings: a sense of greater self-assurance and poise may be counterbalanced with a sense of apprehension. A woman of 40 is frequently thought of as middle-aged, settled, and mature. This set of role expectations may frustrate her, especially if she does not see herself conforming to that model. Involvement in a career may be a source of strength for a woman, as work brings its own rewards and sense of personal accomplishment and her identity is not entirely tied up with her family. It may also be a source of strain as demands from both work and family may be very high. Women

in the work world who may already have experienced some discrimination can find promotions increasingly rare and even resented by a husband who has not been similarly recognized. A woman who has devoted years to home and family may be eager to get into the outside world of school, business, or involvement in community activities.

Weight may become an eminent concern: a battle against weight gain may also be a battle against aging, the loss of physical attractiveness, and all that that implies in our culture. Difficulties in this area may well depend on the amount of self-esteem that has been previously derived from physical attractiveness. Gray hair is yet another manifestation of a physical change accompanying aging and may be a source of distress.

A woman confronted with her own concerns about aging might find these reinforced by her husband's behavior if he appears to be dissatisfied with the marriage. If divorce results, new friends and a new lifestyle must be developed. If the marital storms are weathered, a closer bond may be forged. Expectations of each spouse for the other may become more based in the facts than the fantasies of the relationship, and mutual dependence is accepted as well as the individual strengths and differences.

Single persons may experience a change in their relationships with married couples; aloneness may become a more prominent theme, despite the positive aspects of independence. The previous choice of career over marriage may be reconsidered, particularly if the parents have died.

Menopause, which normally occurs during the 40s or early 50s, involves both physical and psychological changes. The hormonal imbalance may result in episodes of emotional instability, rapid mood shifts, nervousness, irritability, insomnia, and fatigue. Some depression may be involved, but many women react with equanimity. The reaction to menopause may depend on how other developmental crises have been handled. Menopause may be followed by a heightened sexual drive and enjoyment of sex as concerns about pregnancy are diminished.

During the "new" middle years, generally ages 50 to 70, individuals have an opportunity to define and integrate the emotional and intellectual growth that has occurred during the earlier adulthood years. It may be a time of changes within the outside of the family resulting in the time and energy to develop new areas of interest. In the work world, many have attained much or most of what they can, although for a few, advancement is still possible. In certain arenas, such as in legislative, business, governmental, religious, and community service areas, these years may be the prime years of activity. Many of the highest positions in these areas are occupied by people in the new middle years. Within the family setting, spouses may be back to the couple stage, or fast approaching it, and need to readjust to the contracted nuclear family or to life alone if a spouse should die. Grand-parenting is a new role often acquired during this stage. Parents need to reassess their relationships with their children and move from the adult-child type of interactions to adult-adult interactions with their offspring who have reached adulthood. Men may become more aware of, less fearful of, and more accepting of their tendencies to provide care and nur-turance, while women may accept and develop more fully their assertiveness through an interest in busi-ness, politics, or other organizations and activities outside the home. The aging parents of 50 to 70-year olds often require assistance emotionally, physically, and/or financially. It continues to be important to help both the older and younger generations continue their own development and not to stifle either with overwhelming controls.

People in this age group, as in any age group, are confronted with rapid changes in technology and in the social environment. However, they often prefer to advise some caution and restraint in the type and rate of change. Life experiences have, hopefully, brought some sense of wisdom and judgment to the middleaged; and while some younger people may view them as overly cautious and nonprogressive, the balance between the two views is important. At the same time, openness and flexibility continue to be important characteristics to health and well-being. Those who stay current with new ideas and trends will have a more positive approach to life and less need of maintaining a defensive posture and will probably be able to communicate more effectively with younger individuals.

Preparation for retirement is a very important task, perhaps especially for people who have been em-ployed outside the home, but also for those who have maintained the housework. Both must readjust to more shared time. Preparation through adult educa-tion or development of new or latent skills can pave the way for a refocusing of talent. In a way, prepara-tion for retirement is lifelong, in that a person brings to retirement all that he has become throughout the years. Specific planning for retirement should not be delayed until retirement is imminent.

Late adulthood

As is the case with other stages of adulthood, the parameters of later adulthood and old age are not easy to define. Almost everyone is acquainted with some-one who seems "old" at 40 and with someone else who seems "young" at 65. Some gerontologists have attempted to deal with this situation by setting apart the years from 60 to 75 as early old age and the years from 75 on as later old age.

Later adulthood has become a subject of increasing interest to more people over the past several years. Factors influencing this increased interest include the longer life span and the decline in death rates in Western society, leading to increased numbers of the elderly in the population. However, changes in the social and family structure of this society, along with attitudes toward aging and the aged, have created many problems for these ever-larger numbers of old people. Institutional forms of care have been devel-oped but have often proved unsatisfactory; major pieces of legislation have been passed on behalf of the elderly, but often this has not eased the passage of time and the financial, social, and emotional problems that develop. The emphasis on youth and their cul-ture, behavior, and attitudes is accompanied by a negative attitude toward those on the other end of the age spectrum. If is often said that in this culture, all wish to live long but no one wishes to grow old. This is in marked contrast to other cultures, where old age is respected and even revered.

Later adulthood is similar to all other develop-mental stages in that certain adaptations are necessary and certain developmental tasks need to be achieved. Yet these developmental tasks are different from earlier ones in that these are the final ones in life.

Among the most significant developmental and ad-justive tasks in later adulthood are:
1. Maintaining or developing activities that en-hance self-image, contribute to a sense of worth in society, and help to retain functional capacity
2. Developing new roles as in-laws and/or grand-parents
3. Adapting to numerous losses—economically, socially, emotionally (such as job, friends, spouse)

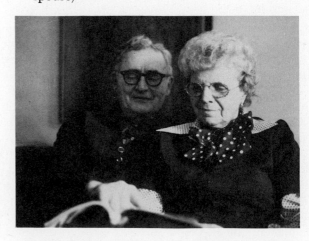

Middle adulthood—the preparation for retirement.

4. Adapting to physical changes
5. Performing a life review
6. Preparing for one's own death

As both demands from work and family and living arrangements change somewhat with the onset of retirement, time to do other things becomes more available. It is very important that preparation be made for the use of time far in advance of the retirement years. Failure to do so can make the change in time utilization and availability come as a shock and the hours may seem empty, heavy, or endless. If, on the other hand, preparation has been made, time can be used to advantage in the development of new careers, hobbies, sporting skills, or community activities. This should enhance both self-worth and functional capacity. Educational opportunities for adults of all ages are increasing. For the older adult, continuing education can provide an opportunity to learn again simply for the pleasure of learning or to enable them to develop another set of skills or an avocation. It is important to both physical and mental well-being that individuals continue to be involved in and contributing to society. If one or both spouses of an elderly couple have been employed they must also learn to adjust to having more time together and to intermeshing their lives effectively.

New roles emerge for older adults as their children marry and have children of their own. Acceptance of their children's spouses into the family network is very instrumental in the ongoing interaction of the family. Interaction with grandchildren can be a very pleasant aspect of aging if it does not become too time-consuming or burdensome. Grandparents need to be able to enjoy their grandchildren without having to be overly responsible for them. Another family role that may continue or may begin in early later adulthood is the caretaking of elderly parents who may be ill or at least more dependent. Individuals need to reevaluate personal identity in light of these new roles in life.

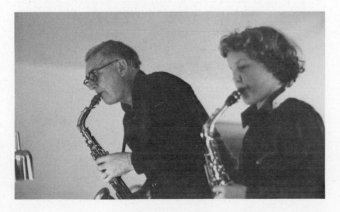

Later adulthood—grandparenting.

It is abundantly evident that numerous losses do accompany the later years of life. Retirement and its consequences must be dealt with. The loss of a job after many years of employment may be one of the greatest developmental and situational crises in the life of an individual. As stated earlier, it is very important to plan far in advance for postretirement activities that enhance self-respect. The loss of a job often includes the loss of the social relationships that were a part of that setting. It may also mean the loss of opportunities for certain kinds of recognition and achievement.

Couples or individuals must learn to adapt their life-style to a retirement income. As retirement incomes become relatively smaller in an inflationary era, this lowered income becomes more of a loss. Homes, entertainment styles, and life long travel plans may have to be given up or diminished in scope in order to meet the costs of necessities for food, housing, and health care.

Other losses may include the deaths of friends, a spouse, or other family members. These losses are among the most difficult aspects of later adulthood. Coping with bereavement for one with whom one has shared life experiences, memories, and plans leaves a great personal void; it is important to experience the profound emotions that accompany the loss and then to go on living one's own life and fostering the development of new relationships.

Adaptation to physical changes may also be viewed as a series of losses. Physical strength and vigor do tend to decline gradually over the years. In the 60s and 70s this change is often accompanied by diminishing sensory acuity of the eyes, ears, and taste. The emergence of one or several chronic illnesses may also impinge on strength, self-image, and independent status. The older population does become more dependent on the health care system for more frequent intermittent care and, for a small percentage of them, for full institutional care in various types of nursing homes. The majority of the elderly do continue to live at home and to receive some care from family or significant others; however, their more independent status is decreased. Major tasks are to accept physical changes and their limitations and to conserve strength and resources as necessary.

The process of performing a life review is an important developmental task of later adulthood. Most older persons do spend some time reflecting on their accomplishments and failures, satisfactions, and disappointments in an effort to integrate and evaluate the diverse elements of a life lived so that a reasonable positive view of their life's worth can be reached. Failure to accomplish this task may lead to serious psychological problems. The life review process is far

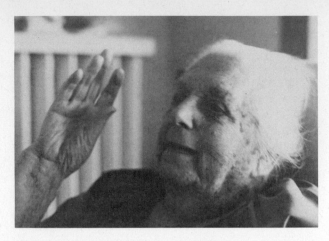

Later adulthood—the life review.

more than useless reminiscence. It allows for some gratification and also for the revision in understanding and clarification of experiences that may have been poorly understood or accepted at the time of their occurrence. It is an inventory that helps put past successes and failures into some perspective. It is often important for the older person to share some of this material with others, particularly with the younger generation. This can be mutually beneficial because it gives the older person a sense of usefulness and some credit for their age and wisdom and can provide the younger person with a sense of history. Today's older Americans have lived through more changes than any other single group in human history. This life developmental task is well described by Erikson (1963) as the eighth cycle of man: ego integrity vs despair. "It is the acceptance of one's one and only life cycle as something that had to be and that, by necessity, permitted of no substitutions" (p. 268).

Preparation for one's own death, views on death, and the possibility of an afterlife may very likely evolve from the life review process. For many, if not all, it is important to consider the issue of their own death and to prepare for it in terms of finishing one's business or setting one's affairs in order. This takes many forms: finalizing a will, achieving some goal, resolving some or many interpersonal relationships, and saying one's farewells to significant family members and friends. If the dying process is prolonged in the presence of some chronic illness, the individual will go through several phases of dealing with their eventual death. Both popular and professional literature are making available knowledge and information about the process of dying as the final phase of life. To die in a way as close as possible to what the individual desires may be thought of as life's final developmental task.

Although there are few tools to assess life changes and their effects on adults, two that have been developed are the Recent Life Change Questionnaire and the Life Experiences Survey. Both of these are an attempt to assess life stresses and to indicate a possible relationship between life stresses and susceptibility to physical and psychological problems or illnesses.

The Recent Life Changes Questionnaire (Rahe, 1975) is a self-administered questionnaire containing a list of events that subjects respond to by checking those events that they have experienced in the previous 6 months to 1 year (Table 4-2). To determine the scores for these events the researchers had a large group of subjects rate each of the items, with "marriage" assigned an arbitrary value, with regard to the amount of social readjustment each event required. Mean values for each item were taken to represent the average amount of social readjustment required. The values, called Life Change Units, were added to yield a life stress score. Studies using this tool have shown correlations between high recent life change scores and the development of health problems. This tool does combine a life stress score based on both desirable and undesirable events and it may be important to take these differences into account in the assessment of an individual's life change and its impact on health. It is also important to consider an individual client's own assessment of both the intensity of the life changes and his assessment of the strength of his coping abilities.

The Life Experiences Survey (Sarason, Johnson, and Siegel, 1978) is a self-report tool that allows respondents to indicate events they have experienced over the past year (Table 4-3). It includes events that occur fairly frequently and allows respondents to weigh the desirability or undesirability of events. Ratings are on a seven-point scale from extremely negative (−3) to extremely positive (+3). A positive change score is obtained by adding those events rated as positive, the negative change score is obtained by adding the negatively rated events, and a total change score is obtained by adding those two values. Studies by Sarason and others (1978) suggest that there is a relationship between negative life change as measured by the Life Experiences Survey and problems of a psychological nature. Although the cause-effect relationship is often unclear between life changes and health status, and the effect of life changes or stresses differs from person to person depending on their unique characteristics, including the degree of perceived control over events and the degree of psychosocial assets, yet these tools may be useful ones to the clinician in obtaining some assessment of the active and recent change factors, some of which may be considered developmental tasks, and their importance in a client's life.

Table 4-2. Recent life changes questionnaire*

Scoring weight	

Health

Within the time periods listed, have you experienced:

53   1. An illness or injury which:
         (a) Kept you in bed a week or more, or took you to the hospital?
         (b) Was less serious than described above?
15   2. A major change in eating habits?
16   3. A major change in sleeping habits?
19   4. A change in your usual type and/or amount of recreation?
    †5. Major dental work?

Work

Within the time periods listed, have you:

36   6. Changed to a new type of work?
20   7. Changed your work hours or conditions?
29   8. Had a change in your responsibilities at work:
         (a) More responsibilities?
         (b) Less responsibilities?
         (c) Promotion?
         (d) Demotion?
         (e) Transfer?
23   9. Experienced troubles at work:
         (a) With your boss?
         (b) With co-workers?
         (c) With persons under your supervision?
         (d) Other work troubles?
39   10. Experienced a major business readjustment?
45   11. Retired?
47   12. Experienced being:
         (a) Fired from work?
         (b) Laid off from work?
    †13. Taken courses by mail or studied at home to help you in your work?

Home and family

Within the time periods listed, have you experienced:

20   14. A change in residence:
         (a) A move within the same town or city?
         (b) A move to a different town, city or state?
15   15. A change in family "get-togethers"?
44   16. A major change in the health or behavior of a family member (illnesses, accidents, drug or disciplinary problems, etc.)?
25   17. Major change in your living conditions (home improvements or a decline in your home or neighborhood)?
100   18. The death of a spouse?
63   19. The death of a:
         (a) Child?
         (b) Brother or sister?
         (c) Parent?
         (d) Other close family member?
37   20. The death of a close friend?
    †21. A change in the marital status of your parents:
         (a) Divorce?
         (b) Remarriage?

*From Rahe, R. H.: Epidemiological studies of life changes and illness, Int. J. Psychiatry 6(½):133-146, 1975. © Baywood Publishing Co., Inc.

†New questions.

[ ] Scaling weight derived from an earlier (military) scaling study.

Continued.

Table 4-2. Recent life changes questionnaire—cont'd

Scoring weight	

Home and family—cont'd

(NOTE: Questions 22-32 concern marriage. For persons never married go to Item 33.)

50	22. Marriage?
35	23. A change in arguments with your spouse?
29	24. In-law problems?
	25. A separation from spouse:
[45]	(a) Due to work?
65	(b) Due to marital problems?
45	26. A reconciliation with spouse?
73	27. A divorce?
39	28. A gain of a new family member?
	(a) Birth of a child?
	(b) Adoption of a child?
	(c) A relative moving in with you?
26	29. Wife beginning or ceasing work outside the home?
40	30. Wife becoming pregnant?
29	31. A child leaving home:
	(a) Due to marriage?
	(b) To attend college?
	(c) For other reasons?
	†32. Wife having a miscarriage or abortion?
	†33. Birth of a grandchild?

Personal and social

Within the time periods listed, have you experienced:

28	34. A major personal achievement?
24	35. A change in your personal habits (your dress, friends, life-style, etc.)?
39	36. Sexual difficulties?
26	37. Beginning or ceasing school or college?
20	38. A change of school or college?
13	39. A vacation?
19	40. A change in your religious beliefs?
18	41. A change in your social activities (clubs, movies, visiting)?
11	42. A minor violation of the law?
63	43. Legal troubles resulting in your being held in jail?
	†44. A change in your political beliefs?
	†45. A new, close, personal relationship?
	†46. An engagement to marry?
	†47. A "falling out" of a close personal relationship?
	†48. Girlfriend (or boyfriend) problems?
	†49. A loss or damage of personal property?
	†50. An accident?
	†51. A major decision regarding your immediate future?

Financial

Within the time periods listed, have you:

17	52. Taken on a moderate purchase, such as a T.V., car, freezer, etc.?
31	53. Taken on a major purchase or a mortgage loan, such as a home, business, property, etc.?
30	54. Experienced a foreclosure on a mortgage or loan?
38	55. Experienced a major change in finances:
	(a) Increased income?
	(b) Decreased income?
	(c) Credit rating difficulties?

Table 4-2. Recent life changes questionnaire—cont'd

Subjective life change unit (SLCU) instructions

Instructions for scoring your adjustment to your recent life changes

Persons adapt to their recent life changes in different ways. Some people find the adjustment to a residential move, for example, to be enormous, while others find very little life adjustment necessary. You are now requested to "score" each of the recent life changes that you marked with an "X" as to the amount of adjustment you needed to handle the event.

Your scores can range from 1 to 100 "points." If, for example, you experienced a recent residential move but felt it required very little life adjustment, you would choose a low number and place it in the blank to the right of the question boxes. On the other hand, if you recently changed residence and felt it required a near maximal life adjustment, you would place a high number, toward 100, in the blank to the right of that question's boxes. For immediate life adjustment scores you would choose intermediate numbers between 1 and 100.

Please go back through your questionnaire and for each recent life change you indicated with an "X", choose your personal life change adjustment score (between 1 and 100) which reflects what you saw to be the amount of life adjustment necessary to cope with or handle the event. Use both your estimates of the intensity of the life change and its duration to arrive at your scores.

Table 4-3. The life experiences survey*

Listed below are a number of events which sometimes bring about change in the lives of those who experience them and which necessitate social readjustment. *Please check those events which you have experienced in the recent past and indicate the time period during which you have experienced each event.* Be sure that all check marks are directly across from the items they correspond to.

Also, for each item checked below, *please indicate the extent to which you viewed the event as having either a positive or negative impact on your life* at the time the event occurred. That is, *indicate the type and extent of impact that the event had.* A rating of −3 would indicate an extremely negative impact. A rating of 0 suggests no impact either positive or negative. A rating of +3 would indicate an extremely positive impact.

	0 to 6 mo	7 mo to 1 yr	Extremely negative	Moderately negative	Somewhat negative	No impact	Slightly positive	Moderately positive	Extremely positive
1. Marriage			−3	−2	−1	0	+1	+2	+3
2. Detention in jail or comparable institution			−3	−2	−1	0	+1	+2	+3
3. Death of spouse			−3	−2	−1	0	+1	+2	+3
4. Major change in sleeping habits (much more or much less sleep)			−3	−2	−1	0	+1	+2	+3
5. Death of close family member:									
a. Mother			−3	−2	−1	0	+1	+2	+3
b. Father			−3	−2	−1	0	+1	+2	+3
c. Brother			−3	−2	−1	0	+1	+2	+3
d. Sister			−3	−2	−1	0	+1	+2	+3
e. Grandmother			−3	−2	−1	0	+1	+2	+3
f. Grandfather			−3	−2	−1	0	+1	+2	+3
g. Other (specify)			−3	−2	−1	0	+1	+2	+3
6. Major change in eating habits (much more or much less food intake)			−3	−2	−1	0	+1	+2	+3
7. Foreclosure on mortgage or loan			−3	−2	−1	0	+1	+2	+3
8. Death of close friend			−3	−2	−1	0	+1	+2	+3
9. Outstanding personal achievement			−3	−2	−1	0	+1	+2	+3

*From Sarason, I. G., Johnson, J. H., and Siegal, J. M.: Assessing the impact of life changes: development of life experiences survey, J. Consult. Clin. Psychol. **46**(5):932-946, 1978.

Table 4-3. The life experiences survey—cont'd

	0 to 6 mo	7 mo to 1 yr	Extremely negative	Moderately negative	Somewhat negative	No impact	Slightly positive	Moderately positive	Extremely positive
10. Minor law violations (traffic tickets, disturbing the peace, etc.)			−3	−2	−1	0	+1	+2	+3
11. *Male:* Wife/girlfriend's pregnancy			−3	−2	−1	0	+1	+2	+3
12. *Female:* Pregnancy			−3	−2	−1	0	+1	+2	+3
13. Changed work situation (different work responsibility, major change in working conditions, working hours, etc.)			−3	−2	−1	0	+1	+2	+3
14. New job			−3	−2	−1	0	+1	+2	+3
15. Serious illness or injury of close family member:									
a. Father			−3	−2	−1	0	+1	+2	+3
b. Mother			−3	−2	−1	0	+1	+2	+3
c. Sister			−3	−2	−1	0	+1	+2	+3
d. Brother			−3	−2	−1	0	+1	+2	+3
e. Grandfather			−3	−2	−1	0	+1	+2	+3
f. Grandmother			−3	−2	−1	0	+1	+2	+3
g. Spouse			−3	−2	−1	0	+1	+2	+3
h. Other (specify)			−3	−2	−1	0	+1	+2	+3
16. Sexual difficulties			−3	−2	−1	0	+1	+2	+3
17. Trouble with employer (in danger of losing job, being suspended, demoted, etc.)			−3	−2	−1	0	+1	+2	+3
18. Trouble with in-laws			−3	−2	−1	0	+1	+2	+3
19. Major change in financial status (a lot better off or a lot worse off)			−3	−2	−1	0	+1	+2	+3
20. Major change in closeness of family members (increased or decreased closeness)			−3	−2	−1	0	+1	+2	+3
21. Gaining a new family member (through birth, adoption, family member moving in, etc.)			−3	−2	−1	0	+1	+2	+3
22. Change of residence			−3	−2	−1	0	+1	+2	+3
23. Marital separation from mate (due to conflict)			−3	−2	−1	0	+1	+2	+3
24. Major change in church activities (increased or decreased attendance)			−3	−2	−1	0	+1	+2	+3
25. Marital reconciliation with mate			−3	−2	−1	0	+1	+2	+3
26. Major change in number of arguments with spouse (a lot more or a lot less arguments)			−3	−2	−1	0	+1	+2	+3
27. *Married male:* Change in wife's work outside the home (beginning work, ceasing work, changing to a new job, etc.)			−3	−2	−1	0	+1	+2	+3
28. *Married female:* Change in husband's work (loss of job, beginning new job, retirement, etc.)			−3	−2	−1	0	+1	+2	+3
29. Major change in usual type and/or amount of recreation			−3	−2	−1	0	+1	+2	+3
30. Borrowing more than $10,000 (buying home, business, etc.)			−3	−2	−1	0	+1	+2	+3
31. Borrowing less than $10,000 (buying car, TV, getting school loan, etc.)			−3	−2	−1	0	+1	+2	+3
32. Being fired from job			−3	−2	−1	0	+1	+2	+3
33. *Male:* Wife/girlfriend having abortion			−3	−2	−1	0	+1	+2	+3
34. *Female:* Having abortion			−3	−2	−1	0	+1	+2	+3
35. Major personal illness or injury			−3	−2	−1	0	+1	+2	+3
36. Major change in social activities, e.g., parties, movies, visiting (increased or decreased participation)			−3	−2	−1	0	+1	+2	+3

Table 4-3. The life experiences survey—cont'd

	0 to 6 mo	7 mo to 1 yr	Extremely negative	Moderately negative	Somewhat negative	No impact	Slightly positive	Moderately positive	Extremely positive
37. Major change in living conditions of family (building new home, remodeling, deterioration of home, neighborhood, etc.)			−3	−2	−1	0	+1	+2	+3
38. Divorce			−3	−2	−1	0	+1	+2	+3
39. Serious injury or illness of close friend			−3	−2	−1	0	+1	+2	+3
40. Retirement from work			−3	−2	−1	0	+1	+2	+3
41. Son or daughter leaving home (due to marriage, college, etc.)			−3	−2	−1	0	+1	+2	+3
42. Ending of formal schooling			−3	−2	−1	0	+1	+2	+3
43. Separation from spouse (due to work, travel, etc.)			−3	−2	−1	0	+1	+2	+3
44. Engagement			−3	−2	−1	0	+1	+2	+3
45. Breaking up with boyfriend/girlfriend			−3	−2	−1	0	+1	+2	+3
46. Leaving home for the first time			−3	−2	−1	0	+1	+2	+3
47. Reconciliation with boyfriend/girlfriend			−3	−2	−1	0	+1	+2	+3
Other recent experiences which have had an impact on your life. List and rate.									
48. _____			−3	−2	−1	0	+1	+2	+3
49. _____			−3	−2	−1	0	+1	+2	+3
50. _____			−3	−2	−1	0	+1	+2	+3

BIBLIOGRAPHY

Barnard, K. E., and Powell, L.: Teaching the mentally retarded child; a family care approach, St. Louis, 1972, The C. V. Mosby Co.

Beard, R. M.: Piaget's developmental outline, New York, 1969, The New American Library, Inc.

Bier, W. C.: Aging; its challenge to the individual and to society, New York, 1974, Fordham University Press.

Birchenall, J., and Streight, M. E.: Care of the older adult, Philadelphia, 1973, J. B. Lippincott Co.

Bowlby, J.: Attachment and loss, vol. 1, Attachment, New York, 1969, Basic Books, Inc.

Brantl, V. M., and Brown, M. L., editors: Readings in gerontology, St. Louis, 1973, The C. V. Mosby Co.

Brazelton, T. B.: The neonatal behavioral assessment scale, Philadelphia, 1973, J. B. Lippincott Co.

Burnside, I. M., editor: Nursing and the aged, New York, 1976, McGraw-Hill Book Co.

Busse, E. W., and Pfeiffer, E., editors: Behavior and adaptation in late life, Boston, 1969, Little, Brown and Co.

Butler, R. N., and Lewis, M. I.: Aging and mental health, ed. 2, St. Louis, 1977, The C. V. Mosby Co.

Carey, W. B., and McDevitt, S. C.: Revision of the Infant Temperament Questionnaire, Pediatrics **61**:735, 1978.

Comfort, A.: A good old age, New York, 1976, Crown Publishers.

Cook, R. E., editor: The biological bases of clinical pediatrics, New York, 1968, McGraw-Hill Book Co.

Davitz, J., and Davitz, L.: Making it from 40 to 50, New York, 1976, Random House.

DeAngelis, C.: Basic pediatrics for the primary care providers, Boston, 1976, Little, Brown and Co.

Drumwright, A., and others: The Denver Articulation Screening Examination, J. Speech Hear. Disord. **38**(1):3, 1973.

Dubowitz, L., Dubowitz, V., and Goldberg, C.: Clinical assessment of gestational age in the newborn infant, J. Pediatr. **77**:1, 1970.

Elkind, D.: Children and adolescents, ed. 2, New York, 1974, Oxford University Press.

Ellison, J.: Life's second half: the pleasures of aging, Old Greenwich, Conn., 1978, The Devin-Adair Co.

Erickson, M. L.: Assessment and management of developmental changes in children, St. Louis, 1976, The C. V. Mosby Co.

Erikson, E. H.: Childhood and society, ed. 2, New York, 1963, W. W. Norton & Co., Inc.

Erikson, E. H.: Identity: youth and crises, New York, 1968, W. W. Norton & Co., Inc.

Erikson, E. H.: Toys and reason, New York, 1977, W. W. Norton & Co., Inc.

Erikson, E. H., editor: Adulthood, New York, 1978, W. W. Norton & Co., Inc.

Frankenburg, W. K., and Camp, B. W., editors: Pediatric screening tests, Springfield, Ill., 1975, Charles C Thomas Publisher.

Frankenburg, W. K., and Dodds, J. B.: The Denver Developmental Screening Test, J. Pediatr. **71**(2):1967.

Friedenberg, E. Z.: The vanishing adolescent, Boston, 1959, Beacon Press. Copyright © 1959 by Edgar Z. Friedenberg. Reprinted by permission of Beacon Press.

Gesell, A., and Amatruda, C.: Developmental diagnosis, ed. 2, New York, 1947, Paul B. Hoeber, Inc.

Gesell, A., Ilg, F. L., and Ames, L. B.: Youth: the years from ten to sixteen, New York, 1956, Harper & Row, Publishers.

Green, M., and Haggerty, R. J., editors: Ambulatory pediatrics, Philadelphia, 1968, W. B. Saunders Co.

Havighurst, R.: Developmental task and education, New York, 1952, David McKay Co., Inc.

Havighurst, R.: Human development and education, St. Louis, 1953, Warren H. Green, Inc.

Haynes, U.: A developmental approach to casefinding with special reference to cerebral palsy, mental retardation and related disorders, 1969, Washington, D.C., U.S. Department of Health, Education, and Welfare, Bureau of Community Health Service.

Holmes, T. H., and Rahe, R. H.: The social readjustment rating scale, J. Psychosom. Res. 11:213-218, 1967.

Illingworth, R. S.: The normal child, ed. 5, Baltimore, 1972, The Williams & Wilkins Co.

Illingworth, R. S.: The development of the infant and young child, normal and abnormal, ed. 6, Edinburgh, 1975, Churchill Livingstone.

Kaluger, G., and Kaluger, M. F.: Human development: the span of life, St. Louis, 1979, The C. V. Mosby Co.

Katchdourian, H. A.: Medical perspectives on adulthood. In Erikson, E. H.: Adulthood, New York, 1978, W. W. Norton & Co., Inc.

Kempe, C. H., Silver, H. K., and O'Brien, D., editors: Current pediatric diagnosis and treatment, ed. 5, Los Altos, Calif., 1978, Lange Medical Publications.

Knoblock, H., and Pasamanick, B.: Predicting intellectual potential in infancy, Am. J. Dis. Child. 43:106, 1963.

Levinson, D. J., and others: The seasons of a man's life, New York, 1978, Ballantine.

Neugarten, B. L., and others: Personality in middle and late life, New York, 1964, Atherton Press.

Pfeiffer, E.: Successful aging: a conference report, Durham, N. C., 1973, Duke University Press.

Piaget, J.: The construction of reality in the child, New York, 1954, Basic Books, Inc.

Piaget, J.: Piaget's theory. In Mussen, P. H., editor: Carmichael's manual of child psychology, New York, 1970, John Wiley & Sons.

Provence, S.: Developmental assessment. In Green, M., and Haggerty, R. J., editors: Ambulatory pediatrics, Philadelphia, 1968a, W. B. Saunders Co.

Provence, S.: Developmental history. In Cooke, R., editor: Biological basis of pediatric practice, New York, 1968b, McGraw-Hill Book Co.

Rahe, R. H.: Life changes and near-future illness reports. In Levi, L., editor: Emotions—their parameters and measurement, New York, 1975, Raven Press.

Rahe, R. H.: Epidemiological studies of life changes and illness, Int. J. Psychiatry 6(½):133-146, 1975.

Redl, F.: When we deal with children: selected writings, New York, 1966, The Free Press.

Riley, M. W., and Foner, A.: Aging and society, vol. 1, An inventory of research findings, New York, 1968, Russell Sage Foundation.

Riley, M. W., Johnson, M., and Foner, A.: Aging and society, vol. 3, A sociology of age stratification, New York, 1972, Russell Sage Foundation.

Riley, M. W., Riley, J. W., and Johnson, M.: Aging and society, vol. 2, Aging and the professions, New York, 1969, Russell Sage Foundation.

Sarason, I. G., Johnson, J. H., and Siegel, J. M.: Assessing the impact of life changes: development of the life experiences survey, J. Consult. Clin. Psychol. 46(5):932-946, 1978.

Sheehy, G.: Passages, New York, 1974, E. P. Dutton and Co., Inc.

Smart, M. S., and Smart, R. C.: Children; development and relationships, ed. 2, New York, 1972, Macmillan, Inc.

Spencer, M. G., and Dorr, C. J., editors: Understanding aging; a multidisciplinary approach, New York, 1975, Appleton-Century-Crofts.

Standards of child health care, ed. 3, Evanston, Ill., 1977, American Academy of Pediatrics.

Stevenson, J. S.: Issues and crises during middlescence, New York, 1977, Appleton-Century-Crofts.

Thomas, A., and Chess, S.: Temperament and development, New York, 1977, Brunner/Mazel, Inc.

Williams, R. H., and Wirths, C. G.: Lives through the years, New York, 1965, Atherton Press.

Working with older people; a guide to practice, U.S. Department of Health, Education, and Welfare, Pub. No. HSM 72-6005, vols. 1-4, 1969-1972; vol. 1, The practitioner and the elderly; vol. 2, Biological, psychological and sociological aspects of aging; vol. 3, The aging person—needs and services; vol. 4, Clinical aspects of aging.

5 Nutritional assessment

SAVITRI KAMATH, Ph.D., R.D.*

Although the widespread occurrence of malnutrition has been recognized in developing countries for more than a quarter of a century, its occurrence in the "affluent" United States has been publicized only recently. Following the publication of *Hunger U.S.A.* by the Citizens Board of Inquiry into Hunger and Malnutrition in 1968 and the CBS television program *Hunger in America*, there was a great deal of concern about the nutritional problems in this country. Senate hearings on nutrition and human needs from 1968 to 1974 and the White House Conference on Food, Nutrition, and Health in 1969 are the outcome of this revelation. Many nutrition intervention programs have been planned and implemented at the national and local levels to combat hunger and malnutrition in the United States. Examples of such programs are the School Lunch Program, the Special Milk Program, the School Breakfast Program, and the Commodity Distribution Program.

How were the needs for these programs identified? How will the efficacy of these programs be evaluated? The best way is to assess the nutritional status of the population periodically, before and following the implementation. A comprehensive attempt to assess the nutritional status of the American people resulted in the National Nutrition Survey. A detailed discussion of the results of this survey is found in the Health, Education, and Welfare (HEW) publication *Ten-State Survey, 1968-1970.* The results do indicate the existence of severe primary nutritional disorders, such as kwashiorkor; however, the incidence is very, very low when compared to that of developing countries. But more rampant are the subclinical deficiencies of certain nutrients such as iron and vitamin A, as judged by biochemical parameters. How these chronic subclinical deficiencies affect one's health in

the long run is not known at this time. It is important to control the deficiency at early stages; otherwise, severe deficiency may occur in a situation of stress, such as surgery or infection. Therefore, nutritionists are concerned with developing sensitive techniques to identify marginal deficiencies so that preventive measures can be undertaken to avoid further aggravation of the conditions.

Much concern has recently been expressed about evidences of malnutrition in hospitalized clients. Several concerned researchers have brought to attention the occurrence of poor nutritional care of hospitalized clients and the resulting malnutrition in this population. This is particularly unnecessary, since many products and techniques are available through which nutritional support can be given to clients who are unable, for a variety of reasons, to consume adequate amounts of the usual foods served. Some of these nutritional problems are of a secondary nature, such as maldigestion or malabsorption; increased requirements, as in fever or infection; or inadequate intake as a result of trauma or alcoholism. As a result, adult kwashiorkorlike or marasmuslike syndromes develop. In some conditions, intervention techniques are more effective when the subject is well nourished than otherwise. A good example is that of cancer patients, most of whom are malnourished for various reasons. This further emphasizes the importance of periodic nutritional assessment.

Currently, drug-induced malnutrition is another cause of concern. Subacute deficiencies of nutrients as a result of drug interference in the bioavailability of the nutrient to the cell are sometimes encountered in clients receiving prolonged drug therapy.

In consideration of these factors, it would appear very desirable to make every health professional aware of the existing and potential nutritional problems in their communities and institutions. Every individual in the United States has a right to receive

*Associate Professor, Department of Medical Dietetics, University of Illinois at the Medical Center, Chicago.

adequate health care, and an integral part of health care is nutritional care.

Nutritional care is a problem-solving process involving assessment before implementation of the care plan and during the period that the plan is carried out. So that nutritional care may be provided to each individual, as many health professionals as possible should be trained to evaluate the nutritional status of individuals or populations. This assessment is one of the techniques necessary to the implementation of the preventive aspects of health care.

Nutritional status may be defined as the state of health enjoyed as a result of nutrition. The World Health Organization (WHO) has defined health as a state of "complete physical, mental and social well being and not merely the absence of disease or infirmity."

Nutritional assessment aids in (1) the identification of malnutrition in an individual or in a population, of current nutritionally high-risk groups in the community, and of factors related to the cause of malnutrition; (2) providing information on resources available in planning efforts to overcome malnutrition; and (3) evaluating the efficacy of the nutritional care provided to the individual or the efficacy of the nutritional programs implemented in the community.

DEVELOPMENT AND NATURE OF MALNUTRITION

Malnutrition results from faulty or imperfect nutrition. At its fundamental level, it represents an inadequate supply of nutrients to the cell. A series of factors may be responsible for cellular malnutrition. Psychosocial, economic, and political factors and personal likes and dislikes of foods may contribute to inadequate intake of food or nutrients, resulting in *primary malnutrition*. On the other hand, factors such as inadequate digestion, improper absorption, faulty utilization, and increased requirement or excretion of nutrients may lead to decreased bioavailability of the nutrient to the cell, causing *secondary malnutrition*. Fig. 5-1 should be helpful in determining factors related to the bioavailability of nutrients.

Although both primary and secondary malnutrition ultimately result in similar manifestations, the cause needs to be identified in order to treat the condition. For instance, the vitamin A deficiency resulting from a lack of intake could be overcome by administering this nutrient through foods or supplements. However, the secondary deficiency of this vitamin observed in severe protein deficiency can be alleviated only by instituting protein therapy. Malnutrition may be *acute*, that is, the result of temporary adverse conditions that can be rapidly overcome, leaving no long-standing effects. Malnutrition may also be *chronic*, that is, the result of adverse conditions continued without relief over a period of time. Chronic malnutrition may lead to irreparable losses, such as blindness and growth retardation, and occasionally may even lead to death.

Fig. 5-2 describes the steps in the development of a nutrient deficiency. As to how fast and to what degree the deficiency of a nutrient would proceed is determined by the level of dietary intake and by the previous nutritional status, reflecting the extent of body stores and the body's ability to adapt to lower levels of the nutrient intake. Irrespective of the rate of progression, the general pattern in which the disease develops is similar to the one shown.

In the gradual development of a nutrient deficiency, tissue reserves are first mobilized in an effort to maintain the necessary supply of the nutrient to the cells. This is reflected in a reduced concentration of the nutrient in the blood or tissues as well as in decreased urinary excretion of the nutrient. As the deficiency progresses, the tissue reserves are depleted, resulting in an inadequate supply of the nutrient to the cell. This leads to biochemical lesions such as changes in enzymes, coenzymes, and metabolites, the levels of which would be altered in the blood and in the tissues. Further progression of the deficiency is manifested in the anatomical lesions and clinical symptoms detectable in a thorough physical examination by an alert practitioner. Clinical manifestation of vitamin deficiencies such as beriberi, pellagra, and scurvy are easily recognized.

In summary, it is possible to identify the development of a nutrient deficiency at the intake level, at the blood and tissue level, and during a physical examination. This is the principle on which the major methods of nutritional assessment, namely food intake studies, biochemical parameters, anthropometric measurements, and clinical examinations, are based.

PROCEDURES FOR ASSESSMENT

Whether the assessment is of a single individual or of a group of people in a population, the procedures are basically the same. However, when individual cases are considered, a more thorough nutritional assessment can be made, including an accurate nutritional history and sophisticated laboratory studies. When population groups are assessed, general methods, simple and fast, perhaps with less accuracy and precision, may have to be resorted to because of limitations of time, personnel, and facilities.

The nutritional profile of a community can be determined from various sources, such as food balance sheets, vital statistics, and agricultural data. Although

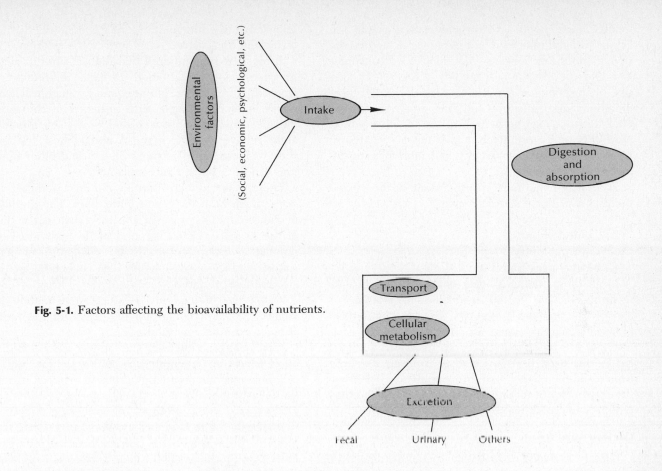

Fig. 5-1. Factors affecting the bioavailability of nutrients.

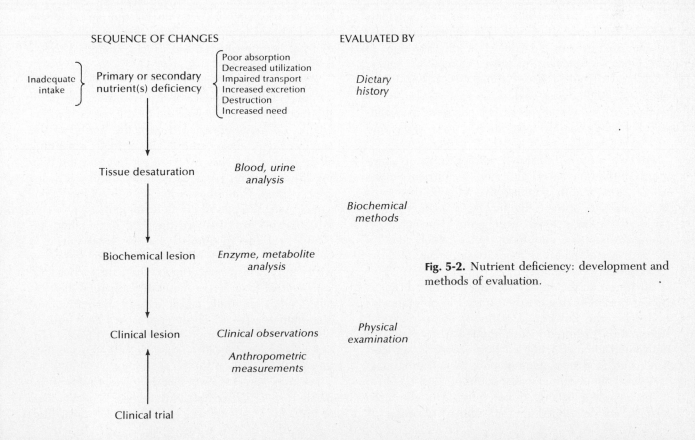

Fig. 5-2. Nutrient deficiency: development and methods of evaluation.

food balance sheets provide information on the per capita availability of food and nutrients to the population, it does not consider individual food consumption and the variation in intakes as a result of age, sex, socioeconomic condition, personal preference, or other factors affecting the food intake. Likewise, vital statistics may be helpful in the identification of morbidity and mortality but may not be reliable in terms of tracing the mortality and morbidity to the nutritional status.

Four major methods are important in the assessment of nutritional status:
1. Dietary surveys
2. Clinical appraisal
3. Anthropometry
4. Biochemical appraisal

In all these methods, data obtained from various techniques have to be evaluated in relation to "norms" or standard guidelines. Uses and limitations of individual guidelines are discussed under each method. However, one point worth stressing is that the norms used here are statistical norms obtained from a sample of the "healthy" population. Whether these are identical with the biological norms compatible with good health is a matter of debate.

Dietary surveys

Dietary surveys, or food intake studies, deal with collecting information on the dietary practices of people, including intakes of specific foods or nutrients over a known period of time. Populations subsisting on marginal intakes may not show physical signs of deficiency, or lesions. For these "subclinical" states, food intake studies have advantages because biochemical methods are extensive in comparison. In addition, this method serves as a check on the validity of the biochemical and clinical observations and vice versa.

Dietary surveys, if carried out appropriately, provide information on (1) the food or nutrient intake of the individual or population group, (2) the nutritional practices of the individual or population group, (3) ration allowances in emergency situations, (4) menu preparation and food procurement, and (5) the nutritional quality of foods available and of those foods actually consumed.

In communities, dietary surveys also help in identifying resources that can be utilized in programs for improving the nutritional status of the population. Information gathered is also applied when plans are developed for modifying existing economic, agricultural, and food management policies and programs.

A word about ethnic foods would be in place here. Many people partially, if not fully, still adhere to food habits developed in the country of origin. A knowledge of ethnic/cultural food is essential in analyzing the diets as well as in nutrition education.

It must be remembered that dietary surveys yield information of the situation during a limited time, whereas much of the clinical and biochemical evidence reflects the long-term nutrition of the individual. A recently improved diet would not immediately relieve the biochemical and clinical lesions; thus, a discrepancy between dietary and other findings can be expected and explained.

Dietary surveys are carried out in a number of ways. Each has merits and limitations. The method of choice depends on several factors, such as the size of the sample; the background of the individual or population group surveyed; the availability of personnel; and the provisions for data collection, analysis, and interpretation.

Two types of food intake studies are mainly in vogue: the family or group method, and the individual food intake method.

Family or group method. The family or group method is useful in obtaining information on the intake of a homogenous population, such as persons in the same institution or in a family sharing a common kitchen. Common methods of gathering information include the food record method and the food list method. In both methods, full cooperation from the individual in charge of the food service is essential. One of the drawbacks is in the need for estimating the food wastage occurring during the period of the study. Approximately 10% of the energy value of the diet has been estimated as this loss, though it varies from study to study.

FOOD RECORD METHOD. The food record or inventory method consists of keeping a record of all the foods in the kitchen at the beginning of the survey, of all foods obtained during the period of the survey (2 to 4 weeks), and of all the foods remaining at the end of the survey. Food waste occurring during the study and foods eaten away from home also are recorded. From these lists, amounts of foods consumed over the period are determined.

FOOD LIST METHOD. In the food list method, an estimate of the quantities of foods used during a given period of time is obtained through an interview with the person responsible for the food service.

Individual food intake method. Individual food intake studies generally consider both qualitative and quantitative aspects. Three approaches have usually been in practice. These include the food intake record, the 24-hour recall method, and the dietary history method.

FOOD INTAKE RECORD. Food intake at each of the meals is recorded concurrently over a known period of time by means of weights, household measures, or estimates of quantities of specific foods. How many days this survey should last and which of the weekdays is to be included are debatable points. In view of the fact that the day-to-day diet varies in the United States, a 1-day intake is not representative of the usual intake. It is desirable to include more than 1 day. The longer the duration, the better the reliability; however, since subjects tend to lose interest in keeping records after a while, it is advantageous to limit the record keeping to short periods.

A 3-day food intake record appears to be quite satisfactory, both in terms of the subject's cooperation and in terms of obtaining reliable information. Since a person's eating pattern tends to change during the weekend, inclusion of a weekend day may be advocated. Some researchers have found that inclusion of a weekend day along with 3 weekdays provides a satisfactory record.

Weighed-food records are a modified version of the food intake method and involve weighing all the foods consumed by the subject. The subject may be trained to weigh the foods accurately, or an investigator may be assigned to do this. This version is expensive and is mainly used in metabolic research studies.

In general, the food intake record has the disadvantage of making the subject conscious of his eating pattern, and this consciousness might make him modify his intake. When the subject is asked to estimate his intake, discrepancies related to the concept of serving size might also occur.

TWENTY-FOUR HOUR RECALL METHOD. The 24-hour recall method is very practical and useful in nutrition clinics. Intake of specific foods is recalled in terms of either estimates or quantities determined by means of weights or household measures. In view of the importance of enteral and parenteral feeding, particularly in the hospitals but becoming more common at home for certain patients, the intake through these routes also should be considered. From the memory point of view, the best recall period appears to be the immediate past 24 hours. A trained interviewer, generally a dietitian, usually carries out this method. To improve the reliability of the informant's memory, cross-check methods have been devised. The same questions are asked in different ways at different times in the interview. However, this procedure is time consuming and expensive and may be used only when the interviewer's time is not a limiting factor.

The accuracy of this method will vary. Women appear to be more accurate than men, and younger people more than elderly people, in giving data. Intake determined by the 24-hour method tends to be higher than that reported in a 7-day record. The day-to-day variation in meal pattern and in food intake make the 24-hour recall method not entirely representative of the individual's usual intake. Validity of the data obtained from the recall method has also been questioned. However, for all practical purposes, this method seems to provide sufficient information. It has been shown that for group comparisons, 24-hour recall records on a larger number of people provide better criteria than long-term studies on a limited population.

DIETARY HISTORY METHOD. The dietary history method yields qualitative information on long-standing food habits. This information is useful in interpreting the biochemical and clinical findings because the latter are indicative of long-standing food habits. The individual is asked to report his current or past intake in terms of frequency of occurrence of food items, changes in meal pattern, methods of food preparation, food likes and dislikes, shopping practices, and any other pertinent information. The history not only reflects the individual's food behavior but also is informative in terms of identifying the cause of nutritional problems. The dietary history also is a check for the validity of the intake reported in the 24-hour recall method. Dietary histories in conjunction with a 24-hour recall enhance the accuracy of the information. Nutrient intake calculated from food records is generally lower than that calculated from diet histories.

Tactics for eliciting data. Since individuals' food habits are of a very intimate nature, much of the success in eliciting suitable information on food habits depends on the interview. All the tactics described for an effective interview would be helpful here, also. Rapport between the interviewer and the informant is of utmost importance. A positive environment enhances the interaction between the interviewer and the interviewee. On an individual basis, a 30- to 45-minute interview using a suitable questionnaire or nutrition history form will yield useful information. Highly trained personnel can obtain very reliable information if the proper interview techniques are used.

To facilitate communication, the interviewer may use various sizes of glasses, spoons, bowls, and food models to help the subject estimate food quantities more accurately. Repetition may be necessary to cross-check information. Data on meal patterns over weekends and holidays help in deciding the days to be included for the food intake study. Observation of food intake, if possible, would further help cross-check the information given by the individual. This is possible only if one visits the home or institution.

Eliciting an accurate diet history and food intake is an art. Food habits are so personal to people that they may not be telling the truth for a variety of rea-

Table 5-1. Data collected and implications from diet history

Factor	Information sought	Implication
Host		
Demographic	Age; sex	Determine nutrient needs
Food intake	Actual foods consumed; frequency of foods; food likes and dislikes; vitamin and other supplements—dosage	Judge dietary pattern and adequacy; gross check information, help plan diets and counsel (megavitamin therapy)
Type of feeding	Oral; enteral; parenteral	Supplement intake data
Appetite	Taste and smell perception; loss or gain of appetite; anorexia	Help plan diet; aid in identifying nutrient deficiencies or disease conditions
Physical activity	Occupation; length and types of exercise; duration of sleep	Determine caloric needs (of particular importance in obesity)
Food avoidances	Allergies and intolerances; reasons for avoiding foods	Help plan diet; identify conditions needing intervention (of particular importance for children)
Dental/oral health	Teeth and gum health; fitting dentures; salivation; swallowing	Help plan diet; identify conditions needing intervention (of particular importance for elderly)
Gastrointestinal	Heartburn; bloating; gas; distention; diarrhea; constipation; GI fistula	Help plan diet; identify conditions needing intervention
Medications	Antacids and laxatives; other medications—frequency of usage, dosage	Help plan diet; drug-nutrient interaction (of particular importance in hospitalized patients and elderly)
Home life-style	Who shops; who cooks; type of cooking and storage facilities; number in household	Aids in family counseling in relation to life-style at home; referral if needed
Economic condition	Source of income and food dollars	Help plan diet, particularly in relation to economic priorities; educate to wise use of food dollars
Ethnicity	Ethnic, cultural, religious background; if migrants, which generation	Determine food habits; help plan diets in accordance with their choice

sons, for example, embarrassment or apprehension. The interviewee oftentimes likes to tell the interviewer what the interviewer would like to know rather than the truth. This might lead to a tendency to over- or underestimate the serving sizes. The combined problems of reliability and accuracy make it apparent that the quality of data obtained is determined by the skill, personality, and sensitivity of the interviewer as well as the honesty of the client.

A diet history may be brief or detailed. A detailed diet history not only helps in assessing the nutritional status but also is useful in identifying factors that affect food behavior and cause malnutrition. This, in turn, is helpful in nutrition planning. For this reason, a diet history could also include information on the client's medical and social background in addition to the data on food intake and habits.

Analysis and evaluation of data. Food intake data are evaluated in terms of either the foods in the diets or the nutrients, or both. Tools used for analysis and evaluation include the Basic Four food guide, food consumption tables, and chemical analysis.

BASIC FOUR FOOD GUIDE. The Basic Four food guide, though not perfect, serves as a practical tool

Table 5-2. Basic Four food guide (1956)

Food group	Essentials of an adequate diet
Milk and mild products	Children, 3 to 4 cups
	Adults, 2 or more cups
Fruits and vegetables	4 servings
Green and yellow vegetables	1 serving
Citrus fruits or raw cabbage	1 serving
Potatoes, other vegetables, and fruits	
Meat, poultry, fish, and eggs	2 or more servings
Bread, flour, and cereal (enriched or whole grain)	4 or more servings

for rapid analysis and evaluation of diets. The guide was recommended by the United States Department of Agriculture (USDA), based on the essentials of an adequate diet. Table 5-2 describes the Basic Four food guide. The intake of the recommended number of servings of determined amounts from each of the food groups is assumed to provide an optimal diet. The 24-hour intake is divided into foods of the four groups: milk, meat, fruits and vegetables, and cereals

Table 5-3. Mean heights and weights and recommended energy intake*

| Age and sex group | Weight | | Height | | Energy | | |
	kg	lb	cm	in	Needs MJ	Needs Kcal	Range in kcal
Infants							
0.0-0.5 yr	6	13	60	24	kg. × 0.48	kg. × 115	95-145
0.5-1.0 yr	9	20	71	28	kg. × 0.44	kg. × 105	80-135
Children							
1-3 yr	13	29	90	35	5.5	1,300	900-1,800
4-6 yr.	20	44	112	44	7.1	1,700	1,300-2,300
7-10 yr.	28	62	132	52	10.1	2,400	1,650-3,300
Males							
11-14 yr.	45	99	157	62	11.3	2,700	2,000-3,700
15-18 yr.	66	145	176	69	11.8	2,800	2,100-3,900
19-22 yr.	70	154	177	70	12.2	2,900	2,500-3,300
23-50 yr.	70	154	178	70	11.3	2,700	2,300-3,100
51-75 yr.	70	154	178	70	10.1	2,400	2,000-2,800
76+ yr.	70	154	178	70	8.6	2,050	1,650-2,450
Females							
11-14 yr.	46	101	157	62	9.2	2,200	1,500-3,000
15-18 yr.	55	120	163	64	8.8	2,100	1,200-3,000
19-22 yr.	55	120	163	64	8.8	2,100	1,700-2,500
23-50 yr.	55	120	163	64	8.4	2,000	1,600-2,400
51-75 yr.	55	120	163	64	7.6	1,800	1,400-2,200
76+ yr.	55	120	163	64	6.7	1,600	1,200-2,000
Pregnancy						+300	
Lactation						+500	

*From Recommended Dietary Allowances, revised 1980, Food and Nutrition Board, National Academy of Sciences–National Research Council, Washington, D.C. The data in this table have been assembled from the observed median heights and weights of children, together with desirable weights for adults for mean heights of men (70 in) and women (64 in) between the ages of eighteen and thirty-four years as surveyed in the U.S. population (DHEW/NCHS data).

Energy allowances for the young adults are for men and women doing light work. The allowances for the two older age groups represent mean energy needs over these age spans, allowing for a 2 per cent decrease in basal (resting) metabolic rate per decade and a reduction in activity of 200 kcal per day for men and women between fifty-one and seventy-five years; 500 kcal for men over seventy-five years; and 400 kcal for women over seventy-five. The customary range of daily energy output is shown for adults in the range column and is based on a variation in energy needs of ±400 kcal at any one age, emphasizing the wide range of energy intakes appropriate for any group of people.

Energy allowances for children through age eighteen are based on median energy intakes of children of these ages followed in longitudinal growth studies. Ranges are the tenth and nintieth percentiles of energy intake, to indicate range of energy consumption among children of these ages.

and cereal products. The servings in each group are compared to the recommended ones for judging the dietary adequacy. A discussion of the uses and limitations of the Basic Four food guide may be found in any textbook on nutrition.

Currently, ethnic foods and vegetarian diets are becoming popular. It is advisable to be knowledgeable about the nutritive value of these foods and diets. The ingredients that go into the combination dishes is important. Once the foods are identified, Basic Four analysis follows the same principle. In a vegetarian diet, meat substitutes (nuts, legumes, and lentils) will take the place of meat foods.

FOOD COMPOSITION TABLES. It is possible to calculate the amount of nutrients provided by a diet from food composition tables if the food is described in the table. The standard food composition table is the *Agriculture Handbook No. 456* (Adams). Data compiled from various laboratories sometimes consider the variety of foods, the method of preparation, and other factors that affect the nutritive value of foods.

With the influx of convenience foods in the market, it is rather hard to analyze diets with these tables because so many of the foods are not listed. Sometimes it may be necessary to obtain the information from the manufacturer.

A short method of dietary analysis could be resorted to if one uses tables in which similar foods are grouped in broad categories and an average value for the nutrient represents the whole group.

Table 5-4. Recommended Dietary Allowances, Revised 1980* (Designed for the maintenance of good nutrition of Sciences–National Research Council)

Age and sex group	Weight		Height		Protein (gm)	Fat-soluble vitamins			Vitamin C (mg)	Thiamin (mg)
	kg	lb	cm	in		Vitamin A (µg R.E.†)	Vitamin D (µg‡)	Vitamin E (mg αTE§)		
Infants										
0.0-0.5 yr.	6	13	60	24	kg. × 2.2	420	10	3	35	0.3
0.5-1.0 yr.	9	20	71	28	kg. × 2.0	400	10	4	35	0.5
Children										
1-3 yr.	13	29	90	35	23	400	10	5	45	0.7
4-6 yr.	20	44	112	44	30	500	10	6	45	0.9
7-10 yr.	28	62	132	52	34	700	10	7	45	1.2
Males										
11-14 yr.	45	99	157	62	45	1,000	10	8	50	1.4
15-18 yr.	66	145	176	69	56	1,000	10	10	60	1.4
19-22 yr.	70	154	177	70	56	1,000	7.5	10	60	1.5
23-50 yr.	70	154	178	70	56	1,000	5	10	60	1.4
51+ yr.	70	154	178	70	56	1,000	5	10	60	1.2
Females										
11-14 yr.	46	101	157	62	46	800	10	8	50	1.1
15-18 yr.	55	120	163	64	46	800	10	8	60	1.1
19-22 yr.	55	120	163	64	44	800	7.5	8	60	1.1
23-50 yr.	55	120	163	64	44	800	5	8	60	1.0
51+ yr.	55	120	163	64	44	800	5	8	60	1.0
Pregnancy					+30	+200	+5	+2	+20	+0.4
Lactation					+20	+400	+5	+3	+40	+0.5

*The allowances are intended to provide for individual variations among most normal persons as they live in the United States under usual ments have been less well defined. (From Recommended Dietary Allowances, Revised 1980, Food and Nutrition Board, National Academy

†Retinol equivalents: 1 retinol equivalent = 1 µg. retinol or 6 µg. β-carotene.

‡As cholecalciferol: 10 µg. cholecalciferol = 400 I.U. vitamin D.

§α tocopherol equivalents: 1 mg. d-α-tocopherol = 1 α T.E.

||1 N.E. (niacin equivalent) = 1 mg. niacin or 60 mg. dietary tryptophan.

¶The folacin allowances refer to dietary sources as determined by *Lactobacillus casei* assay after treatment with enzymes ("conjugases") to

#The RDA for vitamin B$_{12}$ in infants is based on average concentration of the vitamin in human milk. The allowances after weaning are based

**The increased requirement during pregnancy cannot be met by the iron content of habitual American diets or by the existing iron stores of ferent from those of nonpregnant women, but continued supplementation of the mother for two to three months after parturition is advisable

With the limitations of food composition tables, nutritive values should not be considered as accurate figures but as estimates of intakes.

Also, with food composition tables, as well as with the Basic Four food guide, the inaccuracy generated in the description of the food consumed is reflected in the analysis.

CHEMICAL ANALYSIS. Chemical analysis of food eaten is sometimes carried out to accurately determine the nutrient intake. This is an elaborate and expensive method and, as such, is employed only for research purposes. The food intake is weighed accurately, excluding the plate waste. A representative sample is then analyzed for nutrients in the laboratory.

Standards for evaluating the nutrient intake. Once the diet is analyzed for nutrients, the next step is to judge the intake for adequacy. Guidelines used for this in the United States are the Recommended Dietary Allowances (RDA) set by the Food and Nutrition Board of the National Research Council of the National Academy of Sciences. The RDA are numerical expressions of the quantities of certain nutrients believed to be adequate to meet the known nutritional needs of practically all healthy persons in the United States. Tables 5-3 to 5-5 present 1980 RDA for various nutrients in relation to age and sex.

The RDA do not represent minimal requirements. Intakes lower than the RDA do not necessarily mean nutrient deficiency. In fact, intakes of two-thirds or

of practically all healthy people in the U.S.A. Food and Nutrition Board, National Academy

| | Water-soluble vitamins | | | | Minerals | | | | | |
Ribo-flavin (mg)	Niacin (mg NE‖)	Vitamin B⁶ (mg)	Folacin¶ (µg)	Vitamin B¹² (µg)	Calcium (mg)	Phosphorus (mg)	Magnesium (mg)	Iron (mg)	Zinc (mg)	Iodine (mg)
0.4	6	0.3	30	0.5#	360	240	50	10	3	40
0.6	8	0.6	45	1.5	540	360	70	15	5	50
0.8	9	0.9	100	2.0	800	800	150	15	10	70
1.0	11	1.3	200	2.5	800	800	200	10	10	90
1.4	16	1.6	300	3.0	800	800	250	10	10	120
1.6	18	1.8	400	3.0	1,200	1,200	350	18	15	150
1.7	18	2.0	400	3.0	1,200	1,200	400	18	15	150
1.7	19	2.2	400	3.0	800	800	350	10	15	150
1.6	18	2.2	400	3.0	800	800	350	10	15	150
1.4	16	2.2	400	3.0	800	800	350	10	15	150
1.3	15	1.8	400	3.0	1,200	1,200	300	18	15	150
1.3	14	2.0	400	3.0	1,200	1,200	300	18	15	150
1.3	14	2.0	400	3.0	800	800	300	18	15	150
1.2	13	2.0	400	3.0	800	800	300	18	15	150
1.2	13	2.0	400	3.0	800	800	300	10	15	150
+0.3	+2	+0.6	+400	+1.0	+400	+400	+150	**	+5	+25
+0.5	+5	+0.5	+100	+1.0	+400	+400	+150	**	+10	+50

environmental stresses. Diets should be based on a variety of common foods in order to provide other nutrients for which human require-
of Sciences–National Research Council, Washington, D.C.)

make polyglutamyl forms of the vitamin available to the test organism.
on energy intake (as recommended by the American Academy of Pediatrics) and consideration of other factors, such as intestinal absorption.
many women; therefore, the use of 30 to 60 mg. supplemental iron is recommended. Iron needs during lactation are not substantially dif-
in order to replenish stores depleted by pregnancy.

more of the RDA have been interpreted as adequate in nutritional surveys. An intake of less·than this amount is considered suboptimal intake. Because of individual variations in nutrient needs, care should be taken to interpret the individual intake on the basis of the RDA.

A second standard, used mostly in the International Survey, is the Suggested Guide to Interpretation of Nutrient Intake Data, developed by the Interdepartmental Committee on Nutrition for National Defense (ICNND) (Table 5-6). This guide applies only to the 25-year-old, 67-inch tall, physically active man who weighs 143 lb. In order to overcome this problem of age and sex, yet another standard has been developed for the National Nutrition Survey. This stan-dard is derived from the ICNND guidelines and the RDA and is outlined in Table 5-7.

Because of the limitations of these standards, interpretation of dietary data is not diagnostic but only indicative of a deficiency.

Clinical appraisal

Clinical appraisal is concerned with the physical examination of certain parts of the body, such as the eyes, hair, mucous membranes, skin, and oral cavity (lips, teeth, gums, and tongue), in order to detect the symptoms of nutritional deficiency. Generally, this examination is carried out by a physician. However, auxiliary health workers may be trained in nutritional diagnosis based on clinical appraisal. The

Table 5-5. Estimated safe and adequate daily dietary intakes of additional selected vitamins and minerals*

Age group	Vitamins			Trace elements†						Electrolytes		
	Vitamin K (μg)	Biotin (μg)	Pantothenic acid (mg)	Copper (mg)	Manganese (mg)	Fluoride (mg)	Chromium (mg)	Selenium (mg)	Molybdenum (mg)	Sodium (mg)	Potassium (mg)	Chloride (mg)
Infants												
0.0-0.5 yr.	12	35	2	0.5-0.7	0.5-0.7	0.1-0.5	0.01-0.04	0.01-0.04	0.03-0.06	115-350	350-925	275-700
0.5-1.0 yr.	10-20	50	3	0.7-1.0	0.7-1.0	0.2-1.0	0.02-0.06	0.02-0.06	0.04-0.08	250-750	425-1,275	400-1,200
Children and adolescents												
1-3 yr.	15-30	65	3	1.0-1.5	1.0-1.5	0.5-1.5	0.02-0.08	0.02-0.08	0.05-0.1	325-975	550-1,650	500-1,500
4-6 yr.	20-40	85	3-4	1.5-2.0	1.5-2.0	1.0-2.5	0.03-0.12	0.03-0.12	0.06-0.15	450-1,350	775-2,325	700-2,100
7-10 yr.	30-60	120	4-5	2.0-2.5	2.0-3.0	1.5-2.5	0.05-0.2	0.05-0.2	0.1-0.3	600-1,800	1,000-3,000	925-2,775
11+ yr.	50-100	100-200	4-7	2.0-3.0	2.5-5.0	1.5-2.5	0.05-0.2	0.05-0.2	0.15-0.5	900-2,700	1,525-4,575	1,400-4,200
Adults	70-140	100-200	4-7	2.0-3.0	2.5-5.0	1.5-4.0	0.05-0.2	0.05-0.2	0.15-0.5	1,100-3,300	1,875-5,625	1,700-5,100

*From Recommended Dietary Allowances, Revised 1980. Food and Nutrition Board, National Academy of Sciences–National Research Council. Because there is less information on which to base allowances, these figures are not given in the main table of the RDAs and are provided here in the form of ranges of recommended intakes.

†Since the toxic levels for many trace elements may be only several times usual intakes, the upper levels for the trace elements given in this table should not be habitually exceeded.

auxiliary health worker would then alert the physician to the presence or absence of clinical symptoms.

Clinical appraisal is the least sensitive technique among the methods used in the nutritional assessment. Some reasons for this are:

1. Subjectivity of the examiner or examiner bias is involved in the judgment. Different evaluators differ regarding the identification and degree of malnutrition of the same lesion. The more nonspecific a lesion is, the more differing are the opinions. An example of this is seen in the examiner variability observed in the recordings of three examiners in an area included in the recent Ten-State Nutrition Survey (Table 5-8). Another example is that of the examiner who judges the leanness of a male subject's body in relation to his own and that of the female subject's in relation to the contour of his wife. Therefore, standardization of examiners' parameters must be carried out often. Color slides would be very useful in the identification and standardization of signs of deficiency.

2. Because of the nature of the development of nutrient deficiencies, clinical assessment may or may not correlate well with the food intake data or with the biochemical parameters.

3. The nonspecific nature of clinical lesions encountered may complicate the diagnosis. The same lesion could be traced to a deficiency of one or more nutrients. The lesion could also be due to some other reason, such as allergy or trauma.

In spite of its drawbacks, clinical appraisal does have a definite role in the total assessment procedure:

1. It provides information to supplement that obtained in anthropometric, dietary, and biochemical methods.

2. As seen in Fig. 5-2, anatomical lesions do not appear until the deficiency is far advanced. The presence of clinical symptoms in some individuals of a community would indicate the possibility of a subclinical deficiency in others. This identification could lead to correction at earlier stages.

3. Clinical assessment may reveal a host of other diseases not diagnosed earlier but which merit diagnosis and treatment.

4. A physical examination may detect nutritional deficiency not detected by dietary or biochemical methods.

Table 5-9 summarizes certain of the symptoms associated with specific nutrient deficiencies in human beings. Some of the observations made on specific tissues that are useful in the assessment procedure are briefly discussed here. One should note,

Table 5-6. Suggested guide to interpretation of nutrient intake data*

	Deficient	Low	Acceptable	High
Protein (gm/kg)	<0.5	0.5-0.9	1.0-1.4	>1.5
Iron (mg/day)	<6.0	6-8	9-11	>12
Calcium (gm/day)	<0.3	0.30-0.39	0.4-0.7	>0.8
Vitamin A (IU/day)	<2,000	2,000-3,499	3,500-4,999	>5,000
Ascorbic acid (mg/day)	<10	10-29	30-49	>50
Thiamine (mg/100 kcal)	<0.2	0.20-0.29	0.3-0.4	>0.5
Riboflavin (mg/day)	<0.7	0.7-1.1	1.2-1.4	>1.5
Niacin (mg/day)	<5	5-9	10-14	>15

*From Manual for nutrition surveys, ed. 2, Washington, D.C., 1963, Interdepartmental Committee on Nutrition for National Defense.

Table 5-7. Dietary standards used by the U.S. Public Health Service in evaluating dietary intake in the National Nutritional Survey, 1970*

Age	Energy (kcal/kg)	Protein (gm/kg)	Calcium (mg)	Iron (mg)	Thiamine	Riboflavin	Vitamin A (IU)	Ascorbic acid (mg)
6-7 years	82	1.3	450	10	0.4 mg/1,000 kcal	0.55 mg/1,000 kcal	2,500	30
10-12 years								
Male	68	1.2	650	10	0.4 mg/1,000 kcal	0.55 mg/1,000 kcal	2,500	30
Female	64	1.2	650	18	0.4 mg/1,000 kcal	0.55 mg/1,000 kcal	2,500	30
17-19 years								
Male	44	1.1	550	18	0.4 mg/1,000 kcal	0.55 mg/1,000 kcal	3,500	30
Female	35	1.1	550	18	0.4 mg/1,000 kcal	0.55 mg/1,000 kcal	3,500	30
Adults								
Male	38	1.0	400	10	0.4 mg/1,000 kcal	0.55 mg/1,000 kcal	3,500	30
Female	38	1.0		18	0.4 mg/1,000 kcal	0.55 mg/1,000 kcal		
Pregnant	+200	+20	800	18	0.4 mg/1,000 kcal	0.55 mg/1,000 kcal	3,500	30
Lactating	+1,000	+25	900	18	0.4 mg/1,000 kcal	0.55 mg/1,000 kcal	4,500	30

*From Guthrie, H. A.: Introductory nutrition, ed. 4, St. Louis, 1979, The C. V. Mosby Co.

however, that although prolonged and severe deficiencies of nutrients are manifested in anatomical lesions, not all the changes observed can be traced to nutritional origin.

Sometimes complaints from patients who have deficiencies of specific nutrients aid in diagnosing the symptoms faster. Examples of these complaints are general weakness, chronic fatigue, loss of appetite, loss of weight, bleeding gums, and soreness of the eyes and mouth.

Eyes. Dryness of the cornea and conjunctiva and corneal opacity (xerophthalmia) are usually associated with vitamin A deficiency. Infiltration of the cornea by blood vessels is associated with vitamin B_2, or riboflavin, deficiency.

Skin. Some of the dermatitides are associated with certain vitamin deficiencies. In niacin deficiency, dermatitis of skin exposed to sunlight is observed. In vitamin A deficiency, xerosis or roughness of skin caused by the hardness of papillae at the base of the hair follicle is seen. Nasolabial dermatitis is often con-

Table 5-8. Percentage of adult clinical findings by three examiners in a selected area of the Ten-State Nutrition Survey*

	Examiners		
	1	2	3
Number of examinations	1,123	1,127	589
Filiform papillary atrophy	4.1	1.1	11.2
Follicular hyperkeratosis	4.0	0.6	6.8
Swollen red gums	2.8	3.7	4.1
Angular lesions	0.4	0.4	1.2
Glossitis	0.6	0.4	0.5
Goiter	3.6	6.6	3.6

*From Laboratory tests for assessment of nutritional status, Sauberlich, H. E., Dowdy, R. P., and Skala, J. H., CRC Crit. Rev. Clin. Lab. Sci. 4:215, 1973. © CRC Press, Inc., 1973. Used by permission of CRC Press, Inc.

Table 5-9. Clinical syndromes associated with deficiencies of specific nutrients*

Calories: Underweight, underheight, weight loss, lethargy, anemia, edema, marasmus

Protein: As above, fatty liver, kwashiorkor

Fat: Dermatoses in infants (essential fatty acid deficiency), deficiencies of the fat soluble vitamins A, D, E, and K

Vitamin A: Growth failure, follicular hyperkeratosis, night blindness, xerophthalmia, keratomalacia

Vitamin D: Rickets, tetany, osteomalacia

Vitamin E: Unknown, macrocytic anemia

Vitamin K: Decreased plasma prothrombin activity with prolonged coagulation time and hemorrhages

Thiamine: Anorexia, beriberi, polyneuropathy, toxic amblyopia, heart disease, the ophthalmoplegia of Wernicke's syndrome

Riboflavin: Photophobia, corneal vascularization, angular stomatitis, glossitis, dermatitis

Niacin: Pellagra, dermatitis, glossitis, diarrhea, mental confusion and deterioration, encephalopathy

Pyridoxine: Anemia, convulsions (infants), polyneuropathy, seborrheic eczema

Pantothenic acid: Nutritional melalgia (burning feet syndrome)

Folic acid: Glossitis, archrestic anemia, megaloblastic anemis of infancy, megaloblastic anemia of pregnancy, nutritional macrocytic anemia, sprue

Vitamin B$_{12}$: Glossitis, macrocytic anemia, peripheral neuropathy, combined system disease (posterolateral column degeneration), mental changes and deterioration

Biotin: Seborrheic dermatitis

Choline, inositol, and carnitine: Unknown

Ascorbic acid: Scurvy, scorbutic gums, subperiosteal hemorrhages, petechial hemorrhages, anemia, impaired wound healing

Iron: Anemia, achlorhydria, glossitis

Iodine: Simple goiter

Fluorine: Dental caries

Calcium: Osteomalacia, a role in the production of senile osteoporosis has been suggested but not proven

Magnesium: Neuromuscular irritability, tetany

Potassium: Alkalosis, muscle weakness and paralysis, cardiac disturbances

Salt (NaCl): Anorexia, nausea, vomiting, lassitude, asthenia, muscle cramps, circulatory collapse

Water: Thirst, dehydration, oliguria, mental changes progressing to coma

*From Goodheart, R. S., and Wohl, M. G.: Manual of clinical nutrition, Philadelphia, Lea & Febiger, 1964.

sidered a pyridoxine deficiency. Essential fatty acid deficiency results in eczematic skin, particularly in infants. Ascorbic acid deficiency resulting in capillary fragility is the cause of perifollicular petechiae.

Oral cavity. Riboflavin deficiency is considered to be the cause of cheilosis or angular stomatitis, that is, cracks and fissures in the lips, particularly at the corners of the mouth. Often this is followed by redness, swelling, and ulceration of the lips. Riboflavin deficiency sometimes causes the tongue to have a magenta hue, which could also be caused by folic acid or vitamin B$_2$ deficiencies. A scarlet, raw appearance of the tongue with a loss of papillae is a sign of niacin deficiency. Bleeding gums are associated with ascorbic acid deficiency; and mottled teeth, with excessive intakes of fluorides. Dental caries may be a result of fluoride deficiency or faulty nutritional practices after tooth eruption.

Hair. Lack of luster, depigmentation, and decreased hair diameter are often the outcomes of protein deficiency.

Glands. Enlargement of the thyroid gland, goiter, is a manifestation of a lack of iodine availability to the thyroid cells.

Anthropometry

Anthropometry deals with the measurements of a part or whole of the body. Because nutrition is one of the determinants of growth and development, it is not surprising that over the decades researchers have attempted to establish this criterion as a measure of nutritional adequacy. Anthropometry is of particular interest in the nutritional assessment during the growing years. However, the nonspecificity of this method should be kept in mind in light of present findings that the ultimate growth and development of an individual is the result of a complex web of factors, such as genetic tendencies, maternal and childhood nutrition, infections and diseases influencing the growth process from the time of conception to maturity, and environmental factors.

The most commonly used parameters in anthropometry are height; weight; skinfold thicknesses; and the circumference of the arm, chest, and head.

HEIGHT AND WEIGHT

Data collection. Exact height and weight data depend on the accuracy of instruments used, as well as on correct techniques. Weighing machines are convenient. Regular checking and recalibration of the scales may be necessary. Lever balances are more reliable than spring balances. In practice, however, many modifications to accuracy need to be made, depending on the situation. Ideally, the nude weight of the individual should be considered, but this is often impractical. An indirect and practical method of determining the nude weight is to recommend that similar amounts of clothing be worn by the individual each time he is weighed. The deduction of this weight from the total weight would yield an estimate of the nude weight.

Standing height should be measured on a standard scale. The individual should stand erect, and a sliding headpiece may be helpful in judging accuracy. With infants, recumbent length is considered. Here again, innovative methods are often employed when measuring is carried out in developing countries.

Norms. Efforts to correlate height and weight in relation to age and sex with nutritional status have been met with limited success, mainly because of the norms used for comparison. If the standards for height and weight consider body builds without defining the builds—small, medium, or large frame —as was done in the 1959 Build and Blood Pressure Study by the Society of Actuaries, a great deal of subjectivity enters the evaluatory mechanism. On the other hand, if stature is not considered, too high a degree of homogeneity may be assumed, which would also contribute to errors in assessment. The lateral bony chest measurement by roentgenographic determination may be used as a stature reference, but the procedure is expensive and may not be practical in population studies.

The most commonly used standard height and weight tables for age 25 and over were published in 1960 (Tables 5-10 and 5-11). These were derived from the Build and Blood Pressure Study and give ideal or desirable weights in relation to heights for different statures (frames). The ranges of weight given in the tables are those that were associated with lowest mortality. It should be remembered that these tables are based on people who buy insurance and may not be a representative example of the population.

Smoothed average weights for adult men and women by age and height are given in Table 5-12. Published by the National Center for Health Statistics, U.S. Public Health Service, these data on height, weight, and selected body dimensions were collected in 1960-1962 and were based on a nationwide probability sample. They are, therefore, more representative of the adult civilian, noninstitutionalized population in the United States than are data from the Build and Blood Pressure Study, which represents an insured population.

Height and weight standards used for children are the Harvard growth charts and the Iowa growth charts, which mainly reflect the growth rate of middle-class white children. The more recent standards by Falkner (Table 5-13) include the fifth, fiftieth, and ninety-fifth percentile heights and weights for

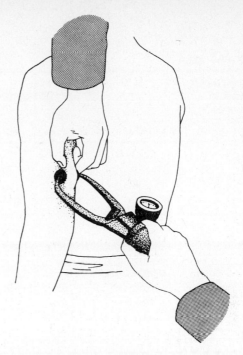

Fig. 5-3. Measuring triceps skinfold with calipers. From Guthrie, H. A.: Introductory nutrition, ed. 3, St. Louis, 1975, The C. V. Mosby Co.

white North American children from birth to 18 years. Falkner suggests that children falling outside the fifth and ninety-fifth range may have to be further assessed for nutritional imbalances.

Many factors, such as secular trends and healthier mothers with better nutrition giving birth to larger babies, have contributed to significant increases in average heights and weights of the present generation. In view of this, height and weight norms developed a decade or more ago would tend to become obsolete.

Again, growth charts developed for a specific population may or may not be applicable for another population. However, unavailability of reliable standards have often made these charts useful for practical purposes in nutritional surveys.

SKINFOLD THICKNESS

The rising incidence of obesity has necessitated the screening of obese individuals from those that are of above-average weight. Obesity is the excessive accumulation of fat in the adipose tissue as a result of caloric surplus in the system. Therefore, efforts are directed toward evolving methods to measure body fat. Fatness can be determined from such variables as body density, lean body mass, and soft tissue roentgenograms; but the most inexpensive and simple, and therefore practical, method of assessing body fat is to measure the skinfold thickness. Skinfold mea-

Table 5-10. Desirable weights for men 25 years of age and over*†

Height with shoes on (1-inch heels)		Small frame	Medium frame	Large frame
Feet	Inches			
5	2	112-120	118-129	126-141
5	3	115-123	121-133	129-144
5	4	118-126	124-126	132-148
5	5	121-129	127-139	135-152
5	6	124-133	130-143	138-156
5	7	128-137	134-147	142-161
5	8	132-141	138-152	147-166
5	9	136-145	142-156	151-170
5	10	140-150	146-160	155-174
5	11	144-154	150-165	159-179
6	0	148-158	154-170	164-184
6	1	152-162	158-175	168-189
6	2	156-167	162-180	173-194
6	3	160-171	167-185	178-199
6	4	164-175	172-190	182-204

*Courtesy Metropolitan Life Insurance Co.: How to control your weight, New York, 1960 supplement. Based on 1959 Build and Blood Pressure Study.
†Weight in pounds, according to frame (in indoor clothing).

Table 5-11. Desirable weights for women 25 years of age and over*†

Height with shoes on (2-inch heels)		Small frame	Medium frame	Large frame
Feet	Inches			
4	10	92-98	96-107	104-119
4	11	94-101	98-110	106-122
5	0	96-104	101-113	109-125
5	1	99-107	104-116	112-128
5	2	102-110	107-119	115-131
5	3	105-113	110-122	118-134
5	4	108-116	113-126	121-138
5	5	111-119	116-130	125-142
5	6	114-123	120-135	129-146
5	7	118-127	124-139	133-150
5	8	122-131	128-143	137-154
5	9	126-135	132-147	141-158
5	10	130-140	136-151	145-163
5	11	134-144	140-155	149-168
6	0	138-148	144-159	153-173

*Courtesy Metropolitan Life Insurance Co.: How to control your weight, New York, 1960 supplement. Based on 1959 Build and Blood Pressure Study.
†Weight in pounds, according to frame (in indoor clothing).

Table 5-12. Smoothed average weights for men and women (by age and height: United States 1960-1962)*

Height	Weight (in pounds)						
	18-24 years	25-34 years	35-44 years	45-54 years	55-64 years	65-74 years	75-79 years
Men							
62 inches	137	141	149	148	148	144	133
63 inches	140	145	152	152	151	148	138
64 inches	144	150	156	156	155	151	143
65 inches	147	154	160	160	158	154	148
66 inches	151	159	164	164	162	158	154
67 inches	154	163	168	168	166	161	159
68 inches	158	168	171	173	169	165	164
69 inches	161	172	175	177	173	168	169
70 inches	165	177	179	181	176	171	174
71 inches	168	181	182	185	180	175	179
72 inches	172	186	186	189	184	178	184
73 inches	175	190	190	193	187	182	189
74 inches	179	194	194	197	191	185	194
Women							
57 inches	116	112	131	129	138	132	125
58 inches	118	116	134	132	141	135	129
59 inches	120	120	136	136	144	138	132
60 inches	122	124	138	140	149	142	136
61 inches	125	128	140	143	150	145	139
62 inches	127	132	143	147	152	149	143
63 inches	129	136	145	150	155	152	146
64 inches	131	140	147	154	158	156	150
65 inches	134	144	149	158	161	159	153
66 inches	136	148	152	161	164	163	157
67 inches	138	152	154	165	167	166	160
68 inches	140	156	156	168	170	170	164

*Estimated values from regression equations of weights for specified age groups. (From Obesity and health; a source book for professional health personnel, U.S. Department of Health, Education, and Welfare, U.S. Public Health Service. Adapted from National Center for Health Statistics: Weight by height and age of adults, United States, 1960-1962, *Vital Health Statistics.* PHS Pub. No. 1000—Series 11, No. 14, May 1966.)

surements are indicative of subcutaneous fat and of the caloric status. However, this variable appears to be more useful in assessing normal and moderately fat people rather than really obese people.

Data collection. Calibrated calipers are used in measuring skinfold thickness. Langes calipers and Herpenden's calipers are examples. The calipers allow most of the assessors to obtain reasonably reliable numerical values, provided the inter- and intrapersonnel variabilities in measurement are overcome. Standardization with the instrument and with the assessor are needed. The skinfold is pinched up to the point where the sides are parallel. Care should be

Table 5-13. Height and weight of children 4 to 18 years of age*

Ages (years)	Height (inches) 5th P†	50th P	95th P	Weight (pounds) 5th P	50th P	95th P
Boys						
4	38.3	40.8	43.3	30.0	36.1	42.2
5	40.3	43.4	46.4	33.0	40.3	47.6
6	42.8	45.9	49.0	36.0	44.7	53.4
7	44.8	48.1	51.4	40.3	50.9	61.5
8	46.9	50.5	54.1	44.4	.57.4	70.4
9	48.8	52.8	56.8	48.0	64.4	80.4
10	50.6	54.9	59.2	51.4	71.4	91.4
11	51.9	56.4	60.9	53.3	78.9	102.5
12	53.5	58.6	63.7	60.0	86.0	113.5
13	55.2	61.3	67.4	65.3	98.6	131.9
14	57.5	64.1	70.7	75.5	111.8	148.1
15	61.0	66.9	72.8	88.0	124.3	160.6
16	63.8	68.9	74.0	97.8	133.8	169.8
17	65.2	69.8	74.4	106.5	139.8	174.0
18	65.9	70.2	74.5	110.3	144.8	179.3
Girls						
4	38.1	40.7	43.3	28.8	36.1	43.4
5	40.6	43.4	46.2	32.2	40.9	49.6
6	42.8	45.9	49.0	35.5	45.7	55.9
7	44.5	47.8	51.1	38.3	51.0	63.7
8	46.4	50.0	53.6	42.0	57.2	72.4
9	48.2	52.2	56.2	45.1	63.6	82.1
10	49.9	54.5	59.1	48.2	71.0	95.0
11	51.9	57.0	62.1	55.4	82.0	108.6
12	54.1	59.5	64.9	63.9	94.4	124.9
13	57.1	62.2	66.8	72.8	105.5	138.2
14	58.5	63.1	67.7	83.0	113.0	144.0
15	59.5	63.8	68.1	89.5	120.0	150.5
16	59.8	64.1	68.4	95.1	123.0	150.1
17	60.1	64.2	68.3	97.9	125.8	153.7
18	60.1	64.4	68.7	96.0	126.2	156.4

*From Falkner, F.: Some physical growth standards for white North American children, Pediatrics **29**:448, 1962.
†P, percentile.

Table 5-14. Percentiles for midarm circumference for whites of the Ten-State Nutrition Survey, 1968-1970*

Age group	Age midpoint, years	Triceps skinfold percentiles, mm 5th	15th	50th	85th	95th
Males						
0.0-0.4	0.3	4	5	8	12	15
0.5-1.4	1	5	7	9	13	15
1.5-2.4	2	5	7	10	13	14
2.5-3.4	3	6	7	9	12	14
3.5-4.4	4	5	6	9	12	14
4.5-5.4	5	5	6	8	12	16
5.5-6.4	6	5	6	8	11	15
6.5-7.4	7	4	6	8	11	14
7.5-8.4	8	5	6	8	12	17
8.5-9.4	9	5	6	9	14	19
9.5-10.4	10	5	6	10	16	22
10.5-11.4	11	6	7	10	17	25
11.5-12.4	12	5	7	11	19	26
12.5-13.4	13	5	6	10	18	25
13.5-14.4	14	5	6	10	17	22
14.5-15.4	15	4	6	9	19	26
15.5-16.4	16	4	5	9	20	27
16.5-17.4	17	4	5	8	14	20
17.5-24.4	21	4	5	10	18	25
24.5-34.4	30	4	6	11	21	28
34.5-44.4	40	4	6	12	22	28
Females						
0.0-0.4	0.3	4	5	8	12	13
0.5-1.4	1	6	7	9	12	15
1.5-2.4	2	6	7	10	13	15
2.5-3.4	3	6	7	10	12	14
3.5-4.4	4	5	7	10	12	14
4.5-5.4	5	6	7	10	13	16
5.5-6.4	6	6	7	10	12	15
6.5-7.4	7	6	7	10	13	17
7.5-8.4	8	6	7	10	15	19
8.5-9.4	9	6	7	11	17	24
9.5-10.4	10	6	8	12	19	24
10.5-11.4	11	7	8	12	20	29
11.5-12.4	12	6	9	13	20	25
12.5-13.4	13	7	9	14	23	30
13.5-14.4	14	8	10	15	22	28
14.5-15.4	15	8	11	16	24	30
15.5-16.4	16	8	10	15	23	27
16.5-17.4	17	9	12	16	26	31
17.5-24.4	21	9	12	17	25	31
24.5-34.4	30	9	12	19	29	36
34.5-44.4	40	10	14	22	32	39

*From Frisancho, A.: Triceps skinfold and upper arm muscle size norms for assessment of nutritional status, Am. J. Clin. Nutr. **27**: 1052, 1974.

taken not to touch the muscle or the bone. The thickness is then measured by means of standard calipers, using constant pressure. Selection of the site for measurement is critical, since not all the sites are practical or reliable as indicators of fatness. The lower thoracic site appears to be ideal but impractical. The most commonly selected sites are the deltoid triceps, the subscapular region, and the upper abdomen. Measurement of triceps skinfold (TSF) with Herpenden's calipers is shown in Fig. 5-3. According to some researchers, a single skinfold measurement of the triceps is useful in diagnosing obesity.

Norms. Normal values for this variable are presented in Table 5-14. These norms are derived for the American white population and are more applicable to this specific group. If used for other groups, discretion is indicated. However, these norms are invariably used for all groups because of the unavailability of any other standard.

MEASUREMENT OF CIRCUMFERENCES

HEAD. With the present concern, though controversial, over the relationship between nutrition and mental development, the need for methods to assess brain growth is being recognized. Measurement of head circumference is being utilized as a tool for this purpose.

This parameter is of importance in infancy because it is an indicator of brain development, most of which is complete in the first year of life. Head circumference is more satisfactory if taken with the infant lying on his back. The measuring tape is passed around the head. The largest circumference is measured by placing the tape anteriorly over the lower forehead just above the supraorbital ridges and by passing it posteriorly over the most prominent part of the occiput. Values ranging from 31 cm to 37 cm at birth have been considered normal. Lower values should be a matter of concern.

ARM. Midarm circumference (MAC) measurement is a useful criterion for the musculature and therefore in determining the extent of protein calorie malnutrition. A soft tape measure calibrated in centimeters is placed around the arm, usually the left arm at its midpoint. The tape should be firmly wrapped around without compressing the underlying muscle. Table 5-15 gives the standard values for this variable. For further discussion refer to Jellife (1966).

MIDARM MUSCLE. Midarm muscle circumference (MAMC) has been a more useful criteria to assess the somatic protein—muscle mass—status of an individual. This is of particular importance in assessing the protein calorie status of hospitalized patients because the muscle mass is reflective not only of the protein calorie status of the individual but also of the general exercise and increased usage of certain muscle groups (Jellife, 1966).

MAMC can be calculated from the formula:

$$C_2 = C_1 - \pi S$$

where C_2 = MAMC in cm
  C_1 = MAC in cm
  S = TSF in cm
  π = 3.143

C_1 and S can be measured as already discussed and C_2 calculated. Table 5-16 gives the standards for

Table 5-15. Percentiles for upper arm circumference for whites of the Ten-State Nutrition Survey, 1968-1970*

Age group	Age midpoint, years	No.	Arm circumference percentiles, mm				
			5th	15th	50th	85th	95th
Males							
0.0-0.4	0.3	41	113	120	134	147	153
0.5-1.4	1	140	128	137	152	168	175
1.5-2.4	2	177	141	147	157	170	180
2.5-3.4	3	210	144	150	161	175	182
3.5-4.4	4	208	143	150	165	180	190
4.5-5.4	5	262	146	155	169	185	199
5.5-6.4	6	264	151	159	172	188	198
6.5-7.4	7	309	154	162	176	194	212
7.5-8.4	8	301	161	168	185	205	233
8.5-9.4	9	287	165	174	190	217	262
9.5-10.4	10	315	170	180	200	228	255
10.5-11.4	11	294	177	186	208	240	276
11.5-12.4	12	294	184	194	216	253	291
12.5-13.4	13	266	186	198	230	270	297
13.5-14.4	14	207	198	211	243	279	321
14.5-15.4	15	179	202	220	253	302	320
15.5-16.4	16	166	217	232	262	300	335
16.5-17.4	17	142	230	238	275	306	326
17.5-24.4	21	545	250	264	292	330	354
24.5-34.4	30	679	260	280	310	344	366
34.5-44.4	40	616	259	280	312	345	371
Females							
0.0-0.4	0.3	46	107	118	127	145	150
0.5-1.4	1	172	125	134	146	162	170
1.5-2.4	2	172	136	143	155	171	180
2.5-3.4	3	163	137	145	157	169	176
3.5-4.4	4	215	145	150	162	176	184
4.5-5.4	5	233	149	155	169	185	195
5.5-6.4	6	259	148	158	170	187	202
6.5-7.4	7	273	153	162	178	199	216
7.5-8.4	8	270	158	166	183	207	231
8.5-9.4	9	284	166	175	192	222	255
9.5-10.4	10	276	170	181	203	236	263
10.5-11.4	11	268	173	186	210	251	280
11.5-12.4	12	267	185	196	220	256	275
12.5-13.4	13	229	186	204	230	270	294
13.5-14.4	14	184	201	214	240	284	306
14.5-15.4	15	197	205	216	245	281	310
15.5-16.4	16	187	211	224	249	286	322
16.5-17.4	17	142	207	224	250	291	328
17.5-24.4	21	836	215	233	260	297	329
24.5-34.4	30	1153	230	243	275	324	361
34.5-44.4	40	933	232	250	286	340	374

*Frisancho, A.: Triceps skinfold and upper arm muscle size norms for assessment of nutritional status, Am. J. Clin. Nutr. **27**:1052, 1974.

Table 5-16. Percentiles for midarm muscle circumference for whites of the Ten-State Nutrition Survey, 1968-1970*

Age group	Age midpoint, years	Midarm circumference percentiles, mm				
		5th	15th	50th	85th	95th
Males						
0.0-0.4	0.3	81	94	106	125	133
0.5-1.4	1	100	108	123	137	146
1.5-2.4	2	111	117	127	138	146
2.5-3.4	3	114	121	132	145	152
3.5-4.4	4	118	124	135	151	157
4.5-5.4	5	121	130	141	156	166
5.5-6.4	6	127	134	146	159	167
6.5-7.4	7	130	137	151	164	173
7.5-8.4	8	138	144	158	174	185
8.5-9.4	9	138	143	161	182	200
9.5-10.4	10	142	152	168	186	202
10.5-11.4	11	150	158	174	194	211
11.5-12.4	12	153	163	181	207	221
12.5-13.4	13	159	169	195	224	242
13.5-14.4	14	167	182	211	234	265
14.5-15.4	15	173	185	220	252	271
15.5-16.4	16	186	205	229	260	281
16.5-17.4	17	206	217	245	271	290
17.5-24.4	21	217	232	258	286	305
24.5-34.4	30	220	241	270	295	315
34.5-44.4	40	222	239	270	300	318
Females						
0.0-0.4	0.3	86	92	104	115	126
0.5-1.4	1	97	102	117	128	135
1.5-2.4	2	105	112	125	140	146
2.5-3.4	3	108	116	128	138	143
3.5-4.4	4	114	120	132	146	152
4.5-5.4	5	119	124	138	151	160
5.5-6.4	6	121	129	140	155	165
6.5-7.4	7	123	132	146	162	175
7.5-8.4	8	129	138	151	168	186
8.5-9.4	9	136	143	157	176	193
9.5-10.4	10	139	147	163	182	196
10.5-11.4	11	140	152	171	195	209
11.5-12.4	12	150	161	179	200	212
12.5-13.4	13	155	165	185	206	225
13.5-14.4	14	166	175	193	221	234
14.5-15.4	15	163	173	195	220	232
15.5-16.4	16	171	178	200	227	260
16.5-17.4	17	171	177	196	223	241
17.5-24.4	21	170	183	205	229	253
24.5-34.4	30	177	189	213	245	272
34.5-44.4	40	180	192	216	250	279

*From Frisancho, A.: Triceps skinfold and upper arm muscle size norms for assessment of nutritional status, Am. J. Clin. Nutr. **27:**1052, 1974.

adults for midarm muscle circumference measurement.

Invariably, anthropometrists have attempted to construct formulas based on various anthropometric measurements to provide an index of nutritional status. In some cases they have proved useful in the nutritional diagnosis; however, in others they have been less satisfactory. Therefore, height and weight are still the choice criteria in community assessment. Depending on the resources and enthusiasm of the assessor, other criteria could be included.

Biochemical appraisal

The biochemical method—or laboratory assessment, as it is sometimes called—measures levels of nutrients; their metabolites; and enzymes associated with or even compounds clearly related to the nutrient under consideration in blood or other body fluids, urine, or tissues such as liver and bone. Because tissue biopsies are hazardous and difficult techniques are involved, tissues are rarely used for analysis; rather, blood or urine is used.

Biochemical assessment is more objective than clinical and dietary methods. In addition, this method detects marginal or subclinical deficiencies before overt clinical lesions appear. It can also indicate metabolic alterations caused by a deficiency of the detected nutrient. Generally, two types of tests are used: (1) measurement of the circulating nutrient in blood or urine and (2) a functional test to evaluate biochemical functions that are dependent on an adequate supply of nutrients. Whereas the former aids in detecting the presence of the problem in earlier stages, the latter indicates the severity.

Specimen collection, handling, and storage are of critical importance, as is the standardization of various laboratory methods in order to overcome the interpersonal and interlaboratory variabilities. A detailed discussion of this can be found in the manual by the ICNND. Recent changes in the quantity and quality of the diet may result in variations in blood and urine composition. The composition of nutrients in blood and urine has also been noted to vary during the day. Therefore, blood samples are usually collected for analysis from a fasting subject.

Parameters. Although nutritional status cannot be completely assessed by the biochemical method, different parameters may be used to assess the status of specific nutrients. The parameter to be chosen for a specific nutrient depends on the physiological significance of the test and also on the facilities and resources available, including the cost. Some test methods are still in the experimental stages. Some are utilized only in research or in individual assessments.

Table 5-17. Assessment of nutritional status

Nutrient	Blood	Urine*	Others
Protein	Protein (P)†	Total nitrogen	
	Albumin (P)	Urea	
	Albumin (S)	Creatinine	Creatine-height index
	Transferrin (S)	Hydroxyproline	
	RBP (S)‡		
	Amino acids (P)		Nitrogen balance
	Lymphocyte counts		
Iron	Hemoglobin		Complete blood count (CBC);
	Hematocrit		size and color of cells
	Transferrin (S)		
	Iron (S)		
Vitamin A	Vitamin A (P)		
	Carotene (P)		
Vitamin C	Vitamin C (S)	Vitamin C	Vitamin C load test
	Vitamin C (WBC)		
Thiamine	Transketolase (E)	Thiamine	
Riboflavin	Glutathione reductase (E)	Riboflavin	
Niacin		N-methyl nicotinamide	
Vitamin B_6	GOT (E)§	Xanthurenic acid	Tryptophan load test
	GPT (E)§	Pyridoxine	
Folic acid	Folic acid (S)	FIGLU (formiminoglutamic acid)	
Vitamin B_{12}	Vitamin B_{12} (S)		CBC; size and color of cells
Iodine		Iodine	

*Urinary values are often considered per unit weight of creatinine excreted.
†P, plasma; S, serum; WBC, white blood cell; E, erythrocyte.
‡ Retinol binding protein.
§ Glutamic-oxalacetic transaminase; glutamic-pyruvic transaminase.

However, the parameter should be sensitive enough to assess the status of the particular nutrient. Table 5-17 describes some of the parameters used to assess the status of certain specific nutrients.

Biochemical parameters have also been used to identify and screen certain diseases. For instance, elevated levels of serum cholesterol and triglycerides have been implicated in heart disease. Efforts are being continued to evolve more sensitive parameters and newer and more accurate techniques. Hair biopsy sample analysis for certain trace minerals and protein status is being considered. Urinary hydroxyproline as an index for detecting protein-calorie malnutrition is another more recent parameter being used. However, the need for large numbers of parameters is being questioned. Whether fewer variables could be utilized for screening population groups is also being debated. Much more experimentation and study are necessary before a decision can be made.

Methods. The biochemical methods utilized vary in cost, reliability, and the degree of technical expertise. They are also constantly being revised and improved. Analytical techniques for evaluating constituents of blood have been adopted for use with very small samples. These microtechniques have enabled the determination of 15 to 20 biochemical constituents in as small a sample as 1 ml of blood. Microtechniques have not only added to the convenience of the individual being tested but have also facilitated the usage of more biochemical parameters in the nutritional assessment. The selection of a test and method and the interpretation of results depend on resources available and on the preference of the researcher.

Norms. Norms for biochemical parameters that are frequently used have been developed by the Interdepartmental Committee on Nutrition for National Defense (ICNND). These standards refer to the adult male only. Therefore, in the National Nutrition Survey, standards referring to all age groups are derived on the basis of research findings and the ICNND standards (Table 5-18).

The norms used are often criticized. The arbitrarily chosen cut-off points, indicative of some degree of risk (deficient, marginal, and acceptable), are a matter of controversy. This is not surprising in view of the fact that the specificity of laboratory evaluation of nutrients and the physiological significance of the tests used are still not conclusive.

Table 5-18. Criteria for evaluating some frequently used biochemical measures of nutritional status (levels indicative of a deficiency state)*

	Adult males	Children 2-5 years	Children 6-12 years
Blood data			
Hemoglobin (gm/dl)	<12	<10	<10
Hematocrit (% packed cell volume)	<37	<30	<30
Serum albumin (gm/dl)	<2.8	†	†
Serum ascorbic acid (mg/dl)	<0.1	<0.1	<0.1
Plasma vitamin A (μg/dl)	<10	<10	<10
Serum iron (μg/dl)	<60	<40	<50
Transferrin saturation (%)	<20	<20	<20
Serum folacin (mg/ml)	<2	<2	<2
Serum vitamin B_{12}	<100	<100	<100
Plasma vitamin E (mg/dl)	<0.2	<0.2	<0.2
Urinary data			
Thiamine (μg/g creatinine)	<27	<85	<70
Riboflavin (μg/g creatinine)	<27	<100	<85
Tryptophan load (100 mg/kg) (mg xanthurenic acid/24 hr)	>75	>75	>75

*From Guthrie, H. A.: Introductory nutrition, ed. 4, St. Louis, 1979, The C. V. Mosby Co. Modified from Christakis, G., editor: Nutritional assessment in health programs, Am. J. Public Health 63 Supplement, Nov. 1973.
†No values available.

Interpretation. Biochemical data indicate the deviation from the norm but not always the cause of the deviation. Further difficulty in interpretation is encountered when the body's homeostatic mechanisms, which could cause a nutrient deficiency, are considered. Only when the body's homeostatic mechanisms fail do deficiencies in specific nutrients become apparent.

Currently, immune response of the host is also being considered in assessing nutritional status. Cell-mediated immunity (CMI), as judged by a failure to develop cutaneous hypersensitivity to various allergens, is depressed in protein-calorie malnutrition. Lymphocyte counts are also reduced in this condition.

Conclusion

More positive correlation between biochemical parameters and dietary intake data have been found in nutrition surveys than between laboratory and clinical findings. This is not surprising in consideration of the nonspecific nature of clinical lesions and the development of biochemical variations before physical abnormalities are apparent.

This does not mean that the clinical method is not of importance or that one method of assessment is better than the other. The data from all the methods should be collected, integrated, and then interpreted to be assured of a reasonable degree of diagnostic accuracy and sensitivity.

Nutritional assessment is an expensive procedure. Presently, the need for large numbers of variables is being questioned. Christakis states that all the variables discussed before do not always have to be considered every time. The screening procedures could be determined by the levels of approach. In some cases, such as a well baby clinic, a minimal level of assessment inclusive of simple indices such as height, weight, hemoglobin level, and food habits may be sufficient. In some situations an "in-depth" approach may be necessary. For detailed discussion see Christakis.

Efforts are being made to reduce the number of tests necessary to identify nutritionally vulnerable individuals and groups without reducing the diagnostic potential. Statistical analysis (factor analysis) of the data collected on more than 25 variables in the Ten-State Survey indicated that perhaps as few as 8 to 10 of these parameters would provide as much information as that provided by all the variables together. For example in children, consumption of as few as two nutrients, calories and iron, seem to reflect that of all the nutrients. With this, time, effort, and money may be efficiently and effectively used.

An example of a simple data-gathering form for nutritional assessment follows.

Sample data-gathering form for nutritional assessment

GENERAL INFORMATION

Name: _____ Date of interview: _____

Address: _____ Interviewer: _____

Age: _____ Sex: _____ Marital status: _____

Occupation (type): _____

Educational attainment: _____

Primary diagnosis (if hospitalized) (include medical history): _____

_____

_____

Chronic conditions, if any (diabetes, PVK, etc.): _____

_____

Living arrangements: ☐ Family ☐ Alone ☐ Institution ☐ Other (specify): _____

Number in the household: _____

Ethnic background: _____

Religion (food restrictions, if any): _____

Economic conditions

   Amount of money spent on food: _____

   Participation in food programs: ☐ WIC ☐ Food stamps ☐ Other (specify): _____

Physical activity (specify type, duration, and frequency)

   Sleep _____ hours/day

   Feeding problems (if any) (chewing, swallowing, dependent feeding, others [specify]) _____

_____

   Food allergies/intolerances: _____

   Food preferences: _____

   Vitamin/mineral supplement (specify type and amount): _____

_____

24-HOUR FOOD INTAKE

(can be completed by the interviewer or interviewee)

Meal	Time	Foods consumed (specify type, additions, ingredients, recipes, etc.)
Breakfast		
Snack(s)		
Lunch		
Snack(s)		
Dinner		
Snack(s)		

Sample data-gathering form for nutritional assessment—cont'd

ANTHROPOMETRIC MEASUREMENTS

Height (cm) _____

Weight (kg) _____

Tricep skinfold (TSF) (mm) _____

Midarm circumference (MAC) (cm) _____

Midarm muscle circumference (MAMC) (cm) _____

LABORATORY DATA OF IMPORTANCE
(depends on the nutrients in which you are interested)

Hemoglobin _____g/ml

Hematocrit _____%

Serum albumin _____g/dl

Serum transfusion _____ g/dl

You can transfer these data from medical chart.

AFTER COLLECTION OF DATA

1. Assess the adequacy of diet using
   a. Basic-Four food guide
   b. RDA (after calculating the nutrient intake using food composition table):

   Caloric intake: _____ cals

   Protein intake: _____ g
   Other nutrients according to the nature of assessment.
2. Compare the anthropometric measurements to standards:
   Weight for height (% standard)
   MAC: Percentile rank
   MAMC: Percentile rank
3. Compare the laboratory values to appropriate norms:
   From the data gathered, identify the nutritional need(s) of the subject.
   To cross-check information, gather data on frequency of foods consumed. This list can be concise or detailed depending on the nature of assessment.

Food	Amount	Frequency of consumption		
		Daily	Weekly	Monthly
Milk group				
Meat group				
Fruit and vegetable group				
Bread and cereal group				
Other				

BIBLIOGRAPHY

Adams, C. F.: Nutritive value of American foods in common units, Agriculture Handbook No. 456, Washington, D.C., 1976, Agriculture Research Service, U.S. Department of Agriculture.

Arroyave, G.: Biochemical evaluation of nutritional status of man, Fed. Proc. **20:**39, 1960.

Beal, V. A.: The nutritional history in longitudinal research, Am. J. Diet Assoc. **51:**426, 1967.

Bollet, A. J., and Owens, S.: Evaluation and nutritional status of selected hospitalized patients, Am. J. Clin. Nutr. **26:**931, 1973.

Butterworth, G., and Blackburn, G.: Hospital malnutrition, Nutr. Today **10:**8, 1975.

Christakis, G. M., editor: Nutritional assessment in health programs, Am. J. Pub. Health (suppl.) **63:**1, 1973.

Food and Nutrition Board: Recommended dietary allowances, Revised 1980, Washington, D.C., 1980, National Academy of Sciences–National Research Council.

Frisancho, A.: Triceps skinfold and upper arm muscle size norms for assessment of nutritional status, Am. J. Clin. Nutr. **27:**1052, 1974.

Garn, S. M.: The applicability of North American growth standards in developing countries, Grad. Med. Assoc. J. **93:**914, 1965.

Grant, A.: Nutritional assessment guidelines. Available from A. Grant, Box 25057, Northgate Station, Seattle, Wa. 98125.

Gueney, M. J., and Jellife, D. B.: Arm anthropometry in nutritional assessment; monogram for rapid calculation of muscle circumference and cross sectional muscle and fat areas, Am. J. Clin. Nutr. **26:**912, 1973.

Guthrie, H. A., and Guthrie, G. M.: Factor analysis of nutritional status data from Ten-State Survey, Am. J. Clin. Nutr. **29:**1238, 1976.

Guthrie, H. A., Owens, G. M., and Guthrie, G. M.: Factor analysis of measures of nutritional status of preschool children, Am. J. Clin. Nutr. **26:**497, 1973.

Hillman, R. W.: Concordance among clinical signs suggestive of malnutrition, Am. J. Clin. Nutr. **20:**1118, 1967.

Hollingsworth, D.: Dietary determination of nutritional status, Fed. Proc. **20:**50, 1960.

Howells, G. R., Wharlon, B. A., and McCance, R. A.: Value of hydroxyproline indices in malnutrition, Lancet **1:**1082, 1967.

Interdepartmental Committee on Nutrition for National Defense (ICNND): Manual for nutrition surveys, Bethesday, Md., 1963, ICNND.

Jellife, D. B.: The assessment of the nutritional status of the community, WHO Monogr. Ser. 53, 1966.

Kelsey, J. L.: A compendium of nutritional status studies and dietary evaluation studies conducted in the United States, 1957-1967, J. Nutr. (suppl. 1, part II) **99:**123, 1969.

Klevay, L. M.: Hair as a biopsy material; assessment of zinc nutriture, Am. J. Clin. Nutr. **23:**284, 1970.

Krehl, W. A., and Hodges, R. E.: The interpretation of nutrition survey data, Am. J. Clin. Nutr. **17:**191, 1965.

Leevy, C. M., and others: Incidence and significance of hypovitaminemia in a randomly selected municipal hospital population, Am. J. Clin. Nutr. **19:**259, 1965.

Medical assessment of nutritional status; report of the Joint FAO/WHO Expert Committee, WHO Techn. Rep. Ser. 258, 1963.

Pearson, W. N.: Biochemical appraisal of the vitamin nutritional status in man, J.A.M.A. **180:**49, 1962.

Pekkarinen, M.: Methodology in the collection of food consumption data, World Rev. Nutr. Diet **12:**145, 1970.

Plough, I. C., and Bridforth, E. B.: Relations of clinical and dietary findings in nutritional surveys, Public Health Rep. **75:**699, 1960.

Selzer, C. C., Goldman, R. F., and Mayer, J.: The triceps skinfold as a predictive measure of body density and body fat in obese adolescent girls, Pediatrics **36:**212, 1965.

Standard, K. L., Lovell, H. G., and Garrow, J. S.: The validity of certain physical signs as indices of generalized malnutrition in young children, J. Trop. Pediatr. **11:**100, 1966.

Suaberlich, H. E., Dowdy, R. P., and Skala, J. H.: Laboratory tests for the assessment of nutritional status, CRC Crit. Rev. Clin. Lab. Sci. September, 1973, p. 215.

U.S. Department of Health, Education, and Welfare Ten-state nutritional survey, 1968-1970, vols. 1-5, Atlanta, Ga., Health Services and Mental Health Administration.

Wilson, C. S., and others: A review of methods used in nutrition surveys conducted by the Interdepartmental Committee on Nutrition for National Defense (ICNND), Am. J. Clin. Nutr. **15:**29, 1964.

6 Assessment of sleep-wakefulness patterns

BIOLOGICAL RHYTHMS

Normal human beings are characterized as organisms that adapt bodily functions in such a way as to have a different physiochemical and psychological makeup for each hour of the day. Yet each of these changes is carefully regulated for the given hour. This ability to maintain a relative internal constancy has been termed *homeostasis* or, more precisely, *homeokinesis*. Thus, healthy individuals represent the integration of a myriad of cyclical alterations of psychophysiological functions.

Since the cyclical nature of human function has been defined, a good deal of experimentation has been focused on determining whether one or more factors in the environment are the cause of the rhythms. Further work has been devoted to locating receptors in humans that sense these external factors and are responsible for the establishment of the rhythms.

Human beings adapt to environmental cues of an immediate nature as well as to external sequences or cycles of regularly changing conditions. Examples of regular external periodicities that are known to be incorporated into organisms' adaptive behavior are the tides, the light-dark cycle, the lunar cycle, and the seasons. This adaptive process involves the establishment of an endogenous rhythm that approximately corresponds to the environmental stimulus. These rhythms are known as the biological clocks that allow the organism to adjust to the changes occurring outside. Once the internal rhythm is established, the environmental cue that caused the change becomes a synchronizing stimulus and is called a *Zeitgeber* (Ger. *Zeit*, time; and *Geber*, giver).

Biological rhythms have been described for all levels of biological functions. It has been shown that cells may be influenced directly by gravity and electrostatic and magnetic fields. The nervous sytem seems important to the control of rhythms in higher organisms, particularly as related to photoperiodicity. At least one researcher has hypothesized different levels of rhythm organization: neural, endocrine, and cellular. In this system, the neural system is thought to be entrained by dominant synchronizers and the cellular elements by weaker synchronizers. In human beings it is necessary to include a fourth level, psychosocial organization, which may serve to modify rhythmical trends.

The influence most frequently observed in plants and animals is the day-night, or light-dark, cycle. Such circadian (L. *circa*, about; and *dies*, day) rhythms have been identified for all cells and functoons of the human body from enzyme levels to complex neural events. Because most human rhythms are 23 to 25 hours in length, they are termed circadian. However, although most human functions are entrained by a period approximating 24 hours, the peaks (high-function point) and troughs (low-function point) of daily rhythms for various functions can occur at different times; and although these functional records show phase relationships to each other, it is not known if all the rhythms for the various functions are entrained by *Zeitgeber* stimuli or by other rhythms internal to the person.

It has been hypothesized that functions such as the sleep-wakefulness cycle are weakly entrained whereas functions such as urinary output, body temperature, cortical secretion, enzyme production, and cellular division are more strongly incorporated. Data to support this hypothesis are those from experiments wherein subjects are placed in light- and soundproof enclosures for weeks to months. As many stimuli as possible are removed, and this is termed the free-running condition, which means that cyclical events occur in the absence of their respective *Zeitgeber*. The sleep-wakefulness cycle becomes desynchronized to 30 to 33 hours. The more deeply entrained cycles, the vegetative functions, retain a 25-

Table 6-1. Time of maximum amplitude of physiological rhythms in a person whose sleep cycle is 11 PM to 7 AM

	Peak of cycle*
Vital signs	
Temperature (rectal)	4-6 PM
Heart rate	4 PM
Respiratory rate	2-3 PM
Blood pressure	7-10 PM
Cardiac output	Midnight
Venous pressure	Midnight
Oxygen consumption	Midnight
Physical vigor	3-4 PM
Optical reaction time	3 AM
Grip strength	2-8 PM
Blood	
Sodium	4-5 PM
Calcium	9-10 PM
17-hydroxycorticosteroid	7-8 AM
Hematocrit	9-10 PM
Polymorphonuclear cells	12-1 PM
Lymphocytes and monocytes	11-3 AM
Urine	
Sodium	12-1 PM
Potassium	12-1 PM
Calcium	3-4 PM
Magnesium	1 AM
Dopamine	3 PM
Catecholamines	5-7 PM
Vanillylmandelic acid	5-7 PM
17-hydroxycorticosteroid	9-10 AM
Rate of excretion	8-9 AM
Mitosis-epidermal	11-12 PM
Body weight	6-7 PM

*The valley or low period for these values occurs approximately 12 hours later.

hour cycle. Thus, many endogenous cycles may be in new phase relationships.

The 24-hour temperature rhythm was defined soon after the development of the clinical thermometer in the 18th century. However, a refined experimental approach to the study of biological rhythms in human physiology had its origin in the 1920s when it was shown that rhythms occur even in metabolism. Table 6-1 reflects some of the data useful to the health care professional in this still relatively unknown field.

It has been shown that the sensitivity to many pharmacological agents, such as morphine and ethanol, to bacteria, and to carcinogens varies over the 24-hour period. Thus, the time the client takes a given medication may influence the effectiveness of the drug.

Some cycles appear to be significantly related to one another; for instance, the pulse rate and respiratory rate in the normal adult demonstrate a 4:1 ratio,

and any long-term deviation from this ratio may be the diagnostic feature of abnormal function.

Nocturnal diuresis has been given as an example of a phase change (180 degrees) in a biological rhythm; the change in time for this function was recognized as abnormal and given diagnostic significance long before circadian rhythms were well defined.

Periodic mood changes are described in both normal mental states and in emotional illnesses. Dramatic changes in affect occur in manic-depressive illness. One group has reported that some hormonal functions may free run whereas other rhythms adhere to the 24-hour cycle and has correlated depression with the times when hormonal functions are out of phase.

A good deal of work has been devoted to determining whether interference with circadian rhythms results in disorders in the affected individual. Two particularly fruitful areas for this study have been work situations requiring a change in the sleep-wakefulness pattern and rapid travel across time zones.

Industrial shift workers demonstrate changes in accuracy and accident proneness. Workers who change shifts give an indication of some imbalance in rhythms through a higher incidence of ulcers and nervousness. Temperature fluctuations in the individual who works at night are reduced in amplitude.

Translongitudinal passage or long-distance travel across time zones results in a derangement of rhythms, so that several days are required to adapt to local time. A 5-hour flight westward results in a readjustment period of 2 days for the sleep-wakefulness cycle, 5 days for body temperature, and 8 days for cortisol secretion.

The health professional is faced with the responsibility for establishing exact limits of normal values for human beings. Experimental data have allowed the establishment of separate sets of norms for men and women, accounting for individual differences in size, various age groups, and various levels of activity. More precise diagnosis will be possible when data are also available for all the body functions, particularly those that will allow the limits of normal to be established for changes that occur throughout the day, seasons, and year. The changing resistance of the body to disease phenomena must be defined, as well as the changing susceptibility to pharmaceutical agents. What is needed is a 24-hour tolerance test for the circadian range of values for each bodily parameter.

SLEEP-WAKEFULNESS PATTERNS

During sleep, the individual shows a greatly increased threshold for external stimuli. Thus, sleep is a normal, physiological condition that can be regarded as an altered state of consciousness from which the subject can be aroused by stimuli of sufficient magnitude. Although the precise function of sleep has not been made clear, most persons agree that the act of sleep is refreshing, that it is a time of physiological and psychosocial reintegration.

The primary care provider is the most appropriate person to evaluate the client with sleep problems. It has been shown that sleep disorders are related for the most part to situational stresses or crises, by medical pathophysiology, by psychosocial illness, by drug-related disorders (particularly withdrawal), and by the effects of the aging process. Furthermore, it has been recorded that one-fifth to one-third of clients who seek health care complain of a difficulty related to sleep and will want a prescription to help them obtain a sleep pattern they would consider more desirable. Clients may complain of disordered sleep as a primary problem or as a concomitant of another condition. Often the client complains that lack of sleep is making him so "nervous and irritable" that his job is in jeopardy and his friends are deserting him. Thus, the magnitude of sleep problems can be appreciated both in the numbers of individuals involved and in the degree to which a client may be incapacitated. The primary care practitioner must assess the client's sleep pattern in order to determine if a problem related to sleep exists.

Sleep habits vary markedly from one individual to another. However, any one person's sleep period may demonstrate consistency.

Factors identified as those that influence the length of time an individual will spend sleeping and the quality of that sleep are (1) anxiety related to the need to meet a task, such as finishing a paper or going to work; (2) the promise of pleasurable activity, such as starting a vacation; (3) the conditioned patterns of sleeping; (4) physiological makeup, such as the metabolic level; (5) age; and (6) physiological alteration, such as disease or alcoholism.

The affective response to sleep, that is, whether the individual feels he had a "good night's sleep," has been found to be dependent on the number of times he was awakened as well as on the total number of hours of sleep.

The practitioner needs to be aware of the unique rest and sleep needs of the individual client.

Sleep research

Sleep research has been systematically conducted for only the past 20 years. The reported findings of this research have shown the diagnostic value of having the client report his sleep-wakefulness pattern as part of the history. This data will indicate the need for further intervention. The electroencephalographic (EEG) tracings of subjects who are asleep have been analyzed by many researchers. Their findings have been correlated with physiological alterations that accompany various EEG sleep patterns as well as with affective phenomena reported by the subjects when they awaken naturally or are awakened by the observers. These studies have indicated that clients' complaints of inability to sleep well may have their basis in organic diseases.

Furthermore, observation for signs of sleep disturbance may yield valuable data for the ongoing assessment and management of the hospitalized client. It has been shown that sleep consists of cyclic patterns of physiological signs that recur periodically throughout the night.

The physiological measurements most valuable to defining the sleep pattern are (1) the recordings of electrical potential made from electrodes placed on the surface of the head (EEG), (2) the tracing made from sensors (electro-oculogram [EOG]) of ocular movement made from both eyes, and (3) the record derived from sensors for skeletal muscle tone (electromyogram [EMG]), these sensors are generally placed beneath the client's jaw.

The differentiation of sleep stages from the EEG tracing is based on alterations in the frequency and amplitude of the brain wave tracings recorded from subjects who are asleep (Fig. 6-1). Waves of 8 to 12 cycles per second (cps) are called alpha activity and are the typical waveforms of a person at rest. Sleep spindles are defined as waves of 12 to 16 cps, and those greater than 16 cps are called beta activity. Slower waves of 4 to 7 cps are called theta activity, and those of 1 to 3 cps are described as delta activity (see Table 6-2).

The normal adult has low-amplitude, fast-frequency activity in the waking state. Alpha activity is the most frequent type of activity recorded during what the subject believed was a period of rest.

Some authorities refer to the awake and resting states as stage zero of the sleep cycle. During sleep, five characteristic tracings can be isolated; these make up the stages of sleep called 1, 2, 3, 4, and rapid eye movement (REM). These five stages constitute the sleep cycle (see Table 6-3).

The sleep cycle

In the critical stage of falling asleep, alpha waves decrease in the EEG record. Sleep spindle waveforms appear within 1 to 2 minutes and herald the beginning of stage 2. As noted, these spindle forms occur at 12- to 16-second intervals, superimposed on a base of low-amplitude, fast-frequency activity. The duration of stage 2 sleep is 5 to 10 minutes, and its termination marks the end of light sleep. Stage 3 is identified on the EEG record as the appearance of delta activity. These slow waves make up

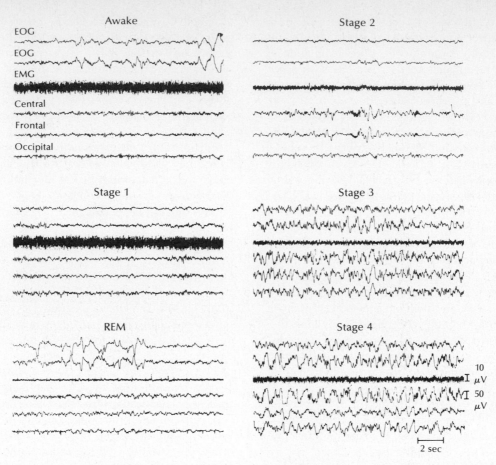

Fig. 6-1. Sleep stages. The same six channels are used throughout, as labeled in the *awake* record. EOG: eye movements; EMG: muscle tonus from beneath the chin. Note the high EMG and eye movements in the awake state, the absence of REMs in stage 1 (NREM), and REMs with decreased muscle tonus during REM sleep. Stages 2, 3, and 4 show progressive slowing of frequency and an increase in amplitude of the EEG. (From Kales, A.: Ann. Intern. Med. **68:**1078, 1968.)

20% to 50% of the EEG sleep record. This is the transition stage between light and deep sleep and may last about 10 minutes. As stage 4 sleep is entered, sleep spindles disappear and high-voltage slow waves occupy 50% or more of the EEG record. This stage lasts from 5 to 15 minutes.

During these four stages of sleep, eye movements are not observed and skeletal muscle tone is only slightly less in amplitude than during the waking state. Calling these four stages non-REM (NREM) allows for categorization of sleep into two categories: NREM and REM (see Table 6-3).

During a normal sleeping period, the client experiences stage 1 sleep followed by stages 2, 3, and 4 sleep. Then there is a reverse from stage 4 sleep to stages 3 and 2. After about 60 to 90 minutes of this pattern of sleep, the first period of REM sleep occurs. The EEG is characterized by lower voltage and by the absence of big, slow waves and sleep spindles. Gross eye movements can be seen and can be re-

Table 6-2. Differentiation of brain wave tracings

EEG pattern	CPS	Sleep-wakefulness cycle
Beta	>16 cps	Alert wakefulness, REM sleep
Sleep spindles	12-16 cps	Stage 2
Alpha	8-12 cps	Relaxed wakefulness; stage 1
Theta	4-7 cps	
Delta	1-3 cps	Stages 3 and 4

corded (EOG). The first REM period of sleep lasts approximately 10 minutes and is demonstrated by a lack of body movement. This period is thought to be the time that most dreaming occurs. The client may only recall the dream if awakened during the REM stage. Dreaming associated with REM sleep is not easily correlated with waking activities and is therefore less realistic. The remembered ideation occurring in NREM sleep seems more like the thinking that surrounds daily life activities.

Table 6-3. The initial sleep cycle*

Stages of sleep	EEG brainwaves	Time span	Approximate percentage of total night's sleep	Affective aspects	Physiological alterations
NREM sleep—slow-wave sleep					
Stage 1	Alpha activity	1-2 min	5%-10%	Fleeting thoughts; may be un- aware of being asleep	Light sleep, easily awakened; pulse rate decreased 10-30 beats per min; BMR decreased 10%-15%; temperature and respiration decreased; muscle tone mini- mal; knee jerks abolished; slight decrease in blood pressure
Stage 2	Sleep spindles	5-10 min	50%		
Stage 3	Delta activity appears	10 min	10%-20%		Transition sleep
Stage 4	Delta activity pre- dominates	5-15 min			Deep sleep; difficult to awaken
REM sleep	Desynchronized pattern of low- voltage beta ac- tivity—similar to waking EEG	10 min, first cycle; 10-12 min, sec- ond cycle; 20- 30 min as length of total sleep increases	20%-25%	Dreams believed to occur	Physiologically active; paradoxical muscle movements, that is, rapid eye movements; increase in cerebral blood flow, brain temperature, and body oxygen consumption (most skeletal muscle tone depressed; tendon reflexes depressed)

*The sleeper, on falling asleep, goes through stages 1 through 4 and then returns to stage 3 and then to stage 2, followed by a period of REM sleep. This pattern is considered a sleep cycle and usually takes 90 minutes (see Fig. 6-2). Further sleep involves stages 2, 3, and sometimes 4, returning to stage 3 and then to stage 2 with another slightly longer REM period.

At the end of the initial REM period, the sleeper returns to stages 2, 3, and sometimes 4, returning again to stage 3 and then to stage 2. This second period of NREM sleep lasts about 60 to 90 minutes. This is followed by another, slightly longer REM period (10 to 12 minutes). The transition from stage to stage is accompanied by body movement. A healthy adult probably experiences 30 to 40 turns during a night's sleep. The mobility of sleep pro- tects the sleeper from the hazards of remaining mo- tionless, that is, pressure changes in the microcircu- lation, thrombus formation, or diminished respira- tion, possibly leading to pneumonia.

As the sleep period continues, the length of the NREM sleep periods decrease and the REM periods increase. In addition, the depth of sleep, usually that of stages 2 and 3, decreases. Thus, the client achieves the greatest amount of stages 3 and 4 sleep early in the sleep period, whereas most of the REM sleep occurs in the later cycles of the sleep period (Fig. 6-1).

The total number of cycles in a normal sleep peri- od range from four to six, depending on the total length of the sleep period.

REM sleep. Phasic activity that occurs during REM sleep may be considered that of an arousal state generated by bursts of central nervous system (CNS) activity resulting in muscle twitches, eye move- ments, phasic changes in pupil size, and cardiopul- monary irregularities.

REM sleep has been described as a physiologically active period. The forebrain appears to be aroused. Animal studies have demonstrated that there is an increase in cerebral blood flow as well as in brain temperature. Lability of cardiopulmonary parame- ters is the rule with REM sleep. That is, there is a marked variation in heart and respiratory rate as well as in blood pressure.

Tonic inhibition of skeletal muscles occurs during REM sleep. The absence of EMG activity, particu- larly as recorded from the digastric or neck muscles, has been cited in support of the statement that there is generalized, skeletal motor inhibition. This large muscle paralysis has been conjectured to be a mecha- nism for preventing the dreamer from acting out his dreams. Tendon reflexes are also suppressed.

On the other hand, some muscles are not sup- pressed. These are the diaphragm, extraocular, middle ear, intercostal muscles, some facial muscles, and the muscles of the pharynx and larynx.

This stage is also referred to as paradoxical rhombencephalic, emergent, dream, or desynchronized sleep. Although data show that most REM sleep occurs during the last half of the sleep period, REM can occur during naps if the sleep period has sufficient duration. For the night sleeper, morning naps contain largely REM sleep, whereas afternoon naps are largely made up of stage 4 sleep. Several investigators have posited that REM sleep serves to reprogram the brain, particularly through the assimilation of new experiences into the existing personality structure. Some theorists contend that the function of REM sleep is to keep disturbing or threatening information from reaching the waking consciousness. Another theory is that the REM arousal periods are the mechanism for vigilance during the rest period that may have contributed to our distant ancestors' survival.

NREM, or slow-wave, sleep. An afternoon nap can be regarded as the beginning of NREM sleep, which represents 80% of the total sleeping time and is also called slow-wave sleep. NREM sleep is characterized by a decrease in tempo of the body's physiological processes. The basal metabolism rate (BMR) is decreased 10% to 15%, resulting in a decrease in body temperature of approximately 1° F. The pulse rate is decreased 10 to 30 beats, and the respiratory rate shows compensatory slowing. The blood pressure is slightly decreased. Muscle tone is minimal. Knee jerks are abolished. All of these characteristics represent an acute inhibitory process. Reflexes are weaker and slower to appear. The pupils of the eye are constricted in sleep and, with relaxation of the extraocular muscles, appear to "roll," that is, are not aligned. Growth hormone is known to be secreted in stage 4. Penile erection occurs in stage 4. The presence of erections during sleep rule out pathophysiological etiology from psychogenic causes of impotence.

Significance of the sleep stages in health assessment. The clinical significance of the presence or absence of the sleep stages in humans is still not clearly understood. Furthermore, it is difficult to make a judgment from the client's explanations of his sleep patterns whether he is more REM or NREM sleep deprived. Some investigators have reported, however, that loss of REM sleep is more likely to cause agitation and irritability, or in some persons, apathy and depression. Most clients report malaise or tiredness when the REM sleep period is shortened.

The EEG pattern may provide support to other data in differentiating such conditions as depression, narcolepsy, endocrine abnormality, or drug dependency.

Sleep patterns throughout the life cycle

Over the life cycle decrements are noted in the time spent in total sleep, in stage 4 sleep, and in REM sleep.

Sleep patterns in the young adult. The young, physically active and healthy adult spends 20% to 25% of sleep time in REM sleep, 50% in stage 2 sleep, and 5% to 10% in stage 1 sleep. The remaining 10% to 20% of sleep time is spent in a combination of stages 3 and 4 sleep (Fig. 6-2). Although most adults sleep 7 to 9 hours a day, many normal individuals sleep more than 9 hours, and another group of normal individuals sleep 6 hours or less in a 24-hour period. One study showed that the long sleepers had a high incidence of mild to moderate anxiety, depression, and social introversion, whereas the short sleepers were predominantly healthy, efficient, and energetic persons who tended to work hard or otherwise keep busy and who were satisfied with themselves and their lives.

Sleep patterns in the infant and child. The newborn

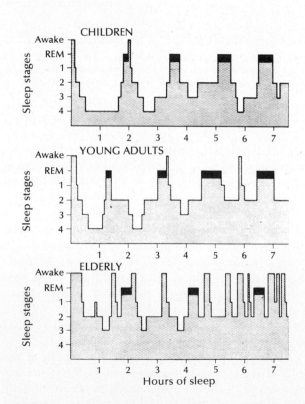

Fig. 6-2. Sleep cycles of normal subjects. The sleep of children and young adults shows early preponderance of stages 3 and 4, progressive lengthening of the first three REM periods, and infrequent awakenings. In elderly adults there is little or no stage 4 sleep, REM periods are fairly uniform in length, and awakenings are frequent and often lengthy. (From Kales, A.: Ann. Intern. Med. **68:**1078, 1968.)

infant spends 50% of his sleep time in REM sleep. By the age of 1 year, this is reduced to 20% to 30%, which is the adult value. Stage 4 sleep is greater in amount during childhood. Sleep cycles in the neonate are 45 to 60 minutes in length and increase as the individual approaches maturity. The total sleep time for the normal newborn may be 14 to 18 hours a day. The child develops normal sleep cycles between 2 and 5 years of age.

Sleep patterns in the aged. "Nap most of the day; can't sleep at night," is a frequent description of the sleep of the elderly client. Stage 4 sleep is markedly decreased and sometimes absent in the aged adult. The total sleeping time is diminished as a result of frequent and prolonged waking periods. This is distinguished from the early morning awakening depression.

Although REM sleep continues to occupy 20% to 25% of the total sleep time, REM latency at every period (the time from the onset of sleep to the first REM activity) is decreased, and the first REM period is longer. The EEG record may show poorly formed spindles that occur at a lower frequency. Insomniacs who are less than 50 years of age generally have difficulty in falling asleep; those over 50 complain of difficulty in staying asleep or in awakening early in the morning. It has been shown that these age-related sleep changes may begin at age 30 in men and age 50 in women.

The sleep-deprived elderly client shows deficits in stages 3 and 4 and REM activity. A question to elicit a description of sleep pattern changes relevant to the aging process might be "Is your sleep the same as it has always been?"

BEHAVIORS AND/OR DISORDERS RELATED TO SLEEP
Effects of sleep deprivation

The affective description associated with sleep loss includes tiredness or fatigue, the sensation of a tight band around the head, and eye problems such as burning or heaviness of the eyelids.

Neurological changes associated with sleep loss have included muscle tremor, particularly of the hands; skeletal muscle weakness, such as neck flexion; lack of coordination of motor movements; dysarthria and decreased facial expressive movement; and decreased attention span. Prolonged sleep deprivation has been accompanied by visual distortion; the individual may see halos around light sources or cobwebs on the floor. The sleep-deprived individual may appear apathetic. The individual functions more poorly during the time that he would normally be asleep. The poorest performance of the sleep-deprived individual occurs in monotonous and prolonged tasks.

Accurate assessment of functioning on short-term tasks is difficult because these individuals appear capable of concentrating effectively for short periods of time. The amount of sleep that an individual caring for a sleepless person gets may affect his coping strengths. Child abuse has been correlated to sleep loss of parents.

Sleep laboratory experiments have been conducted to determine the effects of sleep loss in human beings. The loss of 60 to 200 hours of sleep resulted in the following observations: feelings of fatigue, irritability, difficulty in concentrating, difficulty in maintaining orientation, illusions, hallucinations—particularly visual and tactile, decreased psychomotor ability, decreased incentive to work, mild nystagmus, tremor of hands, and increase in glucocorticoid and adrenergic hormone secretion.

Laboratory tests performed on sleep-deprived individuals show an increase in creatinine phosphokinase (CPK), glucose, and cortisol but a decrease in plasma iron and cholesterol.

The individual has an increased total sleep time following total sleep deprivation, with the increment reflected to stages 3 and 4. Although total REM sleep is increased in the first recovery night, the percentage of REM activity shows little actual change. The second night REM sleep is in greater proportion than that of the subject prior to the sleep loss; this is REM rebound. Animals that are selectively deprived of REM sleep for several nights are hyperactive and have excessive appetite for food and sexual activity. Animals selectively deprived of NREM sleep are less responsive than normal.

Most sleeping pills decrease REM sleep and, therefore, dreaming. Withdrawal of the medication is followed by an increase in REM sleep and dreaming.

Psychotropic drugs—or those that alter the function of the CNS—sedatives or tranquilizers, hypnotic antidepressants, and stimulants, have been observed to alter the course of sleep.

Night terrors and dream anxiety attacks

Two types of frightening dreams have been described as night terrors and dream anxiety attacks. Night terrors occur during slow-wave sleep and are accompanied by autonomic anxiety symptoms. Children who experience night terrors generally do not display daytime anxiety, whereas adults are likely to have anxiety symptoms. Dream anxiety attacks are the most common and are considered to be milder than night terrors. Autonomic anxiety signs may or may not accompany these episodes. Mental confusion frequently occurs, particularly if the sleeper is awakened suddenly.

Primary sleep disorders

Primary sleep disorders are those in which disordered sleep is the only symptom or sign of a problem. These disorders include sleeping periods in excess of less than what is considered a normal sleeping period. Insomnia is the general term for a shortened sleeping period. Hypersomnia and narcolepsy are examples of conditions wherein the client sleeps longer than the normal individual.

Insomnia. The term insomnia, which literally means a complete lack of sleep in common usage, includes the inability to fall asleep, frequent or prolonged awakening, or shortened sleep periods (early morning awakening).

EEG studies of insomniacs have shown the affected individuals to have varying sleep spindle production, longer sleep latencies, shorter sleep periods, and less efficient sleep. These individuals are believed to have greater levels of REM sleep than other persons.

GENERAL CAUSES OF INSOMNIA. Transient insomnia may occur with changes of shift at work or with travel across time zones. Insomnia often accompanies health problems, for example, pain, physical discomfort, fear, or depression. Poor sleep may accompany stressful periods such as the loss of a loved one or pressures from school or job. Environmental factors such as noise or cold can interrupt sleep. Drugs have been shown to be a cause of insomnia, for example, amphetamines, steroid preparations, central adrenergic blockers, and bronchodilating drugs. Insomnia may follow the withdrawal of short-acting benzodiazepine hypnotics. An excess of caffeine in coffee, tea, or colas may interfere with sleep. Insomnia is known to occur more commonly in those over 30 years of age than in younger individuals and is most likely to occur in females older than 50.

Individuals with insomnia have been shown to have higher levels of physiological arousal before and during the sleep period. The poor sleeper has more body movements during sleep. Both heart rate and temperature are increased prior to and during sleep.

Several subgroups of insomniacs have been cited based on the pattern of sleep loss. They are described as follows:

1. *Initial insomnia:* Inability to fall asleep, usually as a result of either rumination on situational stress, sleep phobia, or anxiety. Autonomic activity is higher during sleep in these persons as compared to the normal sleeper. The normal individual falls asleep in 10 to 15 minutes.

    The cause of sleep latency may be apparent from the history. Examples of questions that might reveal situational stress or anxiety as the cause of initial insomnia include: "How are

things going at work?" "Have you had a lot of worries lately?" or "How are you getting on with your wife?" Initial insomnia is the most common type of sleep loss in young adults.

2. *Maintenance or intermittent insomnia:* Disruption of sleep occurring during midcycle as a result of a startle reaction from internal or external stimuli. This is the most common type of insomnia.

3. *Terminal insomnia:* Early awakening; may be due to aging or may be an important sign of depression; could also mean the person is napping during the day or retiring early.

4. *Imaginary insomnia:* Subjective insomnia; the person appears to have slept but claims he has not.

Both the shift worker who has incurred a change in working hours and the traveler who has crossed a time zone have disrupted circadian rhythms and may suffer insomnia. They complain of daytime sleepiness, anxiety, and/or depression and have somatic symptoms and impaired psychomotor ability.

NOCTURNAL MYOCLONUS. Nocturnal myoclonus is a condition characterized by marked muscle contraction resulting in jerking of one or both legs. The jerking has a periodicity of approximately 28 seconds. When the contractions are pronounced, EEG arousal is noted and the client may be aroused to consciousness (1 out of 10 cases). Nocturnal myoclonus has been observed in 10% to 20% of chronic insomniacs. The client's sleeping partner may complain of being kicked at night.

RESTLESS LEGS SYNDROME. Restless legs syndrome is a problem incurred during the waking state; the affected individual is unable to keep his body, particularly the legs, at rest for the period of time necessary for falling asleep. The client complains of discomfort when the legs are immobile or when he lies down for more than 15 to 20 seconds. Paresthesias are also common. These symptoms may prevent the client from falling asleep.

Insomniacs often show an improved sleeping pattern following a judicious increase in activity and exercise during the waking period. However, activity just before bedtime has an excitatory effect in most instances. A thorough assessment of a client who reports insomnia includes a description of his activities of daily living. It is important, particularly, to determine the amount and vigorousness of exercise subscribed to by the client who has difficulty sleeping.

Some investigators have suggested that most insomniacs have problems in sexual adjustment or functioning. The client's description of sexual activity is therefore assessed.

Hypersomnia. Hypersomnia is the term used to

describe the condition wherein an individual has a tendency to sleep for excessive periods. In some clients the sleep period may be extended to 16 to 18 hours a day. The episodes of hypersomnia may be acute or chronic. The EEG sleep patterning is normal. Victims of hypersomnia are found to have higher pulse and respiratory rates than normal individuals during both sleep and wakefulness.

Perihypersomnia is a condition that is described as an increased need for sleep (18 to 20 hours a day) that lasts for only a few days, following which the client is fine.

Hypersomnia has been correlated with uremia, increased intracranial pressure, and diabetic acidosis. The hypothyroid client may report longer hours spent in sleep and sleepiness when awake.

In some cases hypersomnia may be a conversion symptom. The severely anxious client may be escaping discomfort in sleep. The hysterical personality and the depressed individual are predisposed to conversion symptoms. This mechanism should be looked for particularly when the need to sleep occurs repeatedly in conjunction with potentially troublesome experiences, such as "Whenever my mother-in-law comes for a visit."

Narcolepsy. Narcolepsy ("sleep attacks") is the term used to describe the uncontrolled onset of sleep. Although the pathophysiology of narcolepsy is not clearly understood, it is safe to say that the condition is a disorder in the sleep regulatory mechanism. The episode of sleep occurs when the client is engaged in what are considered to be work-time activities. Some 10% of diagnosed narcoleptics have described situations of falling asleep while driving and causing accidents. Others have fallen asleep in such unusual activities as standing at attention while in the military service or while eating. It is particularly important to be alert to the evidence that will establish the diagnosis so that treatment may be instituted, since the untreated narcoleptic is dangerous to himself and to others.

The episodes of involuntary sleep may begin just before puberty, that is, at approximately 12 years of age in girls and 14 years of age in boys. The range of age for the first attack may occur any time between 10 and 40, however. The familial involvement should be explored, since family members show an incidence of narcolepsy 20 times that of the general population.

Clinical records indicate that affected individuals may have the condition for as long as 15 years before it is diagnosed. This is particularly reprehensible since the attacks can be eliminated by amphetamines or methylphenidate (Ritalin) hydrochloride.

Because most normal people feel sleepy from time to time during the day, particularly at quiet times, such as during a dull lecture or television broad-

cast, a careful history is necessary to differentiate this dozing phenomenon from narcolepsy.

Automatism is sometimes reported by the narcoleptic victim's relatives. He appears to be awake but may act irrationally. The client does not remember the episode.

Diagnosed narcoleptics are observed to sleep fewer hours than their normal counterparts, and the sleep they do obtain is interrupted and restless. They fall asleep remarkably quickly, sometimes within 15 seconds after lying down, and complain of difficulty in waking up.

Narcolepsy has been described as a tetrad of four symptoms: sleep attacks, cataplexy, hypnagogic hallucinations, and sleep paralysis. The final two symptoms occur in the transition period between sleep and wakefulness and are only indicative of narcolepsy when accompanied by the preceding symptoms.

SLEEP ATTACKS. The uncontrolled sleep in the early stages of the disorder occurs infrequently and under conditions that are described by normal people as sleep inducing. The episodes increase in number and occur in increasingly bizarre circumstances. Eventually the episodes occur 3 to 5 times a day, lasting 5 to 15 minutes. Some of these victims fall asleep without warning, whereas others feel sleepy for minutes or hours before succumbing to sleep.

CATAPLEXY. Approximately 4 to 5 years after the disorder is initiated, cataplexy may be experienced by the client. Cataplexy is abrupt weakness or paralysis of voluntary muscles and is seen predominantly in the muscles of the arms, legs, and face. There are many gradations of the loss of voluntary skeletal contraction. The episode may be experienced as only a fleeting weakness or as the inability to move quickly. On the other hand, all the skeletal muscles may be paralyzed. The intraocular muscles are a frequent exception. The client may still be capable of perceiving his external environment. He may describe the attacks as "My knees buckled," "My jaws sagged," "I couldn't speak," "The muscles of my neck were twitching," or "I couldn't walk."

The cataplectic attack may last from a half second to 10 minutes, and the client may experience them only once or twice a year or as often as 100 times a day. The attacks appear to be triggered by strong emotion, loud noise, a startle reaction, or sudden fright. Hearty laughter has frequently been implicated as a stimulus to the episodes.

HYPNAGOGIC HALLUCINATIONS. These attacks may be described as dream episodes. They are generally disturbing or frightening dreams that occur as the client is falling asleep. The client describes the dream as very real—"As if I were right there"—and the feeling as one of being awake. This can occur in the normal individual.

SLEEP PARALYSIS. The phenomenon of sleep paralysis is a skeletal muscle paralysis of varying degrees that occurs when the client awakes or is falling asleep. The client describes the arousal as one of waking and being aware of external conditions but unable to move or speak. If undisturbed, the client recovers gradually. However, if he is stimulated, as by touching, paralysis ameliorates quickly. It must be borne in mind that sleep paralysis may occur in as many as 2% to 3% of the normal population.

RELATION TO REM SLEEP. Although narcolepsy has been linked to epilepsy in the past becuase of similar EEG patterning, it is not the same; nor can narcolepsy be logically attributed to depression or schizophrenia. More acceptable in the light of research findings is that narcolepsy is related to REM sleep. REM activity can be recorded during sleep attacks. The victim has a REM period at the beginning of his long sleep period. Some individuals with cataplexy experience REM sleep prior to recovery. Both hypnagogic hallucinations and sleep paralysis in normal individuals has been associated with REM activity.

Secondary sleep disorders

Secondary sleep disorders are those sleep disturbances that occur in individuals who have clinical disorders. Those clinical entities most often accompanied by sleep disorders are alterations in thyroid hormone secretion, chronic renal insufficiency, depression, schizophrenia, alcoholism, and anorexia nervosa.

Alterations in thyroid hormone secretion. Individuals with both hypo- and hypersecretion of the thyroid have derangements of stage 3 and 4 sleep. Individuals with hypothyroid conditions have decreased stages 3 and 4 sleep time while persons with hyperthyroid conditions show increases. Sleep patterns return to normal with adequate treatment to bring the client into the euthyroid range.

Chronic renal insufficiency. The client who undergoes dialysis treatments for chronic renal insufficiency has been observed to have sleep disturbances that occur with greatest frequency just before dialysis and are improved after the dialysis. Investigation has shown that sleep disturbances correlate with the uremic condition.

Depression. Depression is both a mental illness and a symptom. Depression is seen in the grieving process over significant loss or when things otherwise go badly. The depressed client has prolonged latency in achieving sleep, more rapid transition from stage to stage, more frequent awakening, less slow-wave sleep, less total sleep time, and more REM activity.

Depression as a mental illness is that which is incurred without significant loss. A subgroup of depressives is made up of those individuals who alternate between periods of depression and mania. The classical clinical description of the sleep pattern in depression is that of early morning awakening. Stage 4 sleep decreases in both manic and depressive clients. During the manic phase the client is observed to have decreased total sleep time and decreased REM activity. Depressed periods are associated with normal sleep time.

Schizophrenia. Some investigators have reported anorexia and a reduction in REM sleep in the early phases of schizophrenia. Stages 3 and 4 sleep are also significantly reduced in the schizophrenic. Greater eye movement has been reported in hallucinating schizophrenics than in nonhallucinating individuals.

Alcoholism. Studies have shown that the subject who has drunk 6 oz of 95% alcohol prior to sleep shows REM deprivation during his sleep period, whereas the person who drinks small amounts of alcohol may not show changes in his sleep pattern.

Table 6-4. Sleep disorders

Conditions associated with excessive daytime sleepiness	Conditions associated with chronic insomnia
Sleep apnea	Pain
Narcolepsy	Sleep apnea
Stimulant dependency	Restless legs syndrome
Shift change ⎫ Circadian	Nocturnal myoclonus
Change of ⎬ rhythm	Alpha sleep
time zone ⎭ disruption	Depression—nonpsychotic,
Secondary to:	i.e., loss of a loved one
Hypothyroidism	Exercise just before sleep
Brain tumor	Caffeine
	Coffee > 4 cups
	Tea
	Colas
	Secondary to:
	Aging
	Hyperthyroidism
	Anorexia nervosa
	Psychoses:
	Depression
	Manic-depressive illness
	Schizophrenia
	Change of ⎫ Circadian
	time zone ⎬ rhythm
	Shift change ⎭ disruption
	Pain
	Environmental discomfort
	Noise
	Cold
	Drug dependency and drug
	withdrawal
	Steroid administration
	Alcoholism

The client who drinks three to four drinks a day may feel tremulous in the morning and "need" a drink to calm down. Because alcohol is a CNS depressant, it may help the client get to sleep; but because it is a short-acting drug, it does not affect sleep maintenance. Furthermore, it may diminish REM sleep in the early hours of the sleep period and therefore contribute to a rebound increase of REM activity in the latter hours of sleep. Withdrawal studies of chronic alcoholics showed that sleep periods were made up almost entirely of REM sleep. These alcoholics frequently awakened from REM to experience hallucinations.

Both slow-wave and REM sleep appear to be decreased in acute alcoholic psychosis. Initially, slow-wave activity appears to increase, whereas REM sleep is suppressed. As the condition progresses both may disappear. As mentioned above, REM rebound has been employed as an explanation for the hallucinations that occur on withdrawal of alcohol. The rebound of slow-wave sleep has been cited as the harbinger of recovery from the psychosis.

Anorexia nervosa. The individual experiencing anorexia nervosa has a protein calorie deficiency that is accompanied by a patterned sleep disturbance. There is a reduction of the deeper sleep stages, 3 and 4, as well as of REM sleep. Although stage 1 sleep is increased, there is a reduction in total sleep time (see Table 6-4).

Parasomnias

Parasomnia is the term used for those patterns of waking behavior that appear during sleep. Some of those most common behaviors are somnambulism (sleepwalking), sleep talking, bruxism (teeth grinding), nocturnal erection, and enuresis (bedwetting).

Somnambulism. Sleepwalking and night terrors occur more often in children than in adults. Furthermore, boys are affected more frequently than girls. Both of these conditions occur during stages 3 and 4 sleep. The sleepwalker may not awaken during the episode if he is active less than 3 to 4 minutes but will show an awakening pattern if he stays up longer. The somnambulist is amnesic for the episode whether he wakens spontaneously or is aroused by someone else. During ambulation the sleeper functions at a low level of awareness and critical skill.

Sleep talking. Articulation during sleep appears to be a frequent occurrence. Talking during sleep generally occurs during NREM sleep and during body movement.

Nocturnal erections. Nocturnal erections occur during REM sleep and are said to occur at a frequency of approximately 80% in young men. While there is considerable variation in the frequency of penile erection in men in their 70s, with some individuals showing a marked decrement in REM sleep erection, many of these older men maintain the young adult frequency to age 80. The penile circumference during REM sleep erection is markedly decreased as frequency wans. Frequently the client who is impotent in the awake state can achieve an erection during sleep. However, the erection abates soon after awakening.

Although clients may report that the sleep they obtain following sexual intercourse is more relaxed and restful, no significant changes in EEG patterning have been noted.

Bruxism. The grinding of the teeth during the sleep period, called bruxism, may occur in as many as 15% of the population. Evidence of the practice may be seen in damaged teeth or supporting structures. EEG studies demonstrate that bruxism generally is seen during stage 2 sleep.

Enuresis. The problem of enuresis has long been considered a genitourinary problem, though pathology of this system is seldom found. Primary enuresis is bedwetting during sleep. It persists from birth to at least the age of 6. Secondary enuresis refers to bedwetting during sleep by an individual who has physiological control of micturition. This is primarily a disorder of childhood that is identified in 5% to 15% all preadolescent children, and it may have a familial pattern. Enuresis has been observed to exist in some sample adult groups at a rate of 1% or 2%.

Enuresis occurs more frequently in boys than in girls. Research has demonstrated more frequent bladder contractions and greater heart rate during the entire sleep period of those individuals affected, although the act of urination occurs in stage 2. The episode of bedwetting occurs during slow-wave sleep. Children with enuresis are generally described as deep sleepers, that is, difficult to rouse from sleep. Whereas primary enuresis may be the result of a pathophysiological defect, secondary enuresis may be reflected to psychological factors.

In assessing the enuretic child, one should explore the affective state surrounding this condition with both the child and his parents. Although data from sleep laboratories demonstrate that 90% of enuretic children are asleep when bedwetting occurs, in most cases studied the parents believed that the child had control over the occurrence. The parents punished the child, producing shame, embarrassment, guilt, or anxiety. To investigate how the episodes have been dealt with, the following questions might be used.

To the parents: "How have you felt about your child's wetting the bed?" If this question is nonproductive, more specific information might be gained by asking, "Do you feel he (she) could prevent the bedwetting?" or "Do you punish him (her) when he (she) wets the bed?"

To the child: "How do you feel when you wake up after wetting the bed?"

Sleep apnea. Sleep apnea is a periodic cessation of breathing that occurs during sleep. A cessation of diaphragmatic movement may occur. This is called central of diaphragmatic. Obstructive apnea is obstruction as a result of the relaxation of muscles of the nasopharynx, hypopharynx, and pharynx, which also occurs during sleep. Enlarged adenoids or tonsils predispose to this disorder. The bed partner may describe breathing of the affected individual as labored with long periods of apnea or as heavy snoring. The period of apnea leads to progressive hypercapnia, hypoxemia, increased pulmonary arterial pressures, sinus bradycardia, and other arrhythmias. This is known as upper-airway sleep apnea. A mixed form of apnea is both central and upper airway. Sleep apnea is thought to play a role in sudden infant death syndrome (SIDS). Serious arrhythmias are associated with sleep apnea. The syndrome occurs most frequently in people over 40 and predominantly in men.

Sleep-provoked disorders: sleep patterns in chronic illness

The sleep-provoked disorders include symptoms and signs of chronic clinical diseases that are elicited during sleep.

Pain. Clients who experience chronic pain may complain of "tossing and turning all night." These clients awaken frequently and stay awake for long periods of time. What has been shown through observation of individuals with angina pectoris is that they tend to underestimate their actual number of movements. Clients with angina experience pain during REM sleep. On awakening they may or may not report an upsetting dream. A direct cause-and-effect relationship has not been established.

Duodenal ulcer. Clients with duodenal ulcer often awaken in the night and complain of epigastric pain, which is relieved by food or antacid. It has been shown that these incidents are correlated with an increased secretion of gastric hydrochloric acid (3 to 20 times greater than normal), particularly related to REM sleep; normal subjects studied did not demonstrate this increase in secretion.

Cardiovascular symptoms. The pain of myocardial ischemia frequently accompanies REM sleep. Observations of patients with myocardial infarctions have shown that premature ventricular contractions (PVCs) are increased during or immediately following REM sleep. The horizontal position generally assumed during sleep results in an increased plasma volume as gravity effects on the fluid compartments are ob-

Table 6-5. Clinical observations associated with stages of sleep

Stage of sleep	Associated clinical condition
NREM sleep	
Stage 1	Myoclonic jerks
	Bruxism
Stage 2	Bruxism
	Enuresis most likely to occur
Stage 3	Night terrors
	Sleepwalking
	Sleep talking
	Hypothyroidism—metabolic rate most depressed
All stages	Enuresis
	Bronchial asthma—except stage 4 in childhood
REM sleep	Nocturnal erection or emission
	Migraine headaches
	Gastric acid secretion increased
	Duodenal ulcer—incidence of epigastric pain
	Coronary atherosclerosis
	ECG changes
	Anginal attacks
	Bronchial asthma in children

viated. The increased cardiac onput may lead to left ventricular failure, resulting in pulmonary edema and dyspnea. Because many of the manifestations of heart disease do occur during the sleep period, many clients express a fear of going to sleep. This is particularly true of the client with angina pectoris or cardiac arrhythmia.

Respiratory alterations. Clients with emphysema have increased carbon dioxide tension and decreased oxygen saturation during sleep.

Children with asthma have been shown to have a decreased amount of stage 4 sleep as compared to normal children. In children asthmatic attacks originate in the late part of the sleep period, when the child is not in stage 4 sleep. In adults they may occur in any sleep stage. There is a decrease in total sleep time as well as frequent awakenings.

Asthmatics frequently have bronchial spasm during REM sleep periods.

Metabolic disorders. Individuals with diabetes mellitus have been shown to have variable levels of blood glucose during the sleep period. Thus, diabetic individuals who are being regulated for the first time or who are out of control may need special surveillance during sleep.

Rheumatoid arthritis. Early morning stiffness is a frequent symptom of the victim of rheumatoid arthritis. Short periods of disuse lead to stiffness.

Table 6-6. Effects of pharmaceutical agents on the sleep cycle

Decrease time		Increase time		Allow normal time	
Drug	**Dosage**	**Drug**	**Dosage**	**Drug**	**Dosage**
REM sleep					
Placidyl	500 mg	Reserpine	1-2 mg	Chloral hydrate	0.5 g
Doriden	500 mg	LSD	30 μg		1.0 g
Seconal	100 mg				1.5 g
Phenobarbital	200 mg				
Nembutal	100 mg			Dalmane	15-30 mg
Quaalude	300 mg			Quaalude	150 mg
Benadryl	50 mg			Librium	50-100 mg
Scopolamine	0.006 mg/kg			Valium	5-10 mg
Morphine				Caffeine	
Heroin					
Alcohol	1 g/kg				
Tofranil	50 mg				
Elavil	50-75 mg				
Miltown	1,200 mg				
Amphetamine	15 mg				
Stage 4 sleep					
Doriden	500 mg	Antidepressants in the			
Nembutal	100 mg	presence of depression			
Valium	10 mg				
Librium	50 mg				
Reserpine	0.14 mg/kg				
Chloral hydrate	1.5 g				

Migraine headaches. Individuals with migraine headaches and with cluster headaches who suffered severe headache on awakening were monitored by EEG, which showed that the headache began during REM sleep.

ASSESSMENT OF SLEEP HABITS

In most cases it is more productive to allow the client to describe his sleep habits in his own words. An open-ended question may provide the stimulus to the client to give all the information pertinent to assessment. Examples of such questions are:

"How have you been sleeping?"
"Can you tell me about your sleeping habits?"
"Are you getting enough rest?"
"Tell me about your sleep problem."

An adequate history includes a general sleep history, a psychological history, and a drug history. The description obtained of the sleep problem should include the 24-hour pattern of sleep and wakefulness.

There are times when the practitioner will have to ask more specific questions to understand the client's sleep habits. The suggested questions (see upper right column and p. 87) may serve as a guide for this assessment. Only those questions need be used that will elicit the information not given by the more general query.

A technique that might more clearly define the sleep-activity cycle of the client is to provide him with a graph form on which to record his hours of sleep. He should be encouraged to keep a record over a long enough period that the pattern is well demonstrated on the graph.

He might be taught to color code his various activities in order to give the examiner as well as himself a clearer picture of his circadian rhythm. Even a simple written daily record of the sleep-activity cycle may prove helpful. At any rate, a diary of several days' sleep-activity cycles will allow the examiner a broader data base from which to advise the client.

The medication the client has been taking must be assessed. Cases of insomnia resulting from drug interaction have been recorded, and many drugs currently prescribed for induction of sleep may change the EEG activity pattern. Some of these changes are summarized in Table 6-6. The drugs listed in this table should be given particular attention in assessing the client's sleep pattern.

Aspects of sleep pattern	Questions to elicit sleep pattern
Time retired	"What time do you usually go to bed?"
Initial insomnia	"Do you fall asleep right away?" "How long does it take you to fall asleep?" "How often do you have trouble falling asleep? Does it occur every night? Every other night? Just the weekend? Every Monday?" "How do you feel before you fall asleep?"
Maintenance insomnia	"Do you wake up in the night? How often does this occur?" "What wakes you up once you have fallen asleep? Is there something that helps you get back to sleep?"
Arousal-terminal insomnia	"What time do you wake up? How often do you get up this early? What wakes you up at this early hour?" "What do you do once you wake up?"
Quality of sleep (affective response)	"How do you feel when you get up?" "Do you feel rested after a night's sleep?"
Naps	"Do you nap during the day?"
Dreams, night terrors	"Do you dream at night?" "Are your dreams ever frightening?" "Do your dreams ever wake you?" "How do you feel when you wake up from a bad dream?"
Bruxism	"Has anyone ever told you that you grind your teeth in your sleep?"
Somnambulism	"Has anyone ever told you that you walk in your sleep?" "Have you ever awakened in some place different than the one in which you went to sleep?" "Have you ever awakened to find furniture or other objects moved around in your home?"
Daytime activity work pattern	"What kind of work do you do?"
Shift change	"What hours do you work?"
Recreation, exercise	"What kind of activity is involved?" "What do you do for fun?" "Are you engaged in any exercise?"
Home responsibilities	"Do you work at home? What kind of work do you do at home?"
Sleep environment	
Bedding (mattress, pillows, blankets)	"Do you need any special bedding to help you sleep?" "How many pillows do you use?"
Light	"Do you sleep with the lights off?" "Does having a light on at night bother you?"
Noise	"Do you have to have it very quiet to sleep?" "Do noises keep you awake at night? Wake you up?"
Ventilation	"Do you open the window at night?"
Temperature	"Do you need the bedroom to be cold [warm] in order to sleep well?"

Aspects of sleep pattern	Questions to elicit sleep pattern
Special activities associated with sleep	
Bath, massage	"What do you do just before going to bed?"
Food	"Do you eat before you go to bed?" "Do you like to have a snack before bed?"
Drink (warm milk, water)	"Do you like a drink before going to bed?" "What do you prefer as your bedtime beverage?"
Medication	"Do you take any medicine to help you sleep?" "Are you taking any medicine at all?"
Personal beliefs about sleep	"How much sleep do you think you should have to stay healthy?" "What will happen if you don't get enough sleep?"
Internal stimuli	"How does the way you sleep affect your family?"
Psychiatric disorders (anxiety, depression, schizophrenia)	"How have your spirits been?" "Have you had a lot of worries lately?"
Alteration due to physical condition (stimulus, electrolyte imbalance)	"How have you been sleeping?"

BIBLIOGRAPHY

Aschoff, J.: Circadian systems in man and their implications, Hosp. Pract. 11:51, 1976.

Aschoff, J., and others: Reentrainment of circadian rhythms after phase-shifts of the zeitgeber, Chronobiologica 2:22, 1975.

Baker, R. M., and others: Lots of things you should know (and probably were never taught) about sleep, Patient Care 4:24, 1970.

Brown, C. C., and others: Sleep disorders; help for the patient who can't sleep, Patient Care 4:24, 1970.

Brown, F. A.: The "clocks" timing biological rhythms, Am. Sci. 60:756, 1972.

Bünning, E.: The physiological clock, London, 1973, The English Universities Press Ltd.

Conroy, R. T., and Mills, J. N.: Human circadian rhythms, London, 1970, J. and A. Churchill.

Folk, G. E.: Biological rhythms. In Folk, G. E., editor: Textbook of environmental physiology, Philadelphia, 1974, Lea & Febiger.

Frankel, B., Patten, B., and Gillin, C.: Restless legs syndrome, J.A.M.A. 230(9):1302, 1974.

Freemon, F. R.: Sleep research: a critical review, Springfield, Ill., 1972, Charles C Thomas, Publisher.

Guilleminault, C., Tilkian, A., and Dement, W. C.: The sleep apnea syndromes, Ann. Rev. Med. 27:465, 1976.

Hartmann, E. L.: The functions of sleep, New Haven, 1973, Yale University Press.

Kales, A., editor: Sleep physiology and pathology, Philadelphia, 1969, J. B. Lippincott Co.

Kales, A., and Kales, J.: Sleep disorders, N. Engl. J. Med. 290:487, 1974.

Kales, A., and others: Sleep and dreams; recent research on clinical aspects, Ann. Intern. Med. **68:**1078, 1968.

Kales, J. D.: Aging and sleep. In Goldmann, R., and Rockstein, M., editors: Physiology and pathology of human aging, New York, 1975, Academic Press, Inc.

Kales, J. D., and others: Resource for managing sleep disorders, J.A.M.A. **241:**2413, 1979.

Kiester, E., Jr.: I keep falling asleep; what's wrong with me? Today's Health **54:**40, 1976.

Luce, G. C.: Biological rhythms in psychiatry and medicine, U.S. Department of Health, Education, and Welfare, National Institute of Mental Health, Public Health Service Publ. No. 2088, 1970, U.S. Government Printing Office.

Rechtschaffen, A., and Kales, A.: A manual of standardized terminology, techniques and scoring for sleep stages in human subjects (National Institute of Health Publ. No. 204), Washington, D.C., 1968, U.S. Government Printing Office.

Soldatos, C. R., Kales, A., and Kales, J. D.: Management of insomnia, Ann. Rev. Med. **30:**301, 1979.

Sollberger, A.: Biological rhythm research, New York, 1965, Elsevier Publishing Co.

Usdin, G., editor: Sleep research and clinical practice, New York, 1973, Brunner/Mazel, Inc.

Webb, W.: Sleep; an experimental approach, New York, 1968, Macmillan Inc.

Wever, R.: Internal phase-angle differences in human circadian rhythms; causes for changes and problems of determinations, Int. J. Chronobiol. **1:**371, 1973.

Williams, R. L., Karacan, I., and Hursch, C. J.: Electroencephalography (EEG) of human sleep; clinical applications, New York, 1974, John Wiley & Sons, Inc.

Zarcone, V.: Narcolepsy, N. Engl. J. Med. **288:**1156, 1973.

7 General assessment, including vital signs

Having concluded the general remarks about health assessment and the discussion of methods of obtaining subjective data from the client, the examiner proceeds to those techniques that allow the *objective* measurements of health assessment—the physical examination. The recognition and localization of the pathological phenomena occur through the synergism of the client's and examiner's efforts. Symptoms can be elicited only in the interview. The client's description allows the examiner to look at the nature of the complaint from the vantage point of the client's perception. The examiner often gains valuable insights from the client's presentation as to whether pathology of tissue or function exists. Furthermore, indications of the client's cooperation, motivation, and objectives may be obtained. However, the observations of the examiner are essential to verification of the client's descriptions and the identification of signs of which the client was unaware. Furthermore, the tools of physical assessment allow exploration of facets unavailable to the client. It is from the synthesis of information from both of these data sets that conclusions about an individual's health may be drawn.

SURVEY OR GENERAL INSPECTION

The survey or general inspection begins with those observations made of the client as he enters the room, during introductions, and as he follows instructions for seating before the interview begins. It is the over-the *overall impression of the client's general state of health* and *outstanding characteristics*.

The general observations continue throughout the interview. In some cases this initial impression sets the focus of the interview and of the physical examination. For instance, some feature of the client's appearance may point immediately to his problem; sparse, fine hair, for example, may indicate the need to look further for the edema, the slow speech, the hoarse voice, and the sluggish movement of the hypothyroid individual.

There are certain characteristics that typically are noted in this section of the physical examination record: apparent age; sex; race; body type (constitution), stature, and symmetry; weight and nutritional status; posture and motor activity; mental status; speech; general skin condition; apparent state of health and signs of distress or disorder. These are factors that are not limited to a single system of the body but are instead parameters for the total or whole person—the general appearance, head to toe.

In general, the survey proceeds in a cephalocaudal direction. The examiner observes thoroughly and discerningly. Many professionals experience some difficulty in gazing at the client without doing some task simultaneously. However, total absorption in the process of looking and perceiving must be achieved.

The practitioner perceives only that to which he has prepared himself to attend. Therefore, a plan should be kept in mind for the stimuli that should be perceived, associated, and responded to by the practitioner. Although the term inspection implies restriction to the visual stimuli, the examination may include smell, hearing, and touch, as well.

An example of the record of the general survey might read:

Mr. A. is an alert, loquacious, asthenic 25-year-old white male who appears younger than his stated age and exhibits no indication of distress. He does not appear acutely or chronically ill.

Accurate observations can only be made in good light. This is particularly important in assessing skin color.

Although this initial survey may be considered a scanning procedure, the highlights gathered by the astute practitioner may be used as the basis for establishing the client's problem list.

The client as a whole

The general impression of wellness should be assessed. Historically, health and illness have been defined as opposites. For instance, the World Health Organization has defined health as "a state of complete physical, mental, and social well-being and not merely the absence of disease." By implication, any other condition is defined as illness. More recently, health and illness have been described in terms of a continuum. This conceptualization expresses the philosophy that the human being is never in a state of absolute wellness, or nonillness; that the person, in fact, varies from conditions of high-level wellness to markedly poor health, close to death. Illness is considered to exist when there is a disturbance or failure in either the biophysical or psychosocial function or development, so that observable (signs) of felt (symptoms) changes in the body are present. Mental or emotional illness is said to exist when the individual demonstrates inappropriate or inadequate behavior in a given social context. Essentially, wellness for an individual means that his health is such that he functions optimally.

Some terse but typical kinds of descriptions that have appeared as survey summaries are:

He appears acutely ill.
He appears chronically ill.
He appears frail.

The supporting documentation for these general terms makes the description more meaningful. For instance, the description of *chronically ill* might include terms such as *cachectic* or *dehydrated*, or other, more descriptive terms.

The practitioner should be aware of signs of distress in the patient. Detection of distress may predicate dealing with the underlying problem immediately and curtailing the full interview and physical examination for the present. Some of the signs that might require intervention are (1) anxiety that may be indicated by anxious or tense facies, fidgety movements, cold, moist palms, and an apparent inability to process questions normally; (2) pain that may be indicated by drawn features, moaning, writhing, or guarding of the painful part; or (3) cardiopulmonary distress that may be signaled by labored breathing, wheezing, or coughing. Since the color of the skin is determined by the amount of oxygen-carrying hemoglobin and by the constriction or dilatation of the capillary beds, cyanosis and pallor are excellent indications of cardiopulmonary distress.

OBSERVATION OF THE FACE

The attention of the examiner is generally drawn to the face first. The face is observed for symmetry, contour, and normal facial expression. Individuals suffering from Parkinson's syndrome tend to have motionless faces. Limited movement of the musculature leads to a paucity of facial expression. In addition, the blinking rate is slowed so that the client appears to stare. The facial changes that occur with acromegaly include a prominent supraorbital ridge, jutting jaw, and enlarged nose and lips. In myxedema (hypothyroidism) the features are flattened because of the swelling occasioned by fluid retention secondary to the accumulations of mucopolysaccharides. The face appears heavy and coarse. The individual with Bell's palsy has paralysis of muscles served by the facial nerve. He is unable to close the eye, the face appears flaccid, and the mouth droops on the affected side. (Also see the section on nonverbal communication in the interview.)

Body type and stature

A concise description of the client's bodily proportions should be included in the written record of the general survey.

NORMAL BODY TYPES

Although the constitution is to some degree genetically determined in the sense that endocrine control is inherited, the environment may play a significant role in altering the physiognomy. Descriptions of several normal body types (constitutions) by Draper, Dupertuis, and Caughey (1944) may help the examiner understand the variation of anatomy seen in groups of normal individuals.

Sthenic type. The sthenic constitution is one of average height, well-developed musculature, wide shoulders with a subcostal angle that is approximately a right angle, and a flat abdomen. The most frequently observed type of face is ovoid in shape, and the dental arch is round and wide.

Hypersthenic type. The hypersthenic body build is short and stocky and the most likely of the body types to be obese. The chest is shorter and broader than is the sthenic build. The costal margin is a wider angle (obtuse). The heart is likely to lie in a transverse position. The abdominal wall is thicker than in the sthenic constitution. Roentgenographic examination reveals the stomach to be higher in the abdomen and more or less in a transverse configuration. The face is more rectangular in shape, as is the dental arch.

Hyposthenic type. The hyposthenic body build is often characterized as tall and willowy. The musculature is poorly developed. The subcostal angle is more acute than in the sthenic type. The chest is long and flat, with the heart in a more midline and vertical position. Since abdominal muscles are not as well developed, the abdominal wall may sag outward. The stomach is observed to be lower in the abdomen and more vertical in position. The neck is long. The face is triangular in shape (narrower and more pointed), as is the dental arch.

Asthenic type. The asthenic body build is an exaggeration of the hyposthenic constitution.

An essential part of the assessment of children, or for that matter anyone who has not completed the growth cycle, is the accurate, serial measurement of height and weight. Growth charts (see Chapter 24) assembled from data gathered from large populations allow a comparison of the pattern of growth of an individual child with national standards. Children with inherited disorders of growth are known to deviate from the normal standards throughout most of the growth period; for example, children who have genetically determined tall stature grow at a normal rate and thus their growth curves are parallel to the normal curve but higher. An acquired alteration in growth would be deduced from a curve that followed the normal growth curve for some time and subsequently deviated. Chronic diseases of a nonendocrine nature known to cause short stature include diseases of the heart, lungs, kidneys, liver, gastrointestinal tract, bones and cartilage, blood-forming organs, and central nervous system. Lack of psychosocial stimulation may also lead to growth retardation (failure to thrive). Endocrine diseases known to cause inhibition of the growth processes are hypothyroidism, glucocorticoid excess, and growth hormone deficiency. Because it is possible to treat those individuals who have a growth hormone deficiency, it is necessary to differentiate this disorder from other growth patterns. Children who were known to have intrauterine growth retardation or who have a family history of less than normal height or a family pattern of delayed growth are generally not referred unless they are three standard deviations below the mean height for their age.

GROSS ABNORMALITIES IN BODY BUILD

Marfan's syndrome. Elongated arms and limbs as compared to the trunk may indicate hypogonadism or Marfan's syndrome, a genetic disorder.

Two rules of thumb that have been suggested in comparing body parts for appropriate development are (1) the distance from fingertip to fingertip of outstretched arms should equal the height; and (2) the distance from the crown to the pubic symphysis should roughly equal the distance from the pubic symphysis to the sole. Normally the ratio of the upper segment measurement to that of the lower segment is about 0.92 in whites and 0.85 in blacks.

In Marfan's syndrome, an inherited generalized disorder of connective tissue, the tubular bones are elongated and the ratio is lower. In addition, the arm span exceeds the height.

Hyposomatotropism. Dwarfism is the general term that has been used to mean an abnormally small person who has normal body proportions. Achondroplastic dwarfism refers to that individual who has abnormally small limbs but a normal-size trunk and head. This is the result of a disorder of cartilagenous growth.

PITUITARY HYPOSOMATIC DWARFISM. Pituitary dwarfism is the consequence of hyposecretion of growth hormone (GH). That deficiency in GH has little effect over fetal growth is evidenced by the relatively normal size at birth of babies who have no pituitary gland. However, the length at birth of the infant with hyposecretion of GH is less than that of the normal infant. The rate of growth declines in the first months of life and may be noticeable by the sixth month but more frequently is diagnosed between that age and around 3 years, at which time physical growth is half that of normal. However, because the epiphyseal closure is retarded, growth continues into the 40s and 50s, ending at the height of 4 or 5 feet. General health is maintained, and normal immune mechanisms are present. Mental development is usually normal for the chronological age. Males are affected twice as often as females. Many of the children appear obese, with adipose depositions over the iliac crest and lower abdomen. The eruption of secondary teeth is late. In adult life these dwarfs often develop wrinkles about the eyes and mouth and appear prematurely old.

LARON DWARFISM. Laron dwarfism is a genetically transmitted (mendelian recessive) form of dwarfism that occurs in Oriental, Jewish, and other Middle Eastern peoples. The condition is characterized by high levels of GH and low levels of somatomedin (SF), though metabolic response to exogenous GH hormones is subnormal.

AFRICAN PIGMY. The condition known as *African pigmy* is polygenically transmitted and is characterized by resistance to both GH and SF.

• • •

Growth failure can follow any serious illness or nutritional deficiency in childhood. Prolonged corticosteroid therapy has been associated with early epiphyseal closure and growth lag. Some of the diseases associated with growth failure are Laurence-Moon-Biedl syndrome, mongolism, achondroplasia, neurofibromatosis, severe congenital heart disease, congenital hemolytic anemia, and progeria.

FAILURE TO THRIVE. Growth failure occurs in some children who suffer parental neglect or deprivation of love and affection. These children are characterized by distortions of appetite-feeding patterns and by the eating of food not usually considered nourishing or edible (pica). Bloating may be present, and clinical symptoms like those of malabsorption may be present.

HYPOTHYROIDISM. Hypothyroidism, beginning in infancy, is called cretinism and is characterized by retarded bone maturation and multiple abnormal areas of epiphyseal ossification. Juvenile myxedema is also a cause of retarded growth.

GONADAL DYSFUNCTION. Gonadal dysplasia should be suspected in short girls with primary amenorrhea and congenital anomalies such as webbing of the neck, short metacarpal or metatarsal bones, or increased carrying angle of the elbows. (X chromosome defect may be noted on cytological examination.)

Hypersomatotropism. Hypersomatotropism is characterized by abnormally enhanced secretion of GH.

Tall stature may be genetic and may be a cause for concern in girls. Treatment with estrogen has been shown to accelerate epiphyseal closure. However, the long-term effects of estrogen therapy are not known and controversy surrounds the advisability of treatment with this hormone.

GIGANTISM. The hypersecretion of GH occurring before puberty and prior to the ossification of the epiphyseal plates causes overgrowth of the long bones and gigantism results. The length of time of long-bone growth is also lengthened, since the gonadal secretion is depressed. ACTH and/or TSH secretion may be deficient.

Excessive growth hormone in children is caused by an actively secreting pituitary tumor. Because the tumor may be treated by radiation or surgery these individuals are referred to specialists.

Cerebral gigantism (Soto's syndrome) is a growth disorder wherein the individual is abnormally tall at birth and continues to grow at a more rapid than normal rate until the second or third year, after which growth is normal. The disorder is not thought to be hormonally engendered and may be genetic. The affected children are generally mentally retarded.

ACROMEGALY. Acromegaly is a disease caused by hypersecretion of GH; it is evidenced clinically in the fourth or fifth decade. In most instances, growth of the acral (small) parts proceeds so slowly that their appreciation may not occur until the changes are well advanced. Bony and soft tissue growth is apparent clinically. Bony changes in the skull are most apparent. The mandible is increased in length and width. Prognathism or overbite of the lower incisors beyond the upper incisors by as much as a half inch is a characteristic of acromegaly. There is little increase in height since the epiphyseal plates have closed. The

teeth become separated as the jaw elongates. The features are exaggerated as a result of the expansion of the facial, molar, and frontal bones. The skull itself, as well as the sinuses, may be markedly enlarged. However, in some individuals only a single feature appears grossly enlarged, such as the jaw of the supraorbital ridge. Arthralgia and arthritis are commonly present in acromegaly.

With the increased total mass of connective tissue that occurs concomitantly with retention of interstitial fluid, the skin appears coarse and leathery and the pores and markings of the skin appear enlarged. In addition, the hands are large with broad fingers and wide palms, thereby earning the description "spade hand." The tongue is frequently enlarged and furrowed. The body hair is coarse and increased in amount. On physical examination both cardiomegaly and hepatomegaly may be found.

Symmetry

The arrangement of most structures of the human body is symmetrical; that is, there is a correspondence in size and shape of parts. Inspection that reveals obvious areas of lack of symmetry should be noted and investigated later.

Weight

The patient should be weighed and his height measured in order to compare these parameters to actuarial tables prepared by insurance companies of average weights and heights (refer to Tables 5-7 and 5-8).

Unexplained weight loss frequently accompanies acute and chronic disease and may be one of the early signs of illness. Weight loss may occur as a result of fever, infection, neoplastic disease, endocrine or metabolic disorders, drug intoxication, disorders of the mouth and pharynx, and psychiatric disorders.

Patterns of adiposity are described here in order that the typical fat deposits of obesity may be differentiated from those of disease states.

A sex difference is apparent in adipose deposition. Women are observed to have fat deposits over the shoulders, breasts, buttocks or lateral aspect of the thighs, and pubic symphysis. The fat deposits in men are more evenly dispersed throughout the body.

The fat deposition that is characteristic of Cushing's syndrome (hyperadrenalism) or administration of the glucocorticoid hormone is found in the facial, nuchal, truncal, and girdle areas. This kind of obesity has been termed centripetal "buffalo" obesity.

In addition to fat deposition patterns, there are other differences between simple obesity and Cushing's syndrome that may be helpful in establishing the diagnosis.

Obesity	Cushing's syndrome
Thick skin	Thin skin
Pale striae	Purplish striae
Absence of plethora	Plethora
Preservation of muscle strength	Protein wasting resulting in muscle weakness
No evidence of osteoporosis	Evidence of osteoporosis
Uniform distribution of fat—sex related	Redistribution of fat deposits
	Truncal obesity
	"Buffalo hump"—cervicodorsal fat
	"Moon facies"
	Thin extremities

Growth is arrested in Cushing's syndrome; therefore, the obese child who is growing rapidly probably does not have this disease.

It is well to remember that the increased serum levels of the glucocorticoids may be due to delayed metabolism of these hormones by the liver or to increased production of estrogen.

Apparent age

There is great disparity in the apparent age of individuals at the same chronological age. These differences arise as a result of such influences as heredity, sex, past medical history, and life experiences.

Physical changes that have been associated with the aging process are elevations in blood pressure, decreased cardiac output and stroke volume, as well as lessened pulmonary reserve. However, those changes, like the "aches and pains" of old age, may be preventable or at least treatable with judicious exercise and hormone replacement. The kyphosis in women that once indicated the presence of osteoporosis may be prevented with postmenopausal hormones and calcium balancing through diet and medication.

There are some indications that may help the practitioner in estimating the apparent age. Elastic fibers in the corium of the skin decline in number with advancing age. As the individual advances in age, the skin loses turgor, that is, its ability to return to its normal contour when released after being picked up between the examiner's fingers. The skin appears dull, moves less readily, sags, and wrinkles. These changes are noticeable in middle age and are first observable in the anterior neck and chin.

Hair begins to decline in amount in the middle years as the sex hormones decrease in amount.

Progeria is the term for premature senility occurring in childhood. The stature is small; the face looks old and wizened; the skin is dry and thin, and the hair is scanty; sexual organs are infantile.

Precocious puberty is the term for premature maturation of the gonads accompanied by secondary sexual characteristics.

Posture

"Harmonious movement leads to harmonious thought" (Plato). Posture is a part of body image. It is customary to correlate good body alignment with good health. Good posture is dependent on a normal sense of balance—muscular coordination as well as conditioned learning. Appropriate posture in any circumstance is that which requires the least investment of energy.

Minimal muscular effort is required to maintain an upright posture when the line of the center of gravity bisects the principal weight-bearing joints and is the same distance from each foot. Upright posture requires the contraction of the antigravity muscles. Specifically, these muscles are erector spinae, gluteals, quadriceps, and calf muscles. Other muscles contributing to upright posture are the abdominal muscles.

PROPRIOCEPTION AND POSTURE

Eye muscles. The extraocular muscles of the eye and the vestibular function are integrated to maintain the upright individual's eyes in a horizontal plane and to maintain fixation of the eye on the selected object. Eye muscles play a role in proprioception, whereas the exteroceptive impulses are received via the retina. It is important to note that a normal person can balance in the dark when all other neural functions are adequate.

Vestibular organs. Disorders of the vestibular system are known to lead to loss of balance. However, an individual can learn to balance even when all vestibular function is lost. An individual with no vestibular function cannot adjust to rapid postural adjustments or maintain eye fixation in a moving vehicle.

Muscle, tendon, and joints. Proprioceptive impulses from the muscles, tendons, and joints provide information about the body's position in space and are major influences in the maintenance of posture. These impulses are integrated in the midbrain and cerebellum.

EXTEROCEPTION AND POSTURE

Stimulation of the retina of the eye results in the head turning and fixation of the eye.

POSTURE OF THE ELDERLY

Bone and joint changes contribute to the bent posture that has been ascribed to the elderly in the literature of all eras. Joint degeneration and osteoporosis occur with aging. The intervertebral discs decrease in height and osteoporotic changes are noted, particularly in the vertebrae. Thus, changes are correlated with the waning of estrogens levels in the female and testosterone in the male. As a result of these changes any given individual may be as much as an inch shorter than his usual adult height.

While it is generally observed that all muscles decline in girth and strength with aging, the muscles of the trunk are particularly affected. Thus, weakness of the abdominal muscles contributes to the slumped posture.

There is some correlative evidence that appropriate exercise may aid the person to maintain erect posture. The Chinese shadow boxing exercises are purported to maintain body awareness and posture in spite of advancing years. Abnormal posture is most likely to result from pathology of the muscles, bones, joints, or neurological system.

Poor posture maintained over a long period of time results in painful joints, ligaments, and muscles. Occupations requiring positions that deviate from normal alignment may result in chronic pain or deformity, for example, bent shoulders in mine workers and painful shoulders in sewing machine operators.

Frequent changes of posture are necessary to comfort.

Bent or disordered body alignment may lead to changes of the surrounding soft tissue. An example of this is the changes in long volume and ventilation as well as in circulation that occurs with scoliosis.

Certain pathological conditions are characterized by specific postures, for example, the deviation of the spine toward the affected side in sciatica and the maintenance of a position that elevates the clavicles, such as leaning forward on extended arms, by the client with chronic obstructive lung disease.

The practitioner should develop a protocol for accurately observing the main postures of the body in all its common acts. Beginning observations are made by watching the client come into the room and seat himself and by observing the client while he is lying on the examining table. It is important to note whether the client sits tensely or slumps in the chair. Rigid positioning of the neck may be the result of a fixated spine. Respiratory distress may result when the patient tries to lie flat. Hyperextension of the

Table 7-1. Diagnostic patterns of gait

Form	Description	Associated disorders
Spastic	Leg held stiffly—does not flex freely; jerking movements; poorly coordinated; short steps dragging all of foot over floor	Multiple sclerosis, syringomyelia, cerebral spastic diplegia
Scissors	Spasticity of adductor muscles of legs with legs held close together; feet further separated	Spastic paraplegia; paresis; cerebral palsy (choreoathetosis)
Atactic (cerebellar gait)	Staggering, reeling; steps uncertain; some shorter or longer than intended; may lurch to one side	Acute disease of cerebellum, cerebellar tracts of brain; severe alcohol and barbituate intoxication
Sensory atactic	Uncertainty, irregularity, and stamping of feet Depends on vision for clues	Interruption of afferent fibers for proprioception—takes dorsalis Pernicious anemia
Slapping (steppage); weak muscles of dorsiflexion (foot-drop)	Walks on broad base with feet wide apart; raises foot abnormally high (steppage)—slapping noises as foot strikes floor; eyes on floor to observe where to place foot	Peripheral nerve disease; paralysis of pretibial and peroneal muscles; posterior column disease; tertiary syphilis
Foot dragging (hemiplegic gait)	Affected foot dragged in semicircle with toes outward; arms on affected side held rigidly against chest wall	Hemiplegia and paraplegia
Festinating (parkinsonian gait)	Body rigid, trunk bend forward—flexion; short, mincing steps barely clear ground—shuffling; arms carried ahead of body in abduction; wrists extended, fingers flexed at metacarpal joints—do not swing; may make sudden hastening forward movement (propulsion) or backward movement (retropulsion)	Parkinsonism
Waddling or rolling (dystrophic gait)	Proximal muscle weakness Steps regular, but uncertain; often lumbar lordosis; exaggerated elevation of one hip, depression of other	Muscular dystrophy

neck and muscular rigidity may indicate meningitis. Leaning to one side may be a response to a fractured rib. Carcinoma of the tail of the pancreas may result in complaints of pain over the lower thoracic spine when the client is asked to lie flat.

GAIT

The characteristics of the client's walk often provide clues to the pathophysiology involved in the client's problems. The client with a disorder in gait should be observed for his natural stance and for the attitude and dominant positions of the trunk, legs, and arms. The patient may be asked to walk a straight line. The rapidity or slowness of step may be noteworthy, as well as the style of movement. Table 7-1 presents various types of gait that are readily recognized.

Normal gait. The phases of normal gait are stance and swing. The components of stance are described in reference to the pressure exerted by the part of the foot contacting the surface beneath it: (1) heel strike, (2) full foot, (3) midstance of the foot, and (4) metatarsal pushoff.

The normal heel strike is quiet and smoothly coordinated. The knee is in extension during the heel strike. The movement to full contact of the foot with the floor should be complete and proceed smoothly. The midstance of the foot is the shift of weight onto the foot. The weight should be supported evenly by all aspects of the foot. The hip will be displaced 2 to 5 cm over the weight-bearing foot. The knee is slightly flexed during weight bearing. During metatarsal pushoff, a smoothly coordinated lift off the floor is observed. The metatarsal joint is extended. In the swing phase following the contact of the foot with the floor, three components are acceleration, midswing, and deceleration. The acceleration component is the contraction of the quadriceps muscle to initiate extension of the leg and forward swing of the leg. Knee flexion results in elevation of the foot, which is accompanied by dorsiflexion of the foot to allow ground clearance. The foot remains in dorsiflexion in midswing. Deceleration involves a contraction of the hamstring muscles to inhibit forward swing of the leg in preparation for the subsequent heel strike.

Symmetry of arm swing. In normal gait the shoulders rotate 180 degrees out of phase with the pelvis. This is seen as an equal and symmetrical arm swing.

Body movements

Bodily movements are observed for lack of coordination and tremor occurring at rest or stimulated by voluntary movement. The amplitude of tremor or involuntary movement may be fine or coarse and may be confined to a single muscle or be generalized to the entire body. Examples of generalized involvement of skeletal muscles in involuntary contraction include the convulsive movements of epilepsy and the choreiform movements of Huntington's chorea. Asymmetry of body movement frequently occurs with damage to the central nervous system or with peripheral nerve damage.

Hair and hair growth patterns

Inspection for hair growth is made on the following body regions: scalp, beard, mustache, ears, hypogastric area, thoracic area, lower limbs, genital area, lumbosacral area, upper back, midphalangeal area, pubis, and axillae.

The hair is assessed for growth characteristics, distribution, density of growth, appearance, and hygiene.

In the present evolutionary state of *Homo sapiens*, hair growth patterns have a great deal of social value. Whereas in lower animals the skin covering of hair may afford warmth and protection of exposed body parts from friction during motion, in human beings hair serves a decorative function.

Hair growth is influenced by hereditary and racial factors. Excessive hairiness is thought to be a dominant hereditary trait in the presence of androgens, whereas thinning or absence of hair is a recessive trait.

Although hair growth is continuous in some animals, in most animals, including humans, hair growth is cyclic. Hair growth occurs in what is known as an anagen phase; it then enters a telogen, or resting, phase before it is pushed out and new hair grows in the follicle.

The anagen phase may continue for years in areas such as the scalp. This long phase of growth contributes to longer hairs. Pubic hair, on the other hand, grows for only a few months.

Hair growth can be described in terms of cycle, rate of growth, size, and density.

Hair grows at various rates. The most rapid rate of growth is that of the beard, followed by that of the scalp, axillae, thighs, and eyebrows. Long hairs regenerate most rapidly. In the male, more rapid regrowth is noted in scalp hair than for the female, but regrowth is slower in the axillae and on the thighs.

The rate of hair growth is affected by environmental temperature as well as by the general state of health. Extremely cold temperatures such as those experienced in the Antarctic impede hair growth, whereas hot climates appear to promote increased length.

General protein production is inhibited in starvation, and this is reflected in reduced hair growth and dullness in appearance. Chemotherapeutic drugs inhibit cell division and thereby inhibit hair growth. X-ray radiation causes hair to switch to the telogen phase as well as atrophy of perifollicular structures, resulting in hair loss.

White persons have more abundant and coarser bodily hair growth than do Asians. Facial hirsutism has been described for more than 40% of white women. Japanese women, on the other hand, do not develop excessive facial hair growth; and Japanese men have sparser beards than do white men. Blacks have kinky hair, whereas whites have straight or wavy to curly hair, and Mongolians and American Indians have straight hair.

A heavier distribution of hair is correlated with darker skin pigmentation; that is, the brunette individual is more likely to have more hair than the blonde person.

Some male hair growth characteristics may be normal for women of certain ethnic or familial groups, for instance, hair growth on the upper lip; sideburns; and hair growth on the intermammary periareolar area, abdomen, and lower limbs.

Because of the variations in hair growth patterns among individuals, it is more important to note marked changes in hair growth characteristics. Hair growth increases in normal sites have been associated with adrenal tumors.

Hair has been classified into three categories: primary, secondary, and terminal hair. Primary hair is the very fine, thinly pigmented short hair of the fetus. Secondary hair resembles primary hair structurally but appears postnatally. This secondary hair is generally distributed over the body and is the hair type involved in hypertrichosis. This hair is often termed lanuginous or vellus and is not hormonally influenced. Terminal hair is a coarser and more heavily pigmented growth that appears at the time of puberty. Axillary and pubic terminal hair is called ambosexual hair. Adrenal hormones initiate the growth of this coarse hair, which is also influenced by ovarian and testicular hormones. True sexual hair is that which grows on the face, chest, abdomen, back, and extremities.

The hair may also be classified by the types of hormonal influences the growth receives:

1. Hair dependent on GH is that which grows on the head, eyelashes, eyebrows, midphalangeal area, distal portions of limbs, and to some extent, on the lumbosacral area.
2. Hair dependent on female hormones is that which grows on the pubic area, axillary limbs, and hypogastric area. The male hypogastric or pubic hair configuration is that of a diamond with its superior angle at the umbilicus, whereas

Table 7-2. Morphological hair types in humans

Growth site	Description	Length
Head	Relatively small root; tapered tip; many variations	1,000 mm
Eyebrow and eyelash	Curved; smooth; coarse; punctate tip	10 mm
Beard and mustache	Relatively longer root than scalp hair; blunt tip	300 mm
Body	Fine; long tip	Up to 60 mm
Pubic	Coarse; irregular; asymmetrical; usually curved but may be spiral tufted	Up to 60 mm
Axillary	Coarse; straighter than pubic hair; may be spiral tufted in blacks	Up to 50 mm

the female pubic hair pattern is triangular with the base over the mons.

3. Hair dependent on male hormones is that of the beard, mustache, nasal tip, and ear, and body hair (particularly on the back).

Morphological characteristics of the hair found in various anatomical sites are described in Table 7-2.

Hirsutism. Hirsutism, the appearance of excessive hair in normal and abnormal sites, can be most disturbing to the affected female client. The degree of overgrowth need not be marked to pose a threat to the client's feelings of femininity.

On noting hirsutism in the female client, the examiner is alerted to note the presence of other virilizing signs, which include a deepening of the voice, clitoral enlargement, and changes in fat distribution.

Hirsutism has been observed in the following pathophysiological conditions: bilateral polycystic ovary, Cushing's syndrome, and ovarian tumor.

Because of the identity confusion that may exist in the presence of hirsutism, the examiner approaches the investigation of the problem with sensitively phrased queries.

Description of the hirsute condition may be facilitated by Table 7-3.

Balding. Balding (alopecia) is more frequently noted in those individuals with abundant growth of coarse, or terminal, hair on the body and is thought to be related to testosterone production.

Generally, the man with a hairline that is low in the forehead does not bald. As a rule, women do not bald unless androgens are present in relatively increased amounts or the baldness occurs secondary to another disease.

Table 7-3. Classification of hirsutism

Stage	Site	Symbols for recording quantity, quality*
1	Languous hair Not in virilizing sites	D_1Q_1
2	Coarser hair as in men Distribution sites: Upper lips Sideburns Intermammary area Periareolar area Midabdomen	D_1Q_2
3	Same sites as stage 2, as well as: Upper back Shoulders Inner thighs Ears, nose Supragluteal and gluteal areas Temporal recession	D_2Q_2 to D_3Q_3
4	Same sites as stage 3; in addition shows other signs of virilization	D_3Q_3

*D, quantity: D_1, mild; D_2, moderate; D_3, profuse, Q, quality: Q_1, fine; Q_2, coarse; Q_3, very coarse.

Odors

The odor of the body and breath should be noted. The smell of alcohol on the client's breath alerts one to look for other effects of this CNS depressant. The fruity odor of acetone indicates that diabetes and starvation must be ruled out, whereas a fetid breath points to the possibility of an oral or pulmonary infection or may simply be the result of poor oral hygiene but may indicate infection or foreign body with infection. The odor of ammonia may be detectable in the patient with uremia. Body odor may be related to the activities of the sweat and sebaceous glands and to the general cleanliness of the body.

Nails

The nails may be an indication of the level of concern and care the person has for his appearance. The nails are inspected with reference to the length, cleanliness, neatness of filing, and if a woman, the presence and condition of polish. The examiner further notes the texture recording thickness and ridging when present.

Personal hygiene

General cleanliness of the body is an important indication of the individual's self-esteem and of the availability of necessary supplies to maintain good body care. Again, this is a socioculturally flavored value. It is important to note that deodorants are not used in all cultures. Although shaving of the legs is a norm in some groups of women in the United States, it is not practiced by other women.

Manner of dress

The fit of the clothing should be noted, as well as the attendance to current style. In addition, the general cleanliness and press of clothing may provide further clues to the cultural or socioeconomic status, as well as to the ego strength of the individual. The unshaven or unwashed signs of neglect by relatives or others for the dependent client or of self-neglect should be carefully noted.

Speech*

The manner of speech is the cornerstone to diagnosis of both emotional and physical illness. The characteristics that should be noted include:
1. *Pace:* A fast or rapid-fire manner of delivery may indicate hyperthyroidism, whereas slow speech and a thick, hoarse voice are typical of hypothyroidism.
2. *Clarity:* The ability to enunciate clearly may be lost in motor nerve disease of the tongue, jaws, or lips. Slurred speech can result from CNS damage.
3. *Vocabulary:* The choice of words may indicate the level of education of the client, and the accent he uses may indicate his socioeconomic class or the region of the country from which he comes.
4. *Sentence structure:* The client's sentences may give some indication of his cortical associative abilities.
5. *Tone of voice:* The voice should be observed for hoarseness, whining, or squeaky characteristics.
6. *Strength of voice:* Voice strength is evaluated in terms of loudness or softness in delivery of speech.

Some typical observations might be:
1. *Aphasia:* Inability to express oneself through speech (motor or expressive) or loss of verbal comprehension (receptive or sensory).
2. *Anarthria, dysarthria:* Loss of motor power to speak distinctly (stammering or stuttering).
3. *Aphonia, dysphonia:* Inability to produce sounds from the larynx. This is not due to a brain lesion. A possible cause might be laryngitis or malignancy.

In addition to observing the client's speech, one may find it useful to assess a sample of the client's writing for intactness of structures coordinating this complex act and for the client's ability to express his thoughts in this medium.

---

*See Chapter 8 on assessment of mental status.

Mental status*

The focus in this survey is to determine the client's problems in living and the psychodynamics underlying them. It is important that the client's own words be used in describing the problems.

The kind of information that is relevant will include the client's state of awareness form alertness to dullness to unconsciousness or coma. His ability to comprehend what he is told is described, as well as his level of education. The speed of responses to questions and reaction time in following instructions for motor activity may provide valuable clues. The length of attention span should be recorded. The facial expression should be observed at rest and during the early verbal interaction with the client for indications of anxiety, depression, apathy, and pain.

The client who slumps slowly into the chair should be observed for further indications of depression, such as carelessness in grooming and in dress.

The levels of cooperation can be described on a continuum from passive acceptance to rigid resistance. The level of aggressiveness may be described by descriptive terms relative to the client's relationship to things around him.

Mood has been described by such terms as hostility, resentment, depression, fearfulness, distrustfulness, elation, and euphoria. The difficulty in using these terms is that they may mean different things to the people who use them and to those who read the history. For instance, the client who sits looking at his hands while being interviewed might be described as "depressed," "withdrawn," "serious," or "thoughtful" by different observers. To obviate this confusion, it is best to describe the behavior that is observed.

The client's use of vocabulary and the complexity of sentence structure should be recorded, as well as his use of medical or other professional terminology.

Awareness is recorded in descriptive terms, relating the client's apparent perception of external stimuli and response to physiological stimuli.

The client's orientation for person, place, and time is assessed. It should be borne in mind that orientation usually is initially lost in the sphere of time, followed by place, and finally by person. Deviation from this order should be reported.

ASSESSMENT OF VITAL SIGNS

The clinical assessment of temperature, pulse, respiratory rate, and blood pressure are the most frequent clinical measurements made by the health practitioner. These measures of neural and circulatory function provide valuable data in the diagnosis of disease states. Irregularity of these parameters

---

*See Chapter 8 on assessment of mental status.

warrants further investigation. Because of the importance of these indicators in predicting the effectiveness of bodily function, they have been termed the *vital* or *cardinal* signs. Vital signs are assessed as the initial maneuver in any examination.

The history should be carefully attended for symptoms that would indicate alterations in the vital signs. These might include "pounding" of the heart, faintness, or dizziness.

The techniques utilized in the assessment of vital signs include inspection, palpation, and auscultation.

Inspection may reveal changes in color such as the flush of fever, the pallor in response to cold, or the dusky blueness of cyanosis. The bluish color observed as cyanosis results from an increased amount of reduced hemoglobin in superficial blood vessels. It is most readily identified in the vessels beneath the tongue or in the buccal mucosa. The examiner observes the chest for morphological changes that may indicate a pathological condition. For instance, in those individuals with chronic obstructive pulmonary disease, the anteroposterior diameter is often as great as the transverse diameter, and the ribs are observed to flare in the horizontal plane rather than downward. This structural change is thought to be the result of the long period of overinflation of the lungs.

The chest is also observed for defects of the thoracic cage that might change the nature of respiration. Some of these are pigeon or chicken breast (the sternum is markedly protuberant, as in a bird), funnel chest or *pectus excavatum* (sternal retraction), and scoliosis.

Symmetry of thoracic expansion is noted. Bulging or retraction of the interspaces is recorded.

In addition to the assessment of pulsations, *palpation* may be used to determine temperature. Since the dorsal aspect of the hand is more sensitive to temperature variation, it is recommended that the backs of the fingers be used in this rough measure of temperature. Palpation may also reveal moisture and texture variations as well as the vibration of shivering.

Auscultation of the precordial area is employed to further evaluate the irregular pulse. Listening over the heart while simultaneously palpating a peripheral pulse is helpful in detecting a pulse deficit. Auscultation is the technique used to evaluate the sounds produced as a result of sphygmomanometer (Gr. *sphygmos*, pulse) manipulation.

The examiner must bear in mind that the assessment of vital signs is done in the interest of establishing a data base so that on future occasions the client may be compared to his own values—may be his own control.

Measurements of clinical significance are those that reveal variation from the client's basal value or from his last measurement. This is important in view of the considerable variability noted among individuals. The ranges of normal for temperature, for example, are 97° to 99.6° F (36.7° to 37.6° C).

The examiner must bear in mind the fact that his manner of approach to the client may alter the vital signs should the client react emotionally to the examiner's actions. For instance, a brusque, impatient, rude interaction or awkward handling of the instruments may prove upsetting to the client, increasing pulse rate, respiration, blood pressure, and even temperature if the interaction is prolonged.

Temperature

The optimal temperature for metabolic function of all cells of the human body is considered to be 98.6° F (37° C) for most individuals, and the core temperature of the human body is maintained at this level within very narrow limits. Although some individuals have a normal core temperature of 97° F and the range of normal extends to 99.6° F, the temperature of the individual shows little variation.

Temperature regulation is an excellent example of both homeostasis and biological rhythms. The accomplishment of the reasonably steady core temperature is a function of the hypothalamus, which serves as the thermostat. Two hypothalamic centers trigger heat-dissipating or heat-conserving mechanisms. The delivery of overwarmed blood to thermoreceptors in an anterior hypothalamic site results in sweating and redistribution of blood, so that surface capillaries are dilated (flushing). The loss of temperature from the skin is related to the delivery of blood flow to the skin and to the evaporation of sweat. This loss of heat is related to the difference in temperature between the skin and the external environment.

Conduction, convection, radiation, and evaporation are the physical phenomena involved. Heat is lost from the object of higher temperature to the object of lower temperature by *conduction*. *Convection* is the loss of heat to the molecules of air. Warm air rises, carrying the heat away. Conduction and convection cannot occur when external objects and ambient temperature are greater than that of the body.

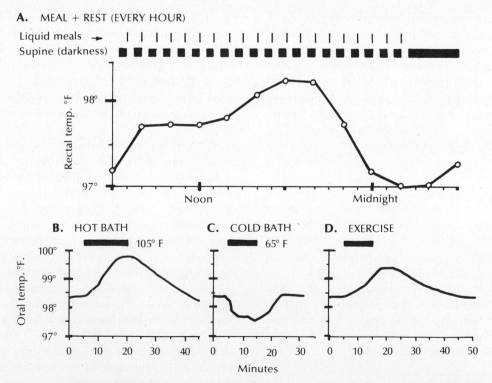

Fig. 7-1. Factors influencing the body temperature of human beings. The body temperature is nicely regulated, but exact maintenance is altered by many factors, such as hot baths, cold water, and exercise. Also, there is a daily resetting of temperature regulation that persists in a resting individual if the influence of exercise or meals is removed. If standardized exercise is carried out at noon and at midnight, the day-night regulation is still apparent in the exercise body temperature. (From Folk, G. E.: Textbook of environmental physiology, ed. 2, Philadelphia, 1974, Lea & Febiger; in part from Green, J. H.: An introduction to human physiology, ed. 4, Oxford, 1976, Oxford University Press.)

Radiation is the loss of heat by electromagnetic infrared waves. The radiation does not heat the air through which it passes.

Evaporation is the conversion of liquid to gaseous form. The liquid involved is sweat. Perspiration in humans is the insensible, thermal sweat from the eccrine glands and the autonomic, or emotional, sweat arising from the palms and soles. Insensible perspiration is moisture of diffusion principally noted from the corneum, from the sweat glands of the skin, and from the lungs. Insensible perspiration and thermal sweat are the most important in terms of heat loss. Evaporation of thermal sweat from the body requires 0.58 calorie per 1 ml of sweat. Vaporization of perspiration is dependent on ambient humidity and does not occur when air is highly saturated with water.

When overcooled blood is delivered to thermoreceptors in a posterior hypothalamic site, heat-conserving mechanisms are instituted. These functions include reduction of blood flow to the distal extremities as a result of shunting via venae comitantes from large arteries to similar veins and constriction of peripheral capillary beds (blanching). Compensatory heat production is enhanced both at the metabolic level (nonshivering thermogenesis) and through voluntary muscle contraction and shivering. Shivering occurs when vasoconstriction is ineffective in preventing heat loss.

Thermoreceptors in the skin sense ambient temperature and transmit neural signals to the spinal cord at all levels for relay through the spinothalamic tracts to the thalamus. These neural messages are thought to act as stimuli to the hypothalamic centers.

FACTORS INFLUENCING TEMPERATURE

Biological rhythms are reflected in temperature assessment (Fig. 7-1). Diurnal variations of 1.0° to 1.5° F are observed; the trough occurs in the hours before waking and the peak in the late afternoon or early evening.

Secretion of hormones affects the body temperature. Increased secretion of thyroid hormones is associated with increased heat production. Progesterone secretion at the time of ovulation is correlated with temperature increases of 0.5° to 1.0° F, which continues to the time of the menses. Both estrogen and testosterone may increase the rate of cellular metabolism.

There are some *environmental effects* on temperature. Although body temperature may be little altered by seasonal changes in environmental temperature, hot and cold baths are known to produce temporary changes in temperature, as shown in Fig. 7-1.

The physiological changes incurred in *exercise* are also known to increase body temperature (Fig. 7-2). The temperature rise associated with the *eating of food* is said to be a result of the specific dynamic activity (SDA) of the food.

Drugs that alter circulation or metabolism will also affect body temperature.

Age is a factor in temperature assessment. Because heat control mechanisms are not as well established in the child as in the adult, considerable variation in temperature may occur.

TEMPERATURE RECORDING

Body temperature is recorded in degrees centigrade (°C) or in degrees Fahrenheit (°F) according to the protocol of the agency. Because the United States is committed to the future adoption of the metric system, the practitioner would do well to think of temperature in degrees centigrade. Scales may be

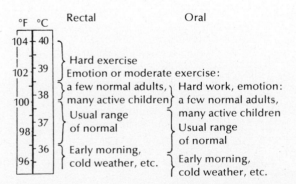

Fig. 7-2. Estimate of ranges in rectal and oral temperatures found in normal persons. This suggests that it would be wise to replace the red arrow on the clinical thermometer with a red band covering the space between 96.5° and 99.3° F (35.9° to 37.8° C). (From DuBois, E. F.: Fever and the regulation of body temperature, American Lecture Series, Publ. No. 13, 1948. Courtesy of Charles C Thomas, Publisher, Springfield, Ill.)

Table 7-4. Metric-Fahrenheit equivalents for possible range of human temperature

Fahrenheit (degrees)	Centigrade (degrees)
93.2	34.0
95.0	35.0
96.8	36.0
98.6	37.0
100.4	38.0
102.2	39.0
104.0	40.0
105.8	41.0
107.6	42.0
109.4	43.0

readily converted through the use of the following formulas:

$$°C = \frac{5}{9} (°F - 32)$$
$$°F = \frac{9}{5} °C + 32$$

Table 7-4 equates Fahrenheit and centigrade temperatures in the range compatible with survival in the human being.

TEMPERATURE REGULATION

Temperature control may be altered in such a way that the mechanisms of control may be effective at a higher or lower level. An example of this might be seen in the individual exposed to marked exercise. During the first few days the core temperature may reach values of 102° F (38.9° C), but with adaptation the individual may undergo a decrease to 100° F (37.8° C), which will be maintained as long as the exercise is carried on.

Fever, or elevation of temperature because of the effect of pyrogens on the hypothalamus, also affects this type of core temperature resetting.

Temperature regulation becomes impaired or lost when extreme variations of temperature occur (Fig.

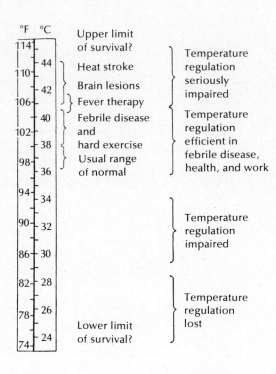

Fig. 7-3. Extremes of human body temperatures with an attempt to define the zones of temperature regulation. (From DuBois, E. F.: Fever and the regulation of body temperature, American Lecture Series, Publ. No. 13, 1948. Courtesy of Charles C Thomas, Publisher, Springfield, Ill.)

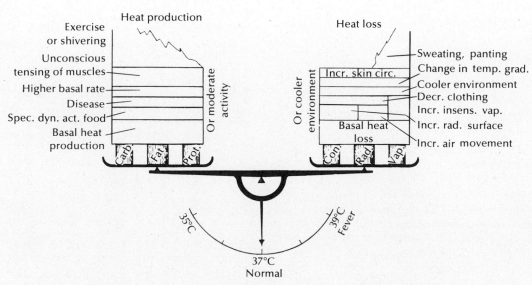

Fig. 7-4. Balance between factors increasing heat production and heat loss. (From DuBrois, E. F.: Heat loss from the human body, Harvey Lecture, Bull. N.Y. Acad. Med. **15:**143, 1939.)

7-3). It results from the balance of heat loss and heat conservation functions. These are summarized in Fig. 7-4.

TEMPERATURE ACCLIMATIZATION

Clients who have spent a good deal of time in very cold climates show an increased ability to tolerate cold. Changes that have been measured in these individuals are (1) increased metabolic rate with increased rates of secretion of thyroid hormones, (2) reduction in shivering, and (3) growth of hair.

Adaptation to heat involves changes in the secretion of sweat. The amount of sweat produced declines from the profuse, dripping early response to a quantity that will evaporate on reaching the air.

THERMOMETRY

Glass thermometry. The clinical glass thermometer has been in use since the 15th century. The thermometer reflects heat changes through the expansion of mercury. The accuracy of the instrument is determined by the amount and quality of the mercury and by the calibrations identified on the glass tube.

Recent studies have shown the glass thermometer to be subject to inaccuracy. Furthermore, in most subjects the oral thermometer must be left in place for 8 to 9 minutes in order to obtain full registration of the instrument. Thus, the readings obtained must be considered to be approximations of the actual temperature of the client.

Other disadvantages in the use of the glass thermometer are frequent breakage and danger to the client through the use of the rigid glass rod. Several instances of perforation of the rectal wall have occurred through inappropriate placement of a glass thermometer.

The examiner may also build in error through improper reading of the thermometer. The eyes must be at a 90 degree angle to the meniscus of the mercury to avoid parallax error.

Electronic thermometry. The electronic thermometer has been in use over the past decade. The advantages to be realized with the fully charged, correctly calibrated instrument are speed and accuracy of measurement. The probes used in these thermometers are unbreakable, thus obviating damage from broken glass and mercury ingestion, which are hazards with the traditional clinical thermometer.

ORAL, RECTAL, AND AXILLARY TEMPERATURE ASSESSMENT

Differences in temperatures recorded from the mouth, rectum, or axilla have been shown to reflect the length of time the thermometer is allowed to register rather than actual variation in temperature from one site to another.

Oral temperature. The oral temperature registration is the most convenient method for the client. This site for temperature determination is the one used unless the client is an infant, unconscious, confused, or has shown erratic behavior.

A 5- to 15-minute wait is recommended before temperature assessment if the client has ingested hot or iced liquids, to allow the temperature to stabilize. Small increases will occur if the client has smoked in the 2 minutes preceding the temperature assessment. The oral thermometer may take as long as 8 to 9 minutes to reach maximum registration. Other assessment procedures may be done at this time.

RECTAL TEMPERATURE

The rectal site for temperature registration is preferable for the confused or comatose client, the individual who is unable to close his mouth, the client who is receiving oxygen or the client who may bite the thermometer for other reasons.

The rectal temperature is routinely ordered as the general mode of temperature registration in some agencies.

The thermometer placed in the rectum will register adequately within a 2-minute time span in adults and within 3 minutes in premature infants.

AXILLARY TEMPERATURE

Eleven minutes has been shown to be the maximum length of time necessary for the full retistration of axillary temperature. This method has been shown to be safe and accurate for infants and small children.

Correlation of pulse and temperature

It should be noted that marked increases in temperature are accompanied by increments in pulse and respiratory rates because oxygen requirements are known to increase 7% for every 1° F (10% for every 1° C) rise in temperature. Since reducing cellular temperatures results in a decreased rate of cell metabolism, oxygen consumption is lessened in hypothermia; therefore, pulse and respiratory rates also decline.

Fever

Fever, or pyrexia, is the elevation of body temperature above normal limits as compared to a given individual's basal data. Fever may be a valid diagnosis when the temperature is found to be 98.6° F for a specific client if his normal temperature ranges about 97° F.

Not all causes of fever are related to disease. Exercise may cause a temporary elevation of temperature, which subsides when the activity is stopped.

It has been suggested that a temperature above 97° F in a client who has been lying in bed (whose metabolism is basal) indicates the presence of disease. The association of an elevated temperature with disease is called a fever.

Fever is caused by those conditions that contribute to heat production, that prevent heat loss, or that affect the heat-regulating centers of the CNS.

Fevers are described according to the chronological pattern of occurrence and amplitude. Frequently, the recognition of the pattern may help to establish the diagnosis. The following paragraphs present descriptions of fever.

A *continuous* or *sustained* fever is one in which there is a persistent elevation of temperature without a return to normal values for that individual. This pattern is typical of typhoid or typhus fever.

An *intermittent fever* is one in which there are major diurnal variations, so that there is a daily elevation of temperature with a drop to subnormal or normal values in the same 24-hour period. When there is a marked difference between the peaks and the troughs of the temperature, the fever is called *hectic* or *septic*. This type of fever is seen in pyrogenic infection.

Remittent fever is characterized by a temperature elevation that does not return to normal level but shows marked spikes of even further increased temperature on the febrile baseline. This appears in sustained or continuous fever, in which there are only slight variations from the elevated set point.

Relapsing fever is one in which febrile periods alternate with periods of normal temperature. This pattern of fever is seen in malaria, relapsing fever, and the Murchison-Pel-Ebstein fever of Hodgkin's disease.

Fever may also be described by the rate pattern of dissolution. *Lysis* is the gradual disappearance of fever, whereas *crisis* is the rapid (less than 36 hours) decrease of temperature to normal.

Stages or chronology of fever. The development of the febrile condition and its abatement have been described in three stages, called cold, hot, and defervescence.

The period of a developing increase in core temperature is characterized by heat conservation reactions. The affected individual has diminished cutaneous circulation, and the skin looks blanched and feels cold. Heat production is attested to by shivering and piloerection ("goose pimples"). Chills and rigor are the extremes of shivering that produce rapid increases in temperature.

The hot stage is the period after the fever has peaked (regulated at the new set point). During this stage blood flow to the periphery is increased. The affected individual's body radiates excess heat, feels hot, and is flushed.

The stage of defervescense is the period of fever abatement and is characterized by heat loss mechanisms; particularly prominent is vasodilation and sweating. Diaphoresis is diffuse perspiration, which may accompany fever abatement.

Respiratory pattern

The assessment of the respiratory pattern is discussed in Chapter 15, "Assessment of the Respiratory System."

Pulsation

The assessment of central pulses discussed in Chapter 16, "Cardiovascular Assessment: the heart and neck vessels," should be read before this section.

Assessment of the peripheral arterial pulse has been a part of the health professional's routine procedure throughout recorded medical history. The peripheral arterial pulse is a pressure wave transmitted from the left ventricle to the root of the aorta to the peripheral vessels.

Examination of the peripheral (radial) arterial pulsation gives less information concerning left ventricular ejection or aortic valvular function than does the assessment of the more central (carotid) arteries because the normal arterial pulse expands normal peripheral arteries only slightly. The information obtained is a necessary part of the data base, however, because the nature of the peripheral pulse gives an indication of cardiac function and of perfusion of the peripheral tissues. These peripheral pulsations are evaluated in terms of rate, amplitude (indicating volume), rhythm, and symmetry regularity. They may also be auscultated for the presence of bruits.

Arterial pulses are most accurately examined while the client is reclining with the trunk of the body elevated about 15 to 30 degrees.

PARAMETERS OF ARTERIAL PULSATION

Visual and palpable pulsations result from diameter changes incurred through vessel filling as well as through straightening of the vessel. These pulsations are referred to as arterial pulse waves.

Pressure changes in the wall of the artery are felt through the overlying skin and subcutaneous tissue. The arterial pressure pulse wave is sensed through the pressure receptors in the pads of the examiner's fingers, which are superimposed on the vessel wall, as in pressure of paired arterial pulses exerted against the wall. The pulse is best palpated over arteries that are close to the surface of the body and that lie over a bony surface. The arteries that are palpated during the health examination include the superficial temporary artery, carotid, brachial, ulnar, radial, femoral, popliteal, dorsal pedal (dorsalis pedic), and posterior tibial.

Rate. As defined by the American Heart Associa-

Table 7-5. Chronological variations in pulse rate

Age	Pulse rate (beats per minute)
Birth	70-170
Neonate	120-140
1 year	80-140
2 years	80-130
3 years	80-120
4 years	70-115
Adult	60-100
Conditioned athlete	$\cong 50$

tion, the heart rate is normal when it is between 50 and 100 beats per minute.

The pulse rate is counted for 1 full minute in order to evaluate rate, rhythm, and volume accurately. Some authorities recommend counting for 15 to 30 seconds for those pulses that are normal on palpation and to extend the period of evaluation only when irregularities are detected.

A diurnal rhythm is noted for pulse rate. The lowest rate is seen in the early morning hours, and the most rapid rates are observed in the late afternoon and evening.

Chronologically the pulse rate decreases from infancy through the middle years; there is a tendency for it to increase in the older client (Table 7-5).

A sex difference is noted in that women have demonstrated a rate 5 to 10 beats per minute faster than men.

Volume. Pulse volume is estimated from the feel of the vessel as blood flows through it with each heartbeat. Bounding is the descriptive term used to describe the full pulse that is difficult to depress with the fingertips. The normal pulse is easily palpable and does not fade in and out and is not easily obliterated. Weak, feeble, and thready and descriptive words for the pulse of a vessel that has low volume. The artery in this case is readily compressed. The absent pulse is not palpable.

Amplitude. The strength of the left ventricular contraction is reflected in the amplitude of the pulsation. This may be recorded as follows:

3+ Bounding, hyperkinetic
2+ Normal
1+ Weak, thready, hypokinetic
0 Absent

ELASTICITY OF THE ARTERIAL WALL

Elasticity of the arterial wall is reflected by the expansibility or deformability of the artery as it is palpated by the examiner's fingers. The normal artery is soft and pliable, whereas the sclerotic vessel may be more resistant to occlusion, even hard and cordlike.

The artery may feel beaded and tortuous to touch in the individual with arteriosclerosis.

PALPATION OF ARTERIAL PULSES—PULSE POINTS

Superficial temporal pulse. The superficial temporal artery is accessible to palpation anterior to the tragus of the ear and upward to the temple and is frequently used in the clinical evaluation of pulsation (Figs. 7-5 and 7-6).

Carotid pulse. Examination of the carotid and jugular pulse is described in Chapter 14. Fig. 7-7 shows one method of palpation of the carotid artery.

The carotid pulse is easily accessible and is frequently the pulse evaluated in emergency situations.

The easiest method of locating the carotid is by placing the fingers lightly over the trachea and allowing them to slide into the trough between the trachea and the sternocleidomastoid muscle. The carotid will be felt immediately below the examining fingers. The pulse is palpated in the lower half of the artery in order to avoid pressure on the carotid sinus. Care should be taken to avoid undue pressure on the carotids in order to avoid stimulation of the baroreceptors of the carotid sinus and a resultant slowing of the heart and a decrease in blood pressure. All symmetrical pulses except the carotid may be measured simultaneously. The carotid pulses should not be measured simultaneously. Excessive biarterial pressure may dangerously occlude the blood supply to the brain.

Radial pulse. The radial pulse is the one most frequently used as an initial indication of the rate and rhythm of pulsation, the pattern of pulsation, and the shape (consistency) of the arterial wall. This pulse is easily accessible to the examiner, and its evaluation causes little inconvenience to the client. Other pulses easily evaluated in the upper extremity are the ulnar and brachial pulses (Fig. 7-8).

The radial pulse is readily assessed by placing the pads of the examiner's second and third (or first, second, and third) fingers on the palmar surface of the relaxed and slightly flexed wrist medial to the radial styloid process (Fig. 7-9). Occasionally the arteries run a deeper and more lateral course. Both radial pulses should be felt simultaneously for an assessment of symmetry. The fingers should exert sufficient pressure to occlude the artery during diastole, yet allow the vessel to return to normal contour during systole.

Ulnar pulse. The ulnar artery may be compressed against the ulna on the palmar surface of the wrist. It is not used as frequently as the radial artery in evaluation.

Brachial pulse. Brachial pulse assessment by auscultation is a part of the blood pressure evaluation. The pulse is palpated as it passes through the upper half

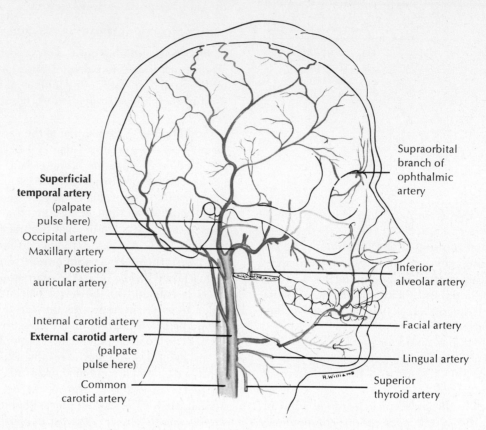

Superficial
temporal artery
(palpate
pulse here)

Occipital artery

Maxillary artery

Posterior
auricular artery

Internal carotid artery

External carotid artery
(palpate
pulse here)

Common
carotid artery

Supraorbital
branch of
ophthalmic
artery

Inferior
alveolar artery

Facial artery

Lingual artery

Superior
thyroid artery

H. Williams

Fig. 7-5. Arteries of the head and neck. (Modified from Francis, C. C., and Martin, A. H.: Introduction to human anatomy, ed. 7, St. Louis, 1975, The C. V. Mosby Co.)

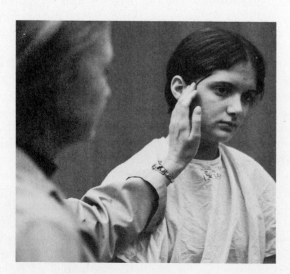

Fig. 7-6. Palpation of the superficial temporal artery.

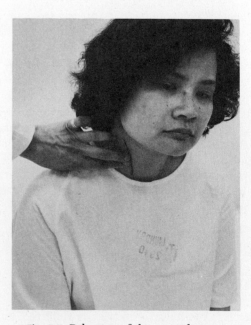

Fig. 7-7. Palpation of the carotid artery.

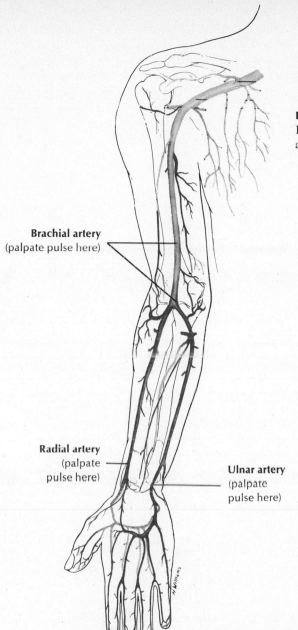

Brachial artery
(palpate pulse here)

Radial artery
(palpate
pulse here)

Ulnar artery
(palpate
pulse here)

Fig. 7-8. Arteries of the upper extremity. (Adapted from Francis, C. C., and Martin, A. H.: Introduction to human anatomy, ed. 7, St. Louis, 1975, The C. V. Mosby Co.)

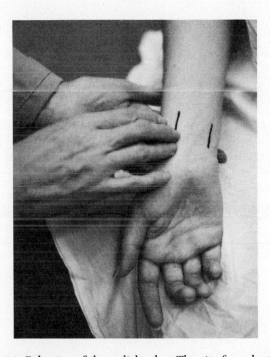

Fig. 7-9. Palpation of the radial pulse. The site for palpation of the ulnar artery is also marked.

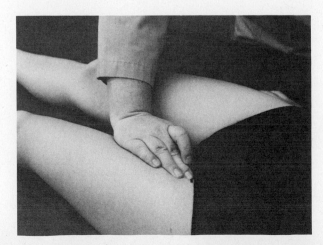

Fig. 7-10. Palpation of femoral pulse.

of the cubital fossa at the midline (anterior surface of the elbow joint) because halfway through the fossa it bifurcates into the radial and ulnar arteries. The brachial artery is palpated medial to the biceps tendon. The brachial artery may be used to determine the arterial waveform, as can the carotid artery. The waveform of more peripheral arteries may be distorted and therefore provide less valuable data.

Femoral pulse. The pads of the examiner's fingers explore the groin in the area just inferior to the midpoint of the inguinal ligament. This is also approximately midway between the anterior superior iliac

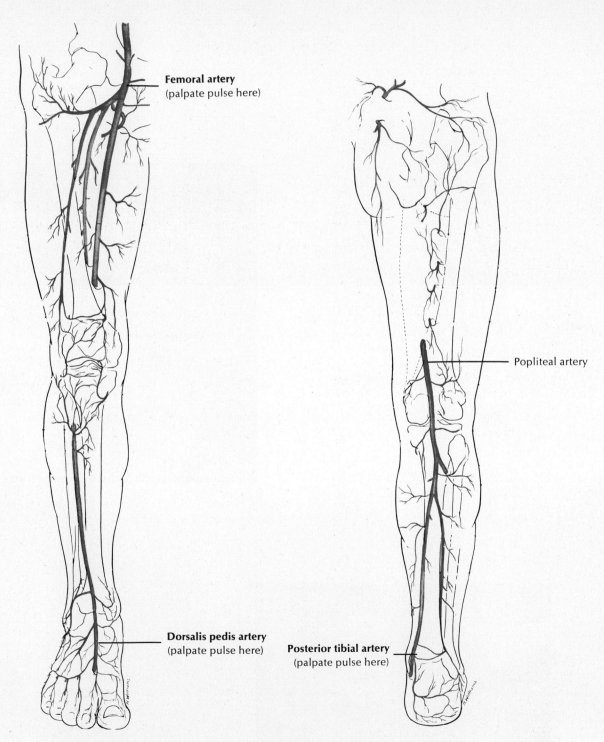

Femoral artery
(palpate pulse here)

Popliteal artery

Dorsalis pedis artery
(palpate pulse here)

Posterior tibial artery
(palpate pulse here)

Fig. 7-11. Arteries of the lower extremity. (Adapted from Francis, C. C, and Martin, A. H.: Introduction to human anatomy, ed. 7, St. Louis, 1975, The C. V. Mosby Co.)

spine and the symphysis pubis (Figs. 7-10 and 7-11).

Popliteal pulse. Since the popliteal artery is situated relatively deeply in the soft tissues behind the knee, the knee should be flexed for examination of the pulsation in this artery. The pulse may be readily examined with the client in either the dorsal recumbent (Fig. 7-12) or prone position (Fig. 7-13). The fingertips are pressed deeply into the popliteal fossa.

Dorsal pedal pulse. The pads of the examining fingers examine the dorsum of the foot. The foot should be dorsiflexed to obviate traction on the artery, preferably to 90 degrees (Fig. 7-14).

When the dorsal pedal pulse is congenitally absent, pulsation may sometimes be discerned in the lateral tarsal artery, located in the proximal dorsum of the foot, or in the peroneal artery, anterior to the lateral malleolus.

Although only one pedal pulse can occasionally be palpated, this need not necessarily indicate arterial insufficiency; it may be due to clinically insignificant congenital variation in the arteries to the foot.

One or both dorsal pedal pulses have been noted to be absent in 12% of children and in 17% of adults. Whereas whites seldom show an absence of the posterior tibial pulse, a 9% incidence of absence has been found in black adults.

Posterior tibial pulse. The pads of the examining fingers palpate posterior or inferior to the tibial medial malleolus while the client's foot is dorsiflexed, preferably to 90 degrees (Fig. 7-15).

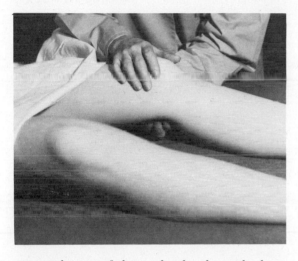

Fig. 7-12. Palpation of the popliteal pulse with client in the dorsal recumbent position.

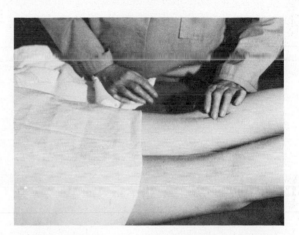

Fig. 7-13. Palpation of the popliteal pulse with client in the prone position.

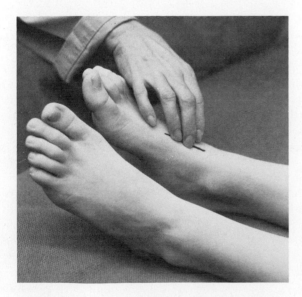

Fig. 7-14. Palpation of the dorsal pedal pulse.

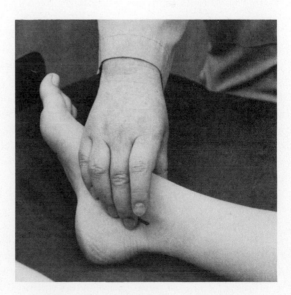

Fig. 7-15. Palpation of posterior tibial pulse.

POSSIBLE ETIOLOGY

Partial arterial occlusion
Myocardial infarction
Myocarditis
Pericardial effusion shock
Stenosis of valves: aortic,
   mitral, pulmonic, tricuspid

Systole| Diastole   Dicrotic notch

NORMAL PULSE

Graphic recording of pulse pressure as obtained from electrical transducer. The normal pulse is easily palpable but may be obliterated by pressure. The wave of a single pulsation rises in systole, reaches a summit, and descends more slowly in diastole. The secondary rise in pressure, noted in diastole is associated with closure of the aortic valve. The point at which the increase in pressure changes the downward slope is known as the dicrotic notch. This may not be palpable. The difference in pressure from the endpoint of diastole to the summit is the amplitude. Normal amplitude (30 to 40 mm Hg) is recorded as 2+. A pulse of greater amplitude is called strong and one of lesser amplitude is weak or faint.

Hypovolemia
Physical obstruction
   to left ventricular
   output, e.g., aortic
   stenosis

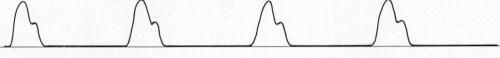

SMALL, WEAK PULSE

A weak pulse may be difficult to feel and the vessel may be obliterated easily by the fingers. The pulse may "fade out" (be impalpable). This pulse is recorded as 1+. The pulsation is slower to rise, has a sustained summit, and falls more slowly than the normal. A pulse that is weak and variable in amplitude is called thready.

Exercise
Anxiety
Fever
Hyperthyroidism
Aortic rigidity or
   atherosclerosis

LARGE, BOUNDING PULSE

The large, bounding (also called hyperkinetic or strong) pulse is readily palpable. It does not "fade out" and is not easily obliterated by the examining fingers. This pulse is recorded as 3+.

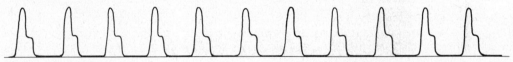

Patent ductus arteriosus

WATER-HAMMER PULSE

Aortic regurgitation

The water-hammer pulse (also known as collapsing) has a greater amplitude than the normal pulse, a rapid rise to a narrow summit, and a sudden descent.

Fig. 7-16. Table of pulses.

The examination of the pulses of an extremity begins with the most distal pulse point. Normal pulses in the dorsal pedal and posterior tibial arteries indicate that that is no disruption of flow to the extremity, whereas a weak or absent pulse is expected to be found distal to an obstruction. However, the observation of an indication that an individual has a disease known to produce a peripheral vascular change, such as circulatory impairment or diabetes, dictates the examination of all the superficial pulse points. A thorough assessment includes assessment of all pulse points.

IRREGULARITIES IN PULSATION (Fig. 7-16)

Tachycardia. Rates persistently over 100 beats per minute (tachycardia) suggest some abnormality (Table 7-6). However, hyperkinetic heart action can be the result of exercise, anger, anxiety, or fear in the nor-

mal client. Heart rates are increased during fever, anemia, hypoxia, and low volume states (shock).

Bradycardia. A slow heart rate less than 50 beats per minute is known as bradycardia (Table 7-7). These slow rates may indicate stimulation of the parasympathetic system or failure in the electrical conduction system of the heart. Bradycardia may be iatrogenically produced through overdoses of digitalis.

The well-trained athlete may have cardiac rates less than 50 beats per minute.

Irregular rhythm—pulse deficit. Cardiac arrhythmias, that is, atrial fibrillation, atrial flutter with block, and second degree heart block resulting in dropped beats, irregular sinus depolarization, and premature complexes result in an irregular rhythm of the pulse.

Pulse deficit means that the number of pressure waves palpable at the peripheral pulse point is less

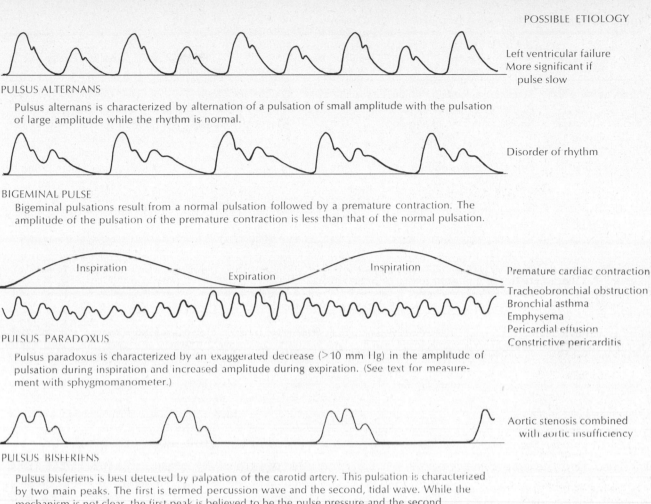

PULSUS ALTERNANS

Pulsus alternans is characterized by alternation of a pulsation of small amplitude with the pulsation of large amplitude while the rhythm is normal.

Left ventricular failure
More significant if
    pulse slow

Disorder of rhythm

BIGEMINAL PULSE

Bigeminal pulsations result from a normal pulsation followed by a premature contraction. The amplitude of the pulsation of the premature contraction is less than that of the normal pulsation.

Premature cardiac contraction

Inspiration   Expiration   Inspiration

PULSUS PARADOXUS

Pulsus paradoxus is characterized by an exaggerated decrease (>10 mm Hg) in the amplitude of pulsation during inspiration and increased amplitude during expiration. (See text for measurement with sphygmomanometer.)

Tracheobronchial obstruction
Bronchial asthma
Emphysema
Pericardial effusion
Constrictive pericarditis

PULSUS BISFERIENS

Aortic stenosis combined
    with aortic insufficiency

Pulsus bisferiens is best detected by palpation of the carotid artery. This pulsation is characterized by two main peaks. The first is termed percussion wave and the second, tidal wave. While the mechanism is not clear, the first peak is believed to be the pulse pressure and the second, reverberation from the periphery.

Irregular pulse rhythm

Pulse deficit means that the number of pressure waves palpable at the peripheral vessel is less than the cardiac contractions.

Cardiac arrhythmia
Atrial fibrillation
Atrial flutter with block
Second-degree heart block
Irregular sinus depolarization
Premature complexes
Weak, premature
    ventricular contractions

Fig. 7-16, cont'd. Table of pulses.

than the actual number of muscular contractions of the heart. Pressure waves initiated by weak, premature ventricular contractions may not be transmitted to the periphery. Simultaneous measurement at the precordium and peripheral pulse point reveals this deficit.

Bigeminal pulse. A pulse that alternates in amplitude from beat to beat may be produced by a small, premature ventricular beat after a strong beat, resulting from normal electrical cardiac conduction. The strong pulse occurs after a long diastolic filling

phase following the premature beat. The pulse is irregular. This condition is called bigeminal pulse and can be identified by simultaneously palpating the radial pulse and listening at the precordium.

Pulses alternans. Pulsus alternans is a pulse that alternates between strong and weak beats while the rhythm is regular. When the variation is marked, the alternation from weak to strong beats is palpable. However, it may be necessary to use the sphygmomanometer and stethoscope to determine minor changes. The examiner will hear the alternation of

Table 7-6. Characteristics of common forms of tachycardia

Type	Rhythm, amplitude	Most common ventricular rate (beats/min)	Onset	Termination	Effect of carotid sinus massage
Sinus tachycardia	Regular; constant amplitude	Usually 170	Gradual	Gradual	Gradual slowing and return to previous state
Paroxysmal atrial tachycardia (PAT)	Regular; constant amplitude	170	Abrupt	Abrupt	Sudden slowing of heart rate or no change
Paroxysmal atrial flutter	Flutter, regular; uniform amplitude	170	Abrupt		Sudden diminution of rate or temporarily irregular rhythm
Ventricular tachycardia	Irregular; variable amplitude	140	Sudden		No effect

Table 7-7. Characteristics of common forms of bradycardia

Type	Rhythm, amplitude	Most common ventricular rate (beats/min)	Effect of exercise
Sinus bradycardia	Regular; constant amplitude	40	Rate increases appropriately through varying degrees of exercise
Incomplete heart block	Constant amplitude	40	May double or become irregular in response to exercise
Complete heart block		40	Increases only slightly in response to exercise

Table 7-8. Guide to causes of palpitations

Possible cause	Signs and symptoms
Menopausal symptom	Associated with heat "flashes" or perspiration
Drugs known to produce a hyperkinetic heart	History of ingestion of monamine oxidase inhibitors, thyroid replacement or stimulatory drugs, adrenergic drugs, alcohol, tea, coffee
Hemorrhage, hypoglycemia, pheochromocytoma	Sudden occurrence of palpitation not related to exercise or emotional arousal
Psychopathology	Clinical examination reveals no evidence of hyperkinetic heart or irregularity of rate
Postural hypotension	Palpitations occur when individual stands
Anemia, fever, atrial fibrillation, thyrotoxicosis, exposure to environmental heat	Clinical examination reveals hyperkinetic heart
Extra systoles	Irregular "skips"

loud and soft sounds in pulses alternans. (See assessment of pulsus alternans in the section on blood pressure in this chapter.)

Pulsus paradoxus. Arterial pressure is known to fluctuate physiologically with the respiratory cycle, falling with inspiration and rising with expiration. This variation is detectable at normal respiratory amplitude, but is more marked during forced respiratory volumes. Two mechanisms appear to explain this effect. One, the changes in pleural pressure during respiration appear to affect the arteries and veins as they enter or leave the thoracic cage, altering the gradients whereby blood enters or leaves the thorax. Second, the relationship between the ventricles of the heart is such that distention of one results in alteration of the filling characteristics (distensibility or compliance) of the other. Reduction in pleural pressure during inspiration increases the return of systemic venous blood to the right ventricle. The increase in right ventricular filling pressure results in a shift of the interventricular septum leftward, thus reducing the amount of blood that is accepted by the left ventricle. The resultant decrease in left ventricular end diastolic pressure decreases the stroke work of the subsequent left ventricular systole. Thus, while there is an increase in right ventricular output, left ventricular output is decreased. In conditions charac-

Differentiation of arterial insufficiency from venous stasis

	Client's response	
	Arterial insufficiency (intermittent claudication)	Venous stasis
Interview		
When does the pain occur?	Walking	Standing
What makes the pain worse?	Cold	
What helps to get rid of the pain?	Standing	Elevation
	Stopping to rest	
Do you notice swelling in your feet or legs?	No	Yes
Inspection of involved extremity		
Pulses	Decreased amplitude or absent	
Skin	Cool to touch	Brownish pigmentation
	Pallor, rubor on elevation	
	Shiny	
	Hair loss	
	Nails thickened, ridged	
If ulcer present	Irregular edges	Shallow exudate covering
	Pale, boggy, granulation tissue	
	Eschar covering	Located on side of ankle
	Gangrene possible	No gangrene
	Located on toes or sites of trauma	

terized by distention of the venous system, for example, right ventricular failure as a result of severe obstructive lung disease or pericardial tamponade, a greater fall in pleural pressure and, thus, arterial pressure occurs. This is called pulsus paradoxus.

The variation in arterial pressure may be objectively measured only through the use of stethoscope and sphygmomanometer. Following detection of systolic pressure, the first noted Korotkoff sound, the pressure is allowed to decrease very slowly until sounds can be heard throughout the respiratory cycle. The decrease in arterial pressure during inspiration in the normal individual may be 10 ± 5 mm Hg. A difference greater than 15 mm Hg is indicative of pulsus paradoxus.

Palpitations. In the resting state the normal individual is unaware of the beating of his heart. *Palpitation* is the term used to record a description given by the client of his perception of the feeling of his heartbeat (Table 7-8). Such expressions as "pounding," "thudding," "fluttering," "flopping," and "skipping" are common descriptive terms used by clients to describe this phenomenon. Palpitation is more common just before falling asleep or during sleep.

Physiological palpitations may be experienced by the normal individual following strenuous exercise or when he is aroused emotionally or sexually. In this case the cardiac contraction is of greater rate and amplitude. Several pathophysiological states are also associated with a hyperkinetic heart (anemia, fever, hypoglycemia, and thyrotoxicosis). Irregularities in cardiac rhythm have also been associated with palpitations, particularly extra systoles and ectopic tachycardia. The chief complaint of palpitations is frequently correlated with psychopathology.

A common feature of the anxiety state, palpitations may be related to the increased adrenergic activity that is present in this arousal state. This relationship creates some problem for the examiner; since the presence of palpitations frequently creates anxiety, careful questions will be necessary to minimize this effect.

ARTERIAL INSUFFICIENCY

Assessment of the arterial pulsation is particularly important in those individuals suspected or diagnosed as having diseases known to compromise the arterial circulation. Some of these pathophysiological conditions are diabetes, atherosclerosis, Buerger's disease, Raynaud's disease, and arterial aneurysm.

Signs and symptoms of arterial insufficiency include intermittent claudication, increased pallor on elevation of the extremity, a prolonged venous filling time following elevation of the extremity, flush incurred by gravitational effect if the extremity is below the level of the heart, and tissue death (gangrene). Symptoms may also include easy fatigability. Ischemic pain may be incurred by simple resistance exercises. Intermittent claudication is the transient ischemic pain encountered by the client in his arms when he is working with them or in his legs when he is walking.

The impaired flow of arterial insufficiency may be adequate to serve the metabolic activities of the muscle at rest but does not maintain the circulation necessary to the increased metabolic rates of exercise. The pain is theorized to be the result of the the buildup of metabolic acids that stimulate the sensory nerves. It is described as cramping or "tightness" and sometimes likened to being in a vise. Many clients, however, do not recognize the discomfort as pain but describe aching, cramping, burning, tiredness, numbness, or weakness of the calf muscles.

Intermittent claudication in the arms may be confused with the pain of angina pectoris. The examiner must carefully define the fact that the pain occurred with work and disappeared with rest. Subclavian arterial insufficiency may result in dizziness and faintness.

In both arterial insufficiency and venous stasis calf pain is experienced that is relieved during sleep.

Physical examination of the client thought to have arterial insufficiency includes auscultation of the arteries, palpation of the pulses, and observations of cutaneous color; examination should be done before and after exercise.

Absence of pulsation in the femoral artery and at least one peripheral vessel is a criterion for the diagnosis of arterial insufficiency.

Arterial insufficiency in the arm, although generally thought to be less frequent than that of the leg, may frequently be demonstrated through changes in murmurs, pulses, and skin color after exercise.

Importance of exercise testing in determining arterial insufficiency of the extremities. Exercise testing of the poorly perfused limb is based on the inability of the occluded vessel to increase blood flow to meet the increased demands for oxygen. Bruits that were present only in systole continue into diastole since there is a relatively decreased diastolic pressure distal to the obstruction, which promotes forward flow (Figs. 7-17 and 7-18).

In clients with intermittent claudication the pulses diminish in amplitude following exercise. Cutaneous ischemia may be apparent.

The amount of exercise needed to produce these vascular changes is usually not more than that which is part of daily living. Flexion—extension exercises of the arms and legs (deep knee bends)—or walking may produce these changes.

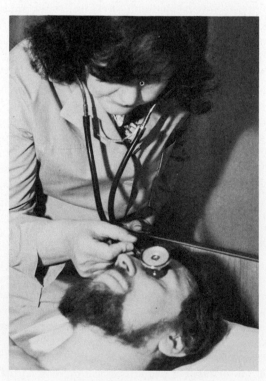

Fig. 7-17. Auscultation for bruits over the supraorbital branch of the ophthalmic artery.

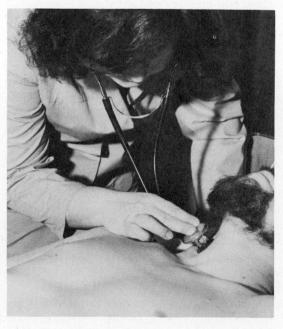

Fig. 7-18. Auscultation for bruits over the carotid artery.

Homan's sign. Thrombosis of the deep veins of the calf muscles may be detected by forced dorsiflexion of the foot. This maneuver compresses the veins and causes pain. The complaint of pain by the client when this maneuver is performed indicates Homans' sign. It is important to remember that deep venous thrombosis may be silent, that is, not give rise to pain.

AUSCULTATION FOR ARTERIAL MURMURS

All accessible arteries should be auscultated in the client suspected of arteriovascular disease. Murmurs are not present over major arteries in the normal adult, and only faint ones are heard in the normal child.

Arterial murmurs may result from hyperdynamic cardiac states or from irregularity of arterial walls.

The bell of the stethoscope is utilized to detect bruits over major vessels. The instrument is lightly held to avoid occluding the underlying vessel. Should the examiner detect a murmur, the limb is exercised if no contraindication exists, and the auscultation is repeated. The auscultation of a systolic murmur that extends into diastole in the postexercise state connotes some degree of arterial obstruction.

SPHYGMOMANOMETER DETECTION OF ARTERIAL FLOW

Failure to palpate pedal pulsation may indicate the use of the sphygmomanometer for detection of arterial flow. The pneumatic cuff is inflated to a pressure between the systolic and diastolic blood pressure. Oscillation of the needle (aneroid) or mercury column (mercury) on synchrony with the ventricular contraction is indicative of blood flow to the extremity. A disadvantage of this method is that it does not indicate the adequacy of the flow volume.

Blood pressure

Arterial blood pressure is the force exerted by the blood against the wall of the artery as the heart contracts and relaxes. *Systolic arterial blood pressure* is the force exerted against the wall of the artery when the ventricles are contracted and *diastolic arterial blood pressure* is the force when the heart is in the filling or relaxed phase. *Pulse pressure* is the difference between the *systolic* and *diastolic* blood pressures.

The blood pressure is determined by the cardiac output and peripheral resistance. Thus, the blood pressure reflects the volume of fluid in the cardiovascular system and elasticity of the arterial walls.

The screening examination is especially important to the recognition of the client who has a disorder in blood pressure, particularly hypertension (persistently elevated blood pressure). Because hyper-

tension may be present without symptoms, it is known as the silent disease. The client who does not fell ill does not usually present himself for health care. Thus, this examination may be instrumental in getting the hypertensive client into the therapeutic milieu in time to prevent some of the sequelae of hypertension.

A measure of the functions of the cardiovascular system may be accomplished through the assessment of peripheral arterial blood pressure. The peripheral blood pressure is the force exerted against the walls of the vessels and the force responsible for the flow of blood through the arteries, capillaries, and veins. The pressure is the result of the interaction of cardiac output and peripheral resistance and is dependent on the velocity of the arterial blood, the intravascular volume, and the elasticity of the arterial walls.

Stephen Hale made the first recorded direct measurement of blood pressure in 1733 when he cannulated the artery of a horse, allowing the blood to rise in a glass tube. He was also able to demonstrate the changes in blood pressure that occur in systole and diastole as he watched the blood rise and fall in the tube with each heartbeat. Almost a century later (1828), Poiseuille attached a mercury-filled tube to a cannulated artery. Since mercury is 13.6 times heavier than blood or water, the column in the tube was much shorter. Several instruments for the indirect method of blood pressure measurement were devised in the late 1800s.

The systemic arterial blood pressure may be assessed either by direct or indirect methods. The direct method requires cannulation of the artery but is the trusted method of measurement. Routine, direct arterial blood pressures are not measured, because of the potential sequelae, though the risks are small. Indirect blood pressure measurement can be made without opening the artery. The valid methods of indirect measurement are those that are closest in values to those made from direct techniques. Direct blood pressure standards are used to calibrate indirect pressure instruments.

INDIRECT MEASUREMENT

Indirect methods of blood pressure measurement involve the following three physiological facts: (1) the arterial wall may be occluded by direct pressure, resulting in the obliteration of the pulse distal to the compression; (2) oscillations that vary directly with the amount of pressure being applied may be measured from the compressed artery; and (3) the normal extremity blanches (pales) when its arterial blood supply is occluded by pressure, and there is flushing or return of color when the pressure is removed.

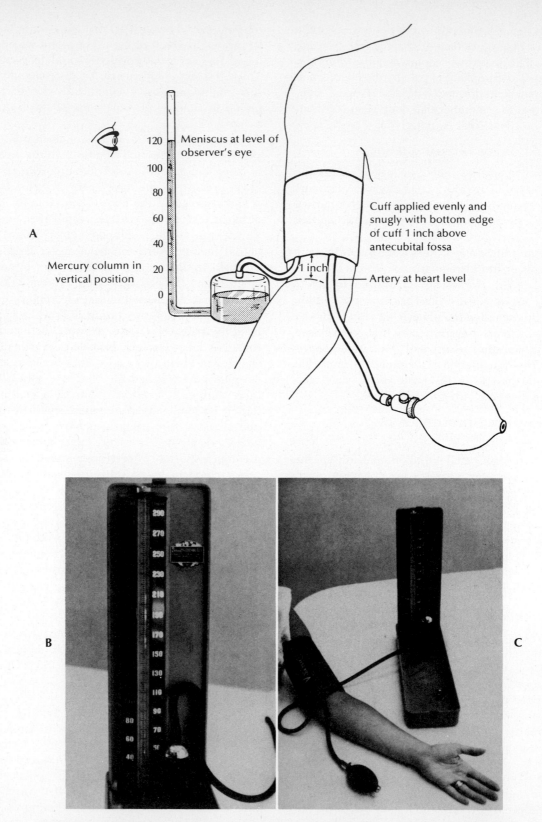

Fig. 7-19. A, Mercury gravity manometer (diagrammatic). **B,** Mercury manometer. **C,** Mercury sphygmomanometer applied to client. (**A** from Burch, G. E., and DePasquale, N. P.: Primer of clinical measurement of blood pressure, St. Louis, 1962, The C. V. Mosby Co. **B** and **C** reproduced with permission from *Blood pressure measurement: a handbook for instructors,* © 1979, Chicago Heart Association.)

The most commonly used method of indirect assessment of blood pressure is the auscultatory technique. For the procedure a sphygmomanometer and a stethoscope are used.

The two types of sphygmomanometers used in the assessment of arterial blood pressure are the mercury gravity and the aneroid instruments. Each instrument includes a pressure manometer, and inflatable rubber bladder encased in a cloth cuff, and a rubber hand bulb with a pressure control valve.

The air distensible bladder encased in the cloth cuff is used to occlude an artery. The cuff is long enough to encircle the extremity and be fastened securely in place. The covering cuff must be made of an elastic material so that pressure will be applied evenly to the limb.

The mercury gravity manometer (Fig. 7-19) is made up of a straight glass tube connected to reservoir of mercury. The reservoir in turn is connected to the pressure bulb, so that pressure created on the bulb causes the mercury to rise in the tube. Because the weight of mercury is dependent on gravity, a given amount of pressure will always support a column of mercury of the same height, given the tube is straight and of uniform diameter. The mercury manometer does not need further calibration after the initial setting.

The aneroid sphygmomanometer (Fig. 7-20) is made up of a metal bellows connected to the compression cuff. Changes in pressure within the apparatus cause the bellows to expand and collapse. The movement of the bellows rotates a gear that moves a pointer across the calibrated dial. The aneroid sphygmomanometer is calibrated against a mercury manometer, since the more complex mechanisms have been shown to need frequent adjustment. This is simply done by using a connecting Y tube between the manometers.

Measurement of blood pressure by palpation. The brachial artery is palpated below the cuff, and the cuff is inflated to 30 mm Hg beyond the point at which the pulse is obliterated. The air pressure in the bladder is released at a rate of 2 to 3 mm Hg per heartbeat, and systemic blood pressure is recorded

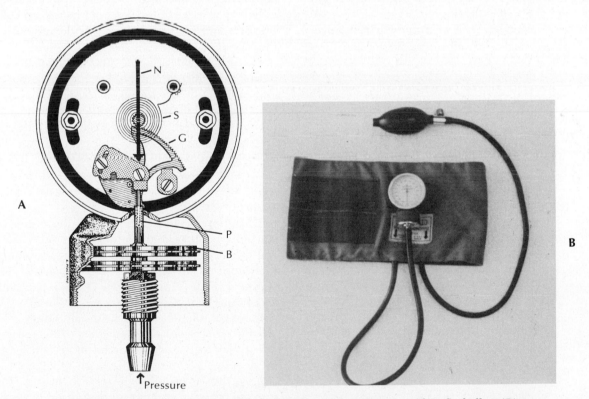

Fig. 7-20. A, Aneroid sphygmomanometer (diagrammatic). Variations within the bellow *(B)* activate a pin *(P)*, which sets a gear *(G)* into motion. The gear, in turn, operates the spring *(S)*, which causes the needle *(N)* to move across the face of a calibrated dial. **B,** Aneroid sphygmomanometer. (**A** from Burch, G. E., and DePasquale, N. P.: Primer of clinical measurement of blood pressure, St. Louis, 1962, The C. V. Mosby Co. **B,** Reproduced with permission from *Blood pressure measurement: a handbook for instructors,* © 1979, Chicago Heart Association.)

at the point at which pulsations first become palpable. The diastolic pressure is said to coincide with the cessation of vibrations in the artery. The diastolic value is difficult to obtain. In a test situation, more than 79% of the values obtained were within ±4 mm Hg of those obtained by auscultatory procedures.

Auscultatory method of arterial blood pressure assessment. When the cuff is properly placed on the limb, the arterial blood can flow past the cuff only when arterial pressure exceeds that in the cuff. Partial obstruction of arterial blood flow disturbs the laminar flow pattern, creating turbulence. This turbulence produces sounds called Korotkoff sounds and can be heard over arteries distal to the cuff through a stethoscope (Fig. 7-21).

The bell of the stethoscope is more effective than the diaphragm in transmitting the low-frequency Korotkoff sounds. The bell is applied snugly over the artery; care is taken not to press hard enough to close the artery.

The deflated cuff is applied, without wrinkles, snugly around the upper arm so that the edge of the cuff is 2 to 3 cm above the site at which the bell of the stethoscope is to be placed. The artery is palpated, and the cuff is inflated at a rate of 12 to 20 mm Hg per second to a peak of 30 mm Hg higher than the point at which the pulse was obliterated. The

cuff is then deflated at a rate of 2 to 3 mm Hg per heartbeat. The level of the meniscus of the mercury column at which the Korotkoff sounds are changed is noted.

The *systolic blood pressure* is recorded for that point at which the Korotkoff sounds are initially heard. This is also the beginning of *phase 1*, which starts with faint, clear, and rhythmic tapping or thumping noises that gradually increase in intensity. At this point the intraluminal pressure is the same as the cuff pressure but not great enough to produce a radial pulse.

Phase 2 is characterized by a murmur or swishing sound heard as the vessel distends with blood, creating eddies and producing vibration of the vessel wall. *Phase 3* is the period during which the sounds are crisper and more intense. In this phase the vessel remains open in systole but obliterated in diastole.

The *muffling* of the Korotkoff sounds is the guidepost for the beginning of *phase 4* and the pressure at this point is believed by many authorities to be the closest to the *diastolic arterial pressure* measured by a direct method. At this point the cuff pressure falls below the intraluminal pressure. It is frequently called the first diastolic pressure. The second diastolic pressure and *phase 5* are said to be present when the Korotkoff sounds are no longer heard. Phase 5 marks the period wherein the vessel remains open during the entire cycle.

If muffling of the Korotkoff sounds is established as indicative of diastolic level, the value will be about 8 mm Hg greater than that obtained by the direct method.

Disappearance of the Korotkoff sounds is a risky criterion for diastolic pressure, since the sounds do not abate in some individuals until a pressure well below the diastolic value is reached.

Thus, three values are recorded: the systolic pressure, the point of muffling of the Korotkoff sounds, and the disappearance of the sounds. An example of the record might be 120/78/54. This method has the approval of the World Health Organization and the American Heart Association.

Korotkoff sounds may be heard all the way to zero on the sphygmomanometer scale. This occurs frequently in normal children and in certain hyperdynamic states such as the aftermath to vigorous exercise, in thyrotoxicosis, or in severe anemia. In this case the pressure at the beginning of phase 4 is noted and recorded as well as a description of sound heard to 0 mm Hg.

CUFF SIZE. If the cuff is too narrow, the blood pressure reading will be erroneously high. A wide cuff increases the risk of an erroneously low reading.

The sphygmomanometer cuff should be 20% to

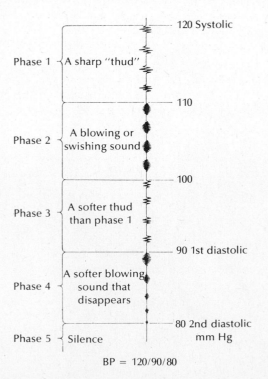

Fig. 7-21. Phases of the Korotkoff sounds. (From Burch, G. E., and DePasquale, N. P.: Primer of clinical measurement of blood pressure, St. Louis, 1962, The C. V. Mosby Co.)

25% wider than the diameter of the extremity in which the blood pressure is being taken. Another recommendation is that the bladder width be equal to two-fifths of the circumference of the limb. A more liberal approximation suggests that the cuff should cover two-thirds of the upper arm. Ideally, the bladder should completely encircle the extremity and should be snugly applied. Cuffs may be obtained in the following sizes:

> 2.5 × 22.5 cm (neonate)
> 5 × 22.5 cm (toddler)
> 7 × 22.5 cm (1 year to 4 years)
> 9 × 22.5 cm (4 years to 8 years)
> 13 × 22.5 cm (standard adult)
> 14 × 40   cm (obese arm)
> 17.5 × 35   cm (thigh cuff and markedly obese arm)

Caution: The cuff size is determined by the diameter of the limb, not the age of the client.

The examiner's eye must be at a direct line with the level of the meniscus of the mercury column to avoid parallax error, and the mercury column must be kept in a vertical position.

The cuff should be deflated completely (0 mm Hg) between successive readings. At least a 15-second interval is allowed between readings, with the cuff completely deflated, to avoid spurious readings due to venous congestion.

The bladder and the pressure bulbs should be monitored for leaks. Erratic inflation or deflation usually indicates a leak.

MEASUREMENT OF BLOOD PRESSURE IN THE LEG. The blood pressure in the leg may be measured with the client in either the supine or prone position. The Korotkoff sounds are evaluated over the popliteal artery.

In the popliteal artery the systolic arterial blood pressure is higher (10 ± 5 mm Hg) than in the brachial artery, whereas the diastolic pressure is generally lower. This difference is magnified in aortic insufficiency and in some hyperdynamic states such as after exercise.

INCREASING AUDIBILITY OF THE KOROTKOFF SOUNDS IN INFANTS AND THE FLUSH TEST. Occasionally the Korotkoff sounds are not heard over the brachial artery in infants. A suggestion for making the sounds audible is to hold the infant's arm upright for 1 to 2 minutes with the cuff in place. The pressure is measured immediately on lowering the arm.

In the event that the Korotkoff sounds cannot be obtained, a flush pressure that approximates the mean blood pressure may be measured in the upper or lower extremity. The procedure for this test is as follows: The properly sized cuff is placed around the infant's wrist or ankle. An elasticized bandage is placed around the extremity distal to the cuff to promote vascular emptying. The bladder pressure of the sphygmomanometer is raised to approximately 150 mm Hg. The bandage is removed, and the cuff pressure is decreased at a rate of 2 to 3 mm Hg per heartbeat until a vascular flush (rubor) is observed. The appearance of the flush is correlated with the sphygmomanometer reading.

AUSCULTATORY GAP. Occasionally, as the pneumatic cuff is being deflated, the Korotkoff sounds disappear and then are heard 10 to 15 mm Hg later. This is called auscultatory gap. The examiner records systolic blood pressure at the onset of the first sound. Thus, the auscultatory gap will not be cause for error if the cuff was inflated to 20 mm Hg above the point at which the artery was occluded as determined by palpation.

Normal systolic and diastolic pressures. The systolic blood pressure shows a normal range of 95 to 140 mm Hg; 120 mm Hg is cited as average (when measured in the brachial artery).

Normal diastolic pressure ranges from 60 to 90 mm Hg; 80 mm Hg is average.

The systolic blood pressure in the neonatal period has a normal range of 20 to 60 mm Hg but then gradually increases until adolescence, when an accelerated rise is incurred. Thus, at about 17 or 18 years, blood pressure reaches adult levels.

The proper application of the auscultatory method yields values that are within ±4 to 5 mm Hg of the direct method of measurement.

Normal variations in blood pressure recordings. The blood pressure in a normal individual varies continually with respiration, autonomic state, emotional levels, and biological rhythms. Furthermore, successive readings of indirect measures of blood pressure by the same or different observers may differ by as much as 10 mm Hg.

In the normal individual, the *change from a supine to an erect position* causes a slight decrease in systolic blood pressure (less than 15 mm Hg) as well as in diastolic (less than 5 mm Hg) pressure. Marked drops in pressure (greater than 30 mm Hg) incurred when the individual stands may be indicative of a vasopressor defect or of hypovolemia.

The blood pressure also shows a *24-hour, or circadian, pattern.* Consistent with the other vital signs, the blood pressure has higher values in the afternoon and evening hours and lower values in the late hours of sleep.

Because blood pressure is readily altered by *stressful events,* an effort should be made to relax the client as much as possible before taking the blood pressure.

Food and exercise also affect the blood pressure. It is recommended that the individual should not eat or exercise in the 30 minutes before the determination is made. The extremity should be at heart level for a period of approximately 5 minutes.

Differences in blood pressure indicating disease. The initial examination of blood pressure should include a measurement in both arms and one from the leg. Differences in blood pressure between the two arms may be caused by aortic stenosis or by obstruction of the arteries of the upper arm.

Constriction or obstruction of the aorta may be suspected when the pressure assessed in the client's arms exceeds that in the legs, particularly when the differences are great.

Coarctation of the aorta must be suspected when the brachial pressure markedly exceeds that of the popliteal artery. This reversal of gradient may also accompany other obstructive lesions of the aorta or obstructive lesions in proximal arteries of the leg.

Assessment of pulsus paradoxus. Arterial blood pressure in normal human beings is known to vary as much as 10 mm Hg during relaxed respiration. The decrease with respiration may be 10 ± 5 mm Hg, whereas on inspiration a proportionate increase is noted. A difference greater than 15 mm Hg is indicative of pulsus parodoxus. These fluctuations may be more accurately assessed by allowing the cuff to deflate very slowly.

Assessment of pulsus alternans. Although the presence of pulsus alternans may be determined from palpation of the pulse, it may be more accurately assessed through the use of the sphygmomanometer. The cuff is inflated to 20 mm Hg above the systolic pressure as determined via palpation. On deflation to phase 1, only alternate beats are heard. Later all beats are audible and palpable. After still further deflation all beats are of equal intensity. The difference between this point and the peak systolic level is often used in determining the degree of pulsus alternans.

Pulse pressure. The pulse pressure is the difference between systolic and diastolic pressure. The normal value is generally 30 to 40 mm Hg. The heart rate may influence the pulse pressure. With a slowly beating heart the period of flow or "runoff" from the aorta to the periphery is lengthened, lowering the diastolic pressure. The net result is an increase in pulse pressure.

A wide pulse pressure accompanied by bradycardia frequently indicates increased intracranial pressure. The pulse pressure is also increased in hyperkinetic states such as hyperthyroidism or after vigorous exercise. Although the stroke volume may be greater, rapid runoff may result in low diastolic recordings.

With increased peripheral resistance, runoff to the peripheral circulation is less; thus, more blood accumulates in the aorta, and both systolic and diastolic blood pressure increase.

A small stroke volume will tend to decrease the pulse pressure.

HYPERTENSION AND HYPOTENSION

Hypertension. The World Health Organization defines hypertension as a persistent elevation of blood pressure greater than 140/90. The American Heart Association recommends that 160/95 be the defining point for hypertension in the client over 40 years of age. Elevation of either systolic or diastolic blood pressure is an indication for further diagnostic tests.

If the definition of hypertension in the adult is accepted as a diastolic pressure in excess of 90 mm Hg, then about 15% of whites and 30% of blacks in the United States have hypertension. One study estimated that one-half of these persons have not been identified.

The structures most frequently observed to suffer damage as peripheral resistance is increased are the heart, the kidneys, and the brain. Vessel changes are best observed in the retina. Sclerosis, hemorrhage, and exudates typify the alterations seen in hypertension.

The incidence of cardiovascular accident (CVA) is increased by high pressure in the vessels in the brain.

Increased cardiac work is required to pump the blood against the increased peripheral resistance. Thus, congestive heart failure, left ventricular hypertrophy, or angina pectoris may result from hypertension.

The examiner must bear in mind other signs and symptoms that accompany hypertension. These might include severe headache, blurred vision, and signs of renal disease.

CLINICAL ASSESSMENT OF HYPERTENSION IN CHILDREN. Although it is accepted that the routine measurement of blood pressure in all children from newborn through adolescence is imperative to the diagnosis of hypertension, this practice is frequently neglected. The screening examination may yield an incidence of hypertension of approximately 2.3% in children 4 to 15 years of age. Early detection of these hypertensive children may mean that diagnosis and treatment may be initiated in time to prevent the sequelae of the underlying disease process. It has been shown that 90% of adults are subject to essential or idiopathic hypertension, whereas this is true only for 20% of children. The blood pressure is recorded each time the child is seen and is considered with other developmental data.

Hypertension is said to exist in children when either the systolic or diastolic blood pressure is greater than the ninety-fifth percentile for age, that is, two standard deviations above the mean. Fig. 7-22 shows the range of blood pressures obtained in children.

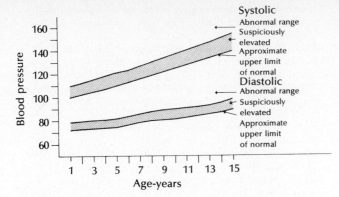

Fig. 7-22. Range of blood pressures measured in children. (From Gruskin, A.: Clinical evaluation of hypertension in children, Primary Care **1:**233, 1974.)

The blood pressure as measured by Doppler technique has demonstrated that blood pressure rises rapidly from between 4 days and 6 weeks and then remains reasonably stable until the first year. The ninety-fifth percentile for blood pressure between 6 weeks and 6 years is about 115 mm Hg. Note the progressive increase in blood pressure that is incurred from 1 year to age 15.

The observation of a brachial blood pressure of 150 mm Hg or more may be indicative of secondary hypertension resulting from renal or endocrine disease or coarctation of the aorta. Coarctation of aorta is also suspected when the blood pressure in the arms exceeds that in the legs by 30 mm Hg. The normal difference in the infant is that the brachial blood pressure is 17 ± 10 mm Hg greater than in the legs.

The findings of an elevated blood pressure in the pediatric client alert the examiner to look for indications of hypertensive encephalopathy (hyperactivity, excitability, and fundal changes).

Hypotension. Hypotension has been defined as a persistent blood pressure less than 95/60.

Hypotension in the absence of other signs or symptoms is generally innocent. In fact, lower blood pressures may be considered beneficial because the heart does not have to pump as hard to circulate the blood. The blood pressure must be high enough to assure an adequate blood supply to the kidneys, brain, and other body tissues.

However, sudden changes in blood pressure may produce changes in body function. Sudden drops in normal blood pressure may result in fainting. This is observed in orthostatic hypotension. In this case, the blood pressure may be normal when the individual is reclining but drops when the individual rises to a sitting or standing position, particularly when the position change is a rapid one. Faintness and dizziness from orthostatic hypotension is common in individuals who have been confined to bed or have diseases of the nervous system.

Blood pressure drops may also follow severe injury, hemorrhage, and endotoxin-producing infections. In hypovolemic or in endotoxic shock, the Korotkoff sounds will be less audible or absent. Since the peripheral blood pressure is an important parameter for determining the method of treatment, ultrasonic direct or invasive techniques of blood pressure assessment may be used. Some other signs of shock might include increased pulse and respiratory rates, dizziness, confusion, blurred vision, diaphoresis, and cold and clammy skin.

Respiratory rate, volume, and rhythm assessment are described in Chapter 13 on assessment of the respiratory system.

BIBLIOGRAPHY

Atkins, E., and Bodel, P.: Fever, N. Engl. J. Med. **286:**27, 1972.

Barnhorst, D. A., and Barner, H. B.: Prevalence of congenitally absent pedal pulses, N. Engl. J. Med. **278:**264, 1969.

Blood pressure measurement: a handbook for instructors, Chicago, 1979, Chicago Heart Association.

deSwiet, M., and others: Blood pressure in infancy. In Harper, P., and Muir, J., editors: Advanced medicine, 15, Bath, England, 1979, Pitman Press.

Draper, G., Dupertuis, C., and Caughey, J., Jr.: Human constitution in clinical medicine, New York, 1944, P. B. Hoeber, Inc.

DuBois, E. F.: Heat loss from the human body, Harvey Lecture, Bull. N.Y. Acad. Med. **15:**143, 1939.

DuBois, E. F.: Fever and the regulation of body temperature, Publ. No. 13, American Lecture Series, Springfield, Ill., 1948, Charles C Thomas, Publisher.

DuBois, E. F.: The many different temperatures of the human body and its parts, West. J. Surg. **59:**476, 1951.

Folk, C. E.: Temperature regulation. In Folk, G. E., editor: Textbook of environmental physiology, Philadelphia, 1974, Lea & Febiger.

Fowler, N. O.: Inspection and palpation of venous and arterial pulses, New York, 1970, American Heart Association.

Garn, S. M.: Types and distribution of hair on man, Ann. N.Y. Acad. Sci. **53:**498, 1951.

Garrison, G. E., Floyd, W. L., and Orgain, E. S.: Exercise and the physical examination of peripheral arterial disease, Ann. Intern Med. **66:**587, 1967.

Geddes, L. A.: The direct and indirect measurement of blood pressure, Chicago, 1970, Year Book Medical Publishers, Inc.

Gold, J. J.: Hirsutism and virilism. In Gold, J. J., editor: Gynecologic endocrinology, New York, 1975, Harper & Row, Publishers.

Gruskin, A.: Clinical evaluation of hypertension in children, Primary Care **1:**233, 1974.

Hochberg, H. M., and Salomon, H.: Accuracy of an ultrasound blood monitor, Curr. Ther. Res. **13:**129, 1971.

Hurst, J. W., editor: The heart, ed. 4, New York, 1974, McGraw-Hill Book Co.

Karvenen, N. J., Telivuo, L. J., and Jarvinen, E. J.: Sphygmomanometer cuff size and accuracy of indirect measurement of blood pressure, Am. J. Cardiol. **13:**688, 1964.

King, G. E.: Errors in clinical measurement of blood pressure in obesity, Clin. Sci. **32:**233, 1967.

King, G. E.: Taking the blood pressure, J.A.M.A. **209:**1902, 1969.

Leon, M., and others: Biosynthesis of testosterone by a Stein-Leventhal ovary, Acta Endocrinol. **39:**411, 1962.

Londe, S.: Blood pressure in children as determined under office conditions, Clin. Pediatr. **5:**71, 1966.

Londe, S., and others: Hypertension in apparently normal children, J. Pediatr. **78:**569, 1971.

McCutcheon, E. P., and Rushmer, R. F.: Korotkoff sounds, Circ. Res. **20:**149, 1967.

McGregor, M.: Pulsus paradoxus, N. Engl. J. Med. **301**(9):480, 1979.

Meninger, K.: A psychiatrist's world; the selected papers of Karl Meninger, M.D., New York, 1959, The Viking Press, Inc.

Nichols, G. A.: Taking adult temperatures; rectal measurement, Am. J. Nurs. **72:**1092, 1972.

Nichols, G. A., and Kucha, D. H.: Taking adult temperatures; oral measurements, Am. J. Nurs. **72:**1090, 1972.

O'Rourke, M. F.: The arterial pulse in health and disease, Am. Heart J. **82:**687, 1971.

Recommendations for human blood pressure determination by sphygmomanometer, New York, 1967, American Heart Association.

Roaf, R.: Posture, New York, 1977, Academic Press, Inc.

Simpson, J. A., and others: Effect of size of cuff bladder on accuracy of measurement of direct blood pressure, Am. Heart J. **70:**208, 1965.

Sphygmomanometers; principles and precepts, Copiague, N.Y., 1965, W. A. Baum Co.

Ur, A., and Gordon, M.: Origin of Korotkoff sounds, Am. J. Physiol. **218:**524, 1970.

Williams, R.: Textbook of endocrinology, Philadelphia, 1974, W. B. Saunders Co.

Wu, R.: Behavior and illness, Englewood Cliffs, N.J., 1973, Prentice-Hall, Inc.

8 Assessment of mental status

The major focus of the mental status examination is the identification of the individual's strengths and capabilities. While it is important to detect the weaknesses and maladaptations that hamper daily living, the examiner must assess the individual's resources for environmental and social adjustment. The information to be obtained includes educational development, occupation, economic status, marital status, responsibilities for the family, stresses in living, and goals toward which the client is striving.

The objective of the mental status examination is to assess those thoughts or mental processes that interfere with the individual's ability to reach optimal level of function. Thus, the examiner is alert to behaviors that may interfere with happiness, life satisfaction, or social adjustment. The examiner further seeks to understand the origin of those behaviors and the development of them to the present time. The developmental history plays an essential role in the mental status examination. The three categories of information assessment include the individual, his experience, and socioeconomic factors. From a *neurological viewpoint* the examiner is assessing *cerebral function.*

The interview is the initial and most important tool in health assessment for obtaining data about the client's behavior and interactions with his environment. While the client's self-report may not be entirely factual, the client's report and/or those of significant others are often the only data base available to the examiner from which to analyze the client's behavior.

The interview is a richer source of behavioral data than questionnaires or interactive computer methods. The examiner has a good deal more flexibility, such as being able to devote more time to exploring specific areas of importance to the client. In addition, the interviewer has the advantage of being able to observe the client's nonverbal behaviors.

The method of interviewing most frequently observed, that is, eliciting feelings and facts for the history, is a combination of asking questions and waiting while appearing alert and interested as the client provides the answers in his own language. This method allows for an observation of awareness, cognitive function, and affect. The questions asked the client are aimed at obtaining more data about symptoms, family and medical history, the parameters of the client's life situation, and an evaluation of his support systems.

The choice of words used to describe behavior during the interview should be carefully selected. The interviewer would do well to avoid words that are semantically unacceptable to the client. For instance, the individual may find it acceptable to be termed hypersensitive but not irritable, or meticulous but not compulsive.

The record should be kept as simple and direct as possible; hazy terminology should be avoided. Words such as *anxious, cheerful,* and *suspicious* are loaded words, fraught with individual variation in connotation. They mean different things to different readers. A more meaningful record describes observations of appearance and behaviors of the client.

The appraisal of mental status is a process that may be built into the interview and the physical examination. However, the client who demonstrates dysfunction in affect or thought processes may indicate further exploration.

In assessing the mental status of the client, the examiner usually deals with symptoms—the thought processes or behavior and how the client feels about them. Some signs may be available, such as behavior that is disturbing to others. The examiner elicits the evolutionary history of the client's complaints and makes his own observations. Because what the client reports may change with each examination and because the client's words may have different connotations for different examiners, it is difficult to obtain agreement in the terminology of the assessment of behavioral symptoms. The most helpful record is one that describes the *client's behaviors and words accurately and succinctly.*

A full mental status examination is indicated when loss of memory or aphasia are encountered in the client.

The only materials that may be helpful in the examination of mental status are a pencil, paper, and a newspaper.

PHYSICAL APPEARANCE AND BEHAVIOR

The examiner carefully observes the client's physical appearance, manner of dress, facial expression, and body posture as a measure of mental function. In essence, assessment of neural status will be the composite of the way the client looks, acts, and feels. (See also Chapter 7 on general assessment.)

Assessment of motor behavior—movement
POSTURE AND BEHAVIOR

The posture is important in providing clues to the client's feelings. The client who walks slowly into the room, barely lifting his feet, and who slumps in the chair while avoiding the examiner's glance may be eloquently describing a lack of affect or depression. On the other hand, the person who bounds into the room, energetically shaking the examiner's hand while rapidly glancing around the room may be demonstrating significant overreaction. The tense muscles and furrowed forehead or the furtive, darting eyes, coupled with the wet handshake of the individual with anxiety should alert the examiner to look for further symptoms to corroborate this impression. With each interchange the speed and appropriateness of reaction are evaluated.

General coordination of movement may be assessed through observation of the gait. To assess the complex acts of coordination, the examiner may give the client simple phrases to write and simple geometric figures to draw. The client is asked to draw more fundamental figures such as a circle, square, or triangle followed by more complex figures such as a house or flower.

GROOMING AND APPAREL

Failure of the client to give attention to personal cleanliness is a clue to underlying emotional problems. Thus, dirty hair or a dirty body, uncombed hair, or unkempt nails warrant further exploration. The nails are examined for evidence of nail biting by the client. The female client with carelessly or bizarrely applied cosmetics should also be examined further. (On the other hand, lack of makeup may have no significance, since the client may have an allergy to the chemicals in cosmetics or her makeup may look so natural that it is not detected by the examiner.

What is looked for in the behaviors is a pattern.) The clothing is examined to determine its appropriateness to the occasion (place, time) and the client's position in life. Bright yellow and red have been associated with euphoria, whereas drab olive green and black have been associated with depression. Attention is given to the amount and type of jewelry worn by the client. The sexual impression conveyed by the clothing may also have diagnostic value. The female client who appears dressed in masculine clothing with closely cropped hair may be giving a message of her sexual identity (or may just be exhibiting the unisex nature of dress popular in the 1970s).

SPEECH

The manner of speech may give clues of the status of thought processes. Comprehension of and ability to use the spoken language may be readily assessed during the interview and the assessment procedure. The answers to the examiner's questions and the ability to follow instructions ("Change into this gown," "Please sit on this chair") give valuable data about the client's comprehension and willingness to cooperate.

The nature of responses to the examiner's questions is important. The normal individual answers questions frankly. Failure to answer a question, circumlocution, or other evasive replies should be noted. Criticism given to the examiner by the client and whether the client talks up or down to the examiner may be recorded.

Rapid-fire conversation should be noted as well as slow and halting delivery. The client who monopolizes the interview should also be noted. Slow monotonous speech is characteristic of parkinsonism. The client, just as the professional, chooses the words he feels best suited to his companion of the moment. In addition, the words chosen by the client usually give a good idea of his general intelligence, educational level, social level, and level of functioning.

Articulation is assessed. This includes fluency, ease of expression, rhythm, hesitancies, stuttering, and repetitiousness. The omission or addition of letters, syllables, and words, or their transposition, and the misuse of words suggest aphasia. In addition, the client may be observed to practice circumlocution or to attempt to express his thoughts nonverbally (pantomime) in order not to reveal that he has forgotten a word. Repetitious, abnormal thought patterns revealed in speech are recorded. These would include neologisms, verbigeration, or echolalia.

Disorders of the structures responsible for speech may be evident during conversation with the client. These include:

1. *Dysphonia:* Difficulty or discomfort in making laryngeal speech sounds, such as hoarseness. *Dysphonia puberum* is difficulty in controlling laryngeal speech sounds that occur as the larynx enlarges in puberty.

2. *Dysarthria:* Difficulty in articulating single sounds or phonemes of speech; individual letters (*f, g, r*); labials—sounds produced with the lips (*b, m, w,* rounded vowels) (cranial nerve [CN] VII); gutterals—sound produced in the throat (CN X); and linguals—sounds produced with the tongue (*l, t, n*) (CN XII). Dysarthria may be demonstrated by asking the client to repeat a phrase such as "Methodist Episcopal" or by asking him to read a short paragraph containing all of these letters.

Clinical indications of aphasia involving speech

Hesitations
Omission or addition of letters, syllables, or words
Substitution of words with inappropriate implication
Circumlocution
Neologism
Using some words again and again—lack of variety in vocabulary
Use of nonverbal language to substitute for a word
Syntactical error (disturbance of balance or rhythm of words in sequence); can write better than speak
Semantic errors (inability to interpret metaphors, the connotation of words)
Severe aphasia:
  Inability to speak
  Repetition of single word or phrase

Table 8-1. Classification of aphasias

Type of aphasia	Site of lesion	Speech or language disorder
Broca's aphasia (expressive speaking)	Left inferior third frontal convolution (Broca's area) (Fig. 8-1)	Nonfluent Agrammatical Difficulty in finding words to no oral expression skills—apraxia Writing generally impaired Comprehension retained
Wernicke's aphasia (auditory receptive)	Posterior portion superior temporal gyrus Part of second temporal gyrus	Normal to hyperfluent Emphasis on verbs Neologism Jargon Jibberish Impaired auditory comprehension Does not recognize his own speech errors Difficulty in repeating phrases after the examiner
Global	Diffuse, large lesion May involve both Broca's and Wernicke's areas	Language skills inconsistent Recurrent repetition of phrases—fluent
Anomia	Area of angular gyrus	Fluent Grammatical Reduced rate due to difficulty in finding words Pauses Circumlocution Impaired comprehension of isolated nouns and verbs General auditory comprehension retained
Transcortical sensory	Lesion isolating angular gyrus from the remainder of brain	Echos interviewer's speech Does not initiate speech Increased ability to preserve and recite memorized material Markedly impaired reading and writing
Transcortical motor	Frontal lobe, anterior to Broca's area	Does not initiate speech No spontaneous speech—short answers to questions Repetition intact Comprehension preserved

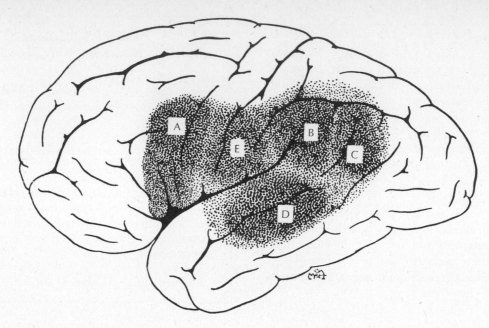

Fig. 8-1. Aphasic zone of the left cerebral hemisphere. Neurological deficits include: *A*, Middle and inferior frontal gyri and lower precentral gyrus: anarthria, alexia, contralateral facial weakness. *B*, Supramarginal gyrus: generalized aphasia, hemianesthesia, hemianopia. *C*, Angular gyrus: aphasia with reading disturbance, quadrantanopia, hemiplegia, hemianesthesia. *D*, Posterior superior and middle temporal gyri: sensory aphasia, paraphasia, jargon aphasia. *E*, Includes island of Reil: severe aphasia, anarthria, right hemiplegia. (Modified from Bailey: Intracranial tumors, Springfield, Ill., 1933, Charles C Thomas Publisher.)

3. *Dysprosody:* Difficulty in speech such that inflection, pronunciation, pitch, and rhythm are impaired.

Aphasia. Aphasia is a general term for a dysfunction or loss of ability to express thoughts by speech, writing, symbols, or signs or to interpret sensory input (Table 8-1). These disorders are due to lesions of the brain. The term aphasia excludes those disturbances of expression related to pathology of neurons to the muscles of speech, disorders of the anatomical structures that participate in the production of speech and mental deficiency. Aphasia encompasses *agnosia*, the impaired ability to recognize once-familiar objects, and *apraxia*, the impaired ability to carry out purposeful activity related to language. The most common cerebral pathology associated with aphasia is vascular in origin. While the cerebral hemispheres share equal responsibility in controlling the two sides of the body in general, language requires the simultaneous input of both and is controlled by one. The hemisphere in which language is controlled is called the dominant hemisphere. It has been shown that 95% of these individuals who are right-handed and have a language deficit have lesions of the left cerebral hemisphere, while 70% of left-handed individuals with language impairment have a lesion of the left cerebral hemisphere.

Aphasia may be evaluated during the initial inter-

Table 8-2. Speech types that may be retained in aphasia

Speech type	Description of speech type
Emotional speech	Swearing, exclamations, oaths
Automatic speech	Nursery rhymes, poems, other series of words learned in early life, days of the week
Singing	Singing may be possible while speech is not

view with the client. The ability of the client to comprehend auditory verbal stimuli may be tested against the client's ability to answer questions and carry out instructions. Visual verbal ability is assessed from the client's ability to read and to explain the content he has read. Further data may be obtained by asking the client to identify familiar objects or geometric figures.

The client may be able to express himself in some forms of speech when his free-flowing conversational speech is impaired. Some of these are included in Table 8-2.

Agnosia. Agnosia is a general term for the dysfunction or loss of ability to interpret sensory stimuli. These disorders have been termed receptive aphasia. Individuals with visual agnosia have the primary reception of the visual image but are unable to associate

Table 8-3. Test for agnosia

Type	Description	Test	Site of lesion
Olfactory	Inability to recognize once-familiar smells	Identify volatile, easily recognized substances: Coffee Vanilla Oil of lemon	Prepiriform lobe
Visual	Inability to recognize once-familiar colors	Identify: color, geometric figures, pictures, sides of body, parts of body	Occipital and adjacent parietal lobe
Auditory	Inability to recognize once-familiar tones, music, sounds	Identify: musical melody, ringing of bell	Temporal lobe—lateral and superior and adjacent to parietal lobe (Wernicke's area)
Tactile	Inability to recognize once-familiar objects by feeling them (stereognosis)	Identify object held in hand such as: coins, key, comb	Superior parietal lobe
Body parts	Inability to recognize body part (somatopaganosia) or to determine laterality (individual may ignore or not use the part)	Identify body parts by name as right or left	Posteroinferior parietal lobe

the previous experience that allows interpretation of what is being viewed. Specific cerebral cortical regions make it possible for the individual to recognize visual, auditory, and tactile stimuli. Testing for tactile interpretation is a part of the sensory examination of the neurological examination.

Apraxia. Comprehension is normal in apraxia. *Ideational apraxia* is the term for dysfunction or loss of ability to formulate the ideational concepts necessary to carry out a skilled motor act. The individual is unable to conceive the idea or retain it. This disability accompanies diffuse cerebral disorders, for example, arteriosclerosis.

Motor apraxia is decline of kinesthetic motor patterns necessary to a motor act. This disability may be related to a lesion of the precentral gyrus.

Ideomotor apraxia is the term that is used to define the situation in which an individual has lost the skills for a given complex act but may retain conditioned habits. These old patterns may be performed repetitiously (perseverance). This may be dissociated with disease of the supramarginal gyrus of the parietal lobe on the dominant side of the brain. Apraxias not related to language are tested at the time of the neurological assessment (Table 8-3).

ABILITY TO WRITE

The client may be asked to write his name or address or may be allowed to write whatever he likes. As with verbal expression, aphasia may be indicated by the omission or addition of letters, syllables, or words. Mirror writing has been interpreted as a symptom of dysfunction related to cerebral dominance. A recently completed letter or other example of writing by the client may give valuable information regarding his thought processes. Agraphia is the term used to describe a disturbance in writing. When agraphia is the only symptom present, it may be the result of a cerebral lesion of the second frontal convolution or the region of the angular gyrus and occipital lobe.

Sensorium

The sensorium is assessed for consciousness, orientation, attention span, recent and remote memory, insight, and judgment.

STATE OF CONSCIOUSNESS, AWARENESS

The first step in the evaluation of the client's sensorium is the determination of the state of consciousness, that is, the individual's awareness and responsiveness to his life's experiences.

Consciousness may be regarded as the individual's awareness of the stimuli from his environment and within himself. Clinical appraisal is more reliable for assessing the awareness of the client to external variables, since these can be checked against the examiner's impressions. However, the client may give a very informative discussion of his internal feelings.

The levels of conscious perception are thought to be a function of the conscious ego. The awareness of self and environment, which is called consciousness, may be affected by the nature and the amplitude of the stimuli received by the individual. Thus, the awareness of feelings and reactions have been de-

Table 8-4. Levels of consciousness (responsiveness)

	Behaviors
Conscious	Appropriate response (rate and quality) to external and internal stimuli
	Oriented to *time, place,* and *person*
Confusion	Inappropriate response to stimuli and decrease in attention span and memory
	Reactions to simple commands may be retained
Lethargy (hypersomnia)	Drowsiness or increased sleeping time
	Can be aroused responds appropriately
	May fall immediately asleep again
Delirium	Confusion associated with disordered perception and decreased attention span, motor and sensory excitement
	Reactions to stimuli are inappropriate
	May have marked anxiety
Coma	Loss or lowering of consciousness
Stage I (stupor)	Arousable for short periods to verbal, visual, or painful stimuli
	Simple motor and verbal response to stimuli (shutting eyes, protruding tongue)
	Responses slow
	Corneal and pupillary reflexes sluggish
	Deep tendon reflexes and superficial reflexes unaffected
	Pathological reflexes may be obtained
Stage II (light coma)	Simple motor and verbal (moaning) response to painful stimuli
	Motor response generally flexion (avoidance) or mass movement
Stage III (deep coma)	Decerebrate posturing to painful stimuli (extension of body and limbs and pronation of arms)
Stage IV	Muscles flaccid
	Eyes do not react to light
	Apneic; on ventilator
	Superficial and some spinal reflexes (deep tendon reflexes) may be present
Brain death	Two EEG tracings 24 hours apart indicate absence of brain waves ⎫
	Cerebral function absent 24 hours ⎬ All must be present
	Expert opinion rules out hypothermia or drug toxicity ⎭
Syncope	Temporary loss of consciousness (partial or complete) associated with increased rate of respiration, tachycardia, pallor, perspiration, coolness of skin
Fugue state	Dysfunction of consciousness (hours or days) wherein the individual carries on purposeful activity that he does not remember (afterward)
Amnesia	Memory loss over a period of time or for specific subjects
	Individual affected responds appropriately to external stimuli

scribed to be different for those excluded from external stimuli and reacting to signals from the self only; that is, for those individuals with perceptual deprivation. Consciousness may also be impaired by internal stimuli (fear, rage) and by some pathophysiological changes (fever, pain). The unconscious ego may also interfere with the client's level of consciousness. Clients with hysteria neurosis may dissociate or fail to perceive both internal and external stimuli.

More precise description of consciousness is obtained by differentiating between field of consciousness and clarity of consciousness. *Field of consciousness* is the range or area of stimuli perceived. *Clarity of consciousness* is the intensity or clarity of perception. An example of the differences in these two aspects is seen in the depressed individual. Although the depressed individual may not attend to all of the events in his milieu, he is clear in his perceptions of those he does describe. Thus, his field of consciousness is narrowed, but his clarity of consciousness remains intact.

A disturbance in consciousness results in lack of clarity or in confusion of the client's awareness of self or the environment. The examination of consciousness may focus on four areas of awareness: awareness of one's internal state, subject-object differentiation, clarity of ego boundaries, and body awareness.

If the normal client is able to describe how he is feeling—his *internal state*—in words that are clear and logical to the examiner, his awareness of inner life experience is considered intact.

The client who is confused concerning time and place may have poor *subject-object differentiation*, frequently confusing one object for another or persons for inanimate objects.

Disruption of *ego boundaries* implies that the individual involved is hazy about his perception of the origin of stimuli—whether they are of an external,

Table 8-5. Glasgow coma scale—record of individual recovering from coma

	Score		Day				
			1	2	3	4	5
Eye opening response	Spontaneous opening	4					X
	To verbal stimuli	3				X	
	To pain	2	X	X	X		
	None	1					
Most appropriate verbal response	Oriented	5					X
	Confused	4					
	Inappropriate words	3				X	
	Incoherent	2		X	X		
	None	1	X				
Most integrated motor response (arm)	Obeys commands	5				X	X
	Localizes pain	4		X	X		
	Flexion to pain	3					
	Extension to pain	2	X				
	None	1					
TOTAL SCORE			5	8	8	11	14

subconscious, or conscious origin. This is normal in the developing child. This lack of clarity of ego boundaries is also typical of some religious rituals practiced by adults.

The normal person is alert to the *parameters of his body* and its performance. Although there is considerable variation from one individual to another, the normal client can distinguish himself from the environment. The nursing infant is not always able to make this distinction, regarding the mother's breast as an extension of his own body.

Levels of consciousness. The following sections deal with alterations in levels of consciousness including assessment of the individual in coma. The reader may prefer to study this material after learning more about health assessment, particularly neurological assessment.

The levels of consciousness (responsiveness) are generally described according to the behavior exhibited by the individual. Table 8-4 includes a useful categorization of the levels of consciousness.

Clinical states frequently mistaken for coma include:

"Locked-in state"—client's face and limbs are totally paralyzed but may be differentiated by other signs

Hysteria

Catatonic state—increased limb tone to passive motion (waxy flexibility) is a sign that may help to differentiate this condition

Negativism

Many systems of classification of coma have been devised. The Glasgow Coma Scale (1974) is an assessment tool that relies totally on behavioral evaluation. The advantage in the use of such a tool is that words

Table 8-6. Etiology of coma

Toxic and metabolic	Disorders involving physical damage to the brain
Exogenous toxins	Tumor
Alcohol	Edema
Drugs	Stroke
	Intracerebral hemorrhage
	Contusion
Metabolic	
Uremia	
Hepatic failure	
Hypoxia	
Hypercapneia	
Hypercalcemia	

having different meanings to various individuals are avoided, for example, "stupor," "semicomatose," or "obtunded." Thus, reliability in evaluation of coma is enhanced. A score is obtained by weighting of behaviors (Table 8-5). A person with normal consciousness would obtain a score of 14.

Response to pain may be the only indication of sensory stimulation. Painful stimuli include pinching of skin, pricking with a pin, pressure over supraorbital notches (oculosensory reflex), pinching the skin of the neck (ciliospinal reflex), pressure over knuckles, pressure (squeezing muscle masses or tendons), particularly the gastrocnemius. The client may respond by extension of limbs, facial grimacing, or withdrawal. Flexion responses are considered withdrawal responses and therefore purposeful. Nonpurposeful responses are mass reactions or extension of limbs. This scale is particularly useful in the ongoing care of hospitalized clients in coma (Tables 8-6 and 8-7).

Table 8-7. Assessment of the individual in coma

Assessment category	Examination	Possible findings	Possible underlying conditions
General inspection	Appearance	Chronic or acute illness	
		Emaciation	
		Dehydration	
	Odor	Fruity breath	Ketosis
		Alcohol	Alcoholic intoxication
	Position	Opisthotonos	Meningitis
Skin	Color	Pallor	Hemorrhage; anemia
		Florid	Hypertension; polycythemia
		Flushing	Fever; acute alcoholic intoxication
		Cyanosis	Cardiorespiratory
		Cherry red	Carbon monoxide poisoning
		Sweating	Hypoglycemia; lysis of fever
		Uremic frost of nose and lips	Uremia
		Jaundice	Hepatic or biliary disease
		Petechiae	Blood dyscrasias
		Dependent edema on ankles	Cardiac, renal disease
		Signs of injury—especially head bruises, Battle's sign, hematoma, laceration	Injury
			Trauma—most frequent cause of coma
Vital signs	Blood pressure	Increase	Hypertension; renal disease
		Decrease	Shock
	Temperature	Increase	Infection
		Decrease	Increased intracranial pressure
	Pulse	Tachycardia	Fever; hyperthyroidism
		Bradycardia	Increased intracranial pressure
			Heart block
		Bounding	Hypertension
	Respiration	Cheyne-Stokes	Neural lesion; central respiratory structures
		Kussmaul's ventilation	Diabetic acidosis
		Posthyperventilation apnea of 15 to 30 seconds	Brain damage
		Respiratory ataxia	Lesion of medulla
		Hyperventilation	Hypoxia; acidosis; lesion of brain, reticular area
Neurological	Sensory	Impairment of orientation, attention span, memory	
		May have illusions, delusions, hallucinations	
		Pain response—purposeful avoidance; withdrawal of limbs moving away from midline; arms triple flexed	
Cranial nerves	CN II, optic	Ophthalmoscopic examination of fundus	
		Papilledema	Increased intracranial pressure
		Hemorrhages and exudates	Uremia
	CN III, oculomotor	Palpebral fissure decreased	CN III paralysis
	PERRLA (pupils equal, round, reactive to light and accommodation)	Pupils pinpoint in size	Toxic states, especially morphine; thrombosis or hemorrhage of basilar artery; lesion of the pons

Table 8-7. Assessment of the individual in coma—cont'd

Assessment category	Examination	Possible findings	Possible underlying conditions
		Miosis	Unilateral lesions of brain stem
		Unequal pupil size	Head trauma; alcohol toxicity; diabetic coma; uremia; carbon monoxide poisoning
		Diminished light reflex	
		Aniscoria such that pupil dilated and not reactive to light on side of lesion due to increased intracranial pressure	Supratentional lesion, that is, brain tumor, abscess, subdural hematoma, skull fracture with middle cerebral artery hemorrhage
		Mydriasis	
	CN V, sensory motor	Diminished response to painful stimuli	
		Diminished response of corneal reflex	
		Diminished response of jaw jerk reflex	
	CN VII, motor	Diminished response to corneal reflex	
		Chvostek's sign	Tetany
		Facial paresis, palpabral fissure increased in width in deep coma; eyes open; shallow nasolabial fold; droop of mouth; puffing of cheek on expiration and retraction on inspiration	
	CN VIII, auditory (auditory-palpebral reflex) vestibular	Diminished response to sound	
		Diminished blinking in response to loud noise	
		Nystagmus at rest	
		Diminished caloric nystagmus	
	CN IX, X	Diminished palatal and pharyngeal reflexes—causes stertorous respiration, swallowing difficulties	
		Impaired laryngeal function; tone of voice altered	
		Diminished cough reflex	
Motor status	Involuntary movement	Tremors, twitches, spasms, convulsions	Epilepsy, cerebral lesions
	Symmetry of motion		
	Paralysis	One side flaccid, becoming spastic with hyperactive stretch reflexes	Cerebral lesions
		Face—lower portion only	Cerebral lesion
	Position of limbs	Flaccid, decreased tone	Recently paralyzed
		Spasticity	Cerebral lesions
		1. Early flaccid paralysis, deep tendon reflexes and superficial reflex normal or diminished extensor plantar	

Continued.

Table 8-7. Assessment of the individual in coma—cont'd

Assessment category	Examination	Possible findings	Possible underlying conditions
		2. Later—deep tendon responses hyperactive, superficial reflexes absent, extension of arms, legs, plantar	
Reflexes	Deep tendon reflexes (DTRs)	Diminished or abolished DTRs	Deep coma
		First, flaccid paralysis	
		Tonic neck reflex, decerebrate rigidity	Brain stem lesions
Meningeal involvement		Nuchal rigidity	Meningeal irritation
		Kernig's sign	Infection
		Brudzinski's sign	

ORIENTATION

Orientation is assessed from the client's awareness of person, place, and time.

A typical kind of protocol used in obtaining this information is:

Person

"What is your name? Address? Telephone number?"

"Do you know who I am?"

"Do you know what my job is?"

Place

"Tell me where you are. What is the name of this place?"

"Do you know the name of the town you are in?"

"Who brought you here?"

Time

"Do you know what day this is? Month? Year?"

The degree of disorientation is recorded. Descriptions should include enough data to allow the reader to know if the client has no awareness of a particular parameter, limited or dysfunctional awareness, or exact perception.

Time orientation is the one most frequently disordered in clients with mental disease. The feeling that time is passing slowly is characteristic of anxious or depressed patients who tend to underestimate the passage of time. On the other hand, obsessive-compulsive individuals are highly cognizant of the exact time. A disturbance in time orientation is an early finding in organic brain syndrome as well as toxic or metabolic central nervous system alterations.

A disturbance of place orientation may accompany organic brain syndrome or schizophrenia. An individual may not be oriented as to person in the aftermath of cerebral trauma or seizures or in amnesic fuguelike conditions.

Loss, disappointment, and suffering are associated with withdrawal and isolation in normal persons. They may complain of feelings of depersonalization and deny the reality of what is happening to them. The normal person is able to accept the circumstances causing his pain when the stress abates. The less integrated individual may become progressively more depersonalized or develop amnesia.

The individual with schizophrenia may have behavior characterized by marked withdrawal and isolation, symbolism, and grandiose gesture. In addition, body image may be distorted as to shape and movement, as well as feelings of weight.

ATTENTION SPAN

An appraisal of the individual's attention span is a worthwhile task of the mental status examination. This includes the examiner's description of the client's ability to maintain interest and his ability to concentrate.

The attention span is one of the first functions of the sensorium to suffer disturbance. Allowing the client to talk over a short period of time gives evidence of his stream of consciousness. The continuity of ideas is evaluated. The client's response to questions and directives will provide evidence of his attentiveness to external conditions. When a new idea is introduced in the interview, the normal client processes this alteration and responds appropriately. The client may be given a series of numbers to repeat immediately or two or three sentences that he is asked to memorize and repeat at a later time in the interview. Sometimes a fictitious name and address are employed.

Attention span may be impaired in normal individuals who are fatigued, anxious, or drugged. In many pathological states attention span is shortened. The client may be easily distractible, confused, or negativistic.

MEMORY

Memory is a function of general cerebral competence. Impairment of memory occurs in both neurological and psychiatric disorders. Some general questions that may help the examiner establish a disorder in memory are:

"Have you noticed any loss of memory?"
"How well do you remember what you are told? What has happened to you?"
"Do you remember those things that happened years ago best or those that happened today or yesterday?"

Immediate memory (verbalized remembering immediately after presentation). Immediate memory is tested by digit recall.

Recent memory (verbalized remembrances after several minutes to an hour). Examples of questions and exercises for assessing recent memory are:

"How long have you been here?"
"Why did you come here?"
"What were you doing before you came here?"
"What time did you get up today?"
"How many meals have you eaten today?"
"What did you eat for breakfast today?"
"Please allow me to test your memory skills. I'd like you to repeat these numbers after me:
7, 4
9, 6, 5, 3
8, 9, 4, 1, 5
3, 8, 7, 4, 1, 6."
"I will say some numbers; you say them backward. For instance, I say 8, 2; you say 2, 8:
3, 8
7, 2, 0
5, 9, 2, 7."

The normal individual can generally repeat five to eight digits forward and four to six digits backward.

Recent memory may be impaired in temporal lobe trauma, senile dementia, and Korsakoff's psychosis.

Remote memory (verbalized remembrances after hours, days, or years). The client may also be given three to five unrelated words to remember and repeat back. Examples of questions for assessing remote memory are:

"Where were you born?"
"Tell me the name of the high school you attended."
"What was your mother's maiden name?"

Remote memory is lost in widespread cortical damage. It may be dysfunctional in schizophrenic illnesses.

In testing for memory the examiner does not ask questions for which he does not have access to answers. Memory loss in organic dementia may involve disorders for immediate and recent events while clients may be able to recall events from childhood with accuracy. Memory disturbances are observed in febrile and toxic conditions as well as in mania and hysteria. Frontal lobe lesions are often associated with memory loss.

Amnesic conditions are those in which memory is lost for a specific period of time or for certain life situations. In spite of memory loss the individual with amnesia remains aware of his environment. Amnesia is frequently associated with the posttrauma periods and epileptic disorders.

Confabulation is an attempt by the client to "fill in the gaps" with fabricated or made-up answers when he is unable to remember.

COGNITIVE SKILLS

Abstraction ability. To assess abstraction ability, the examiner may ask the client to give the meaning of familiar proverbs:

"A bird in the hand is worth two in the bush."
"People in glass houses should not throw stones."
"When the cat's away, the mice will play."
"Don't count your chickens before they hatch."
"A rolling stone gathers no moss."
"A stitch in time saves nine."

Individuals with schizophrenia or organic brain syndrome may give concrete explanations. Inability to provide an explanation may indicate lack of intelligence, brain damage, or organic brain syndrome.

Similarities. The following exercises may be used to assess the client's ability to determine similarities:

"Tell me how the following are like each other: bird and butterfly; dog and goldfish; fish and plankton; window and door; German person and Swiss person; pencil and typewriter."
"Try to finish these comparisons for me: beer is to glass as coffee is to _____; engine is to airplane as pedal is to _____."

The assessment of the ability to define the fine but essential differences between objects or between events is the objective in testing the perception of dissimilarities. Some examples of items that may be used to assess this ability follow:

"Tell me how these objects differ: a bush and a tree; a rock and a plant."

Lesions of the left hemisphere may impair the client's ability to recognize similarities and to discriminate objects and events.

Ability to learn (comprehension). The ability to learn includes abilities in perception retention, association (interpretation), and recent memory. These processes are thought of as registration, storage, and retrieval. The client is given an address or a sentence that does not contain familiar associations. The material may be presented in writing or may be spoken. The client is asked to remember the content verbatim:

> "Listen to me carefully, I am going to give you an address that I want you to remember. Later on, I will ask you to repeat it for me: Apartment 13, Dover Hill Building."

Or the client might be given a sentence such as the Babcock sentence:

> "One thing a nation must have in order to become rich and great is a large and secure stock of wood."

Or the rest may consist of four unrelated words. An approximate 5- to 10-minute interval is allowed before the client is asked to repeat the material.

Computation. The following exercise may be used to assess the client's computational abilities:

> "Subtract 7 from 100. Continue on subtracting 7 from the resulting remainder."

The ability to calculate may be impaired in diffuse brain disease and lesions of the angular gyrus. The normal individual is able to complete the computation in 1½ minutes with less than four errors. Organic brain syndrome may be the reason for slowness in computation or increased numbers of errors.

Ability to read. A copy of a current newspaper or popular periodical is generally available and may be used to determine the client's reading skills. The examiner should be certain that the client is wearing corrective lenses if they are needed for reading.

Impairment of the ability to read is called dyslexia.

GENERAL KNOWLEDGE—GENERAL INFORMATION

Health assessment may include an evaluative estimate of what the client has learned in school and an estimate of his awareness of current events. The examiner should *match* his *inquiries* to the *educational* and *sociocultural* and *life experiences of the client*. The client might be asked questins about well-known national leaders such as the president, capitals of countries, or names of oceans. The questions of current events should include generally known phenomena. The examiner might base these questions on recent newspaper headlines that dealt with important current issues.

INTELLECTUAL LEVEL

The examiner has obtained several criteria that are a part of human intellectual capacity: vocabulary, memory, calculation, reading, writing, and general knowledge. There is no need, in a screening assessment, to administer intelligence tests. However, the incorporation of selected items from the Stanford-Binet test may provide enough information to allow the examiner to further assess whether referral is necessary. It has been suggested that test items be selected from the 10-year-old level for initial presentation and then move to progressively more difficult tasks.

The intellectual level of the client may be deduced from his perceptive grasp of the comments and questions directed toward him, his level of general information and vocabulary, his exercise of logic, range and originality of thought, and cultural attainments.

Higher intellectual functions of judgment, analysis, and synthesis as well as abstraction are impaired in acute brain injury even when specific receptive, expressive, or memory functions are intact. On the other hand, cognitive abilities may remain operant when specific expressive and memory functions are dysfunctional.

Expressive functions are speaking, drawing, writing, and other physical movement, including nonverbal behaviors. All mental activity must be inferred from the expressive functions. Disorders of the expressive functions are known as apraxias.

JUDGMENT

Judgment is a term that encompasses all the cognitive processes that include the processes of evaluation, assessment, and decision making, particularly those in which two or more experiences are related to one another. The individual who is able to evaluate a situation and determine the appropriate reaction(s) is said to have good judgment or reasoning ability. Assessment of judgment is accomplished through evaluation of the client's expressed attitudes to his social, physical, vocational, and domestic status and his plans for the future. Judgment may be inferred to be intact if the client's business affairs are in order and he is meeting social (including family) obligations. The client might also be asked to tell the examiner how he would respond in certain social situations.

Simple tests of reasoning power include an explanation indicating the meaning of abstractions. Judgment has been observed to be impaired in emotional states, mental retardation, organic brain syndrome, and schizophrenia.

THOUGHT PROCESSES

The thoughts expressed by the client are evaluated in reference to his ability to be logical, coherent, and relevant. Thought processes are the subjective ideations, comprehensions, and interpretative experiences of the client. The examiner must rely on what the client expresses verbally and nonverbally in drawing conclusions concerning the client's thought processes. The examiner should consider affect, insight, and the content of communication.

EMOTIONAL STATUS, AFFECT

The examiner is generally able to develop an estimate of the client's mood and emotional status or affective state from his verbal and nonverbal behavior.

Affective responses, the feelings associated with ideas, are noted throughout the interview process. The examiner notes appropriateness and degree of affect to a given idea as well as the range of affect to a variety of situations. The depressed individual may have blunted affect. The depressed individual who expresses suicidal feelings needs immediate attention. Extreme emotional responses may be observed in manic behavior. Bizarre behavior may be seen in the person with schizophrenia.

An interview protocol to help the examiner bring out the feelings of the client when he does not offer spontaneous data might contain the following:

"How do you feel inside?"
"How have your spirits been?"
"Do you feel this way most of the time?"
"Are you in good spirits, happy [unhappy] most of the time?"
"Do you let people know how you feel?" *If no,* "Are you afraid to let people see how you feel?"
"Can you control how you feel?"
"When do you feel the best, in the morning or in the evening?"
"How do you feel life has treated you?"
"Do you enjoy your life?"
"Is life worth living for you?"
"What does the future look like?" *If a negative reply,* "Does everything look hopeless? Do you think you will see tomorrow?"
"What plans have you made for your future?"
"Have you ever considered hurting yourself?" *If yes,* "Did you follow through and actually hurt yourself?"
"Do you think about dying?"

Some adjectives used to describe mood include:

appropriate Feelings correspond to situation
inappropriate Mood does not match culturally normal feeling state that would accompany client's life situation or what he is saying
flat Unresponsive, constricted
depressed Sad, feels deserted without help, hopeless, feels a burden to others
anxious Worried and concerned, fearful, alarmed, apprehensive
agitated Feels in turmoil, perturbed, disturbed
elated Lively, joyful, high spirits
manic Excitation, euphoria, irritability possible (accompanied by hyperactivity, rapid speech rate, and other signs of an excited state)

The client's mood may be altered in both organic and psychogenic disorders.

INSIGHT

Insight is the client's ability to perceive himself realistically and to understand himself. The evaluation of insight involves the assessment of the client's understanding of and attitude toward the cause and nature of his illness. Simple questions such as "Why did you decide to come here (name of health care facility) at this time?" allow the client to explain in his own words his comprehension of his health status and his realization of physical and mental symptoms.

It is important to elicit the individual's attitude and willingness to accept professional advice and treatment. When an apparent lack of insight is found, the examiner should attempt to determine if a real loss has occurred or whether the client may be attempting to hide his problems. Insight may be lost in the euphoria of mania. Difficulties may be ascribed to external sources in paranoia.

The elicitation of the chief complaint and the data of present illness may provide information about the client's insight to the examiner. Helpful questions with which to conclude the analysis of the chief complaint are:

"Have you noticed any change in yourself or in your outlook on life?"
"Have you noticed any change in your feelings?"

The appraisal of emotional status includes an investigation of the client's life situation and personality (general coping behavior). An interview protocol to elicit this information might be similar to the one below.

Queries	Frequently recorded responses
Present (chief) complaint	
"Tell me why you are here."	
Present illness	
"When did you last feel well?"	
"What changes have you noted in yourself?"	
"When did you first notice the problem?"	
"How long did it last?"	
"What do you feel is causing the problem?"	
"Have you had any other troubling bodily or psychological feelings (symptoms)?"	
"How are you sleeping? Eating?"	
"Do you feel better in the morning or in the evening?"	
"Have you gained or lost any weight?"	
Family history	
"How old is your father? Is he employed?"	
"What does [did] he do for a living?"	
"How old is your mother? Is [was] she employed?"	
"Did either your father or your mother have any other marriages?"	

Queries	Frequently recorded responses	Queries	Frequently recorded responses
Family history—cont'd		**Drug history**	
"How well did they get along?"		"Have you ever been given a prescrip-	
"Tell me about their personality [tem-	Affectionate, warm, easy	tion for medicine by a doctor?" *If*	
perament]?"	going, strict, cold, al-	*yes*, "Tell me about it."	
"How did you feel about your par-	ways worried, always	"Have you ever used drugs available in	Grass (marijuana), up-
ents?"	in debt, drunk all the	the street?" *If yes*, "How much?	pers, downers, hash,
"Was your home a comfortable place?"	time	How long? Are you taking drugs	tic (phencyclidine
"Did any of your family have any emo-		now?"	[PCP]), horse (heroin)
tional problems? Ever need to see a		"Do you drink beer? Wine? Whiskey?	
doctor because of a nervous prob-		How much? How long?" *or* "How	
lem?"		much and what are you drinking	
		these days?"	
Childhood and premorbid personality		"Do you drink soda pop? How much?"	
"What were you like as a child?"	Friendly; happy; ner-		
"How did your parents [brothers, sis-	vous; jumpy; shy; self-	**Marital history**	
ters] describe you to others?"	conscious; delicate;	"How old is your wife [husband]?"	
"What did your teachers think of you?"	enuresis; nail biting;	"How long have you been married?"	
"Did you like to be with people?"	fears—of the dark,	"How do you feel about your mar-	Hate to go home, often
"Tell me how you would describe	small rooms, open	riage?"	go out with the guys
yourself."	spaces, high places,	"How many children do you have?"	
	crowds; depressed;	"Were there any other pregnancies?"	
	loner; read all the	"How do you get along with your chil-	
	time; hated sports;	dren?"	
	successful; unsure of	"What kinds of things do you do as a	
	self	family?"	
Medical history		"How many times were you engaged?"	
"Have you ever been diagnosed as		"Were you ever married before?" *If*	
having a disease?" *If yes*, "Explain		*yes*, "Tell me about it."	
this to me."		"Is your sexual relationship satisfactory	Masturbation, homosex-
		to you?" *If no*, "How do you man-	uality, extramarital
Psychological history		age?"	intercourse
"Have you ever been in counseling or		"Do you have any extramarital rela-	
treatment for an emotional prob-		tionships?"	
lem?"			
		Social milieu	
Recent stress		"Tell me about your friends."	
"Have you had any recent cause for			
grief?"		**Support systems**	
"Have you been bereaved over the loss		"Who would you turn to if you were in	
of a loved person?"		trouble?"	
"Are all of your relatives and friends in		"Do you feel that you need someone	
good health?"		to turn to?	
"Are there any problems with your			
job?"		**Insight**	
"Is money a problem for you?"		"Do you consider yourself different	
"Are there problems in your marriage?		now than before your problem be-	
Love life?"		gan?"	
		"What do you think about your prob-	
Education		lem?"	
"Where did you go to school?"		"Do you think you are sick?" *If yes*,	
"What was the highest grade you at-		"Do you think you will get over it?"	
tended?"		"Do you think you need help?"	
"How did you feel about school?"		"In what way would you change if you	
"How well did you do in school?"	Overachievement, tru-	had a choice?"	
	ancy, suspension	"Do you think the same way now that	
		you always have?"	
Employment		"Do your thoughts come slower	
"What kind of work do you do?"		[faster] than they used to?"	
"Tell me where you have worked and	Long periods of unem-		
how long you worked at each job?"	ployment, frequent		
"Have you ever served in a military	job turnover		
service?"			
"Do you enjoy working?"			
"How do you get along with your boss?			
People who work for you?"			

Delinquency
"Have you ever been in trouble with
school? The police?"

Self-drawings made by the client on blank pieces of paper may help the examiner in his examination of body image. ("Draw yourself for me.") The drawing is inspected with special reference to size of image, the facial expression (affect), the activity of the figure, the amount and nature of detail, and the diminution or exaggeration of body parts. Another useful device is that of asking the client to fill in an outline of the human body. ("Draw your insides.") The heart, lungs, and intestines are the structures most frequently added. The placement and size of the organs drawn by the client may provide clues of their meaning to him.

Once a symptom has been identified as a chief complaint (that is, phobia, depression, compulsion, psychosomatic dysfunction) the history relevant to its development is explored. The individual's previous personality (characteristic behavior pattern) is explored in relation to behaviors that led to the exacerbation of the symptom in response to stress. In addition, the potential for resolution of the problem is identified. That is, the individual's personal, social, and environmental resources are determined.

COPING BEHAVIORS

In an evaluation of the individual's resources for adjusting to life's experiences, it is valuable to know the coping behaviors he has found helpful in reducing stress, such as contact sports, jogging, meditation, and reading.

Defense mechanisms. Unconscious defense mechanisms include:

projection Attribution of one's feelings, attitudes or desires to others, that is, blaming others for one's faults

rationalization Creation of self-satisfying but erroneous reasons for one's behaviors

denial Failure to recognize internal or external reality

displacement Transposition of feelings such as anger from an appropriate to an inappropriate (less threatening) object

The examiner must be aware of thoughts expressed by the client indicating the exercise of these defenses.

Mental dysfunction

Mental dysfunction or psychiatric symptoms are referred if some relief of symptoms can be anticipated. The symptoms that are most worthy of attention are those that are uselessly repetitive in nature, uncomfortable for the client, and disabling.

The common disorders of emotion and thought processes are defined here. Familiarity with this symptomatology may help the examiner focus questioning and recognize a cluster of symptoms. As with the physical examination, the examiner is looking for a pattern.

delusion A false belief of great magnitude, not influenced by experience, improbable in nature, and not related to the cultural and educational background of the client.

depersonalization Feelings that one is not real or has lost his identity may occur alone. Some individuals describe feeling mechanical.

derealization Feelings that environmental objects or the world around one is unreal; almost always associated with depersonalization.

eidetic imagery Vivid imagery of past event, present in some artists; original experience more intense, however; 50% to 60% of children up to age 12 able to visualize previously perceived object.

hallucination Perception for which no external stimuli can be ascertained. An endogenous experience in an individual whose sensorium is clear. *Simple hallucination:* simple perception, such as seeing light. *Complex hallucination:* more detailed experiences, such as seeing figure of a person.

ideas of reference Falsely interpreting external events as relating to oneself. Normal individuals often voice this symptom, that is, suspecting that a partially overheard conversation refers to oneself.

illusion Perception based on an actual external stimulus with misinterpretation or distortion of the event.

paranoid ideation Feeling that one is being persecuted or plotted against; feeling that one is controlled or manipulated by others (influence); feeling that one is being communicated with or controlled from the outside (reference).

Hallucinations occur in many mental illnesses and brain disorders. The most frequently reported hallucinations is the one of hearing voices that occurs most often in schizophrenia. Highly organized and detailed hallucinations like "watching television" are recounted most often by individuals with hysteria. Hallucinations or perceptual disturbances are a part of the effect of psychedelic drugs, that is, the tryptamine group, the phenylethylamine group, Ditran, tetrahydrocannabinol (the active principle of *Cannabis*), phencyclidine, lysergic acid diethylamide (LSD).

ORGANIC BRAIN SYNDROME

Organic brain syndrome is a diagnostic term used to describe those individuals with signs indicating

Table 8-8. Organic brain syndrome: characteristic symptoms and signs

Acute delirium	Dementia
Impairment of consciousness	May be disoriented
Delusions possible	Attention span impaired
Hallucinations possible	Judgment impaired
May be disoriented	Recent memory impaired
Attention span impaired	Mood swings
Judgment impaired	Irritability
Mood swings	
Recent memory impaired	
Restlessness	
Anxiety	
Fear	

medical or neurological dysfunction causing an impairment of orientation, memory, or other mental functions (Table 8-8). Affective symptoms, delusions, hallucinations, and obsessions may also be present. An acute brain syndrome (delirium) is one of short duration that is usually reversible. A chronic brain syndrome (dementia) is long standing and often progressive in nature; its prognosis is less favorable.

AFFECTIVE DISORDERS

The client with an effective disorder runs the gamut from depression to exaggerated euphoria or mania. The highs and lows show little correlation with the life situation (Table 8-9).

During the down mood period the client evidences such symptoms as anorexia, insomnia, sense of worthlessness, sense of being a burden, and thoughts of

self-destruction. On the high mood cusp the client may describe flights of ideas or hyperactivity.

Primary affective disorders are those observed in a client who has had no previous psychiatric disorders. *Secondary affective disorders* are those seen in a client who has been previously diagnosed as having psychiatric illness.

A *bipolar affective disorder* is diagnosed when mania is present whether or not depression occurs. Depression occurring in the absence of mania is known as a *unipolar affective disorder*.

The client with an affective disorder often tells the examiner that "something is wrong with my mind."

Paranoid ideations have been reported in clients with affective disorders. These thoughts appear to be augmented ideas of reference related to the feeling of worthlessness.

The periods of illness may last from a few days to several years, and the client appears to function well in the interim.

Primary affective disorders are most frequently first diagnosed when the client is about 40, whereas the client with a bipolar affective disorder may be in his 30s.

Clients being treated with tricyclic antidepressant drugs may have complaints of side effects, such as tremor, dry mouth, or orthostatic hypotension. Thus, a precise record of the client's drug history is important.

Table 8-9. Affective disorders: characteristic symptoms and signs

Mania

Euphoria	*Somatic*
Irritability (sometimes)	Hyperactivity
Flight of ideas—generally comprehensible	Rapid speech rate
	Rhyming
Distractibility	Punning
Delusions possible (may be of grandeur)	Decreased sleep
Passivity—sensation that body is under external control	
Depersonalization	

Depression

Dejection	*Somatic*
Discouragement	Pain
Despondency	Tachycardia
Depression	Dyspnea
Feeling of being down in the dumps, blue	Gastrointestinal dysfunction
Irritability	Anorexia
Fearfulness	Constipation
Loss of interest in daily activities	Sleep disorders
Social withdrawal	Insomnia
Guilt	Hypersomnia
Inability to focus thoughts	Lack of energy
Indecisiveness	Psychomotor retardation
Recurring preoccupation with suicide, death	Frequent crying
Thoughts of self-destruction	Impotence (in men)
Hopelessness	Restlessness
Feeling of gloomy future, impending doom	Pacing, wringing of hands
Loss of interest in sexual activity	
Delusions possible (frequently involving self-deprecation)	

SCHIZOPHRENIC DISORDERS

Hallucinations and delusions are the diagnostic signposts of schizophrenia. These symptoms are the criteria by which mental disorders are classified as schizophrenic disorders (Table 8-10). Both delusions and hallucinations represent an internal modification of the environment in order to meet the desires or needs of the client. The presence of hallucinations

Table 8-10. Schizophrenia: characteristic symptoms and signs

Poor prognosis	Good prognosis
Delusions	Delusions
Hallucinations (most common of persecution), auditory	Hallucinations
Clear sensorium	Clear sensorium
Chronic disorder	Symptoms transitory
Blunted, shallow (flat), or inappropriate affect	Symptoms develop abruptly
Catatonic motor behavior	More likely to show affective responses, usually depression
Waxy flexibility; periods of immobility	Recovery is usual
Repeated grimacing, posturing	
Disordered thought processes	

may be suspected in the person who adopts listening attitudes or appears preoccupied.

Two classifications of these disorders are described in the literature related to prognosis. Schizophrenic disorders with a poor prognosis include *chronic schizophrenia, nuclear schizophrenia,* and *process schizophrenia.* Schizophrenic disorders with a good prognosis include *schizophreniform* and *schizoaffective disorders* and *acute, reactive,* or *remitting schizophrenia.*

The client's use of language is a valuable identifying characteristic of the individual who is schizophrenic. Individuals with schizophrenia have been noted to use the same set of syntactic, semantic, and discourse patterns as normal individuals but not as proficiently. Furthermore, those who are schizophrenic appear to ignore the listener. Normal individuals generally base the organization and content of their remarks on the last remark(s) of the person with whom they are talking. Schizophrenic individuals tend not to maintain this relationship and to ignore the lack of awareness of his listener to the subject that he has newly introduced.

The development of schizophrenia may occur over a long period of time.

A schizoid personality is said to exist in the client who is markedly shy, who withdraws from social relationships, and who is unable to establish close personal relationships. This behavior is generally noted in adolescence, though delusions and hallucinations generally start in the 20s.

The schizophreniform disorders are abrupt in onset and occur without a psychiatric history prior to the present illness.

NEUROSES

Anxiety neurosis. The client with an anxiety neurosis has recurrent periods of abrupt onset anxiety that terminate without intervention. The client complains of fright. The autonomic nervous system is activated. Characteristic symptoms and signs include:

Palpitations	Headache
Breathlessness, smothering	Fatigue, weakness
Dyspnea	Paresthesias
Nervousness	Tremors, shakiness
Dizziness	Sighing
Faintness	Nausea and vomiting
Feeling of impending doom	Abdominal cramps
	Diarrhea
	Flatus

The age of onset extends from midadolescence through the early 30s.

Hysteria. Hysteria is a disorder characterized by multiple somatic symptoms. Examples of such complaints include gastrointestinal disturbances, pains (dysmenorrhea, headaches, back pain), anxiety, sexual problems, and conversion symptoms. The symptoms often defy the boundaries of what is commonly known about pathophysiology. The descriptions are often vividly portrayed or markedly exaggerated, or both, so that these clients often spend a good deal of time in hospitals and undergo many surgical procedures. Because there are often many vague symptoms, the history may be difficult to complete and to organize for the record. The examiner would do well to record the complaints verbatim. Conversion symptoms are idiopathic symptoms that indicate neurological disorder. These might include amnesia, unconsciousness, paralysis, anesthesias, or blindness.

Hysteria is most commonly first seen in the teens. The incidence is higher in men than in women.

Compulsional or obsessional neurosis. *Obsessions* are long-lasting, upsetting thoughts or impulses that usually do not interest the individual and serve no purpose but cannot be ignored. *Compulsions* are the behaviors that are the result of obsessions. Thus, an obsessional neurosis is said to exist in the presence of obsessions and compulsions when no other disorder is evident. Other terms for this neurosis include psychasthenia, phobic-ruminative state, and obsessional state.

DEFINITIONS

obsessional convictions Magical formulations. ("If I have my purse here, nothing can happen to me.")

obsessional fears Repeated feelings of fright, particularly of disease, filth, sharp instruments.

obsessional ideas Words, phrases, or rhymes that recur in the thought processes of the individual, frequently interrupting other thought sequences.

obsessional images Recurrent imagined scenes, often dealing with sexual acts or excreta.

obsessional impulses Irresistible thoughts related to self-injury, to injury of others, or to some other embarrassing behavior.

obsessional rituals Recurrent, stylized actions; protocols for washing or combing hair, eating.

obsessional rumination Prolonged reflection on a subject without reaching a decision.

phobia A highly disturbing, recurring, and unrealistic fear; may relate to any situation or object.

SOCIOPATHIC, ANTISOCIAL PERSONALITY

The sociopathic personality is a synonym for the antisocial personality of an individual who has displayed a pattern of antisocial, delinquent, or criminal behavior. The disorder has its inception in adolescence. Early symptoms include restlessness, a short attention span, and defiance of discipline. A history of poor school and work adjustment is the rule. Promiscuous sexual behavior is a frequent observation.

Conversion symptoms are frequently observed in the sociopathic personality.

The acute appearance of psychiatric symptoms in an individual whose history indicates that affect and behavior had been normal prior to this occurrence is commonly seen in frontal and temporal lobe tumor, hydrocephalus, and cortical atrophy. The most common symptom found in these individuals is depression.

SAMPLE PROTOCOL FOR ELICITING PSYCHIATRIC SYMPTOMS

Questions leading to the elucidation of psychiatric symptoms might include the following:

Disturbing events
"How did you feel at the time?"

Hallucinations
"Have you heard [sounds, voices, messages], seen [lights, figures], smelled [strange, bad, good odors], tasted [strange, bad, good tastes], or felt [touching, warm, cold sensation] anything that others who were present did not? If no one was present, would I have been able to have the same impressions from the experience?"

Delusions
"Do you feel that someone or something outside you is controlling you in some way? Are you able to control other people?"
"Do you feel that you are being watched? Followed?"
"Are people talking about you?" *If yes,* "Explain to me how you know."
"Do you have anything to feel guilty about?"
"Do you feel you are a bad person?"

Obsessions
"Do you have some thoughts that keep coming back again and again?" *If yes,* "Tell me about them. How often? Are they pleasant [frightening] thoughts? Can you make them stop?"

Compulsions
"Are there some things you find yourself doing over and over?" *If yes,* "Tell me about them. How often? Can you stop doing these things?"
"Do you have someone or something outside you that is forcing you to do these things?"
"Do you find yourself checking and rechecking to make sure water is turned off? Gas? To make sure the doors are locked?"

Somatic symptoms
"Do you ever feel a lump in your throat?"
"Do you have difficulty swallowing? Speaking?"
"Have you ever been paralyzed?"
"How do your bowels function?"
"How is your appetite?"
"Do you have headaches?"
"Do you have enough energy to do all the things you would like to do?"

SUMMARY

I. Physical appearance and behavior
  A. Motor ability (observation)
    1. Posture
    2. Grooming and apparel
    3. Body movement (gait)
    4. Nonverbal behaviors
  B. Ability to use language
    1. Speech patterns
      a. Speed
      b. Omissions
      c. Neologisms
      d. Circumlocution
      e. Vocabulary
      f. Disarthria
    2. Writing ability
    3. Aphasia
    4. Agnosia
    5. Apraxia
  C. Sensory ability (client's appraisal)
    1. Smell
    2. Taste
    3. Sight
    4. Hearing
    5. Touch
    6. Awareness of body parts
II. Sensorium
  A. Level of consciousness
    1. Responds
      a. To verbal stimuli
      b. To touch stimuli
      c. To painful stimuli
    2. Does not respond
  B. Orientation
    1. Person
    2. Place
    3. Time
  C. Attention span
  D. Memory
    1. Immediate (seconds)
    2. Recent (several minutes)
    3. Remote (hours, days, or years)
  E. Cognitive skills
    1. Abstractions
    2. Similarities
    3. Dissimilarities
    4. Computation
    5. Reading
  F. General knowledge—current information
  G. Intellectual level
  H. Judgment
  I. Thought processes

        1. Logical
        2. Coherent
        3. Relevant
    J. Emotional status, affect, mood
    K. Insight
III. Mental dysfunction
    A. Disorders
        1. Delusion
        2. Illusion
        3. Depersonalization
        4. Derealization
        5. Paranoid ideation
        6. Hallucination
        7. Obsession
        8. Compulsion
        9. Phobia
    B. Addictive behaviors
        1. Smoking (packs/day/time)
            a. Nicotine
            b. Marihauna
        2. Alcohol
        3. Coffee
        4. Caffeine containing, carbonated drinks
        5. Prescription and nonprescription drugs
    C. Coping behaviors—defense mechanisms
    D. Affect
    E. Life situation

BIBLIOGRAPHY

Chusid, J. G.: Correlative neuroanatomy and functional neurology, ed. 16, 1976, Los Altos, Calif., Lange Medical Publications.

Daube, J. R., and Sandok, B. A.: Medical neurosciences, 1978, Boston, Little, Brown and Co., 1978.

Dawson, D. F. L., Bartolucci, G., and Blum, H. M.: Language and schizophrenia: toward a synthesis, Compr. Psychiatry 21(1):81, 1980.

DeJong, R. N.: The neurologic examination, ed. 4, New York, 1979, Harper and Row, Publishers, 1979.

Dreikurs, R.: Psychodynamics, psychotherapy and counseling, Chicago, 1967, Alfred Adler Institute.

Fieve, R. R., and Dunner, D. L.: Unipolar and bipolar affective states. In Flach, F. F., and Draghi, S. C., editors: The nature and treatment of depression, New York, 1975, John Wiley & Sons, Inc.

Lewis, A.: Mechanisms of neurological disease, Boston, 1976, Little, Brown and Co.

Lezak, M.: Neuropsychological assessment, New York, 1976, Oxford University Press.

Masserman, J. H., and Schwab, J. J.: The psychiatric examination, New York, 1974, Intercontinental Medical Book Corp.

Mayo Clinic and Foundation: Clinical examinations in neurology, ed. 4, Philadelphia, 1976, W. B. Saunders Co.

Schmidt, R. F.: Fundamentals of sensory physiology, New York, 1978, Springer-Verlag.

Strahl, M. O., and Lewis, N. D., editors: Differential diagnosis in clinical psychiatry, New York, 1972, Science House.

Strub, R. L., and Black, F. W.: The mental status examination in neurology, Philadelphia, 1979, F. A. Davis Co.

Teasdale, G., and Jennett, B.: Assessment of coma and impaired consciousness: a practical scale, Lancet 2:81, 1974.

Woodruff, R. A., Goodwin, D. W., and Guze, S. B.: Psychiatric diagnosis, Oxford, 1974, Oxford University Press.

9 Assessment of the skin, hair, and nails

The skin is an organ system readily accessible to examination. As a membrane barrier between the individual and his external environment, the skin responds to changes in the external environment and also reflects changes in the internal environment. A careful examination of the skin may yield valuable information about the client and his general health, along with specific information that will aid in the identification of a systemic disease or a specific problem of the skin. It is important to describe the skin of the healthy client, as well as the skin of the client with a health problem, paying special attention to any deviation from normal. (The examination of the sclera and conjunctiva is discussed in Chapter 11 and the examination of the oral mucosa is discussed in Chapter 10.)

The examination of the skin requires some understanding of the structure and function of the system and familiarity with the appearance of the skin, hair, nails, and mucous membranes in health and disease. This chapter includes a brief discussion of the anatomy and function of the skin, methods for conducting a systematic examination of the skin and appendages, and an approach to the description and classification of skin lesions.

ANATOMY AND FUNCTION

The skin has many important functions, including (1) assistance in maintaining an internal environment by providing a barrier to loss of water and electrolytes, (2) protection from external agents injurious to the internal environment, (3) regulation of body heat, (4) a sense organ for touch, temperature, and pain, (5) self-maintenance and wound repair, (6) maintenance of buffered protective skin film by eccrine and sebaceous glands, (7) participation in production of vitamin D, and (8) delayed hypersensitivity reaction to foreign substances.

The skin is divided into three layers: the epidermis, the dermis, and the subcutaneous tissues (Fig. 9-1).

The epidermis is an avascular, cornified, cellular structure. It is stratified into several layers and is composed chiefly of keratinocytes, cells that produce keratin. Keratin makes up much of the horny material in the outermost epidermal layer of dead cells and is the principal constituent of the harder, keratinized structures of nails and hair. The innermost layer of the epidermis contains melanocytes, the source of melanin, the pigment that gives color to the skin and hair.

Epidermal appendages include the hair, nails, eccrine sweat glands, apocrine sweat glands, and sebaceous glands. These are formed by invagination of the epidermis into the underlying dermis. The hair and nails are keratinized appendages and have no significant function in human beings. The eccrine, sebaceous, and apocrine appendages are glandular. The sebaceous glands usually arise from the hair follicles and produce sebum, which has a lubricating effect on the horny outer layer of the epidermis. The eccrine sweat glands are widely distributed and have an important function in the dissipation of body heat as sweat is produced and evaporated. The apocrine sweat glands are found in the axillary and genital areas and usually open into the hair follicles. The sweat produced by the apocrine glands decomposes when contaminated by bacteria, resulting in the characteristic body odor.

The dermis underlying the epidermis constitutes the bulk of the skin. It is a tough connective tissue that contains lymphatics and nerves and is highly vascular. It supports and nourishes the epidermis.

The subcutaneous layer immediately under the dermis is distinguished by the storage of fat and is important in temperature insulation.

EXAMINATION

The examination of the skin and appendages begins with a general inspection, followed by a detailed examination. A good source of illumination is neces-

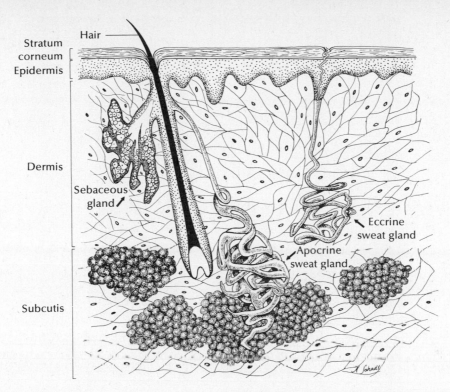

Fig. 9-1. Anatomy of the skin and its appendages. (From Prior, J. A., and Silberstein, J. S.: Physical diagnosis; the history and examination of the patient, ed. 5, St. Louis, 1977, The C. V. Mosby Co.)

sary; indirect natural daylight is preferred. A small magnifying glass will aid in the examination of individual lesions of the skin.

The examination may begin with an observation of the entire integument with the client disrobed; or a more simple approach may be taken: the skin that is exposed may be surveyed, followed by inspection of the skin, mucous membranes, and epidermal appendages of each body part as it is examined. Comparison of symmetrical anatomical areas is made throughout the examination.

The skin is inspected for color and vascularity and for evidence of perspiration, edema, injuries, or skin lesions. During the examination the practitioner should think about the underlying structures, the thinness of the skin, and the particular kind of exposure of a body part. It is also helpful to note those changes in the skin that are indicative of past injuries and habits, such as calluses, stains, scars, needle marks, and insect bites, and to note the grooming of hair and nails.

Skin color

Skin color varies from person to person and from one part of the body to another but is normally a whitish pink or a brown shade, depending on race. The exposed areas of the body, including the face, ears, back of neck, and backs of hands and arms, are noticeably different and may be more damaged after long exposure to the sun and weather. The vascular flush areas are the cheeks, the bridge of the nose, the neck, the upper chest, the flexor surfaces of the extremities, and the genital area. These areas may be involved in a vascular disturbance or may demonstrate increased color caused by blushing or temperature elevation. They should be compared with areas of less vascularity. The pigment labile areas are the face, the backs of the hands, the flexors of the wrists, the axillae, the mammary areolae, the midline of the abdomen, and the genital area. These areas may demonstrate normal systemic pigmentary changes, such as occur during pregnancy.

There are other changes in skin color that should be noted as evidence of systemic disease. Cyanosis, a dusky blue color, may be observed in the nailbeds and in the lips and the mouth area. It results from decreased oxyhemoglobin binding, or decreased oxygenation of the blood, and can be caused by pulmonary or heart disease, by abnormalities of hemoglobin, or by cold. The yellow or green hue of jaundice occurs when tissue bilirubin is increased and may be noted first in the sclerae and then in the mucous membranes and the skin. Pallor, or decreased color in the skin, results from decreased blood flow to the superficial vessels or from decreased amounts of hemoglobin in the blood; it is most evi-

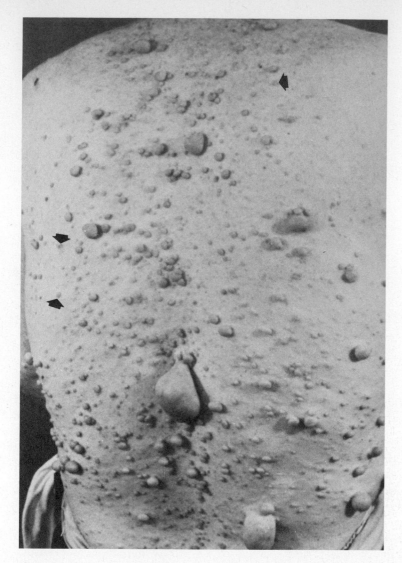

Fig. 9-2. Neurofibromatosis. Note café au lait spots (arrows). (Courtesy American Academy of Dermatology and Institute for Dermatologic Communication and Education, Evanston, Illinois.)

dent in the face, the conjunctiva, the mouth, and the nails. Generalized redness of the skin may be caused by fever, while defined areas of redness may be the result of a localized infection or sunburn. Other localized changes in color may indicate a problem such as edema, which tends to blanch skin color. Alterations in the normal pattern of pigmentation result from changes in the distribution of melanin or in the function of the melanocytes in the epidermis; hyperpigmentation or depigmentation can occur. The nevus, or birthmark, is an example of a defined area of hyperpigmentation that may be an innocent manifestation, such as the mongolian spots found on infants, or may be a more serious finding, such as the numerous café au lait spots of neurofibromatosis (Fig. 9-2). Depigmentation of the skin, which is seen in vitiligo, may involve only one or few areas, or it may be more generalized. Common sites of vitiligo

are the face, neck, axillae, groin, anogenital area, eyelids, hands, and wrists. Table 9-1 lists other conditions causing variations in pigmentation.

The color changes in the skin of dark-skinned or black clients are more difficult to assess. Color should be observed in the sclera, conjunctiva, buccal mucosa, tongue, lips, nail beds, palms, and soles (Fig. 9-3). Normal variations are found in the sclera and the oral mucosa. Jaundice is observable in the sclera but should not be confused with the normal yellow pigmentation of the dark-skinned black client. The oral mucosa may have a normal freckling pigmentation, evident in the gums, the borders of the tongue, and the lining of the cheeks. The gums sometimes have a dark blue color that may be blotchy or evenly distributed. Pallor or cyanosis can be difficult to determine. The lips, earlobes, or nail beds can be gently pinched to see how quickly the color returns. The

Table 9-1. Variation in pigmentation

Condition	Characteristic color	Location
Diffuse hyperpigmentation		
Addison's disease, ACTH-producing tumors	Tan to brown	Generalized, more marked on exposed areas, flexures, mucous membrane of mouth
Arsenic toxicity	Dusky, diffuse, paler spots	Trunk, extremities
Chloasma (mask of pregnancy), phenytoin ingestion	Tan to brown	Forehead—adjacent to hair line, malar prominence, upper lip, chin
Hemochromatosis	Bronze to grayish brown, deposits of hemosiderin	Generalized
Ichthyosis	Tan, fine to coarse scaling	Generalized
Malabsorption syndrome (sprue)	Tan to brown patches	Any area of body
Scleroderma	Yellow to tan (may also have depigmentation)	Generalized
Uremia (chronic renal failure)	Yellow-brown, retention of urinary chromogens	Generalized
Lack of pigmentation		
Vitiligo	Circumscribed lack of pigmentation	
Albinism—hereditary	Complete or partial lack of melanin	Generalized (universal albinism), skin, hair, eyes

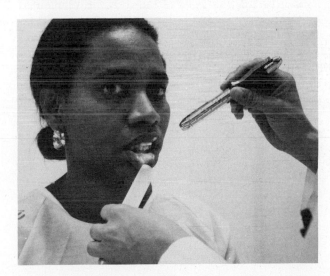

Fig. 9-3. In black individuals pallor and cyanosis are best detected by examining the mucosa of the mouth (above) and the palpebral conjunctiva of the eye.

color usually returns quickly, but if the delay is prolonged, there may be decreased oxygenation of the blood or decreased blood flow to the skin.

Skin palpation

Palpation of the skin is used to amplify the findings observed on inspection and is usually carried out simultaneously as each body part is examined. Changes in temperature, moisture, texture, and turgor are detected by palpation.

Temperature of the skin is increased when blood flow through the dermis is increased. Localized areas of skin hyperthermia are noted in the presence of a burn or a localized infection. Generalized skin hyperthermia involving all of the integument may occur when there is fever associated with a localized or systemic disease. Temperature of the skin is reduced when there is a decrease in blood flow in the dermis. Generalized skin hypothermia occurs when the client is in shock, whereas localized hypothermia occurs in conditions such as arteriosclerosis.

The moisture found on the skin will vary from one body area to another. It is normal to find the soles of the feet, the palms of the hands, and the intertriginous areas—where two surfaces are close together—containing more moisture than other parts. The amount of moisture found over the entire integument also varies with changes in the environmental temperature, with muscular activity, and with the body temperature. The skin functions in the regulation of body temperature and produces perspiration that evaporates and cools the body when the temperature is increased. The skin is normally drier during the winter months, when environmental temperatures and humidity are decreased, and with the increase in age of the individual. Abnormal dryness of the skin occurs with dehydration; the skin will feel dry even when the temperature is increased. Dryness of the skin is also found in conditions such as myxedema and chronic nephritis.

Texture refers to the fineness or coarseness of the skin, and changes may indicate local irritation or trauma to defined skin areas or may be associated with problems of other systems. The skin becomes soft and smooth in hyperthyroidism and rough and dry in hypothyroidism.

Turgor refers to the elasticity of the skin and is most easily determined by picking up a fold of skin over the abdomen and observing how quickly it returns to its normal shape. There is a loss of turgor associated with dehydration, and the skin demonstrates a laxness and a loss of normal mobility, returning to place slowly. Loss of turgor is also associated with aging; the skin becomes wrinkled and lax. Increased turgor is associated with an increase in tension, which causes the skin to return to place quickly when pinched.

Hair

The hair over the entire body is examined to determine the distribution, quantity, and quality. There is a normal male or female hair pattern that evolves after puberty, and a deviation may be indicative of an endocrine problem. Changes in the quantity of the hair are of importance. Hirsutism, increased hair growth, is found in conditions such as Cushing's syndrome and acromegaly. Decreased hair growth or loss of hair may be associated with hypopituitarism or a pyogenic infection. Types of alopecia, or hair loss, are listed in Table 9-2. The quality of the hair is determined by the color and texture. Changes in color such as graying occur normally with aging, but patchy gray hair may develop following nerve injuries. Changes in texture of hair associated with hypothyroidism include dryness and coarseness, and changes associated with hyperthyroidism include increased silkiness and fineness.

Nails

The assessment of the nails is important to determine not only their condition but also possible evidence of systemic diseases. The nails are examined for shape, normal dorsal curvature, adhesion to the nail bed, regularity of the nail surface, color, and thickness. The skin folds around the nails are examined for any color changes, swelling, increased temperature, and tenderness (Fig. 9-4).

The nails are keratinized appendages of the epidermis, as are hairs. The nails consist of (1) the nail matrix (root), wherein the nail plate is developed, (2) the nail plate, (3) the nail bed, which is attached to the nail plate, and (4) the periungual tissue, including the eponychium and the perionychium.

The nail matrix is not visible. The lunula, located at the base of the visible nail, has the shape of a half moon. The whiter color of the lunula compared to the more distal nail is caused by the uptake of keratojalinic granules and by the lunula's looser connection to the underlying vascularized derma. A bluish hue

Table 9-2. Alopecia—hair loss

Type of alopecia	Description
Androgen (in female)	Thinning of scalp hair; male pattern hirsutism on body
Areata	Circumscribed bald areas; sudden onset, usually reversible
Chemical	Hair brittle; breaks off
Cicatricial	Permanent localized loss of hair associated with scarring
Drug or radiation	Loss of hair caused by antineoplastic agents, such as gold, thallium, and arsenic, or by radiation
Male pattern	Regression of anterior hairline, temples, and vertex; hereditary
Mucinosa	Erythematous papules or plaques without hair
Syphilitic	Generalized thinning of hair or baldness; mucous patches without hair

is observed in the nails of more darkly pigmented subjects. The size of the lunula is variable and may not be visible in older subjects.

The nail plate is a horny, semitransparent structure with a dorsal convexity. The nail bed lies distal to the lunula and is not known to participate in nail formation. The visible nail has a roughly rectangular shape. Normal thickness of the nail is 0.3 to 0.65 mm, being somewhat thicker in males.

The free edge of the nail fold is continuous with the cuticle, which is an extension of the stratum corneum of the dorsum of the finger. The eponychium lies below this and is the anterior extension of the roof of the nail fold on the nail plate. The hyponychium is the portion of the fingertip underlying the free portion of the nail. The perionychium is the epidermis bordering the nail.

NAIL GROWTH

The nail plate is formed continuously and uniformly at all points in the matrix. The plate is pushed forward by cells of the germinative layer of the matrix. The fingernail growth rate in the normal adult has been reported variously as 0.1 to 1 mm. The rate varies with nutrition, age, and activity level.

Nail growth also has a circadian and seasonal rhythm. It is greater in the morning, lessening progressively in the afternoon and the night. Nail growth is greater in warm seasons than in cold, and accelerated growth has been observed in warm climates. The growth rate slows with aging. The total time required for reaching the free margin of the nail from the lunula is called the migration time and is normally 130 days. The time required for complete re-

TRANSVERSAL SECTION

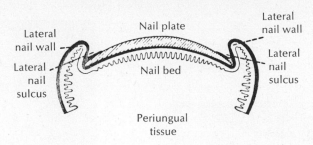

LONGITUDINAL SECTION

Fig. 9-4. Scheme of nail anatomy in transversal and longitudinal sections. (Diagram based on Achten, 1959. From DeNicola, P., and Morsiani, M.: Nail diseases in internal medicine, Springfield, Ill., 1974, Charles C Thomas, Publisher.)

newal of the fingernail (regeneration time) is 170 days, while that of the toenail is 1 to 1½ years.

NAIL ABSENCE

Anonychia is the complete absence of the nail. This condition is usually congenital.

CHANGES IN NAIL CURVATURE

Platyonychia is flattening of the nails, although color, consistency, and thickness are not altered. This may be hereditary or may be the forerunner of koilonychia.

Koilonychia describes a nail that has the general shape of a spoon. The color is generally white, and the nail is opaque. The concave portion of the nail is particularly fragile. When all of the nails are not involved, the etiology may be chronic eczema or a tumor of the nail bed. Systemic diseases associated with koilonychia are hypochromic anemias, chronic infections, malnutrition, pellagra, and Raynaud's disease (Fig. 9-5).

Racket nail is a flattened and expanded nail, usually the thumb. It has been considered a sign of secondary syphilis.

CHANGES IN NAIL ADHESION

Onycholysis is separation of the nail from the nail bed originating at the free edge and progressing proximally. While the condition may be congenital, it has also been associated with disorders of the thy-

roid—both hypothyroidism and hyperthyroidism—repeated trauma, peripheral arteriospasm (as in Raynaud's disease), hypochromic anemias, syphilis, eczema, and acrocyanosis (Fig. 9-6).

Onychomadesis is the separation of the nail starting at the roof of the nail and progressing to the free margin. This condition is the result of a lesion of the matrix and the hyponychium. The separation may be the result of peripheral neuritis, amyotrophy, hemiplegias, thrombosis, vascular disease, frostbite, exanthemas (scarlet fever, measles), or hypocalcemia.

Paronychia is an inflammation of the folds of tissue surrounding the nails leading to erythema, with inflammation, swelling, and induration of the nail fold accompanied by pain and tenderness. It is the most common complaint related to the nails. Drops of pus may be extruded from beneath the nail fold ulceration. The ulceration tends to involve surrounding tissues. The lesion generally involves the distal third of the nail, which may be broken or destroyed as necrosis progresses. This condition is common in diabetic persons. *Candida albicans*, staphylococci, and streptococci are the organisms most frequently involved. Both third-stage syphilis and leprosy may lead to paronychia (Fig. 9-7).

CHANGES IN THE NAIL SURFACE

Beau's lines (Beau's striations, transverse sulci) are striations approximately 1 mm deep and 0.1 to 0.5 mm wide running across the entire nail perpendicu-

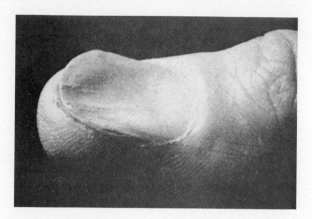

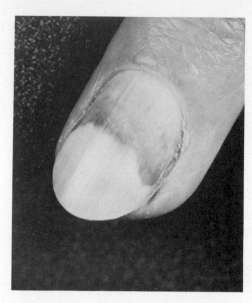

Fig. 9-5. Koilonychia. (From Samman, P. D.: The nails in disease, London, 1978, William Heinemann Medical Books Ltd.)

Fig. 9-6. Onycholysis. (From Samman, P. D.: The nails in disease, London, 1978, William Heinemann Medical Books Ltd.)

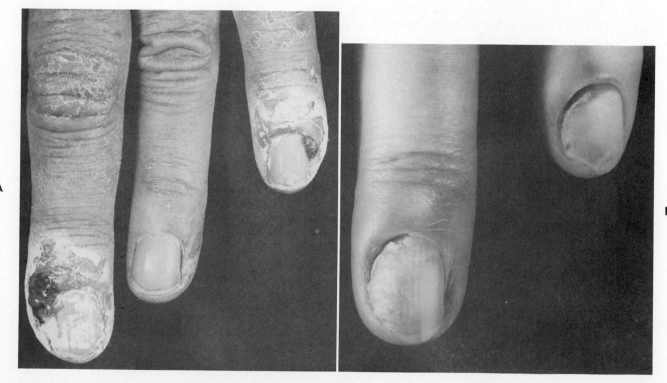

Fig. 9-7. A, Acute paronychia. **B,** Chronic paronychia—early stage. Note loss of cuticle and bolstering of posterior nail fold. (From Samman, P. D.: The nails in disease, London, 1978, William Heinemann Medical Books Ltd.)

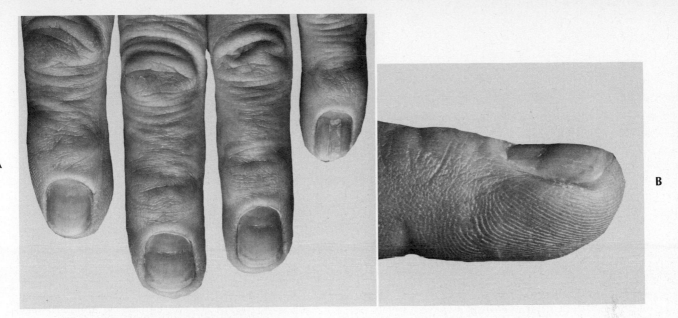

Fig. 9-8. A, Beau's lines. **B,** Beau's lines, side view. (From Samman, P. D.: The nails in disease, London, 1978, William Heinemann Medical Books Ltd.)

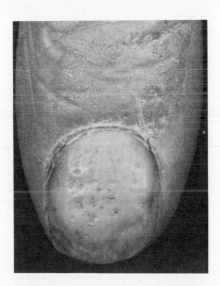

Fig. 9-9. Psoriasis—nail pitting. (From Samman, P. D.: The nails in disease, London, 1978, William Heinemann Medical Books Ltd.)

lar to the longitudinal axis. Beau's lines appear on all fingers. The color is the same as the remainder of the nail. Beau's lines are thought to be caused by an arrest of nail growth at the matrix. If the retardation of growth is repeated another line may result. Because the nail grows at a rate of approximately 0.1 mm per day and the eponychium is about 3 mm long, it is possible to calculate the point in time at which the hiatus in nail production occurred. Beau's lines have been associated with the acute phase of infectious diseases, malnutrition, and anemia (Fig. 9-8).

Pitting deformities of the nail may vary from pinpoint to pinhead size and may be linear or irregular in distribution. These depressions have been observed in psoriasis, peripheral vascular disease, diabetes, and infectious diseases such as syphilis and tuberculosis (Fig. 9-9).

Mee's lines are crescent-shaped transverse lines similar in color to the lunula. They have been observed in arsenic poisoning.

Striated nails are characterized by longitudinal ridges running the length of the nail and are associated with increased fragility. Nail striations have been observed in malnutrition, anemia, defective peripheral circulation, chronic infections, and psoriasis. Nail striations are frequently observed in the elderly.

CHANGES IN NAIL COLOR

Leukonychia is characterized by white striations or 1- to 2-mm dots that progress to the free edge of the nail as growth proceeds. The white areas may result from trauma, infections, vascular disease, psoriasis, and arsenic poisoning.

Leukonychia totalis (white nails) is a condition in which the entire nail plate is white. While the white nail may be congenital, this type of nail has been associated with hypocalcemia, severe hypochromic anemia, leprosy, hepatic cirrhosis, and arsenic poisoning. Paired narrow white bands parallel to the lunula have been associated with hypoalbuminemia. These white lines affect the nail bed rather than the nail plate.

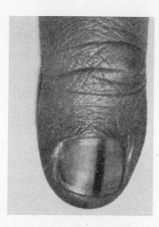

Fig. 9-10. Pigment band probably caused by a junctional nevus. (From Samman, P. D.: The nails in disease, London, 1978, William Heinemann Medical Books Ltd.)

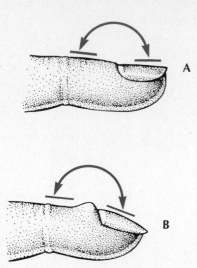

Fig. 9-11. A, Normal angle of the nail. **B,** Abnormal angle of the nail seen in late clubbing.

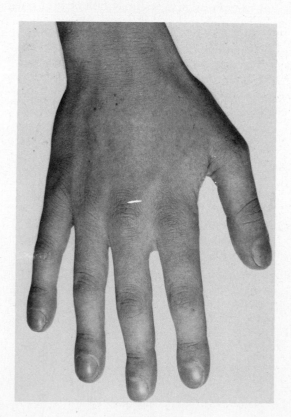

Fig. 9-12. Finger clubbing. (From Samman, P. D.: The nails in disease, London, 1978, William Heinemann Medical Books Ltd.)

Melanonychia is the presence of brown color in the nail plate resulting from a melanin redistribution in the melanophore cells. Normal nails in white persons are not pigmented, but the nails are pigmented in black persons from adolescence. An increase in pigment of the nails may be seen in Addison's disease and malaria.

Pigment band is a single black or brown streak in the nail of a white person. The development of such a line may be caused by junctional nevus in the nail matrix. Brown striations are common in black persons (Fig. 9-10).

Bluish nails are observed in cyanosis and venous stasis. Sulfhydric acid poisoning results in the formation of sulfhemoglobin, which creates a blue tinge as it circulates in the capillary bed beneath the nail. Wilson's disease has been associated with a bluish tint of the lunula. *Pseudomonas aeruginosa* infection is associated with a bluish gray color of the entire nail.

CHANGES IN NAIL THICKNESS

Thickening or hypertrophy of the nail is generally caused by trauma. The nail of the small toe is often the only one affected; it takes on a clawlike shape. Thickening of the nails has been associated with psoriasis, fungal infection, defective vascular supply, and trauma. Thinning of the nail has been linked to defective peripheral circulation and nutritional anemias.

Brittleness of the nails is a common sign. Systemic diseases associated with brittle nails are nutritional anemias and impaired peripheral circulation. Prolonged exposure to water and alkaline substances has also been associated with brittle nails.

CLUBBING OF FINGERS

Clubbing of fingers (drumstick fingers) is associated with a decrease of oxygen supply in general. The resultant changes in the nail have been called *hippocratic* or *watch-glass* nails. The watch-glass nail is longer in the longitudinal axis than in the transverse axis, and the dorsal convexity is increased (Fig. 9-11). The nail is thickened, hard, shiny, and curved at the free end. The matrix atrophies. Early in the process the normal angle of the nail to the nail base (160 degrees) is lost. The nails are flatter and may be at a 180-degree angle to the nail base. In advanced cases the entire nail is pushed away from the base at an angle greater than 180 degrees and feels "spongy." (The student may simulate this spongy feel by grasping the distal phalanx on the lateral aspects of a finger at the level of the nail bed of one hand firmly between thumb and middle finger of the opposite hand. After a second or two the lunula will feel spongy when

pressed down by the nail of the index finger of the examining hand.) The distal phalanx becomes enlarged as the condition progresses. Clubbing is associated with respiratory (emphysema, chronic obstructive lung disease, carcinoma of the lung) and cardiovascular diseases and cirrhosis (Fig. 9-12).

Sebaceous glands

The sebaceous glands, which are more numerous over the face and scalp areas, normally become more active during adolescence, resulting in increased oiliness of the skin. A sudden increase in the oil of the skin at other ages would not be normal and may be suggestive of an endocrine problem.

SKIN LESIONS: DESCRIPTION AND CLASSIFICATION

The initial examination of any skin lesion should be carried out at a distance of 3 feet or more in order to determine the general characteristics of the eruption. This first observation should provide the opportunity to determine the body areas affected and the configuration of the lesions. A closer examination is required next to determine the particular characteristics of the individual lesions. The examiner should then be able to give a concise description of a lesion or lesions in terms of location and distribution, configuration, and morphological structure.

The examiner should also obtain a history of the eruption, such as, how long it has been present, whether it itches, and whether it appeared abruptly or seemed to start in a specific area and spread.

It is not possible to discuss the particular manifestations of the many skin problems that the examiner may find in practice. This discussion is limited to a few examples that demonstrate some of the different characteristics of skin lesions that will assist the examiner in describing the problem when consulting a dermatologist or a textbook on dermatology.

The distribution of skin lesions is fairly simple to describe according to the location or body region affected and the symmetry or asymmetry of findings in comparable body parts. The examiner must keep in mind that there are characteristic patterns that provide the major clue in the diagnosis of a specific skin problem. Fig. 9-13 illustrates a few distribution patterns manifested by specific problems.

The configuration of skin lesions is equally important in defining the problem. Configuration refers to the arrangement or position of several lesions in relation to each other. For example, the skin lesions of tinea corporis, ringworm of the body, have an annular configuration that is circular. Fig. 9-14 illustrates some of the different configurations that occur.

Text continued on p. 199.

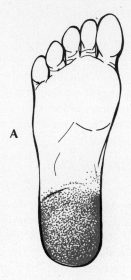

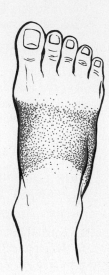

Fig. 9-13. Distribution of lesions in selected problems of the skin. **A,** Contact dermatitis (shoes). **B,** Contact dermatitis (cosmetics, perfumes, earrings).

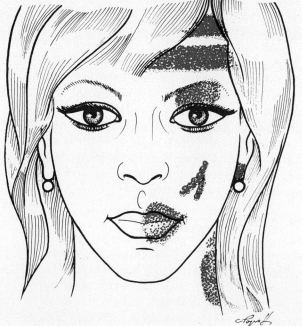

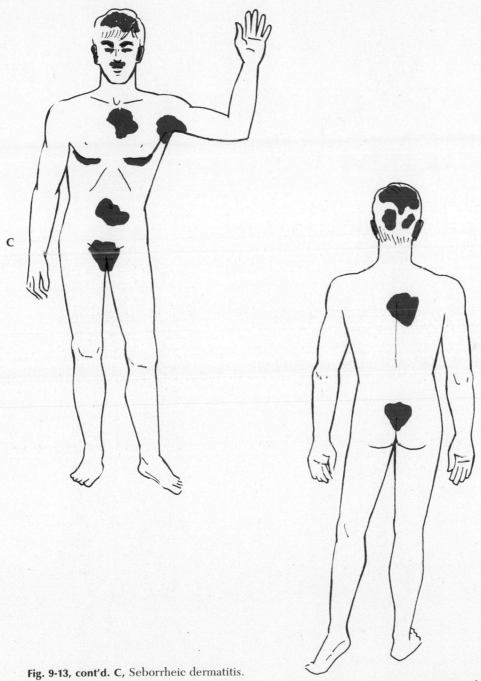

C

Fig. 9-13, cont'd. C, Seborrheic dermatitis.

Continued.

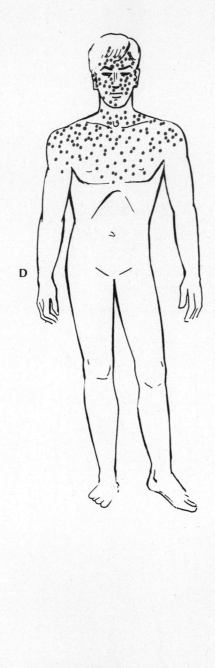

D

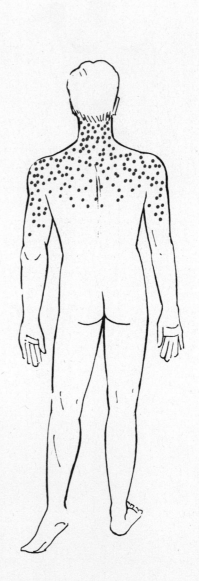

Fig. 9-13, cont'd. D, Acne.

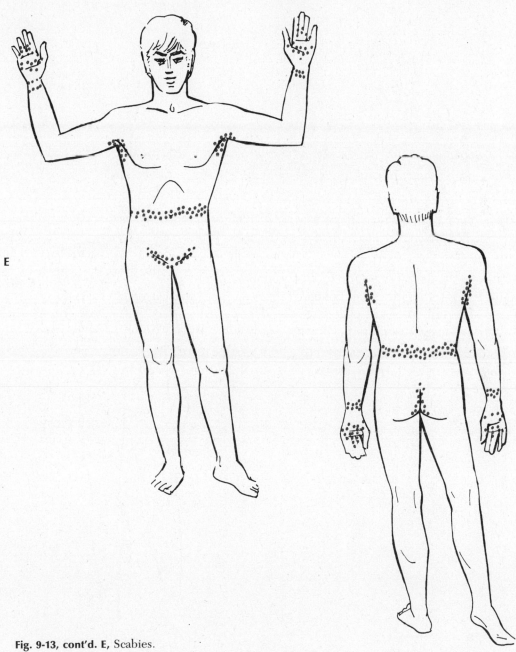

E

Fig. 9-13, cont'd. E, Scabies.

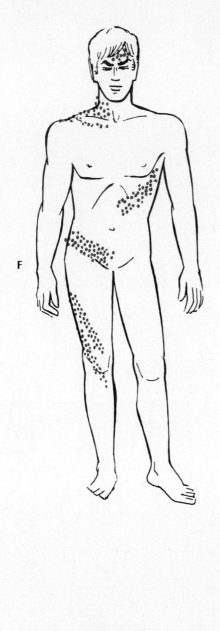
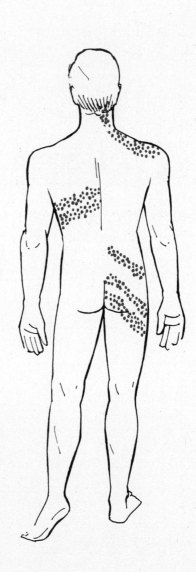

F

Fig. 9-13, cont'd. F, Herpes zoster.

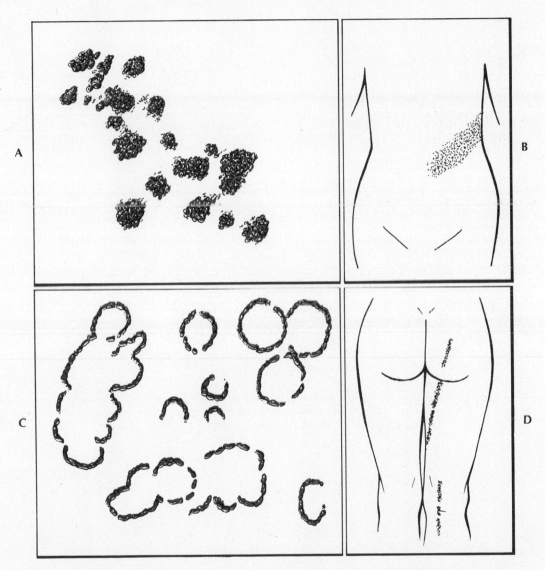

Fig. 9-14. Examples of different configurations of skin lesions. **A,** Grouped. **B,** Zosteriform. **C,** Annular and polycyclic. **D,** Linear.

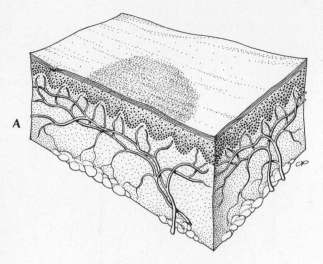

MACULE—circumscribed change in skin color without elevation or depression of the surface. Less than 1.0 cm in size. Such a lesion larger than 1.0 cm is called a patch.

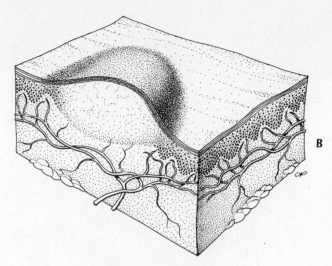

PAPULE—solid elevated area that varies in size but is usually less than 1.0 cm in diameter. Such a lesion larger than 1.0 cm is called a plaque.

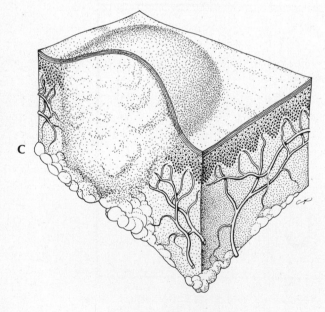

NODULE—small lesion in the dermal or subcutaneous tissue.

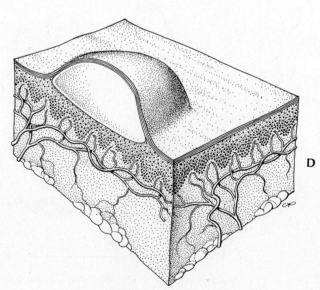

VESICLE—circumscribed elevated lesion containing serous fluid and less than 1.0 in diameter. Such a lesion larger than 1.0 cm is called a tumor.

Fig. 9-15. Primary lesions.

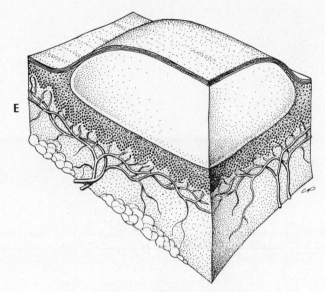

BULLA—vesicle larger than 1.0 cm in diameter.

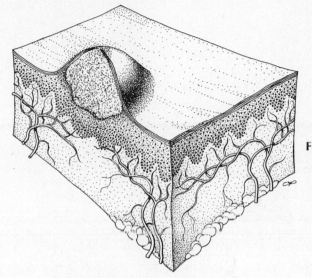

PUSTULE—vesicle or bulla containing purulent exudate.

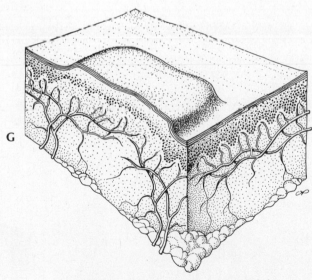

WHEAL—circumscribed, flat-topped, firm elevation of the skin with a well-defined palpable margin.

Fig. 9-15, cont'd. Primary lesions.

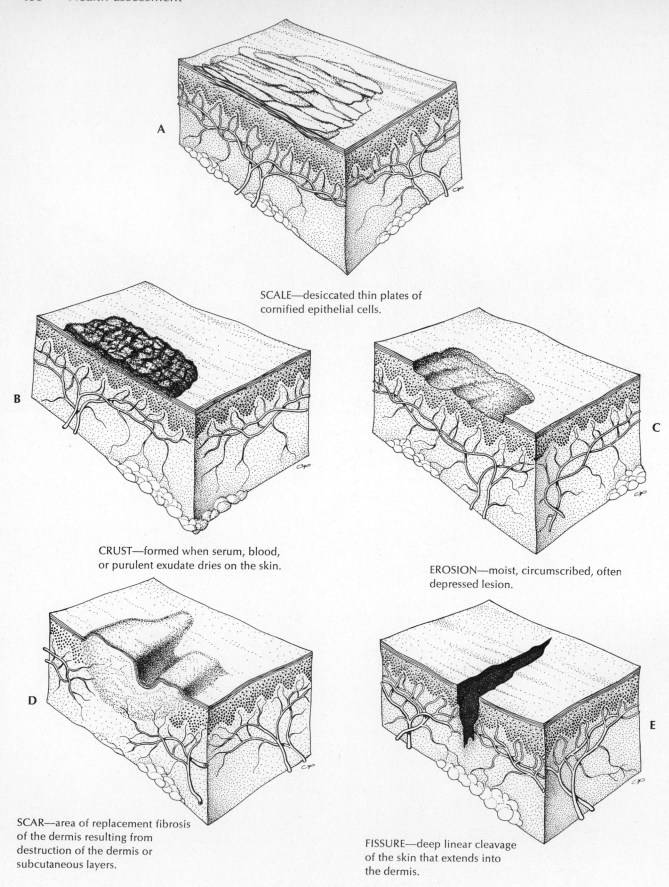

A SCALE—desiccated thin plates of cornified epithelial cells.

B CRUST—formed when serum, blood, or purulent exudate dries on the skin.

C EROSION—moist, circumscribed, often depressed lesion.

D SCAR—area of replacement fibrosis of the dermis resulting from destruction of the dermis or subcutaneous layers.

E FISSURE—deep linear cleavage of the skin that extends into the dermis.

Fig. 9-16. Secondary lesions.

Table 9-3. Identification of skin lesions

History: How long has it been present? ——————————————————————— Does it itch? ————
Type of lesion:

	Description	Name of lesion	
		<1 cm	>1 cm
Primary	Flat, circumscribed discoloration	Macule (Fig. 9-15, *A*)	Patch (Fig. 9-15, *A*)
	Solid, elevated lesion	Papule (Fig. 9-15, *B*)	Plaque (Fig. 9-15, *B*)
	Solid, elevated lesion also has depth	Nodule (Fig. 9-15, *C*)	Tumor (Fig. 9-15, *D*)
	Fluid filled, superficial, elevated	Vesicle (Fig. 9-15, *D*)	Bulla (Fig. 9-15, *E*)

	Description	Name of lesion
Primary of varying size	Vesicle or bulla containing pus	Pustule (Fig. 9-15, *F*)
	Lesion caused by cutaneous edema irregular in shape, elevated, transient	Wheal (Fig. 9-15, *G*)
	Dilated capillary fine red line(s)	Telangiectasia

	Description	Name of lesion
Secondary	Accumulation of loose surface epithelium	Scale (Fig. 9-16, *A*)
	Dried surface fluids: serum or pus	Crust (Fig. 9-16, *B*)
	Scratch mark	Excoriation
	Superficial denuded lesion	Erosion (Fig. 9-16, *C*)
	First red, then pale smooth hyaline wound repair; may be flat, depressed, elevated, or hypertrophic (keloid)	Scar (Fig. 9-16, *D*)
	Loss of tissue from a surface caused by destruction of a superficial lesion	Ulcer
	Thinning of skin, loss of hair and sweat glands	Atrophy
	Linear crack in skin that extends to dermis	Fissure (Fig. 9-16, *E*)
	Thickening of skin caused by chronic scratching	Lichenification

Shape of lesion: ☐ Round ☐ Oval ☐ Annular ☐ Archiform ☐ Linear ☐ Umbilicated
Color of lesion. ☐ Red ☐ Brown ☐ Black ☐ Gray-blue ☐ White ☐ Purple ☐ Orange ☐ Yellow
☐ Circumscribed? ☐ Diffuse? ☐ Change with diascopy*?
Configuration: ☐ Isolated ☐ Grouped: ☐ Herpetiform ☐ Linear ☐ Annular ☐ Archiform ☐ Reticular

Distribution pattern: Symmetry, sites of pressure, opposed surfaces of skin (intertriginous), exposed areas

———

*Diascopy consists of the application of firm pressure against a microscope slide or clear plastic placed over a skin lesion, allowing identification of capillary dilatation and thus differentiating telangiectasia from purpura. The technique also makes lymphoma, sarcoidosis, and tuberculosis of the skin appear yellow-brown.

Table 9-4. Stages of dermatitis

Stage	Lesions
Acute	Erythema; edema; vesicles; exudate; crusting
Subacute	Erythema; residual crusting; scaling
Chronic	Scaling; hyperpigmentation; lichenification; fissuring

Finally, there is a morphological classification of skin lesions that classifies lesions in terms of structure. It is important to identify the morphological structure of the individual lesion in order to identify the specific problem (Table 9-3). Lesions are classified as primary or secondary. *Primary lesions* are those that appear initially in response to some change in the external or internal environment of the skin. *Secondary lesions* do not appear initially but result from modifications in the primary lesion. For instance, the primary lesion may be a vesicle, which is a small, circumscribed, elevated lesion containing clear fluid. The vesicle will rupture, leaving a small moist area, which is classified as a secondary lesion called an *erosion*. Figs. 9-15 and 9-16 illustrate some of the primary and secondary lesions. Tables 9-4 to 9-6 identify various skin lesions.

Table 9-5. Common flat lesions of the skin

Condition	Lesion	Location
Actinic keratosis	Macule; scaling; red	Areas exposed to sunlight; scalp; ears
Atopic dermatitis	Dry, scaling inflammation, pruritus, excoriated lichenification, abnormally sensitive to environmental irritants	Forehead; cheeks; flexure regions; may be generalized
Contact dermatitis	Erythema; pruritus due to environmental irritant	Area of contact
Discoid lupus erythematosus	Discrete with hyperkeratotic plugs; scaling; central atrophy; scarring, red	Paranasal area; eyebrows; upper midback
Eczema		
Allergic	Erythema to exudate	Scalp; nose; forehead; eyelids; neck (from shampoo or hair dye); feet (from shoes); ears (from hearing aids or glasses); hands (from rubber gloves)
Chronic hereditary	Laminated silvery scales, tiny bleeding spots if scale pulled off	Points of trauma; genitalia
Nummular	Round lesions; moist surface; crusting; excoriation	Extensor surfaces of arms and legs
Intertrigo	Moist patches or erosions; borders well demarcated; red; associated with friction; macerated	Skin folds (warm and moist); breasts; axilla; inguinal regions, between toes, marked in obesity
Pityriasis rosea (unknown etiology)	Macules; scaling, oval shape; long axis follows lines of cleavage; red	Herald patch; then generalized
Psoriasis	Early lesion discrete; deep red patches; scaling; later discrete or confluent patches; plaques; gray-white thick scale; scale may appear shiny (disorder of keratin synthesis, hereditary)	May arise in one skin area or may appear as generalized skin involvement
Rosacea	Papules; pustules; oiliness; erythema; telangiectasia may be present	Face
Seborrhea	Noninflammatory dryness and scaling "dandruff" or oiliness	Scalp; face
Seborrheic dermatitis	Inflammation; dryness; scaling (loose, flaky); oiliness; pruritus may be crusted; eczematous	Scalp; ears; face (nasolabial fold, temples, eyelids); shoulders; navel; perianal region
Seborrheic keratosis	Early lesion—tan macule; progresses to papules, plaques; surface brown, rough	Any area; common on trunk
Scleroderma	Indurated; atrophic; shiny; skin appears tight, fastened down; hyperpigmentation or depigmentation	Generalized; tight facies; claw fingers
Systemic lupus erythematosus	Purpuric lesions; erythema; telangiectasia	Malar prominence over joints
Vascular		
Nevus flammeus (port wine stain)	Plaque; plexus of capillaries may have rough surface; red or purple	Present at birth; 50% on nuchal area
Nevus vasculosus	Capillary hemangioma; single tumor; rough surface; bright or dark red	75% in head region; appear in first or second month; most disappear by age 7
Spider nevus (arteriolar spider or spider angioma)	Small branching; arteriole, red; blanches on pressure	
Telangiectasia	Capillary dilatation; red; blanches on pressure	
Extravasation of blood		
Senile purpura	Ecchymoses; large areas blue-black, then green-yellow, then yellow; lesions do not blanch	

Table 9-5. Common flat lesions of the skin—cont'd

Condition	Lesion	Location
Neoplasia		
Paget's disease	Crusted dermatitis; moist veruccous surface; pruritus	Nipple and areola (manifestation of deeper intraductal malignancy)
Scar		
Striae	Linear; depressed; red-blue first, then silvery white	
Bacterial infection		
Erysipelas	Acute; edematous; red; tender	Face; limbs; abdomen
Impetigo	Yellow crusts; erythematous base; rapid spreading	Facial area; may be localized or may spread
Leprosy	Macules—tan to pink; nodules—yellowish; may ulcerate; incubation about 3 years	
Scarlet fever	Confluent, diffuse, blanching dermatitis; erythematous 1-7 days after—sore throat, fever	Generalized
Syphilis (secondary)	Macules; papules; lymphadenopathy; malaise, myalgia; low-grade fever	Mucous membranes; palms; soles
Syphilitic chancre	Small, round, red macule; erodes to indurated ulcer (1-2 cm); regional lymphadenopathy	Breast; vulva; penis
Trichomonas infection		
Trichomoniasis	Granular vaginal mucosa; bright red; petechiae may be present; discharge "foamy"	Vagina; labia
***Candida* infection**		
Candida	Patch borders well demarcated; flaccid pustules; patches creamy white; erythematous base; curdlike white discharge; pruritus patches; erythema	Inguinal region; vagina; glans penis
Viral infection		
Rubella, rubeola, roseola	Macules; discrete; erythematous; fever; lymphadenopathy (rubella); Koplik's spots (rubeola); 2-3 week incubation (rubella); then malaise, fever	Appear on trunk first; spread peripherally
Varicella (chickenpox)	Papule; vesicle; erythematous base; first clear fluid, then turbid; crusting on fourth day; 2-week incubation; 24-hour fever; malaise	First on chest and back; then face, arms, and legs
Variola (smallpox)	Macules; erythematous; progress to umbilicated lesions; then pustules, firm, round; then crusting; 2- to 3-week incubation; 5-day prodromal; toxic myalgia; fever	More lesions on face, extremities
Fungal infection		
Tinea corporis (ringworm)	Scaling; red with pale center; vesicular border; pruritic	Face; neck; extremities
Tinea cruris	Scaling; crescentic; red-brown	Axilla; inguinal region
Tinea pedis (fungal infection of foot)	Scaling; circular; vesicular border; red; chronic-hyperkeratotic	Feet
Infestations		
Pediculosis capitis	Pruritus; white concretions on hair—nits	

Continued.

Table 9-5. Common flat lesions of the skin—cont'd

Condition	Lesion	Location
Variation in pigmentation		
Hyperpigmentation		
Café au lait spots	Patches; light tan (six or more larger than 1.5 cm indicative of neurofibromatosis)	
Freckle (ephelis)	Discrete; macule; tan to brown	Pigmenting increased in areas exposed to sun
Lentigo		
Juvenile	Discrete macule; brown	Not affected by sun exposure
Senile	Single-macule; scaling; yellowish-brown; may be dark brown	Exposed surfaces, forehead, cheeks, extensor surfaces of limbs
Malignant	Mottled; irregular macule; enlarging; tan-brown, black-white; may ulcerate—then red	
Mongolian spots	Patch; irregular; dark blue or purple (chromophobe-like cell in skin)	Sacrum; present at birth; more common with darker pigmented individuals; disappear spontaneously by age 4
Nevus	Macule; pigmented or nonpigmented; may be present at birth or arise later	
Peutz-Jeghers syndrome	Brown spots; abdominal pain	Lips; fingers; toes
Depigmentation		
Vitiligo		
Addison's disease	Circumscribed patch(es) of depigmentation	
Pernicious anemia		
Thyrotoxicosis		

The following are examples of the recording of selected abnormal skin findings.

1. **Measles (rubeola).** Skin is hot and dry with an erythematous, confluent, maculopapular rash covering the neck, trunk, arms, and abdomen but fading from the face. Discrete erythematous maculopapular lesions are densely scattered over the lower extremities.
2. **Impetigo.** Skin is dark brown, warm, moist, elastic, and smooth, except for four irregularly grouped, moist, honey-colored crusted pustular lesions, 1 to 2 cm in diameter, inferior to the right lower lip.
3. **Vitiligo.** Skin is light brown, warm, moist, elastic, and smooth, with several nontender, macular, depigmented, roughly oval-shaped areas varying in size from 1 by 2 cm to 3 by 4 cm and scattered over dorsal surfaces of both hands.
4. **Ecchymosis.** Skin is light pink, warm, elastic, and smooth with a tender, 8 by 10-cm, irregularly shaped, dark purple to green-yellow macular area over extensor surface of left shoulder.

SUMMARY

I. General observation while client is standing, if possible, and with the examiner 3 feet or more away.

A. General skin color
B. Hair distribution, texture, and quantity over body
C. Sun-exposed areas (face, ears, back of neck, dorsum of hands and arms) compared with less-exposed areas
D. Pigmented labile areas (dorsal flexor surfaces of hands and wrists, face around mouth, axillae, areolae, midline of abdomen, and genital area)
E. Vascular flush areas (from cheek to cheek across bridge of nose, neck, upper chest, flexor surface of extremities, and genital area)
F. Location and distribution of any rash, birthmarks, scratches, bruising, or swelling

II. Closer observation and palpation of skin while client is sitting or lying down
A. Nails
1. Color, contour, and thickness of nails and their adherence to the nail beds
2. Temperature, color, shape, and tenderness of skinfolds around nails
3. Grooming
B. Hair of scalp
1. Quantity
2. Color
3. Texture
4. Grooming

Table 9-6. Common raised lesions

Condition	Lesion	Location
Acne vulgaris	Comedones; papules; pustules; cysts; scars	Face; back; shoulders; upper arms
Dermatitis herpetiformis (chronic)	Macules; papules; vesicles; excoriated vesicles; pruritus (intense); residual hyperpigmentation; hereditary	Scalp; interscapular; sacral
Leukoplakia	Plaque; thick; indurated; white	Mucous membrane; mouth; labia; vagina
Lichen planus (unknown etiology)	Maculopapular lesion; deep red to purple; pruritus; hyperkeratotic	Flexor surfaces of wrists; palms; soles; ankles; abdomen; sacrum
Lichen simplex (chronic)	Plaque; dry; lichenification; hyperpigmentation	Scalp; labia
Seborrheic keratosis	Single plaque; soft lesion with rough surface; brown	
Lipid disorder		
Xanthelasma	Papules or plaques; yellow; lipid deposits	Eyelids
Cysts		
Epidermoid and sebaceous cysts	Fluctuant, globular lesions	
Milia	Pinhead (1-2 mm) white, sebaceous cyst	Infraorbital skin, nose, chin; common in newborn
Neoplasia		
Achrochordon (skin tag)	Pedunculated skin tag; skin color	Neck; axilla; groin
Basal-cell carcinoma	Nodule—rolled edge; tendency to ulcerate in center	
Basal-cell epithelioma	May follow actinic keratosis; papule or nodule—rolled edge; ulcer—nonhealing	
Squamous-cell carcinoma	Nodule; indurated; ulcer—nonhealing; history of overexposure to sun, x-rays	Often on face
Dermatofibroma	Tumor; discrete; dome-shaped; brown; less than 1 cm	
Lipoma	Fatty tumor; soft	
Malignant melanoma	Arises from pigmented nevus; indurated	
Neurofibroma	Pedunculated; soft; flaccid lesion; skin color black, brown, rose, white	
Pigmented nevus	Single or multiple dome-shaped lesions; may be hairy; brown to black; present at birth	
Vascular		
Angioma (sometimes called senile angioma)	Papule; vascular; cherry red; pinhead (1-3 mm); most adults after climacteric	.
Hyperkeratosis		
Clavus (corn)	Hyperkeratosis; hard; tender; shape—inverted cone	Dorsum of toes; most common on fifth toe
Cutaneous horn	Horn projection of hyperkeratotic lesion	
Wheals		
Dermographism	Wheal in response to scratch or pressure; (histamine easily released)	
Erythema multiforme (varied causes)	Wheallike, round darker depressed center (target appearance)	Arms and legs first; then on body
Urticaria	Wheal; pale on erythematous base; pruritus; transient	
Bullae		
Pemphigus	Bullae; flaccid, moist, fluid-filled rupture easily bleeds; erythematous base; from lack of mucopolysaccharide protein for intercellular cement	Skin—all parts mucous membrane

Continued.

Table 9-6. Common raised lesions—cont'd

Condition	Lesion	Location
From bacterial infection		
Chancroid	Vesicopustule; ulcer; ragged, undermined edges; shallow; may be multiple; red; lymphadenopathy	Genitalia—male and female
Folliculitis	Discrete perifollicular papules and pustules; erythematous	
Furuncle	Swelling becomes pustular; red; tender, painful	
From viral infection		
Herpes simplex	Vesicles; grouped; may be recurrent	Lips; anywhere on face
Herpes zoster	Tenderness; burning; pruritus; vesicles later crusting; erythematous base; hypersensitivity; localized lymphadenopathy	Pathway of a peripheral nerve, may have postherpetic neuralgia
Molluscum contagiosum	Multiple, discrete globules; waxy depression in center	Trunk
Verruca acuminata	Papillary (cauliflower-like); red; soft	Penis; vulva; perianal area
Verruca plantaris (plantar wart)	Circumscribed callus; surrounded by hyperkeratosis; black dots; tender	Plantar surface of foot or toes
Verruca vulgaris (wart)	Single or multiple; tan	Hands
From infestation		
Pediculosis corporis (body lice)	Wheal; central hemorrhagic spot; linear excoriations; later dry, scaly pigmentation	
Pediculosis pubis (pubic lice)	Papules; discrete; excoriated; gray-white dots at base of hair—nits; lice may be seen at base of hairs	Genital region; lower abdomen; chest; axillae; eyebrows; eyelashes
	Gray-blue macules	May be present on abdomen; thighs; axillae
Scabies	Vesicles; papules; pruritus	Skin folds

C. Mucosa of nose and mouth
  1. Color
  2. Moisture
  3. Texture
D. Each part of the body as examined
  1. Color
  2. Temperature
  3. Moisture
  4. Texture
  5. Turgor
E. Abnormal changes or lesions of the skin
  1. Color
  2. Configuration and arrangement
  3. Morphological structure of individual lesions
  4. Size of individual abnormality, such as a lesion, birthmark, or bruise (to be measured)
  5. Moisture
  6. Number (count when possible)
  7. Depth and consistency
  8. Temperature
  9. Tenderness

BIBLIOGRAPHY

DeNicola, P., and Morsiani, M.: Nail diseases in internal medicine, Springfield, Ill., 1974, Charles C Thomas, Publishers.

Fitzpatrick, T. B.: Dermatology in general practice, New York, 1971, McGraw-Hill Book Co.

Lazarus, G. S., and Goldsmith, L. A.: Diagnosis of skin disease, Philadelphia, 1980, F. A. Davis Co.

Lewis, G. M., and Wheeler, C. E.: Practical dermatology, ed. 3, Philadelphia, 1967, W. B. Saunders Co.

Rook, A., and Wilkerson, D. S.: Textbook of dermatology, vol. 1, ed. 2, Oxford, 1972, Blackwell Scientific Publications Ltd.

Samman, P. D.: The nails in disease, London, 1978, William Heinemann Medical Books Ltd.

Saver, G. C.: Manual of skin diseases, ed. 3, Philadelphia, 1973, J. B. Lippincott Co.

Stewart, W. D., Danto, J. L., and Maddin, S.: Dermatology: diagnosis and treatment of cutaneous disorders, ed. 4, St. Louis, 1978, The C. V. Mosby Co.

10 Assessment of the ears, nose, and throat

The examination of the ears, nose, and throat is an important part of every physical examination because it provides the opportunity to inspect directly or indirectly most parts of the upper respiratory system and the first division of the digestive system. The clinical examination of these body orifices can provide information about the client's general health as well as information about significant local disease. The methods of examination are primarily inspection and palpation.

The client should be seated for the ear, nose, and throat examination with the examiner's head at approximately the same level as that of the client. The necessary equipment includes an otoscope with various sizes of speculums, tongue blades, 4 by 4 gauze sponges, rubber gloves or finger cots, and a tuning fork (512 cycles per second [cps]). A good light source such as a gooseneck lamp with a 100- to 150-watt bulb is helpful but if not available a penlight can be used. A dental mirror and a nasal speculum may also be helpful.

Discussion is focused on each of the three areas: the ears, the nose and paranasal sinuses, and the mouth and oropharynx. The portion of the chapter on each area includes a brief review of the anatomy and physiology, a description of the methods to be used in the examination, and some of the common findings of which the examiner should be aware when examining the particular area.

EARS
Anatomy and physiology

The ear is a sensory organ that functions both in hearing and in equilibrium. It has three parts: the external ear, the middle ear, and the inner ear. Fig. 10-1 illustrates the structures of the ear.

The external ear has two divisions, the flap called the auricle or pinna and the canal called the external auditory canal or meatus. Stretching across the proximal portion of the canal is the tympanic membrane, which separates the external ear from the middle ear. The auricle is composed of cartilage, closely adherent perichondrium, and skin. The main components of the auricle are the helix, antihelix, crus of helix, lobule, tragus, antitragus, and concha (Fig. 10-2). The mastoid process is not part of the external ear but is a bony prominence found posterior to the lower part of the auricle.

The external auditory canal, which is about 1 inch in length, has a skeleton of cartilage in its outer third and a skeleton of bone in its inner two-thirds. It has a slight curve with the outer one-third of the canal directed upward and toward the back of the head, while the inner two-thirds is directed downward and forward. The skin of the inner ear is exceedingly thin and sensitive.

The tympanic membrane, which covers the proximal end of the auditory canal, is made up of layers of skin, fibrous tissue, and mucous membrane (Fig. 10-3). The membrane is shiny, translucent, and a pearl gray color. The position of the ear drum is oblique with respect to the ear canal. The antero-inferior quadrant is most distant from the examiner, which accounts for the cone of light or the light reflex. The membrane is slightly concave and is pulled inward at its center by one of the ossicles, the malleus, of the middle ear. The short process of the malleus protrudes into the eardrum superiorly, and the handle of the malleus extends downward from the short process to the umbo, the point of maximum concavity. Most of the membrane is taut and is known as the pars tensa. A small part superiorly is less taut and is known as the pars flaccida. The dense fibrose ring surrounding the tympanic membrane, with the exception of the anterior and posterior malleolar folds superiorly, is the annulus.

The middle ear is a small, air-filled cavity located in the temporal bone. It contains three small bones called the auditory ossicles: the malleus, the incus, and the stapes. The middle ear cavity contains sev-

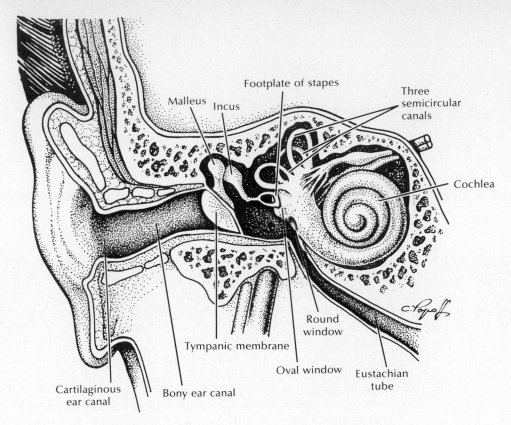

Fig. 10-1. External auditory canal, middle ear, and inner ear.

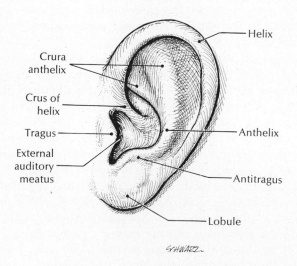

Fig. 10-2. Structures of the external ear.

eral openings. One is from the external auditory meatus and is covered by the tympanic membrane. There are two openings into the inner ear, the oval window into which the stapes fits and the round window covered by a membrane. Another opening connects the middle ear with the eustachian tube. The middle ear performs three functions: (1) it transmits sound vibrations across the ossicle chain to the inner ear's oval window, (2) it protects the auditory apparatus from intense vibrations, and (3) it equalizes the air pressure on both sides of the dividing tympanic membrane to prevent the tympanic membrane from being ruptured.

The inner ear is made up of two parts, the bony labyrinth and, inside this structure, a membranous labyrinth. The bony labyrinth consists of three parts: the vestibule, the semicircular canals, and the cochlea. The vestibule and the semicircular canals comprise the organs of equilibrium. The cochlea comprises the organ of hearing. The cochlea is a coiled structure that contains the organ of Corti, which transmits stimuli to the cochlear branch of the auditory nerve (cranial nerve [CN] VIII).

Hearing occurs when sound waves enter the external auditory canal and strike the tympanic membrane, causing it to vibrate at the same rate as the sound waves striking it. The auricle does not direct or amplify sound and has little apparent usefulness. The vibrations are transmitted through the auditory ossicles of the middle ear to the oval window. From the oval window the vibrations travel via the fluid of the cochlea, winding up at the round window, where they are dissipated. The vibrations of the membrane cause the delicate hair cells of the organ of Corti to

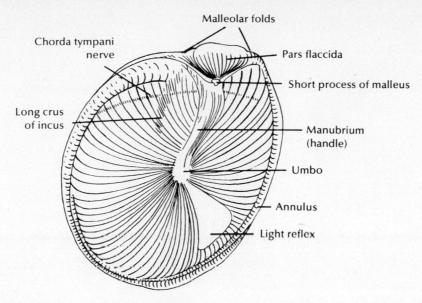

Chorda tympani nerve

Long crus of incus

Malleolar folds

Pars flaccida

Short process of malleus

Manubrium (handle)

Umbo

Annulus

Light reflex

Fig. 10-3. Right tympanic membrane. (From Prior, J. A., and Silberstein, J. S.: Physical diagnosis: the history and examination of the patient, ed. 5, St. Louis, 1977, The C. V. Mosby Co.)

impact against the membrane of Corti, acting as a stimuli setting up impulses in the sensory endings of the cochlear branch of the auditory nerve (CN VIII).

Hearing loss

There are several types of hearing loss. However, almost every form may be classified under one of three headings: conductive hearing loss, sensorineural or perceptive hearing loss, or mixed hearing loss.

Conductive hearing loss occurs when there are external or middle ear disorders such as impacted cerumen, perforation of the tympanic membrane, serum or pus in the middle ear, or a fusion of the ossicles. The vibrations are not adequately transmitted to the inner ear through the ear canal, tympanic membrane, middle ear, and ossicular chain; and a partial loss of hearing occurs.

Sensorineural, or perceptive, hearing loss occurs when there is a disorder in the inner ear, the auditory nerve, or the brain. Vibrations are transmitted to the inner ear, but an impairment of the cochlea or auditory nerve attenuates the nervous impulses from the cochlea to the brain.

Mixed hearing loss is a combination of conductive and sensorineural loss in the same ear.

Examination

The examination of the external ear begins with an inspection of both auricles to determine their position, size, and symmetry. Then the lateral and medial surfaces of each auricle and the surrounding tissues are inspected to determine the skin color and the presence of deformities, lesions, or nodules. The auricles and mastoid areas are palpated for evidence of swelling, tenderness, or nodules. Although fairly simple, this part of the examination is frequently neglected.

Examination of the external auditory canal and tympanic membrane requires additional lighting. It is suggested that the examiner become acquainted with the use and maintenance of the electric otoscope. For the otoscope to be effective, the batteries should be changed frequently to ensure optimal efficiency. The focus of light should be directed out of the end of the speculum. Some speculum carriers are movable and can be out of alignment with the bulb carrier. Some older models have a bulb carrier that can be bent, causing the light to be deflected to one side of the speculum.

Before insertion of the speculum in the ear, the opening of the auditory canal should be carefully inspected for evidence of external otitis, furunculosis, a foreign body, or a discharge. Any discharge should be described in terms of appearance and odor. A putrid odor is usually indicative of mastoid disease with bone destruction. After this inspection, the speculum can be inserted. The following points should, however, be remembered:

1. Use the largest speculum that can be inserted in the ear without pain.
2. The client's head should be tipped toward the opposite shoulder for easy examination of the canal and tympanic membrane.
3. In adults the ear canal may be straightened by pulling the auricle upward and backward; in

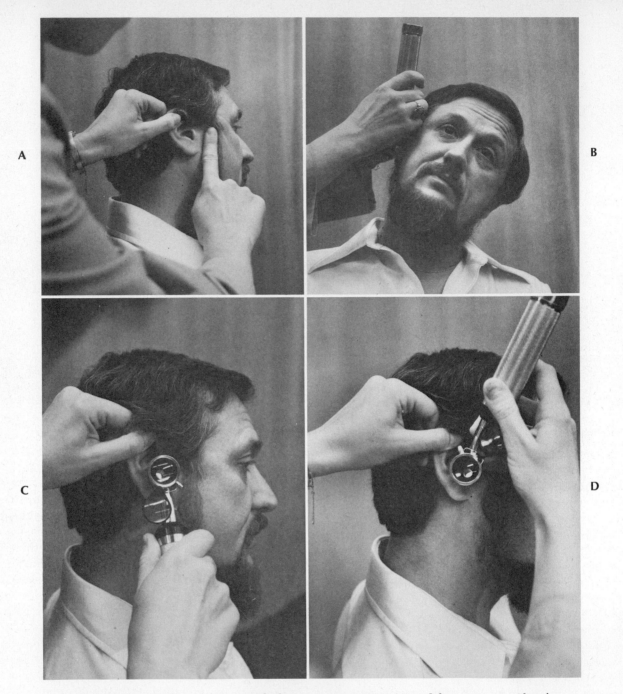

Fig. 10-4. Examination of the ear with the otoscope. **A,** Inspection of the meatus. **B,** Client's head is tipped toward the opposite shoulder. **C** and **D,** Two ways of holding the otoscope.

young children and infants it may be straightened by pulling the auricle downward.

4. The inner two-thirds of the external meatus, which has a bony skeleton, is sensitive to pressure. Insert the speculum gently and not too far to avoid causing pain.

5. The angle at which the speculum is inserted into the meatus must be varied, or only a limited area of the tympanic membrane will be seen.

The auditory canal should be inspected for cerumen, redness, or swelling. The appearance of the normal canal varies in diameter, shape, and growth of hairs. Hair growth is limited to the outer third of the canal, but the hairs may be numerous.

Another aspect of the examination of the auditory canal is the evaluation of cerumen, which is produced by the sebaceous glands and the apocrine sweat glands in the canal. There are apparently racial variations in color, and black or brown cerumen will be noted in the client with darker skin coloring. There is also some difference in the color of fresh cerumen as compared to older, drier cerumen; the former is a lighter, yellow or even pink color, and the latter is a darker, yellowish brown color. A small amount of cerumen will not interfere with the examination; the examiner can look past it and visualize the tympanic membrane. However, if the wax is excessive, it may be necessary to remove it.

Two of the methods that can be used for the removal of wax are currettement and irrigation. *Currettement* is appropriate if the wax is soft or there is a question of perforation of the tympanic membrane. However, it should not be done except by a skilled clinician. The closeness of the blood vessels and nerves to the surface make it easy to cause bleeding and pain. There is also a risk of perforating the tympanic membrane if the client moves or the curette is used with too much vigor. *Irrigation* may be used when the wax is dry and hard but should not be carried out if there is a possibility that the membrane is perforated. Lukewarm water is used for the irrigation, which is done by repeatedly injecting the water from a syringe toward the posterosuperior canal wall. This procedure will cause the client to feel dizzy.

The examination of the tympanic membrane (Fig. 10-3) requires a careful assessment of the color of the membrane and the identification of landmarks. The membrane is usually a translucent pearl gray color; in disease the color may be yellow, white, or red. Some membranes have white flecks or dense white plaques that are the result of healed inflammatory disease. The landmarks are identified, beginning with the light reflex, which is a triangular cone of reflected light seen in the anteroinferior quadrant of the membrane. A diffuse or spotty light is not normal. At the top point of the light reflex toward the center of the membrane is the umbo, the inferior point of the handle of the malleus. Anterior and superior to the umbo is the long process of the malleus, which appears as a whitish line extending from the umbo to the juncture of the malleolar folds, where the small white projection of the short process of the malleus can be seen. The malleolar folds and the pars flaccida, the relaxed portion of the membrane, are superior and lateral to the short process. Finally, an attempt should be made to follow the annulus around the periphery of the pars tensa. It is in the areas close to the annulus that perforations are frequently noted.

Bulging of the tympanic membrane may occur when pus forms in the middle ear. The pressure increases, and the membrane may bulge outward in one part, or the entire membrane may bulge, resulting in obliteration of some or all of the landmarks. The light reflex is usually lost, and the membrane appears dull.

Retraction of the tympanic membrane occurs when pressure is reduced due to obstruction of the eustachian tube, usually associated with an upper respiratory system infection. The retraction of the membrane causes the landmarks to be accentuated. The light reflex may appear less prominent.

Normal tympanic membranes vary to some extent in size, shape, and color. It is only by examining many normal, healthy membranes that the ability to recognize the abnormal membrane is acquired.

TESTING OF AUDITORY FUNCTION

Clinical testing of auditory function is a process that starts early in the physical examination of the client. Understanding the spoken word is the principal use of hearing, and it may become apparent during the interview that there is an impairment or loss of auditory function. The actual testing of auditory function should be delayed until the end of the examination, after obvious problems related to hearing may have been identified. A precise measurement of hearing requires the use of the audiometer, but a good estimate of hearing can be made during the physical examination with the use of the tests discussed in this section.

Simple assessment of auditory acuity requires that only one ear be tested at a time. Therefore, it is necessary to mask the hearing in the ear not being tested. The examiner may occlude one of the client's ears by placing a finger against the opening of the auditory canal and moving the finger rapidly but gently.

Voice tests are frequently used in estimating the client's hearing. The testing is begun with a very low whisper; the lips of the examiner should be 1 or 2 feet away from the unoccluded ear. The examiner exhales and softly whispers numbers that the client is to repeat. If necessary, the intensity of the voice is increased to a medium whisper, and then to a loud whisper; then to a soft, then medium, then loud voice. To prevent lipreading during the voice tests, the examiner may stand behind the client. If it is more convenient to be in front of the client, the client should be asked to close his eyes.

The watch tick is useful in testing but should not be used exclusively, because it provides only a high-frequency sound. The ticking watch is moved away from the ear until the client can no longer hear the sound.

Tuning fork tests are useful in determining whether the client has a conductive or a perceptive hearing loss. A fork with frequencies of 500 to 1,000 cps is

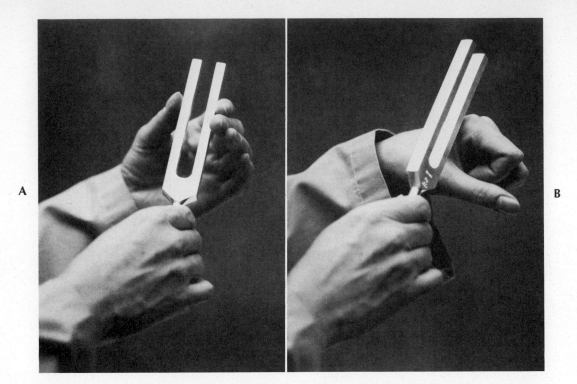

Fig. 10-5. Activating the tuning fork. **A,** Stroking the fork. **B,** Tapping the fork on the knuckle.

used because it can provide an estimate of hearing loss in the speech frequencies of roughly 500 to 2,000 cps. The tuning fork is held by the base without the fingers touching either of the two prongs. The sound vibrations are softened or stopped entirely when the prongs of the fork are touched or held. The fork is activated by gently stroking or tapping on the knuckles of the opposite hand (Fig. 10-5). It should be made to ring softly, not harshly.

The terms bone conduction and air conduction need to be clearly understood in the discussion of tuning fork tests. *Air conduction* implies the transmission of sound through the ear canal, tympanic membrane, and ossicular chain to the cochlea and auditory nerve. *Bone conduction* implies that sound is transmitted through the bones of the skull to the cochlea and auditory nerve. The client with normal auditory function will hear sound twice as long by air conduction, when the tuning fork is held opposite the external meatus, as he will by bone conduction, when the base of the tuning fork is placed on the mastoid bone.

The Rinne test makes use of air conduction and bone conduction. The tuning fork is used to compare the conduction of sound through the mastoid bone and the conduction of sound through the auditory meatus. There are two different methods of performing the Rinne test but the principle remains the same:

the sound will be heard twice as long by air conduction as by bone conduction when there is no conductive hearing loss. The most common method is to place the activated tuning fork against the mastoid bone until the client can no longer hear the sound and then move the fork to a distance of ½ to 1 inch from the auditory meatus. The client with no conductive hearing loss will continue to hear the sound by air conduction.

The second method merely reverses the order. The activated tuning fork is held 1 inch from the auditory meatus and when the client can no longer hear the sound, the base of the fork is placed immediately on the mastoid bone. If the client cannot hear the sound when the fork is placed on the mastoid bone, his Rinne test is considered positive and he does not have a conductive hearing loss. If the opposite is true and the client can hear the sound better by bone conduction, his Rinne test is negative and there is a conductive hearing loss. A positive Rinne with *an overall reduction in the time* where the sound is heard and normal ratio of air conduction to bone conduction is maintained results when there is a sensorineural hearing loss. This demonstrates that the client does not hear well by either air conduction or bone conduction.

The *Weber test*, which makes use of bone conduction, is carried out by placing the base of the

Table 10-1. Hearing tests using tuning forks

Hearing	Weber (bone conduction)	Rinne (air and bone conduction)

Normal

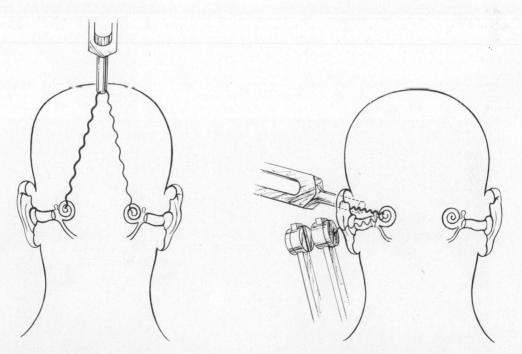

Normal hearing
Sound does not lateralize to either side; heard equally well in both ears

Normal hearing
"Positive Rinne." Sound is heard twice as long by air conduction as by bone conduction

Conduction loss (problem of external or middle ear)

Conductive deafness in right ear
Sound lateralizes to defective ear as few extraneous sounds are carried through external or middle ear

Conductive deafness in right ear
"Negative Rinne." Sound heard longer by bone conduction than by air conduction

Continued.

Table 10-1. Hearing tests using tuning forks—cont'd

Hearing	Weber (bone conduction)	Rinne (air and bone conduction)
Sensorineural loss (perceptive problem of inner ear or nerve)	**Perceptive deafness of right ear** Sound lateralizes to the better ear	**Perceptive deafness of right ear** "Positive Rinne." Sound is heard longer by air conduction than by bone conduction

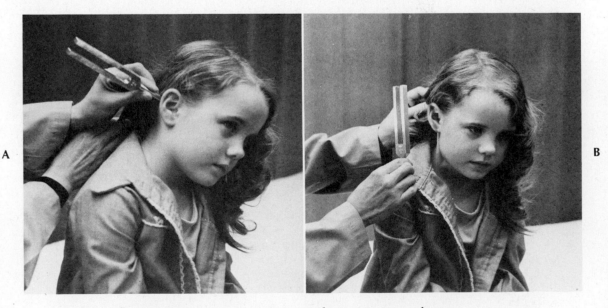

Fig. 10-6. Rinne test. **A,** Bone conduction. **B,** Air conduction.

Plate 1. Some common dermatoses and cutaneous manifestations of systemic disorders.

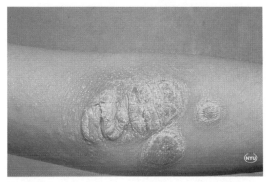

Psoriasis

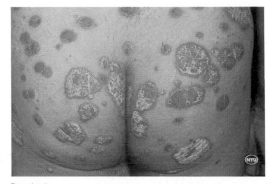

Psoriasis

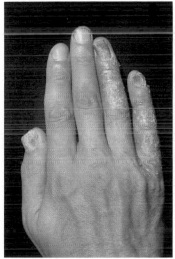

Psoriasis

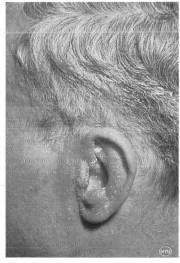

Seborrheic dermatitis

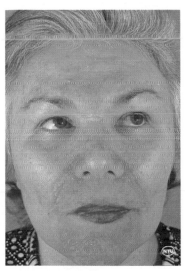

Seborrheic dermatitis

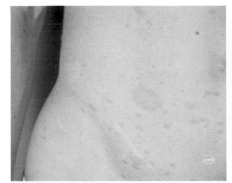

Pityriasis rosea

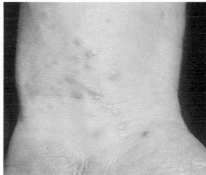

Lichen planus

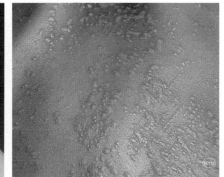

Lichen planus

Continued.

Plate 1, cont'd. Some common dermatoses and cutaneous manifestations of systemic disorders.

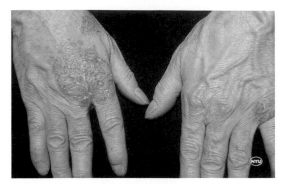

Nummular eczema

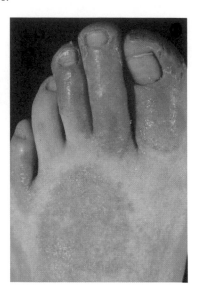

Atopic dermatitis

Allergic contact dermatitis—shoe

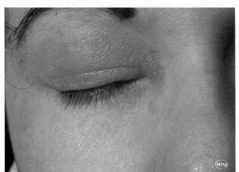

Allergic contact dermatitis—shampoo

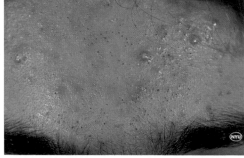

Acne

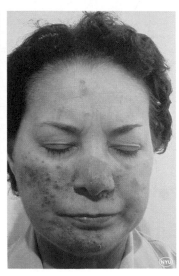

Rosacea

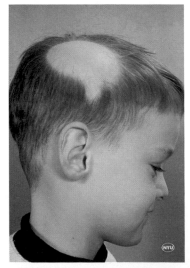

Alopecia areata

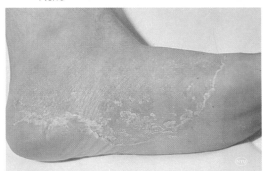

Tinea pedis

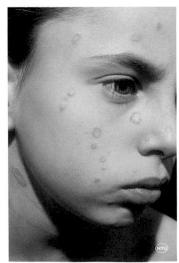

Tinea faciale

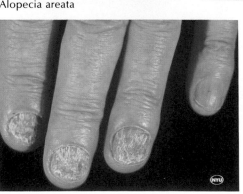

Tinea unguium

Plate 1, cont'd. Some common dermatoses and cutaneous manifestations of systemic disorders.

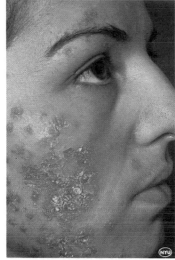

Impetigo contagiosa

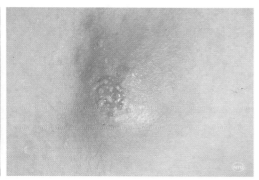

Folliculitis

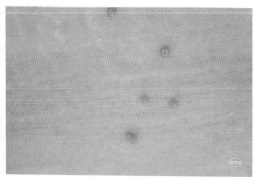

Carbuncle

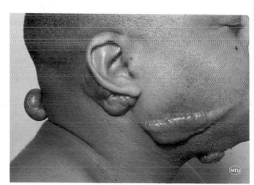

Keloids

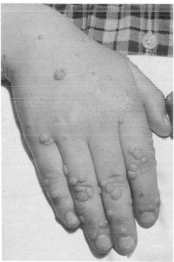

Verruca vulgaris

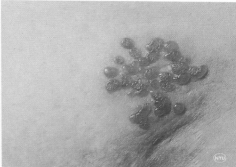

Molluscum contagiosum

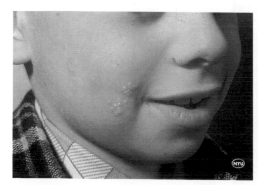

Herpes simplex

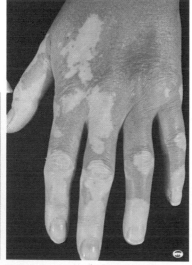

Herpes zoster

Vitiligo

Continued.

Plate 1, cont'd. Some common dermatoses and cutaneous manifestations of systemic disorders.

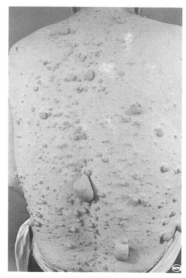

Neurofibromatosis

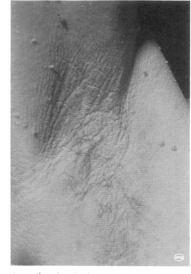

Acanthosis nigricans

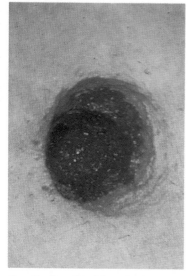

Paget's disease of the nipple
(Courtesy of Stewart, W. D., et. al.:
Dermatology, 1978, The C. V. Mosby Co.)

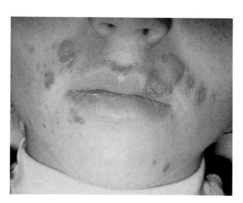

Impetigo (bullous)

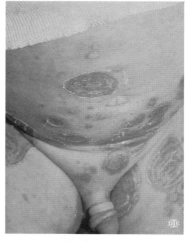

Impetigo (bullous)

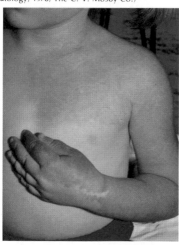

Nevus flammeus

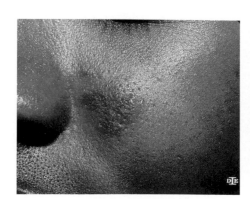

Discoid lupus erythematosus

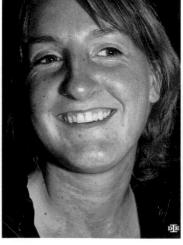

Systemic lupus erythematosus

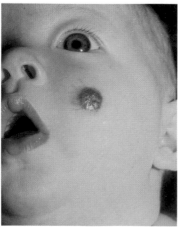

Hemangioma

Plate 1. Courtesy American Academy of Dermatology and Institute for Dermatologic Communication and Education, Evanston, Illinois.

Plate 2. Ear.

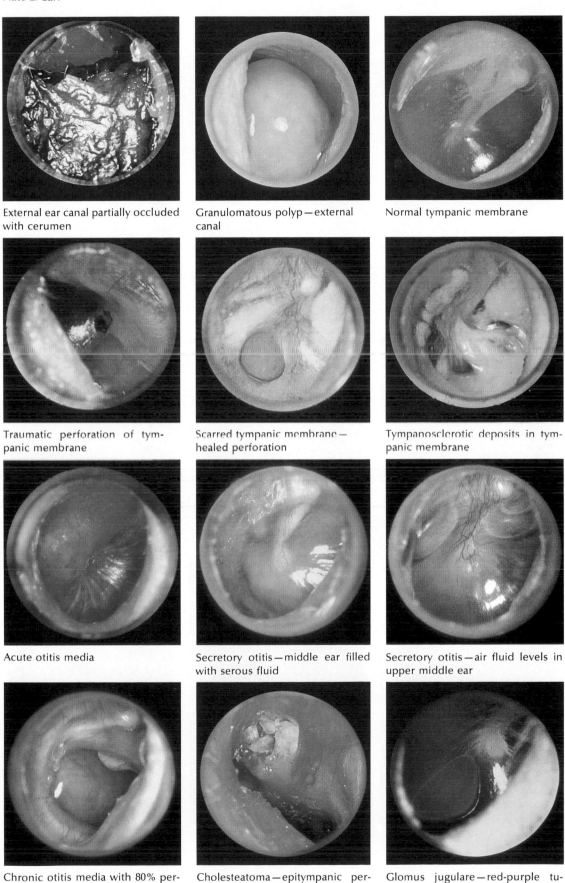

External ear canal partially occluded with cerumen

Granulomatous polyp—external canal

Normal tympanic membrane

Traumatic perforation of tympanic membrane

Scarred tympanic membrane—healed perforation

Tympanosclerotic deposits in tympanic membrane

Acute otitis media

Secretory otitis—middle ear filled with serous fluid

Secretory otitis—air fluid levels in upper middle ear

Chronic otitis media with 80% perforation of tympanic membrane

Cholesteatoma—epitympanic perforation with epithelial debris

Glomus jugulare—red-purple tumor in contact with tympanic membrane

Plate 2. Courtesy Dr. Richard A. Buckingham, Clinical Professor, Otolaryngology, Abraham Lincoln School of Medicine, University of Illinois, Chicago, Illinois.

Plate 3. Nose.

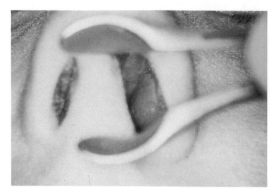

Allergic rhinitis

Plate 4. Mouth.

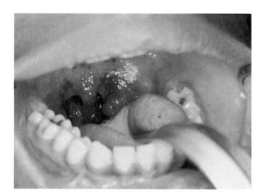

Acute viral pharyngitis

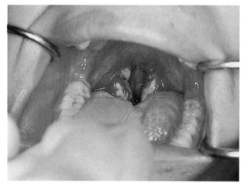

Tonsillitis, pharyngitis

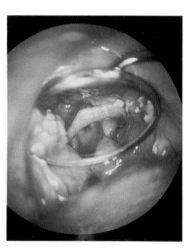

Yeast infection, lingual tonsil, hypopharynx

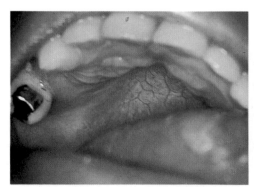

Leukoplakia

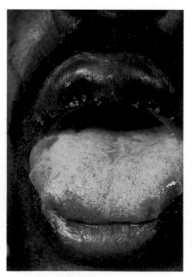

Acute bacterial stomatitis

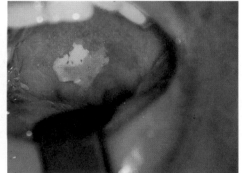

Vincent's angina

Continued.

Plate 4, cont'd. Mouth.

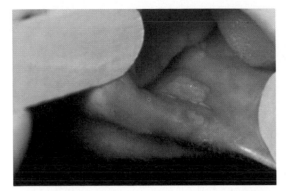

Herpes zoster

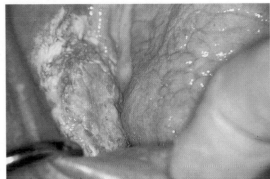

Squamous cell carcinoma

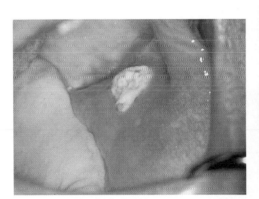

Carcinoma of oral mucosa

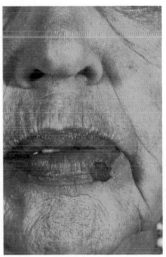

Senile keratosis—lip

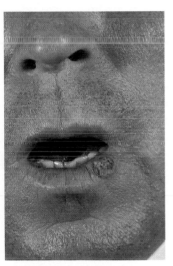

Epidermal carcinoma—lip

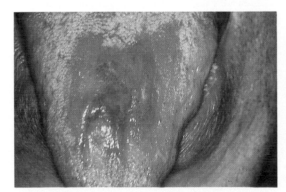

Drug reaction—tongue

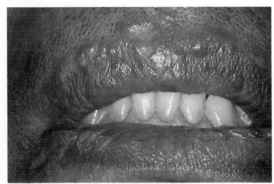

Drug reaction—lip

Plate 4. Courtesy Dr. Edward L. Applebaum, Head, Department of Otolaryngology, University of Illinois Medical Center, Chicago, Illinois.

Plate 5. Eyes.

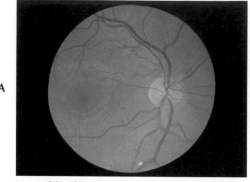

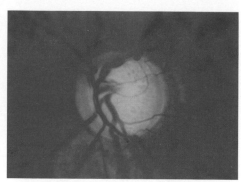

Normal fundus of a right eye. Note the optic disc, retinal arterioles and veins, macular area, and retinal background.

Deep physiologic cupping of glaucoma. Note course of vessels at rim of optic disc.

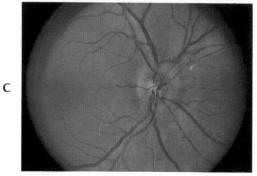

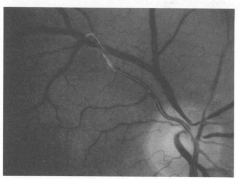

Papilledema. Note blurred margins of the optic disc.

Hypertensive retinopathy. Note increased light reflex and narrowing of arterioles and the arteriovenous crossing change.

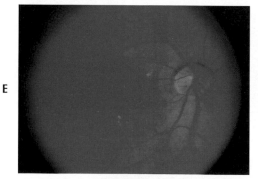

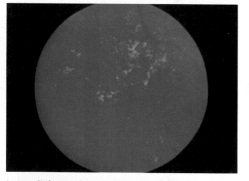

Early diabetic retinopathy. Note microaneurysms, blotlike hemorrhages, and small exudates.

Later diabetic retinopathy. Note blotlike hemorrhages and hard exudates.

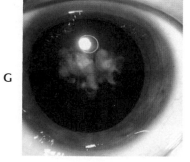

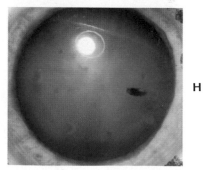

Senile cataract.

Snowflake cataract of diabetes.

A to **F** from Thomas, B. A., editor: Introduction to ophthalmoscopy, Kalamazoo, Mich., 1976, The Upjohn Co. **G, H** from Donaldson, D. D.: Atlas of diseases of the eye. The crystalline lens, vol. V, St. Louis, 1976, The C. V. Mosby Co.

vibrating tuning fork on the vertex of the skull, on the forehead, or on the front teeth and asking the client if he hears the sound better in one ear or in the other (Fig. 10-7). In conductive deafness, the sound is referred to the deafer ear. This happens because the cochlea on that side will be undisturbed by extraneous sounds in the environment; these sounds are not transmitted, because of a problem or defect in the ear canal or middle ear. In perceptive deafness, the sound is referred to the better ear because the cochlea or auditory nerve is functioning more effectively.

Another test is the Schwabach test, which allows the examiner to compare the client's bone conduction with his own, presuming that the examiner has normal bone conduction. The tuning fork is moved back and forth and placed on the client's mastoid bone and then on the examiner's. Both should be able to hear the sound for an equal length of time if the client's hearing is normal. If the client has a conductive hearing loss, he will hear the sound longer. If the client has a sensorineural hearing loss, he will hear the sound for a shorter time.

The caloric tests that measure labyrinthine function of the inner ear are discussed in Chapter 24 on neurological assessment.

NOSE AND PARANASAL SINUSES
Anatomy and physiology

The nose is the sensory organ for smell. It also warms, moistens, and filters the air inspired into the respiratory system.

The functions of the paranasal sinuses are not definitely known, but they may perform the same functions as the nose—that of warming, moistening, and filtering air. They also aid in voice resonance.

The nose is divided into the external nose and the internal nose or nasal cavity (Fig. 10-8). The upper third of the nose is bone; the remainder of the nose

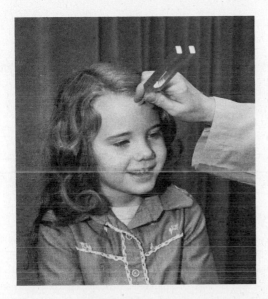

Fig. 10-7. Weber test.

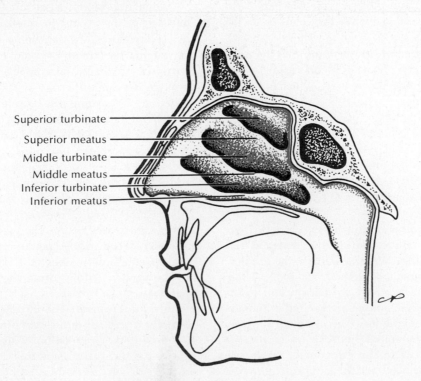

Superior turbinate
Superior meatus
Middle turbinate
Middle meatus
Inferior turbinate
Inferior meatus

Fig. 10-8. Lateral view of the left nasal cavity.

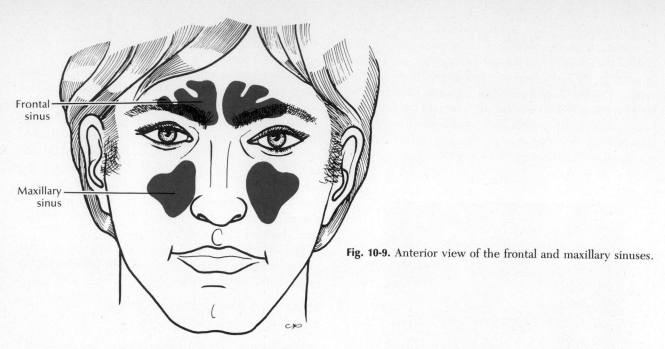

Frontal
sinus

Maxillary
sinus

Fig. 10-9. Anterior view of the frontal and maxillary sinuses.

is cartilage. The nasal cavity is divided by the septum into two narrow cavities. The cavities have two openings: the anterior cavity is the vestibule where the naris is located and is thickly lined with small hairs; the posterior opening, or choana, leads to the throat. The nasal septum forms the medial walls. The lateral walls are divided into the inferior, middle, and superior turbinate bones, which protude into the nasal cavity. The turbinates are covered by a highly vascular mucous membrane. Below each turbinate is a meatus named according to the turbinate above it. The nasolacrimal duct drains into the inferior meatus, and most of the paranasal sinuses drain into the middle meatus. There is a plexus of blood vessels in the mucosa of the anterior nasal septum, which is a common site for epistaxis.

The receptors for smell are located in the olfactory area in the roof of the nasal cavity and upper third of the septum. The receptor cells, grouped as filaments, pass through openings of the cribiform plate, become the olfactory nerve (CN I), and transmit neural impulses for smell to the temporal lobe of the brain.

The paranasal sinuses are air-filled, paired extensions of the nasal cavities within the bones of the skull. They are the frontal, the maxillary, the ethmoidal, and the sphenoidal sinuses (Fig. 10-9). Their openings into the nasal cavity are narrow and easily obstructed. The frontal sinuses are located in the anterior part of the frontal bone. The maxillary sinuses, the largest of the paranasal sinuses, are located in the body of the maxilla. The ethmoidal sinuses are small and occupy the ethmoidal labyrinth between the orbit of the eye and the upper part of the cavity

of the nose. The sphenoidal sinuses are found in the body of the sphenoid.

Examination

The external portion of the nose is inspected for any deviations in shape, size, or color; the nares are inspected for flaring or discharge. The ridge and soft tissues of the nose are palpated for displacement of the bone and cartilage and for tenderness or masses.

Examination of the nasal function includes determination of the ability to smell and the patency of the nasal cavities. To determine if the nasal cavities are patent, the client is asked to close his mouth, exert pressure on one naris with a finger, and breathe through the opposite naris. The procedure is repeated to determine the patency of the opposite naris. To determine the adequacy of function of the olfactory nerve (CN I), the client is asked to close his eyes and occlude one naris again. The examiner places an aromatic substance, such as coffee or alcohol, close to the client's nose and asks the client to identify the odor. Each side is tested separately.

The examination of the nasal cavities may be carried out in several ways. The electric otoscope with the short, broad nasal speculum may be used or the nasal speculum with a penlight. The examination can also be carried out by using the thumb of the left hand to push the tip of the nose upward while shining a light into the naris. The last method is the easiest to perform and the most comfortable for the client. If the otoscope or speculum is used, the instrument is held in the left hand, and the index finger is placed on the side of the nose to stabilize the position of the speculum and prevent displacement (Fig. 10-11).

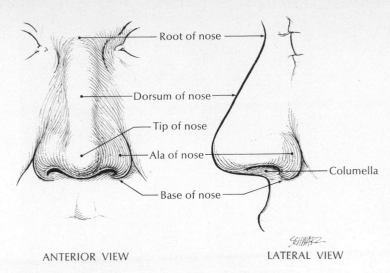

Root of nose

Dorsum of nose

Tip of nose

Ala of nose

Columella

Base of nose

ANTERIOR VIEW   LATERAL VIEW

Fig. 10-10. External structure of the nose.

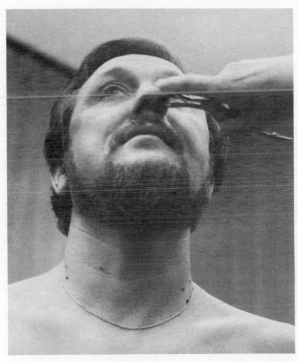

Fig. 10-11. Proper position for insertion of nasal speculum.

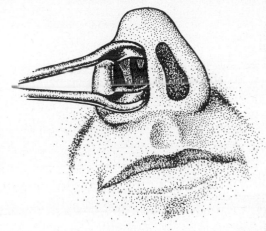

Fig. 10-12. Examination of the anterior nasal cavity. View of the inferior and middle turbinates.

The right hand is used to position the head and hold the light. Care must be taken not to apply pressure on the nasal septum because of its great sensitivity; but if a nasal speculum is being used, the blades must be opened as far as possible.

Examination of the nasal cavity through the anterior naris is limited to the vestibule, the anterior portion of the septum, and the inferior and middle turbinates. It is necessary to change the position of the head several times during the examination to inspect the various areas. With the client's head tipped back, the inferior and middle turbinates can be seen (Fig. 10-12). The septum is inspected for

deviation, exudate, and perforation. The septum is rarely straight. The lateral walls of the nasal cavities and the inferior and middle turbinates are examined for polyps, swelling, exudate, and change in color. The nasal mucosa is normally redder than the oral mucosa. Increased redness indicates infection; pale, boggy turbinates are typical of allergy. Any drainage from the middle meatus, which drains several of the paranasal sinuses, is important and should be described. The floor of the vestibule should be carefully inspected for evidence of a foreign body.

Examination of the paranasal sinuses is made indirectly. Information about their condition is gained by inspection and palpation of the overlying tissues or by transillumination. Only the frontal and maxillary sinuses are accessible for examination. Palpation for examination of the maxillary sinuses is performed on the maxillary areas of the cheeks, where tenderness may be elicited. By palpating both cheeks si-

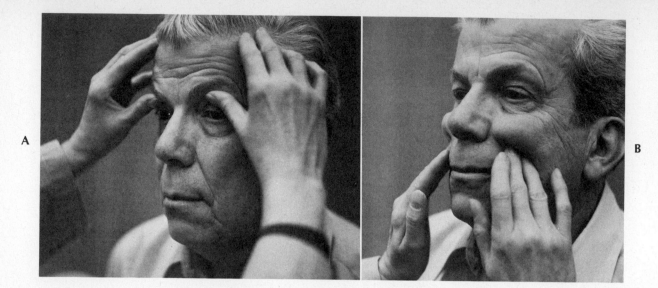

Fig. 10-13. Palpation of the frontal **(A)** and maxillary **(B)** sinuses.

multaneously, one can determine differences in tenderness. Swelling of the cheek rarely occurs in maxillary sinusitis. The frontal sinuses can be palpated by finger pressure below the eyebrows. Palpation of the sinuses is demonstrated in Fig. 10-13. Both the maxillary and the frontal sinuses may also be percussed by lightly tapping with the index finger to determine if the client feels pain.

Transillumination of the maxillary sinuses is accomplished in a completely darkened room by shining a bright light in the client's mouth. The frontal sinus is transilluminated by shining a light through the medial aspect of the supraorbital rim.

Transillumination has limitations as a diagnostic tool and is not highly successful, since even normal sinuses will show differences in the amount of transillumination.

MOUTH AND OROPHARYNX
Anatomy and physiology

The mouth is the first division of the digestive tube and an entry site to the respiratory system. The oropharynx conducts air to and from the larynx and food to the esophagus from the mouth. The structures of the mouth and oropharynx are illustrated in Fig. 10-14.

The boundaries of the mouth are the lips anteriorly and the soft palate and uvula posteriorly. The floor is formed by the mandibular bone, which is covered by loose, mobile tissue. The roof of the oral cavity is formed by the hard and soft palates. They are distinctly different in color; the soft palate is pink, and the hard palate is white. The uvula is a muscular organ that hangs down from the posterior margin of the soft palate. The muscles of mastication are innervated by

two main nerves: the trigeminal nerve (CN V) and the facial nerve (CN VII).

The mouth contains the tongue, gums, teeth, and salivary glands. The tongue is composed of a mass of striated muscles interspersed with fat and many glands. The dorsal surface is rough due to the presence of papillae. The ventral surface toward the floor of the mouth is smooth and shows large veins. The fold of mucous membrane that joins the tongue to the floor of the mouth is the frenulum. The tongue is innervated by the hypoglossal nerve (CN XII). The sensory receptors for taste are the glossopharyngeal nerve (CN IX) and the facial nerve (CN VII).

The gums are composed of fibrous tissue covered with a smooth mucous membrane and are attached to the alveolar margins of the jaws and to the necks of the teeth. In the adult there are 32 teeth, 16 in each arch.

Three pairs of salivary glands secrete into the oral cavity. They are the parotid, submandibular, and sublingual salivary glands. The largest is the parotid gland, which lies in front of and below the external ear. The parotid (Stensen's) duct opens into the buccal membrane opposite the second molar. The submandibular gland lies below and in front of the parotid gland. The submandibular (Wharton's) duct opens at the side of the frenulum on the floor of the mouth. The sublingual gland is the smallest salivary gland and lies in the floor of the mouth. It raises the mucous membrane, covering its superior surface to form the sublingual fold. It has numerous small openings, which open on the sublingual fold.

The oropharynx is the section of the pharynx that is posterior to the oral cavity and most accessible to examination. The nasopharynx lies behind the

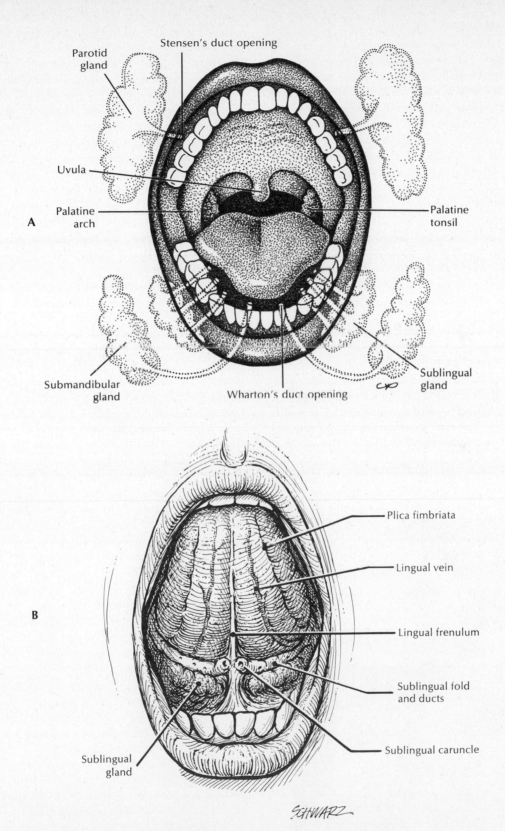

Fig. 10-14. Structures of the mouth.

nasal cavities and is superior to the oropharynx. The laryngopharynx is inferior to the oropharynx. Along both lateral walls of the oropharynx are two palatine arches, and between them are the tonsils. The tonsils are usually the same color as the surrounding tissue and do not normally extend beyond the pillars. Tonsillar tissue in children enlarges until puberty and then shrinks back into the folds of the arches. Consequently, a child's tonsils may normally be larger than an adult's. The posterior pharyngeal wall that is visible during the clinical examination may show many small blood vessels and small areas of pink or red lymphoid tissue.

Examination

The examination is conducted from the anterior to the posterior areas of the mouth and begins with the external components of the mouth and jaw.

The lips are inspected for symmetry, color, edema, or surface abnormalities. The client is asked to open and close his mouth to demonstrate the mobility of the mandible and the occlusion of the teeth. The temporomandibular joint is palpated while the mouth is opened wide and then closed, for any tenderness, crepitus, or deviation (Fig. 10-15). Pressure applied to the joint during closing of the mouth may result in referred pain to the ear; a common cause of the referred pain is malocclusion. The lips are palpated for induration.

The client is asked to remove dentures, if worn,

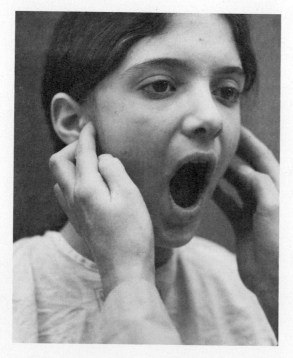

Fig. 10-15. Palpation of the temporomandibular joint.

for the rest of the mouth and throat examination. A good source of additional light is essential in examination of the mouth and throat.

The oral mucosal surfaces are normally light pink and are kept moist by saliva. The surfaces are examined systematically to ensure that all areas are inspected (Fig. 10-16). The examiner may use two tongue depressors or the fingers as retractors. With the client's mouth partially open, the mucosa in the anteroinferior area between the lower lip and gum is examined. With the mouth wide open, the buccal mucosa and Stensen's duct (the opening to the parotid gland, opposite the upper second molar) of the right cheek are examined. The maxillary mucobuccal fold between the upper lip and gum is examined next; then the mucosa and Stensen's duct of the left cheek are examined.

The examination of the tongue begins with inspection of the dorsum for any swelling, variation in size or color, coating, or ulceration. The client is asked to extend the tongue in order to demonstrate any deviation, tremor, or limitation of movement; any of these would be indicative of impairment of the hypoglossal nerve (CN XII). To inspect the posterior and lateral areas of the tongue, a 4 by 4 piece of gauze is wrapped around the tip of the extended tongue and the examiner's hand is used to hold and position the tongue (Fig. 10-17). The tongue is swung to the left, and the right lateral border is inspected. The position is reversed, and the left lateral border is examined. The tongue is released, and the client is asked to touch the tip of the tongue to the palate. The ventral surface is observed for swelling or varicosities. The floor of the mouth is inspected for abnormalities or swelling; Wharton's ducts (the openings of the submandibular glands), the frenulum, and the sublingual ridge are identified. The entire tongue and the floor of the mouth are carefully palpated, because some diseases or tumors cause little change in the surface and can only be detected by palpation. A rubber glove or finger cots may be used if there is evidence of infection.

The examination of the teeth and gums is not a substitute for a dental examination but should reveal gross problems that need attention. A dental mirror can be used productively as a retractor and to reflect some of the surfaces of the teeth and gums that are not readily accessible. The teeth are inspected for caries, missing teeth, and malocclusions. The examination is conducted systematically so that each tooth of one arch is visualized before those of the other arch. Any soft discolorations on the crown of a tooth should be suspected as carious. The teeth are counted, taking into consideration the client's age in determining the number of primary teeth, 20, or permanent teeth, 32, that are present and the number missing. Malocclusions, such as two teeth in the space for one, overlapping of teeth, and missing teeth with wide spaces should be noted. The palpation of the temporomandibular joint with opening and closing of the mouth, described in the beginning of the oral examination, is helpful in demonstrating normal or abnormal occlusion such as the lower teeth biting outside the upper teeth (underbite) or the upper front teeth protruding and hanging over the lower front teeth (overbite).

The gums are inspected in the same systematic way as the teeth with the completion of one arch and then the other arch. Any signs of inflammation and hemorrhage of the gums (gingivitis) may indicate more serious periodontal disease (pyorrhea) involving the bones and ligaments that anchor the tooth in its socket (Fig. 10-18). Any stains, tartar (calculus), or loose teeth are noted as signs of periodontal disease. Fig. 10-19 is a form that can be used in recording observations made during the examination of the teeth and gums.

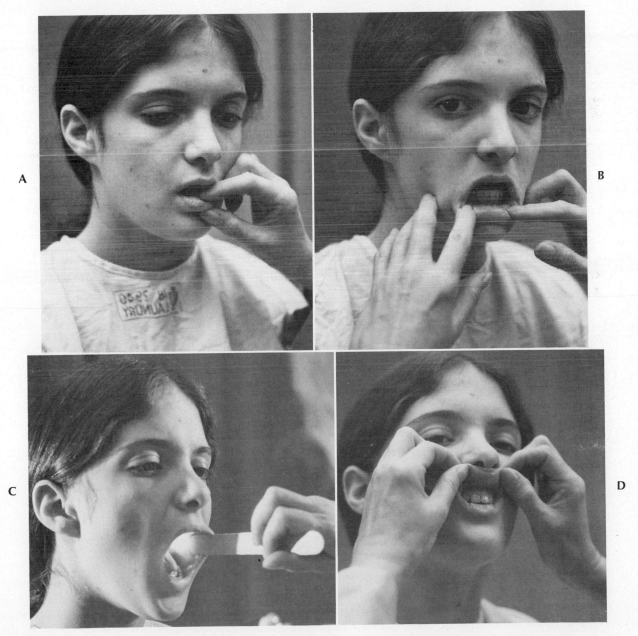

Fig. 10-16. Examination of the lips and oral mucosa. **A,** Palpation of the lips. **B,** Inspection of the mucosa of the lower anterior area. **C,** Inspection of mucosa of each cheek with identification of Stensen's duct opening. **D,** Inspection of mucosa of the upper anterior area.

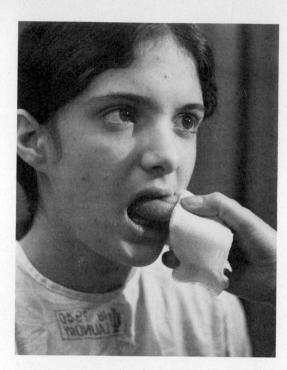

Fig. 10-17. Examination of the tongue.

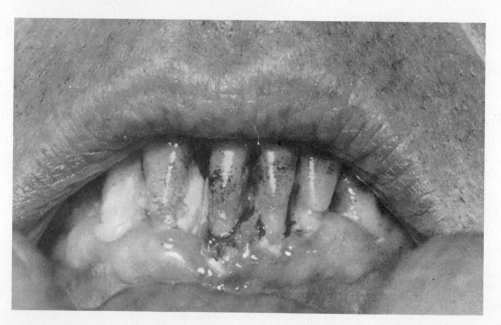

Fig. 10-18. Advanced pyorrhea. (From Prior, J. A., and Silberstein, J. S.: Physical diagnosis: the history and examination of the patient, ed. 5, St. Louis, 1977, The C. V. Mosby Co.)

With the client's head back, the palate and uvula are inspected. It may be necessary to depress the base of the tongue with a tongue depressor. The difference in color of the hard and soft palate is noted, as is any abnormality of architecture. An exostosis (torus palatinus) is frequently found in the midline of the posterior two-thirds of the hard palate (Fig. 10-20). This is a smooth, symmetrical bony structure resulting from the down-growth of the pala-

tal processes. Such bony growths are benign. The uvula may be bifid and part of a submucosal cleft palate. The client is asked to say, "Ah," and the rise of the soft palate and uvula is noted. Any deivation or lack of movement indicates impairment of the vagus nerve (CN X).

The oropharynx is inspected while the client's head is back, and the base of the tongue is gently depressed with a tongue depressor. The anterior pala-

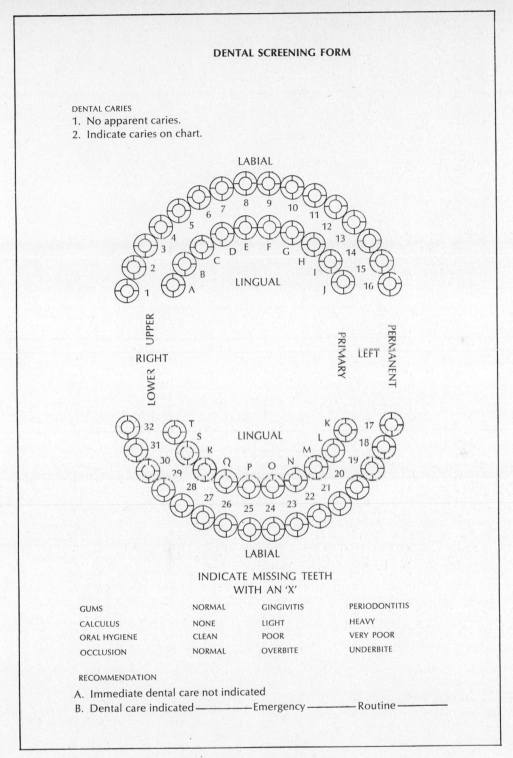

DENTAL SCREENING FORM

DENTAL CARIES
1. No apparent caries.
2. Indicate caries on chart.

LABIAL

LINGUAL

UPPER

RIGHT

LOWER

PRIMARY LEFT PERMANENT

LINGUAL

LABIAL

INDICATE MISSING TEETH
WITH AN 'X'

GUMS	NORMAL	GINGIVITIS	PERIODONTITIS
CALCULUS	NONE	LIGHT	HEAVY
ORAL HYGIENE	CLEAN	POOR	VERY POOR
OCCLUSION	NORMAL	OVERBITE	UNDERBITE

RECOMMENDATION
A. Immediate dental care not indicated
B. Dental care indicated ———— Emergency ———— Routine ————

Fig. 10-19. Dental screening form.

tine arches and the posterior arches are inspected for inflammation or swelling. The size of the tonsils is estimated, and any exudate is noted. The posterior wall of the oropharynx is examined for any change in color. The glossopharyngeal nerve (CN IX) and the vagus nerve (CN X) are tested by touching the posterior wall of the pharynx on each side. The normal response is a gag reflex. A unilaterally impaired gag reflex usually indicates impairment of glossopharyngeal as well as vagal function.

Throughout the examination of the mouth and throat, attention should be given to mouth odors, which may result from systemic as well as oral disease.

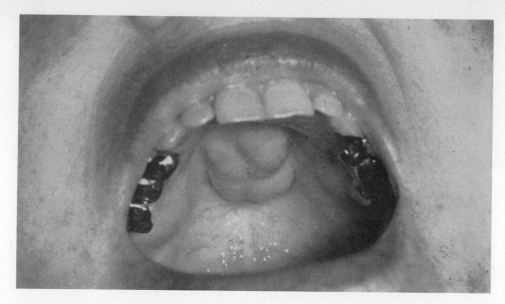

Fig. 10-20. Exostosis. (From Prior, J. A., and Silberstein, J. S.: Physical diagnosis: the history and examination of the patient, ed. 5, St. Louis, 1977, The C. V. Mosby Co.)

SUMMARY

I. Ears
  A. Inspect auricles and mastoid area
  B. Palpate auricles and mastoid area
  C. Inspect auditory meatus
  D. Perform otoscopic examination of auditory canal
    1. Skin color
    2. Cerumen
    3. Exudate
  E. Perform otoscopic examination of tympanic membrane
    1. Color
    2. Landmarks
  F. Hearing tests
    1. Tests for hearing acuity
      a. Voice tests
      b. Watch tick
    2. Rinne
    3. Weber
II. Nose and paranasal sinuses
  A. Inspect external portion of nose
  B. Palpate external portion of nose and test for patency
  C. Test olfactory nerve (CN I)
  D. Inspect nasal cavities
    1. Mucosa
    2. Septum
    3. Inferior and middle turbinates
  E. Palpate paranasal sinuses
    1. Frontal sinuses
    2. Maxillary sinuses
III. Mouth and oropharynx
  A. Inspect lips and facial structure
  B. Palpate temporomandibular joint
  C. Palpate lips
  D. Test hypoglossal nerve (CN XII)
  E. Inspect buccal mucosa
  F. Inspect teeth and gums
  G. Inspect tongue and floor of mouth
  H. Inspect hard and soft palate
  I. Inspect tonsillar areas
  J. Inspect posterior pharyngeal wall
  K. Test glossopharyngeal nerve (CN IX) and vagus nerve (CN X)
    1. Movement of uvula
    2. Gag reflex
  L. Palpate tongue and floor of the mouth

BIBLIOGRAPHY

Ballantyne, J., and Groves, J.: Scott-Brown's diseases of the ear, nose and throat, vols. 1-4, Philadelphia, 1971, J. B. Lippincott Co.

DeWeese, D. D., and Saunders, W. H.: Textbook of otolaryngology, ed. 5, St. Louis, 1977, The C. V. Mosby Co.

Foxen, E. H. M.: Lecture notes on diseases of the ear, nose and throat, ed. 3, Oxford, 1972, Blackwell Scientific Publications Ltd.

Romanes, G. J.: Cunningham's manual of practical anatomy, vol. 2, ed. 13, New York, 1973, Oxford University Press, Inc.

11 Assessment of the eyes

Examination of the eyes is fascinating, although it seems quite difficult at first. With much practice and great patience, the fundamentals of this complex examination can be mastered; the rewards for this effort are great. A thorough examination of the eyes can reveal something of the emotional status of the client, as well as information on both local and systemic health and disease processes.

The eye examination involves multiple components; students learning it should learn a reasonable arrangement of the various components in order to remember all portions. The ordering of these parts should focus both on completeness of the examination and on the comfortable positioning of the client.

This examination encompasses measurement of visual acuity, evaluation of visual fields, testing of ocular movements, inspection of the ocular structures, testing of nerve reflexes, and the ophthalmoscopic, or funduscopic, examination. Tonometry should also be included, especially for persons over 40 years of age. The technique of inspection is the principal physical examination technique involved.

Because of the complexity of the eye examination, instead of presenting examination techniques with normal and abnormal findings together, the chapter is arranged as follows: first, a brief review of the anatomy of the eyes and the normal appearance of the various structures is presented; then the examination technique and a method of organizing the examination are suggested; finally, some of the more common abnormal eye findings are discussed. The equipment and the environmental requirements are listed at the beginning of the section on examination.

ANATOMY AND NORMAL FINDINGS
Ocular structures

The structures of the eyelid and the globe of the eye are shown in Figs. 11-1 and 11-2.

Eyelids and eyelashes. The eyelashes are evenly distributed along the margin of the lids and curve outward. The eyelids serve a protective function, covering the anterior aspect of the eye and lubricating its surface. The lids should be able to close completely, so that the upper and lower lid margins approximate. When the eyes are open, the upper lid normally covers a small portion of the iris and the cornea overlying it, coming about midway between the limbus and the pupil. The margin of the lower lid lies at or just below the limbus. The limbus is the junction line where the cornea and sclera meet. The distance between the lid margins, called the palpebral fissure, should be equal in both eyes. The tarsal plates are thin strips of connective tissue that lie within the lid and give the lid some form and consistency.

Conjunctiva. Lining the lids and covering the anterior portion of the eyeball is the conjunctiva. This is a continuous, transparent structure that is divided into two portions: the palpebral portion and the bulbar portion. The palpebral portion lines the lids and appears shiny pink or red because it overlies the fleshy vascular structures of the lids; the bulbar portion lies over the sclera.

The palpebral conjunctiva recesses into the folds of the lids and is continuous with the bulbar conjunctiva, which lies loosely over the sclera to the limbus, where it merges with the corneal epithelium. This portion of the conjunctiva is normally clear; the white color comes from the sclera below. The bulbar portion does, however, contain many small blood vessels; these are normally visible and may become dilated, producing varying degrees of redness. A small fleshy elevation, the caruncle, is located in the nasal corner of the conjunctiva. Yellowish, triangular deposits called pinguecula, may occur in the bulbar conjunctiva near the limbus. These are essentially normal senile changes caused by a hyaline degeneration of fibrous tissue. The meibomian glands, which secrete an oily, lubricating substance, appear as vertical yellow striations on the palpebral conjunctiva.

Sclera. The sclera is the white portion of the eye visible anteriorly. Normally, several small, distinct conjunctival vessels are visible over the sclera, particularly around the periphery. In some dark-com-

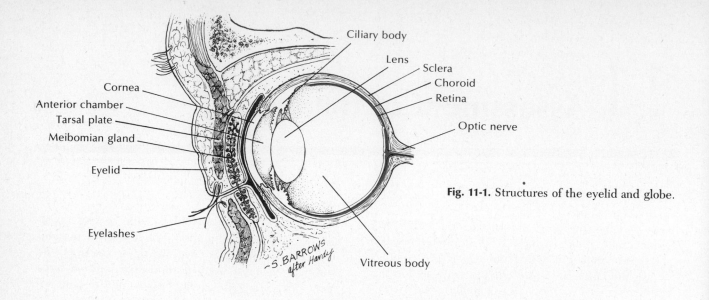

Fig. 11-1. Structures of the eyelid and globe.

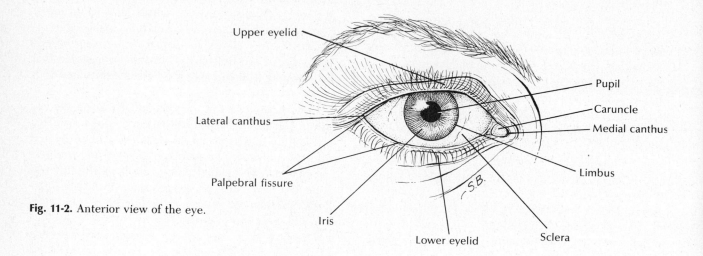

Fig. 11-2. Anterior view of the eye.

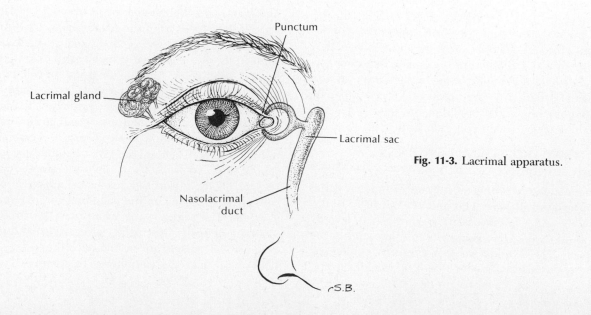

Fig. 11-3. Lacrimal apparatus.

plected persons, small, dark-pigmented dots may be visible on the sclera near the limbus.

Cornea. The cornea, like the bulbar conjunctiva, is a smooth, moist, transparent tissue. It covers the area over the pupil and iris and merges with the conjunctiva at the limbus. It is normally invisible except for the light reflections from its surface. The cornea is quite sensitive to touch; this sensation is transmitted by the ophthalmic branch of the trigeminal nerve (cranial nerve [CN] V). Stimulation of either cornea causes a blinking reflex in both eyes, which is transmitted by the facial nerve (CN VII).

Anterior chamber. The anterior chamber is bounded anteriorly by the cornea, laterally by the sclera and the ciliary body, and posteriorly by the iris and that portion of the lens within the pupillary opening. It is filled with aqueous, which is constantly produced by the ciliary body. The function of the anterior chamber is very important, because the relation between the rate of aqueous production and the resistance to aqueous outflow at the anterior chamber angle determines the intraocular pressure.

Lacrimal apparatus. The components of the lacrimal apparatus are illustrated in Fig. 11-3. The lacrimal gland, located above and slightly lateral to the eye, produces tears, which moisten and lubricate the conjunctiva and cornea. The tears are washed across the eye and then drain through the puncta, which are located on the nasal end of both upper and lower lids. The tears then pass into the nasolacrimal sac, located in the medial portion of the orbit, and from there through the nasolacrimal duct to the nose. Of these several components of the lacrimal system, only the puncta are normally visible.

Iris. The iris is a circular pigmented structure containing two involuntary muscles. It is located in front of the anterior chamber and behind the lens. The iris functions as a diaphragm within the image-forming portion of the eye. The diaphragm has a variable aperture—the pupil. The aperture's size, or pupillary opening, varies with the amount of light striking the retina. The surface of the iris is composed of numerous fibrils that vary in color within a given iris as well as from person to person. Posterior to the layer of fibrils are the dilator and sphincter muscles. The deepest layer of the iris is the pigment epithelium.

Pupils. The pupils are normally round in shape and equal in size. A small percentage of individuals (about 5%) do have a slight but noticeable difference in the size of their pupils. Although this may be normal, the finding should be regarded with some suspicion. The size of the pupils is controlled by the autonomic nervous system. Stimulation of the parasympathetic fibers leads to constriction of the pupils; stimulation of the sympathetic fibers produces dilatation. The amount of ambient light influences the size; normally, increasing illumination causes pupillary constriction, whereas diminishing illumination causes dilatation. The pupils also constrict in response to accommodation, which is the change in focus from a distant to a near object.

The size of the pupils does vary in individuals exposed to the same degree of ambient light. Pupils tend to be smaller in infants and older persons; myopic (nearsighted) persons tend to have larger pupils, whereas hyperopic (farsighted) persons tend to have smaller pupils.

The constricting response of the pupils to a bright direct light, a pupillary reflex, consists of both a direct and a consensual reaction. The direct reaction refers to the constriction of the pupil receiving the increased illumination. The constriction of the pupil that is not receiving increased illumination is the consensual reaction. The optic nerve (CN II) mediates the afferent arc of this reflex from each eye, and the oculomotor nerve (CN III) mediates the efferent arc to both eyes; thus, the presence of both direct and consensual responses indicates the functioning of these two cranial nerves.

The accommodation response of the pupils consists of convergence of the eyes and constriction of the pupils as the glance is shifted from a distant to a near object.

The rapidity of the responses to both light and accommodation varies in normal persons. What is important is the presence of the responses and the equality of the responses in both eyes.

Lens. Directly behind the iris and at the pupillary opening lies the lens, the center of the refracting system of the eye. It is normally transparent and has no blood vessels, nerves, or connective tissue. It is composed of epithelial cells within an elastic membrane, the lens capsule. The thickness of the lens is controlled by muscles of the ciliary body, and it is the changes in thickness of the lens that enable the eye to focus on objects both far and near. Thus, the coordinated functions of the muscles of the iris and the muscles of the ciliary body acting on the lens control the amount of light permitted to reach the neurosensory elements of the retina and the focusing of objects on the retina.

Retina. The eyeball is a spherical structure lined from the inside toward the outside by the retina, the choroid, and the sclera. Within this sphere lies yet another transparent fluid structure, the vitreous body.

The layers of the eyeball accessible to physical examination are the sclera anteriorly and the retina interiorly; the retina is visible by means of the ophthalmoscope.

The color of the retina is reddish orange because

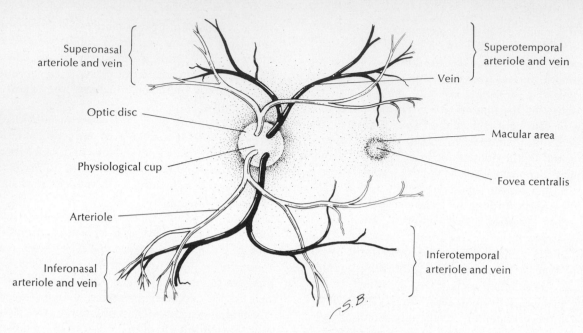

Superonasal arteriole and vein

Superotemporal arteriole and vein

Vein

Optic disc

Macular area

Physiological cup

Fovea centralis

Arteriole

Inferotemporal arteriole and vein

Inferonasal arteriole and vein

S.B.

Fig. 11-4. Retinal structures of the left eye.

of the deeper vascular supply and the deeper-pigmented layers. The pigment present in the posterior layers of the retina also accounts for the slightly stippled appearance of the retina. Normally, the color of the retina is quite uniform throughout, with no patches of light or dark discoloration.

Observable on the retina are several important structures, including the optic disc, or nerve head of the optic nerve, with its physiological cup; the four sets of retinal vessels, which emerge from the optic disc and travel medially and laterally around the retina; the macular area, where central vision is concentrated; and the retinal background itself (Fig. 11-4).

OPTIC DISC. The optic disc is located on the nasal half of the retina. Important characteristics of the disc include its size, shape, color, the nature of the margins, and the physiological cup. The optic disc is about 1.5 mm in diameter, and its shape is round to vertically oval. Its color ranges from creamy yellow to pink; it is lighter in color than the surrounding retina. The color of both the disc and the retinal background vary from one individual to another; it is somewhat lighter in fair-complected, light-haired people and slightly darker in dark-complected, dark-haired people.

The margins of the disc are usually sharp and are clearly demarcated from the surrounding retina, though there are several normal variations that deserve comment. The nasal outline may normally be somewhat more blurred than the temporal outline. Dense pigment deposits may be situated about the disc margins, particularly in dark-complected peo-

ple. A whitish to grayish crescent of scleral tissue may be present immediately adjacent to the disc, particularly on the temporal side.

Most discs have a small depression just temporal to the center of the disc; slightly lighter in color than the rest of the disc, this depression is yellowish white and is called the physiological cup or physiological depression. In normal individuals it does not extend completely to the disc margins but may occupy one-fourth to one-third of the area of the disc.

RETINAL VESSELS. As shown in Fig. 11-4, four sets of retinal vessels emerge from the optic disc and wind outward, becoming smaller at the periphery. Each set includes an arteriole and a vein and is known by the quadrant of the retina that it supplies: superonasal, inferonasal, inferotemporal, or superotemporal. Important characteristics of the vessels include color, size, regularity of caliber, arteriolar light reflex, and the characteristics where one vessel crosses another.

The vessel walls are normally quite transparent, and the "color" of the vessels describes the oxygenated or deoxygenated blood they carry. Thus, the arterioles are a brighter red than the veins, which are dark red. The arterioles are about 25% smaller than the veins; thus, an arteriole-to-vein (A:V) ratio of 2:3 or 4:5 is normal. When observed, arterioles have a narrow light reflex from the centerline of the vessel. Pulsations are sometimes visible in the veins near the optic disc and are caused by the forcing of blood out of the eye through the vein with each systole. Veins do not show a light reflex. Normally, both arterioles and veins show a gradually and regularly diminished diameter as they go from the disc to the periphery. They normally cross and intertwine each other; but where the vessels cross one another, there should be no change in the course or caliber of either vessel.

RETINAL BACKGROUND AND MACULAR AREA. The neurosensory elements, rods and cones, are contained in the retina. At a point temporal to the disc at the posterior pole of the eye, there is a slight depression in the retina, known as the fovea centralis. The cones are most heavily concentrated here, making this the point of central vision and acutest color vision. The retinal area immediately around this is called the macula. The macular area has no visible retinal vessels; it is nourished by choroidal vessels and appears slightly darker than the rest of the retinal background.

Visual pathway and visual fields

For a clear visual image to be perceived, light reflected from an object must pass through the cornea, the anterior chamber, the lens, and the vitreous fluid and then be focused on the retina. The images formed on the retina are reversed right to left and are upside down; thus, an object in the upper nasal field of vision will be formed on the lower temporal quadrant of the retina. The light stimulates neuron impulses that are conducted through the retina, the optic nerve, and the optic tract to the visual cortex of the occipital lobes.

The layout (spatial arrangement) of the nerve fibers in the retina are maintained in the optic nerve; that is, temporal (lateral) fibers run along the lateral side of the nerve, and nasal (medial) fibers run along the medial portion of the nerve. However, as the optic chiasm, the nasal or medial fibers cross over and join the temporal or lateral fibers of the opposite optic tract. Thus, the left optic tract contains fibers only from the left half of each retina (the right half of each field of vision), and the right optic tract contains fibers only from the right half of each retina (left half of each field of vision). By this sequence of pathways and events, conscious vision is produced. The relationship of visual pathways and fields of vision is illustrated in Fig. 11-5.

Neuromuscular aspects

Six muscles of each eye, working in a coordinated "yoked" fashion with the other eye, control eye movement, which normally occurs in conjugate, parallel fashion except during convergence, when a very close object is visualized. These six muscles include the superior, inferior, lateral, and medial rectus muscles; the superior oblique muscle; and the inferior oblique muscle. This parallelism of the axis of the eye makes

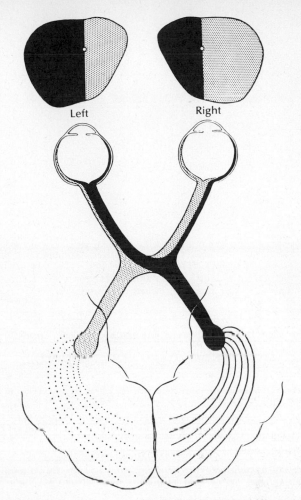

Left   Right

Fig. 11-5. Representation of the visual field in the optic pathways. (From Havener, W. H.: Synopsis of ophthalmology, ed. 4, St. Louis, 1975, The C. V. Mosby Co.)

possible single-image, binocular vision. Thus, the yoked muscles are the muscles in each eye that work together to move the eyes in parallel motion to any given position of gaze. For example, the left lateral rectus and the right medial rectus are yoked muscles working concurrently to move the gaze to the left. The attachment of the muscles to the globe of the eye and the direction of their action are illustrated in Fig. 11-6.

These six eye muscles are innervated by three cranial nerves. The oculomotor nerve (CN III) innervates four muscles: the superior, inferior, and medial rectus muscles and the inferior oblique muscle. The trochlear nerve (CN IV) innervates the superior oblique muscle, and the abducens nerve (CN VI) innervates the lateral rectus muscle. A mnemonic device helpful for remembering this innervation is: LR_6SO_4.

Six of the 12 cranial nerves and portions of the cerebral hemispheres are involved in the total neurologi-

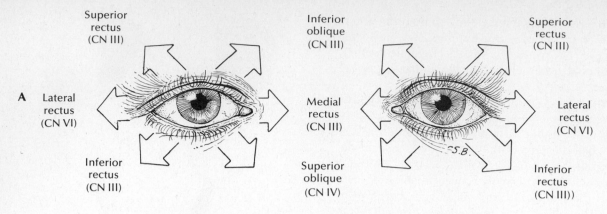

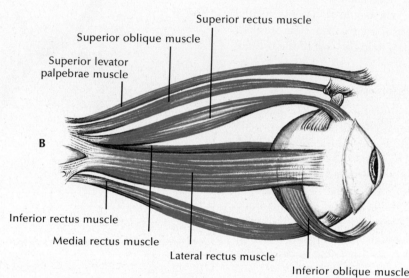

Fig. 11-6. A, Movement generated by the six extraocular muscles. **B,** Muscles of the right orbit as viewed from the side. (**B,** From Anthony, C. P., and Kolthoff, N. J.: Textbook of anatomy and physiology, ed. 9, St. Louis, 1975, The C. V. Mosby Co.)

cal innervation of the eye and related structures. Table 11-1 summarizes the relationship of the six cranial nerves to the eye structures.

EXAMINATION

Examination of the functions and the structures of the eyes involves multiple procedures and should be performed in a manner that provides efficient access to physical findings while maintaining the greatest degree of comfort for the client. There are, of course, numerous ways to organize this examination; the method suggested here is to examine initially the functions of visual acuity (central and peripheral) and ocular motility. This assessment of function is followed by the examination of ocular structures, starting with the outermost structures and working toward the retina. Finally, the estimation of intraocular tension should be performed as appropriate. The method allows the examiner to perform much of the ocular examination before touching any of the

rather sensitive eye structures and reserves the somewhat uncomfortable procedures of ophthalmoscopic examination and tonometry until last.

Several pieces of equipment are required for the eye examination. These should be organized before the examination is begun:

Visual acuity chart

Newspaper clipping with several sizes of print for assessing near vision

Opaque card or eye cover for assessing visual acuity, visual fields, and muscle function

Penlight for assessing pupillary reflexes and external structures

Cotton-tipped applicator for eversion of the upper lid

Wisp of cotton for assessing corneal reflex

Ophthalmoscope for assessing ocular media and for the retinal examination

Tonometer for assessing ocular pressure

In addition to the equipment needed, there is an

Table 11-1. Relationship of cranial nerves to eye structures

Cranial nerve	Activity
II Optic	Mediates vision
III Oculomotor	Innervates medial, superior, and inferior rectus muscles; inferior oblique muscle; musculature elevating the eyelid (levator palpebrae); and muscles of the iris and ciliary body
IV Trochlear	Innervates superior oblique muscle
V Trigeminal, ophthalmic division	Innervates sensory portion of corneal reflex
VI Abducens	Innervates lateral rectus muscle
VII Facial	Innervates lacrimal glands and musculature involved in lid closure (orbicularis oculi)

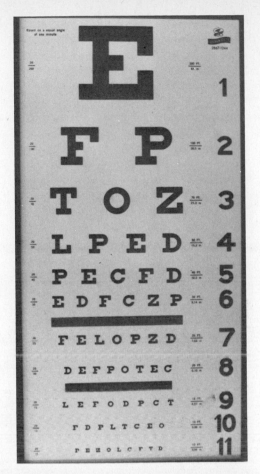

Fig. 11-7. Snellen chart. (Courtesy Graham-Field Surgical Co., Inc., New Hyde Park, N.Y.)

important environmental requirement, a room where the amount of lighting can be controlled by the examiner. A darkened room enables the examiner to assess the pupillary reflexes and to perform the funduscopic examination with greater ease.

In examination of the eye, the range of normal is broad and the variations from normal are numerous. Much time, patience, and practice are required to begin to assess the normal and the common abnormal eye patterns.

Visual acuity

The assessment of visual acuity is a simple and rewarding test of ocular function. Findings in a normal range of visual acuity give the examiner an indication of the clarity of the transparent media (cornea, anterior body, lens, and vitreous body), the adequacy of macular, or central, vision, and the functioning of the nerve fibers from the macula to the occipital cortex.

Traditionally, Snellen's chart, with various sizes of letters or with the letter *E* facing various ways, is utilized (see Fig. 11-7). The chart has standardized numbers at the end of each line of letters; these numbers indicate the degree of visual acuity when measured from a distance of 20 feet. The numerator is 20, the distance in feet between the chart and the client, or the standard testing distance. The denominator is the distance from which the normal eye can read the lettering; therefore, the larger the denominator, the poorer the vision. It is important to note that although the terms numerator and denominator are commonly

used, the measurement is not a fraction or a percentage of normal vision. Measurement of 20/20 vision in a client is an indication of a normal eye and optic pathway. Measurement of less than 20/20 vision is an indication of either a refractive error or some other optic disorder. Only one eye should be tested at a time; the other may be covered with an opaque card or eye cover, not with the client's fingers. The room used for this test should be well lighted. A person who wears corrective lenses may be tested with and without them; this allows for an assessment of the adequacy of the correction. Reading glasses, however, do blur distant vision.

Persons who cannot see the largest letter on the chart (20/200) should be checked to see if they can perceive hand movements about 12 inches from their eyes or if they can perceive the light of the penlight directed into their eyes.

A gross assessment of near vision is performed in the client who complains of reading difficulty and in persons over 40 years of age. A newspaper clipping with various sizes of print or a small, hand-held,

Snellen-type chart may be used for this. With advancing age the lenses may become less flexible, resulting in difficulty with near vision. This condition is known as presbyopia.

Visual fields

The assessment of visual acuity is indicative of the functioning of the macular area, the area of central vision. However, it does not test the sensitivity of the other areas of the retina, which perceive the more peripheral stimuli. The visual field confrontation test provides a rather gross measurement of peripheral vision.

The performance of this test assumes that the examiner has normal visual fields, since the client's visual fields are compared with the examiner's. The

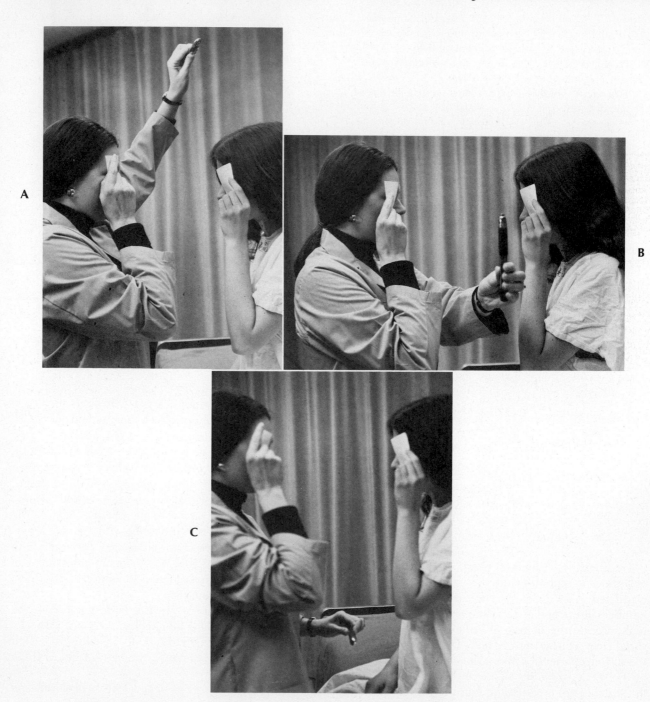

Fig. 11-8. In order to examine the visual fields, the examiner and client cover opposite eyes with an opaque card; the examiner brings in a penlight or other small object from the superior **(A)**, nasal **(B)**, inferior **(C)**, and temporal fields of vision. (Temporal assessment not shown.)

examiner and the client sit or stand opposite each other with their eyes at the same horizontal level at a distance of 1½ to 2 feet apart. The client covers one eye with an opaque card or eye cover, and the examiner covers his own eye opposite the client's covered eye; that is, if the client's right eye is covered, then the examiner's left eye is covered. This leaves the client's and the examiner's same field of vision open for inspection.

The client is asked to stare directly at the examiner's open eye while the examiner stares directly at the client's open eye. Neither looks out at the object approaching from the periphery. The examiner holds a small object, such as a pencil or penlight, in his hand and gradually moves it in from the periphery of both directions horizontally and from above and below. The object should be beyond the limits of the field of vision initially, held equidistant from both persons, and then advanced toward the center. The client and the examiner should be able to visualize the object at the same time. It is often difficult for the examiner to move the test object out far enough so that neither he nor the client can see it, especially in the temporal field. It may be necessary for the examiner to hold the object slightly farther from himself and closer to the client in the temporal field, moving it to a line equidistant between them as it is brought in (Fig. 11-8).

This test provides only a crude estimate of visual fields, and although it would pick up larger field defects, such as hemianopias, quadrantanopias, or large scotomas, it does not ascertain small lesions or changes. (Hemianopia is blindness for one-half of the field of vision in one eye or in both eyes. Quadrantanopia is blindness in one-fourth of the field of vision in one eye or in both eyes. A scotoma is an islandlike blind area in the visual field.) Thus, clinical use of this test is limited to gross screening. Any suspicions of decreasing peripheral vision, such as occurs with glaucoma and some brain lesions, should be referred for the more accurate quantitative measurements that can be performed with a perimeter or tangent screen. These tests are more useful for detecting, evaluating, and following visual pathway damage, whereas the confrontation method may fail to detect early evidence of damage, possibly delaying timely intervention.

Extraocular muscle function

There are three aspects to the assessment of extraocular muscle function: the corneal light reflex, the six cardinal positions of gaze, and the cover-uncover test. Basic to each of these is the observation of the parallelism of the eyes and ocular movements.

Corneal light reflex. The parallelism, or alignment, of the anteroposterior axes of the two eyes can be assessed by observing the reflection of a light from the cornea. The client is requested to stare straight ahead while the examiner shines a penlight on the corneas from a distance of 12 to 15 inches. The bright dot of light reflected from the shiny surface of the corneas should be located at the same spot in each eye, for example, at the 1 o'clock position (Fig. 11-9). An asymmetrical reflex will indicate a deviating eye and a probable muscle imbalance. A weak or paralyzed extraocular muscle is a cause of ocular deviation.

Six cardinal positions of gaze. The second mode of assessing muscle function is movement of the eyes through the six cardinal positions of gaze:

$$SR \to IO \qquad IO \to SR$$
$$\nearrow 6 \qquad 1 \searrow \qquad \nearrow 6 \qquad 1 \searrow$$
$$LR\ 5 \qquad\quad 2\ MR\ 5 \qquad\quad 2\ LR$$
$$\nwarrow 4 \qquad 3 \swarrow \qquad \nwarrow 4 \qquad 3 \swarrow$$
$$IR \leftarrow SO \qquad SO \leftarrow IR$$

Right eye   **Left eye**

These six positions are used because the muscle indicated is weak or paralyzed if the eye will not turn to that particular position. As stated earlier, the normal eye muscles work in yoked fashion, so that when the left eye is moved to the upward and outward position, the right eye moves to the upward and inward position.

The client is asked to follow a small object held by the examiner, which is moved to each position in a clockwise fashion. The client holds his head in a fixed position, and only his eyes follow the examiner's object. The examiner asks the client to fix his gaze momentarily in the extreme position of each of the six positions; and while the client is doing so, the examiner notes any jerking movements of the eye, or

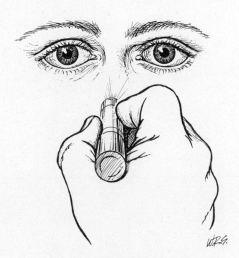

Fig. 11-9. Corneal light reflex.

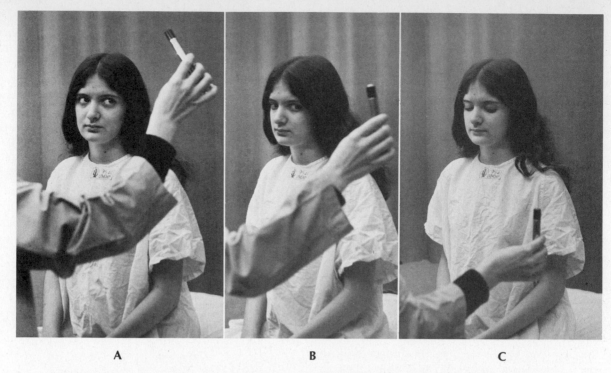

A   B   C

Fig. 11-10. To assess extraocular muscle function, the examiner directs the client's gaze into the six cardinal positions. Shown here: upward and left **(A)**; left lateral **(B)**; and downward and left **(C)**. The client's gaze is then directed to the right in these three positions.

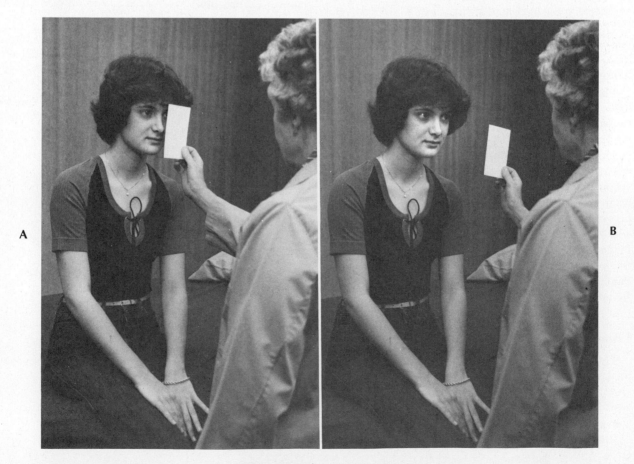

A   B

Fig. 11-11. Cover-uncover test.

nystagmus. On extreme lateral gaze, some eyes will develop a rhythmic twitching motion, known as end-positional nystagmus. A few beats of nystagmus on extreme lateral gaze are normal, but any other nystagmus is abnormal. Three of the six positions of gaze are illustrated in Fig. 11-10.

After examining the extraocular muscles in the six cardinal positions, the examiner observes the relationship of the upper eyelid to the globe while directing the client's eyes from an upward to a downward gaze. The lid should overlap the iris slightly throughout this movement; no sclera should show between the iris and the upper lid.

Cover-uncover test. A third, more delicate method of assessing muscle function is the cover-uncover test. Maintenance of parallel eyes is a result of the fusion reflex, which makes binocular vision possible. If a muscle imbalance is present and the fusion reflex is blocked when one eye is covered, this weakness can be observed.

The examiner asks the client to look at a specific fixation point, such as the examiner's nose, with both eyes. Then the examiner covers one eye with an opaque card or eye cover and while doing so observes the uncovered eye to see if it moves to fix on the object (Fig. 11-11, A). If it does move, then it was not straight before the other eye was covered. The examiner then removes the opaque cover from the covered eye and observes for any movement of the eye just uncovered (Fig. 11-11, B). When an eye is covered, the appearance of an object on that retina is suppressed. The eye relaxes, and if there is a weak tendency in one of the extraocular muscles, the eye drifts to another resting position. Then, when the client's eye is uncovered, the eye jerks back into the position where the visual image again appears on the retina.

The examiner then repeats this procedure on the other eye.

Ocular structures

The ocular structures to be examined include the eyelashes and eyelids, the conjunctiva, the cornea, the anterior chamber, the lacrimal apparatus, the sclera, the iris, the pupil, the lens, the vitreous body, and the retina.

EXAMINATION OF OUTERMOST STRUCTURES

Eyelids and eyelashes. The functions of the lids are to protect and lubricate the anterior portions of the globe. They are inspected for the ability to close completely, for position and color, and for any lesions, infection, or edema. When the lids do not close properly, drying of the cornea may result in serious damage.

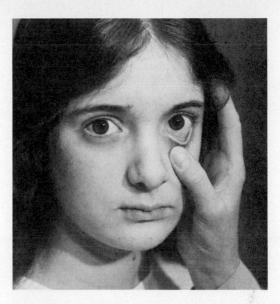

Fig. 11-12. The examiner inspects the conjunctiva by moving the lower lid downward over the bony orbit.

The examiner observes for equality in the height of the palpebral fissures. The margins of the upper lids normally fall between the superior pupil margin and the superior limbus.

Raised yellow plaques, xanthelasma, may appear on the lids near the inner canthi; these grow slowly and may disappear spontaneously.

At this time the position of the globe, whether normal, prominent, or sunken, can be observed.

The distribution, condition, and position of the eyelashes are noted. The eyelashes should be evenly distributed and should curve outward.

Conjunctiva. The bulbar and palpebral portions of the conjunctiva are examined by separating the lids widely and having the client look up, down, and to each side. When separating the lids, the examiner should exert no pressure against the eyeball; rather, the examiner should hold the lids against the ridges of the bony orbit surrounding the eye (Fig. 11-12). The client is then instructed to direct his gaze upward and to each side. Many small blood vessels are normally visible through the clear conjunctiva. The white sclera is, of course, visible through the bulbar portion.

Although eversion of the upper lid is not a necessary part of the normal or screening examination, the beginning examiner should learn a careful technique for performing lid eversion when it is indicated. The entire procedure should be explained to the client before it is begun, and reassurance should be given during the process. In the absence of gentleness, carefulness, and reassurance, the client is very likely to become tense when the sensitive eye structures are manipulated, thereby making the examination much more difficult for both himself and the examiner.

Eversion of the upper eyelid is performed as follows (Fig. 11-13):

1. Ask the client to look down but to keep his eyes slightly open. This relaxes the levator muscle, whereas closing the eyes contracts the orbicularis muscle, preventing lid eversion.
2. Gently grasp the upper eyelashes and pull gently downward. Do not pull the lashes outward or upward; this, too, causes muscle contraction.
3. Place a cotton-tipped applicator about 1 cm above the lid margin on the upper tarsal border and push gently downward with the applicator while still holding the lashes. This everts the lid.

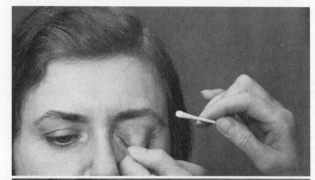

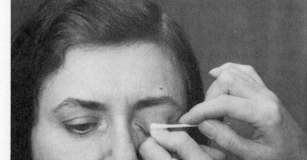

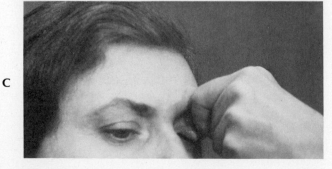

Fig. 11-13. Eversion of the upper eyelid. The examiner grasps the upper lid lashes, gently pulling downward and outward **(A)**, then places the cotton-tipped applicator near the lower lid margin **(B)**, and gently pulls the lashes upward over the applicator **(C)**.

4. Hold the lashes of the everted lid against the upper ridge of the bony orbit, just beneath the eyebrow, never pushing against the eyeball.
5. Examine the lid for swelling, infection, a foreign object, and so on.
6. To return the lid to its normal position, move the lashes slightly forward and ask the client to look up and then to blink. The lid returns easily to a normal position.

Sclera. The sclera is easily observed during assessment of the conjunctiva. It is normally white, though some pigmented deposits are within the range of normal.

Cornea. The cornea is best observed by directing the light of a penlight at it obliquely from several positions. The cornea should be transparent, smooth, shiny, and bright. There should be no irregularities in the surface, and the features of the iris should be fully visible through the cornea. In older persons the appearance of arcus senilis is normal. Arcus senilis is a white ring located around the periphery of the cornea; it is composed of lipid deposits.

Testing of the corneal reflex may be reserved for later in the eye examination, after the observation of all external structures is complete, but is discussed here as part of the complete assessment of the cornea. Corneal sensitivity is tested by bringing a wisp of cotton from the lateral side of the eye and brushing it lightly across the corneal surface (Fig. 11-14). The normal response is lid closure of both eyes when either eye is brushed.

Anterior chamber. The anterior chamber is easily observed in conjunction with the cornea. The tech-

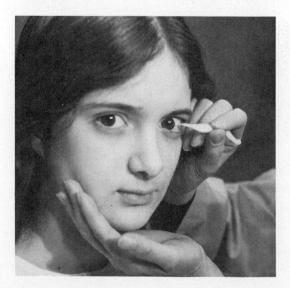

Fig. 11-14. Testing for corneal sensitivity, the examiner brings in a wisp of cotton from the side and lightly brushes it over the cornea.

nique of oblique illumination is also useful in assessing the anterior chamber. This, too, is a transparent structure. Any visible material in it is abnormal. The depth of the chamber should be noted by looking at the eye from the side instead of from directly in front. The depth is the distance between the cornea and the iris. From a side view, the iris should appear quite flat and should not be bulging forward (see Fig. 11-24, *A*).

Lacrimal apparatus. Of the various components of the lacrimal apparatus, including the lacrimal gland, the puncta, the lacrimal sac, and the nasolacrimal duct, only the puncta can normally be observed. These are located on the upper and lower nasal margins of the lids.

Blockage of the nasolacrimal duct can be checked by pressing against the lacrimal sac with the index finger inside the lower inner orbital rim, not against the side of the nose (Fig. 11-15). In the presence of blockage, this will cause regurgitation of material through the puncta.

Iris. The iris should be observed for shape and coloration.

Pupils. Examination of the pupils involves several observations, including assessment of their size, shape, reaction to light, and accommodation.

The pupils are normally round in shape and equal in size. The pupillary response to light consists of both a direct and a consensual reaction. The beam of a penlight is brought in from the side and directed on one eye at a time. The eye toward which the light is directed is observed for the direct response of constriction. Simultaneously, the other eye is observed for a consensual response of constriction. Each eye is observed for both the direct and consensual response. Normally, both responses are present; however, the rapidity with which the pupils respond does vary. A room that can be darkened to facilitate dilatation is helpful in assessing constriction in response to light; a sunny, well-lighted room can make the assessment of constriction responses very difficult.

The test for pupillary accommodation is the examination for change in pupillary size as the gaze is switched from a distant to a near object. It is performed by asking the client to stare at an object across the room. Visualization of a distant object normally causes pupillary dilatation. The client is then asked to fix his gaze on the examiner's index finger, which is placed 5 to 6 inches from the client's nose. The normal response is pupillary constriction and convergence of the eyes. The rapidity of the response in individuals varies; the response is slower in older persons.

The notation *PERRLA* stands for *pupils equal, round, react to light, and accommodate.*

OPHTHALMOSCOPIC EXAMINATION

Examination of other ocular structures includes observation of the lens, the vitreous body, and the retinal structures and is performed with an ophthalmoscope. It is helpful to darken the room while performing the ophthalmoscopic examination, since this causes the pupils to dilate and thus facilitates the examination. If darkening the room does not adequately dilate the client's pupils, 10% phenylephine hydrochloride, 0.5% Mydriacyl, or 1% Cyclogel drops may be instilled in the client's eyes. Before utilizing dilating drops however, it is absolutely essential to rule out any suspicion of glaucoma. If the client wears corrective lenses, the examination may be done either with or without them. It is generally easier to perform the examination without the client's glasses on unless he has a high degree of astigmatism. Contact lenses may be left in place on the cornea. The examiner may choose to perform the retinal examination wearing or not wearing corrective lenses. Both ways should be tried to determine which is more satisfactory to the examiner.

Use of the ophthalmoscope (see also Chapter 1). The head of the ophthalmoscope is equipped with a series of lenses that are changed by moving the round, white wheel. The 0 lens is clear glass; the red, or negative, numbers focus farther away; and the

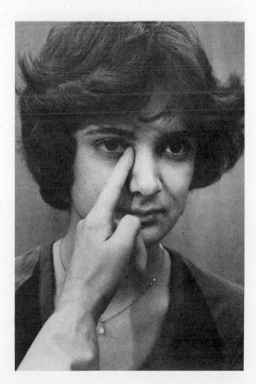

Fig. 11-15. To examine the lacrimal sac, the examiner presses with the index finger against the client's lower inner orbital rim, *not* against the nose.

black, or positive, numbers focus closer to the ophthalmoscope. Several apertures and filters for the light are built into most ophthalmoscopes; however, the round aperture with white light is best for most examinations. The examiner should read the manual accompanying the ophthalmoscope for information on other apertures and filters. The light should be turned to maximum brightness unless the client cannot tolerate it.

The client's cooperation is essential to the performance of this examination. The client is asked to stare directly ahead at some object across the room, such as the light switch or the corner of a picture.

This assists in two ways: staring at a distant point encourages dilatation of the pupils, and staring at one fixed point helps to prevent the eyes from rotating and moving about so much that it is impossible for the examiner to focus on any of the retinal structures.

The client is told that he may blink from time to time during the examination. If the blinking becomes so frequent that it is difficult to visualize the retinal structures, the examiner may elevate the upper lid and hold it against the upper orbital rim.

The examiner holds the ophthalmoscope in the right hand and to the right eye to examine the client's right eye, and in the left hand and to the left eye to

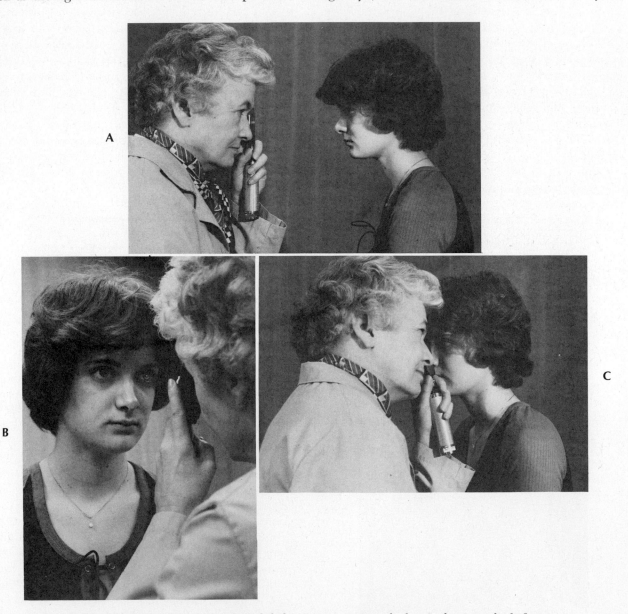

Fig. 11-16. A, The examiner uses the ophthalmoscope to inspect the lens and vitreous body from a distance of about 12 inches. The examiner uses the left eye and left hand to examine the client's left eye. **B,** The light from the ophthalmoscope is flashed on the eye through the pupil. **C,** Moving in closer to the client's eye, the examiner studies the retinal structures.

examine the client's left eye. The examiner initially sets the ophthalmoscope lens at 0, holds the viewing aperture directly in front of the eye with the top of the ophthalmoscope against the forehead, and begins about 12 inches away from the client's eye (Fig. 11-16, *A*). The index finger of the hand holding the ophthalmoscope rests on the lens wheel to permit focusing during the examination. The bright circle of light is flashed on the eye through the pupil (Fig. 11-16, *B*); a red glow, the red reflex, is visible through the pupil of the normal eye. While continuing to focus on the red reflex, the examiner moves close to the eye being examined (Fig. 11-16, *C*). If the examiner loses sight of the red reflex, it is usually because the light is no longer directed through the pupil and is resting instead on the iris or sclera. If this occurs, it is easiest to relocate the red reflex by backing away several inches and redirecting the beam of light. As the examiner moves close to the eye, the lenses are rotated to the positive numbers (+15 to +20), which focus on the near objects. At this setting the anterior chamber and lens are examined for transparency; there should be no clouding or opacities.

Gradually rotating the lens back toward 0, the examiner also observes the vitreous body for transparency. At this setting the examiner begins to look for some retinal structure, such as a vessel or the disc. Once some structure is located, the lens wheel is rotated until it is brought into focus. In a myopic or nearsighted person, whose eyeball is more elongated than normal, the more negative lenses will be needed to focus farther back. In a farsighted client the lens wheel is rotated toward the positive numbers. Focusing is quite individual and does depend on the refractive status of both the client and the examiner.

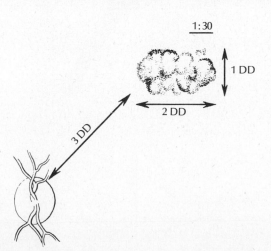

Fig. 11-17. Method of giving position and dimensions of a lesion in terms of disc diameters. (From Havener, W. H.: Synopsis of ophthalmology, ed. 4, St. Louis, 1975, The C. V. Mosby Co.)

Often, a vessel is detected first and can be followed in toward the optic disc. If the examiner directs the beam of light through the pupil in a slightly nasalward direction, the beam will fall on or near the optic disc initially.

Retinal structures. Examination of the various retinal structures should be performed in a consistent and orderly fashion. The following order is recommended: (1) optic disc, (2) retinal vessels, (3) retinal background, and (4) macular area.

The disc is examined for its size, shape, color, the distinctness of its margins, and the physiological cup. The disc is also utilized as a standard measurement device. The distance from the disc and the size of other findings are estimated in terms of disc diameters (DD); for example, an alteration slightly larger than the disc situated in the upper portion of the fundus may be described as being 1 × 2 DD in size and 3 DD away from the disc at 1:30 (clock position) in the left eye (Fig. 11-17).

The retinal vessels are examined for their color, the ratio in size of arterioles to veins is determined, arteriovenous crossings are examined for indentations, and the arterioles are examined for their light reflex. Each set of vessels should be followed out from the disc to the periphery. The retinal background is examined for its color and regularity of appearance and for any areas of light or dark color alterations. The more peripheral reaches of the vessels and retinal background can be examined by having the client direct his gaze upward, downward, and to each side. Observation of the macular area is reserved for last, because having a bright light directed at the center of acutest vision is very uncomfortable for the client. The macula is about 1 DD in size and is located 2 DD temporal to the optic disc. It appears as an avascular area with the bright spot of light reflected from its center, the fovea. This area can be examined by having the client look directly at the examining light. When the client does so, the examiner is visualizing the macula.

Intraocular pressure

Screening for intraocular pressure is best accomplished by using the Schiøtz tonometer. Instructions accompanying the instrument on measurement and cleaning should be followed carefully.

For an accurate tonometry reading, the client should be in either a recumbent position or a reclining position in a chair. A tight collar or tie must be loosened to avoid an artificial increase in intraocular pressure caused by impeded venous return from the jugular system. If contact lenses are worn, they should be removed. Before proceeding, the examiner explains the procedure to the client. The cornea of each eye is then anesthetized by instilling a drop of a topical anesthetic such as proparacaine hydrochloride. Any tearing may be blotted with a tissue, but the eyes should not be rubbed. The client is then asked to fix his gaze directly overhead and to breath regularly. The examiner uses the thumb and index finger of one hand to hold the client's upper and lower lids against the bony orbital rim; with the other hand, the footplate of the vertically held tonometer is placed lightly on the center of the cornea (Fig. 11-18). The reading is taken, and the footplate is lifted, not slid, off the cornea. The lower the reading on the tonometer scale, the greater the pressure. The tonometer should be carefully cleaned after each procedure.

The following conditions are contraindications to performing tonometry:
1. Any ocular infection or discharge
2. Recent ocular injury
3. Herpes on the face or eyelids
4. Corneal edema, distortion, thickening, or scarring
5. Marked nystagmus
6. Uncontrollable coughing
7. Significant apprehension or blepharospasm

It should be remembered that examination of the depth of the anterior chamber, assessment of the visual fields, and examination of the optic nerve head are also components of the examination for increased intraocular pressure, or glaucoma.

Intraocular pressure may be grossly estimated by touch. The client is asked to look down but to keep his eyes open; the examiner then palpates over the sclera with a gentle to-and-fro motion using both index fingers. This maneuver gives only a rough estimate and is much less valuable than tonometry for measurement of intraocular pressure. All persons over 40 years of age should be checked regularly by tonometry. Glaucoma is a major cause of blindness and although it cannot be reversed, it can be halted.

PATHOLOGY
Visual acuity

Limited visual acuity may be an indication of a refractive error or of a more serious pathological condition. The determination of blindness cannot be made unless neither hand movements nor a bright beam of light can be perceived.

Visual fields

Visual field defects may be caused by lesions of the retina, by lesions at any point along the optic nerve or tract, or by lesions in the occipital lobes (Fig. 11-19). Damage to one optic nerve will affect the field of vision in that eye. Lesions occurring at the optic

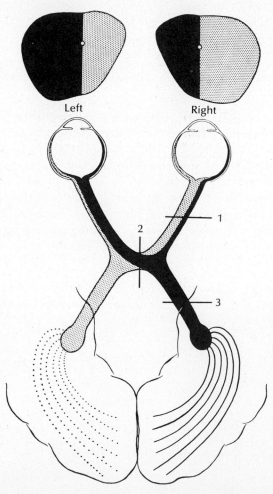

Fig. 11-19. Visual field defects. *1,* Blind right eye; *2,* bitemporal hemianopia—no temporal vision; *3,* left homonymous hemianopia—no vision in left field of either eye. (Adapted from Havener, W. H.: Synopsis of ophthalmology, ed. 5, St. Louis, 1979, The C. V. Mosby Co.)

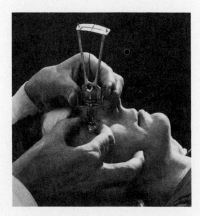

Fig. 11-18. Screening for intraocular pressure. (From Newell, F. W.: Ophthalmology: principles and concepts, ed. 4, St. Louis, 1978, The C. V. Mosby Co.)

chiasm, at the optic tract, or in the brain usually affect the visual fields of both eyes because of the crossing of fibers at the chiasm. Lesions at the optic chiasm, as from a pituitary tumor, cause a loss of vision from the nasal portion of each retina, resulting in a loss of both temporal fields of vision. This condition is termed heteronomous or bitemporal hemianopia.

Since nerves from both eyes mingle behind the chiasm in the optic tracts and in the brain, lesions along the optic tract or in the temporal parietal or occipital lobes will impair the same half of the field of vision in both eyes. For example, a lesion of the right optic tract or right side of the brain will result in visual field defects in the right nasal field and in the left temporal field. This condition is termed homonymous hemianopia and may be caused by occlusion of the middle cerebral artery.

The location of disease on the retina determines the type of resultant visual field defects. Macular defects lead to a central blind area. Localized damage in other areas of the retina will cause a loss of vision corresponding to the involved area. A blind spot is known as a scotoma, that is, an area of blindness surrounded by an area of vision. Advanced diabetic retinopathy may cause macular damage, resulting in a loss of central vision. Glaucoma, or increased intraocular pressure, causes decreased peripheral vision because of the damage caused by the elevated pressure. As the disease advances, it may also cause a loss of central vision. A retinal detachment will cause loss of vision from that portion of the retina.

Extraocular neuromuscular function

An asymmetrical corneal light reflex, an inability of the eyes to move in parallel fashion to the six cardinal positions of gaze, or an abnormal cover test indicates a weakness or paralysis of one or more of the extraocular muscles or a defect in the nerve supplying it. Table 11-2 indicates the muscle and cranial nerve involved when the eye will not turn to one of these six positions.

Examples of the effects of nerve lesions are:
1. *Oculomotor paralysis (CN III):* the eye turns down and out with drooping of the upper lid.
2. *Abducens paralysis (CN IV):* the eye turns in toward the nose because of unopposed action of the medial rectus.

Carrying the fixation point of the six cardinal positions out to the extremes will exaggerate a defect. A disparity of the anteroposterior axes of the eyes is called strabismus. Deviations in these axes may be detected during the cover test, which blocks the fusion reflex of the eyes. A mild weakness of the extraocular muscles is called phoria. If there is a weak tendency during the cover test, a definitely perceptible jerk of the eye is noted when the cover is removed. Tropia is a more pronounced imbalance producing a permanent disparity in the axes of the eyes. A mild outward deviation of the eye is called exophoria; an inward deviation is called esophoria. The rhythmical twitching motion of nystagmus may be normal at the end of the lateral position but is abnormal when the eyes are in any other position.

Ocular structures

Eyelids and eyelashes. Faulty positioning of the eyelids occurs in a variety of ways. The lid margins may fall above or below the middle part of the iris. A drooping lid margin (ptosis) that falls at the pupil or below may indicate an oculomotor nerve lesion or a congenital condition. If the lid margin falls above the limbus so that some sclera is visible, thyroid disease may be present. In the presence of thyroid disease the lid may lag behind the limbus as the gaze moves from an upward to a downward position (Fig. 11-20). Another type of faulty positioning of the lids is improper approximation of the lids to the eyeballs. The lids may be loose or lax and roll outward. This condition is called ectropion. Because the puncta cannot effectively drain the tears, epiphora (tearing) results. The lids may also roll inward because of lid spasm or the contraction of scar tissue. This condition is called entropion. Because the lashes are pulled inward, they may produce corneal irritation.

Table 11-2. Diagnostic clues to dysfunction of extraocular neuromuscular units

Position to which eye will not turn	Muscle	Cranial nerve
Straight nasal	Medial rectus	III
Up and nasal	Inferior oblique	III
Down and nasal	Superior oblique	IV
Straight temporal	Lateral rectus	VI
Up and temporal	Superior rectus	III
Down and temporal	Inferior rectus	III

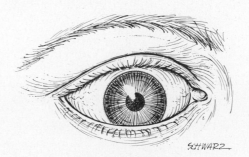

Fig. 11-20. Lid lag.

The tissues within the lids are loosely connnected and collect excess fluid rather readily. Edema of the lids may be a manifestation of local or systemic disease. Examples of systemic problems that may cause lid edema include allergy, heart failure, nephrosis, and thyroid deficiency.

The glands of the lids may be sites of infection. A localized infection of the small glands around the eyelashes in the hair follicle at the lid margin is a hordeolum, or sty (Fig. 11-21). The meibomian glands lying within the posterior portion of the lid may develop an infection or a retention cyst, known as a chalazion (Fig. 11-22); crusting or scaling at the

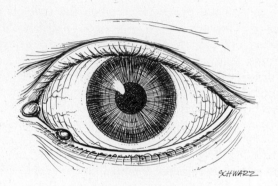

Fig. 11-21. Hordeolum or sty.

lid margins may occur as a result of staphylococcal infection or seborrheic dermatitis. If a lid infection is present or suspected, the lids may be gently palpated by moving the examining finger across the lid surface. Pressure should never be exerted over the eye in an effort to separate the lids. As mentioned earlier, the bony orbital rims should be used as points over which to slide the lids.

Xanthelasma, the raised yellow plaques that may appear on the lids, may have no pathological significance, or they may be associated with hypercholesterolemia.

Conjunctiva. Infectious disease of the conjunctiva typically produces engorgement of the conjunctival vessels and a discharge. The infected vessels are usually more pronounced at the fornices. Small subconjunctival hemorrhages may result from more severe involvement, though in some persons these may also result from sneezing, coughing, or lifting.

Sclera. Changes in the color of the sclera may be indicative of systemic disease. For example, jaundice manifests its presence in the eyes as a yellow discoloration, scleral icterus. Excessive bilirubinemia may be evident as scleral icterus before jaundice of the skin becomes apparent. In the presence of osteogenesis imperfecta the sclera is bluish.

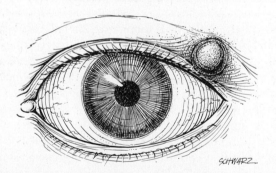

Fig. 11-22. Chalazion.

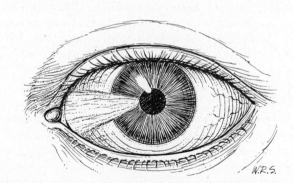

Fig. 11-23. Pterygium.

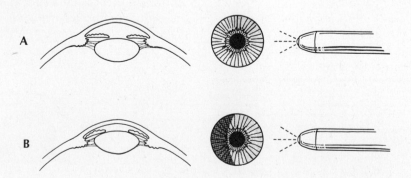

Fig. 11-24. A, Normal anterior chamber. **B,** Shallow anterior chamber. (From Havener, W. H.: Synopsis of ophthalmology, ed. 5, St. Louis, 1979, The C. V. Mosby Co.)

Cornea. The cornea is a very sensitive structure, and pain and photophobia are common manifestations of corneal disease. Any dullness, irregularities, or opacities of the cornea are abnormal. Two of the more frequent abnormalities affecting the cornea are abrasions and opacities. Although an abrasion may cause the surface to look irregular or may cast a shadow on the iris, it may be invisible and detectable only with fluorescein stain. Suspected corneal abrasion should be referred to an ophthalmologist.

Abnormal growth of bulbar conjunctival tissue from the edge toward the center of the cornea, known as pterygium, may interfere with vision (Fig. 11-23).

Although the presence of arcus senilis is normal in elderly people, in younger individuals it may be associated with abnormal lipid metabolism.

Anterior chamber. Abnormalities observable in the anterior chamber are a decrease in depth and any foreign material interrupting the normal transparency. A shallow anterior chamber may be a sign of glaucoma or may predispose the eye to glaucoma (Fig. 11-24). Symptoms typical of glaucoma include pain, redness, and seeing colored halos around lights. As the increased intraocular pressure causes the iris to become displaced anteriorly, there is less distance between the cornea and the iris. As a result of this anterior displacement, light directed obliquely from the temporal side will illuminate only the temporal side, and the nasal side will appear darker or shadowed. The presence of a shallow anterior chamber is a contraindication to the use of dilating drops for the ophthalmoscopic examination.

Any cloudiness of the aqueous fluid or accumulation of blood (hyphema) or purulent material (hypopyon) is abnormal. Hyphema may be caused by trauma or may result from spontaneous hemorrhage. If the hyphema is mild, the red blood cells settle out inferiorly by gravity to a height of a few millimeters. In severe hyphemas, the entire anterior chamber may be filled with blood.

Lacrimal apparatus. Both the lacrimal gland, which produces tears, and the system that drains the tears are subject to certain abnormalities. The lacrimal gland may be swollen as a result of infection or tumor. Infection with consequent blockage of the lacrimal sac or duct may occur with associated findings of swelling, redness, warmth, pain, and purulent discharge. The swelling tends to occur in the area below the inner canthus. The technique for examining for infection in the lacrimal sac is to press with the examining finger against the *inner* orbital rim (not against the nose), then to gently depress the lower lid over the lower orbital rim to observe for regurgitation of fluid through the puncta.

As mentioned earlier, ectropion may cause tearing because of inadequate drainage. Any unusual markings or growths should be noted.

Iris. Iritis, inflammation of the iris, results in throbbing pain and visual blurring and is associated with the findings of circumcorneal injection, a deep pinkish red flush about the cornea, and a constricted pupil. This is in contrast to conjunctivitis, wherein the infected vessels tend to extend from the periphery toward the center. The iris may become inflamed because of bacterial infections, which may also lead to the production of a purulent exudate, as well as to diffuse congestion around the iris. If the lens has been removed, the normal support of the iris is absent and the iris will, with movements of the eye, have a tremulous, fluttering motion.

Pupils. Abnormalities of the pupils include alterations in size and in reflexes. Although a slight but noticeable difference in pupil size does occur in about 5% of the population, this finding should be regarded with suspicion because it can be an indication of central nervous system (CNS) disease. Inequality in the size of the pupils is known as anisocoria. Dyscoria is a congenital abnormality in the shape of the pupils.

Mydriasis, enlargement of the pupils, may result from emotional influences, recent or old local trauma, acute glaucoma, systemic reaction to parasympatholytic or sympathomimetic drugs, or the local use of dilating drops. A unilateral fixed enlarged pupil may be caused by local trauma to the eye or head injury. Fixed dilatation of both eyes occurs with deep anesthesia, CNS injury, and circulatory arrest.

Miosis, constriction of the pupils, is associated with iritis, use of morphine, and glaucoma treatment by pilocarpine and is seen physiologically with sleep.

Any irregularity in pupil contour is abnormal and may result from iritis, trauma, CNS syphilis, or congenital defects.

Failure of the pupils to react to light with preservation of the accommodation reaction is another characteristic of CNS syphilis. This is known as the Argyll-Robertson pupil.

In the case of monocular blindness, the blind eye and optic tract will transmit no response to light, and neither pupil will constrict. However, when the unaffected eye receives illumination, both pupils will constrict because the efferent pupil constriction stimuli are distributed evenly to both eyes.

Lens. Opacities in any of the clear portions of the eye (anterior chamber, lens, or vitreous body) will appear as dark shadows on black spots within the red reflex on ophthalmoscopic examination because they prevent light from being reflected back to the examiner's eye. An opacity within the lens is referred to as a cataract. These opacities vary in appearance; some look like pieces of coral, some look like various-shaped crystals, and others have a stellate, or starlike, appearance. Cataract formation may be associated with various systemic disorders, may occur as the complex of findings in various hereditary syndromes, or may result from senescent changes within the lens. In certain endocrine disorders, such as diabetes mellitus, the metabolic disturbance results in abnormal lens fiber formation and cataracts. Such cataracts typically attack young persons more frequently than older persons, are bilateral, progress rapidly, and have a classical snowflake appearance. Senile cataracts occur as a result of various degenerative processes within the lenticular material. Typical symptoms include cloudiness of vision, particularly in bright light, decrease in the visual field, and occasionally the appearance of black spots with movements of the eyes. Because of the increase in the size of the lens with a maturing cataract, the depth of the anterior chamber may be diminished, thus precipitating glaucoma.

Retinal structures

OPTIC DISC. Three of the major conditions causing alterations of the optic disc are papilledema, glaucoma, and optic atrophy. Papilledema, or swelling of the optic nerve head, causes the margins of the disc to become blurred and indistinct (Fig. 11-25). The nerve head appears out of focus with the surrounding retina. The degree of elevation can be assessed by focusing first on the disc and then on the surrounding retina and noting the difference in diopters on the ophthalmoscope.

Papilledema is a sign of increased intracranial pressure. This causes decreased venous drainage from the eye, hence venous stasis, or the accumulation and leakage of fluid, leading to edematous appearance of the disc. This condition may be associated with malignant hypertension, eclampsia, brain tumor, and hematoma.

The increased intraocular pressure of glaucoma gradually exerts pressure anteriorly against the iris, as mentioned earlier, and posteriorly against the optic disc, causing increased cupping (Fig. 11-26). This may be noted by observing the course of vessels as they emerge from the center and over the disc margins, since glaucoma may cause a vessel to seem to disappear from sight at the disc rim and then reappear at a slightly different site just past the rim. The pressure of glaucoma may also eventually cause pallor of the disc, a sign of optic atrophy. Advanced cupping and optic atrophy are late findings of the disease; the early findings are very subtle and are likely to be very difficult to recognize. Thus, the need for careful tonometry as a far more sensitive indicator is reemphasized.

Death of the optic nerve fibers leads to the disappearance of the tiny disc vessels that give the disc its normal pinkish color and results in optic pallor. The disc appears pale and white, either in a section or throughout. *Note:* The scleral crescent, a normal, crescent-shaped area around the rim of the disc only, should not be mistaken for disc pallor.

RETINAL VESSELS. Changes in caliber and alterations at crossings can occur in the retinal vessels. Changes in these vascular structures are often indicative of systemic diseases, such as hypertension. Because any vessel caliber changes may or may not be evenly distributed along the course of the vessel, vessels should be observed from the disc to the periphery. Arterioles, normally about two-thirds to three-fourths of the diameter of the corresponding veins, are subject to a decrease in diameter as a re-

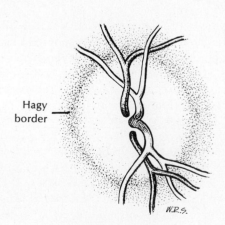

Hagy
border

Fig. 11-25. Papilledema.

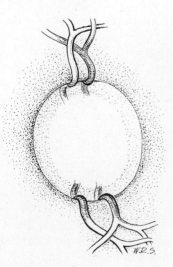

Fig. 11-26. Glaucomatous cupping.

sult of constriction of the vessels or reduced blood flow to the eye. In hypertension, arterioles may become narrowed to a 3:5 or 2:4 or less ratio. More rarely, veins may increase in diameter as a result of conditions causing more blood to circulate to the eye or conditions impeding the exit of blood from the eye.

The condition of the arteriole vessel walls determines their color. Normally, they are transparent and reflect the color of the column of blood within, but they may develop sclerotic or sheathing changes, causing them to become opaque and lighter in color. The width of the light reflex from the arteriolar wall also increases with arteriosclerosis to one-third or more of the width of the vessel. In advanced stages, the vessels may appear as fine, silvery lines.

Changes at arteriolovenous crossings include an apparent narrowing or blocking of the vein where an arteriole crosses over it. This appearance is the result of some degree of concealment of the underlying

veins by an abnormally opaque arteriole wall and occurs with long-standing hypertension; it is initially apparent as venous narrowing and later as a more complete interruption of the vessel. These changes are referred to as arteriovenous nicking (Fig. 11-27).

Emboli in a retinal vessel cause abrupt narrowing of arterioles and abrupt dilatation of a vein as it impedes return flow.

RETINAL BACKGROUND. Among the more common abnormalities to appear on the retinal background are microaneurysms, exudates, and hemorrhages (Fig. 11-28). Microaneurysms, outpouchings in the walls of capillaries, appear as tiny bright red dots on the retina. These are frequently associated with diabetes mellitus.

Exudates are whitish yellow infiltrates that may occur alongside vessel walls. They are rather round, appearing somewhat like a small cumulus cloud, and may have hazy or distinct edges. Exudates may be associated with systemic diseases, including diabetes mellitus and hypertension, and may occur with degenerative or inflammatory diseases of the retina. They may be resorbed over time.

Hemorrhages are bright to dark red, may be small and round, as is commonly found with diabetes mellitus, or linear and flame-shaped, as occurs in hypertension. Bleeding may occur from retinal or chloridal vessels into the preretinal, retinal, or choroidal areas.

In the case of any retinal abnormality, the color, shape, size, and proximity to the disc or vessels should be described.

Problems such as those just described may affect any part of the retinal background, including the

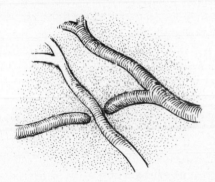

Fig. 11-27. Arteriovenous nicking.

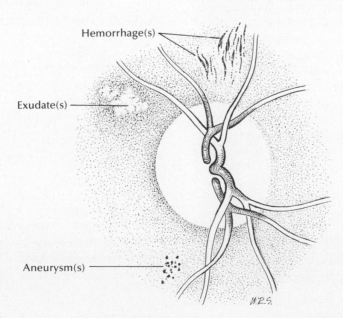

Hemorrhage(s)

Exudate(s)

Aneurysm(s)

Fig. 11-28. Abnormalities of the retinal background: microaneurysms, exudates, and hemorrhages.

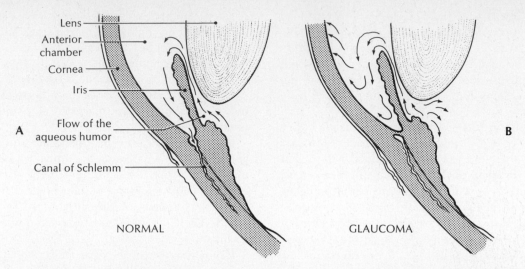

Lens
Anterior chamber
Cornea
Iris
Flow of the aqueous humor
Canal of Schlemm
A
B
NORMAL
GLAUCOMA

Fig. 11-29. A, Normal flow of aqueous. **B,** Closed angle glaucoma: the flow of aqueous is blocked.

macular area. Depending on the area affected, resultant difficulty with central or peripheral vision may occur.

Increased intraocular pressure

Glaucoma is a disease characterized by increased intraocular pressure secondary to an inadequate drainage system for the aqueous fluid. If not treated, it results in damage to the optic nerve, with subsequent loss of peripheral vision and leads eventually to blindness. The disease may be chronic or acute, primary or secondary, painless or painful. It is frequently asymptomatic and proceeds so gradually that it may go unnoticed until well advanced. Primary glaucomas include chronic open-angle, chronic and acute closed-angle, and congenital. Approximately 90% of the primary glaucomas are the chronic open-angle type, where interference with the drainage system of the eye and a resulting imbalance in the normal flow of the aqueous increase the intraocular pressure (Fig. 11-29). Closed-angle glaucoma, which may be acute or chronic, occurs in the individual with an abnormally narrow space or angle formed by the iris and the cornea. The adhesions that form decrease or totally inhibit the normal flow of the aqueous. In congenital glaucoma, certain developmental defects interfere with the flow of aqueous. Secondary glaucoma may result from a number of causes including trauma, drugs, inflammation, and neovascularization.

Persons particularly at risk for glaucoma include those who are diabetic, hypertensive, or black; those who have had eye injuries; large-eyed children; and those with a family history of glaucoma. It is the third major cause of blindness in the United States. It is detectable and treatable and should be a part of a regular screening examination for those at risk and for all persons over the age of 40.

SUMMARY

I. Visual functions
  A. Visual acuity
    1. Snellen chart—far vision
    2. Newspaper—near vision
  B. Visual fields
  C. Extraocular muscles
    1. Corneal light reflex
    2. Six cardinal positions of gaze
    3. Cover-uncover test
II. Ocular structures
  A. Eyelids and eyelashes
  B. Conjunctiva
  C. Sclera
  D. Cornea
  E. Anterior chamber
  F. Lacrimal apparatus
  G. Iris
  H. Pupils
  I. Lens
  J. Vitreous
  K. Retinal structures
    1. Optic disc
    2. Retinal arterioles and veins
    3. Retinal background
    4. Macular area
III. Intraocular pressure measurement

BIBLIOGRAPHY

Albert, D. M.: Jaeger's atlas of diseases of the ocular fundus, Philadelphia, 1972, W. B. Saunders Co.

Becker, B., and Drews, R. C.: Current concepts in ophthalmology, vol. I, St. Louis, 1967, The C. V. Mosby Co.

Blodi, F. C., Allen, L., and Frazier, O.: Stereoscopic manual of the ocular fundus in local and systemic disease, vol. II, St. Louis, 1970, The C. V. Mosby Co.

Donaldson, D. D.: Atlas of external diseases of the eye, vol. IV: anterior chamber, iris, and ciliary body, St. Louis, 1973, The C. V. Mosby Co.

Donaldson, D. D.: Atlas of disease of the anterior segment of the eye, vol. V: the crystalline lens, St. Louis, 1976, The C. V. Mosby Co.

Harrington, D. O.: The visual fields: a textbook and atlas of clinical perimetry, St. Louis, 1956, The C. V. Mosby Co.

Jackson, C. R. S.: The eye in general practice, Baltimore, 1972, The Williams & Wilkins Co.

Mechner, F.: Patient assessment: examination of the eye, part I, Am. J. Nurs. 74(11):1-24, part II, 75(1):1-24, 1974.

Newell, F. W.: Ophthalmology principles and concepts, ed. 4, St. Louis, 1978, The C. V. Mosby Co.

Potts, A. M., editor: The assessment of visual function, St. Louis, 1972, The C. V. Mosby Co.

Thomas, B. A., editor: Introduction to ophthalmoscopy, Kalamazoo, Mich., 1976, The Upjohn Co.

Vaughn, D., Cook, R., and Asbury, T.: General ophthalmology, Los Altos, Calif., 1968, Lange Medical Publications.

12 Assessment of the head, face, and neck

A great variety of structures are located in the head and neck area, including several organs of special sensation. Although the examination of the entire head involves the examination of the special sense organs, those topics are covered in other chapters: Chapter 10 on assessment of the ears, nose, and throat and Chapter 11 on assessment of the eyes. This chapter deals with the remaining structures. Similarly, in the case of the neck examination, multiple structures are involved, some of which are covered in other chapters: Chapter 13 on assessment of the lymphatic system, Chapter 15 on assessment of the respiratory system, and Chapter 16 on cardiovascular assessment: the heart and the neck vessels. This organization is presented so that the learner may better understand the examinations of complete body systems. Having learned this, the beginning practitioner must then proceed to organize and integrate the components of the physical examination by anatomical area.

The assessment techniques of inspection, palpation, and auscultation are utilized in the examination of the head and neck. Equipment requirements include a good light source, a glass of water, and a stethoscope.

HEAD

Those portions of the head examination covered here include assessment of the size and shape of the skull and assessment of the condition of the scalp and hair.

The shape of the skull is generally round with several prominences; the frontal areas are prominent anteriorly. The areas of the head take their names from the underlying bones, including the frontal, parietal, occipital, and mastoid bones; the maxilla; and the mandible (Fig. 12-1). There is a large range of normal-shaped skulls.

The skin overlying the superior, lateral, and pos-

terior portions of the skull is called the scalp and is normally covered with hair.

The size and shape of the skull are assessed by inspection; the examiner also inspects the condition of the scalp by parting the hair in several areas. Obviously, wigs or other hairpieces must be removed to accomplish this assessment. The client should be carefully questioned regarding any previous head trauma, because the hair covering makes it difficult to assess the head and scalp completely. The examiner also notes the texture and amount of hair and the use of coloring or lubricating agents. The condition of the hair may be a useful indication of the client's emotional status, social group identification, and personal hygiene.

Several conditions may result in abnormalities of the skull. For example, an abnormally large head in children may result from the accumulation of fluid in the ventricles of the brain (hydrocephalus). In adults a large head may result from osteitis deformans, wherein the bony thickness increases, or from excessive growth hormone secretion (acromegaly), wherein the skull becomes enlarged and thickened, the length of the mandible increases, the nose and forehead are more prominent, and the facial features appear coarsened. Local deformities of the skull may result from trauma or from the surgical removal of portions of the skull.

Sebaceous cysts may develop on the scalp. These result from the occlusion of sebaceous gland ducts and are palpable as smooth, rounded nodules attached to the scalp. The scalp should also be assessed for dandruff and for the presence of parasites.

The hair is subject to the influence of altered metabolic conditions. The classical examples are the changes caused by thyroid disorders. In hypothyroidism, the hair is coarse, dry, and brittle; in hyperthyroidism, the hair becomes fine, silky, and soft. The thinning or loss of hair (alopecia) may be hereditary, especially in males, or a side effect of drugs used to treat malignant tumors. This condition may also accompany prolonged illness or emotional stress.

FACE

The variations in facial appearance are as numerous as the earth's population. Furthermore, a client's facial expression at any moment is subject to change and often reveals much about his general feeling tone. In general, the examiner should observe the bilateral structures for symmetry in size, position, and movement.

In examining the face, the examiner observes the facial expression, the color and condition of the facial skin, and the shape and symmetry of the facial structures, including the eyebrows, eyes, nose, mouth, and ears. Normally the palpebral fissures, the distance between the eyelids, are equal in size. The nasolabial folds, the creases extending from the angle of the nose to the corner of the mouth, are symmetrical (Fig. 12-2). Within the range of normal, there are many individuals with slightly asymmetrical characteristic expressions.

Sensation of the face is mediated by the trigeminal nerve (cranial nerve [CN]V), which has three sensory divisions. Its function is tested as part of the neurological examination for pain and touch. The muscles of facial expression are supplied by the facial nerve (CN VII). The examiner can test for facial muscle function by asking the client to elevate his eyebrows, frown or lower his eyebrows, close his eyes tightly, puff his cheeks, show his teeth, and smile.

The major accessible artery on the face is the temporal artery, which passes just anterior to the ear over the temporal muscle and into the forehead (Fig. 12-3). It is palpable in the temporal area just anterior to the tragus of the ear. Any thickening, hardness, or tenderness of the vessel should be noted.

Changes in color, shape, symmetry, hair distribution pattern, or movement of the face may occur. In situations where there is an increased amount of unsaturated hemoglobin in the body tissues, as may occur with cardiac or pulmonary disease, or where there is a local stasis of circulation, various facial and head structures, including the lips, nose, cheeks, ears, and oral mucosa, may become bluish, or cyanotic. Facial pallor results from a decrease in circulating red blood cells, as in anemia, or from a decrease in local vascular supply, as in shock. The yellow color of jaundice results from an abnormal increase in bilirubin. Before jaundice is generally evident in the skin, it may be observed in the sclera and in the mucous membranes of the mouth under the tongue and on the palate. Localized color changes result from acne, moles, and scar tissue. More rare conditions associ-

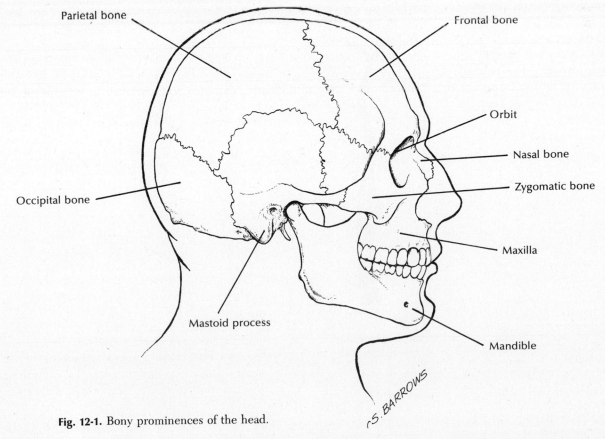

Fig. 12-1. Bony prominences of the head.

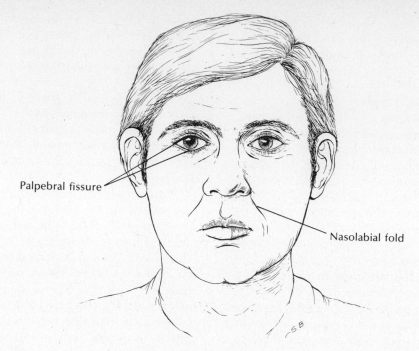

Fig. 12-2. Anterior view of the face showing the palpebral fissures and nasolabial folds.

Palpebral fissure

Nasolabial fold

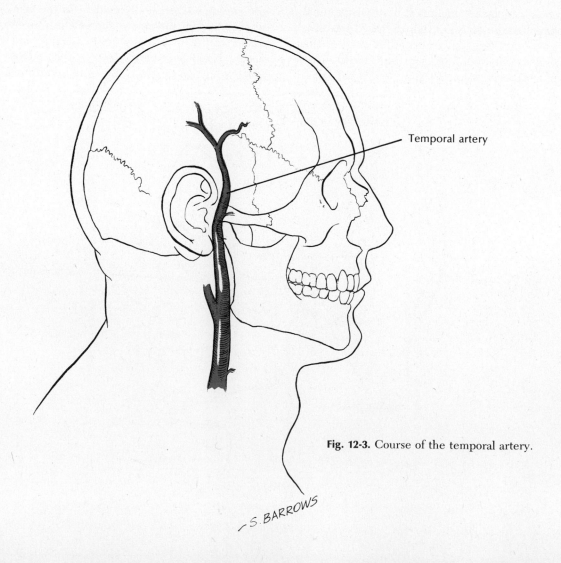

Temporal artery

Fig. 12-3. Course of the temporal artery.

S. BARROWS

ated with color alterations include lupus erythematosus, wherein an erythematous discoloration bridges the cheeks and nose, and conditions that alter the deposition of melanin, resulting in light or dark patchy areas.

Numerous situations may cause a change in facial shape. Edema, often initially evident in the eyelids, may result from cardiovascular or kidney disease. Thyroid disorders also affect the face: excessive function, hyperthyroidism, may be associated with an apparent protrusion of the eyeballs (exophthalmos) and with elevation of the upper lids, resulting in a staring or startled expression; diminished function, hypothyroidism, may lead to "myxedema facies," wherein the face is dull and puffy with dry skin and coarse features. As a result of increased adrenal hormone production (Cushing's syndrome) or secondary to the intake of synthetic adrenal hormones, "moon facies" may be observed, wherein the face is round and the cheeks quite red. Prolonged illness, dehydration, or starvation may produce a cachectic face, wherein the eyes, cheeks, and temples appear sunken, the nose appears sharp, and the skin is dry and rough.

Asymmetry or abnormal movements, or both, may result from facial nerve lesions. In Bell's palsy, a paralysis of the seventh nerve, the eye on the affected side cannot close completely, the lower eyelid droops, the nasolabial fold is lost, and the corner of the mouth droops. Slight weakness may be present but is not evident when the face is at rest, so the examiner should carefully check facial muscle function.

In the women of some ethnic groups, increased facial hair is a normal finding. Elevated production of adrenal hormones may lead to excessive hair growth in the moustache and sideburn areas and on the chin. Myxedema causes thinning of the scalp hair and eyebrows.

NECK

A complete examination of the neck includes assessment of the neck muscles and cervical vertebrae, the trachea, the thyroid gland, the carotid arteries and jugular veins, and the cervical lymph nodes. As mentioned earlier, this chapter covers only the muscles and the thyroid gland because the other structures are discussed elsewhere in the text.

Neck muscles

The major neck muscles are the sternocleidomastoid muscles and the trapezius muscles. Each sterno-

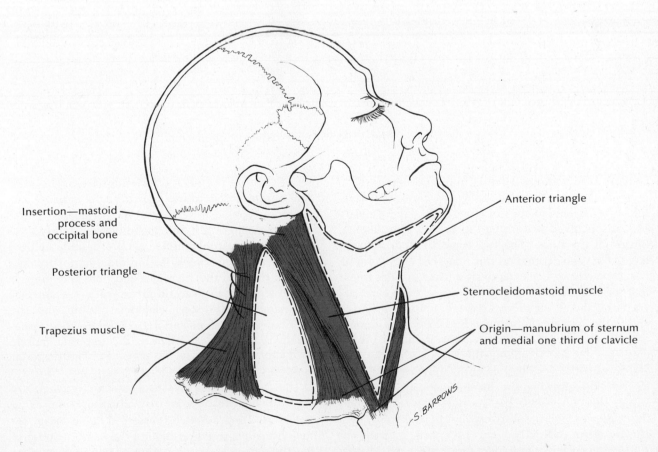

Insertion—mastoid process and occipital bone

Posterior triangle

Trapezius muscle

Anterior triangle

Sternocleidomastoid muscle

Origin—manubrium of sternum and medial one third of clavicle

S. BARROWS

Fig. 12-4. Sternocleidomastoid muscle and the anterior and posterior triangles.

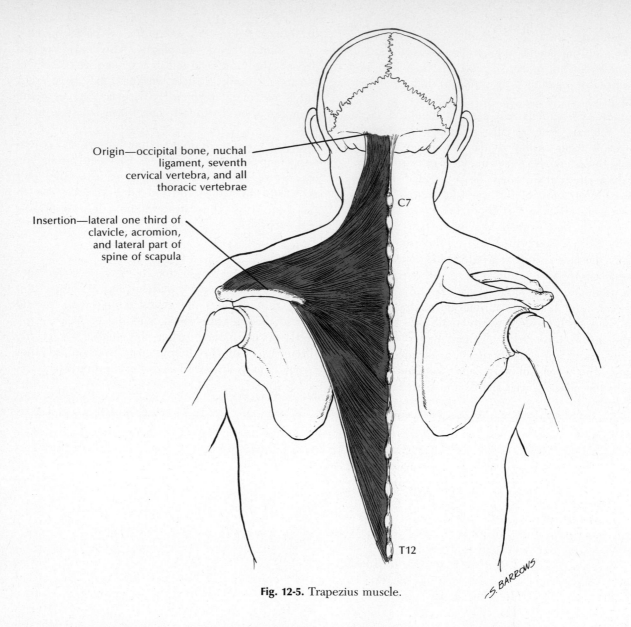

Origin—occipital bone, nuchal ligament, seventh cervical vertebra, and all thoracic vertebrae

Insertion—lateral one third of clavicle, acromion, and lateral part of spine of scapula

C7

T12

S. BARROWS

Fig. 12-5. Trapezius muscle.

cleidomastoid muscle extends from the upper sternum and proximal portion of the clavicle to the mastoid process behind the ear (Fig. 12-4). These muscles are involved in turning the head and in lateral flexion of the head. The two trapezius muscles are large, flat, and triangular, and together they form a trapezoid shape. Each trapezius muscle extends from the occipital bone of the skull, the seventh cervical vertebra, and all the thoracic vertebrae to the clavicle and to the spine of the scapula (Fig. 12-5). The trapezius muscles are involved in the movements of shrugging the shoulders, pulling the scapulae downward and toward the vertebral column, drawing the head to the side, drawing the head backward, and elevating the chin. Both the sternocleidomastoid and the trapezius muscles are supplied by the spinal accessory nerve (CN XI).

The sternocleidomastoid muscles are used to de-

scribe areas of the neck. These muscles divide each side of the neck into two triangles, the anterior and posterior triangles (Fig. 12-4). The parameters of the anterior triangle are the mandible superiorly, the sternocleidomastoid muscle laterally, and the midline of the trachea medially. Within the anterior triangle lie the trachea, the thyroid gland, and the anterior cervical nodes; the carotid artery runs just anterior and parallel to the sternocleidomastoid muscle. The parameters of the posterior triangle are the sternocleidomastoid muscle laterally, the trapezius muscle medially, and the clavicle inferiorly. The posterior cervical lymph nodes are located here.

The neck muscles are inspected for symmetry of the musculature and for any abnormal masses or swellings. Their function is assessed by observing for the normal centered position of the head, by observing the active range of motion of the head, and by

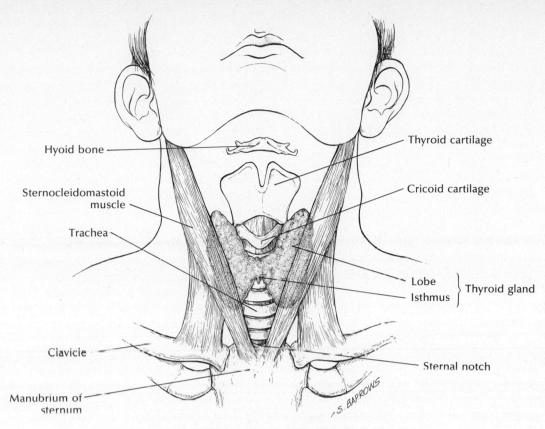

Fig. 12-6. Midline neck structures.

testing muscle strength against resistance. Normally, the head should flex until the chin rests on the chest with the mouth closed; the head should turn about 90 degrees laterally and flex in that position until chin and shoulder touch; the head normally extends about 70 degrees to 80 degrees backward. Strength of the sternocleidomastoid muscles is tested by having the client turn his head to one side and then to the other against the resistance of the examiner's hand. Strength of the trapezius muscles is assessed by asking the client to shrug his shoulders against the resistance of the examiner's hands.

Common abnormalities of the neck muscles include stiffness and pain. In tense individuals, some degree of muscle spasm may occur and tenderness on palpation may be elicited over the affected muscles. Stiffness of the neck may also result from vertebral disease or meningitis. Cercival arthritis produces limitation of motion, and central nervous system disease involving irritation of the meninges is associated with pain on neck motion. *Note:* If there is any suspicion of traumatic neck injury, passive range of motion should never be done.

An abnormal position or tilting of the head may result from shortening of the sternocleidomastoid muscle or may be secondary to visual difficulties. An abnormal up-and-down nodding movement of the head is seen with Parkinson's disease.

Thyroid gland

The thyroid gland is the largest endocrine gland in the body and the only one accessible to direct physical examination.

An awareness of the midline neck structures is important in performing the examination of the thyroid gland (Fig. 12-6). Structures lying in the midline include:

1. The hyoid bone, which lies just below the mandible at the angle of the floor of the mouth.
2. The thyroid cartilage, which is shaped like a shield and which is the largest of the cartilagenous structures in the neck. The upper edge is notched, and its level corresponds to the level of bifurcation of the common carotid artery into the internal and external carotid arteries.
3. The cricoid cartilage, which is the uppermost ring of the trachea. It is palpable just below the thyroid cartilage.
4. The tracheal rings.
5. The isthmus of the thyroid gland, which lies across the trachea below the cricoid cartilage.

The thyroid gland is butterfly-shaped. It has two

lateral lobes and a connecting isthmus that joins the lobes at their lower-third area. The lobes are irregular and cone-shaped, each about 5 cm long, 3 cm in diameter, and 2 cm thick. The average weight of the total gland is about 25 gm. The lobes curve posteriorly around the cartilages; the lateral portions are covered by the sternocleidomastoid muscles. Thyroid arteries supply the highly vascular thyroid tissue.

EXAMINATION

The techniques used to examine the thyroid gland include observation, palpation, and auscultation. Observation of thyroid function or possible dysfunction includes more than observation of the area where the thyroid gland is located. The effects of thyroid activity are widespread; therefore, observations of behavior, appearance, skin, eyes, hair, and cardiovascular status are important.

To inspect the thyroid gland, the examiner stands before the client and observes particularly the lower half of the neck, first in normal position, next in slight extension, and then while the client swallows a sip of water (Fig. 12-7). The movements of the cartilages are easily observed. Any unusual bulging of thyroid tissue in the midline of the lobes or behind the sternocleidomastoid muscles should be noted;

normally, none is seen. A good cross light is helpful for observing subtle neck movements or ascending masses.

Following observation, the neck is palpated for the presence of an enlarged thyroid, for consistency of the gland, and for any nodules. The normal thyroid gland is not palpable. However, in a thin neck, the isthmus is occasionally palpable; and in a short, stocky neck, even an enlarged gland may be difficult to palpate. Palpation may be done with the examiner standing either in front of or behind the client. Although there are several techniques utilized for palpation of the thyroid, the underlying principles for each technique include movement of the gland while the client swallows, adequate exposure of the gland by relaxation and manual displacement of surrounding structures, and comparison of one side of the gland with the other. The thyroid gland is fixed to the trachea and thus ascends during swallowing. This distinguishes thyroid structures from other neck masses.

Posterior approach. The client is seated on a chair or examining table while the examiner stands behind him. The client is requested to lower his chin in order to relax the neck muscles. The examining fingers are curved anteriorly, so that the tips rest on

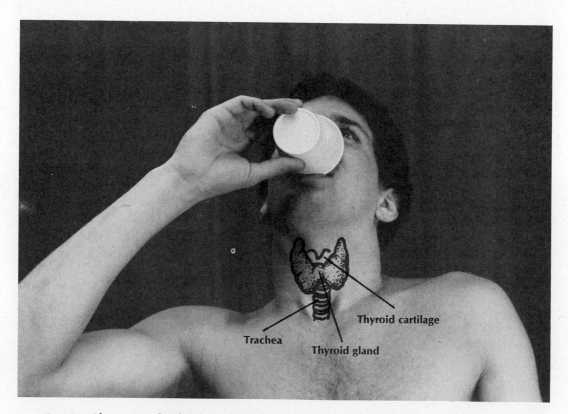

Fig. 12-7. Observation for the thyroid gland with the neck in slight extension. The structures of the thyroid gland are more distinct during swallowing.

Thyroid cartilage

Trachea

Thyroid gland

the lower half of the neck over the trachea (Fig. 12-8). The client is asked to swallow a sip of water while the examiner feels for any enlargement of the thyroid isthmus. To facilitate examination of each lobe, the client is asked to turn his head slightly toward the side to be examined with the chin still lowered. For example, to examine the right thyroid lobe, the examiner has the client lower his chin and turn his head slightly to the right. With the fingers of the left hand, the examiner displaces the thyroid cartilage slightly to the right while the fingers of the right hand palpate the area lateral to the cartilage where the thyroid lobe lies, for any enlargement (Fig. 12-9). The client is asked to swallow a sip of water as this procedure is being done. The examiner may also palpate for thyroid enlargement on the right side by placing

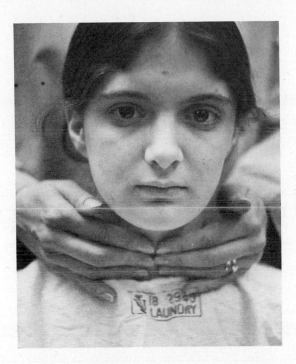

Fig. 12-8. Posterior approach to thyroid examination. Standing behind the client, the examiner palpates for the thyroid isthmus by placing the palmar aspects of the fingertips over the lower portion of the trachea.

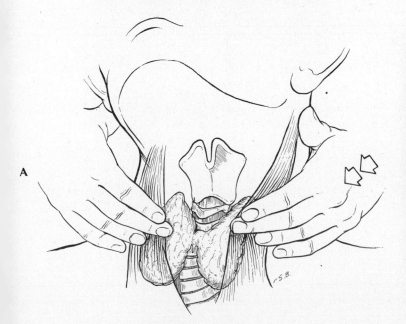

A

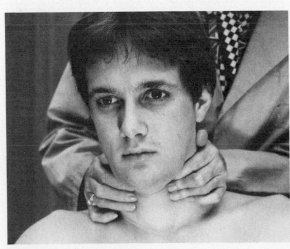

B

Fig. 12-9. Posterior approach to thyroid examination. In order to examine the right lobe of the thyroid gland, the examiner displaces the trachea slightly to the right with the fingers of the left hand and palpates for the right thyroid lobe with the fingers of the right hand.

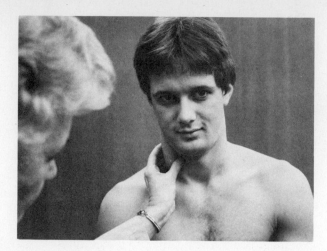

Fig. 12-10. Anterior approach to thyroid examination. Examining for an enlarged right thyroid lobe, the examiner grasps and palpates around and deep to the right sternocleidomastoid muscle.

Fig. 12-11. Anterior approach to thyroid examination. Standing in front of the client, the examiner uses the fingers of the left hand to displace the trachea slightly to the left while the fingers of the right hand palpate for the left thyroid lobe.

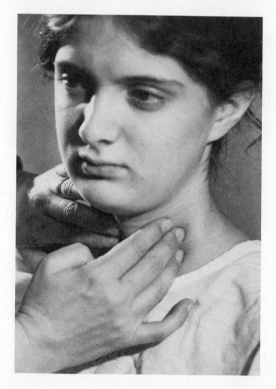

the thumb deep to and behind the sternocleidomastoid muscle while the index and middle fingers are placed deep to and in front of the muscle (Fig. 12-10). This procedure is then repeated for the left lobe; the right hand displaces the cartilage, and the left hand palpates.

Anterior approach. The examiner stands in front of the client and with the palmar surfaces of the index and middle fingers palpates below the cricoid cartilage for the thyroid isthmus as the client swallows a sip of water. In a procedure similar to the one used with the posterior approach, the client is asked to flex his head and turn it slightly to one side and

then the other. The examiner palpates for the left lobe by displacing the thyroid cartilage slightly to the left with the left hand and examining for thyroid enlargement with the right hand (Fig. 12-11). Again, the examiner palpates the area and hooks thumb and fingers around the sternocleidomastoid muscle (Fig. 12-12). The procedure is repeated for the right side.

If enlargement of the thyroid gland is detected or suspected, the area over the gland is auscultated for a bruit. In a hyperplastic thyroid gland, the blood flow through the thyroid arteries is accelerated and produces vibrations that may be heard with the bell

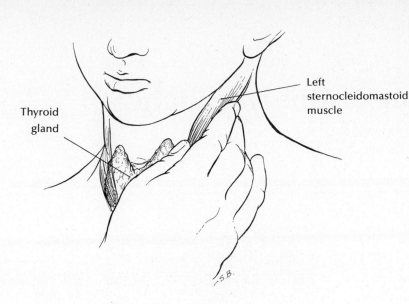 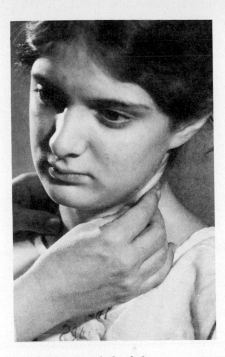

Fig. 12-12. Anterior approach to thyroid examination. The examiner grasps around the left sternocleidomastoid muscle with the right hand to palpate for an enlarged left thyroid lobe.

of the stethoscope as a soft, rushing sound, or bruit. (See Chapter 16, "Cardiovascular Assessment: the Heart and the Neck Vessels" for further discussion of bruits.)

The thyroid gland may incur diffuse or local enlargement. Diffuse enlargement may occur to varying degrees. Symmetrical thyroid enlargement is not uncommon in areas where there is a deficiency of dietary iodine. Localized or nodular enlargement may consist of one or more nodules and may occur in either lobe or in the isthmus. Solitary nodules are suggestive of carcinoma, particularly in younger people.

Thyroid tissue located in the retrosternal area may also become enlarged. This is not discernible by physical examination but should be considered if other physical findings are suggestive of thyroid dysfunction.

SUMMARY

I. Skull, scalp, and hair
   A. Observe size and shape of skull
   B. Observe scalp in several areas; inquire about injuries; palpate
   C. Observe condition of hair

II. Face
   A. Observe symmetry of structures, color, and condition of skin
   B. Test for facial sensation (CN V) and muscular function (CN VII)
   C. Palpate temporal artery

III. Neck
   A. Examine structure and function of neck muscles (CN XI)
   B. Palpate cervical vertebrae
   C. Palpate trachea
   D. Observe and palpate for thyroid gland
   E. Observe, palpate, and auscultate neck vessels, the carotid arteries, and jugular veins (see Chapter 14)
   F. Palpate for cervical lymph nodes (see Chapter 11)

BIBLIOGRAPHY

DeGroot, L. J., and Stanbury, J. B.: The thyroid and its diseases, ed. 4, New York, 1975, John Wiley & Sons, Inc.

Hamburger, J. I.: Your thyroid gland—fact and fiction, ed. 2, Springfield, Ill., 1975, Charles C Thomas Publisher.

Werner, S. C.: Physical examination. In Werner, S. C., and Ingbar, S. H., editors: The thyroid; a fundamental and clinical text, ed. 3, New York, 1971, Harper & Row, Publishers.

13 Assessment of the lymphatic system

The technique of health assessment allow the detection of enlarged lymph nodes (lymphadenopathy) as an indicator of the function of the lymphatic system. Only the superficial lymph nodes (Fig. 13-23) are accessible to palpation. Lymph nodes are not palpable in the normal individual except for occasional small (less than 1 cm), hard ("shotty") nodes usually in the inguinal region. The most common causes of lymphadenopathy are infection and neoplasm. In order to understand the findings of this system a discussion of the physiology of the lymphatic system follows.

The lymphatic capillary bed is very extensive. All tissues supplied with blood vessels also possess lymphatic vessels with the exception of the placenta. The lymphatic system is older in evolutionary history than the circulatory system. The function of the lymph is concerned with metabolic processes that have a slower pace than those of the blood circulatory system. The cardiovascular system was a phylogenetic development for a more active animal life wherein the transport of oxygen was necessary for the rapid processes of oxidation and reduction.

PHYSIOLOGY

The lymphatic system consists of a system of collecting ducts, the lymph fluid, and tissues; this tissue makes up the lymph nodes, the spleen, the thymus, the tonsils, and Peyer's patches in the intestines. Lymphoid aggregates are also found in bone marrow, in the lungs, and in gastric and appendiceal mucosa.

The lymphatic vessels originate as microscopic open-ended tubules termed capillaries. These capillaries merge to form larger collecting ducts, which drain to specific lymphatic tissue centers (nodes). Ducts from these lymph node centers eventually empty as trunks into the venous system at the subclavian veins (Fig. 13-1). The right subclavian vein receives the thin-walled lymphatic trunk, which drains from the right side of the head and neck, from the right arm, and from the right chest wall. The left subclavian vein is joined by the thoracic duct, which drains lymph from the remainder of the body. These vessels then return fluid and protein that has entered the lymphatic system from the interstitial space via the cardiovascular system.

Although the specific functions and properties of the lymphatic system are still imperfectly understood, the lymphocytic tissue has been ascribed responsibility for the immunological and various metabolic processes of the body and is implicated in the formation of corpuscular elements of the blood as well as in the extension of malignant disease.

Included in the functions of the lymphatic system are (1) the transport of lymph fluids, protein, and microorganisms for return to the cardiovascular system; (2) the production of lymphocytes in germinal centers of lymph nodes; (3) the production of antibodies (immune substances may be extracted from lymphocytes; lymphocytes contain at least one globulin identical with blood globulin); (4) phagocytosis by the reticuloendothelial cells lining the sinuses of the lymph nodes; (5) hematopoiesis in some pathological states; and (6) the absorption of fat and fat-soluble materials from the intestine.

Lymphatic tissue in human beings is calculated to be 2% to 3% of the total body weight. Lymphatic capillaries and collecting ducts are the transport ducts of the system. The lymph channel section of the lymphatic system consists of lymphatic capillaries, lymph node precollecting ducts, lymph node postcollecting ducts, lymph nodes, and main lymphatic trunks. Lymphoid tissue is organized in its biological architecture to form nodes that are located at strategic points for filtering the lymph. Structurally the lymph node consists of the capsule, the cortex, and the medulla. The lymph and any substance that enters the lymph, including contrast media injected for lymphography, are filtered by the lymph nodes.

The lymph nodes are seldom found singly but are usually arranged in chains or clusters called lymph centers. The lymph nodes are found either in the subcutaneous connective tissue (superficial lymph nodes) or beneath the muscular fascia and in the cavities of the body (deep lymph nodes). The nodes are disseminated along the course of the collecting ducts and are usually round or oval, though they are often observed as elongated and flattened to a cylindrical shape. Size is variable from small (almost invisible) to the size of a large pea or even an olive. Nodes

found in children are comparatively larger than those found in adults.

Lymphocytes are mobile, spherical, mononuclear cells (6 μm to 8 μm in diameter) derived from reticular cells of the nodes. Lymphocytes may evolve in one of three ways: (1) they may remain in lymphoid tissue and die there, (2) they may differentiate in lymphoid tissue, giving rise to other types of cells, or (3) they may leave lymphoid tissue, entering the lymph and then the blood and various organs.

Some of the processes carried on in this system have been clarified by inspecting the ducts with a radiopaque dye (lymphography). Three stages of lymphography have been described. During the first

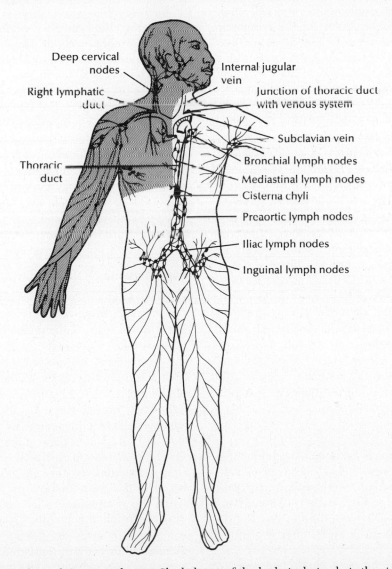

Fig. 13-1. Lymphatic drainage pathways. Shaded area of the body is drained via the right lymphatic duct, which is formed by the union of three vessels: the right jugular trunk, the right subclavian trunk, and the right bronchomediastinal trunk. Lymph from the remainder of the body enters the venous system by way of the thoracic duct. (From Francis, C. C, and Martin, A. H.: Introduction to human anatomy, ed. 7, St. Louis, 1975, The C. V. Mosby Co.)

stage the afferent lymphatics, portions of the lymphoid sinuses, and the efferent lymphatics are filled with the contrast medium. The second stage is characterized by phagocytosis by the reticuloendothelial cell of the lipid soluble contrast media, and the third stage is the period during which the contrast media leaves the node. It can be assumed that all substances entering the lymphatic system undergo this fate.

Factors affecting the movement of lymph are (1) remitting compression of the lymphatic vessels by surrounding structures, especially contracting muscles; (2) respiratory movements that propel lymph from the cisterna chyli—origin of the thoracic duct in the lumbar region—into the thoracic duct; (3) propulsive action of the smooth muscles contained in the walls of the lymphatic vessels, lymph nodes, and collecting ducts; (4) arterial pulsations (most of the lymphatic vessels course with the regional blood vessels; the deep lymphatic vessels accompany not only the veins but also the arteries, the pulsations of which can be transmitted to the lymphatic vessels); (5) negative pressure in the great vessels at the root of the neck, which determines the flow of lymph from the terminal parts of the jugular, subclavian, bronchial, mediastinal, and thoracic ducts into them; (6) peristaltic contractions of the intestines; (7) capillary blood pressure; and (8) force of gravity.

The formation and flow of lymph can be increased by the following processes: (1) an increase in capillary pressure resulting from increased venous pressure from venous stasis or obstruction; (2) an increase in permeability of the capillary walls resulting from an increase in temperature, a decrease in oxygen supply, or the administration of histamine; (3) increases in metabolic activity, the muscular pumping effect, or glandular activity (little lymph is formed when the client is given anesthesia or absolute bed rest); (4) passive movements and massage, which facilitate the flow of lymph through the lymphatic vessels; and (5) administration of hypertonic solutions, such as glucose and sodium chloride solutions.

PATHOPHYSIOLOGY

Pathological findings may be demonstrated for the lymphatic system as a result of (1) localized or systemic infection; (2) disorders in metabolism, particularly of lipids (storage-type adenopathy); (3) metastatic cancer; (4) infiltration of foreign substances; (5) primary hematopoietic disorders; and (6) hypersensitivity reactions.

The lymph nodes are the most significant parameters of the lymphatic system in physical diagnosis. The location and nature of involvement of diseased lymph nodes provide help in determining the site or origin of disease and the identity of the etiological agent.

The archaic term "swollen glands" is widely used by the lay populace. The early anatomists believed the lymph nodes were glands that functioned in a manner similar to true glands, such as the thyroid. Actual structure and function became apparent with the improved visualization afforded by light microscopy, but the continued use of the glandular reference will be apparent in both the chief complaint and the history.

Alterations in lymphatic flow patterns may also indicate disease.

Mechanical stasis of lymph

Any mechanical impediment to the flow of lymph results in deceleration or cessation of flow of lymph from that region. As a result of this impaired drainage, lymphatic vessels become dilated with the trapped lymphatic fluid. The valves become incompetent, causing a backflow of lymph within the interstitial space. Because the lymphatic system functions to return protein to the blood supply, colloid osmotic pressure increases as the interstitial protein concentration rises. Consequently, even more fluid is drawn into the extracellular spaces from the capillaries. In the absence of effective intervention, the extracellular protein precipitates and a fibrin reticulum forms. Proliferation of fibrocytes is stimulated. Subsequently, elastic and collagen fibers are formed and accumulate to give the connective tissue the characteristics of the so-called "brawny edema." This is followed by a fibrosclerotic end stage.

Lymphedema

Mechanical obstruction in the lymphatic system could result from extrinsic and intrinsic pressure, such as sclerosis, inflammation, neoplasm, surgical injuries, and functional lymphospasm. Compensating mechanisms are elicited that may result in complete or partial drainage of the lymph. The excess lymph of the dilated lymphatic vessels may be transuded back through the walls into the interstitial fluid and, as sufficient pressure builds up, back into the vascular system. Another compensating mechanism is the development of collateral anastomotic channels.

Lymphedema is the excessive accumulation of lymph in the interstitial spaces. Lymphedema results when the compensating mechanisms fail to provide drainage of all the lymph. Lymphedema is not accompanied by cyanosis, dilatation of veins, hyperpigmentation, or leathery indentation. It is usually firm and does not pit well. The more common pathological conditions leading to the formation of edema are inflammatory processes resulting from tuberculosis, syphilis or filariasis, thrombophlebitis, and trauma related to ionizing radiation or surgical operations.

Baseline measurement of edema should be as pre-

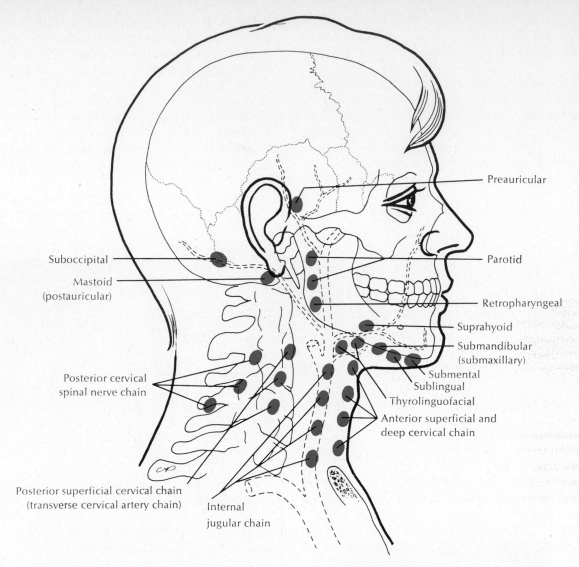

Fig. 13-3. Lymphatic drainage system of the head and neck. If the group of nodes is commonly referred to by another name the second name appears in parentheses.

Labels on figure:

Preauricular

Parotid

Retropharyngeal

Suprahyoid

Submandibular (submaxillary)

Submental

Sublingual

Thyrolinguofacial

Anterior superficial and deep cervical chain

Suboccipital

Mastoid (postauricular)

Posterior cervical spinal nerve chain

Posterior superficial cervical chain (transverse cervical artery chain)

Internal jugular chain

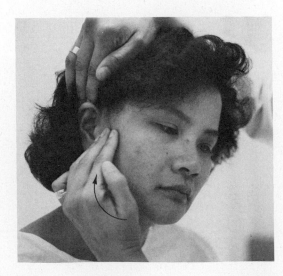

Fig. 13-4. Palpation of the preauricular lymph nodes.

but deeper than the external jugular vein. The nodes are beneath the platysma muscle and superficial cervical fascia and receive lymph from the skin and neck.

The nodes of the *thyrolinguofacial chain* are found between the lower margins of the posterior head of the diagastric muscle and the thyrolinguofacial venous trunk. Lymph draining to this group is from the parotid, submaxillary retrolaryngeal, prelaryngeal, pretracheal, and recurrent areas as well as from the tongue, palate, tonsils, thyroid and submaxillary glands, nose, pharynx, and outer and middle ear.

The *deep cervical chain* is made up of four chains

of lymph nodes: (1) the prelaryngeal chain, located anterior to the larynx; (2) the prethyroid chain, situated anterior to the thyroid gland; (3) the pretracheal and laterotracheal chain, located anterior and lateral to the trachea; and (4) recurrent chains, found along the course of the recurrent laryngeal nerve. These nodes receive lymph via the collecting ducts from the larynx, thyroid gland, trachea, and upper part of the esophagus. The efferent vessels go to the internal jugular chain, mediastinal lymph nodes, and the bracheocephalic trunk.

The finger must be bent or hooked around the sternocleidomastoid muscle to palpate the deep cervi-

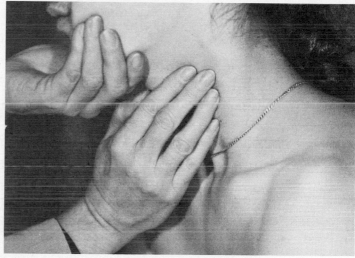

Fig. 13-5. The entire neck is lightly palpated for nodes. The anterior triangle is being palpated in this photograph.

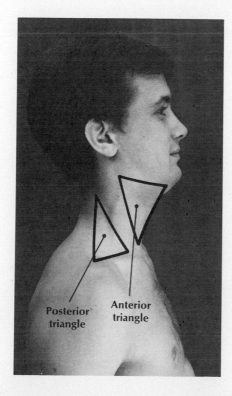

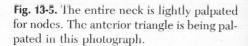

Posterior triangle   Anterior triangle

Fig. 13-6. The conception of the triangles of the neck is useful in defining the location of palpable lymph nodes. The sternocleidomastoid muscle is the division line between the anterior and posterior triangles. The trapezius muscle marks the posterior border of the posterior triangle. (Point of interest: this subject is executing a Valsalva's maneuver in an attempt not to laugh. Note the distention of the jugular vein as it passes over the sternocleidomastoid muscle.)

cal nodes, which are frequently enlarged in rubella, infectious mononucleosis, and hepatitis.

Thus, the *internal jugular chain* is made up of many lymph nodes in contact with the jugular vein. The last of these nodes lie in contact with the thoracic duct.

The *chain of the spinal nerve* consists of four to twelve nodes and follows the external branch of the spinal nerve (CN IX). Collecting ducts from the posterior and lateral regions of the neck reach these nodes as well as those of the occipital and mastoid regions of the head.

The posterior superficial cervical *transverse cervi-*

cal artery chain of six to eight lymph nodes follows the transverse cervical artery and vein (between the anterior scalene muscle and the carotid sheath). This chain terminates in the great lymphatic trunk on the right side and in the thoracic duct on the left side. Lymph from the subclavian, laterocervical, anterothoracic, and internal mammary regions reaches these nodes.

The entire neck is lightly palpated for nodes (Fig. 13-5).

The anterior border of the sternocleidomastoid muscle is the dividing line for the anterior and posterior triangles of the neck. Description of locus may

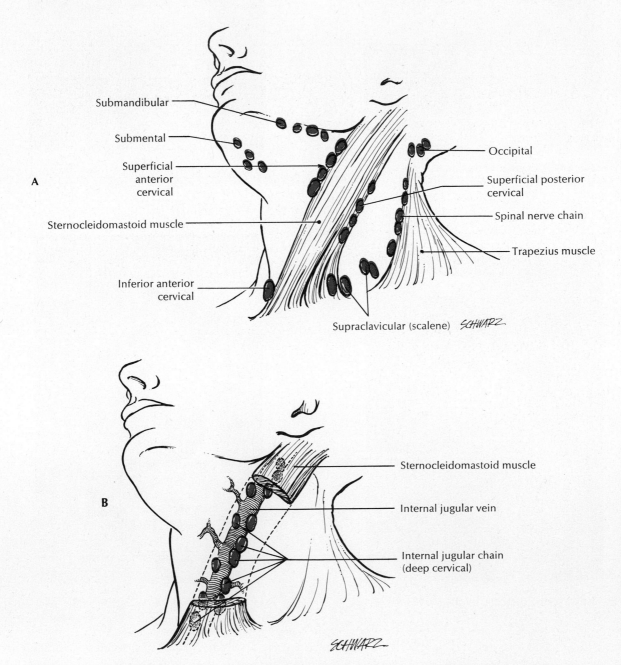

Fig. 13-7. The lymph nodes of the neck. Note relationship to the sternocleidomastoid muscle.

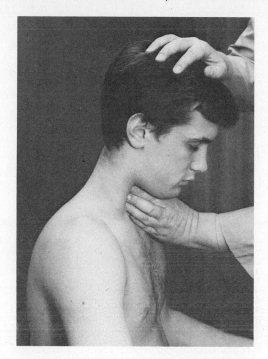

Fig. 13-8. Palpation of the anterior triangle.

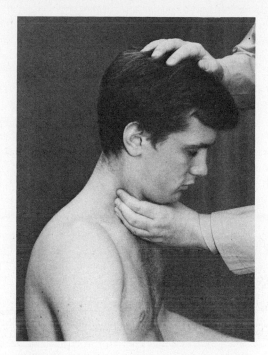

Fig. 13-9. Palpation of the posterior triangle.

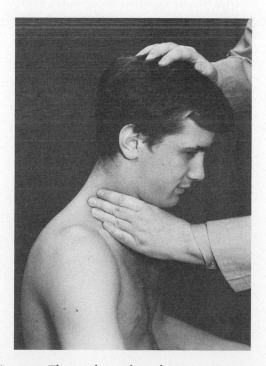

Fig. 13-10. Flexing the neck to obviate tissue tension.

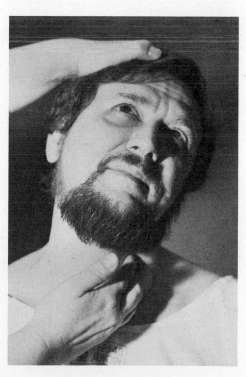

Fig. 13-11. Bending the head toward the side being examined to relax muscles and soft tissue, allowing more accurate palpation for lymph nodes.

be facilitated through the use of these triangles (Figs. 13-6 and 13-7).

Bending the client's head forward (Figs. 13-8 and 13-9) or to the side being examined (Figs. 13-10 and 13-11) will obviate tissue tension and permit more accurate palpation.

EXAMINATION

The following maneuvers may be helpful in examining specific lymph node chains of the head and neck.

The *submental, sublingual,* and *submandibular nodes* can be examined by facing the client and placing the fingertips under the mandible on the side nearest the palpating hand. The skin and subcutaneous tissue are pulled laterally over the ramus of the mandible, and enlarged nodes can be felt as they roll over the mandibular surface beneath the examining fingers.

Another technique for the examination of the submandibular nodes is accomplished by placing one index finger in the floor of the mouth and the other fingers below the ramus of the mandible. The tissue between the fingers is gently rotated.

Palpation of the supraclavicular or *scalene* region (Fig. 13-12) on the client's right side can be done by bending the left index finger over the clavicle and just lateral to the tendinous portion of the sternocleidomastoid muscle. Moving the bent or hooked index finger in a rotary manner should allow nodes in the scalene triangle to be felt. The index finger should probe deeply into the triangle. To facilitate this entry, bending the client's head forward with the right hand will promote relaxation of the sternocleidomastoid muscle. The hand maneuver is reversed for the client's left scalene area.

The client is encouraged to generally relax the musculature of the upper extremities so that the clavicles will be pulled down, allowing the supraclavicular area to be explored thoroughly.

Because of their location in proximity to the termination of the thoracic duct and other terminal lymphatic ducts, the supraclavicular nodes are frequently the sites of metastatic cancer. Virchow first described this phenomenon in 1849. Virchow's nodes are located in the left supraclavicular (scalene) region. However, mediastinal collecting ducts from the lungs go to both sides of the neck and thus may provide an avenue for metastasis of lung cancer to either supraclavicular region. The nodes from the supraclavicular region are frequently biopsied (scalene node biopsy) to search for occult metastases from the lung or esophagus as well as for gastric, pancreatic, or other abdominal structures. The supraclavicular

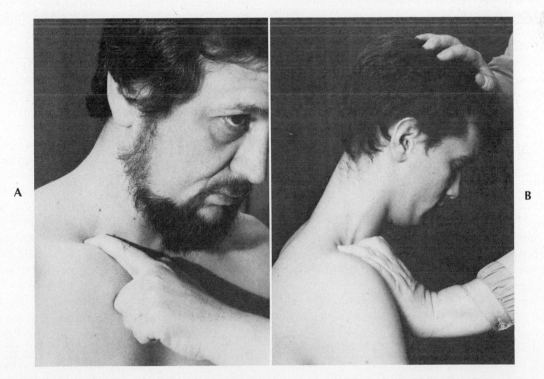

Fig. 13-12. Palpation of the scalene triangle for the supraclavicular lymph nodes. The client is encouraged to relax the musculature of the upper extremities, so that the clavicles are dropped. The examiner's free hand is used to flex the client's head forward in order to obtain relaxation of the soft tissues of the anterior neck. The left index finger is hooked over the clavicle lateral to the sternocleidomastoid muscle.

nodes are the lowermost nodes of the internal jugular and posterior superficial cervical chains.

The posterior cervical nodes are examined from behind or while facing the client and by placing the dorsal surface of the fingertips along the anterior surface of the trapezius muscle and moving them slowly forward in a circular motion against the posterior surface of the sternocleidomastoid muscle (Fig. 13-13).

In some cases it is possible to determine the source of an infection from a characteristic pattern of lymph node involvement. For instance, infections of the tongue might produce enlargement of the submental, submandibular, suprahyoid, thyrolinguofacial, and internal jugular nodes (Fig. 13-14).

Another example would be infections of the ear that typically involve the preauricular, mastoid, parotid retropharyngeal, and deep cervical nodes (Fig. 13-15).

Upper extremity

A system of superficial and deep collecting ducts carry the lymph from the upper extremity to the subclavian lymphatic trunk (Fig. 13-16). The only peripheral lymph center is the epitrochlear center, which receives some of the collecting ducts from the pathway of the ulnar artery and nerve, and is located in a depression above and posterior to the medial condyle of the humerus (Fig. 13-17).

Enlargement of these nodes may be seen in secondary syphilis.

Lymphatics of the ulnar surface of the forearm, the little and ring fingers, and the medial surface of the middle finger drain into the epitrochlear nodes. Efferent ducts drain into the axillary or infraclavicular nodes, or both.

AXILLARY REGION

There are an average of 53 lymph nodes in the axillary fossa. Five groups of lymph nodes are distinguished in this area (Fig. 13-18).

The *center of the axillary or brachial veins*, or *lateral group*, consists of two to seven nodes lying close to the axillary vein. These nodes receive collecting ducts from the upper extremity, deltoid region, and anterior wall of the chest, including the breast. Efferent ducts from this center terminate in the central lymph center, although some are known to connect with the subclavian lymph center.

The *scapular center*, or *posterior group*, consists of four or five nodes in contact with the inferior scapular vessels. The collecting ducts converging on these nodes are from the posterior wall of the chest and the posteroinferior neck. The efferent ducts drain to the central lymph center.

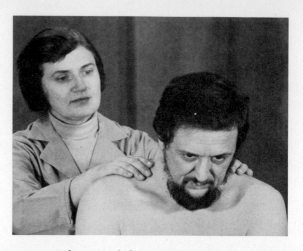

Fig. 13-13. Palpation of the posterior cervical nodes and spinal nerve chain is accomplished while facing the client. The dorsal surfaces (pads) of the fingertips are used to palpate along the anterior surface of the trapezius muscle and then moved slowly forward in a circular movement toward the posterior surface of the sternocleidomastoid muscle.

The *central* or *intermediate center* consists of eight to ten nodes and receives ducts from the brachial and scapular lymph centers as well as from the chest wall, breast, and arm. The ducts leaving these nodes go to the subclavian lymph center.

The *external mammary center*, or *anterior* or *pectoral group*, is a chain of nodes located along the course of the external mammary artery. A superior group of two or three nodes is found in the region of the third rib and the second and third intercostal spaces, and an inferior group is located over the fourth to sixth ribs. The ducts entering these nodes are from the breast and anterolateral chest wall and from the integument and muscles of the abdominal wall superior to the umbilicus. The efferent ducts from these nodes go to the subclavian center.

The *subclavian*, or *infraclavicular*, *center* may contain one to nine nodes situated in the tissues of the upper axilla. It receives lymph from all the other axillary centers, and ducts from this center empty into the venous junction of the jugular and subclavian veins.

Infections of the hand and arm may result in enlargement of these nodes.

Axillary examination is approached by regarding the area as a four-sided pyramid with its apex superior. The apex is located between the first rib and the clavicle. The apex in lay parlance is the armpit. The anterior border of the axilla is formed by the pectoral muscles; the posterior border is made up of back muscles, including the latissimus dorsi and subscapularis muscles; the medial border consists of the rib cage and serratus anterior muscle; and the lateral

Text continued on p. 271.

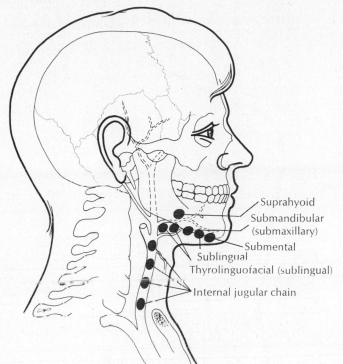

Fig. 13-14. Lymph nodes that may be potentially involved as a result of pathology of the tongue.

Suprahyoid
Submandibular (submaxillary)
Submental
Sublingual
Thyrolinguofacial (sublingual)
Internal jugular chain

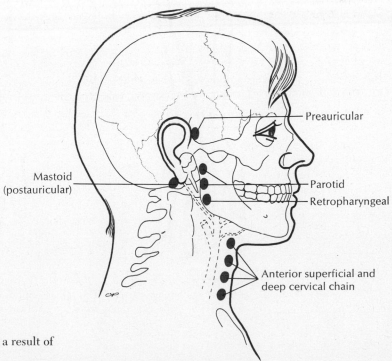

Preauricular
Mastoid (postauricular)
Parotid
Retropharyngeal
Anterior superficial and deep cervical chain

Fig. 13-15. Lymph nodes that may be involved as a result of pathology of the ear.

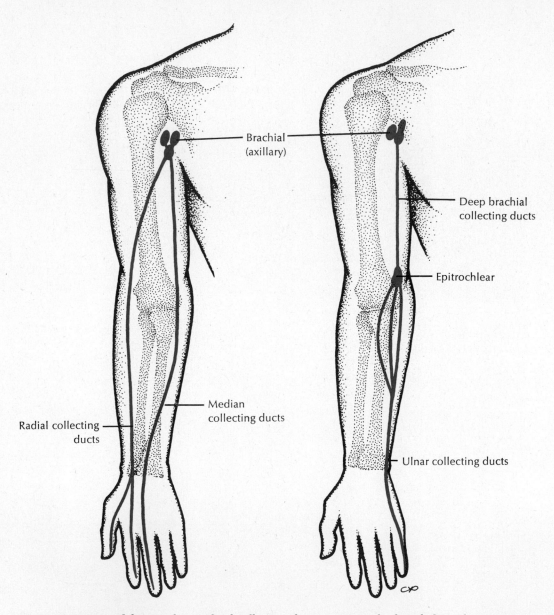

Fig. 13-16. System of deep and superficial collecting ducts, carrying the lymph from the upper extremity to the subclavian lymphatic trunk. The only peripheral lymph center is the epitrochlear, which receives some of the collecting ducts from the pathway of the ulnar and radial nerves.

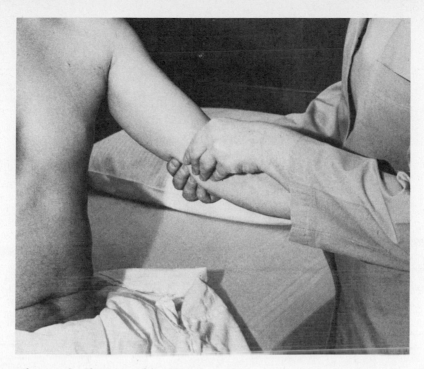

Fig. 13-17. Palpation for the epitrochlear lymph nodes is performed in the depression above and posterior to the medial condyle of the humerus.

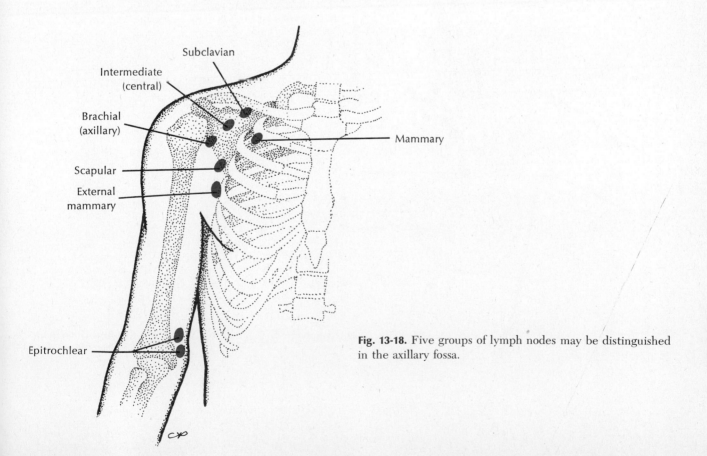

Fig. 13-18. Five groups of lymph nodes may be distinguished in the axillary fossa.

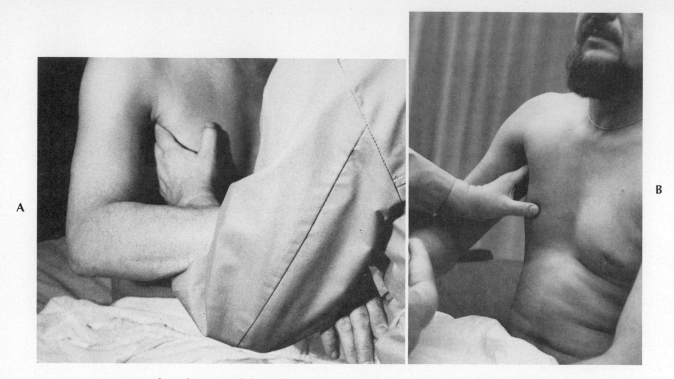

Fig. 13-19. The soft tissues of the axilla are gently rolled against the chest wall and the muscles surrounding the axilla. Note two methods of supporting the client's arm.

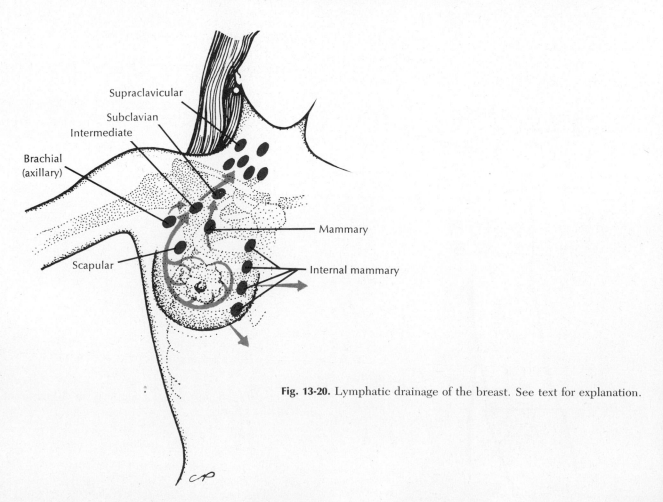

Fig. 13-20. Lymphatic drainage of the breast. See text for explanation.

border, of the upper arm. Thus, the sides are anterior, posterior, medial, and lateral. Inspection and palpation must be done for each of the anatomical sides, first in a position of partial adduction of the subject's arms and then in abduction. The examination of the axillary area is accomplished by gently rolling the soft tissues against the chest wall and the muscles of the axilla (Fig. 13-19). Bimanual palpation is performed anteriorly to encompass the pectoralis muscle, as well as the posterior wall to include the back muscles.

BREAST

The lymphatic system of the breast is particularly abundant. The lymphatic vessels drain to two major sites: the axillary and the internal mammary centers (Fig. 13-20). Lymph from the lower outer quadrant

of the breast drains to the lateroinferior lymph nodes. Lymph from the areolar area, the upper outer quadrant, and the tail of the Spence drains to the mediosuperior axillary nodes. Lymph then courses through efferent ducts to the infraclavicular and supraclavicular nodes. The lymph from the inner aspect of the breast drains to the internal mammary nodes, which are three to four in number and inaccessible to palpation.

Lower extremity

As in the upper extremity, a system of superficial and deep collecting ducts drain the lymph from the leg (Fig. 13-21). Two or three nodes make up the *popliteal lymph center* in the back of the knee near the terminal portion of the saphenous vein. The afferent ducts to these nodes are, in fact, from the

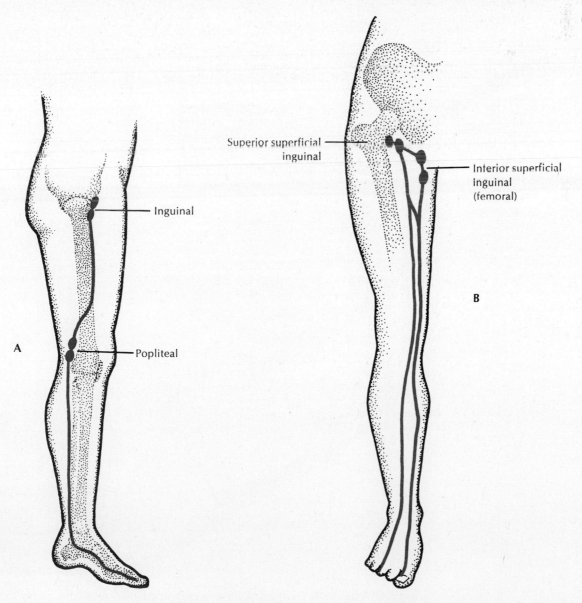

Fig. 13-21. Lymphatic drainage of the lower extremity.

regions surrounding the external saphenous vein, that is, the heel and the outer aspect of the foot. However, the majority of the lymph is delivered to the inguinal nodes.

SUPERFICIAL INGUINAL LYMPH CENTER

A superior and inferior group of superficial inguinal nodes has been described.

The *inferior group* is a group of large lymph nodes that receive lymph from the superficial plexuses of the leg and foot (Fig. 13-22). They are the inguinal nodes below the junction of the saphenous and femoral veins. The superficial nodes lie along the course of the saphenous vein. The deep subinguinal nodes lie medial to the femoral vein and follow the vessel into the abdomen. Cloquet's gland, a node of

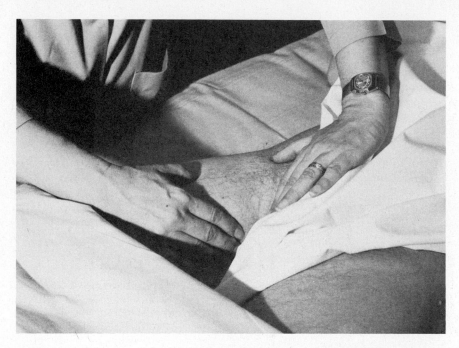

Fig. 13-22. Palpation of the inferior superficial inguinal (femoral) lymph nodes.

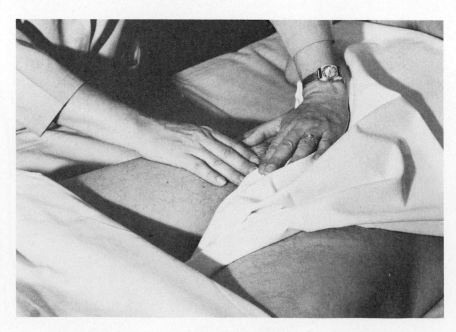

Fig. 13-23. Palpation of the superior superficial inguinal lymph nodes.

this group, lies immediately above the saphenous opening. When this node is enlarged, incarcerated, or strangulated, femoral hernia may result.

The *superior group* is a center containing five or six nodes whose afferent ducts are from the abdominal wall inferior to the umbilicus, the buttocks, and the external genital organs as well as the efferent vessels from the inferior center (Fig. 13-23). These nodes lie along and parallel to the inguinal ligament.

• • •

Fig. 13-24 is a diagrammatic summary of the areas where pathological lymph nodes may be identified by inspection and palpation. These are the sites to be assessed during the physical examination.

PATHOLOGY
Common diseases related to lymph node characteristics

The assessment parameters of pathological lymph nodes may combine to establish the diagnosis of the disease process of the client. Some common findings related to specific diseases are described here.

Acute pyogenic infections. The nodes of acute infections are large, tender, and discrete. These alterations are accompanied by the classical signs of inflammation, which are *tumor* (swelling), *color* (redness and heat), and *dolor* (tenderness). The involvement may lead to limitation of motion.

The nodes may become confluent if the infection becomes chronic.

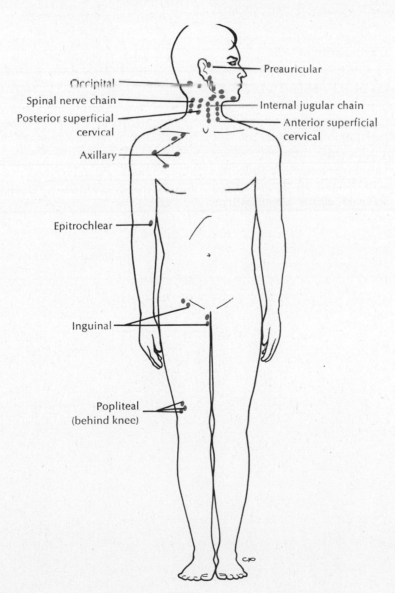

Fig. 13-24. Diagrammatic summary of the areas to be examined for lymph nodes during the course of the physical examination.

Tuberculosis. The lymph nodes of the tubercular client may be soft and matted together. The nodes are generally nontender to the client. Occasionally sinus formation is present.

Metastatic cancer. Lymph nodes of metastatic cancer are described as discrete, nontender, of a firm to hard consistency, and unilateral in focus. They may be small or several centimeters in diameter.

Hodgkin's disease. Hodgkin's disease results in lymph node involvement in which the nodes are large, discrete, nontender, and of a firm, rubbery consistency.

Syphilis. A lymph node in the chain draining a syphilitic chancre is called a bubo. Characteristically, the nodes are enlarged, hard, nonfluctuant, and painless. Such a node in the inguinal chain should prompt the practitioner to inspect thoroughly for a genital chancre.

Common disorders of lymphatic vessels

Acute lymphangitis. The chief complaint of the client may include pain in the affected extremity. Elevation of temperature may be present, and the client may complain of malaise.

Inspection of the affected limb may reveal redness along the course of lymphatic collecting ducts, which appear as fine lines. The tubules may be palpable. The source of infection is sought. In the lower extremity interdigital spaces are carefully examined for cracks, which are often the site of entry for epidermophytosis.

Lymphedema. Congenital lymphedema may result in swelling or distortion of the extremities, caused by hypoplasia and maldevelopment of the system. Trauma to the ducts, leading to blockage, may result in lymphedema. This may be the result of surgery of the regional lymph nodes, as in radical mastectomy or groin dissection. Extension of cancer to the lymphatics may also result in stasis of lymph flow. Infection may also block lymphatic ducts.

Elephantiasis. Elephantiasis is the term used for the massive accumulation of lymphedema. The condition may be the sequelae of congenital or acquired forms of lymphedema. The marked lymphedema predisposes the client to further infection and episodes of cellulitis. Recurrent infectious involvement leads to marked fibrosis of the edematous tissues.

REFERENCES

Battezatti, M., and Donini, I.: The lymphatic system, New York, 1973, John Wiley & Sons, Inc.

Brouse, N. L.: Response of lymphatics to sympathetic nerve stimulation, J. Physiol. **197**:25, 1968.

Haagensen, C. D., and others: The lymphatics in cancer, Philadelphia, 1972, W. B. Saunders Co.

Kinmonth, J. B.: The lymphatic disease; lymphography and surgery, Baltimore, 1972, The Williams & Wilkins Co.

Mayerson, H. S.: Lymph and lymphatic system, Springfield, Ill., 1968, Charles C Thomas, Publisher.

Solnitzky, O. C., and Jeghers, H.: Lymphadenopathy and disorders of the lymphatic system. In McBride, C., and Blacklow, R., editors: Signs and symptoms; applied pathologic physiology and clinical interpretation, Philadelphia, 1970, J. B. Lippincott Co.

Yoffey, J. M., and Courtice, F. C.: Lymphatics; lymph and the lymphomyeloid complex, New York, 1970, Academic Press, Inc.

Zuelzer, W. W., and Kaplan, J.: The child with lymphadenopathy, Semin. Hematol. **12**:323, 1975.

14 Assessment of the breasts

ANATOMY

The breast is a modified sebaceous gland that is paired and located on the anterior chest wall between the second and third ribs superiorly, the sixth and seventh costal cartilages inferiorly, the anterior axillary line laterally, and the sternal border medially.

The functional components of the breast consist of the acini or milk-producing glands, a ductal system, and a nipple (Fig. 14-1, *A*). The glandular tissue units are called lobes and are situated in circular, spokelike fashion around the nipple. There are 15 to 25 lobes per breast. Each lobe is composed of 20 to 40 lobules, each containing 10 to 100 acini.

Much of the bulk of the breast is composed of subcutaneous and retromammary fat. The breast is fairly mobile but is supported by a layer of subcutaneous connective tissue and by Cooper's ligaments (Fig. 14-1, *B*). The latter are multiple fibrous bands that begin at the breast's subcutaneous connective tissue layer and run through the breast, attaching to the muscle fascia.

Knowledge of the lymphatic drainage of the breast is critical because of the frequent dissemination of breast cancer through this system. There are three types of lymphatic drainage of the breast (Fig. 14-2).

Cutaneous lymphatic drainage is of lymph from the skin of the breast, excluding the areolar and nipple areas; this lymph flows into the ipsilateral axillary nodes (the mammary, scapular, brachial, and intermediate nodes). Lymph from the medial cutaneous breast area may flow to the opposite breast. Lymph from the inferior portion of the breast can reach the lymphatic plexus of the epigastric region and subsequently the liver and other abdominal regions and organs.

Areolar lymphatic drainage is of lymph formed in the areolar and nipple areas of the breast; this lymph flows into the anterior axillary group of nodes (the mammary nodes).

Deep lymphatic drainage is of lymph from the deep mammary tissues; this lymph flows into the anterior axillary nodes. Some of this lymph also flows into the apical, subclavian, infraclavicular, and supraclavicular nodes. Also, lymph from the retroareolar areas, medial glandular breast tissue areas, and lower glandular breast tissue areas communicate with lymphatic systems draining into the thorax and abdomen.

The largest portion of glandular breast tissue occurs in the upper lateral quadrant of each breast. From this quadrant there is an anatomical projection of breast tissue into the axilla. This projection is termed the axillary tail of Spence (Fig. 14-3). The majority of breast tumors are located in the upper lateral breast quadrant and in the tail of Spence.

On general appearance the normal breasts are reasonably symmetrical in size and shape, though not usually absolutely equal. This symmetry remains constant at rest and with movement. The skin of the breast is the same as that of the abdomen or back. There may be a small number of scattered hair follicles around the areola. In light-complected persons a horizontal or vertical vascular pattern may be observed. This pattern, when normally present, is symmetrical.

The areolae are pigmented areas surrounding the nipples. Their color varies from pink to brown, and their size varies greatly. Several or many sebaceous glands (termed Montgomery's tubercles or follicles) may be present on the areolar surface.

The nipples are round, hairless, pigmented, protuberant structures whose size and shape vary among women and in an individual woman depending on the state of contraction. Usually nipples are directed or "point" slightly upward and laterally.

Inversion of the nipple is an invagination or depression of its central portion. Inversion can occur congenitally or as a response to an invasive process.

During early embryonic development longitudinal ridges exist, extending from the axilla to the groin. Called "milk lines" (Fig. 14-4), these ridges usually atrophy, except at the level of the pectoral muscles,

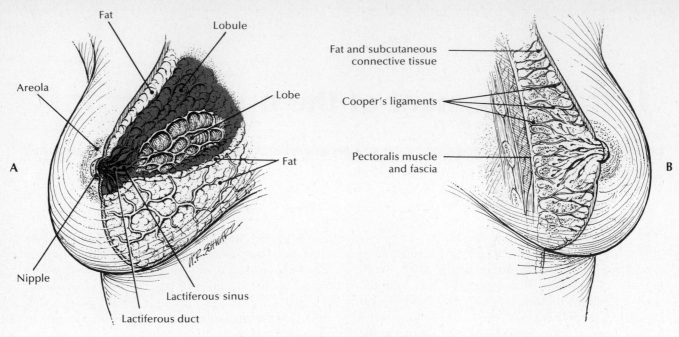

Fat

Lobule

Areola

Lobe

Fat

A

Nipple

Lactiferous sinus

Lactiferous duct

Fat and subcutaneous connective tissue

Cooper's ligaments

Pectoralis muscle and fascia

B

Fig. 14-1. Female breasts. **A,** Internal structures. **B,** Supportive tissue structures.

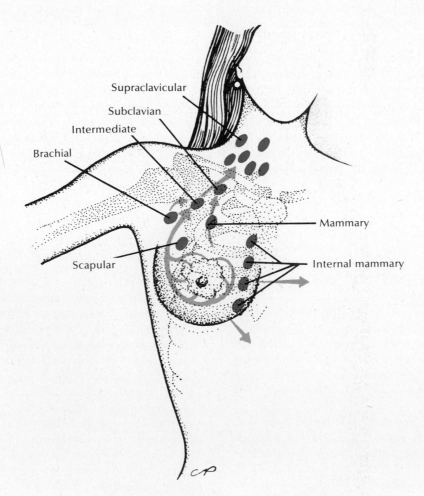

Supraclavicular

Subclavian

Intermediate

Brachial

Mammary

Scapular

Internal mammary

Fig. 14-2. Lymphatic drainage of the breast.

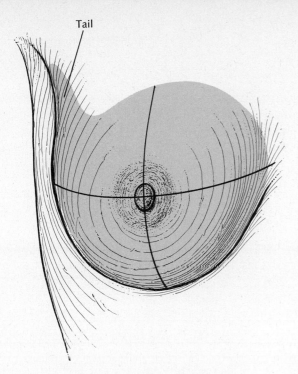

Fig. 14-3. Axillary tail of Spence.

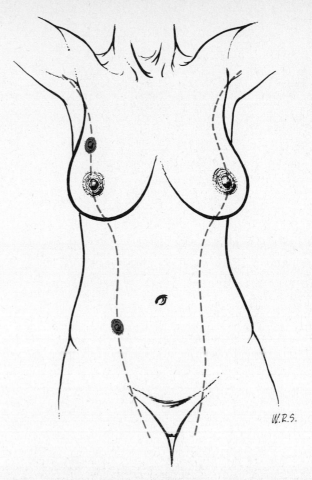

Fig. 14-4. Milk lines.

where a breast will eventually develop. In some women the ridges do not entirely disappear, and portions of the milk lines persist. This existence is manifested in the presence of a nipple, a nipple and a breast, or glandular breast tissue only. This congenital anomaly is termed a supernumerary breast or nipple.

The gross appearance and size of the normal female breast both among individuals and for an individual at various phases of development. The following describes breast development through a woman's life span (Fig. 14-5):

1. *Appearance before age 10:* There is little difference in gross appearance between male and female breasts. The nipples are small and slightly elevated. There is no palpable glandular tissue or areolar pigmentation.
2. *Appearance between the ages of 10 and 12:* The mammary tissues adjacent to and beneath the areola grow, resulting in an increased diameter of the areola and the formation of a "mammary bud." The nipple and breast protrude as a single mound. Breast development may normally begin or progress unilaterally.
3. *Appearance between the ages of 11 and 13:* During this period general mammary growth and increases in diameter and pigmentation of the areola continue, resulting in further elevation of the breasts. The separation of the nipple from the areola begins.

4. *Appearance between the ages of 12 and 14:* Growth continues in the mammary tissues. The nipple and areola form a mound distinct from the globular shape of the rest of the breast.
5. *Appearance between the ages of 14 and 16:* The shape of the adult female breast is gradually formed. The areola recedes into the general contour of the breast, and only the nipple protrudes. The size of the adult female breast is influenced by heredity, individual sensitivity to hormones, and nutrition.
6. *Appearance during the female reproductive years:* In response to hormonal changes during the menstrual cycle, there is a cyclic pattern of breast size change, along with nodularity and tenderness, that is maximal just before menses. The breast is smallest in days 4 through 7 of the menstrual cycle. During days 3 to 4 prior to the onset of menses, mammary tenseness, fullness, heaviness, tenderness, and pain are experienced by many women, and the total breast volume is significantly increased.

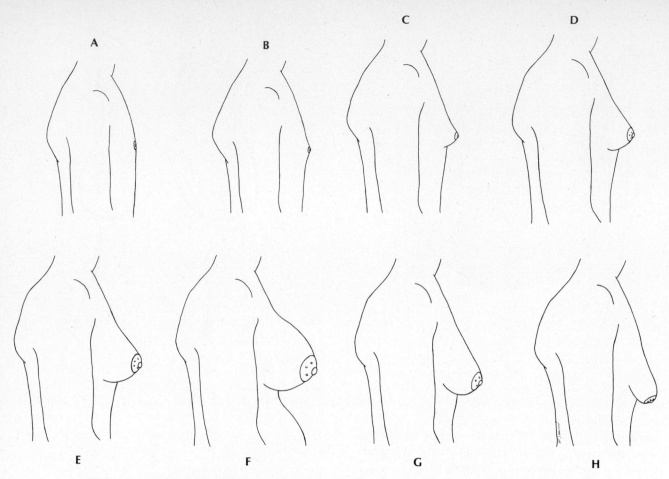

Fig. 14-5. Appearance of the female breast in various life periods. **A,** Appearance before age 10. **B,** Beginning development between ages 10 and 12. **C,** Appearance between ages 11 and 13. **D,** Appearance between ages 12 and 14. **E,** Appearance of the nulliparous, adult, female breast. **F,** Appearance of the breast during pregnancy. **G,** Appearance of the breast in a woman who has had a pregnancy. **H,** Appearance of the breast after menopause.

7. *Changes in pregnancy:* The breast increases in size, sometimes to as large as two or three times the usual size. The areolae and nipples become more prominent and more deeply pigmented. The veins engorge, the Montgomery's glands become more apparent, and striae are often observed.

8. *Menopausal changes.* After menopause, the breast's glandular tissue gradually involutes, and fat is deposited in the breasts. Breast form becomes flabby and flattened.

EXAMINATION
Inspection

Inspection and palpation are the techniques used in the examination of the breast. No special equipment is necessary. The client is uncovered to the waist and is seated on the side of an examining table. The breasts are observed for (1) symmetry of shape, color, size, and surface characteristics; (2) hyperpig-

mentation; (3) moles or nevi; (4) edema; (5) retraction or dimpling; (6) abnormal amount of distribution of hair; (7) presence of focal vascularity; and (8) lesions (Fig. 14-6).

Retraction, or dimpling, appears as a depression or pucker on the skin (Fig. 14-7, *A*). It usually is caused by the fibrotic shortening and immobilization of Cooper's ligament by an invasive process.

Whenever the skin of the breasts is stretched rapidly, damage to the elastic fibers or the dermis may occur and observable striae, or stretch marks, are produced. Newly created striae appear reddish; they become whitish with age.

Edema of the breasts produces exaggeration of the skin pores, creating an orange peel appearance of the breast, called peau d'orange (Fig. 14-7, *B*).

Vascular patterns should be diffuse and symmetrical. Focal or unilateral patterns are abnormal (Fig. 14-7, *A*).

The areolar area is inspected for size, shape, sym-

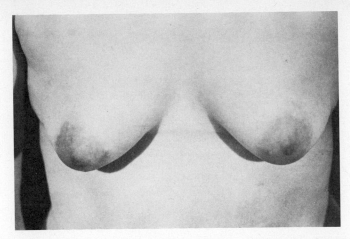

Fig. 14-6. Observation of the breasts. These breasts have several characteristics that are deviations within normal limits: (1) the left breast is slightly larger than the right; (2) the direction of the nipples is slightly different; and (3) there are two indentations in the outer right breast.

metry, color, surface characteristics, bulging, and lesions. As mentioned previously, size, shape, and color can normally vary greatly. Any asymmetry, mass, or lesion should be considered abnormal.

If the breasts are symmetrical, both nipples should be pointing laterally in the same way. The nipple is observed for size, shape, ability to erect, color, discharge, and lesions. The nipples should be round, equal in size, homogeneous in color, and have convoluted surfaces, which give them a wrinkled appearance. Inversion of one or both nipples, if present from puberty, is normal; however, this condition may interfere with breastfeeding. Recent inversion of the nipple is probably retraction (Fig. 14-7, A) and should be investigated.

Paget's disease appears as a red glandular erosion of the nipple or as a nipple that is dry, scaly, or friable. The areola may also be affected. Paget's disease is a malignant condition requiring prompt therapy.

Breast secretions are normal in pregnancy or lactation. Other causes of discharge are mechanical nipple stimulation, drug influence, hypothalamic and pituitary disorders, and malignant and benign breast lesions. The discharge can be milky, watery, purulent, serous, or bloody. The method for determining the site of discharge production is discussed under "Palpation."

There are four major sitting positions of the client used for breast inspection. Every client should be examined in each position (Fig. 14-8):

1. The client is seated with her arms at her sides.
2. The client is seated with her arms abducted over her head.
3. The client is seated and is pushing her hands into her hips, simultaneously eliciting contraction of the pectoral muscles.

4. The client is seated and is leaning over while the examiner assists in supporting and balancing her.

While the client is performing these maneuvers, the breasts are carefully observed for symmetry, bulging, retraction, and fixation. An abnormality may not be apparent in the breasts at rest (Fig. 14-9, A), but a mass may cause the breasts, through invasion of suspensory ligaments, to fix, preventing them from upward or forward movement in positions 2 (Fig. 14-9, B) and 4. Position 3 specifically assists in eliciting dimpling if a mass has infiltrated and shortened suspensory ligaments.

The breasts are also observed with the client lying down, before the examiner palpates.

Palpation

The range of normal breast consistency is wide. The normal breast feels granular. This granularity is generalized and becomes more prominent with age. The breasts feel homogeneous in the young adolescent. The presence of progesterone in pregnancy and premenstrually causes the breasts to feel generally nodular. Hormonally induced nodularity is bilateral and diffuse.

The primary purpose for the palpation of breasts is to discover masses. If a mass is discovered, it is assessed according to the following characteristics:

1. *Location:* Masses are designated according to the quadrant in which they lie: upper outer, lower outer, upper inner, or lower inner (Fig. 14-10, A). When describing the mass in the client's record, one may find it helpful to draw the mass within a diagram of the breast (Fig. 14-10, B). Another method of describing location is to visualize the breast as the face of a clock; the

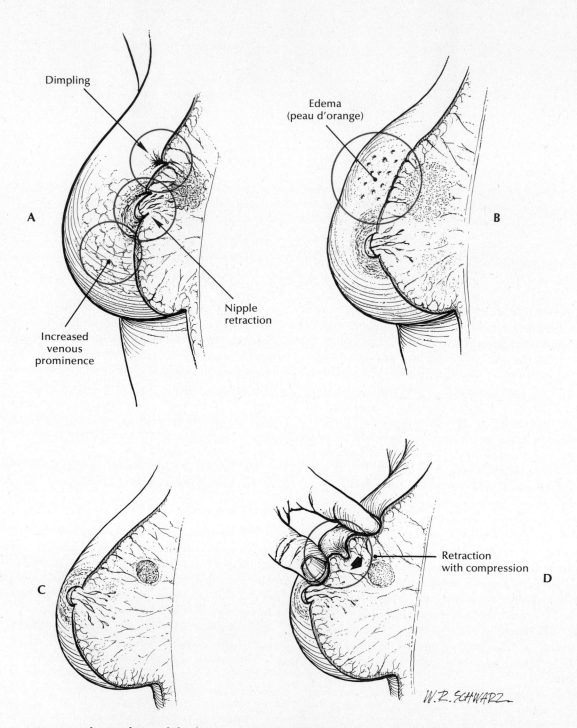

Fig. 14-7. Abnormalities of the breast. **A,** Breast with dimpling, nipple retraction, and increased venous prominence. **B,** Breast with edema (peau d'orange or pigskin appearance). **C,** Breast with tumor; no retraction is apparent. **D,** Breast with tumor; retraction is apparent with compression.

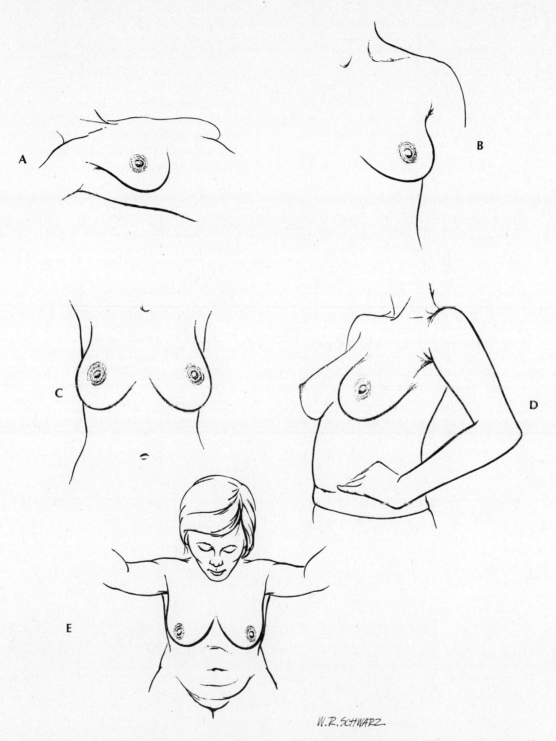

Fig. 14-8. Positions of client for breast examination. **A,** Supine, at rest. **B,** Seated, at rest. **C,** Seated, arms elevated. **D,** Seated, pectoral contraction. **E,** Seated, leaning forward.

nipple is center. A mass can be designated, for example, as being "5 cm from the nipple in the 8 o'clock position."

2. *Size:* The size should be approximated in centimeters in all its planes. For example, a mass may be ovoid, 3 cm wide, 2 cm long, and 1 cm thick.

3. *Shape:* The shape may be round, ovoid, irregular, or matted. Matting occurs in the presence of multiple lesions.

4. *Consistency:* A breast mass may be soft or hard, solid or cystic.

5. *Discreteness:* The borders of the mass are as-sessed to determine if they are sharp and well defined or irregular.

6. *Mobility:* The examiner attempts to move the mass over the chest wall. It is noted as being freely movable, movable, or fixed.

7. *Tenderness:* The client is questioned regarding any discomfort with palpation.

8. *Erythema:* The area of skin overlying the mass is inspected for erythema.

9. *Dimpling over the mass:* The tissue over the mass is compressed to determine if this maneuver produces dimpling (Fig. 14-7, *D*).

The palpation portion of the examination of the

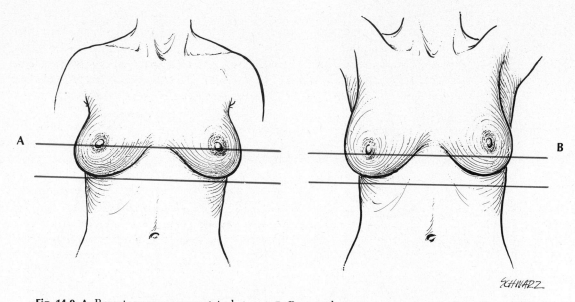

Fig. 14-9. A, Breasts appear symmetrical at rest. **B,** Breasts do not move symmetrically with arm elevation. The right breast is immobilized.

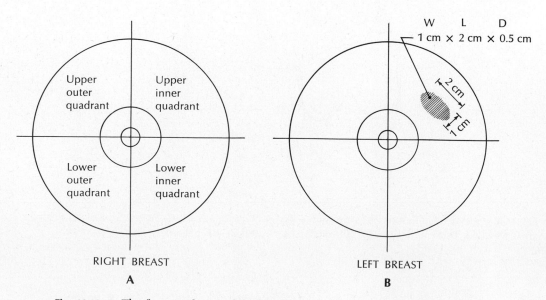

Fig. 14-10. A, The four quadrants of the breast. **B,** Diagram of a mass within a breast.

breast begins with palpation for axillary, subclavicular, and supraclavicular lymph nodes. This is most effectively performed with the client in a sitting position. The location and palpation of the axillary, subclavicular, and supraclavicular nodes are described in Chapter 11 on assessment of the lymphatic system. To emphasize the importance of an adequate axillary area examination with each breast examination, this procedure is reviewed here.

In examining the axilla, the tissues can be best appreciated if the area muscles are relaxed. Contracted muscles may obscure slightly enlarged nodes. To achieve this relaxation while at the same time abducting the arm, the examiner supports the ipsilateral arm (Fig. 14-11).

The examiner should visualize the axilla as a four-sided pyramid and thoroughly palpate the following areas: (1) the edge of the pectoralis major muscle for the mammary group of nodes, (2) the thoracic wall for the intermediate group of nodes, (3) the upper part of the humerus for the brachial axillary group of nodes, and (4) the anterior edge of the latissimus dorsi muscle for the subscapular group of nodes.

The breasts are most effectively palpated with the client in a supine position. Because of time constraints on most physical examinations, it is not advised that all breasts be also palpated with the client in a sitting position. However, several groups of clients should also be examined in the sitting position: women with present or past complaints of breast masses, women at high risk of breast cancer, and women with pendulous breasts.

With the client in a sitting position, small breasts can be examined by using one hand to support the breast while the other hand palpates the tissue against the chest wall. Pendulous breasts are palpated using a bimanual technique (Fig. 14-12). The inferior portion of the breast is supported in one hand while the

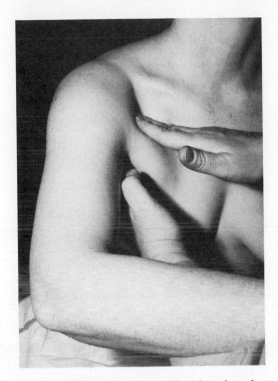

Fig. 14-11. Palpation of the axillary lymph nodes.

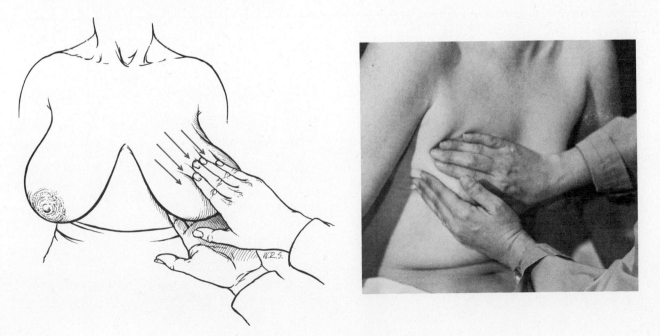

Fig. 14-12. Bimanual palpation of the breasts.

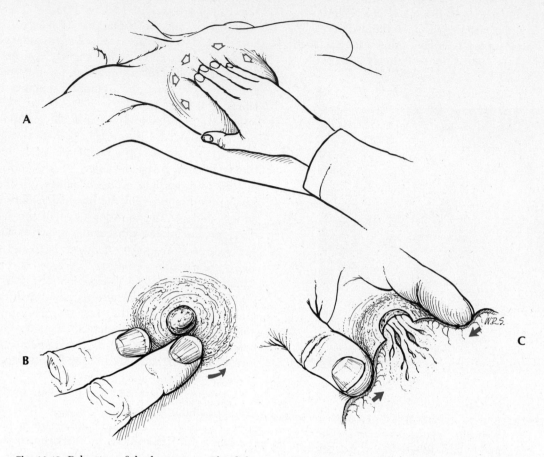

Fig. 14-13. Palpation of the breasts. **A,** Glandular area. **B,** Areolar area. **C,** Compression of the nipple.

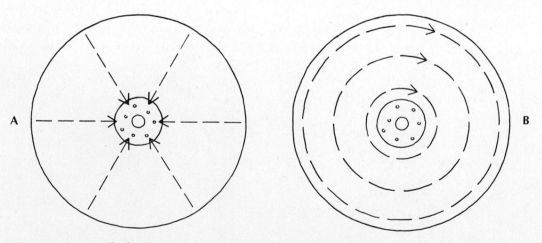

Fig. 14-14. Two methods of systematic breast palpation. **A,** Palpation in wedge sections from breast periphery to center. **B,** Palpation along concentric circles from periphery to center.

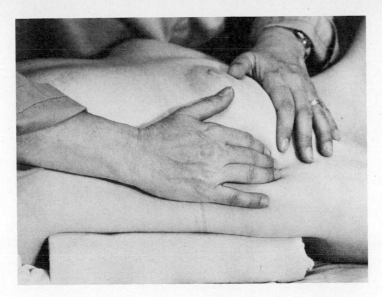

Fig. 14-15. Palpation of the axillary tail of Spence.

other palpates breast tissue against the supporting hand.

The client is then asked to lie down. The breasts are palpated while they are flattened against the rib cage. If the breasts are large, several mechanisms can be employed to enhance this flattening. A pillow can be placed under the ipsilateral shoulder, or the client can abduct the ipsilateral arm and place her hand under her neck. Both maneuvers shift the breast medially. The humerus should be at least slightly abducted to allow for thorough palpation of the tail of Spence.

The breasts are then thoroughly palpated (Fig. 14-13). The examiner should develop a system of breast examination and habitually start and end at a fixed point on the breasts. The starting point is arbitrary. The breasts are palpated with the palmar surfaces of the fingers held together. The movements are smooth, and back and forth or circular. The breast is visualized as a bicycle wheel with six or eight spokes, and palpation occurs along each spoke until the breast has been thoroughly surveyed (Fig. 14-14, *A*). Special attention is focused on the upper outer quadrant area and on the tail of Spence (Fig. 14-15).

An alternate method of breast palpation is to consider the breast as a group of concentric circles with the nipple as the center. Palpation occurs along the circumferences of the circle, starting at the outermost circle, until the total breast area is adequately surveyed (Fig. 14-14, *B*).

The areolar areas are carefully palpated to determine the presence of underlying masses. Each nipple is gently compressed to assess for the presence of masses or discharge (Fig. 14-13, *C*). If discharge is noted, the breast is milked along its radii to identify the lobe from which the discharge is originating. Compression of the discharge-producing lobe will cause discharge to exude from the nipple.

If a client reports a breast nodule, the "normal" breast is examined first so that the baseline consistency of that breast will serve as a control when the reportedly abnormal one is palpated.

Mammary folds, crescent-shaped ridges of breast tissue found at the inferior portions of very large or pendulous breasts, may be confused with breast masses but are nonpathological.

The sequence of the breast examination is illustrated in Fig. 14-16.

Breast self-examination

Many breast masses are found by the clients themselves. Too often the malignant masses are found after extensive development and metastasis. During the examination, the practitioner should review the rationale and process of the examination with the client and advise her to perform the examination at home during the period of the fourth to the seventh menstrual cycle day. During this time the breasts are smallest and the glandular tissue least congested.

The client can perform the breast self-examination in a manner similar to the one used by the examiner. For the axillary examination, it is recommended that she lie down with her arm abducted and supported by a bed.

Special examination procedures

Further evaluation of breast masses is accomplished through the use of several newly developed techniques. However, despite the actual and potential merits of mammographic techniques for supple-

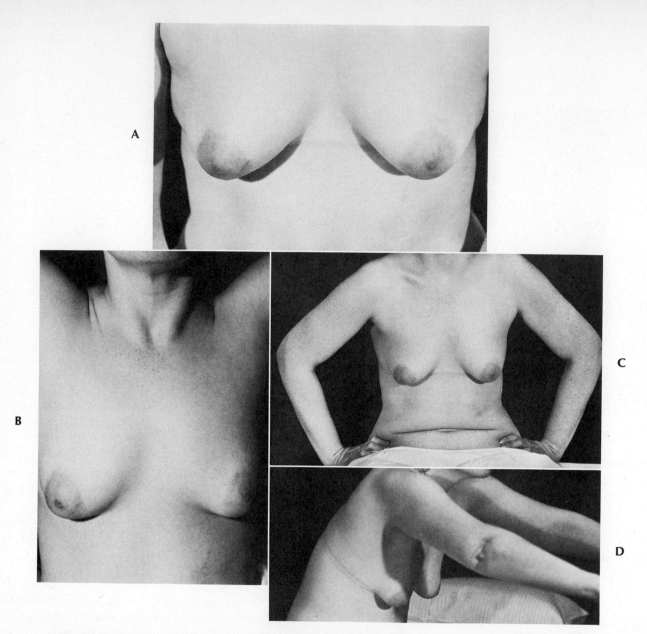

Fig. 14-16. Sequence of the breast examination. **A,** Observation of the breasts at rest. **B,** Observation with client's arms overhead. **C,** Observation with client contracting pectoral muscles. **D,** Observation with client leaning forward.

menting clinical examinations and for screening, recent clinical trials have indicated that the most successful techniques for locating small and early lesions is still clinical examination.

Mammography is the technique of breast examination by the use of low-energy radiography.

Xerography is mammography using a xerographic plate instead of film. The advantages of this technique are that radiation doses are smaller than with conventional mammography and the images produced are more distinct.

Thermography is a technique that measures the temperature distribution of the breast. Malignant lesions appear as "hot spots" in the breast.

PATHOLOGY
Breast cancer

Although certain breast lesions have characteristic findings on inspection and palpation, diagnosis is not made by clinical examination but by surgical procedures and laboratory examinations. The practitioner is encouraged to learn distinguishing characteristics of breast lesions, but not to rely on them for diagnosis.

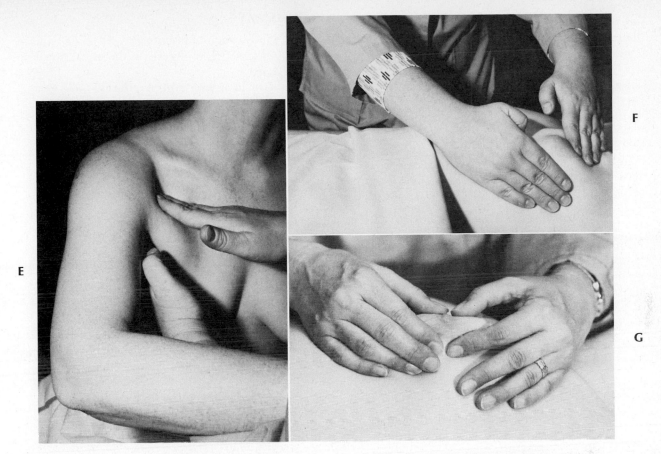

Fig. 14-16, cont'd. E, Palpation of axillary nodes. (Palpation of the supraclavicular and subclavicular areas is not illustrated). **F,** Palpation of the glandular area. **G,** Palpation of the nipple and areolar area.

The lesions of breast cancer are often solitary, unilateral, solid, hard, irregular, poorly delineated, nonmobile, painless, nontender, and located in the upper, outer quadrants.

Breast cancer is a leading cause of death in women in the United States and also a leading cause of cancer morbidity. On the average one out of every 13 women will develop breast cancer. Knowledge of factors indicating that a woman is at a higher than usual risk of cancer can assist in making decisions about screening programs and the frequency of general physical examinations. The following groups of women are at higher than usual risk of breast cancer:

1. Women over age 40
2. Women who have never been pregnant
3. Women whose first full-term pregnancy was at age 34 or older
4. Women with a history of an early menarche (before age 12) or late menopause (after age 50)
5. Women with a history of benign breast disease
6. Women of North American or European descent
7. Women with a previous breast cancer
8. Women with a strong family history of breast cancer
9. Women who have a wet type of cerumen

These women should be taught to perform self-examination and should receive a professional physical examination at least once a year.

The American Cancer Society (1980) recommends the following breast cancer screening test schedule for asymptomatic women:

1. All women over age 20 should perform breast self-examination monthly.
2. Women between the ages of 20 and 40 should have a breast examination by a qualified health care provider every 3 years and women over age 40 should have such an examination yearly.
3. All women should have a baseline mammogram between the ages of 35 and 40.
4. All women over 50 should have a mammogram every year.

The male breast

Occurring most frequently in the areolar area, male breast cancer accounts for approximately 1% of all breast cancers. Every male client should be given a thorough breast examination with an adaptation of the technique used for female clients.

Gynecomastia, enlargement of the male breast, is a frequently occurring multicausal condition. Causes include pubertal changes, hormonal administration, cirrhosis, leukemia, thyrotoxicosis, and drugs.

Benign lesions of the female breast

Benign lesions account for approximately 70% to 80% of breast operations. The most commonly seen benign breast lesions are fibrocystic disease and fibroadenomas.

Fibrocystic disease is an exaggeration of the normal changes in the breasts during the menstrual cycle and is eventually characterized by the formation of single or multiple cysts in the breasts. Fibrocystic disease develops in three stages:

1. The first stage is called *mazoplasia* and occurs in the late teens and early twenties. It is characterized by painful, tender, premenstrual breast swelling (chiefly in the axillary tails) that subsides after menses.
2. The second stage occurs in the late twenties and early thirties. The breasts exhibit multinodular changes, and sometimes a dominant mass can occur, which is usually described as a thickness rather than a lump.
3. Subsequently, cysts develop. The onset of cyst formation is often preceded by sudden, dull pain, a full feeling, or a burning sensation in the breast.

The lesions of cystic disease are commonly bilateral, multiple, painful, tender, well delineated, and slightly mobile. The discomfort from and size of lesions increase premenstrually.

Fibroadenomas are benign lesions that contain both fibrous and glandular tissues. They are usually solitary and unilateral. They are generally palpated as mobile, solid, firm, rubbery, regular, well-delineated, nontender, painless lumps. Fibroadenomas are usually found in women between the ages of 15 and 35 and produce no premenstrual changes.

SUMMARY

I. Observation of breasts at rest
II. Observation of breasts in three additional positions
   A. Client with arms overhead
   B. Client contracting pectoral muscles
   C. Client leaning forward
III. Palpation of axillary node areas
IV. Palpation of supraclavicular and subclavicular areas
V. Palpation of breasts with client in a sitting position, if indicated
VI. Observation of breasts with the client lying down and the breasts shifted medially
VII. Palpation of breasts
   A. Glandular tissue areas
   B. Areolar areas
   C. Nipples
   D. Tail of Spence areas

Every female client should be taught to examine her breasts and should be advised to do this each month on the completion of the menses.

BIBLIOGRAPHY

American Cancer Society report on cancer-related health checkup, CA **30:**194-240, 1980.
Dunphy, J. E., and Botsford, T. W.: Physical examination of the surgical patient, ed. 4, Philadelphia, 1975, W. B. Saunders Co.
Evans, K. T., and Gravelle, I. H.: Mammography, thermography and ultrasonography in breast disease, Sevenoaks, Kent, 1973, Butterworth & Co. (Publishers) Ltd.
Gallager, S., and others: The breast, St. Louis, 1978, The C. V. Mosby Co.
Kishner, R.: Breast cancer; a personal history and an investigative report, New York, 1975, Harcourt Brace Jovanovich, Inc.
Mahoney, L. J., Bird, B. L., and Cooke, G. M.: Annual clinical examination; the best available screening test for breast cancer, N. Engl. J. Med. **301:**315-316, 1979.
Memorial Hospital for Cancer and Associated Diseases: Breast Cancer Monograph, New York, 1973, Memorial Hospital.
Papaioannou, A. N.: The etiology of human breast cancer, New York, 1974, Springer-Verlag New York Inc.
Rush, B.: Breast. In Schwartz, S. I., editor: Principles of surgery, ed. 2, New York, 1969, McGraw-Hill Book Co.
Vorherr, H.: The breast, New York, 1974, Academic Press, Inc.

15 Assessment of the respiratory system

ANATOMY AND PHYSIOLOGY

The major purpose of the respiratory system is to supply the body with oxygen and eliminate carbon dioxide. This is accomplished through complex cooperation of many body systems that, in wellness, act in harmony. The actual transfer of oxygen and carbon dioxide between environmental gas and body liquid occurs in the alveoli, which are obviously not accessible to clinical examination. However, assessment of respiratory efficiency is accomplished by direct and indirect appraisal of structures supporting alveolar function.

The thoracic cage consists of a skeleton of 12 thoracic vertebrae, 12 pairs of ribs, the sternum, the diaphragm, and the intercostal muscles and is semirigid (Fig. 15-1). This cage is perpetually moving in the inspiratory and expiratory phases of respiration (Fig. 15-2). During inspiration the diaphragm descends and flattens. This maneuver produces differences in pressure among the areas of the mouth, the alveoli, and the pleural areas; and air moves into the lungs. The intrathoracic pressure is decreased, the lungs are expanded, and the ribs flare, increasing the diameter of the thorax. The second to the sixth ribs move around two axes in a motion commonly termed the "pump handle" movement. The lower ribs move in a "bucket handle" motion. Because of the length and positioning of the lower ribs and because the lower interspaces are wider, the amplitude of movement is greater in the lower thorax.

Inspiration is opposed by the elastic properties of the respiratory system. At the end of respiration, the volume of inspired air equals the volume exchange of the thoracic cavity, the tidal volume. Expiration is a relatively passive phenomenon. At the completion of inspiration, the diaphragm relaxes and the elastic recoil properties of the lungs expel air and pull the diaphragm to its resting position.

The thoracic cavity is divided into right and left pleural cavities; lined by the pleural layers—the visceral (lung) layer and the parietal (wall) layer—the pleural cavity is the space between the pleura. It contains a lubricating fluid.

The lungs are paired, but not symmetrical, conical organs that conform to the thoracic cavity. The right lung contains three lobes, and the left lung contains two.

Air reaches the lungs via a system of flexible tubes. Air enters through the mouth or nose, traverses the respiratory portion of the larynx, and enters the trachea. The trachea begins at the lower border of the cricoid cartilage and divides into a left and right bronchus, usually at the level of thoracic vertebra 4 or 5 posteriorly and slightly below the manubriosternal joint anteriorly.

The right bronchus is shorter, wider, and more vertical than the left bronchus. The bronchial structures further subdivide into increasingly smaller bronchi and bronchioles. Each bronchiole opens into an alveolar duct from which multiple alveoli radiate (Fig. 15-3). Lungs in the adult contain approximately 300 million alveoli.

The bronchi have both transport and protective purposes. Their cavities contain mucus, which entraps foreign particles and is continuously swept by ciliary action into the throat, where it can be eliminated.

Topographical anatomy

Topographical (surface) landmarks of the thorax assist the examiner in identifying the location of the internal, underlying structures and in describing the exact location of abnormalities (Fig. 15-4).

Manubriosternal junction (Louis's angle). The manubriosternal junction is an extremely useful aid in rib identification. It is a visible and palpable angulation of the sternum. The superior border of the second rib articulates with the sternum at the manubriosternal

289

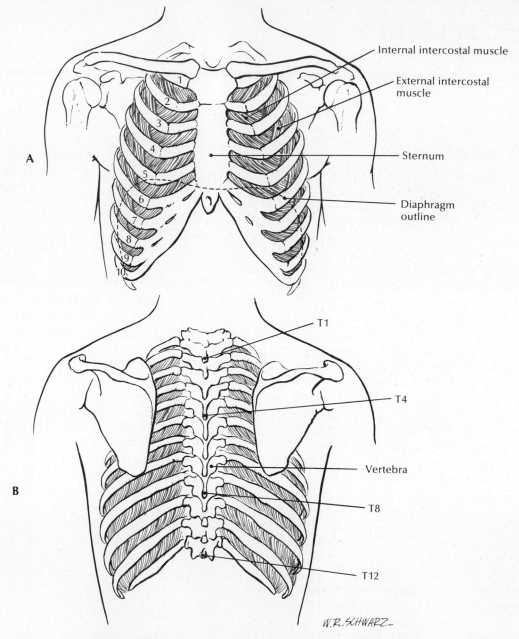

Fig. 15-1. Thoracic cage. **A,** Anterior thorax. **B,** Posterior thorax.

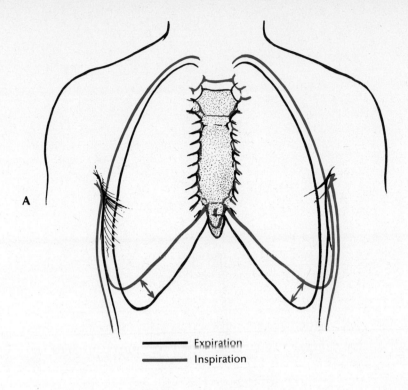

A

———— Expiration

———— Inspiration

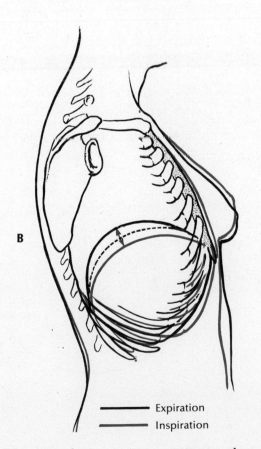

B

———— Expiration

———— Inspiration

Fig. 15-2. Movement of the thorax during respiration. **A,** Anterior thorax. **B,** Lateral thorax.

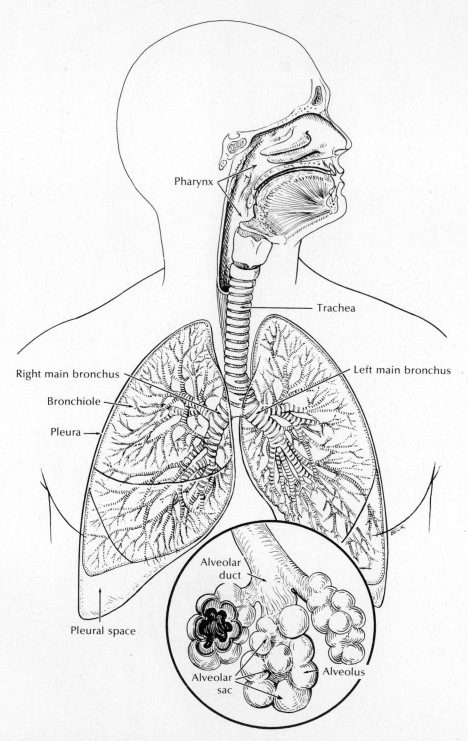

Fig. 15-3. Pharynx, trachea, and lungs. Alveolar sacs in inset. (From Anthony, C. P., and Thibodeau, G. A.: Anatomy and physiology, ed. 10, St. Louis, 1979, The C. V. Mosby Co.)

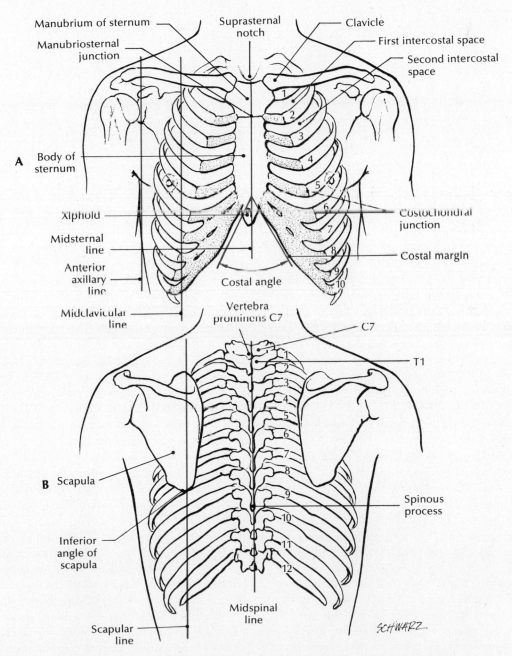

Fig. 15-4. Topographical landmarks. **A,** Anterior thorax. **B,** Posterior thorax.

Continued.

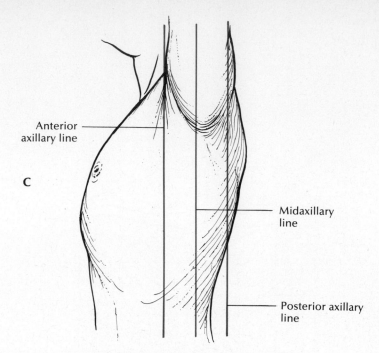

Anterior
axillary line

C

Midaxillary
line

Posterior axillary
line

Fig. 15-4, cont'd. C, Lateral thorax.

junction. The examiner can begin to palpate and count distal ribs and rib interspaces from this point. The intercostal spaces are numbered corresponding to the number of the rib immediately superior to the space. In palpation for rib identification, the examiner should palpate along the midclavicular line rather than at the sternal border because the rib cartilages are very close at the sternum, and the cartilages of only the first seven ribs attach directly to the sternum.

Suprasternal notch. The suprasternal notch is the depression above the manubrium.

Costal angle. The costal angle is the angle formed by the intersection of the costal margins.

Midsternal line. The midsternal line is an imaginary line drawn through the middle of the sternum.

Midclavicular lines. The midclavicular lines are left and right imaginary lines drawn through the midpoints of the clavicles and parallel to the midsternal line.

Anterior axillary lines. The anterior axillary lines are left and right imaginary lines drawn vertically from the anterior axillary folds, along the anterolateral chest, and parallel to the midsternal line.

Vertebra prominens (seventh cervical vertebra). When the client flexes his neck anteriorly and the posterior thorax is observed, a prominent spinous process can be observed and palpated. This is the spinous process of the seventh cervical vertebra. If two spinous processes are observed and palpated, the superior one is C7 and the inferior one is the spinous

process of T1. The counting of ribs is more difficult on the posterior than on the anterior thorax. The spinous processes of the vertebrae can be counted relatively easily from C7 to T4. From T4 the spinous processes project obliquely, causing the spinous process of the vertebra not to lie over its correspondingly numbered rib, but over the rib below it. For example, the spinous process of T5 lies over the body of T6 and is adjacent to the sixth rib.

Midspinal line. The midspinal line is an imaginary line that runs vertically along the posterior spinous processes of the vertebrae.

Scapular lines. The scapular lines are left and right imaginary lines that lie vertically and are parallel to the midspinal line. They pass through the inferior angles of the scapulae when the client stands erect with arms at his sides.

Posterior axillary lines. The posterior axillary lines are imaginary left and right lines drawn vertically from the posterior axillary folds along the posterolateral wall of the thorax when the lateral arm is abducted directly from the lateral chest wall.

Midaxillary lines. The midaxillary lines are imaginary left and right lines drawn vertically from the apices of the axillae. They are approximately midway between the anterior and the posterior axillary lines and parallel to them.

Underlying thoracic structures

When examining the respiratory system, the practitioner must maintain a mental image of the place-

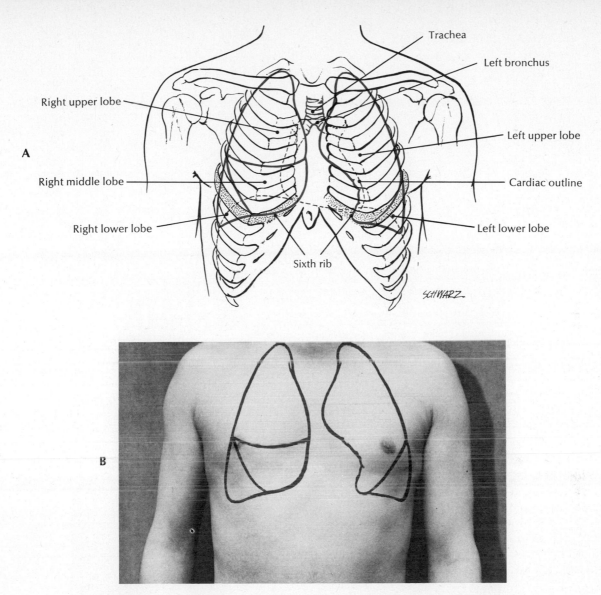

Fig. 15-5. Anterior thorax. **A,** Internal organs and structures. **B,** Lung borders.

ment of organs and organ parts of the respiratory system and other systems sharing the thoracic area (Figs. 15-5 to 15-8).

Lung borders. In the anterior thorax, the apices of the lungs extend for approximately 1½ inches above the clavicles. The inferior borders of the lungs cross the sixth rib at the midclavicular line. In the posterior thorax, the apices extend to T1. The lower borders vary with respiration and usually extend from the spinous process of T10 on expiration to the spinous process of T12 on deep inspiration. In the lateral thorax, the lung extends from the apex of the axilla to the eighth rib of the midaxillary line.

Lung fissures. The right oblique (diagonal) fissure extends from the area of the spinous process of the third thoracic vertebra laterally and downward until

it crosses the fifth rib at the right midaxillary line. It then continues anteriorly and medially to end at the sixth rib at the right and left midclavicular lines. The right horizontal fissure extends from the fifth rib slightly posterior to the right midaxillary line and runs horizontally to the area of the fourth rib at the right sternal border. The left oblique (diagonal) fissure extends from the spinous process of the third thoracic vertebra laterally and downward to the left midaxillary line at the fifth rib and continues anteriorly and medially until it terminates at the sixth rib in the left midclavicular line.

Border of the diaphragm. Anteriorly, on expiration, the right dome of the diaphragm is located at the level of the fifth rib at the midclavicular line and the left dome is at the level of the sixth rib. Posterior-

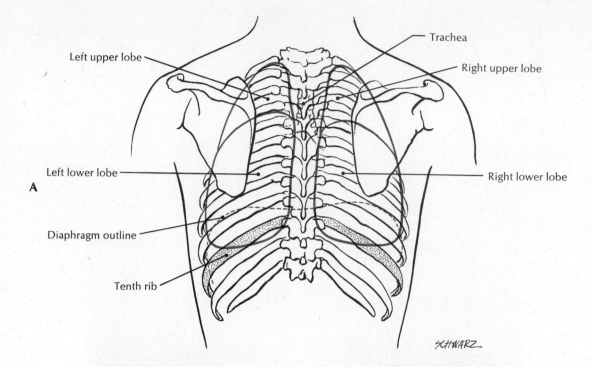

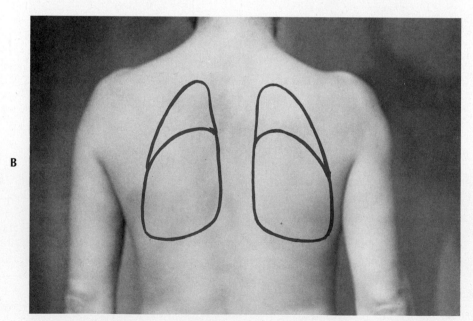

Fig. 15-6. Posterior thorax. **A,** Internal organs and structures. **B,** Lung borders.

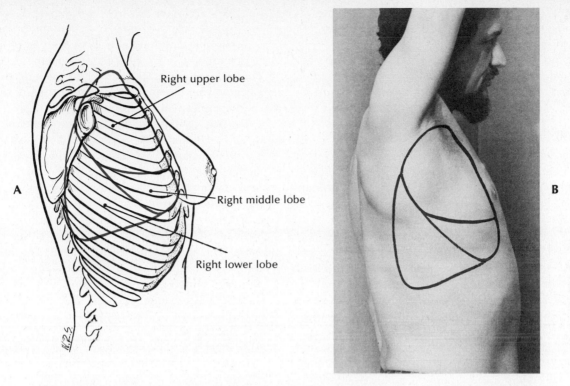

Fig. 15-7. Right lateral thorax. **A,** Internal organs and chest structures. (Note the relationship of the breast to chest organs and structures.) **B,** Lung borders.

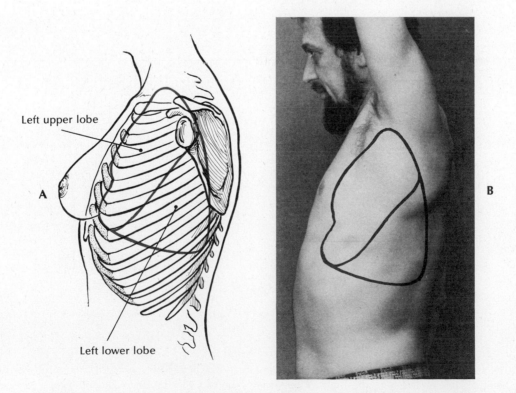

Fig. 15-8. Left lateral thorax. **A,** Internal organs and chest structures. **B,** Lung borders.

ly, on expiration, the diaphragm is at the level of the spinous process of T10; laterally, it is at the eighth rib at the midaxillary line.

Trachea. The bifurcation of the trachea occurs approximately just below the manubriosternal junction anteriorly and at the spinous process of T4 posteriorly.

EXAMINATION

Equipment needed for the respiratory system examination are a stethoscope, a marking pencil, and a centimeter ruler. The examination should be performed in a well-illuminated area that allows for privacy.

Inspection

For adequate inspection of the thorax, the client should be sitting upright without support and uncovered to the waist. It is essential that the room lighting be adequate and that a mechanism for supplementary lighting be available for close inspection of small areas. It is critical that the client be warm and not observed by persons extraneous to the examina-

tion. The examiner first observes the general shape of the thorax and its symmetry. Although no individual is absolutely symmetrical in both body hemispheres, most individuals are reasonably similar side to side. Using the client as his own control whenever paired parts are examined is an excellent habit and will often yield significant findings.

Thoracic configuration. The anteroposterior diameter of the thorax in the normal adult is less than the transverse diameter at approximately a ratio of 1:2 to 5:7 (Fig. 15-9). In the normal infant, in some adults with pulmonary disease, or in aged adults the thorax is approximately round. This condition is called barrel chest. The barrel chest is characterized by horizontal ribs, slight kyphosis of the thoracic spine, and prominent sternal angle. The chest appears as though it were in continuous inspiratory position. Other observed abnormalities of thoracic shape might include:

1. Retraction of the thorax. The retraction is unilateral, or of one side.
2. Pigeon or chicken chest (pectus carinatum)—sternal protrusion anteriorly. The anteroposte-

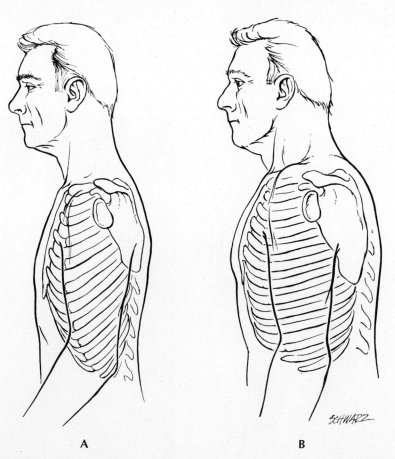

A   B

Fig. 15-9. A, Client with normal thoracic configuration. **B,** Client with increased anteroposterior diameter. Note contrasts in the angle of the slope of the ribs and the development of the accessory muscles of respiration in the neck.

rior diameter of the chest is increased, and the resultant configuration resembles the thorax of a fowl.

3. Funnel chest (pectus excavatum)—depression of part or all of the sternum. If the depression is deep, it may interfere with both respiratory and cardiac function.

4. Spinal deformities. While the client is uncovered and the examiner is behind him, the spine should be examined for deformities. (See Chapter 22 on musculoskeletal assessment for the specific techniques of spinal examination.)

The approach to the physical examination is regional and integrated. The examination of systems is combined in body regions when appropriate. Since the client is uncovered to the waist during the examination, a large portion of skin and tissue is accessible to inspection. The observation of skin and underlying tissue provides the examiner with knowledge of the general nutrition of the patient. Common thoracic skin findings are the spider nevi associated with cirrhosis and seborrheic dermatitis (see Chapter 9 on skin assessment).

Ribs and interspaces. The reaction of interspaces on inspiration may be indicative of some obstruction of free air inflow. Bulging of interspaces on expiration occurs when there is obstruction to air outflow or may be the result of tumor, aneurysm, or cardiac enlargement. Normally the costal angle is less than 90 degrees, and the ribs are inserted into the spine at about a 45-degree angle (Fig. 15-1). In clients with obstructive lung diseases these angles are widened.

Pattern of respiration. Normally, men and children breathe diaphragmatically, and women breathe thoracically or costally. A change in this pattern might be significant. If the client appears to have labored respiration, the examiner observes for the use of the accessory muscles of respiration—the sternocleidomastoid and trapezius muscles—and for supraclavicular retraction. Impedance to air inflow is often accompanied by retraction of intercostal spaces during inspiration. An excessively long expiratory phase of respiration accompanies outflow impedance.

The normal adult resting respiratory rate is 16 to 20 breaths per minute and is regular. The ratio of respiratory rate to pulse rate normally is 1:4. Tachypnea

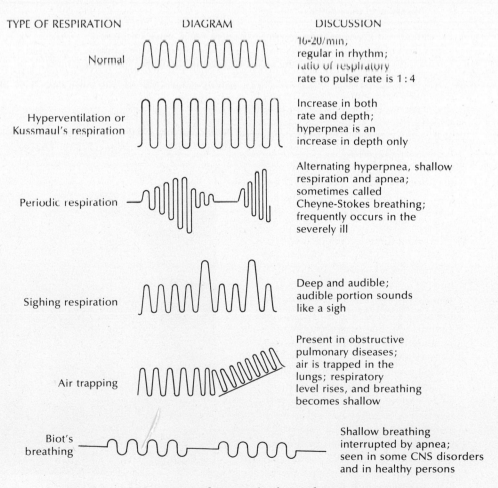

TYPE OF RESPIRATION	DIAGRAM	DISCUSSION
Normal		16-20/min, regular in rhythm; ratio of respiratory rate to pulse rate is 1:4
Hyperventilation or Kussmaul's respiration		Increase in both rate and depth; hyperpnea is an increase in depth only
Periodic respiration		Alternating hyperpnea, shallow respiration and apnea; sometimes called Cheyne-Stokes breathing; frequently occurs in the severely ill
Sighing respiration		Deep and audible; audible portion sounds like a sigh
Air trapping		Present in obstructive pulmonary diseases; air is trapped in the lungs; respiratory level rises, and breathing becomes shallow
Biot's breathing		Shallow breathing interrupted by apnea; seen in some CNS disorders and in healthy persons

Fig. 15-10. Characteristics of commonly observed respiratory patterns.

is an adult respiratory rate of over 20 breaths per minute; bradypnea is an adult respiratory rate of less than 10 breaths per minute.

There are many abnormal patterns of respiration. Some of the commonly seen patterns are listed in Fig. 15-10. Dyspnea is a subjective phenomenon of inadequate or distressful respiration.

Lips and nails. Inspection in the respiratory system examination includes observation of lips and nail beds for color and observation of the nails for clubbing. These phenomena are discussed in Chapter 7 on general assessment and in Chapter 16 on cardiovascular assessment.

Palpation

Palpation is performed to (1) further assess abnormalities suggested by the history or observation, such as tenderness, pulsations, masses, or skin lesions; (2) assess the skin and subcutaneous structures;

Table 15-1. Characteristics of normal and abnormal tactile fremitus

Type of fremitus	Discussion of characteristics
Normal fremitus	Varies greatly from person to person and is dependent on the intensity and pitch of the voice, the position and distance of the bronchi in relation to the chest wall, and the thickness of the chest wall. Fremitus is most intense in the second intercostal spaces at the sternal border near the area of bronchial bifurcation.
Increased vocal fremitus	May occur in pneumonia, compressed lung, lung tumor, or pulmonary fibrosis. (A solid medium of uniform structure conducts vibrations with greater intensity than a porous medium.)
Decreased or absent vocal fremitus	Occurs when there is a diminished production of sounds, a diminished transmission of sounds, or the addition of a medium through which sounds must pass before reaching the thoracic wall as, for example, in pleural effusion, pleural thickening, pneumothorax, bronchial obstruction, or emphysema.
Pleural friction rub	Vibration produced by inflamed pleural surfaces rubbing together. It is felt as a grating, is synchronous with respiratory movements, and is more commonly felt on inspiration.
Rhonchal fremitus	Coarse vibrations produced by the passage of air through thick exudates in the large air passages. These can be cleared or altered by coughing.

(3) assess the thoracic expansion; (4) assess vocal (tactile) fremitus; and (5) assess the tracheal position.

General palpation. The examiner should specifically palpate any areas of abnormality. The temperature and turgor of the skin should be generally assessed. The examiner then palpates the muscle mass and the thoracic skeleton. If the client has no complaints in relation to the respiratory system, a rapid, general survey of anterior, lateral, and posterior thoracic areas is sufficient. If the client does have complaints, all chest areas should be meticulously palpated for tenderness, bulges, or abnormal movements.

Assessment of thoracic expansion (Fig. 15-11). The degree of thoracic expansion can be assessed from the anterior or posterior chest. Anteriorly, the examiner's hands are placed over the anterolateral chest with the thumbs extended along the costal margin, pointing to the xiphoid process. Posteriorly, the thumbs are placed at the level of the tenth rib and the palms are placed on the posterolateral chest. The examiner feels the amount of the thoracic expansion during quiet and deep respiration and observes for divergence of the thumbs on expiration. There should be symmetry of respiration between the left and right hemithoraces.

Assessment of fremitus. Fremitus is vibration perceptible on palpation. Vocal or tactile fremitus is palpable vibration of the thoracic wall, produced by phonation.

The client is asked to repeat "one, two, three" or "ninety-nine" while the examiner systematically palpates the thorax (Fig. 15-12). The examiner can use

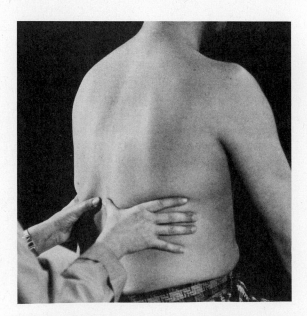

Fig. 15-11. Palpation for thoracic excursion.

the palmar bases of the fingers, the ulnar aspect of the hand, or the ulnar aspect of the closed fist. If one hand is used, it should be moved from one side of the chest to the corresponding area on the other side. If two hands are used for examination, they should be simultaneously placed on the corresponding areas of each thoracic side. Types of fremitus are shown in Table 15-1.

Whenever examining the thorax, the practitioner must be mindful of the four parts for examination: the posterior chest, the anterior chest, the right and left lateral thoracic areas, and the apices. The examiner should move from the area of one hemisphere to the corresponding area on the other (right to left,

left to right) until all four major parts are surveyed. During palpation for assessing fremitus and all subsequent procedures for the examination of the respiratory system, all areas must be meticulously and systematically examined. Usually, the apices, posterior chest, and lateral areas can be examined with the practitioner standing behind the client.

Assessment of tracheal deviation. The trachea should be assessed by palpation for lateral deviation. The examiner places a finger on the trachea in the suprasternal notch, then moves his finger laterally left and right in the spaces bordered by the upper edge of the clavicle, the inner aspect of the sternocleidomastoid muscle, and the trachea. These spaces

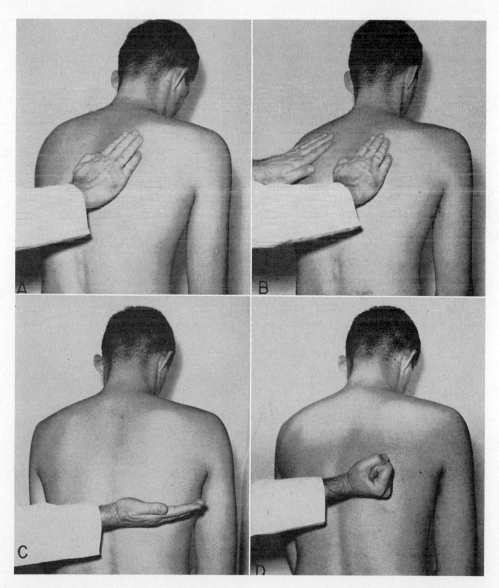

Fig. 15-12. Palpation for assessment of vocal fremitus. **A,** Use of palmar surface of fingertips. **B,** Simultaneous application of the fingertips of both hands. **C,** Use of ulnar aspect of the hand. **D,** Use of ulnar aspect of the closed fist. (From Prior, J. A., and Silberstein, J. S.: Physical diagnosis: the history and examination of the patient, ed. 4, St. Louis, 1973, The C. V. Mosby Co.)

should be equal on both sides. In diseases such as atelectasis and pulmonary fibrosis, the trachea may be deviated toward the abnormal side. The trachea may be deviated toward the normal side in conditions such as neck tumors, thyroid enlargement, enlarged lymph nodes, pleural effusion, unilateral emphysema, and tension pneumothorax.

Crepitations. In subcutaneous emphysema, the subcutaneous tissue contains fine beads of air. As this tissue is palpated, audible crackling sounds are heard. These sounds are termed *crepitations*.

Percussion

Percussion is the tapping of an object in order to set underlying structures in motion and consequently to produce a sound called a percussion note and a palpable vibration. Percussion penetrates to a depth of approximately 5 to 7 cm. Percussion is utilized in the thoracic examination to determine the relative amounts of air, liquid, or solid material in the underlying lung and to determine the positions and boundaries of organs.

Two techniques of percussion are immediate, or direct, percussion and mediate, or indirect, percussion. In *immediate*, or *direct, percussion,* the examiner strikes the object to be percussed directly with the palmar aspect of two, three, or four fingers held together or with the palmar aspect of the tip of the middle finger. The strikes are rapid and downward; movement of the hand from the wrist is in rapid strokes. This type of percussion is not normally utilized in thoracic examination. It is useful in the

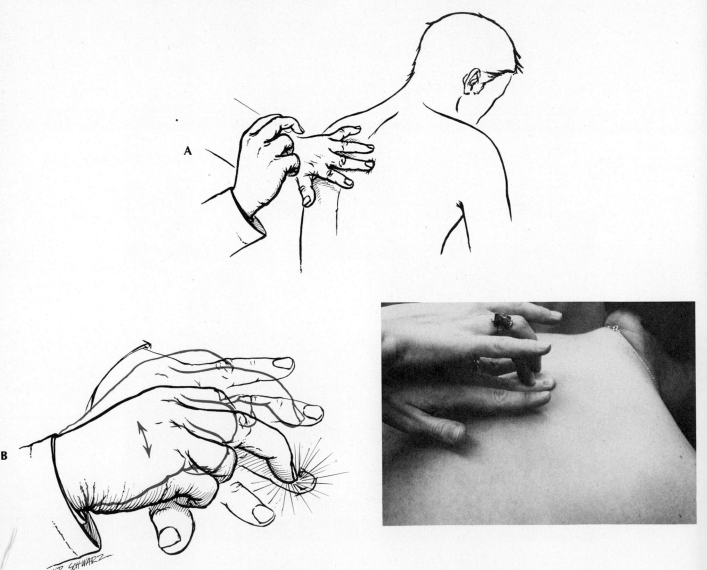

Fig. 15-13. Percussion. **A,** Positioning of the hands. **B,** Hand movement. **C,** Percussion of the posterior thorax.

Table 15-2. Description of percussion notes

Note	Intensity	Pitch	Duration	Quality	Normal location
Resonance	Moderate to loud	Low	Long	Hollow	Peripheral lung
Hyperresonance	Very loud	Very low	Very long	Booming	Child's lung
Tympany	Loud	High	Moderate	Musical, drumlike	Air-filled stomach
Dullness	Soft	High	Moderate	Thudlike	Liver
Flatness	Soft	High	Short	Extreme dullness	Thigh

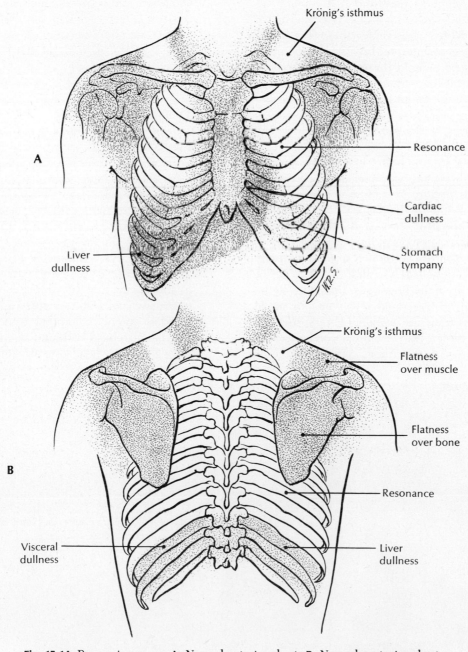

Fig. 15-14. Percussion areas. **A,** Normal anterior chest. **B,** Normal posterior chest.

examination of the thorax in the infant and the sinuses in the adult. *Mediate,* or *indirect, percussion* is the striking of an object held against the area to be examined (Fig. 15-13). The middle finger of the examiner's left hand (if the examiner is right-handed) is the pleximeter. The distal phalanx and joint and the middle phalanx are placed firmly on the surface to be percussed. Although most practitioners usually find that the area of the interphalangeal joint is the most effective pleximeter point for percussion, the quality of the percussion sound and the comfort of the examiner should serve as criteria for the selection of a pleximeter point. The examiner may find that a point between the proximal and the distal interphalangeal joints is more effective and comfortable. This alteration of technique is acceptable. In all cases, the point struck by the plexor should be pressed as tightly as possible against the patient, with all other areas of that hand held off the client's skin. The plexor is the index finger of the examiner's right hand or the index and middle fingers held together. For position see Fig. 15-13.

With the forearm and shoulder stationary and all movement at the wrist, the pleximeter is struck sharply with the plexor. The blow is aimed at the portion of the pleximeter that is exerting maximum pressure on the thoracic surface, usually the base of the terminal phalanx, the distal interphalangeal joint, or the middle phalanx. The blow is executed rapidly and the plexor is immediately withdrawn. The plexor strikes with the tip of the finger at right angles to the pleximeter. One or two rapid blows are struck in each area. Bony areas are avoided; interspaces are used for percussion. The examiner compares one side of the thorax with the other.

With experience and study the practitioner will be able to differentiate among the five percussion tones commonly elicited on the human body. In the study of tones, the determination of four characteristics will assist in assessment and labeling:

1. *Intensity (amplitude):* the loudness or softness of the tone.
2. *Pitch (frequency):* relates to the number of vibrations per second. Rapid vibrations produce high-pitched tones; slow vibrations produce low-pitched tones. The greater the density of an object, the higher the frequency.
3. *Quality:* a subjective phenomena relating to the innate characteristics of the object being percussed.
4. *Duration:* the amount of time a note is sustained.

Table 15-2 describes the commonly used descriptive terms for percussion tones elicited by physical examination.

Fig. 15-14 is a percussion map for the normal chest. The procedure for thoracic percussion is:

1. Percuss the apices to determine if the normal 5-cm area of resonance is present between the neck and shoulder muscles (Fig. 15-14).
2. Position the client with his head bent and his arm folded over his chest (Fig. 15-15). With this maneuver, the scapulae move laterally and more lung area is accessible to examination.
3. On the posterior chest percuss systematically at about 5-cm intervals from the upper to lower chest, moving left to right, right to left, and avoiding scapular and other bony areas; percuss the lateral chest with the client's arms positioned over his head (Fig. 15-16).

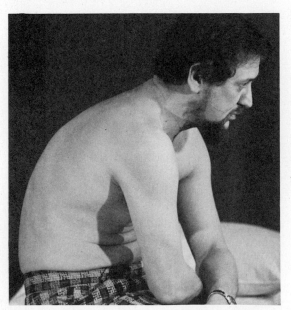

Fig. 15-15. Position of client for examination of the posterior thorax.

4. Measure the diaphragmatic excursion. Instruct the client to inhale deeply and hold his breath in. Percuss along the scapular line on one side until the lower edge of the lung is identified. Sound will change from resonance to dullness. Mark the point of change on each side at the scapular line. Then instruct the client to take a few normal respirations. Next, instruct the cli-

ent to exhale completely and hold his expiration. Proceed to percuss up from the marked point at the midscapular line to determine the diaphragmatic excursion in deep expiration. Repeat the procedure on the opposite side. Measure and record the distance between the upper and lower points in centimeters on each side. The diaphragm is usually slightly higher on the

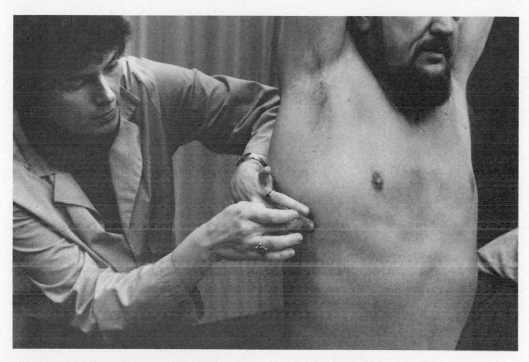

Fig. 15-16. Position of the client for percussion of the lateral thorax.

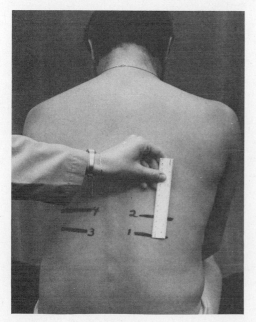

Fig. 15-17. Assessment of diaphragmatic excursion. The numbers indicate a suggested sequence of percussion.

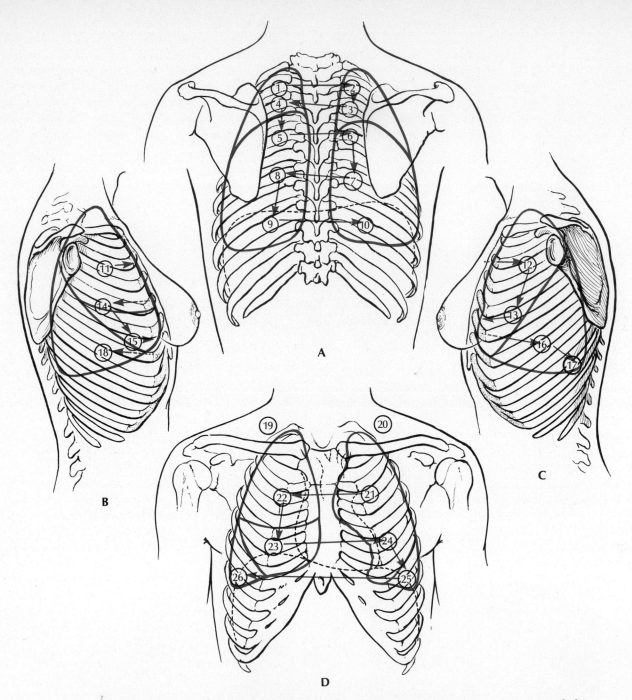

Fig. 15-18. Routine for the systematic percussion of the thorax. Numbers indicate a recommended sequence for percussion and auscultation during a routine screening examination. **A,** Posterior thorax. **B,** Right lateral thorax. **C,** Left lateral thorax. **D,** Anterior thorax.

right side and excursion is normally 3 to 5 cm bilaterally. Diaphragmatic excursion is usually measured only on the posterior chest (Fig. 15-17).

In the actual examination, the practitioner would complete the examination of the apices and the posterior and lateral chest and would then percuss the anterior chest. A recommended sequence for the exam-

ination of the posterior, lateral, and anterior thoracic areas is illustrated in Fig. 15-18.

Auscultation

Through auscultation, the practitioner obtains information about the functioning of the respiratory system and about the presence of any obstruction in the passages. Auscultation of the lungs is accom-

Table 15-3. Characteristics of breath sounds

Sound	Duration of inspiration and expiration	Diagram of sound	Pitch	Intensity	Normal location	Abnormal location
Vesicular	Inspiration > expiration 5:2		Low	Soft	Peripheral lung	Not applicable
Bronchovesicular	Inspiration = expiration 1:1		Moderate	Moderate	First and second intercostal spaces at the sternal border over major bronchi	Peripheral lung
Bronchial (tubular)	Inspiration < expiration 1:2		High	Loud	Over trachea	Lung area

plished by the use of a stethoscope. The diaphragm of the stethoscope is usually used for the thoracic examination because it covers a larger surface than the bell. The stethoscope is placed firmly on the skin. Client or stethoscope movement are avoided because movements of muscle under the skin or movements of the stethoscope over hair will produce confusing extrinsic sounds.

Before beginning auscultation, the examiner should instruct the client to breathe through his mouth and more deeply and slowly than in usual respiration. The examiner systematically auscultates the apices and the posterior, lateral, and anterior chest (Fig. 15-18). At each application of the stethoscope, the examiner listens to at least one complete respiration. The examiner should observe the client for signs of hyperventilation and stop the procedure if the client becomes light-headed or faint. The process of auscultation includes (1) the analysis of breath sounds, (2) the detection of any abnormal sounds, and (3) the examination of the sounds produced by the spoken voice. As with percussion, the examiner should use a zigzag procedure, comparing the finding at each point with the corresponding point on the opposite hemithorax.

Breath sounds. Breath sounds are the sounds produced by the movement of air through the tracheobronchoalveolar system. These sounds are analyzed according to pitch, intensity, quality, and relative duration of inspiratory and expiratory phases. Table 15-3 outlines the types of sounds heard over the normal and the abnormal lung.

The sounds that are heard over normal lung parenchyma are called vesicular breath sounds. The inspiratory phase of the vesicular breath sound is heard better than the expiratory phase and is about three times longer. These sounds have a low pitch and soft intensity.

Bronchovesicular breath sounds are normally heard in the areas of the major bronchi, especially in the apex of the right lung and at the sternal borders. Bronchovesicular breath sounds are characterized by inspiratory and expiratory phases of equal duration, moderate pitch, and moderate intensity. Whenever bronchovesicular breath sounds are heard over the peripheral lung, underlying pathology is likely.

Bronchial breath sounds are normally heard over the trachea and indicate pathology if heard over lung tissue. They are high-pitched, loud sounds, with equal inspiratory and expiratory phases. The inspiratory and expiratory phases are audibly separated by a gap of silence.

Fig. 15-19 shows the various areas for assessing breath sounds of the anterior and posterior thorax.

Absent or decreased breath sounds can occur in (1) any condition that causes the deposition of foreign matter in the pleural space, (2) bronchial obstruction, (3) emphysema, or (4) shallow breathing.

Increased breath sounds, as from vesicular to bronchovesicular or bronchial, can occur in any condition that causes a consolidation of lung tissue.

Abnormal or adventitious sounds. Adventitious sounds are not alterations in breath sounds but sounds superimposed on breath sounds. Classification of these sounds varies among authorities; consequently, nomenclatures are arbitrary. Commonly utilized terms for adventitious sounds are described in Table 15-4.

A rale is a short, discrete, interrupted, crackling or bubbling sound that is most commonly heard during inspiration. Rales are thought to be produced by air passing through moisture in the bronchi, bron-

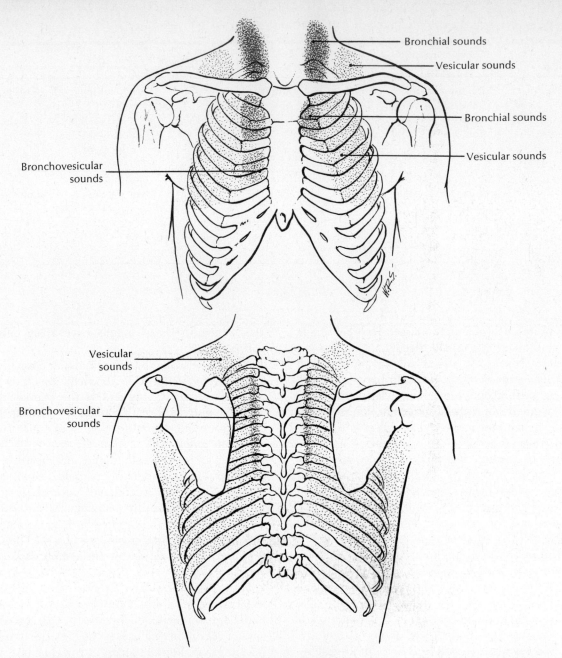

Bronchial sounds

Vesicular sounds

Bronchial sounds

Vesicular sounds

Bronchovesicular sounds

Vesicular sounds

Bronchovesicular sounds

Fig. 15-19. Areas for assessing breath sounds of the anterior and posterior thorax. Areas more darkly colored indicate normal points for the auscultation of bronchial and bronchovesicular breath sounds.

chioles, and alveoli or by air rushing through passages and alveoli that were closed during expiration and abruptly opened during inspiration. The pitch and location in the inspiratory phase of the rales are thought to be indicative of their site of production. Low-pitched, coarse rales occurring early in inspiration are thought to have their origins in the bronchi, as in bronchitis. Medium-pitched rales in midinspiration occur in diseases of small bronchi, as in bronchiectasis. High-pitched, fine rales are found in dis-

eases affecting the bronchioles and alveoli and occur late in inspiration.

Rhonchi are continuous sounds produced by the movement of air through narrowed passages in the tracheobronchial tree. Rhonchi predominate in expiration because bronchi are shortened and narrowed during this respiratory phase. However, rhonchi can occur in the inspiratory as well as the expiratory phase of respiration, suggesting that lumen have been narrowed during both respiratory phases. As with

Table 15-4. Origin and characteristics of adventitious sounds

Sound	Diagram of sound	Origin	Characteristics
Rales—fine to medium		Air passing through moisture in small air passages and alveoli	Discrete, discontinuous; inspiratory; have a dry or wet crackling quality; not cleared by coughing; sound is simulated by rolling a lock of hair near the ear
Rales—medium to coarse		Air passing through moisture in the bronchioles, bronchi, and trachea	As above; louder than fine rales
Rhonchi—sibilant (wheezes)		Air passing through air passages narrowed by secretions, swelling, tumors, and so on	Continuous sounds; originate in the small air passages; may be inspiratory and expiratory but usually predominate in expiration; high-pitched, wheezing sounds
Rhonchi—sonorous		Same as wheezes	Continuous sounds; originate in large air passages; may be inspiratory and expiratory but usually predominate in expiration; low-pitched, moaning or snoring quality; coughing may alter sounds
Friction rubs		Rubbing together of inflamed and roughened pleural surfaces	Creaking or grating quality; superficial sounding, inspiratory and expiratory; heard most often in the lower antero-lateral chest (area of greatest thoracic expansion); coughing has no effect

---

Voice sound assessment techniques

Client vocalization	Normal auscultory finding	Abnormal auscultory finding
"Ninety-nine" spoken	Muffled, nondistinct sound	"Ninety-nine": bronchophony
"e- e- e" spoken	Muffled, nondistinct sound	"a- a- a": egophony
"Ninety-nine" whispered	Barely audible, nondistinct sound	"Ninety-nine": whispered pectoriloquy

---

rales, the pitch and location of rhonchi in the expiratory phase are thought to indicate their origins. Low-pitched rhonchi, sometimes called sonorous rhonchi and usually heard in early expiration, originate in the larger bronchi; high-pitched, sibilant rhonchi, sometimes called wheezes, originate in small bronchioles and often occur in late expiration.

A pleural friction rub is a loud, dry, creaking or grating sound indicative of pleural irritation. It is produced by the rubbing together of inflamed and roughened pleural surfaces during respiration and therefore is heard best during the latter part of inspiration and the beginning of expiration. Because thoracic ex-

pansion is greatest in the lower anterolateral thorax, pleural friction rubs are most often heard there.

If the client has rales, the examiner listens for several respirations in the areas in which the rales are heard to determine the effects of deep breathing. Also, the client is asked to cough, with the changes in adventitious sounds noted after coughing.

If the client has complained of respiratory difficulty and no adventitious sounds are heard, he is asked to cough; often, adventitious sounds are noted in post-tussive breathing.

Voice sounds. Vocal resonance is produced by the same mechanism that produces vocal fremitus. Reso-

Text continued on p. 320.

Table 15-5. Assessment findings frequently associated with common lung conditions

Condition	Illustration*	Breath sound	Description
Normal lung			The tracheobronchial tree and alveoli are clear; the pleurae are thin and close together; the chest wall is mobile
Asthma	Bronchospasm Normal bronchial lumen		Asthma is characterized by intermittent episodes of airway obstruction caused by bronchospasm, excessive bronchial secretion, or edema of bronchial mucosa

*Although some disease conditions are bilateral, one diseased lung and one normal lung will be illustrated for each condition to provide

Inspection	Palpation	Percussion	Auscultation
Good, symmetrical rib and diaphragmatic movement	Trachea—midline Expansion—adequate Tactile fremitus—present Diaphragmatic excursion—3 to 5 cm	Resonant	Breath sounds—vesicular Vocal fremitus—normal Adventitious sounds—none, except for a few transient rales at the bases
Cyanosis Tachypnea with audible wheezing Use of accessory muscles of respiration	Tactile fremitus—decreased	Hyperresonant	Breath sounds—distant Vocal fremitus—decreased Adventitious sounds—sibilant rhonchi

contrast.

Continued.

Table 15-5. Assessment findings frequently associated with common lung conditions—cont'd

Condition	Illustration	Breath sound	Description

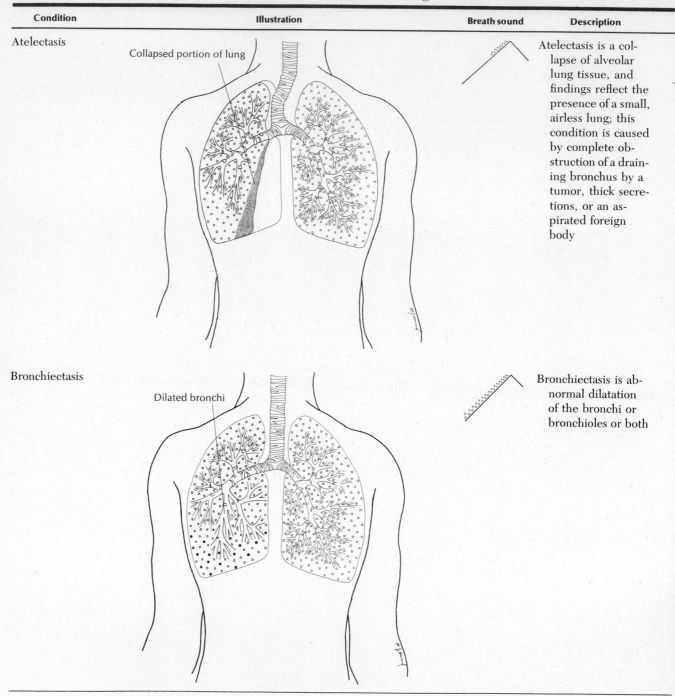

Atelectasis

Collapsed portion of lung

Atelectasis is a collapse of alveolar lung tissue, and findings reflect the presence of a small, airless lung; this condition is caused by complete obstruction of a draining bronchus by a tumor, thick secretions, or an aspirated foreign body

Bronchiectasis

Dilated bronchi

Bronchiectasis is abnormal dilatation of the bronchi or bronchioles or both

Inspection	Palpation	Percussion	Auscultation
Less chest motion on affected side Affected side retracted, with lungs appearing close together Cough	Trachea—shifted to affected side Expansion—decreased on affected side Tactile fremitus—decreased or absent	Dull to flat over collapsed lung Hyperresonant over the remainder of the affected hemithorax	Breath sounds—decreased or absent Vocal fremitus—varies in intensity, usually reduced or absent on affected side Adventitious sounds—fine, high-pitched rales may be heard over the terminal portion of inspiration
If mild, respirations are normal If severe, tachypnea Less expansion on affected side Cough with purulent sputum	Trachea—midline or deviated toward affected side Expansion—decreased on affected side Tactile fremitus—increased	Normal or dull	Breath sounds—usually vesicular Vocal fremitus—usually normal Adventitious sounds—rales

Continued.

Table 15-5. Assessment findings frequently associated with common lung conditions—cont'd

Condition	Illustration	Breath sound	Description
Bronchitis—acute			Acute bronchitis is an inflammation of the bronchial tree characterized by partial bronchial obstruction by secretions or constrictions; it results in abnormally deflated portions of the lung
Emphysema			Emphysema is a permanent hyperinflation of the lung beyond the terminal bronchioles, with destruction of alveolar walls

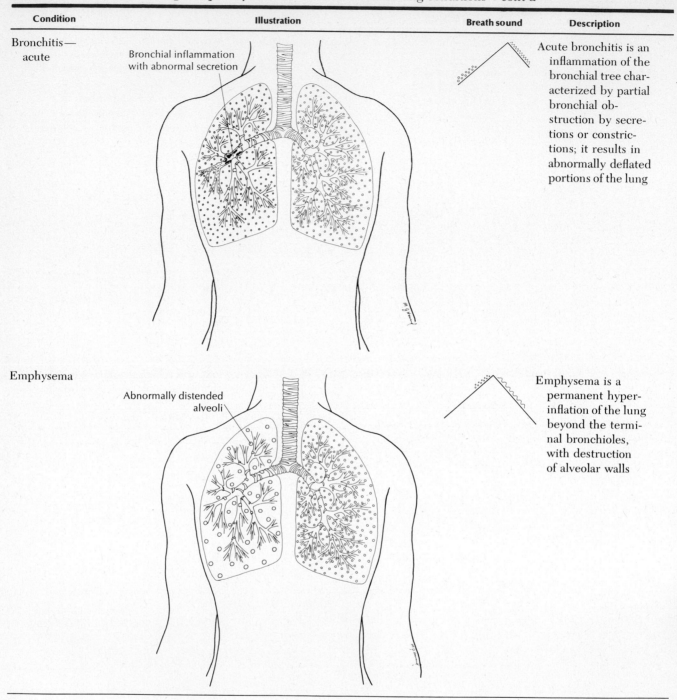

Bronchial inflammation with abnormal secretion

Abnormally distended alveoli

Inspection	Palpation	Percussion	Auscultation
If severe, tachypnea and cyanosis Rasping cough with mucoid sputum	Tactile fremitus—normal or increased	Normal	Breath sounds—vesicular Vocal fremitus—normal Adventitious sounds—localized rales, sibilant ronchi
Dyspnea with exertion Barrel chest Tachypnea Use of accessory muscles of respiration	Expansion diminished Tactile fremitus—decreased	Resonant to hyperresonant Diaphragmatic excursion—small	Breath sounds—decreased intensity; often prolonged expiration Vocal fremitus—normal or decreased Adventitious sounds—occasional sonorous and/or sibilant ronchi; often fine rales in late inspiration

Continued.

Table 15-5. Assessment findings frequently associated with common lung conditions—cont'd

Condition	Illustration	Breath sound	Description
Pleural effusion and thickening			Pleural effusion is a collection of fluid in the pleural space; if pleural effusion is prolonged, fibrous tissue may also accumulate in the pleural space; the clinical picture depends on the amount of fluid or fibrosis present and the rapidity of development; fluid tends to gravitate to the most dependent areas of the thorax, and the overlying lung is compressed
Pneumonia with consolidation			Pneumonia with consolidation occurs when alveolar air is replaced by fluid or tissue; physical findings depend on the amount of parenchymal tissue involved

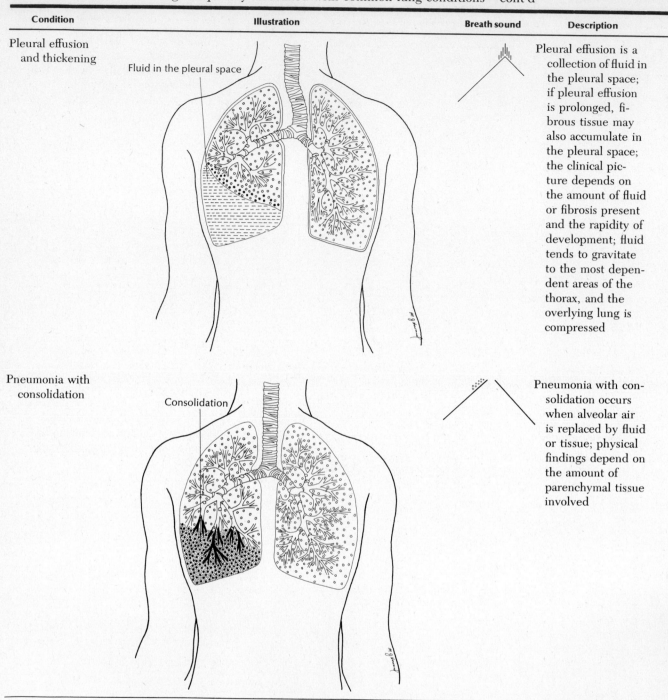

Fluid in the pleural space

Consolidation

Inspection	Palpation	Percussion	Auscultation
Tachypnea Decrease in the definition of the intercostal spaces on the affected side	Trachea—deviation toward normal side Expansion—decreased on affected side Tactile fremitus—decreased or absent	Dull to flat	Breath sounds—decreased or absent Vocal fremitus—decreased or absent; if the fluid compresses the lung, sounds may be bronchial over the compression, and bronchophony, egophony, and whisper pectoriloquy may be present Adventitious sounds—pleural friction rub sometimes present
Tachypnea Guarding and less motion on affected side	Expansion—limited on the affected side Tactile fremitus—usually increased, but may be decreased if a bronchus leading to the affected area is plugged	Dull to flat	Breath sounds—increased in intensity, bronchovesicular or bronchial breath sounds over affected area Vocal fremitus—increased bronchophony, egophony, whisper pectoriloquy present Adventitious sounds—inspiratory rales, terminal third of inspiration

Continued.

Table 15-5. Assessment findings frequently associated with common lung conditions—cont'd

Condition	Illustration	Breath sound	Description

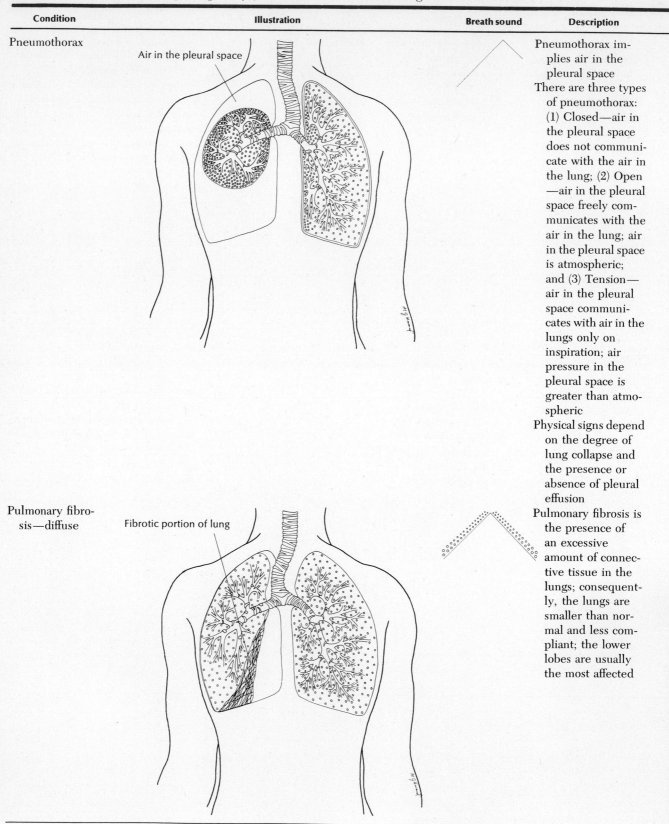

Pneumothorax — Air in the pleural space

Pulmonary fibro-sis—diffuse — Fibrotic portion of lung

Pneumothorax implies air in the pleural space

There are three types of pneumothorax: (1) Closed—air in the pleural space does not communicate with the air in the lung; (2) Open—air in the pleural space freely communicates with the air in the lung; air in the pleural space is atmospheric; and (3) Tension—air in the pleural space communicates with air in the lungs only on inspiration; air pressure in the pleural space is greater than atmospheric

Physical signs depend on the degree of lung collapse and the presence or absence of pleural effusion

Pulmonary fibrosis is the presence of an excessive amount of connective tissue in the lungs; consequently, the lungs are smaller than normal and less compliant; the lower lobes are usually the most affected

Inspection	Palpation	Percussion	Auscultation
Restricted lung expansion If large, tachypnea Bulging in the intercostal spaces on the affected side Cyanosis	Trachea—deviated toward normal side Expansion—decreased on affected side Tactile fremitus—absent	Hyperresonant	Breath sounds—usually decreased or absent; if open pneumothorax, have an amorphic quality Vocal fremitus—decreased or absent Adventitious sounds—none
Dyspnea on exertion Tachypnea Thoracic expansion diminished Cyanosis	Trachea—deviated to most affected side	Resonant to dull	Breath sounds—reduced or absent, bronchovesicular or bronchial Vocal fremitus—increased, whisper pectoriloquy may be present Adventitious sounds—rales on inspiration and expiration

nance is transmitted voice sounds as heard by the stethoscope on the chest wall. Normal vocal resonance is heard as muffled, nondistinct sounds; it is loudest medially and is less intense at the periphery of the lung. Vocal resonance is assessed if there has been any respiratory abnormality detected on observation, palpation, percussion, or auscultation. The routine utilized is the same systematic one previously utilized in the respiratory examination. The client says "one, two, three" or "ninety-nine" while the examiner surveys the thorax.

The increase in loudness and clarity of vocal resonance is termed *bronchophony*. Special vocal resonance techniques are used when resonance is increased. These include tests for whispered pectoriloquy and egophony.

Whispered pectoriloquy is exaggerated bronchophony. The client is instructed to whisper a series of words. The words as heard through the stethoscope on the chest wall are distinct and understandable.

In *egophony*, the intensity of the spoken voice, as heard through the stethoscope applied to the chest wall, is increased and the voice has a nasal or bleating quality. If the client says "e- e- e," the transmitted sound will be "a- a- a."

Decreased vocal resonance occurs in the same clinical situations as when vocal fremitus is decreased and breath sounds are absent. Vocal resonance is increased and whispered pectoriloquy and egophony may be present in any condition that causes a consolidation of lung tissue.

Respiratory distress syndrome

Despite the heavy reliance on laboratory and x-ray findings in the diagnosis of respiratory problems, the examiner can derive reasonably sound diagnostic probabilities by compiling and analyzing the physical assessment data. Table 15-5 outlines the usual assessment findings in a variety of common problems.

SUMMARY

I. Observation
   A. Thoracic configuration
      1. Anteroposterior diameter
      2. Skin and subcutaneous tissue
   B. Ribs and interspaces

   C. Respiratory pattern
      1. Accessory muscles of respiration
      2. Oxygenation
      3. Respiratory rate
II. Palpation
   A. General palpation
      1. Areas of observed abnormality
      2. Tissue and bony structures
   B. Assessment of thoracic expansion
   C. Assessment of tactile fremitus
   D. Assessment of tracheal deviation
III. Percussion
   A. Systematic survey
      1. Apices
      2. Lateral chest
      3. Posterior chest
      4. Anterior chest
   B. Diaphragmatic excursion
IV. Auscultation
   A. Systematic survey (same as for percussion)
   B. Analysis of breath sounds
   C. Identification of adventitious sounds
   D. Vocal resonance (assessed if tactile fremitus or breath sounds are increased)
      1. Test for whisper pectoriloquy
      2. Test for egophony

BIBLIOGRAPHY

Burrows, B., Knudson, R. J., and Kettel, L. J.: Respiratory insufficiency, Chicago, 1975, Yearbook Medical Publishers, Inc.

Capel, L. H.: Lung sounds: a new approach, Practitioner **219**:633, 1979.

Cotes, J. E.: Lung function: assessment and application in medicine, ed. 3, Oxford, 1979, Blackwell Scientific Publications.

Druger, G.: The chest, its signs and sounds, Los Angeles, 1973, Humetrics Corp.

Geschickter, C. F.: The lung in health and disease, Philadelphia, 1973, J. B. Lippincott Co.

Holman, C. W., and Muschenheim, C.: Bronchopulmonary diseases and related disorders, vols. 1 and 2, New York, 1972, Harper & Row, Publishers.

Kao, F.: An introduction to respiratory physiology, ed. 2, Amsterdam, 1972, Excerpta medica.

Mitchell, R. S.: Synopsis of clinical pulmonary disease, ed. 2, St. Louis, 1978, The C. V. Mosby Co.

Pulmonary terms and symbols: A report of the ACCP-ATS Joint Committee on Pulmonary Nomenclature, Chest **67**:583, 1975.

Slonim, N. B., and Hamilton, L. H.: Respiratory physiology, ed. 2, St. Louis, 1971, The C. V. Mosby Co.

16 Cardiovascular assessment: the heart and the neck vessels

This chapter covers those portions of the cardiovascular examination dealing with examination of the heart and the major neck vessels—the jugular veins and the carotid arteries. A brief review of the anatomy and physiology of the heart precedes the description of examination techniques and findings. Assessment of the peripheral pulses and blood pressure measurement, also integral components of the cardiovascular examination, are described in Chapter 7 on general assessment.

The heart

ANATOMY AND PHYSIOLOGY

In the examination of the heart and the subsequent description of findings, several anterior chest wall landmarks are important. These include the midsternal line; the midclavicular line; the anterior, middle, and posterior axillary lines; the suprasternal notch; and the ribs and intercostal spaces. The area of the chest overlying the heart and pericardium is known as the precordium. These landmarks are illustrated in Fig. 16-1.

The heart lies in the thoracic cavity within the mediastinum. The upper portion, consisting of both atria, lies at the top behind the upper portion of the body of the sternum; the lower portion, composed of both ventricles, is directed downward and toward the left. The upper portion is referred to as the base of the heart, and the lower left portion is referred to as the apex. The aorta, pulmonary arteries, and great veins are located around the upper portion, or base, of the heart.

Heart chambers

Most of the anterior cardiac surface consists of the right ventricle, which lies behind the sternum and extends to the left of it. The left ventricle lies posterior to the right ventricle and extends further to the left, thus forming the left border of the heart and making up a small portion of the anterior cardiac surface. The right atrium lies slightly above and to the right of the right ventricle, and the left atrium occupies a posterior portion of the heart (Fig. 16-2). It is the contraction and thrust of the left ventricle that produces the normal apical impulse, sometimes referred to as the point of maximum impulse, that is located at or just medial to the midclavicular line in the fifth left intercostal space.

Heart valves

The atrioventricular (AV) valves lie between the atria and ventricles; the right AV valve is the tricuspid valve, and the left is the mitral valve. The semilunar valves separate the ventricles from the great vessels, the aorta, and the pulmonary artery. On the right the pulmonic valve separates the right ventricle from the pulmonary artery, and on the left the aortic valve separates the left ventricle from the aorta. It is basically the closure of the heart valves that produces the normal heart sounds. (There is much discussion as to the actual mechanism of heart sound production; it is thought that tensing of the muscular structures and flow of blood may be involved, as well as valve closure.)

Although the four valves are actually located rather close to each other in a small area behind the sternum (Fig. 16-3, A), the areas on the chest wall where their closure is best heard are not located directly over the valves (Fig. 16-3, B). The sound produced by closure of the mitral valve is best heard at the apex, at the fifth left intercostal space in the midclavicular line; the sound produced by closure of the tricuspid valve is best heard along the lower left sternal border at the fourth left intercostal space; the sound produced by the aortic valve is heard best at the second right intercostal space at the sternal border; and the sound produced by the pulmonic valve

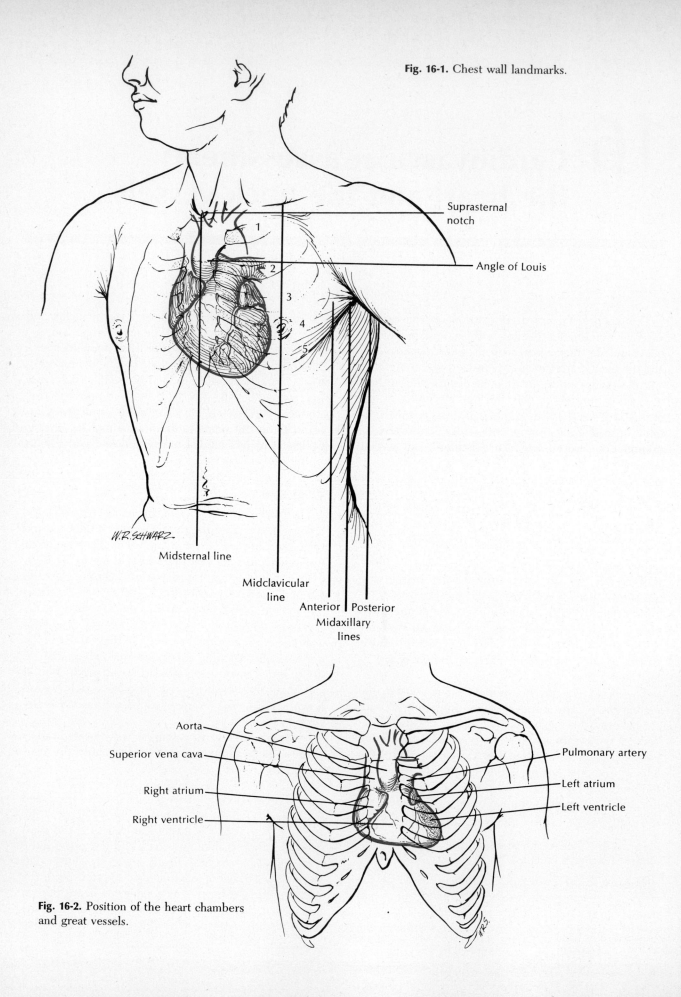

Fig. 16-1. Chest wall landmarks.

Suprasternal notch

Angle of Louis

1

2

3

4

5

W.R. SCHWARZ.

Midsternal line

Midclavicular line

Anterior Posterior

Midaxillary lines

Aorta

Superior vena cava

Right atrium

Right ventricle

Pulmonary artery

Left atrium

Left ventricle

Fig. 16-2. Position of the heart chambers and great vessels.

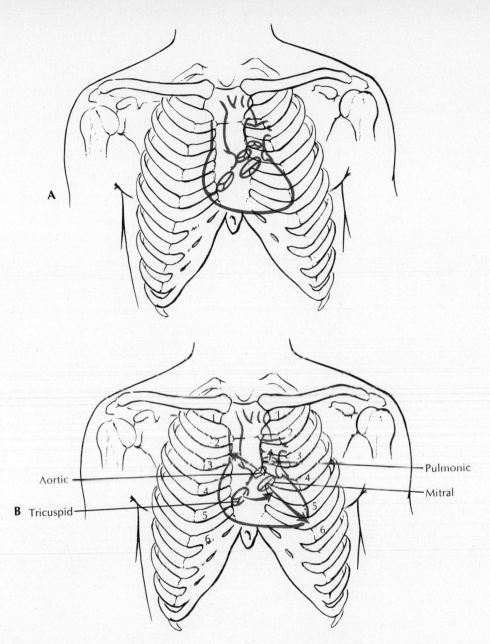

A

B   Tricuspid

Aortic

Pulmonic

Mitral

Fig. 16-3. A, Anatomical location of the heart valves. **B,** Transmission of closure sounds from the heart valves.

is best heard at the second left intercostal space at the sternal border. The ausculatory valve areas can be summarized as follows:

Mitral valve: Fifth LICS at MCL.
Tricuspid valve: Fourth LICS at LSB.
Aortic valve: Second RICS at SB.
Pulmonic valve: Second LICS at SB.

The great vessels

As mentioned earlier, the great vessels lie at the top, or base, of the heart. The pulmonary artery extending from the right ventricle bifurcates quickly into its left and right branches. The aorta, extending from the left ventricle, curves upward over the heart, then backward and down. The superior and inferior vena cava empty into the right atrium, and the pulmonary veins return blood to the left atrium. The relationship of these vessels to the heart chambers is shown in Fig. 16-4.

Pericardium

The pericardium is a tough, double-walled, fibrous sac encasing and protecting the heart. Several cubic centimeters of fluid are present between the inner

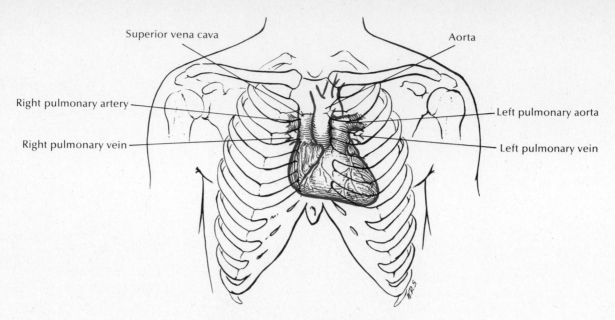

Fig. 16-4. Location of the great vessels.

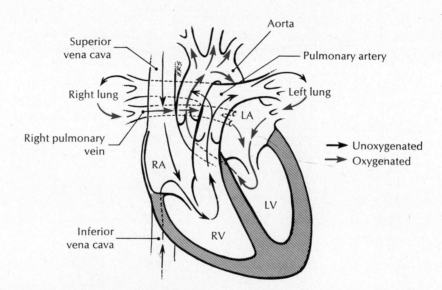

Fig. 16-5. The route of blood flow through the chambers of the heart and the great vessels.

and outer layers of the pericardium, providing for easy, low-friction movement. The outer layer of the pericardium is firmly attached to the diaphragm, sternum, pleura, esophagus, and aorta.

Variable position of the heart

The position of the heart in the thorax has a large range of normal and varies considerably with different body builds, chest configurations, and diaphragm levels. In an average-size person, the heart lies obliquely; one-third of it lies to the right of the midsternal line, and two-thirds of it lies to the left of it. In short, stocky persons the heart may tend to lie more

horizontally; in tall, slender persons it may hang more vertically.

Cycle of cardiac events

The flow of blood, movements of the chambers and valves, pressure relationships, and electrical stimulation are discussed here briefly.

The cardiac cycle may be said to begin with the return of blood from the systemic circulation via the superior and inferior vena cavae to the right atrium and with the return of oxygenated blood from the lungs via the pulmonary veins to the left atrium (Fig. 16-5). Following ventricular systole, during which

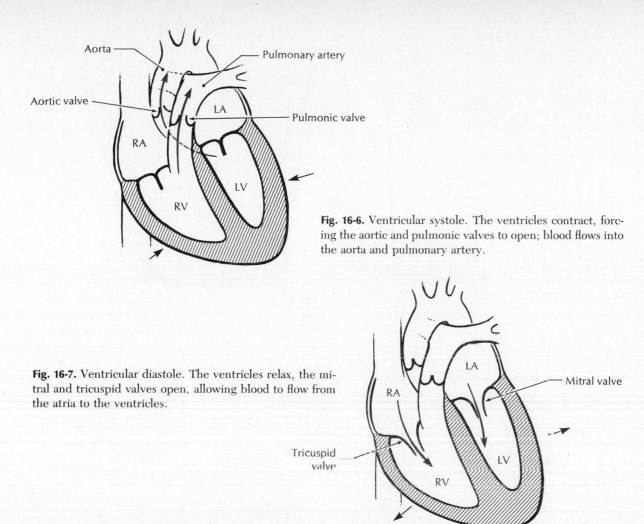

Fig. 16-6. Ventricular systole. The ventricles contract, forcing the aortic and pulmonic valves to open; blood flows into the aorta and pulmonary artery.

Fig. 16-7. Ventricular diastole. The ventricles relax, the mitral and tricuspid valves open, allowing blood to flow from the atria to the ventricles.

blood has been ejected from the ventricles, the AV valves open, allowing blood that has been collected in the atria to flow into the ventricle. Toward the end of this passive filling phase, or ventricular diastole, the atria contract, ejecting the remaining blood into the ventricles. Then ventricular contraction begins. As intraventricular pressure increases, the AV valves are forced closed, preventing regurgitation of blood to the atria and producing the first heart sound (S_1). During the early part of contraction, the volume of blood in the ventricle remains the same; this is called the period of isovolumic contraction. As the pressure continues to rise during ventricular contraction, a point is reached when the pressure in the left ventricle exceeds the pressure in the aorta; the semilunar valves are forced open, and blood is ejected into the aorta (see Fig. 16-6). (Events on the left side of the heart are used for describing the cycle. Right-sided events are similar but occur at much lower pressures.)

At the end of ejection, the ventricle relaxes, the pressure in the ventricle drops below the pressure in the aorta, and the semilunar valves snap shut, producing the second heart sound (S_2). Meanwhile, during ventricular systole the atria have been filling; as the ventricular pressure drops, the AV valves open, permitting the flow of blood into the ventricles once again (Fig. 16-7). Because of the manner in which myocardial depolarization occurs, events on the left side of the heart normally occur slightly before events on the right side. Therefore, in the production of S_1, mitral valve closure briefly precedes tricuspid valve closure. Similarly, in the production of S_2, aortic valve closure precedes pulmonic valve closure. The pressure relationships and points of valve closure are illustrated in Fig. 16-8.

Normally, ventricular systole, the contraction phase, is slight shorter than ventricular diastole, the relaxation or filling phase. At heart rates of about 120 beats per minute, the phases become nearly equal in length.

The electrical events stimulating and coordinating the mechanical events just described begin with an electrical discharge originating at the sinoatrial (SA)

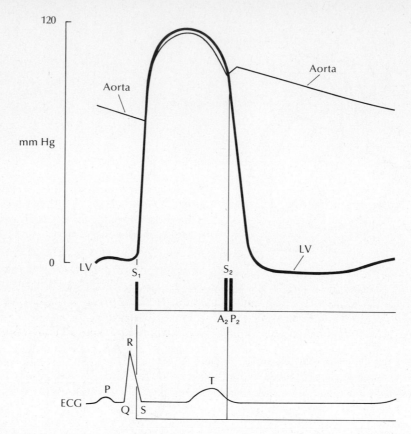

Fig. 16-8. Pressure curves of the left ventricle and aorta, S_1 and S_2, and the ECG.

node, located in the right atrium. This electrical discharge then flows through the atria, producing atrial contraction. The impulse then travels to the AV node, located in the low atrial septum, and on through the bundle of His and its branches in the myocardium, stimulating ventricular contraction. The SA node is the cardiac pacemaker, normally discharging between 60 and 100 impulses per minute. The passage of the electrical impulses is shown in the electrocardiogram (ECG) tracing below the pressure diagram in Fig. 16-8. The P wave represents spread of the impulse through the atria; the P-R interval extends from the beginning of the P wave to the beginning of the QRS complex; it represents the time taken for the original impulse to pass from the SA node, through the atria and the AV node, to the ventricles. The QRS complex represents spread of the impulse through the ventricles; and the T wave represents repolarization of the ventricles. Electrical stimulation briefly precedes the mechanical response.

Characteristics of cardiovascular sounds

All sounds, including those of cardiovascular origin, can be characterized by their frequency (pitch), intensity (loudness), duration, and their timing in the cardiac cycle. All cardiovascular sounds are of rela-

tively low frequency and require special concentration for perception by the human ear. Examples of heart sounds in the lower frequencies include the diastolic murmur of mitral stenosis and a third heart sound (S_3); the normal S_2 is of a slightly higher frequency, and the diastolic murmur of aortic or pulmonic valve insufficiency is of yet a higher frequency.

The intensity of cardiovascular sounds is widely variable. The range extends from sounds that can be heard only with great concentration and by careful "tuning in" to those that can be heard with the edge of the stethoscope barely touching the chest wall.

The duration of most cardiovascular sounds is very brief, usually much less than 1 second. In cardiac auscultation, both the duration of sounds and the periods of silence are important. Normally, S_1 and S_2 are very brief, lasting only fractions of a second; the intervals of silence, that is, systole and diastole, are longer. Diastole is longer than systole at a heart rate below 120 beats per minute; at faster rates the duration of diastole is diminished, and systole and diastole become about equal in duration.

The timing of any additional cardiac sounds is designated as occurring during either systole or diastole. Systole begins with S_1 and extends to S_2; diastole begins with S_2 and extends to the next S_1.

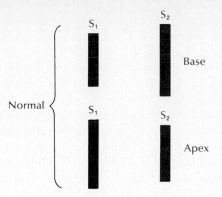

Fig. 16-9. Relative loudness of S_1 and S_2 as heard over the base and apex of the heart.

A helpful method for determining S_1 and S_2 and thus differentiating systole and diastole is to palpate the carotid pulse while auscultating the heart. The carotid pulsation and S_1 are very nearly synchronous; S_1 only briefly precedes the carotid impulse.

Heart sounds are illustrated by vertical bars on a horizontal line. The height of the bar indicates the relative loudness of the sound, and the width of the bar indicates the duration. For example, S_1 and S_2 as heard at the base and apex of the heart are illustrated as shown in Fig. 16-9.

The audibility of cardiac sounds is modified by the amount of interposed tissue between the sound at its point of origin and the outer chest wall. Large amounts of fat, muscle, or air, as in the obese, muscular, or emphysematous client, tend to dampen or diminish the heart sounds and cause them to sound more distant.

THE HEART SOUNDS

First heart sound. The AV valves are forced closed as ventricular pressure rises, producing S_1. This sequence of events is similar on both sides of the heart, but pressures and pressure gradients are much greater on the left side, and the sounds produced by left-sided events are usually louder. Events on the left side usually slightly precede those on the right side because the left ventricular myocardium begins depolarization slightly earlier. S_1 can be heard over the entire precordium but is heard best at the apex and is usually louder than S_2 there (Fig. 16-9). At the base of the heart S_1 is usually louder on the left than on the right and on both sides is quieter than S_2. Usually both components of S_1, mitral and tricuspid valve closure, are heard as one sound. As a result of slight asynchrony in valve closure, however, a split S_1 may be audible and may be heard in the area where tricuspid valve closure is best transmitted, that is, at the

fourth left intercostal space at the sternal border. Tricuspid valve closure may become louder as a result of pulmonary hypertension because of the increased right-sided pressures. Splitting of S_1 is neither as commonly nor as easily heard as splitting of S_2.

The frequency of S_1 is slightly lower than that of S_2, and its duration is slightly longer. Its occurrence can be timed with the apical impulse or with the carotid pulsation; it should not be timed with the radial pulse, because the time lapse is too great and leads to confusion.

ALTERATIONS IN THE FIRST HEART SOUND. Factors altering or influencing the loudness of S_1 may be extracardiac or cardiac. Extracardiac factors usually affect both S_1 and S_2. An increase in the amount of tissue interposed between the heart and the stethoscope, as found in obesity, emphysema, or the accumulation of pericardial fluid will diminish the intensity of both S_1 and S_2. Cardiac factors influencing the intensity of S_1 consist of the position of the AV valves at the time of ventricular contraction, the structure of the valves, and the force and abruptness of ventricular contraction. If ventricular systole begins when the AV valves are still wide open, before they have time to "drift" or "float" close together, a loud S_1 results. This situation occurs when the P-R interval is short, as accompanies hyperkinetic states such as exercise, anemia, fever, and hyperthyroidism. Conversely, a prolonged P-R interval, during which the AV valves may begin to close and ventricular contraction is delayed, may result in a faint S_1. Even with a normal P-R interval, S_1 may be diminished. With forceful atrial contraction into a noncompliant ventricle, a situation that may exist with hypertension, the pressure rise in the ventricle may cause the valve to close sooner; the valve may already be partially closed at the onset of ventricular contraction.

Changes in valve leaflet structure may alter the intensity of S_1. As a result of rheumatic fever, the mitral valve may become so fibrosed and calcified that only limited motion is possible and S_1 is diminished. However, if the valve leaflets retain some mobility, as they may with mitral stenosis, S_1 may be accentuated. Significant mitral stenosis may also increase S_1 because of the greater ventricular pressure needed to overcome the increase in atrial pressure. This produces an increased closing pressure and more abrupt closure. Abrupt ventricular contractions producing a more intense S_1 may also result from the hyperkinetic states mentioned earlier.

In the presence of a complete heart block, where the length of the P-R interval is frequently changing, variation in the intensity of S_1 will occur.

Second heart sound. As ventricular systole is completed, pressure in the aorta and pulmonary artery exceeds ventricular pressure and the semilunar valves close. Vibrations produced by closure of the aortic and pulmonic valves are primarily responsible for S_2. Closure of the aortic valve is the loudest component of S_2 at both the right and left second intercostal spaces and is referred to as A_2; the sound produced by the pulmonic valve, referred to as P_2, is normally heard only in a small area centering around the second left interspace and can be identified as separate from the component of S_2 caused by aortic valve closure only when splitting of S_2 occurs. In children and adolescents P_2 may normally be accentuated, causing an increase in S_2 heard in the pulmonic area. It should be reemphasized that A_2 and P_2 refer to the two components of S_2; they do not refer to any anatomical location on the chest wall.

S_2 is audible over the entire precordium but is best heard at the base of the heart and is louder there than S_1; at the apex it is quieter than S_1 (Fig. 16-9). S_2 marks the beginning of diastole, normally the longer interval. It is slightly higher in frequency and shorter in duration than S_1.

NORMAL PHYSIOLOGICAL SPLITTING OF THE SECOND HEART SOUND. Right ventricular systolic ejection time is very slightly longer than left ventricular systolic ejection time. Therefore, pulmonic valve closure, which marks the end of right ventricular ejection, occurs slightly later than aortic valve closure. This normal asynchrony of valve closure is increased during inspiration because of the decrease in intrathoracic pressure, which facilitates increased venous return to the right side of the heart and a further delay in pulmonic valve closure. During expiration, the disparity between left and right ejection times is decreased and splitting becomes less pronounced or nonexistent as the valves close nearly synchronously, producing a single sound (Fig. 16-10). Inspiratory splitting is commonly most marked at the peak of the inspiratory phase of respiration and is best determined during ordinary respiration. If the breath is held in inspiration, rather than sustaining the splitting, the ejection times again equalize and the split

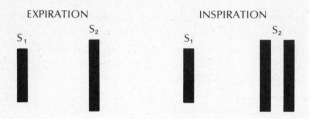

Fig. 16-10. Normal splitting of S_2.

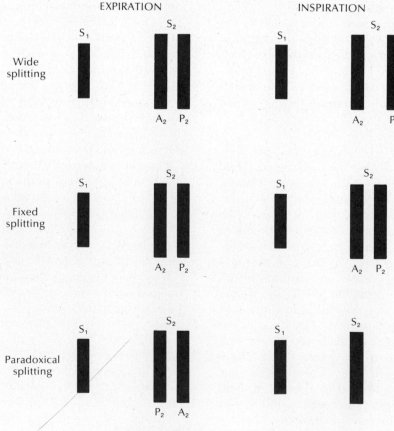

Fig. 16-11. Variations in splitting of S_2.

sound becomes single. Splitting will be evident only where pulmonic as well as aortic closure can be heard, that is, at the second left interspace.

The degree of splitting varies from one individual to another. In some individuals two distinct sounds are quite clear though very close in sequence (the splitting seems more like two parts of a single sound), whereas in others no splitting can be recognized. In some individuals clear splitting may be audible during inspiration and a very slight degree of splitting is audible during expiration.

Variations in S_2 include changes in loudness as well as variations in splitting. In general, louder closure sounds result from higher closing pressure. In systemic hypertension, for example, louder aortic closure sounds occur; S_2 may become ringing or tambourlike in quality and may become louder than S_1 at the apex. Exercise and excitement may also increase the pressure in the aorta and thus increase the aortic S_2. Conditions associated with pulmonary hypertension, including mitral stenosis and congestive heart failure, may produce an increased pulmonic S_2. A fall in systemic blood pressure, as occurs with shock, will produce a diminished aortic S_2. As was the case with S_1, pathological changes in the valves will also affect the intensity of S_2. Semilunar valves that are injured but still flexible may increase S_2, whereas injured valves that have become markedly thickened and calcified may diminish it.

Variations in splitting of S_2 include wide splitting, fixed splitting, and paradoxical splitting (Fig. 16-11). Conditions causing delayed electrical activation, on contraction or emptying, or both, of the right ventricle, for example, right bundle branch block, also cause a delay in pulmonic valve closure. Wide splitting of S_2 exists with expiration; on inspiration, the splitting is even wider. Fixed splitting is associated with large atrial septal defects. Here, pulmonic closure is delayed because with each beat, the right ventricle is ejecting a larger volume than is the left ventricle. Presumably, right-sided filling cannot be further increased by inspiration, so the split sound remains relatively fixed. In contrast to delayed closure of the pulmonic valve with its resultant wide splitting, delayed closure of the aortic valve in a left bundle branch block may result in narrowed splitting

or splitting where the normal sequence of sounds is reversed, so that pulmonic closure precedes aortic closure. This produces a paradoxical situation wherein inspiration results in the two sounds coming closer together and even fusing to a single sound and expiration results in more widely separated sounds. On expiration, pulmonic closure occurs first, followed by aortic closure; then on inspiration, when pulmonary valve closure is normally delayed, the pulmonic sound merges with the aortic sound.

Third heart sound. During diastole there are two phases of rapid ventricular filling. The first is in early diastole and is a passive, rapid filling phase. When the AV valves open, after S_2, the blood stored in the atria flows rapidly into the ventricles. This rapid distention of the ventricles causes vibrations of the ventricular walls to occur. Known as the third heart sound (S_3) (Fig. 16-12), these vibrations are low in frequency and intensity and are best heard at the apex with the bell of the stethoscope. The sound may be accentuated by having the client assume the left lateral decubitus position. This sound is commonly heard in normal children and young adults and in such instances is known as a physiological S_3. However, in other circumstances, an S_3 is abnormal. For example, in an older person with heart disease an S_3 often signifies myocardial failure. In such a case S_3 contributes to the production of a ventricular or protodiastolic gallop.

Fourth heart sound. The second phase of rapid ventricular filling occurs after the first phase of passive filling. In late diastole, with atrial systolic ejection of blood into the ventricle, the second, active rapid filling phase occurs, just before S_1. The inflow of this phase, too, may cause vibrations of the valves, supporting structures, or ventricular walls, resulting in a late diastolic filling, or fourth, heart sound (S_4) (Fig. 16-13). It may be heard physiologically, especially in a young person with a thin chest wall, but is more rare in a normal client than a physiological S_3. An abnormal S_4 results from an increased resistance to filling secondary to either a change in compliance of the ventricle or to an increase in volume. Therefore, it may be associated with hypertensive cardiovascular disease, coronary artery disease, or aortic stenosis, wherein there may be decreased left ven-

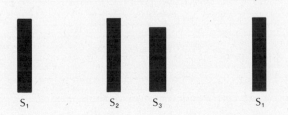

Fig. 16-12. S_3: an early diastolic sound.

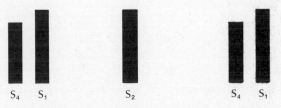

Fig. 16-13. S_4: a late diastolic sound.

tricular compliance. It may be associated with severe anemia or hyperthyroidism, wherein there is an increased stroke volume.

S_4 is also a low-frequency, low-intensity sound, heard best with the bell at the apex shortly before S_1. It may also be well heard at the base. Care must be taken not to confuse an S_4 with a split S_1. The presence of an S_4 produces a sequence of sounds known as a presystolic gallop because of its timing in the cardiac cycle.

Summation gallop. When both phases of rapid ventricular filling become audible events as an S_3 and S_4, a quadruple rhythm results. As the heart rate in-

creases and diastole become shorter, the two sounds come closer together and may be heard as one sound in diastole. Then there are three cardiac sounds: S_1 and S_2 and the summation sound of S_3 and S_4. This is known as a summation gallop.

Abnormal extra heart sounds. There are two extra heart sounds that always indicate an abnormality. Both of these sounds are produced by the opening of diseased valves. They are the opening snap of the mitral valve and the ejection click, or opening snap, of a semilunar valve. Pericardial friction rub also produces an extra cardiac sound.

OPENING SNAP OF THE MITRAL VALVE. Opening of the mitral valve, normally a silent event, may become audible if it becomes thickened or otherwise altered, as by rheumatic heart disease. This sound occurs early in diastole, is high pitched, brief, and of a snapping or clicking quality (Fig. 16-14). It is usually best heard medial to the apex and toward the lower left sternal border and may radiate toward the base. It is always associated with a good, and often accentuated, S_1. It can be differentiated from an S_3 because it occurs earlier (temporally, mitral valve opening is before ventricular filling), is sharper and higher pitched, and radiates more widely. In the pulmonic area, the opening snap must be differentiated from a split S_2. A split S_2 is best heard in the second left intercostal space, and an opening snap is best heard between the apex and the lower left sternal border. Whereas respiration affects the splitting of S_2, an opening snap is not affected by respiration and will remain at a fixed interval after the aortic component of S_2.

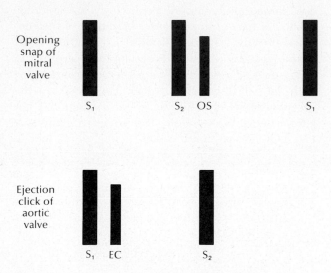

Opening snap of mitral valve

S_1 S_2 OS S_1

Ejection click of aortic valve

S_1 EC S_2

Fig. 16-14. Opening snap of the mitral valve following S_2 and ejection click of the aortic valve following S_1.

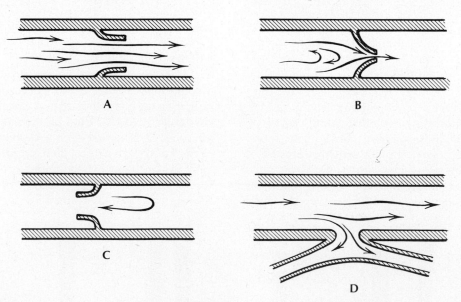

Fig. 16-15. Mechanisms of murmur production. **A,** Increased flow across a normal valve. **B,** Forward flow through a stenotic valve. **C,** Backflow through an incompetent valve. **D,** Flow through a septal defect or arteriovenous fistula.

The loudness of the opening snap is affected by the pressure in the left atrium and by the flexibility of the mitral valve. Higher left atrial pressures increase the loudness of the opening snap. Marked fibrosis and calcification of the valve decrease the mobility, and consequently, the sound produced.

EJECTION CLICK. Semilunar valve changes may also be associated with an opening sound. This sound occurs early in systole at the end of isovolumic contraction when the semilunar valves open (Fig. 16-14). The aortic ejection click, the more common of the two, is heard both at the base and at the apex and does not change with respiration. Pulmonary ejection clicks are heard best at the second left interspace, radiate poorly, and change in intensity with respiration, increasing with expiration and decreasing with inspiration.

PERICARDIAL FRICTION RUB. Inflammation of the pericardial sac causes the parietal and visceral surfaces of the roughened pericardium to rub against each other. This produces an extra cardiac sound of to-and-fro character with both systolic and diastolic components. One, two, or three components of a pericardial friction rub may be audible. A three-component rub indicates the presence of pericarditis and serves to distinguish a pericardial rub from a pleural friction rub, which ordinarily has two components. It resembles the sound of squeaky leather and is often described as grating, scratching, or rasping. The sound seems very close to the ear and may seem louder than or may even mask the other heart sounds. Friction rubs are usually best heard between the apex and sternum but may be widespread.

HEART MURMURS

A variety of conditions may result in the production of the more prolonged sound during systole or diastole known as a murmur. These are abnormal sounds produced by vibrations within the heart or in the walls of the large vessels. They tend to originate in the vicinity of the heart valve and are often best heard around the area of the valve responsible for their production.

Mechanisms of production. Three main factors related to murmur production are (1) increased flow rate of blood across normal valves, (2) forward flow through an irregular or constricted valve or into a dilated vessel or chamber, and (3) backflow or regurgitant flow through an incompetent or insufficient valve, a septal defect, or a patent ductus arteriosus (Fig. 16-15). In addition, a combination of these factors may prevail.

Murmurs are illustrated in a manner similar to the way in which they appear in a phonocardiogram, that is, with a series of vertical lines in systole between S_1 and S_2 or in diastole between S_2 and S_1. The lines are drawn in such a way as to indicate the level of, and increase or decrease in, intensity of the sound. For example, a midsystolic ejection murmur that is crescendo-decrescendo in nature, is shown in Fig. 16-16, A; a holosystolic regurgitant murmur is shown in Fig. 16-16, B.

VALVE ALTERATIONS. The adequacy of opening and closure of the valves and of the orifice size determines many of the characteristics of murmurs. Heart valves that are functioning normally and competently permit the forward flow of blood and prevent backflow or regurgitation. It is essential to understand the stations of the valves and flow patterns during systole and diastole. During ventricular systole, the mitral and tricuspid valves are closed, preventing backflow, and the aortic and pulmonic valves are open, permitting forward flow. During ventricular diastole, the mitral and tricuspid valves are open, permitting forward flow, and the aortic and pulmonic valves are closed, preventing backflow.

Stenotic valves prevent adequate forward flow; thus, a stenosed mitral or tricuspid valve interferes with normal flow during diastole, when the atrium empties blood into the ventricle. Mitral or tricuspid stenosis produces a diastolic murmur (Fig. 16-17, A). A stenosed aortic or pulmonic valve prevents adequate forward flow of blood during ventricular systole, when the blood is being forced from the ventricle into the aorta or pulmonary artery; thus, aortic (or pulmonic) stenosis produces a systolic murmur

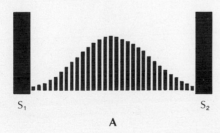

Fig. 16-16. Systolic murmurs. **A,** Crescendo-decrescendo systolic ejection murmur. **B,** Holosystolic regurgitant murmur.

(Fig. 16-17, *B*). Blood flowing through such a narrowed orifice meets resistance and produces vibrations.

Incompetent or insufficient valves fail to close completely during that phase of the cardiac cycle when their leaflets should be firmly approximated; they leave an aperture through which blood flows inappropriately back from the ventricles to the atria or from the aorta or pulmonary artery back to the ventricles.

This regurgitation, or backflow, of blood produces vibrations of the valve and of parts of the myocardium, producing a murmur. An incompetent mitral or tricuspid valve permits the inappropriate backflow of blood from the ventricle to the atrium during ventricular systole, producing a systolic murmur (Fig. 16-18, *A*). An insufficient aortic or pulmonic valve permits the backflow of blood from the aorta or pulmonary artery to the ventricle during ventricular

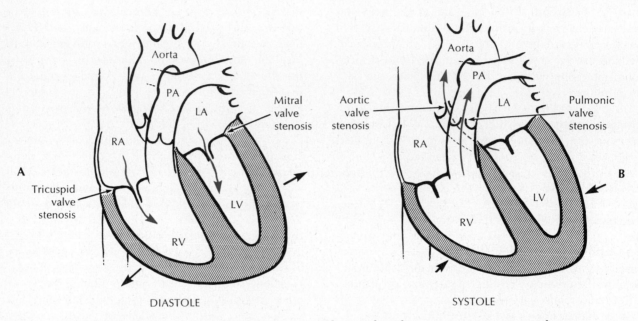

Fig. 16-17. A, Mitral or tricuspid valve stenosis produces a diastolic murmur. **B,** Aortic or pulmonic valve stenosis produces a systolic murmur.

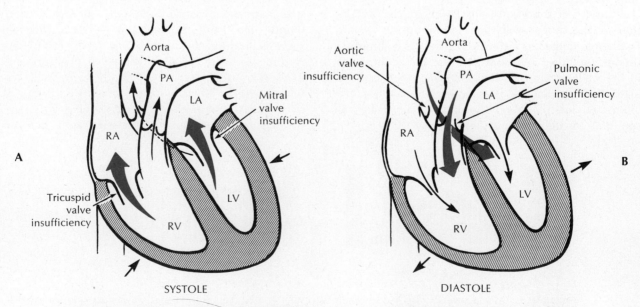

Fig. 16-18. A, Mitral or tricuspid valve insufficiency produces a systolic murmur. **B,** Aortic or pulmonic valve insufficiency produces a diastolic murmur.

diastole, producing a diastolic murmur (Fig. 16-18, *B*).

Characteristics. Murmurs are classified and described according to several characteristics, including timing (systolic or diastolic), frequency, location, intensity, radiation, quality, and effects or respiration.

TIMING. The timing of murmurs is according to their occurrence during either diastole or systole. At times, murmurs may occur during both phases of the cycle. The timing of the murmur may be further characterized as occurring during the entire phase of a cycle, or for instance, during early, mid, or late systole. Murmurs that endure throughout systole are known as holosystolic or pansystolic murmurs; the same is true for diastolic murmurs. Early diastolic murmurs are known as protodiastolic, and late diastolic murmurs are called presystolic.

In general, systolic murmurs are caused by stenosed aortic or pulmonic valves or by incompetent mitral or tricuspid valves, and diastolic murmurs are produced by stenosed mitral or tricuspid valves or by incompetent aortic or pulmonic valves. It is important to remember, however, that not all murmurs result from valve defects; they may also be produced by alteration in the velocity of flow, by changes in the vessels, and by defects in the myocardium.

FREQUENCY. The frequency, or pitch, of murmurs varies from high to low. The main determining factor is the velocity of blood flow. Generally, when the rate of flow is rapid, a high pitch results; when the velocity is slow, the pitch is low. The pitch of a murmur is described as high, medium, or low.

LOCATION. A murmur is described by means of anatomical landmarks according to where it is best heard. Some are localized to small areas, whereas others are heard over large portions of the precordium. The location of a murmur is significant in terms of its size of production. The murmurs originating from valvular alterations are usually best heard in the area to which sounds from that valve are transmitted.

INTENSITY. The loudness of a murmur is described on a scale of one to six; one is the softest, and six is the loudest. The description of each level of loudness is as follows:

Grade I: Barely audible, very faint; can be heard only with special effort.
Grade II: Clearly audible but quiet.
Grade III: Moderately loud.
Grade IV: Loud.
Grade V: Very loud; may be heard with stethoscope partly off the chest.
Grade VI: Loudest possible; audible with the stethoscope just removed from contact with the chest wall.

It is important to note that though the grading of the loudness of a murmur is helpful, it is also a rather subjective description, dependent on the auditory acuity of the listener.

The terms crescendo and decrescendo are used to describe the pattern of intensity reflecting changes in the flow rate. A crescendo-decrescendo murmur, for example, increases from quiet to louder and then decreases again, forming a diamond-shaped pattern. In the case of aortic stenosis, for example, the flow rate increases, reaches a peak, and then decreases, producing a crescendo-decrescendo systolic murmur with a rather harsh quality. The diastolic murmur of aortic insufficiency is a decrescendo, high-pitched, blowing murmur. The flow rate of blood leaking back into the ventricle from the aorta is approximately proportional to the decreasing pressure gradient between the aorta and the ventricle. Although the patterns of the various murmurs may not be that easily determined with the stethoscope, the murmurs do appear that way on the phonocardiogram.

RADIATION. Some murmurs radiate in the direction of the bloodstream by which they are produced. For example, the diastolic murmur of aortic insufficiency may be heard along the left sternal border. In this case, the blood leaks back from the aorta into the left ventricle. Other factors, such as the variation in sound transmission through various tissues, also influence radiation.

QUALITY. Several descriptive terms are often used to characterize a murmur; these include *musical*, *blowing*, *harsh*, and *rumbling*. For example, the murmur of aortic stenosis may be described as harsh; the murmur of mitral insufficiency may be described as a long, blowing sound; and the murmur of mitral stenosis tends to be of a low, rumbling quality.

EFFECT OF RESPIRATION. As mentioned earlier in this chapter, certain events on the right side of the heart are affected by respiration due to intrathoracic pressure changes and right-sided filling changes. Murmurs that originate on the right side of the heart are also subject to influence by these factors. The murmur of tricuspid insufficiency, for example, may increase with inspiration.

Systolic murmurs. Murmurs occurring during ventricular systole are a result of increased flow rate across normal valves or abnormal blood flow patterns across (1) the inflow tract (the AV valves), (2) the outflow tract (the semilunar valves), or (3) ventricle to ventricle (ventricular septal defect). Incompetent or insufficient AV valves do not prevent backflow of blood from the ventricles to the atria during ventricular systole and thus produce systolic regurgitant murmurs. These murmurs may last during all or part of systole. Insufficient AV valves may be the result of rheumatic valvular disease or papillary muscle dysfunction. Stenotic aortic or pulmonic valves make it difficult for the blood to flow from the ventricles to the aorta and pulmonary arteries during ventricular systole and thus produce systolic ejection murmurs. Because there is a short time interval between the closing of the AV valves (S_1) and the opening of the semilunar valves, systolic ejection murmurs will begin after the first heart sound, reflect the ejection of blood during systolic contraction, and end before the second heart sound. They are often called *midsystolic ejection murmurs.* Some systolic ejection murmurs are innocent, while others are pathological. Abnormalities causing a turbulent flow across these semilunar valves may be the result of dilation of narrowing of the pulmonary artery or aorta, aortic or pulmonic valvular or subvalvular stenosis, or high output states such as anemia, thyrotoxicosis, or pregnancy.

Innocent systolic ejection murmurs are commonly heard in children and adolescents. They occur within a normal cardiovascular system and are not the result of any recognizable heart pathology. They reflect the contractile force of the heart that results in greater blood flow velocity during early or midsystole. Smaller chest measurements in the young also increase the audibility of these murmurs. Innocent systolic ejection murmurs may also occur with other high output states including pregnancy, anxiety, anemia, fever, and thyrotoxicosis.

Innocent systolic ejection murmurs are heard best with the bell held lightly against the chest in the pulmonic area (second left intercostal space) or around the lower left sternal border toward but not including the apex. They may radiate to the neck. They tend to be short, rarely extending through the entire systole, but begin shortly after the first heart sound and end well before the second heart sound (Fig. 16-19). They are softer than Grade III, of medium pitch, and have a blowing quality. They increase in held expiration and may be heard best when the client is in the recumbent position. The heart sounds remain unchanged.

These murmurs must be differentiated from pathological systolic ejection murmurs that may result from

mild aortic or pulmonic stenosis or atrial or ventricular septal defects. A pansystolic or late systolic murmur indicates an organic problem.

Stenosis or obstruction of the aortic or pulmonic valves or deformity of the valves or adjacent vessels, the aorta and the pulmonary arteries, may cause *midsystolic ejection murmurs.* The murmur of aortic valve stenosis or deformity begins after the first heart sound when the pressure in the ventricle is high enough to open the aortic and pulmonic valves, ends before the aortic and pulmonic valves close (S_2), and, thus, has a crescendo-decrescendo or diamond shape (Fig. 16-16, *A*). With less aortic deformity present, the murmur reaches a peak earlier in systole. The murmur is medium-pitched and harsh, may be faint to loud, and is best heard with the diaphragm at the first or second right intercostal spaces with the client sitting up and leaning forward with the breath held in expiration. If the murmur is loud it may be heard over the entire thorax and is often accompanied by a thrill. The existence of emphysema may cause the murmur to seem faint. Arythmias, shock, or heart failure cause the murmur to decrease in loudness.

The systolic murmur of aortic stenosis may be associated with a diminished second heart sound, an early ejection click, the thrusting sustained apical impulse of left ventricular hypertrophy, a slowly rising carotid pulse wave, and narrow pulse pressure. Rheumatic fever is the most common cause of aortic stenosis and valve deformity. Congenital deformities are another cause.

A basal systolic murmur associated with hypertension and arteriosclerotic roughening of the aorta and aortic valve are commonly heard in older people. This murmur is best heard at the second right intercostal space, is of medium pitch, has a rough quality, is usually not very loud, and is often transmitted to the apex. It is best heard with the client sitting up and leaning forward. Either the diaphragm of the bell may be used. The second heart sound is of normal or increased loudness.

Murmurs that occupy all of systole are called *holosystolic* or *pansystolic.* They are associated with turbulent blood flow from a high pressure to a low pressure area, such as occurs with regurgitation from a ventricular chamber to an atrial chamber across an incompetent AV valve, or with leakage from the left to the right ventricle through a ventricular septal defect. The murmur will continue as long as there is a sufficient pressure gradient across the incompetent orifice beginning with the first heart sound and lasting up to the second heart sound (Fig. 16-16, *B*).

Mitral regurgitation may result from malfunction of a number of structures including the valve ring or leaflets, the chordae tendineae, papillary muscles,

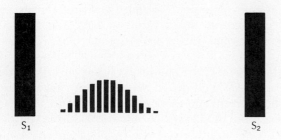

S_1 S_2

Fig. 16-19. Innocent systolic murmur.

and wall of the ventricle. This murmur is usually loudest at the apex; as the loudness increases, the sound may be transmitted to the axilla. It has a high pitch and a blowing quality and is best heard with the diaphragm of the stethoscope. If the murmur is faint, it may be heard better after exercise in the left lateral position or sitting up and leaning forward to the left. This murmur does not increase with inspiration. The first heart sound may be normal, increased, or decreased depending on the condition of the mitral valve. The second sound may be normal or increased. A third heart sound may be present.

The murmur resulting from a ventricular septal defect is best heard at the fourth, fifth, and sixth interspaces at the left sternal border. It may radiate over the precordium but not to the axilla. It is high pitched, harsh, and may be accompanied by a thrill. The size of the septal defect and the resistance in the pulmonary vessels determine the direction and velocity of flow during systole. With a small defect there may be greater resistance to pressure than with a larger defect, thus producing a louder holosystolic murmur.

Diastolic murmurs. Diastole is normally free of murmurs; therefore, a murmur heard during this portion of the cardiac cycle is almost always indicative of heart disease. Causes of diastolic murmurs include insufficiency of the aortic or pulmonic valves, permitting abnormal backflow from the aorta and pulmonary arteries, or stenosis of the mitral or tricuspid valves, preventing an adequate forward flow of blood.

Diastolic murmurs may occur in early, middle, or late diastole. Early diastolic murmurs are usually produced by aortic or pulmonic valvular insufficiency or dilation of the valvular ring. Mid and late diastolic murmurs are usually caused by narrowed, stenosed, mitral or tricuspid valves that obstruct the inflow or by an increased flow rate across the valves.

Aortic valve insufficiency is associated with a diastolic regurgitant murmur that begins with the aortic component of the second heart sound at the time the aortic pressure exceeds the ventricular pressure. As the pressure in the aorta falls and the ventricles fill, the murmur decreases in intensity. This murmur be-

gins loud in early diastole and then fades (Fig. 16-20), giving it a decrescendo character. It is high pitched and blowing and is best heard with the diaphragm with the client leaning forward in deep expiration. If the aorta is dilated, it may be loudest in the second right intercostal space. It may be accompanied by an aortic systolic murmur caused by increased flow, a third heart sound, a sustained thrusting apical impulse, and wide pulse pressure. The second heart sound may be increased or diminished depending on the condition of the aortic valve. This murmur is most commonly caused by rheumatic heart disease, but it may be caused by congenital valve disease.

Mitral stenosis is associated with a diastolic murmur that is produced by the flow of blood from the left atrium into the left ventricle and is most intense when that flow is greatest, that is, after the opening of the mitral valve. This is a middiastolic murmur. As the degree of stenosis increases, contraction of the auricle may force more blood across the valve and produce a presystolic phase of this diastolic murmur (Fig. 16-21). When faint or moderately loud, the murmur is low pitched and rumbling; as it becomes louder, it becomes more harsh. This murmur is generally heard only over a small area just medial to and above the apex, or at the point of maximum impulse. It may be best heard when the client turns from the supine to the left lateral position. Exercise will increase the intensity of the murmur. The bell of the stethoscope should be held very lightly on the skin; heavy pressure on the bell may obliterate the sound of a faint middiastolic murmur.

Mitral stenosis is frequently associated with an increased first heart sound; there may also be an opening snap of the mitral valve. However, the first sound may be decreased and the opening snap absent if the valve and chordae tendineae are very fibrosed.

The *venous hum* is a continuous low-pitched hum heard over the neck in many children and some adults. It is produced by turbulent blood flow in the internal jugular veins. The venous hum is best heard over the supraclavicular spaces, more commonly on the right. It is heard better with the client sitting up and is accentuated on the right by having the cli-

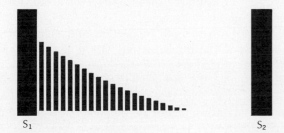

Fig. 16-20. The murmur of aortic valve insufficiency.

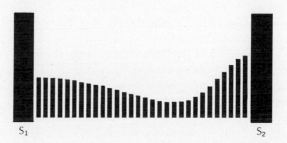

Fig. 16-21. The murmur of mitral stenosis.

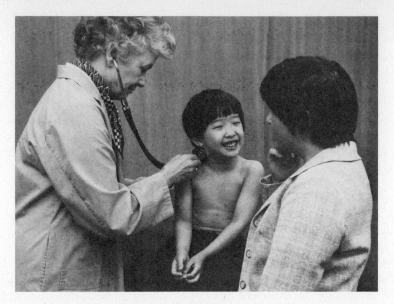

Fig. 16-22. Venous hum. The venous hum is a continuous, low-pitched hum heard over the neck in many children; it is often best heard over the right supraclavicular space.

ent turn his head to the left and slightly upward (Fig. 16-22). The hum is loudest in diastole. Because it is produced by blood flow in the jugular veins, it can be stopped by applying gentle pressure over the internal jugular in the neck between the trachea and the sternocleidomastoid muscle at about the level of the thyroid cartilage.

EXAMINATION

The division of the cardiac examination into the techniques of inspection, palpation, and auscultation is useful. Because the findings of inspection and palpation are closely related and complementary to one another, these techniques are discussed together. Auscultation provides much valuable information about cardiac dynamics, but the practitioner must be cautious not to apply the stethoscope to the chest wall before performing the visual and palpatory examinations.

Several environmental considerations are basic to the cardiac examination. A quiet room is essential, because cardiac sounds are for the most part subtle and low pitched and are thus easily missed if outside noises prevail. A good light source that can be directed tangentially across the chest wall is important for adequate observation.

Examination of the precordium is most effectively performed with the examiner standing on the client's right side. The complete assessment requires that the client be examined in the sitting, supine, and left lateral recumbent positions. Whereas inspection and palpation are performed primarily with the client in the supine position, thorough auscultation should be performed with the client in all three positions. Sitting forward and lying in the left lateral position both bring various parts of the heart closer to the chest wall, thus enhancing certain auditory findings.

It is important to remember that examination of the peripheral pulses, including the radial, brachial, femoral, popliteal, dorsalis pedis, and posterior tibial, is an essential component in the assessment of the cardiovascular system. Also included are the assessment of the abdominal aorta and assessment of the blood pressure in the upper and lower extremities in the sitting, standing, and lying positions. These components may be assessed during this portion of the examination or integrated with other portions of the physical examination.

Inspection and palpation

Inspection and palpation of the precordium should be performed before the stethoscope is applied to the chest wall. It is sometimes tempting to use the stethoscope as the only means of assessing findings over the precordium, but much valuable information can be gained by using visual and tactile assessment procedures. These findings will enhance and may augment the auditory findings.

The purpose of both inspection and palpation is to determine the presence and extent of normal and abnormal pulsations over the precordium. These pulsations may be manifested as the apex beat (or apical impulse) or as heaves or lifts of the chest; they provide some reflection of myocardial and hemodynamic activity. Inspection and palpation together provide a useful method of assessing left, right, and

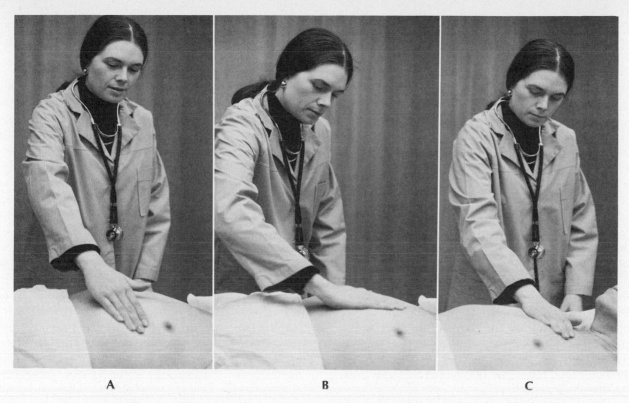

A   B   C

Fig. 16-23. Palpation of the precordium. The examiner palpates three areas of the precordium: **A,** over the apex; **B,** over the left sternal border; **C,** over the base of the heart.

combined ventricular hypertrophy. The visibility and palpability of those movements are affected by the thickness of the chest wall and by the type and amount of tissue through which the vibrations must travel.

INSPECTION

The chest wall and epigastrium are inspected while the client is in the supine position. A tangential light is helpful for observing subtle movements of the chest. The examiner stands to the client's right side and observes the chest for size and symmetry and then for any pulsations, lifts or heaves, or retractions. The location and timing of all impulses should be noted.

Apical impulse. The thrust of the contracting left ventricle may produce a visible pulsation in the area of the midclavicular line in the fifth left intercostal space. This is the normal apical impulse, and it is visibly evident in about half of the normal adult population. It occurs nearly synchronously with the carotid impulse, and simultaneous palpation of a carotid artery is helpful in identifying it.

When visible, the apical impulse helps to identify an area very near the cardiac apex, thus giving some indication of cardiac size. In the case of left ventricular hypertrophy or dilatation, or both, as may occur with systemic hypertension, the apical impulse may be located more laterally or inferiorly, or both; for example, it may be located at the left anterior axillary line in the sixth left intercostal space.

Retractions. A slight retraction of the chest wall just medial to the midclavicular line in the fifth interspace is a normal finding. Marked or actual retraction of the rib is abnormal and may result from pericardial disease. Left ventricular hypertrophy is often accompanied by a systolic thrust, producing a "rocking" movement.

Heaves or lifts. When the work and forcefulness of the right ventricle is greatly increased, a diffuse lifting impulse is often produced along the left sternal border with each beat. This is referred to as a lift or heave; these terms are generally used interchangeably.

PALPATION

The technique of palpation builds on and expands the findings gleaned from inspection. The entire precordium is palpated methodically, beginning at the apex, moving to the left sternal border, and then to the base of the heart (Fig. 16-23). Other areas may also be included if indicated, including the left axillary area, the epigastrium, and the right sternal border. During palpation the examiner is searching for the apical impulse at or near the apex and for any abnormal heaves, thrills, or retractions elsewhere on the precordium, indicating cardiac hypertrophy, dilatation, or murmurs. The abnormal flow of blood resulting in an audible murmur may also result in the palpatory sensation known as a thrill. It is rather like a rushing sensation beneath the fingers and has been likened to the feeling transmitted to the fingers placed over the larynx of a purring cat. As with inspection, the shape and thickness of the chest wall are important variables.

The client is in the supine position for this portion of the cardiac examination. The examiner should take adequate time to "tune in" or "warm up" to movements over the precordium, because many are faint and subtle and are perceived only after a "warming up" period. It is important to describe pulsations in relation to their timing in the cardiac cycle. This is facilitated by simultaneously palpating the carotid pulsation with the left hand while palpating the precordium with the right. All pulsations should be described in terms of their location in an interspace and their distance from the midsternal, midclavicular, or axillary lines.

Apical impulse. Although the thrust noted over the apex of the heart is sometimes referred to as the point of maximum impulse (PMI), this term is not recommended, because the actual point or area of maximum impulse may or may not be located over the apical area. The term apical impulse is preferred. The presence, location, size, and character of the apical impulse should be assessed. The apical impulse is palpable in about half the normal adult population.

Standing to the right of the client and using the finger tips and palmar aspect of his right hand, the examiner palpates first over the apex, particularly in the area of the fifth interspace in the midclavicular line. Normally, the apical impulse is palpable in or just medial to the midclavicular line and is felt as a faint, short-duration, localized tap less than 2 cm in diameter. On occasion the apical impulse may be normally located lateral to the midclavicular line, for example, in association with a high diaphragm, as occurs with pregnancy. The outward movement of the normal impulse is not excessively forceful and is palpable only during the first part of systole. The amplitude of the apical impulse may seem to be increased in normal individuals with thin chest walls. Turning the client to the left lateral position may cause a normal impulse to seem abnormal in both amplitude and duration, since the apex is brought closer to the chest wall, thus accentuating its activities. In obese persons or those with an increased anteroposterior chest diameter, the apical impulse is not likely to be palpable. Conditions such as anxiety, anemia, fever, and hyperthyroidism may produce an

apical impulse increased in force and duration. Normally, systolic ejection may be associated with a slight retraction of the lower left parasternal area.

Apex area: left ventricular hypertrophy. Hypertrophy of the left ventricle typically produces an abnormally forceful and sustained outward movement during ventricular systole. In addition, the apex impulse may be displaced laterally and downward and may be increased in size. For example, the apical impulse may be found 4 cm lateral to the midclavicular line in the sixth intercostal space and may be 4 cm in diameter.

Generally, the degree of displacement of the impulse correlates with the extent of cardiac enlargement. In addition to an alteration in location and size, the impulse may become more diffuse and palpable in more than one interspace; also, the amplitude or forcefulness may be increased. Displacement tends to be maximal when there is both dilatation and hypertrophy. Conditions associated with a volume overload, such as mitral and aortic regurgitation and left-to-right shunts, tend to produce such dilatation and hypertrophy. Hypertrophy of the left ventricle without dilatation, as may occur with aortic stenosis and systemic hypertension, results in an apical impulse that is increased in force and duration but not necessarily displaced laterally; it may still be located in the midclavicular line. In some persons with left ventricular hypertrophy, the increased force and prolonged duration of the apical impulse produces a lifting sensation under the examiner's fingers.

Left sternal border: right ventricular hypertrophy. Right ventricular hypertrophy is less common than left ventricular hypertrophy. It may be detected on palpation as a diffuse, lifting systolic impulse along the lower left sternal border. This finding may be associated with a systolic retraction at the apex, resulting from displacement and rotation of the left ventricle posteriorly by the enlarged right ventricle. A diffuse lift, or heave, along the lower left sternum is associated, for example, with pulmonary valve disease, pulmonary hypertension, and chronic lung disease. A thrill may also be palpated in this area and is associated with ventricular septal defects. The palmar aspect of the examiner's right hand is placed over the left sternal border.

Base of the heart. The examiner's right hand then rests over the base of the heart at the second left and right intercostal spaces at the sternal borders and feels for pulsations, thrills, or the vibrations of semilunar valve closure. Normally, the base is fairly "quiet" to palpation.

Aortic stenosis may be associated with a thrill palpable in the first and third right interspaces as well as in the second right interspace. In persons with systemic hypertension, it may be possible to palpate the accentuated vibration of aortic valve closure at the time of S_2.

Pulmonic valve stenosis may be associated with a thrill in the second and third left interspaces near the sternum. In persons with pulmonary hypertension, pulsations may be palpated in the same area. The most common causes of abnormal pulsations in the pulmonary artery area are increases in pressure or flow in the pulmonary artery, such as in pulmonary hypertension or atrial septal defect. In some normal people with thin chest walls, it is possible to palpate a brief, slight pulsation in this area. Conditions such as anemia, fever, exertion, and pregnancy would accentuate this pulsation.

Percussion

The technique of percussion is of limited value in cardiac assessment. In the past, percussion was used to determine the borders of cardiac dullness, but the actual size of the heart is much more accurately determined by a chest roentgenogram, and ventricular hypertrophy is better determined by combined inspection and palpation. Variations in chest wall configuration and the type and amount of interposed tissue, such as air or fat tissue, alter and limit the accuracy of this procedure. The value of percussion is further limited in the assessment of right ventricular enlargement, since this condition causes substernal and anteroposterior enlargement, which is not accessible to the percussion note.

Auscultation

The stethoscope is a device that gathers and slightly amplifies sound before it is transmitted to the ears. A comfortable and properly fitting stethoscope is essential for adequate auscultation. Although the selection of proper earpieces for comfort and the best sound transmission is a matter of individual preference, there are several general guidelines that are useful in making that selection. The earpieces should be large enough to provide a snug fit in the external canal and to block out extraneous room noises. Enough tension should be present to hold the earpieces tightly in place. The rigid metal tubing leading to the earpieces should be bent so as to angle in the same direction as the ear canal, that is, forward. The flexible tubing may be made of rubber or plastic, and it should be thick enough to keep out extraneous sounds; it should also be reasonably short, about 1 foot, because added length dampens the sound and decreases the efficiency of the stethoscope in transmitting higher frequencies.

The stethoscope chestpiece should be equipped with both a bell and a diaphragm, each of which selectively transmits different frequencies of sound. The valve facilitating a change between the two should be tight fitting, permitting a change without the admission of outside sound. The diaphragm accentuates the higher-frequency sounds. It should be made of a fairly rigid substance and should be pressed firmly against the skin during auscultation, further enhancing faint, high-frequency sounds. In contrast to the diaphragm, the bell brings out the low-frequency sounds and filters out the high-frequency ones. It should be placed very lightly on the chest wall with just enough pressure applied to seal the edge. If greater pressure is applied to the bell against the chest wall, the skin becomes a relatively tight diaphragm, filtering out the lower-pitched sounds. Alternating the application of light and heavy pressure to the bell may be a helpful maneuver when listening to low-pitched murmurs or filling sounds. Most low-pitched sounds are diastolic filling sounds or murmurs and are often best heard with the client lying down, since orthostatic pooling on standing may cause such sounds to diminish in intensity. Although heart sounds are referred to as being of "high" or "low" frequency, these terms are relative. All heart sounds are generally low pitched (low frequency) and are in a range ordinarily difficult for the human ear to hear. Thus, any technique that improves audibility should be carefully utilized.

Satisfactory auscultation requires a quiet room; mechanical and conversational noises must be minimized. The room should be comfortably warm for the client so that shivering and subsequent muscular noises are avoided. The anterior chest should be exposed to the waist. The examining table should be adequately large for the client to change positions from sitting to supine to left lateral recumbent with ease. Auscultation in only one position is not adequate.

A systematic method of auscultation is essential; all precordial areas and each sound and pause must be attended to. One recommended system is to begin at the apex and "inch" the stethoscope toward the left sternal border and up the sternal border to the second left and then to the second right intercostal space. Another method consists of beginning the examination at the base of the heart at the second right intercostal space, where S_2 is always the loudest of the two heart sounds. This is particularly helpful if the heart sounds are heard as nearly equal in intensity at the apex. Auscultation should be performed using both the bell and the diaphragm and should cover the entire precordium and areas of radiation, such as the axillary area or carotid arteries, when indicated.

In each area examined, the examiner listens selectively to each component of the cardiac cycle; as with palpation, this usually requires a period of "warming up" or "tuning in" to the various cardiac

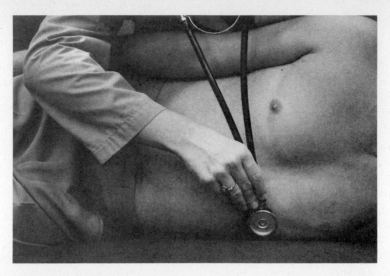

Fig. 16-24. With the client lying in the left lateral position, the examiner listens for low-pitched diastolic sounds using the bell of the stethoscope.

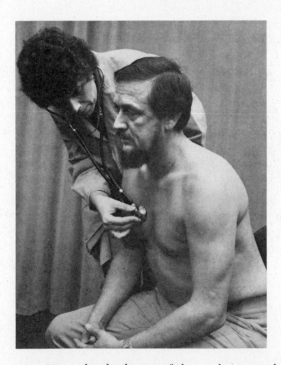

Fig. 16-25. Using the diaphragm of the stethoscope while the client leans forward and holds his breath in full expiration, the examiner listens for high-pitched murmurs at the base of the heart.

events. First, the examiner notes the rate and rhythm of the heartbeat. Then, at each auscultatory area, he concentrates initially on S_1, noting its intensity and variations therein, possible duplication, and the effects of respiration. The examiner then selects out S_2 and focuses on the same characteristics. Next, he concentrates on systole, then on diastole, listening first for any extra sounds and then for murmurs. The

examiner must listen selectively for each component; it is impossible to listen for everything at once.

If the initial part of the examination was done on the client lying in a supine position, the client is now asked to roll to his left side; the examiner applies the bell lightly at the apex and listens for the presence or absence of low-frequency diastolic sounds, such as a filling sound or a mitral valve murmur (Fig. 16-24). The client is then asked to sit up and lean slightly forward. Pressing the diaphragm firmly against the chest, the examiner listens at both the second left and the second right intercostal spaces at the sternal border to detect the presence or absence of high-pitched diastolic murmurs of aortic or pulmonic valve insufficiency (Fig. 16-25). Listening is done during normal respiration and then with the client's breath held in deep expiration.

Neck vessels

The vascular structures of the neck accessible for and included in the cardiovascular examination are the jugular veins and the carotid arteries. Examination of these vessels provides information on local states and also reflects the activity of the heart. The jugular veins are observed for pulse waves and pressure level; the carotid arteries are examined by inspection, palpation, and auscultation to assess the characteristics of their pulsations.

JUGULAR VEINS

Venous pulse waves and venous pressure are assessed at the external and internal jugular veins. The external jugular veins lie superficially and are visible above the clavicle close to the insertion of

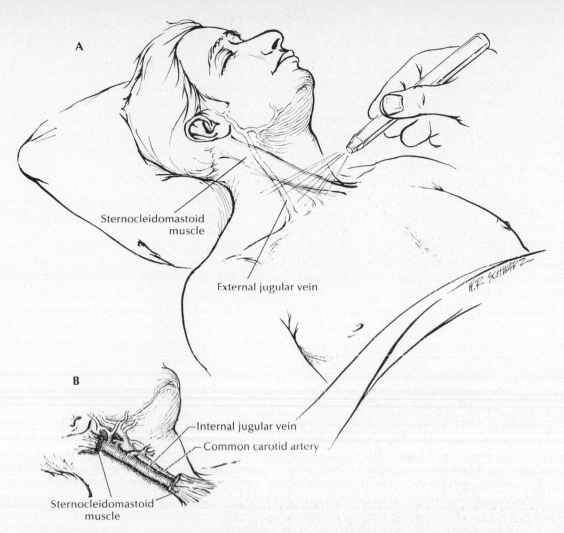

Fig. 16-26. A, Inspection of the external jugular vein. **B,** Location of the internal jugular vein and common carotid artery.

the sternocleidomastoid muscles. The internal jugular veins are larger and lie deep to the sternocleidomastoid muscles near the carotid arteries; reflection of their activity may be visible on the skin overlying these vessels. Blood from the jugular veins flows directly into the superior vena cava. Fig. 16-26 illustrates the location of the external and internal jugular veins.

Venous return and the filling volume are important determinants of cardiac performance. These cannot be directly assessed on physical examination, but a general estimate can be made from observation of the jugular veins. The veins leading to the right side of the heart may be thought of as a system of distensible tubes with partially competent valves. Therefore, some judgment of the filling pressure of the heart may be made by observing the pressure level and the waveforms transmitted from the heart. Observation of the two components of pressure level and pulse waves in the veins gives an indication of the dynamics of the right side of the heart.

When the normal person is in the sitting position, no jugular venous pulsations are visible; with the trunk elevated 45 degrees from horizontal, the jugular venous pulse does not rise more than 1 to 2 cm above the level of the manubrium. When the normal person is in the reclining position, the venous pulse becomes evident because gravity no longer prevents backflow from the heart and the veins become filled.

In the examination of the jugular veins the client is in the supine position. If this position is uncomfortable, the client's trunk may be elevated to a 45-degree angle. If the veins are very distended, it is best to examine them with the client in a sitting position. The veins or venous pulsations are more readily visible if the client's neck is slightly turned away from the side being examined, and the veins are observed with tangential lighting so that small shadows are cast. Clothing should be removed from the neck and upper thorax so that there is no constriction. The head and neck may rest comfortably on a pillow, but the neck should not be sharply flexed.

Jugular venous pulse

The normal venous pulse consists of three positive components—the a, c, and v waves—and two negative slopes—the x and y descents (Fig. 16-27). The a wave is frequently the highest part of the total pulse wave and is produced by atrial contraction. As the right atrium contracts, ejecting blood into the right ventricle, there is also a brief backflow of blood into the vena cava. This retrograde pulse wave is reflected in the jugular veins as the a wave. This wave occurs just before S_1; if an S_4 is present, it occurs at the peak of the a wave.

Two simultaneous events contribute to the production of the c wave: the impact of the adjacent carotid artery pulsation and the retrograde transmission of a pulse wave, caused by right ventricular systole and bulging of the closed tricuspid valve. The c wave occurs at the end of S_1.

The tricuspid valve remains closed during ventricular systole while blood from the systemic circulation continues to fill the vena cava and the right atrium. The increased volume in these structures leads to a pressure increase reflected in the jugular veins as the v, or passive filling, wave. This wave reaches a peak during late ventricular systole. Following this, the pressure in the right atrium begins to fall as the bulging of the tricuspid valve decreases, first during relaxation of the right ventricle and then as the tricuspid valve opens.

The x descent following the c wave is produced by downward displacement of the base of the ventricles (including the tricuspid valve) during ventricular systole and by atrial diastole. The y descent following

the v wave is produced by the opening of the tricuspid valve and the subsequent rapid flow of blood from the right atrium to the right ventricle.

It is usually possible to discern the three positive and two negative waves of the jugular venous pulse when the heart rate is below 90 beats per minute and the P-Q interval is normal. At more rapid heart rates, there is often a fusion or overlapping of some of the waves and analysis of the waveform is difficult.

ABNORMALITIES OF WAVES

The a wave. The a wave, which may be the highest or most pronounced of the three positive waves, is increased when it becomes more difficult for the contracting right atrium to empty into the right ventricle. For example, in tricuspid valve stenosis, the a wave is more prominent. When there is right ventricular enlargement resulting from severe pulmonary stenosis or pulmonary hypertension and the right atrium must contract more forcefully to fill it, an enlarged a wave also results.

Irregularly enlarged a waves result from a complete AV block. When the atrium contracts against a closed tricuspid valve, giant (cannon) a waves are produced. In ventricular tachycardia, the cannon waves may occur irregularly, since the cause of their production—simultaneous atrial and ventricular systole and a closed tricuspid valve—does not accompany each beat.

The x descent, and c and v waves. When the tricuspid valve is insufficient, backflow of blood from the right ventricle to the right atrium occurs during ventricular systole. This causes the x slope to become

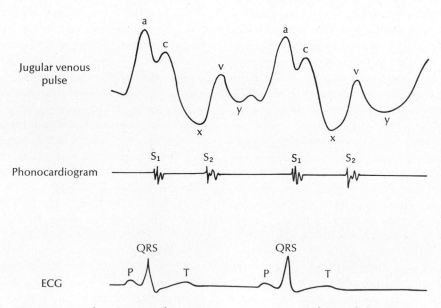

Fig. 16-27. Jugular venous pulse waves in relation to S_1 and S_2 and the ECG.

obliterated or replaced by the positive waves, the c and v waves, which then form the c-v wave. Thus, with the obliteration of a negative slope and the accentuation of the two positive waves, a large jugular venous pulse wave is produced. The c-v wave may become so enlarged as to resemble exaggerated arterial pulsations. Tricuspid insufficiency may be organic, resulting from rheumatic heart disease; or it may be produced in clients with generalized cardiac failure, wherein the right ventricle becomes so dilated that the tricuspid ring is stretched and regurgitation ensues.

The y descent. The tricuspid valve opens shortly after S_2, and the rapid filling phase of ventricular diastole begins. The characteristics of the y descent depend on several factors, including pressure and volume circumstances in the great vessels, the right atrium, and the right ventricle, and resistance to flow across the tricuspid valve. Tricuspid stenosis, therefore, would produce a slow y descent because it presents obstruction to right atrial emptying. In clients with severe heart failure in which the venous pressure is extremely high, a sharp, exaggerated y wave is produced.

DIFFERENTIATION FROM CAROTID ARTERIAL PULSATIONS

Because the internal jugular vein lies deep to the sternocleidomastoid muscle and close to the carotid artery, its pulsations may be confused with those produced by the common carotid artery. There are several means of differentiating these pulsations.

Quality and character of the pulse. In normal sinus rhythm, the jugular venous pulse has three positive waves and the carotid pulse has one positive wave. Usually, the venous pulse waves are more undulating than the brisk arterial waves. The examiner may be assisted in differentiating the two by palpating the carotid pulse on one side of the neck and observing the jugular venous pulse on the other.

Effect of respiration. With normal inspiration, intrathoracic pressure decreases, blood flow into the right atrium increases, and the level of the pulse wave in the neck veins descends. The opposite occurs during expiration. Respiration does not have this effect on the carotid pulsations.

Effect of changing position. Pulsations in the neck veins become more prominent when the client assumes the recumbent position and less prominent when the client is in the sitting position. Carotid pulsations are not affected by posture.

Effect of venous compression. The pulsations of the jugular veins are rather easily eliminated by applying gentle pressure over the vein at the base of the neck above the clavicle. This blocks the retrograde trans-

mission of the venous pulse wave, leaving only the arterial pulsations.

Effect of abdominal pressure. Pressure applied by the examiner's hand over the client's abdomen may cause an increased prominence of the venous pulsations. The examiner presses, using the palm of his hand and applying moderately firm pressure over the upper right quadrant of the abdomen for 30 to 60 seconds. In normal persons there is slight, if any, increase in the venous pulsations. However, if there is right-sided heart failure, the jugular venous pulsations and distention may markedly increase as venous return to the heart is increased. Normally this maneuver produces no change in the carotid pulsations.

Jugular venous pressure

The level of the column of blood in the jugular veins reflects the volume and pressure circumstances on the right side of the heart. Both the external and internal jugular veins can be assessed. Although other mechanical techniques are available for the evaluation of venous pressure, inspection on physical examination remains a useful and reliable maneuver.

In a normal client examined in the supine position, full neck veins are normally visible. When the normal person is examined with the thorax elevated to a 45-degree angle from horizontal, the venous pulses should ascend no more than a few millimeters above the clavicle. With markedly elevated venous pressure, the neck veins may be distended as high as the angle of the jaw, even when the person is in the upright sitting position. The height of venous pressure may be estimated by measuring the distance that the veins are distended above the manubrium sterni.

The examiner should inspect the veins on both

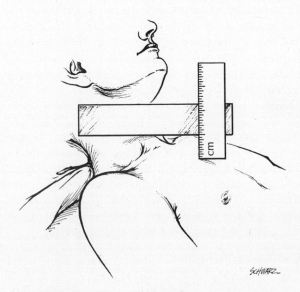

Fig. 16-28. Measurement of jugular venous pressure.

sides of the neck. When the venous pressure is generally increased, distention is noted on both sides; unilateral distention may occur as a result of kinking in the left innominate vein in some older clients. It may be necessary to change the position of the client in order to view the jugular venous pulse and pressure most clearly. The sternal angle, or angle of Louis, is used as a reference point. The vertical distance between the sternal angle and the highest level of the jugular pulsations is measured and recorded in centimeters (Fig. 16-28). The lower the client's head must be placed before the pulsations are visible, the lower the pressure; the higher the client's head must be placed before the upper level of the pulsations can be identified, the higher the venous pressure. Venous pressures greater than 3 to 4 cm above the sternal angle are abnormal. The level to which distention is observed and the position of the client should be noted.

Elevation of venous pressure may be an indication of congestive heart failure, constrictive pericarditis, or obstruction of the superior vena cava. The most common cause of elevated venous pressure is failure of the right ventricle secondary to left ventricular failure. As described earlier, the effect of applying increased abdominal pressure may increase the amount of venous distention in the presence of right-sided heart failure.

CAROTID ARTERIES

The techniques of inspection, palpation, and auscultation are utilized in examining the carotid arteries. The neck is observed for unusually large or bounding carotid pulses. The carotid arterial pulses are then palpated bilaterally, as are all the pulses, for rate, rhythm, equality, amplitude, and contour. The examiner palpates with his forefinger below and just medial to the angle of the jaw (Fig. 16-29). Only one side is examined at a time in order to avoid excessive carotid sinus massage, thus preventing unnecessary slowing of the pulse, and to avoid further embarrassment of borderline circulation in older clients. The head should be rotated slightly toward the side being examined in order to relax the sternocleidomastoid muscle. The heart sounds may be used as reference points, and simultaneous auscultation of the heart is then helpful. S_1 and the carotid impulse are very nearly simultaneous events. The carotid arteries are auscultated with the bell of the stethoscope for bruits indicating local obstruction or for the sound of transmitted cardiac murmurs.

Carotid arterial pulse

The carotid arteries are the best arteries in which to assess several characteristics of the arterial pulse, for example, whether the force is strong or weak, the

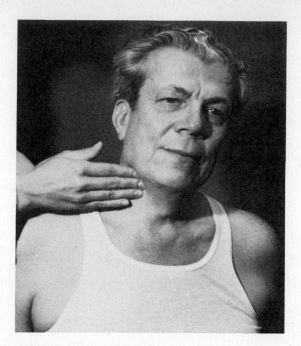

Fig. 16-29. The examiner palpates the carotid pulse below and just medial to the angle of the jaw.

rise and collapse rapid or slow, and the impulse double or single in nature.

The normal carotid pulse consists of a single positive wave followed by a dicrotic notch (Fig. 16-30). The upstroke is smooth and rapid, the summit is dome shaped, and the downstroke is less steep than the upstroke. The dicrotic notch on the downstroke may not be palpable or may be only slightly palpable. It is often definitely felt in the otherwise normal client during exercise, excitement, or fever.

The size or amplitude of the arterial pulse is determined by a variety of factors, including left ventricular stroke volume and ejection rate, peripheral resistance or distensibility, and pulse pressure. Clinically, abnormalities of the pulse size may be divided into two groups: exaggerated, or hyperkinetic, pulses and weak, or hypokinetic, pulses. During palpation, the examiner may gain an impression of the height of the pulse and the rate of change on the upstroke and downstroke.

Situations associated with a widened arterial pulse pressure—an increased stroke volume and a decreased peripheral resistance—produce a hyperkinetic carotid pulse. The pulse may be large and strong with a normal contour (bounding pulse), or it may be characterized by a markedly high and rapid upstroke (water-hammer pulse) or by an extremely rapid downstroke (collapsing pulse). In the latter two cases, the peak of the pulse is short and rapid. The hyperkinetic pulse may be produced as the result of hyperdynamic or high-output states, such as occur with anxiety, exercise, fever, or pregnancy;

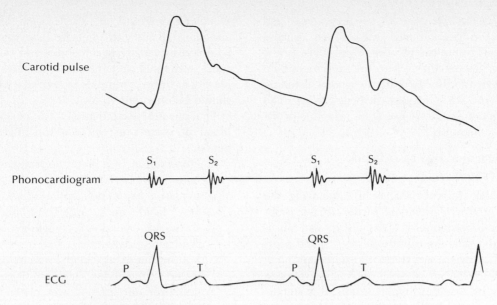

Fig. 16-30. The carotid pulse wave in relation to S₁ and S₂ and the ECG.

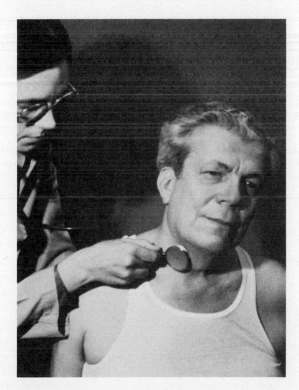

Fig. 16-31. The examiner listens with the bell of the stethoscope for bruits over the carotid artery.

as the result of hyperthyroidism or anemia; or as the result of abnormally rapid runoff of blood from the arterial system, such as occurs with abnormal shunting of blood (patent ductus arteriosus or septal defects) or with aortic insufficiency. Aortic insufficiency is a common organic cause of the hyperkinetic pulse in adults. With severe regurgitation, the pulse is described as water hammer and collapsing; a large volume of blood is rapidly ejected from and then returns to the left ventricle across the incompetent valve. Another cause of the hyperkinetic pulse in adults is a complete heart block with bradycardia and increased stroke volume.

The hypokinetic carotid pulse is associated with conditions wherein there is a diminished stroke volume of the left ventricle, increased peripheral vascular resistance, a narrowed pulse pressure, or resistance to flow across the cardiac valves. Examples of causes of a hypokinetic pulse include left ventricular failure resulting from myocardial infarction, constrictive pericarditis, and moderate or severe valvular aortic stenosis. In aortic stenosis, the pulse may demonstrate a slow upstroke, a delayed peak, and a small volume.

Pulses with double, rather than single, pulsations may be produced by combined aortic stenosis and insufficiency (pulsus bisferiens) or by lowered peripheral resistance and lowered diastolic pressure (dicrotic pulse).

A pulse that occurs at regular intervals but varies in amplitude (pulsus alternans) is produced by alterations in left ventricular contractile force, as may occur with left ventricular failure. Premature ventricular contractions coupled with previous normal beats produce a bigeminal pulse; that is, every alternate beat is premature.

Auscultation

Several conditions may produce a palpable carotid thrill associated with an audible bruit. These conditions include local obstruction of a carotid artery, a jugular vein–carotid artery fistula, and a high-output state, such as occurs with severe anemia and thyrotoxicosis. Aortic valvular stenosis may cause a thrill to be referred to the carotid arteries. The bruits are heard by placing the bell of the stethoscope on the skin overlying the carotid artery and listening while the client holds his breath (Fig. 16-31). The bell of the stethoscope is used because the bruits are low-pitched sounds.

Cardiovascular findings associated with hypertension

To assist the student-clinician in organizing the examination around a prevalent cardiovascular problem, the various components of the history and physical examination of a client with elevated blood pressure, or hypertension, are presented here. Although approximately 90% of persons with hypertension have primary or essential hypertension, it is important to rule out potentially curable secondary causes; findings indicative of those causes are also included here.

Many persons with elevated blood pressure have no observable symptoms related to that abnormality, and it may be identified during a routine examination. Others, however, do describe one or several symptoms, most commonly a headache, which may be present on awakening and subside after the individual has been up for some time. Other early symptoms include lightheadedness, dizziness, tinnitus, fatigue, weakness, nervousness, flushing sensations, and epistaxis. Later symptoms of hypertension are attributable to the effects of sustained high blood pressure on the heart, eyes, cerebral circulation, and kidneys. These symptoms may include, for example, dyspnea, orthopnea, paroxysmal nocturnal dyspnea, palpitations, chest pain, edema, eye fatigue, blurred vision, headache, weakness, numbness, tingling of the hands and feet, polyuria, nocturia, and flank pain.

The examiner should inquire about the presence of any of these symptoms. The client should also be asked about any family history of hypertension, the use of steroids, and, with women, the use of oral contraceptives or any previous hypertension associated with pregnancy.

Secondary causes of hypertension include coarctation of the aorta, primary hyperaldosteronism, Cushing's syndrome, pheochromocytoma, and renal vascular disease. Symptoms related to these causes include: history of leg fatigue with coarctation of the aorta; episodes of muscular weakness, polyuria, nocturia, polydipsia and intermittent paresthesias with primary aldosteronism; alteration of sexual function (amenorrhea, impotence), emotional lability, weakness, and backache with Cushing's syndrome; weight loss, palpitations, headache, nervousness, sweating,

blanching, coldness of skin, nausea, vomiting, and abdominal pain with pheochromocytoma; and flank pain and urinary tract infections and symptoms with renal and renal vascular disease. A careful history for any of these symptoms of secondary hypertension should be obtained.

The physical examination of a person with high blood pressure must include the following components:

1. Observation of general appearance—facial and body expression. Is nervousness, anxiety, or a plethoric expression apparent? Are the round face, head, neck, and trunk obesity, purple striae, or ecchymosis suggestive of Cushing's syndrome present?
2. Measurement of blood pressure in both arms in the sitting, lying, and standing positions and measurement of blood pressure in the lower extremities. A rise in the diastolic pressure when the client changes from the supine to the standing position suggests essential or renal arterial hypertension. Blood pressure that is lower in the legs than in the arms suggests coarctation of the aorta.
3. Examination of the retina. The status of the retina is one of the best indications of the duration and prognosis of the hypertension. Narrowing of the arterioles and an increased light reflex on them may be among the earliest manifestations of hypertension (see color plate of eye). Later, arteriovenous compression may be present. Small, well-defined exudates and isolated hemorrhages may accompany a more benign phase of hypertension. More hemorrhages and soft, poorly defined exudates indicate more severe hypertension. Papilledema (swelling of the optic nerve head) indicates a serious stage of the hypertension.
4. Palpation and auscultation of the carotid arteries for bruits, which give evidence of stenosis or occlusion.
5. Examination of the precordium for evidence of left ventricular hypertrophy, cardiac decompensation, or murmurs. Observe and palpate for lifts and heaves; auscultate for an increased second heart sound, for the presence of third and/or fourth heart sounds, and for murmurs. Coarctation of the aorta may give rise to a systolic murmur and it may be accompanied by aortic valvular disease that may be associated with an ejection click and murmurs of either aortic stenosis or regurgitation.
6. Examination of the lungs for evidence of congestion.
7. Examination of the abdomen by auscultation for

bruits originating in stenotic renal arteries. These bruits may have both systolic and diastolic components and are best heard just to the right or left of the midline above the umbilicus. The abdomen should also be examined by palpation for a pulsating abdominal aneurysm and for enlarged kidneys associated with polycystic renal disease.

8. Palpation of the femoral pulses. A decrease in amplitude and/or a delay in the pulse may accompany coarctation of the aorta.

9. Performance of a neurological examination to search for evidence of cerebrovascular disease (for specifics see Chapter 20 on the neurological examination).

SUMMARY

I. Measure blood pressure in both arms and, if indicated, legs

II. Examine heart
   A. Inspect anterior chest wall
   B. Palpate precordium
      1. Apex
      2. Left sternal border
      3. Base
      4. Other areas as indicated, e.g., right sternal border
   C. Auscultate heart sounds in sitting, supine, and left lateral recumbent positions
      1. Apex
      2. Along left sternal border
      3. Second left intercostal space
      4. Second right intercostal space

III. Examine neck vessels
   A. Jugular veins
      1. Observe jugular venous pulsations
      2. Observe jugular venous pressure
   B. Carotid arteries
      1. Observe carotid arterial pulsation
      2. Palpate carotid pulses, one at a time
      3. Auscultate carotid arteries

IV. Palpate peripheral pulses, including temporal, radial, femoral, popliteal, dorsalis pedis, and posterior tibial (assessment of these pulses may be integrated with other portions of the physical examination.)

V. Palpate and auscultate the abdominal aorta

BIBLIOGRAPHY

Ayres, S. M., Gregory J. J., and Buehler, M. E., editors: Cardiology: a clinicophysiologic approach, New York, 1971, Appleton-Century-Crofts.

Burch, G. E.: A primer of cardiology, Philadelphia, 1971, Lea & Febiger.

Butterworth, J. S., and others: Cardiac auscultations, New York, 1960, Grune & Stratton, Inc.

Carson, P.: Cardiac diagnosis, New York, 1969, McGraw-Hill Book Co.

Examination of the heart (series of four), New York, 1967, American Heart Association.

Fowler, N. O.: Physical diagnosis of heart disease, New York, 1962, MacMillan, Inc.

Friedburg, C. K.: Diseases of the heart, ed. 3, Philadelphia, 1966, W. B. Saunders Co.

Hurst, J. W., editor: The heart, ed. 3, New York, 1974, McGraw-Hill Book Co.

Ravin, A.: Auscultation of the heart, Chicago, 1958, Yearbook Medical Publishers, Inc.

Selzer, A.: Principles of clinical cardiology, Philadelphia, 1975, W. B. Saunders Co.

17 Assessment of the abdomen

Abdomen

Although physical assessment of the abdomen includes all of the four methods of examination (inspection, auscultation, percussion, and palpation), palpation is the technique most useful in detecting abdominal pathological conditions. Inspection is done first, followed by auscultation, since the movement or stimulation by pressure on the bowel occasioned by palpation and percussion are known to alter the motility of the bowel and generally to heighten the sounds.

The only special equipment necessary for examination of the abdomen is a stethoscope; a metal, cloth, or plastic ruler or tape measure that will not stretch; a skin-marking pencil; examining table and light; small pillows; and drapes to cover the client.

INSPECTION

The optimal position of the patient for inspection of the abdomen is supine with the abdominal muscles as relaxed as possible. Tension in these muscles is best avoided by placing the client's arms comfortably at his sides as opposed to extending them upward, as in placing them behind the head. Contraction of the abdominal muscles may be further avoided by placing a small pillow beneath the knee to aid in maintaining the legs in slight flexion. Also, a small pillow placed beneath the head may add to the comfort of the client.

The room should be sufficiently warm that the draped client does not shiver, thereby tensing the abdominal wall. A further advantage may be obtained by instructing the client to relax and to breathe quietly and slowly through the mouth. Explanation of the entire examination prior to beginning and support during the examination may help to ease tension.

The entire abdomen must be free of clothing. An examination gown may be folded up over the chest, or a small towel may be used to cover the breasts of women. A sheet may be folded downward to the level of the mons.

A single source of light is used in inspection of the abdomen (Fig. 17-1). The light may be directed at a right angle to the long axis of the client or may be focused lengthwise over him, shining from the foot to the head. The examiner assumes a sitting position, *generally at the right side of the client;* the examiner's head is only slightly higher than the client's abdomen. The resultant shadow will be high, so that even small changes in contour will be highlighted, thereby increasing the likelihood of detection of a pathological condition. The examiner should carefully focus attention on the abdomen to accurately describe the presence or absence of symmetry, distention, masses, visible peristaltic waves, and respiratory movements. If the presence of peristalsis is in question, the examiner should carefully study the abdomen for several minutes.

The client is instructed to take a deep breath, forcing the diaphragm downward and decreasing the size of the abdominal cavity. In this manner, masses such as the enlarged liver or spleen are made more obvious. The rectus muscles (Fig. 17-2) are prominent landmarks of the abdominal wall. Diastasis recti abdominis is a separation of rectus abdominis muscles. The separation may be palpated and may be observed as a ridge between the muscles when the intraabdominal pressure is increased by raising the head and shoulders. The defect does not pose a threat to the functions of the abdominal structures. Diastasis recti abdominis generally occurs as a result of pregnancy or marked obesity.

The examiner should then inspect the abdomen from a standing position at the foot of the bed or examining table. Asymmetry of the abdominal contour may be more readily detected from this position.

Anatomical mapping

Definitive description of signs and symptoms of the abdomen is facilitated through two commonly used methods of subdivision. The most frequently used method divides the abdomen into four quadrants (Fig. 17-3). An imaginary perpendicular line is

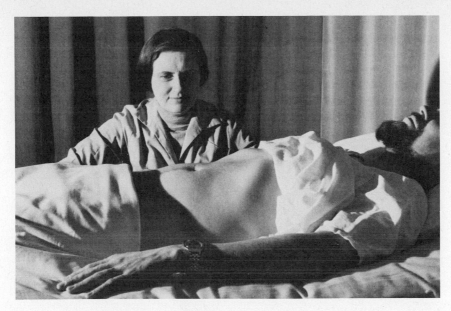

Fig. 17-1. Inspection of the abdomen with the examining light focused to provide the greatest amount of contrast for the abdominal terrain.

dropped from the sternum to the pubic bone through the umbilicus, and a second line is dropped at a right angle to the first through the umbilicus.

For the most part, abdominal structures will be located in these quadrants as shown on p. 351.

Loops of the small bowel are found in all four quadrants. The bladder and the uterus are located at the lower midline.

The second method of establishing zones of the abdomen results in nine sections (Fig. 17-4). This is accomplished by dropping two imaginary vertical lines from the midclavicles to the middle of Poupart's (inguinal) ligament, analogous to the lateral borders of the rectus abdominis muscles. At right angles to these lines, two imaginary parallel lines cross the border of the costal margin and the anterosuperior spine of the iliac bones. Essentially, the abdominal structures correlate with the zones shown in the lower left column.

Certain anatomical structures have been used as landmarks to facilitate the description of abdominal signs and symptoms (Fig. 17-5). The following landmarks have been useful for this purpose: the ensiform (xiphoid) process of the sternum, the costal margin, the midline—drawn from the tip of the sternum through the umbilicus to the pubic bone, the umbilicus, the anterosuperior iliac spine, Poupart's (inguinal) ligament, and the superior margin of the os pubis.

Abdominal structures protected by the rib cage that are examined in health assessment are the liver, stomach, and spleen (Fig. 17-6). These structures are evaluated by palpation and percussion.

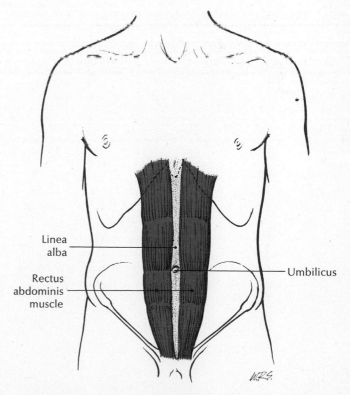

Linea alba

Rectus abdominis muscle

Umbilicus

Fig. 17-2. Rectus abdominis muscles. Separation of these muscles is called diastasis recti and may be detected by observation or palpation.

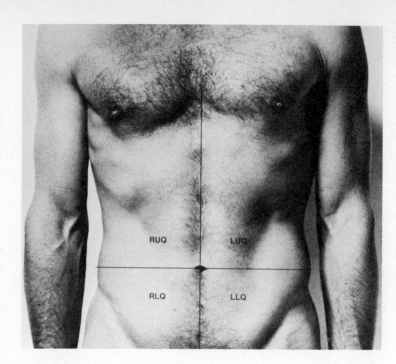

Fig. 17-3. The four quadrants of the abdomen. (From G. I. series; physical examination of the abdomen, part 1, Inspection, Richmond, Va., 1969, A. H. Robins Co.)

Fig. 17-4. The nine regions of the abdomen. *1*, Epigastric; *2*, umbilical; *3*, hypogastric (pubic); *4* and *5*, right and left hypochondriac; *6* and *7*, right and left lumbar; *8* and *9*, right and left inguinal. (From G. I. series; physical examination of the abdomen, part 1, Inspection, Richmond, Va., 1969, A. H. Robins Co.)

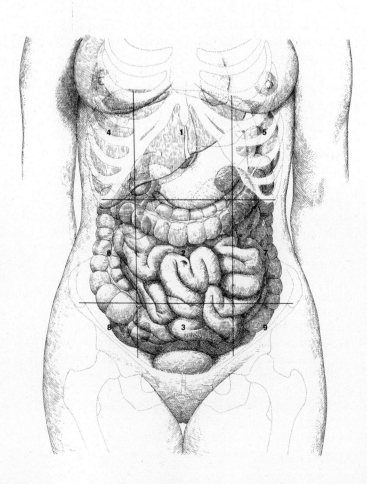

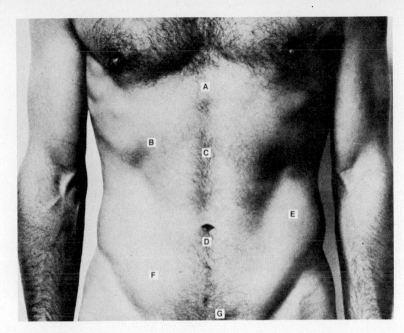

Fig. 17-5. Landmarks of the abdomen. *A*, Ensiform (xiphoid) process of the sternum; *B*, costal margin; *C*, midline; *D*, umbilicus; *E*, anterosuperior iliac spine; *F*, Poupart's ligament; *G*, superior margin of the os pubis. (From G. I. series; physical examination of the abdomen, part 1, Inspection, Richmond, Va., 1969, A. H. Robins Co.)

Right upper quadrant	Left upper quadrant
Liver and gallbladder	Left lobe of liver
Pylorus	Spleen
Duodenum	Stomach
Head of pancreas	Body of pancreas
Right adrenal gland	Left adrenal gland
Portion of right kidney	Portion of left kidney
Hepatic flexure of colon	Splenic flexure of colon
Portions of ascending and transverse colon	Portions of transverse and descending colon

Right lower quadrant	Left lower quadrant
Lower pole of right kidney	Lower pole of left kidney
Cecum and appendix	Sigmoid colon
Portion of ascending colon	Portion of descending colon
Bladder (if distended)	Bladder (if distended)
Ovary and salpinx	Ovary and salpinx
Uterus (if enlarged)	Uterus (if enlarged)
Right spermatic cord	Left spermatic cord
Right ureter	Left ureter

Right hypochondriac	Epigastric	Left hypochondriac
Right lobe of liver	Pyloric end of stomach	Stomach
Gallbladder	Duodenum	Spleen
Portion of duodenum	Pancreas	Tail of pancreas
Hepatic flexure of colon	Portion of liver	Splenic flexure of colon
Portion of right kidney		Upper pole of left kidney
Suprarenal gland		Suprarenal gland

Right lumbar	Umbilical	Left lumbar
Ascending colon	Omentum	Descending colon
Lower half of right kidney	Mesentery	Lower half of left kidney
Portion of duodenum and jejunum	Lower part of duodenum	Portions of jejunum and ileum
	Jejunum and ileum	

Right inguinal	Hypogastric (pubic)	Left inguinal
Cecum	Ileum	Sigmoid colon
Appendix	Bladder	Left ureter
Lower end of ileum	Uterus (in pregnancy)	Left spermatic cord
Right ureter		Left ovary
Right spermatic cord		
Right ovary		

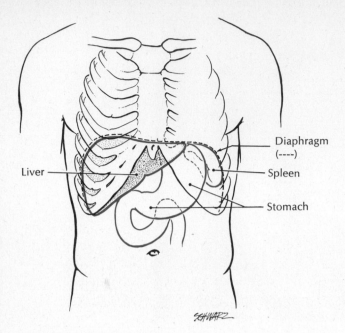

Fig. 17-6. Abdominal structures protected by the rib cage. The liver, stomach, and spleen are examined by palpation and percussion.

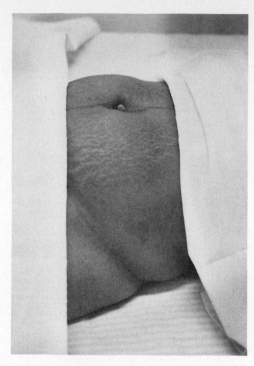

Fig. 17-7. Striae of the abdominal wall resulting from the stretching of the skin from pregnancy.

Skin

The abdomen is an especially valuable area for observation of the skin since it encompasses a relatively large expanse of skin. Inspection of the abdominal skin for pigmentation, lesions, striae, scars, dehydration, general nutritional status, and venous patterns may yield valuable information about the client's general state of health.

Pigmentation. Because the skin of the abdomen is frequently protected from the sun by clothing, it may serve as a baseline for comparison with the pigmentation of the more tanned areas. Jaundice is more readily observed in this less-exposed skin. Irregular patches of faint pigmentation may be due to von Recklinghausen's disease.

Lesions. The observation of skin lesions is of particular significance since gastrointestinal alterations are frequently associated with skin changes.

Generally, the skin lesions are secondary to gastrointestinal disease. However, skin lesions and gastrointestinal disease may arise from the same cause. They may also occur without interrelationship.

Although the presence of small, hard, painless nodules over a wide area of the abdomen may be due to metastasis of malignancy, they are generally not the result of carcinoma of the abdominal viscera.

Tense and glistening skin is often correlated with ascites or edema of the abdominal wall.

Striae. Linea albicantes, or striae, are atrophic lines or streaks that may be seen in the skin of the abdomen following such rapid or prolonged stretching of the skin that the elastic fibers of the reticular layer of the cutis are disrupted. Striae of recent origin are pink or blue in hue but progress to a silvery white color. Striae occurring as a result of Cushing's disease, however, remain purple. The stretching of abdominal skin may occur as a result of pregnancy (Fig. 17-7), an abdominal tumor, ascites, or obesity.

Scars. Inspection of the abdomen for scars may yield valuable data concerning previous surgery or trauma. The size and shape of scars are best described through the use of a drawing of the abdomen on which the landmarks or quadrants are shown and the dimensions noted in centimeters, as in the following:

If the cause of the scar was not elicited in the history, the information is sought during inspection. The fact that the client has experienced a previous surgery should alert the examiner to the possibility that adhesions may be present.

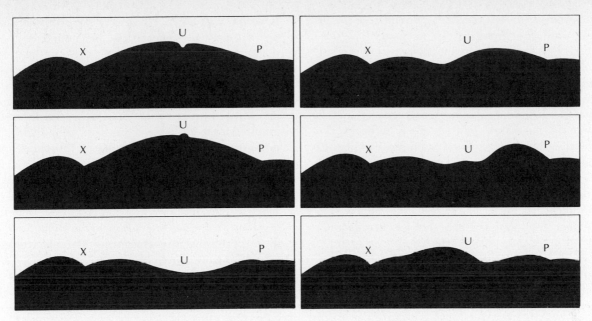

Fig. 17-8. Abdominal profiles. **Left. Top,** Generalized distention, with umbilicus inverted: obesity or recent distention from gas. **Middle,** Generalized distention with umbilicus everted, chronic ascites, tumor, or umbilical hernia. **Bottom,** Scaphoid abdomen from malnourishment. **Right. Top,** Distention of lower half: ovarian tumor, pregnancy, or bladder. **Middle,** Distention of lower third: ovarian tumor, uterine fibroids, pregnancy, or bladder. **Bottom,** Distention of upper half: carcinomatosis, pancreatic cyst, or gastric dilatation. *X,* xiphoid; *U,* umbilicus; *P,* pubis. (From G. I. series; physical examination of the abdomen, part 1, Inspection, Richmond, Va., 1969, A. H. Robins Co.)

Deep, irregular scars may indicate burns. Some individuals produce a dense overgrowth of fibrous tissue in the healing process. This overgrowth is called a keloid and consists of large, essentially parallel bands of dense collagenous material, separated by bands of cellular fibrous tissue. Keloid formation most frequently occurs following a traumatic injury or burn. Increased prevalence of keloid formation has been noted in black individuals and those of Asian extraction.

Contour

Contralateral areas of the normal abdomen are symmetrical in contour and appearance. The contour of the normal abdomen is described as flat, rounded, or scaphoid. Contour is a description of the profile line from the rib margin to the pubic bone, viewed from a right angle to the umbilicus with the client in a recumbent position (Fig. 17-8).

A flat contour is one wherein the abdominal wall is viewed as an essentially horizontal plane from the rib margins to the pubic bone. The flat contour is seen in the muscularly competent and well-nourished individual.

A rounded contour is the description given the convex profile made by the abdominal wall to the horizontal plane. With the individual in the recumbent position, the maximum height of the convexity is at the umbilicus. However, when the individual stands, the convexity has its greatest height between the umbilicus and the symphysis pubis because of the pull of gravity. The rounded abdomen is normal in the infant or toddler, but in the adult it is generally due to poor muscle tone or excessive subcutaneous fat deposits, or both. The rounded abdomen is often called the "spare tire" or "bay window" of middle age.

A scaphoid contour depicts a concave profile to the horizontal plane and may be seen in thin clients of all ages. The scaphoid contour reflects a decrease in fat deposits in the abdominal wall, as well as a relaxed or flaccid abdominal musculature.

If an umbilical or incisional hernia or diastasis recti abdominis is suspected, the client is instructed to raise his head from the pillow, increasing the intra-abdominal pressure, which may cause the hernia to protrude. The rectus muscles will contract, and a separation will be revealed.

Distention. Distention is the term used for unusual stretching of the abdominal wall. The presence of distention generally implies disease and therefore warrants further investigation. *Asymmetrical distention* of the abdominal wall may be due to hernia, tumor, cysts, or bowel obstruction. A mnemonic device for classifying the six common causes of distention are fluid, flatulence, fat, feces, fetus, and fibroid tumor.

Generalized, or *symmetrical, distention* of the abdomen with the umbilicus in its normal inverted position is generally due to obesity or recent pressure of fluid or gas within the hollow viscera. If the umbilicus is observed to be everted (umbilical hernia), ascites or underlying tumor may be the cause. Ovarian tumor, distended bladder, or pregnancy may be suspected if the distention is confined to the area between the umbilicus and the symphysis pubis; distention of the lower third of the abdomen suggests ovarian tumor, uterine fibroid tumor, pregnancy, or bladder enlargement (Fig. 17-8). Possible causes of distention of the upper half of the abdominal wall include pancreatic cyst or tumor and gastric dilatation.

Movement

Respiratory movement. Observation of respiratory movement has more significance in the male client since the female client manages gaseous exchange mainly with costal movement. On the other hand, the male client evidences essentially abdominal respiratory movement at rest. Peritonitis or other abdominal infection and disease may limit this abdominal respiratory action in the male client.

Whereas abdominal breathing is the mode in the child who is less than 6 or 7 years of age, the presence of abdominal respiratory movements in an older child may indicate respiratory problems. The absence of abdominal respiratory movements in the child who is less than 6 is suggestive of peritoneal irritation. Retraction of the abdominal wall on inspiration is called Czerny's sign and is associated with some central nervous system (CNS) diseases, such as chorea.

Visible peristalsis. Motility of the stomach and intestines may be reflected in movement of the abdominal wall in lean individuals, even in the absence of disease. However, when strong contractions are visible through an abdominal wall of average thickness, the possibility of bowel obstruction should be investigated. The abdomen is observed for several minutes from just above the level of the abdominal profile while the examiner sits at the client's side, gazing across the abdomen. Weak peristalsis may be augmented by percussing the abdomen. Peristaltic waves of the stomach and small intestine may be seen as elevated oblique bands in the upper left quadrant that move downward to the right. Several of these peristaltic waves occuring in rapid succession may produce a series of parallel bands or a "ladder effect."

Reverse peristalsis, observed in the upper abdomen in an infant, is seen as an undulation moving from left to right. This observation indicates the presence of pyloric stenosis or, more rarely, duodenal stenosis or malrotation of the bowel.

Before touching the abdomen, the examiner asks the client whether any of the abdominal areas are painful or tender. If the answer is positive, the indicated areas are treated with gentleness.

AUSCULTATION

Auscultation of the abdomen precedes percussion because bowel motility, and thus bowel sounds, will be increased by percussion. The stethoscope and hands should be warmed; if cold, they may initiate a contraction of the abdominal muscles.

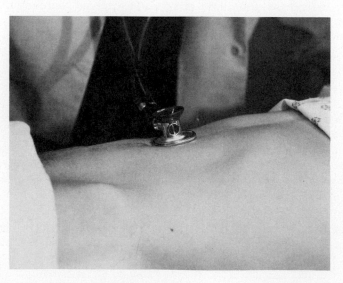

Fig. 17-9. Auscultation for bowel sounds. Intestinal sounds are relatively high pitched; the diaphragm of the stethoscope is used.

Auscultatory findings of diagnostic significance are those sounds originating from the viscera, the arterial system, the venous system, muscular activity, or parietal friction rubs. Light pressure on the stethoscope is sufficient to detect bowel sounds as well as bruits (Fig. 17-9). Because the abdominal intestinal sounds are relatively high pitched, the diaphragm of the stethoscope, which accentuates the higher-pitched sounds, should be used. However, the bell may be used in exploring arterial murmurs and venous hums.

Peristaltic sounds

The use of the diaphragm of the stethoscope to hear the sounds of air and fluid as they move through the gastrointestinal tract can provide valuable diagnostic clues relevant to the motility of the bowel. Normal bowel sounds are high-pitched gurgling noises that occur approximately every 5 to 15 seconds. Some authorities suggest that the number is as high as 15 to 20 per minute, or roughly, 1 bowel sound for each breath sound. However, peristaltic sounds may be quite irregular. Thus, it is recommended that the examiner listen for at least 5 minutes before concluding that no bowel sounds are present. The duration of a single sound may be less than a second or may extend over several seconds. The frequency of sounds is related to the presence of food in the gastrointestinal tract or to the state of digestion. Uninterrupted bowel sounds may be heard over the ileocecal valve 4 to 7 hours following a meal. A silent abdomen, that is, the absence of bowel sounds, indicates the arrest of intestinal motility. Stimulation of peristalsis may be achieved by flicking the abdominal wall with a finger (direct percussion).

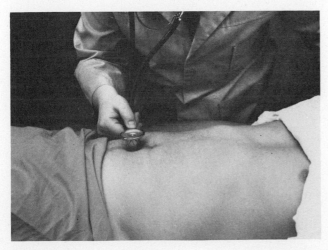

Fig. 17-10. Auscultation for bruits is performed with the bell of the stethoscope held lightly against the abdomen.

Stomach sounds may be heard in a well child by rocking him back and forth. The presence of fluid within the stomach may produce a splash.

The two significant alterations in bowel sounds are (1) the absence of any sound or extremely soft and widely separated sounds; and (2) increased sounds with a characteristically high-pitched, loud, rushing sound.

Decreased bowel sounds. Inhibition of motility of the bowel is accompanied by diminished or absent bowel sounds. Decreased motility occurs with inflammation, gangrene, or reflex ileus. Peritonitis, electrolyte disturbances, the aftermath of surgical manipulation of the bowel, and late bowel obstruction are frequently accompanied by decreased peristalsis. In addition, diminished bowel sounds are often correlated with pneumonia.

Increased bowel sounds. Loud, gurgling borborygmi accompany increased motility of the bowel. Sounds of loud volume also are heard over areas of a stenotic bowel. Sounds resulting from an early bowel obstruction are high pitched. These may be splashing sounds, similar to the emptying of a bottle into a hollow vessel. Fine, metallic, tinkling sounds are emitted as tiny gas bubbles break through the surface of intestinal juices. Increased motility may be the result of a laxative or gastroenteritis. Common pathological conditions associated with increased bowel sounds are gastroenteritis and subsiding ileus.

Vascular sounds

Arterial sounds. A bruit that is heard while the client is in a variety of positions and with the bell of the stethoscope held lightly against the abdomen may indicate a dilated, tortuous, or constricted vessel (Fig. 17-10). Loud bruits detected over the aorta may indicate the presence of an aneurysm. The aorta is auscultated superior to the umbilicus. The locations of the aorta, renal arteries, and iliac arteries are illustrated in Fig. 17-11. Soft, medium- to low-pitched murmurs due to renal arterial stenosis may be heard over the upper midline or toward the flank. For the hypertensive client, particular care is devoted to listening over the center and posterior flank for a bruit in the arterial tree.

Venous hums. A normal hum originating from the inferior vena cava and its large tributaries is continuously audible through the stethoscope. Its tone is medium pitched in quality and is similar to a muscular fibrillary hum. In the presence of obstructed portal circulation, as from a cirrhotic liver, an abnormal venous hum may be detected in the periumbilical region. Pressure on the bell may obscure the hum. The hum may be accompanied by a palpable thrill.

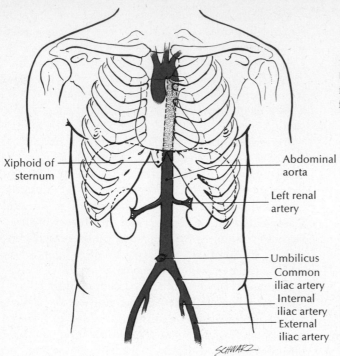

Fig. 17-11. The abdominal aorta. Note location of renal and iliac arteries. These arteries and the aorta are auscultated for bruits.

Xiphoid of
sternum

Abdominal
aorta

Left renal
artery

Umbilicus
Common
iliac artery
Internal
iliac artery
External
iliac artery

Fig. 17-12. Scratch test in assessment of liver size. The stethoscope is placed over the liver while the other hand scratches lightly over the abdominal surface with short, transverse strokes; when the scratch is done over the liver, the sound is magnified.

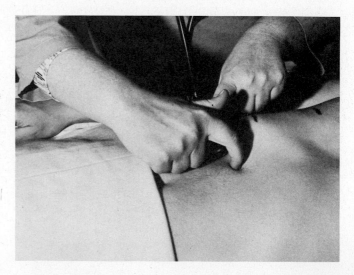

Another pathological hum accompanies the dilated periumbilical circulation of Cruveilhier-Baumgarten disease. The hum may be detected near the midline between the umbilicus and the xiphoid process. Hepatic angiomas may produce hums that can be auscultated over the liver.

Scratch test

The scratch test utilizes the difference in sound over solid as opposed to hollow organs. It is actually a percussion technique. It is occasionally used to assess the size of the liver. The stethoscope is placed over the liver while the opposite hand scratches lightly over the abdominal surface with short, transverse strokes (Fig. 17-12). When the scratch occurs

over the liver, the sound is magnified. Although the test is of questionable accuracy, it is thought to be of some value in assessing the individual with abdominal distention or spastic abdominal muscles.

Peritoneal friction rub

Peritoneal friction rub provides a rough, grating sound that resembles two pieces of leather being rubbed together. Because the liver and spleen have large surface areas in contact with the peritoneum, these two structures are most often the originating sites of the peritoneal friction rubs.

Common causes of friction rubs include splenic infection, abscess, or tumor; these are heard best over the lower rib cage in the anterior axillary line. Deep

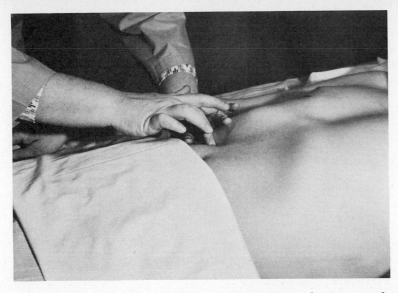

Fig. 17-13. Percussion of the abdomen for evaluation of fluid, gaseous distention, and masses within the abdominal cavity.

respiration may emphasize the sound. Metastatic disease of the liver and abscess are the usual causes of peritoneal friction rubs located over the lower right rib cage.

Muscular activity sounds

A fibrillating muscle produces a hum that can be heard with a stethoscope. Both voluntary and involuntary contraction (as in muscle guarding of a painful area) produces this sound. The hum is often accentuated by palpation of the tender area.

PERCUSSION

Percussion of the abdomen is aimed at detecting fluid, gaseous distention, and masses and in assessing solid structures within the abdomen (Fig. 17-13). The major contribution of this technique, in the absence of disease, is the delineation of the position and size of the liver and spleen.

The entire abdomen should be percussed lightly for a general picture of the areas of tympany and dullness. Tympany will predominate because of the presence of gas in the large and small bowel, while resonance will be heard in some areas. Solid masses will percuss as dull, as will the distended bladder.

To lessen the chance of omitting any portion of the examination, the practitioner should establish a definite pattern or route to use habitually in percussing abdominal structures.

Assessment of the liver span

Percussion to determine the size of the liver is begun in the right midclavicular line at a level below the umbilicus (Fig. 17-14). The percussion is done

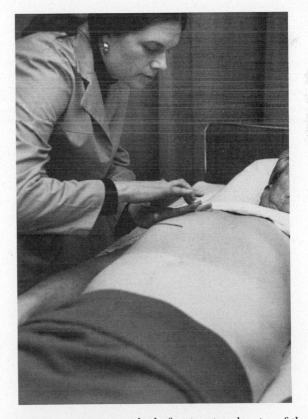

Fig. 17-14. Percussion method of estimating the size of the liver in the midclavicular line. Lower border percussion is begun over a region of air- or gas-filled bowel and carried upward to the dull percussion note of the liver. The spot is marked. Upper border percussion is performed over the midclavicular line from an area of lung resonance to the first dull percussion note (generally the fifth to seventh interspace). The spot is marked.

over a region of gas-filled bowel (tympanitic) and progressed upward toward the liver. The lower border of the liver is indicated by the first dull percussion note, and the site is marked on the abdomen. The upper border of liver dullness is ascertained by

starting the percussion in the midclavicular line and examining caudally from an area of the lung resonance to the first dull percussion note (generally the fifth to seventh interspace) (Fig. 17-15). This spot is duly marked, and the distance between the two marks is measured in centimeters (Fig. 17-16). Other sites for measurement are the anterior axillary line and the midsternal line.

Suggested ranges of values for normal are 6 to 12 cm in the midclavicular line and 4 to 8 cm in the midsternal line (Fig. 17-17).

It is important to note that there is a direct correlation between body size (lean body mass) and liver span. Thus, the mean midclavicular liver span in men is 10.5 cm and 7.0 cm in women. A midclavicular liver span of 11 cm may indicate hepatomegaly in a 5-foot, 100-pound female, but may be within normal limits for a man.

Percussion of liver dullness is important in detecting atrophy of the liver, such as might occur in acute fulminating hepatitis.

A less accurate sign of an enlarged liver is the percussion or palpation of the liver edge 2 or 3 cm below the costal margin in the midclavicular line because the upper border must be considered as well. The liver span is seen to be greater in men than in women and in the tall as opposed to the short individual. Error in estimating the liver span can occur when

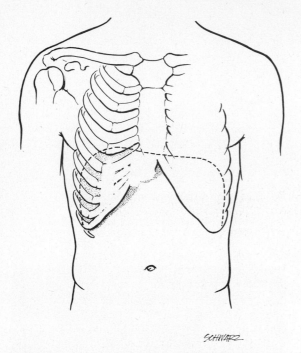

Fig. 17-15. Anatomical characterization of the measurement of liver span.

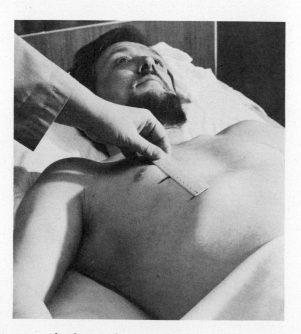

Fig. 17-16. The distance between the two marks measured in estimating the liver span is normally 6 to 12 cm.

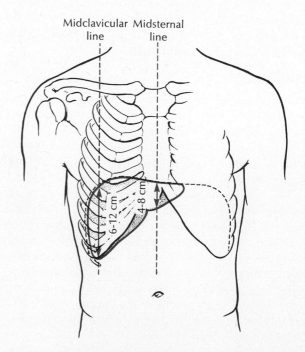

Fig. 17-17. The range of liver span in the midclavicular and midsternal lines. The size of the liver shows a direct correlation to lean body mass. Thus the mean clavicular liver span in men is 10.5 cm and in women 7.0 cm.

pleural effusion or lung consolidation obscures the upper liver border or when gas in the colon obscures the lower border.

On inspiration the diaphragm moves downward; thus, the span of liver dullness will normally be shifted inferiorly 2 to 3 cm. Pulmonary edema may also displace the liver caudally, whereas ascites, massive tumors, or pregnancy may push the liver upward. The liver assumes a more square configuration in cirrhosis of the liver, and the midclavicular and midsternal measurements may approach equality.

Percussion for tympany and dullness

Spleen. Splenic dullness can be percussed from the level of the sixth or ninth to the eleventh rib just posterior to or at the midaxillary line on the left side.

Stomach. A lower-pitched tympany than that of the intestine is typical of the percussion note of the gastric air bubble. Percussion is performed in the area of the left lower anterior rib cage and in the left epigastric region to define the region occupied by the bubble. The percussion sounds of the stomach vary with the time the last meal was eaten.

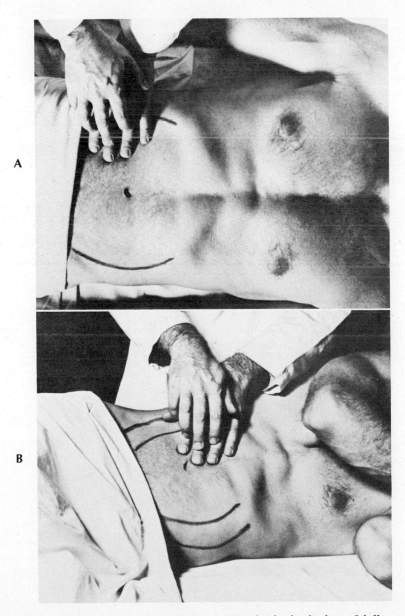

Fig. 17-18. Test for shifting dullness. **A,** With the client on his back, the line of dullness is marked in both flanks. **B,** The client is rotated on one side and then the other, and the new levels of dullness are marked each time. (From G. I. series; physical examination of the abdomen, part 3, Percussion, Richmond, Va., 1972, A. H. Robins Co.)

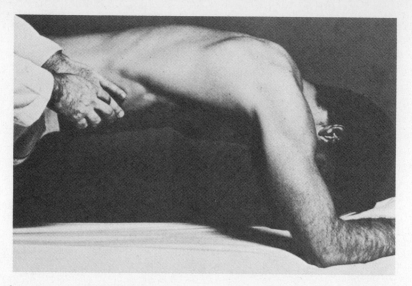

Fig. 17-19. Elicitation of the puddle sign. (From G. I. series; physical examination of the abdomen, part 3, Percussion, Richmond, Va., 1972, A. H. Robins Co.)

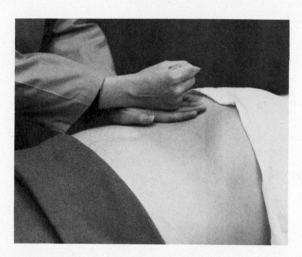

Fig. 17-20. Fist percussion of the liver. The palm of the hand is placed over the region of liver dullness and is struck a light blow with the fisted right hand. Tenderness elicited by this method is usually due to hepatitis or cholecystitis. Fist percussion may be used over the costovertebral junction to elicit renal tenderness.

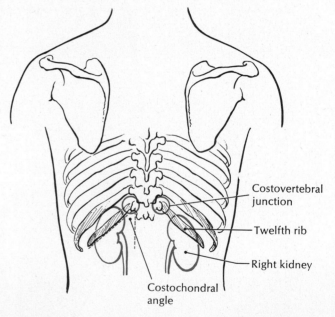

Costovertebral junction

Twelfth rib

Right kidney

Costochondral angle

Fig. 17-21. Relationship of the kidney to the twelfth rib. Note the costovertebral angle.

Percussion for ascites (free fluid)

Test for shifting dullness. A technique for differentiating ascites from cysts or edema fluid in the abdominal wall is the percussion test for shifting dullness (Fig. 17-18).

The client is placed in the supine position, and fluid dullness is percussed laterally in the flank while the abdomen medial to the dullness is tympanitic due to the presence of gas within the bowel. The line of demarcation between the dull and tympanitic sounds is marked, and the client is instructed to lie on his side. The ascites fluid will flow via gravity to shift the line of dullness closer to the umbilicus. A new line is marked, and the change is measured in centimeters. Subsequently, the client is turned to the opposite side and the change recorded. The test enables the examiner to detect free fluid as well as make a rough estimate of the volume.

KNEE-CHEST POSITION. Percussion of the periumbilical region of a client in the knee-chest position

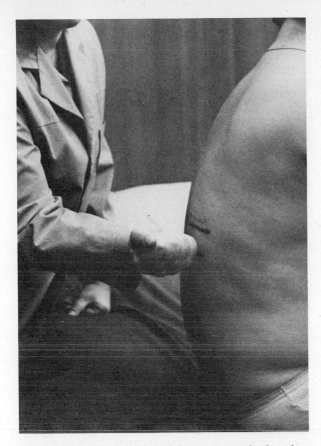

Fig. 17-22. Direct percussion of the costovertebral angle to elicit tenderness related to the kidney.

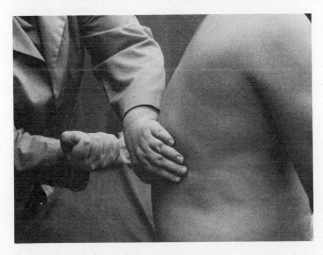

Fig. 17-23. Indirect percussion of the costovertebral angle to elicit tenderness related to the kidney.

enables the examiner to detect smaller amounts of fluid than is possible with the individual supine.

PUDDLE SIGN. After maintaining the client in the knee-elbow position for several minutes so that ascitic fluid puddles over the umbilicus by gravity, the examiner percusses the umbilical area for the dull notes of fluid (Fig. 17-19).

A volume of free fluid in the peritoneal cavity greater than 2 L can be detected by methods of shifting dullness. Ascites is caused by (1) diseases of the liver, such as cirrhosis and hepatitis; (2) diseases of the heart, such as congestive failure and constrictive pericarditis; (3) pancreatitis; (4) cancer, such as peritoneal metastases and ovarian tumors; (5) tuberculous peritonitis; and (6) hypoalbuminemia.

Fist percussion

Another use of percussion in the abdominal examination is the use of fist percussion to vibrate the tissue rather than produce sound (Fig. 17-20). The palm of the left hand is placed over the region of liver dullness and is struck a light blow by the fisted right hand. Tenderness elicited by this method is usually associated with hepatitis or cholecystitis. Fist percussion at the costovertebral junction is also useful in assessing renal tenderness. Fig. 17-21 demonstrates the relationship of the kidney to the costovertebral junction. The technique of direct fist costovertebral percussion is demonstrated in Fig. 17-22, and the indirect method is shown in Fig. 17-23.

PALPATION

Following careful visual scrutiny, auscultation, and percussion, palpation is used to substantiate findings and to further explore the abdomen. Palpation is used to evaluate the major organs of the abdomen; these organs are examined with respect to shape, position, and mobility, size, consistency, and tension. Thorough and systematic screening is performed to detect areas of tenderness, muscular spasm, masses, or fluid.

The client's position is checked to make sure that maximum relaxation has been achieved. The examiner's hands should be warm, and the examiner should use techniques for enhancing bodily and psychological relaxation. Observation that the client does not relax the abdominal muscles in spite of these maneuvers may justify the use of the technique in which the examiner exerts downward pressure on the lower sternum with his left hand while palpating with the other. The deeper inspiration that results inhibits abdominal muscle contraction. A suggestion for achieving relaxation in children is putting them into a tub of warm water, but this is not practical for a screening examination. The examiner is at the right side of the client, and the fingers of the examining hand are approximated. Measurements are more accurately recorded in centimeters. The older method of describing distance in finger breadths invites error since the fingers of examiners are of varying diameters. The abdomen is explored in all four quadrants with both light and deep palpation. Light palpation is always done first.

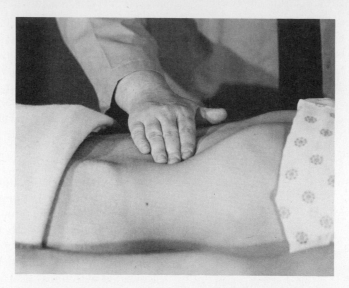

Fig. 17-24. Light palpation is performed with the hand parallel to the floor and the fingers approximated. The fingers depress the abdominal wall about 1 cm. This method of palpation is recommended for eliciting slight tenderness, large masses, and muscle guarding.

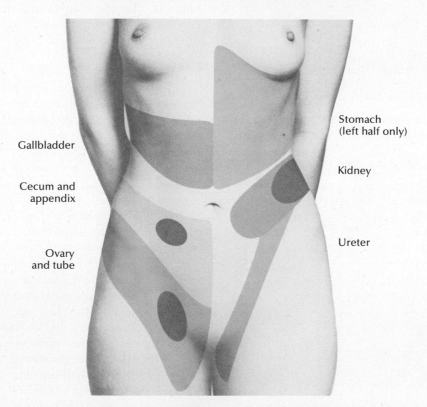

Gallbladder

Cecum and appendix

Ovary and tube

Stomach (left half only)

Kidney

Ureter

Fig. 17-25. Head's zones of cutaneous hypersensitivity. (From G. I. series; physical examination of the abdomen, part 2, Palpation, Richmond, Va., 1972, A. H. Robins Co.)

Light palpation

Light palpation is gentle exploration performed while the client is in the supine position, with the examiner's hand parallel to the floor, the palm lying lightly on the abdomen, and the fingers approximated (Fig. 17-24). The fingers depress the abdominal wall approximately 1 cm without digging. This method of palpation is best for eliciting slight tenderness, large masses, and muscle guarding. Frequently, an enlarged or distended structure may be appreciated with this light touch as a sense of resistance.

Areas of tenderness or guarding, or both, defined by light palpation will alert the examiner to proceed with caution in the application of more vigorous

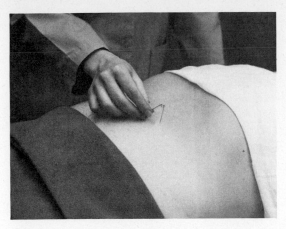

Fig. 17-26. Assessment of superficial pain sensation of the abdomen.

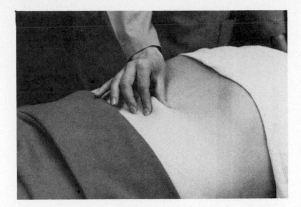

Fig. 17-27. Assessment of hypersensitivity by lifting a fold of skin away from the underlying musculature.

manipulation of these structures during the remainder of the examination.

Assessment of hypersensitivity

Zones of hypersensitivity of sensory nerve fibers of the skin have been described and are thought to reflect specific zones of peritoneal irritation. These are called Head's zones of cutaneous hypersensitivity (Fig. 17-25). Although research has not provided proof for all of the zones, clinical reliance has been demonstrated for the zone shown for the appendix in cases of appendicitis and for the midepigastrium in the individual with peptic ulcer.

Evaluation of this hypersensitivity may be achieved in two ways. One method is to stimulate gently with the sharp end of an open safety pin, a wisp of cotton, or the fingernail (Fig. 17-26). The second method is to gently lift a fold of skin away from the underlying musculature (Fig. 17-27). The alert patient may be able to describe his reaction to this stimulation, or changes in facial expression (grimacing) may indicate the increased sensation the individual is experiencing.

Assessment of muscle spasticity

Involuntary muscle contraction or spasticity may indicate peritoneal irritation. Further palpation is done to determine whether the spasticity is unilateral or on both sides of the abdomen. Generalized and boardlike contraction is thought to be typical of peritonitis. Further definition is achieved by asking the client to raise his trunk from a horizontal position without arm support. The experience of unilateral pain in response to this maneuver may further pinpoint the areas of spasticity. This mechanism may also help to differentiate muscle contraction from abdominal mass; as the head is raised, the hand would be moved away from an abdominal mass. Rigidity

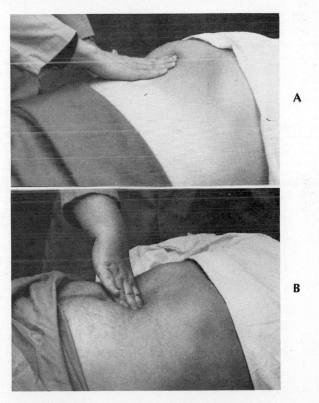

A

B

Fig. 17-28. Moderate palpation is performed with the side of the hand. This method of palpation is particularly useful in assessing organs that move with respiration, such as the liver and spleen.

and tenderness over McBurney's point and in some cases over the entire right side are strongly suggestive of appendicitis. Acute cholecystitis is frequently accompanied by rigidity of the right hypochondrium.

Moderate palpation

The side of the hand rather than the fingertips is used in moderate palpation (Fig. 17-28). This method

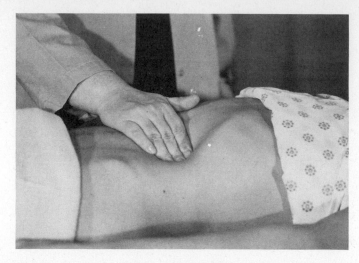

Fig. 17-29. Deep palpation is performed by pressing the distal half of the palmar surfaces of the fingers into the abdominal wall. Deep structures such as the retroperitoneal organs are assessed by deep palpation.

obviates the tendency to dig into the abdomen with the fingertips as well as the resultant discomfort and involuntary guarding that may accompany such focal probing.

The sensation produced by palpating with the side of the hand is particularly useful in assessing organs that move with respiration, such as the liver and the spleen. The organ is felt during normal breathing cycles and then as the client takes a deep breath. On inspiration the organ will be pushed downward against the examining hand.

Tenderness not elicited by gentle palpation may be perceived by the client on deeper pressure.

Deep palpation

Deep palpation is indentation of the abdomen performed by pressing the distal half of the palmar surfaces of the fingers into the abdominal wall (Fig. 17-29). The abdominal wall may slide back and forth while the fingers are moving back and forth over the organ being examined. Deeper structures, such as retroperitoneal organs (the kidneys), or masses may be felt with this method. Tenderness of organs not elicited by light or moderate palpation may be uncovered with this method. In the absence of disease, the pressure produced by deep palpation may produce tenderness over the cecum, the sigmoid colon, and the aorta.

The technique of deep palpation may help to give more specific information concerning a lesion or mass detected by lighter palpation.

Bimanual palpation

Superimposition of one hand. Bimanual palpation with superimposition of one hand may be used when additional pressure is necessary to overcome resistance or to examine a deep abdominal structure. In this method one hand is superimposed over the other, so that pressure is exerted by the upper hand while the lower hand remains relaxed and sensitive to the tactile sensation produced by the structure being examined. Generally, for the right-handed examiner the left hand is the lower, or examining, hand while the right hand applies pressure exerted by the tips of the left fingers on the terminal interphalangeal points of the examining fingers (Fig. 17-30). The technique is recommended because the palpating hand is less sensitive if it has to be used to exert pressure at the same time.

Trapping technique. Both hands may be used to establish the size of a mass. The mass is trapped between the examining hands for measurement.

Detection of a pulsatile mass. Pulsation may be sensed in the fingertips of both hands as they are pushed apart as a pulsatile flow expands a structure such as the aorta; pulsation may also be felt in a mass held between the examining hands. This palpatory finding indicates that the structure being felt is pulsating rather than transmitting pulsation. The normal aorta is approximately 2.5 to 4 cm wide, whereas an aneurysm is a good deal broader. As noted previously, a bruit is generally heard over an aneurysm. The most common physical finding in clients with an abdominal aneurysm is the presence of an expansile, pulsating mass, more than 95% of which are located inferior to the renal arteries but generally at or above the umbilicus. Femoral pulses are usually present but are markedly damped in amplitude. More than half of clients with abdominal aneurysms are asymptomatic; thus, the mass might be discovered during

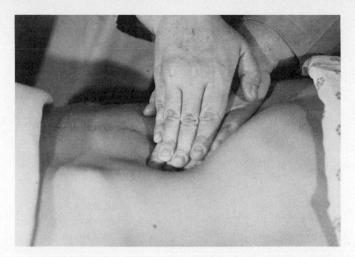

Fig. 17-30. Bimanual palpation with superimposition of one hand. Pressure is exerted by the upper hand while the lower hand remains relaxed and sensitive to tactile stimulation.

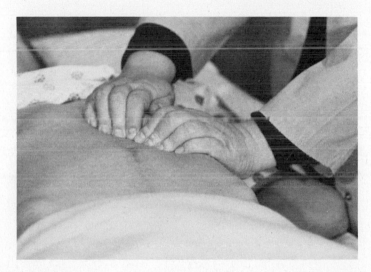

Fig. 17-31. Bimanual palpation with the hands side by side. Descent of the liver or spleen (as above) is often measured by hooking the fingers over the costal margin from above. This technique is called the Middleton technique and is used to examine the spleen.

a screening physical examination. Although more than 80% of abdominal aneurysms can be palpated, small aneurysms in the markedly obese client may not be felt.

Hands approximated (side by side). Minimal descent of the liver or spleen below the costal margin is occasionally detected by hooking the fingers over the costal margin from above while standing beside the thorax, facing the client's feet (Fig. 17-31). This procedure is called Middleton's technique and is used to examine the spleen.

The outline of a tubular structure such as the sigmoid colon or cecum can frequently be more specifically outlined with the hands side by side, rolling the fingers over the structure.

Palpation to elicit rebound tenderness

To provoke rebound tenderness, the approximated fingers are pushed gently but deeply in a region remote from that suspected of tenderness and then rapidly removed. The maneuver as illustrated in Fig. 17-32 is being performed over McBurney's point and might elicit rebound tenderness related to appendicitis. The rebound of the structures indented by palpation causes a sharp stabbing sensation of pain on the side of the inflammation. This sensation of pain following the withdrawal of pressure is a sign of peritoneal irritation. The test may be repeated over to the side of the suspected disease. The test is best performed near the conclusion of the examination, since the production of severe pain or muscle spasm

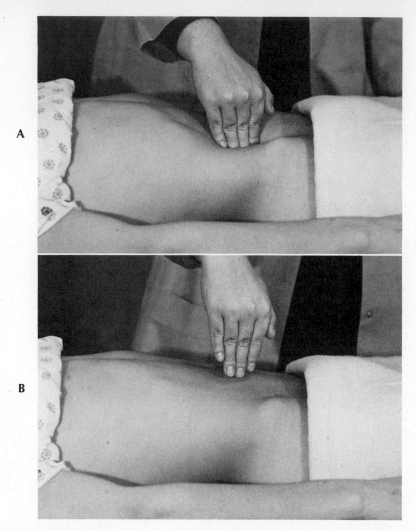

Fig. 17-32. Palpation to elicit rebound tenderness. **A,** Deep pressure is applied to the abdominal wall. **B,** On release of pressure, a sensation of pain would indicate peritoneal irritation. This is a test for appendicitis. In this case, the test for rebound tenderness is being performed over McBurney's point and may elicit tenderness related to appendicitis.

may interfere with subsequent examination. Voluntary coughing by the client may produce the same results.

Ballottement (Fig. 17-33)

Ballottement is a palpation technique used to assess a floating object. Fluid-filled tissue is pushed toward the examining hand so that the object will float against the examining fingers. This is the technique used to determine whether the head or the breech of the fetus is in the fundus of the uterus by abdominal palpation.

Single-handed ballottement. Single-handed ballottement is performed with the fingers extended in a straight line with the forearm and at a right angle to the abdomen. The fingers are moved quickly toward the mass or organ to be examined and held

there. As fluid or other structures are displaced, the mass will move upward and be felt at the fingertips. Some examiners prefer this technique for examination of the spleen.

Bimanual ballottement. Bimanual ballottement is accomplished by using one hand to push on the anterior abdominal wall to displace contents to the flank while the other receives the mass or structure pushed against it and feels the dimensions.

Demonstration of ascites by palpation

The presence of large amounts of fluid within the peritoneal cavity allows the elicitation of a fluid wave (Fig. 17-34). To test for the presence of a fluid wave, the client is placed in a supine position. The examiner places the palmar surface of one hand firmly against the lateral abdominal wall and taps the contralateral

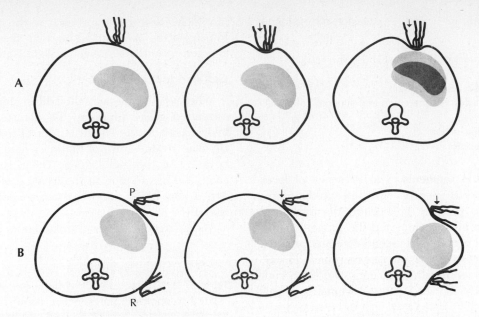

Fig. 17-33. Ballottement. **A,** Single-handed ballottement. **B,** Bimanual ballottement: *P,* pushing hand; *R,* receiving hand. (From C. I. series; physical examination of the abdomen, part 2, Palpation, Richmond, Va., 1972, A. H. Robins Co.)

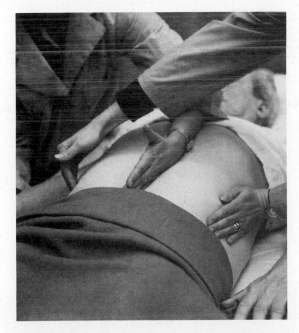

Fig. 17-34. Test for presence of a fluid wave.

wall with the other hand. An assistant places the edge of one hand and lower arm firmly in the vertical midline of the client's abdomen to damp vibrations that might otherwise be transmitted through the tissues of the anterior abdominal wall.

Palpation for abdominal masses

All of the quadrants of the abdomen are examined systematically by palpation. For the most part, bi-

Table 17-1. Characteristics of abdominal masses related to common pathological conditions

Description of mass	Possible pathological condition
Descends on inspiration	Liver, spleen, or kidney mass
Pulsatile mass	Abdominal aneurysm, tortuous aorta
Movable from side to side, not head to foot	Mesenteric or small bowel mass
Complete fixation	Tumor of pancreatic or retroperitoneal origin

manual examination with the hands superimposed is the technique most useful. Initially, light palpation is utilized; the examiner then proceeds to deep palpation.

The characteristics of an abdominal mass are carefully described. Of particular importance are consistency, regularity of contour movement with respiration, and mobility. A sketch of the anterior abdominal wall with all of its bony landmarks and the umbilicus may be the most efficient way to convey location, shape, and size.

Difficulties in determining that a palpable mass is in the anterior abdominal wall rather than in an intraabdominal position may be resolved by asking the client to flex the abdominal muscles. Masses in the subcutaneous tissue will continue to be palpable, whereas those in the peritoneal cavity will be more difficult to feel or will be pushed out of reach altogether.

Normal abdominal structures occasionally mistaken for masses are:

1. Lateral borders of the rectus abdominis muscles
2. Uterus
3. Feces-filled ascending colon
4. Feces-filled descending colon and sigmoid colon
5. Aorta
6. Common iliac artery
7. Sacral promontory

Palpable bowel segments. The presence of feces within the bowel frequently contributes to the examiner's ability to palpate the cecum, the ascending colon, the descending colon, and the sigmoid colon. The feces-filled cecum and ascending colon produce a sensation suggestive of a soft, boggy, rounded mass. The client may complain of cramps resulting from stimulation of the bowel by the movements of palpation.

EXAMINATION OF THE SPECIFIC ABDOMINAL STRUCTURES

Palpation is a useful technique for identification and assessment of the specific abdominal structures. A systematic approach, always beginning at the same area, is suggested in order that the examiner not skip any part of the abdomen. Since most examiners approach the client from the right, the liver may prove to be the most convenient structure to palpate first.

Liver

Two types of bimanual palpation are recommended for palpation of the liver. The first of these is superimposition of the right hand over the left hand. The client is asked to breathe normally for two or three breaths. Then he is asked to breathe deeply. The diaphragm is exerted downward in inspiration and will push the liver toward the examining hand. The liver usually cannot be palpated in the normal adult. However, in extremely thin but otherwise well individuals, it may be felt at the costal margin. When the normal liver margin is palpated, it feels regular in contour and somewhat sharp.

In the second technique, the left hand is placed beneath the client at the level of the eleventh and twelfth ribs and upward pressure applied in order to throw the liver forward toward the examining right hand. The palmar surface of the examiner's right hand is placed parallel to the right costal margin. As the client inspires, the liver may be felt to slip beneath the examining fingers.

Tenderness over the liver may be demonstrated by placing the palm of one hand over the lateral costal margin and delivering a blow to that hand with the ulnar surface of the other hand, which has been curled into a fist (Fig. 17-20).

Whichever technique is chosen, the initial attempt to palpate the liver should be done slowly, carefully, and gently so that the liver margin is not missed.

Gallbladder

Whereas the normal gallbladder cannot be felt, a distended gallbladder may be palpated below the liver margin at the lateral border of the rectus muscle. The cystic nature of the mass helps in the identification of the gallbladder. There is, however, a good deal of variation in the location of the left border; it may be found either more medially or more laterally.

An enlarged, tender gallbladder is indicative of

Table 17-2. Characteristics of hepatomegaly related to common pathological conditions

Description of liver	Possible pathological condition
Smooth, nontender	Portal cirrhosis
	Lymphoma
	Passive congestion of the liver
	Portal obstruction
	Obstruction of the vena cava
	Lymphocytic leukemia
	Rickets
	Amyloidosis
	Schistosomiasis
Smooth, tender	Acute hepatitis
	Amebic hepatitis or abscess
	Early congestive cardiac failure
Nodular	Late portal cirrhosis
	Tertiary syphilis
	Metastatic carcinoma
Hard	Carcinomatosis

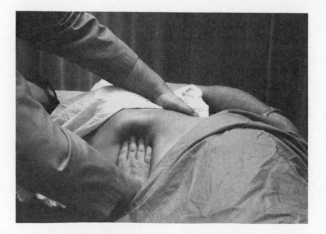

Fig. 17-35. Assessment of the spleen.

cholecystitis, whereas a large but nontender gallbladder portends of obstruction of the common bile duct.

Murphy's sign: inspiratory arrest. Murphy's sign is helpful in determining the presence of cholecystitis through bimanual examination. While performing deep palpation, the examiner asks the client to take a deep breath. As the descending liver brings the gallbladder in contact with the examining hand, the client with cholecystitis will experience pain and stop the inspiratory movement. Pain may also occur in the client with hepatitis.

Spleen

The spleen is generally not palpable in the normal adult. Since the spleen is normally soft and is located retroperitoneally, it is frequently difficult to palpate. Turning the client on his right side (in order to gain gravitational advantage) brings the spleen downward and forward and thus closer to the abdominal wall and is often employed in the examination.

With the client in the supine position, three techniques of palpation are useful. In the first technique, the right hand is placed flat on the client's abdomen in the upper left quadrant with the fingers delving beneath the costal margin and toward the anterior axillary line (Fig. 17-35). The left hand is stretched over the client's abdomen and brought posterior to the client in the flank below the costal margin. This hand is used to exert an upward pressure that will displace the spleen anteriorly.

The Middleton technique for examination of the spleen is performed with the examiner standing on the client's left side, facing the client's feet. The fingers are hooked over the costal margin, pressing upward and inward at the anterior axillary line (Fig. 17-31). On inspiration the spleen may be felt at the fingertips. The client may assist by placing his left fist under the left eleventh rib.

Either of these techniques may be used with the client on the right side to throw the spleen forward and with the knees flexed to relax the abdomen. Some authorities recommend that the client lie on the left side during splenic palpation; they propose that lying on the left side more effectively relaxes the musculature of the abdomen.

The technique of one hand superimposed over the other may also be used to palpate the spleen. Again, the examiner stands at the client's left side, facing the client's feet. The fingers are hooked over the costal margin, and the uppermost hand is used to apply pressure while the lower hand is used as a sensing device. Again, the client is asked to breathe in and out while the examiner focuses on the inspiratory phase in an attempt to feel the contour of the spleen.

Splenic enlargement is described by the number of centimeters the spleen extends below the costal margin: (1) slight is 1 to 4 cm below the costal margin, (2) moderate is 4 to 8 cm below the costal margin, and (3) great is more than 8 cm below the costal margin.

The spleen may also be percussed. Normally, splenic dullness may be percussed from the sixth or the ninth to the eleventh rib in the midaxillary line or posterior to the line. The span of normal splenic dullness does not exceed 7 cm. When the spleen has normal dimensions, resonance may be percussed over the lowest left intercostal space between the anterior

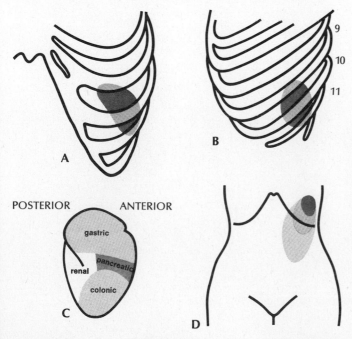

Fig. 17-36. Normal (**A, B, C**) and enlarged (**D**) spleen. **A,** Anterior view. **B,** Left lateral view. **C,** Regions of spleen (anterior view) that touch other viscera. **D,** Directions of splenic enlargement. (From G. I. series; physical examination of the abdomen, part 2, Palpation, Richmond, Va., 1972, A. H. Robins Co.)

and midaxillary lines both during inspiration and expiration. However, a finding of resonance on expiration and dullness on inspiration probably denotes splenic hypertrophy.

Enlargement of the spleen may best be described by a drawing of the anterior abdomen indicating the relative site and shape of the spleen in relation to the costal border and the umbilicus (Fig. 17-36).

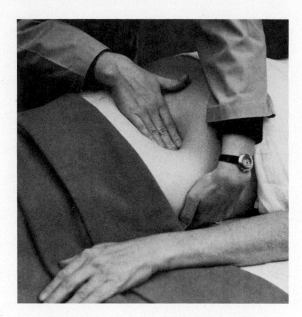

Fig. 17-37. Assessment of the left kidney.

Pancreas

The pancreas cannot be palpated in the normal client because of its small size and retroperitoneal position. However, a mass of the pancreas may occasionally be felt as a vague sensation of fullness in the epigastrium.

Kidney

Palpation of the kidney is best accomplished with the client in the supine position and with the examiner standing on the client's right side. For the left kidney, the examiner reaches across the client with the left arm, placing the hand behind the client's left flank (Fig. 17-37). The left flank is elevated with the examiner's fingers, displacing the kidney anteriorly. With the kidney optimally positioned, the right palmar surface of the examiner's hand is used in deep palpation through the abdominal wall.

The kidneys are not palpable in the normal adult, and only the lower pole of the right kidney can be felt in very thin persons. In the elderly, as muscles lose tone and elastic fibers are lost, the kidneys may be more readily palpated. The left kidney is generally not palpable.

The examiner remains on the client's right side to examine the right kidney. The right flank is similarly elevated with the left hand, and the right hand is used to palpate deeply for the right kidney. The lower pole of the right kidney may be felt as a smooth, rounded mass that descends on inspiration.

Differentiation between splenic and kidney en-

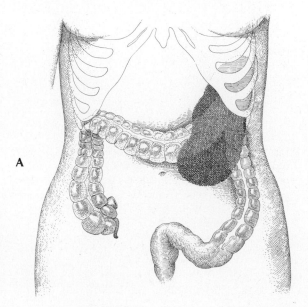
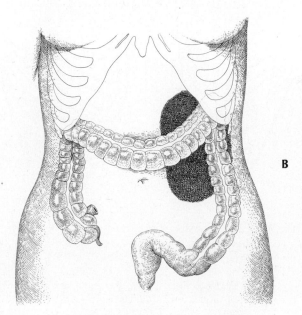

Fig. 17-38. Differentiation of enlarged spleen **(A)** from enlarged left kidney **(B)**. (From G. I. series; physical examination of the abdomen, part 3, Percussion, Richmond, Va., 1972, A. H. Robins Co.)

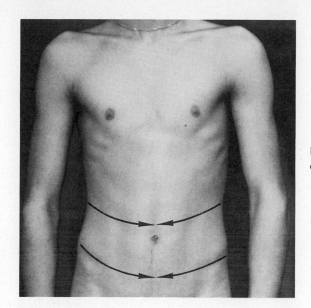

Fig. 17-39. Stimulus sites for abdominal reflexes. All four quadrants must be tested.

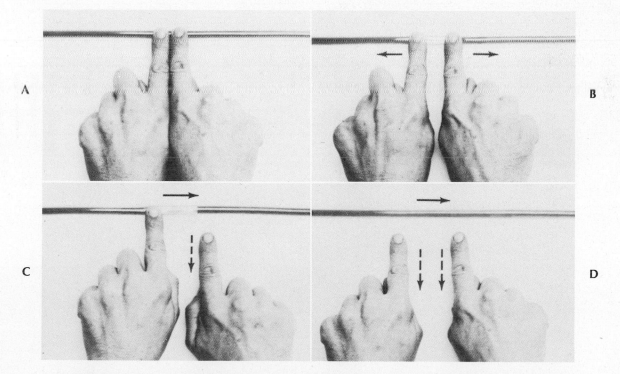

Fig. 17-40. Procedure for detecting the direction of venous flow. **A,** Press the blood from the vein with two index fingers in apposition. **B,** Slide the two index fingers apart, milking the blood from the intervening segment of vein. **C,** Release the pressure from one end of the segment to observe the time for refilling from that direction. **D,** Repeat the procedure, but release the other end to observe the time of filling. The flow of venous blood is in the direction of the faster filling. (From G. I. series; physical examination of the abdomen, part 2, Palpation, Richmond, Va., 1972, A. H. Robins Co.)

largement may be accomplished by percussion. The percussion note over the spleen is dull since the bowel is displaced downward, whereas resonance is heard over the kidney because of the intervening bowel (Fig. 17-38). In addition, the free edge of the spleen is sharper in contour and tends to enlarge caudally and to the right.

Urinary bladder

The urinary bladder is not palpable in the normal client unless it is distended with urine. When the bladder is distended with urine, it may be felt as a smooth, round, and rather tense mass. Percussion may be used to define the outline of the distended bladder, which may extend up as far as the umbilicus.

Umbilicus

The umbilicus is observed for relationship to skin surface, hernia, inflammation, or signs of bleeding. The normal umbilicus is recessed below the skin surface.

Umbilical hernia. Whereas umbilical hernia noted in children is seen directly at the umbilical opening centrally located in the linea alba, the adult defect is often apparent above an incomplete umbilical ring and may be called paraumbilical.

The examination for hernia is done by pressing the index finger into the navel. The fascial opening may feel like a sharp ring, and there is a soft center. The umbilicus may be everted by marked intraabdominal pressure from masses, pregnancy, or large amounts of ascitic fluid.

Sr. Mary Joseph's nodule. Carcinoma originating in the abdomen and particularly in the stomach may metastasize to the navel. The metastatic lesion is called Sr. Mary Joseph's nodule.

Patent urachus. On occasion the urinary tract of the fetus, which extends from the apex of the bladder to the umbilicus, does not fibrose. The result is a umbilicourinary fistula called a patent urachus. The client may report dampness or the smell of urine at the umbilicus.

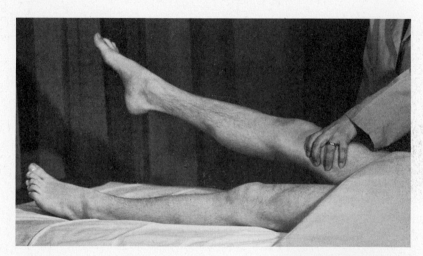

Fig. 17-41. Iliopsoas muscle test.

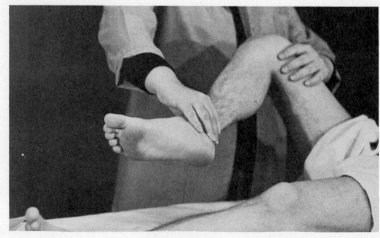

Fig. 17-42. Obturator muscle test.

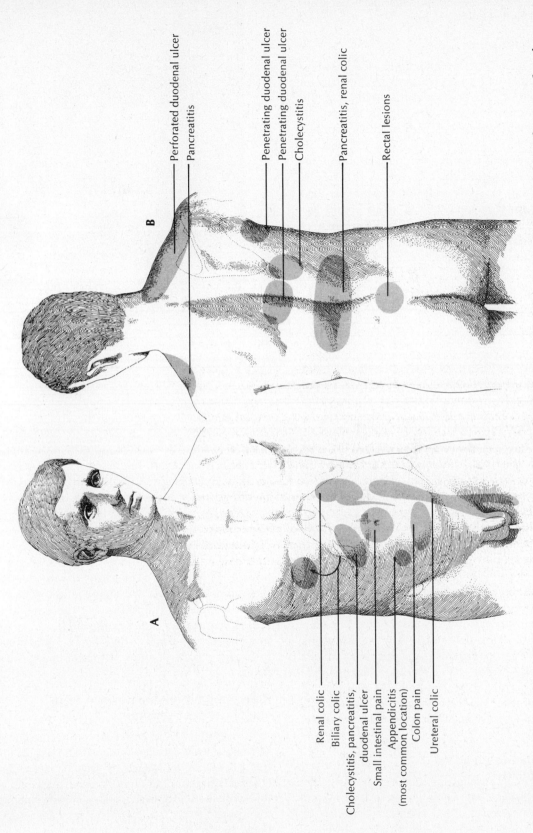

Fig. 17-43. **A,** Common areas where abdominal pain is referred or perceived—anterior view. **B,** Common areas where abdominal pain is referred or perceived—posterior view. (From G. I. series; physical examination of the abdomen, part 2, Palpation, Richmond, Va., 1972, A. H. Robins Co.)

Cullen's sign. Free blood in the peritoneal cavity may produce a blue hue at the umbilical opening, which is known as Cullen's sign.

Abdominal reflexes

The reflex is elicited by using a key, the base end of an applicator, or a fingernail and gently stroking the abdominal skin over the lateral borders of the rectus abdominis muscles toward the midline (Fig. 17-39). This maneuver is repeated in each quadrant. With each stroke, contraction of the rectus abdominis muscles is observed, coupled with pulling of the umbilicus to the stimulated side.

The reflex may be weak or absent in the individual who has sustained a good deal of stretching of the abdominal musculature. Thus, the practitioner may be unable to obtain the abdominal reflex in the multiparous or obese client. The reflex may also be absent in the normal, aging client. Absence of the reflex may indicate a pyramidal tract lesion.

Changes in vascular patterns: venous engorgement

In health, the veins of the abdominal wall are not prominent, but in the malnourished individual the veins are more easily visible because of decreased adipose tissue. The venous return to the heart is cephalad in the veins above the umbilicus and caudal below the navel. Direction of flow may be demonstrated by placing the index fingers side by side over a vein, pressing laterally, and separating the fingers (Fig. 17-40). A section of the vein may be emptied. One finger is removed, and the time for filling is measured. The blood is milked from a short section of the vein, the other index finger is removed, and the time for filling from this side is measured. The flow of venous blood is in the direction of the faster filling.

Reversal of flow or an upward venous flow in the veins below the umbilicus accompanies obstruction of the inferior vena cava, whereas superior vena cava obstruction promotes downward flow in the veins above the navel. A pattern of engorged veins around the umbilicus is called caput medusae and is occasionally seen as an accompaniment to emaciation, obstruction of the superior or inferior vena cava, superficial venous obstruction, or portal vein obstruction.

Tests for irritation resulting from appendicitis

Iliopsoas muscle test. An inflamed or perforated extrapelvic appendix may cause contact irritation of the lateral iliopsoas muscle. To elicit this tenderness, the client is placed in a supine position and asked

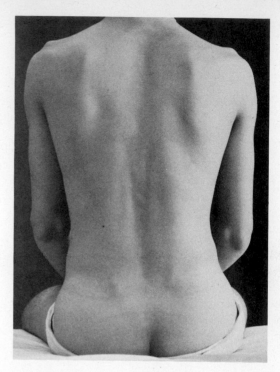

Fig. 17-44. Inspection of the back with the client in the sitting position is the final step in the abdominal examination.

to flex the lower extremity at the hip. The examiner simultaneously exerts a moderate downward pressure over the lower thigh (Fig. 17-41). With psoas muscle inflammation, the client will describe pain in the lower quadrant. A more sensitive test of psoas muscle irritation is performed with the client lying on his left side. Pain is elicited through full extension of the right lower limb at the hip.

Obturator muscle test. A perforated intrapelvic appendix may cause irritation of the obturator internus muscle. This pain is demonstrated with the client in the supine position. The client is asked to flex the right extremity at the hip and at the knee to 90 degrees. The examiner grasps the ankle and rotates internally and externally (Fig. 17-42). A complaint of hypogastric pain denotes obturator muscle involvement.

Referred pain or somatic pain from intraabdominal structures

Pain related to abdominal structures may be sensed in remote body surface regions. The explanation for this phenomenon is that as pain is intensified, increased afferent impulses lower the client's pain threshold and excite secondary sensory neurons in the spinal cord. Thus, contact may be established between afferent visceral fibers and somatic nerves of the same embryological dermatome. An example of this is pain sensed in the top of the shoulder caused by abdominal lesions or peritonitis. The diaphragm, which is irritated in this case, originates in the region of the fourth cervical nerve and derives its nerve supply from the third, fourth, and fifth cervical nerves. The shoulder is innervated by the fourth cerival nerve. Thus, shoulder pain may be a valuable clue in diagnosing perforated ulcer, hepatic abscess, pancreatitis, cholecystitis, ruptured spleen, pelvic inflammation, and hemorrhage into the peritoneum. Other examples of referred pain are noted in Fig. 17-43.

Back

The final step in the abdominal examination is inspection of the back with the client in the sitting position (Fig. 17-44). The flanks in the normal individual will be symmetrical. Fullness or asymmetry may be due to renal disorders.

The costovertebral margin is percussed for tenderness (see fist percussion).

SUMMARY

I. Inspection
  A. Contour
  B. Symmetry
  C. Condition of umbilicus
  D. Musculature
  E. Dilated veins
  F. Skin
    1. Pigmentation
    2. Lesions
    3. Striae
    4. Scars
  G. Respiratory movement
  H. Abnormal movements
II. Auscultation
  A. Peristaltic sounds
  B. Bruits
III. Percussion
  A. Liver span
  B. Spleen
  C. Stomach
  D. Masses
IV. Palpation
  A. Tone of abdominal wall
    1. Resistance—distention
    2. Muscle tone
  B. Tenderness
  C. Masses
  D. Hernia
V. Organ examination
  A. Liver
    1. Palpation
      a. Size, contour, and character of edge
      b. Tenderness
    2. Percussion—midclavicular diameter
  B. Spleen
    1. Palpation
    2. Percussion
  C. Kidneys
    1. Palpation
      a. Location
      b. Mobility
      c. Costovertebral tenderness
    2. Percussion

BIBLIOGRAPHY

Brooks, F. P., editor: Gastrointestinal pathophysiology, New York, 1974, Oxford University Press, Inc.

Castell, D. O.: The spleen percussion sign, a useful diagnostic technique, Ann. Intern. Med. **67:**1265, 1967.

Castell, D. O., and others: Estimation of liver size by percussion in normal individuals, Ann. Intern. Med. **70:**1183, 1969.

Chalmers, T. C.: Centimeters, even inches, but no fingers, N. Engl. J. Med. **282:**397, 1970.

Cope, Z.: The early diagnosis of acute abdomen, ed. 14, New York, 1972, Oxford University Press, Inc.

Dunphy, J., and Botsford, T.: Physical examination of the surgical patient; an introduction to clinical surgery, Philadelphia, 1975, W. B. Saunders Co.

Dworken, H. J.: The alimentary tract, Philadelphia, 1974, W. B. Saunders Co.

Gelin, L., Nyhus, L., and Condon, R.: Abdominal pain; a guide to rapid diagnosis, Philadelphia, 1969, J. B. Lippincott Co.

18 Assessment of the anus and rectosigmoid region

The terminal gastrointestinal tract is a distal section that may be termed the rectosigmoid region and includes the anus, the rectum, and the caudal portion of the sigmoid colon.

ANATOMY

The anal canal is the final segment of the colon; it is 2.5 to 4 cm in length and opens into the perineum (Fig. 18-1). The tract is surrounded by the external and internal sphincters, which keep it closed except when flatus and feces are passed. These sphincters are laid down in concentric layers. The striated external muscular ring is under voluntary control, whereas the internal, smooth-muscle sphincter is under autonomic control. The internal sphincter is innervated from the pelvic plexus; sympathetic stimulation contracts the sphincter; parasympathetic stimulation relaxes it. The distal portion of the external sphincter extends past the internal sphincter and may be palpated by the examining finger. The stratified squamous epithelial lining of the anus is visible to inspection, since it extends beyond the sphincters, where it merges with the skin. The junction is characterized by pigmentation and the presence of hair. From an internal view of the anal canal, columns of mucosal tissue, which extend from the rectum and terminate in papillae, amy be identified; these anal columns, or columns of Morgani, fuse to form the pectinate, or dentate, line. Spaces between these columns are called crypts. The anal columns are invested with cross channels of anastomosing veins, which form mucosal folds known as anal valves. These anastomosing veins form a ring known as the zona hemorrhoidalis. When dilated, these veins are called internal hemorrhoids. The lower section of the anal canal contains a venous plexus, which has only minor connection with the zona hemorrhoidalis and drains downward into the inferior rectal veins. Varicosed veins of this plexus are known as external hemorrhoids. Thus, internal hemorrhoids are encountered superior to the pectinate line and are characterized by the moist, red epithelium of the rectum, whereas external hemorrhoids are located inferior to the pectinate line and have the squamous epithelium of the anal canal or skin as their surface tissue.

The rectum is encountered as the portion of the gastrointestinal tract rostral to the anal canal. It is approximately 12 cm in length and is lined with columnar epithelium. Superiorly, the rectum has its origin at the third sacral vertebra and is continuous with the sigmoid colon. Its distal end dilates to form the rectal ampulla, which contains flatus and feces. Four semilunar transverse folds (Houston's valves) extend across half of the circumference of the rectal lumen. The purpose of the valves is not clear. It has been suggested that the valves serve to support feces while allowing flatus to pass. The rectum ends where the muscle coats are replaced by the sphincters of the anal canal.

The sigmoid colon has its origin at the iliac flexure of the descending colon and terminates in the rectum. It is approximately 40 cm in length. It is accessible to examination via the sigmoidoscope, and examination is limited by the length of the scope. Recently, flexible fiberoptic instruments have made possible inspection of the mucosal surfaces of the entire sigmoid colon as well as of the other portions of the colon.

EXAMINATION

The rectal examination is an important procedure in the physical examination; it is particularly significant when the client's chief complaint includes anal pain or spasm, itching or burning, and a history of black, tarry stools (melena).

The client may give some indication of a problem by his movements; for example, shifting from one buttock to the other often alleviates the discomfort of a thrombosed hemorrhoid.

The purposes of the rectal examination include assessment of anorectal status, assessment of the male prostate gland and seminal vessels (see Chapter 19 for assessment of the male genitalia and assessment of the inguinal area for hernias) and assessment of the accessible pelvic viscera.

Since most patients experience a good deal of embarrassment as well as fear of discomfort at the prospect of the rectal examination, the procedure should be preceded by an explanation and assurance that the examiner will proceed with gentleness. The client should be draped to avoid undue exposure and helped to assume the desired position. The client may be examined in several positions:

1. *Left lateral* or *Sims's position.* The client lies on his left side with the superior thigh and knee flexed, bringing the knee close to the chest. The rectal ampulla is pushed down and posteriorly in this position and thus is advantageously aligned for the detection of rectal masses. However, the upper rectum and pelvic structure tend to fall away in this position and a pathological condition of these structures may be overlooked.

2. *Knee-chest position.* The client is on his knees with his shoulders and head in contact with the examining table. The knees are positioned more widely apart than the hips. The angle at the hip is 75 to 80 degrees. Assessment of the size of the prostate gland is best done in this position.

3. *Standing position.* The client's hips are flexed, and the trunk is resting on a bed or table. Prostate evaluation is facilitated in this position. This is the most commonly used position for examination of the prostate gland.

4. *Lithotomy position.* With the client supine, both knees are drawn up as far as possible toward the chest. It is convenient to perform the rectal examination in the female client immediately following the pelvic examination while her feet remain in stirrups.

5. *Squatting position.* Rectal prolapse may frequently be brought out in this position. Lesions of the rectosigmoid region and pelvis may be felt in this position only.

The equipment needed is a small penlight to facilitate inspection of the perianal and anal area, a finger cot or disposable glove, lubricating jelly, and a guaiac testing kit.

The methods of the rectal examination include inspection and palpation.

Inspection

The buttocks are carefully spread with both hands to examine the anus and the tissue immediately

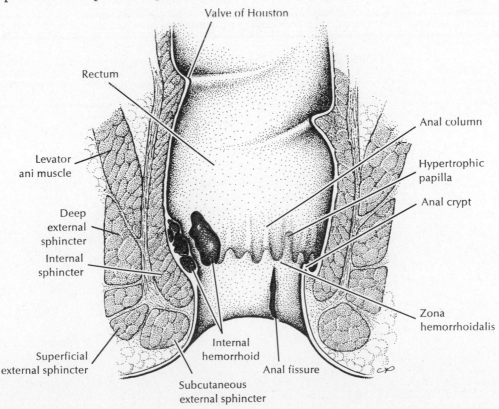

Fig. 18-1. Anorectal structures and common pathological conditions. (Adapted from Dunphy, J. E.: Arch. Surg. **57**:791, 1948.)

around the anus. This skin is more pigmented and coarser than the surrounding perianal skin and is also moist and hairless. The examiner visually assesses the perianal region for skin tags, lesions, scars or inflammation, fissures, external hemorrhoids, or fistula openings and tumors.

Valsalva's maneuver. The client is asked to strain downward as though defecating, so that with slight pressure on the skin, rectal fissures, rectal prolapse, polyps, or internal hemorrhoids might be identified. Abnormal findings are described by locating them in terms of a clock, with the 12:00 position toward the symphysis pubis in the midline of the back over the lower sacrum or coccyx.

The sacrococcygeal area is inspected for pilonidal cyst or sinus. The pilonidal area is inspected for dimples (at the tip of the coccyx), sinus openings, or the presence of inflammation. The pilonidal area is felt for tenderness, induration, or swelling.

The skin of the pilonidal sinus may have abundant hair growth. The accumulation of secretions often leads to infection, which is generally accompanied by a foul-smelling discharge and local tenderness. The sinus may be simply blocked up by secretion, so that a tumescence is observed, which is tender to palpation.

Palpation

While the patient strains downward, the pad of the lubricated, gloved index finger is gently placed against the anal verge; firm pressure is exerted until the sphincter begins to yield, and the finger is then slowly inserted in the direction of the umbilicus as the rectal sphincter relaxes (Fig. 18-2). The patient

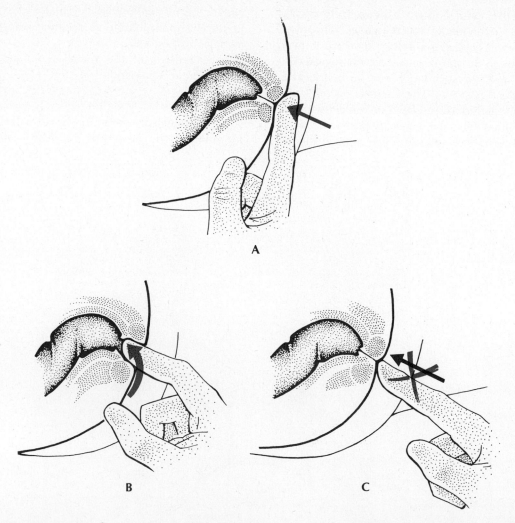

Fig. 18-2. A, Digital pressure is applied against the anal verge until the external sphincter is felt to yield. **B,** The gloved, lubricated finger is slowly introduced in the direction of the umbilicus. **C,** Avoid discomfort for the client by this approach at a right-angle to the sphincter and without promoting relaxation. (Adapted from Dunphy, J. E., and Botsford, T. W.: Physical examination of the surgical patient; an introduction to clinical surgery, ed. 4, Philadelphia, 1975, W. B. Saunders Co.)

is asked to tighten the sphincter around the examining finger to provide a measurement of muscle strength of the anal sphincter. Hypertonicity of the external sphincter may occur with anxious, voluntary or involuntary contraction or as a result of an anal fissure or other local pathological condition. A relaxed or hypotonic sphincter is seen occasionally after rectal surgery or may be due to a neurological deficiency. The subcutaneous portion of the external sphincter is palpated on the inner aspect of the anal verge. The palpating finger is rotated to examine the entire muscular ring. The intersphincteric line is marked by a palpable indentation. Palpation of the deep external sphincter is performed through the lower part of the internal sphincter, which it surrounds. Assessment of the levator ani muscle is accomplished by palpating laterally and posteriorly where the muscle is attached to the rectal wall on one side and then the other (Fig. 18-3).

The posterior wall of the rectum follows the curve of the coccyx and sacrum and feels smooth to the pal-

pating finger. The mucosa of the anal canal is palpated for tumor or polyps. The coccyx is palpated to determine mobility and sensitivity.

The examining finger is able to palpate a distance of 6 to 10 cm of the rectal canal. A bidigital palpation of the sphincter area may yield more information than would be obtained by probing with the index finger alone. This is accomplished by pressing the thumb of the examining hand against the perianal tissue and moving the examining index finger toward it. This is a useful technique for detecting a perianal abscess and for palpating the bulbourethral (Cowper's) glands.

Rectal valves may be misinterpreted as protruding intrarectal masses, especially when they are well developed.

The lateral walls of the rectum may be palpated by rotating the index finger along the sides of the rectum. The ischial spines and sacrotuberous ligaments may be identified through palpation.

The prostate gland is situated anterior to the rec-

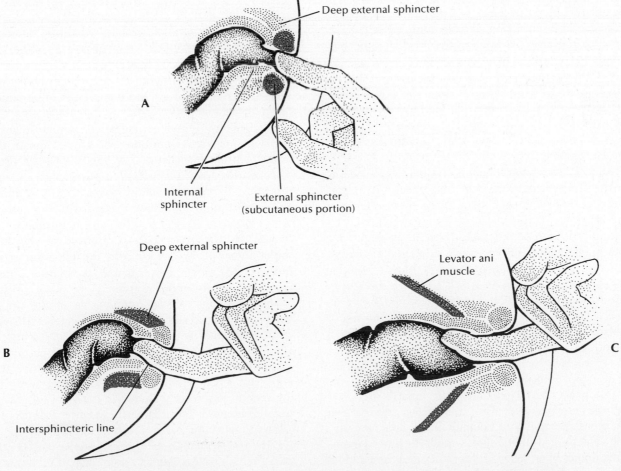

Fig. 18-3. The subcutaneous portion of the external sphincter is palpated, **A,** followed by digital exploration of the deep external sphincter, **B. C,** Palpation of the levator ani muscle. (Adapted from Dunphy, J. E., and Botsford, T. W.: Physical examination of the surgical patient; an introduction to clinical surgery, ed. 4, Philadelphia, 1975, W. B. Saunders Co.)

tum; therefore, palpation through the mucosa of the anterior wall of the rectum allows the examiner to assess the size, shape, and consistency of the prostate gland. The client is asked to bear down so that a mass not otherwise reached might be pushed downward into the range of the examining finger.

The prostate gland, a bilobed structure, has a normal diameter of approximately 4 cm. The palpating finger indentifies the smooth lateral lobes separated by a central groove. The prostate is approximately 2.5 cm in length, and the presence of nodules is noted. The prostate should feel firm and smooth. The client should be asked to report tenderness to touch. (See Chapter 19 for assessment of male genitalia.)

The normal cervix can be felt as a small round mass through the anterior wall of the rectum. (See Chapter 20 for assessment of the female genitalia.)

Examination of the stool

On withdrawal of the examining finger, the nature of any feces clinging to the glove should be examined (Table 18-1). The presence of pus or blood is noted. Bright red blood in small or large amounts may be from the large intestine, the sigmoid colon, the rectum, or the anus. However, the stool may be burgundy in color if the bleeding occurred in the ascending colon. Colonic bleeding may be suspected when blood is mixed with the feces, whereas rectal bleeding is probably occurring when the blood is observed on the surface of the stool. The presence of a good deal of blood in the stool may be associated with marked malodor.

A black, tarry stool (melena) results from bleeding in the stomach or small intestine; the blood is partially digested during its passage to the rectum. On the other hand, the black color may result from ingested iron compounds and bismuth preparations.

A small quantity of the feces is subjected to a chemical test for the presence of occult blood. Minimal abrasions of the gastrointestinal tract are thought to be responsible for blood loss of 1 to 3 ml daily in the feces. The loss of more than 50 ml from the upper gastrointestinal tract will produce melena. To detect quantities less than 50 ml or to determine whether black stools actually do contain blood, several reagents may be used.

The guaiac test is the most frequently used test for routine screening. The gum guaiac solution can identify 0.5% to 1% of hemoglobin in aqueous solution. The procedure involves wiping the gloved examining finger on a piece of filter paper and then adding 1 to 2 drops of guaiac solution, glacial acetic acid, and hydrogen peroxide. A positive reaction is denoted by the solution turning blue or dark green

Table 18-1. Characteristics of the stool related to the possible pathological conditions

Description of the stool	Possible pathological condition
Light tan, gray	Absence of bile pigments—obstructive jaundice
Greasy, pale, and yellow; increased fat content (steatorrhea, sprue)	Malabsorption syndromes
Tarry, black (melena)	Gastrointestinal tract bleeding; ingestion of iron compounds or bismuth preparations
Small flakes of jellylike mucus mixed with stool	Inflammation

within 30 seconds (Fig. 18-4). Orthotoluidine is also useful in the detection of occult blood and is more sensitive than guaiac solution (it detects 0.01% to 0.1% of hemoglobin in aqueous solution).

The most common cause of occult bleeding is cancer of the colon.

Endoscopic procedures

The presence of a pathological condition detected by the digital examination is further explored by endoscopy.

Anoscopy. The Hirshman or Brincker-Hoff anoscope may be used for a more complete examination of the anal canal and internal hemorrhoidal zone.

Proctoscopy. Direct visualization of anal or lower rectal pathological conditions (or 9 to 15 cm of the lower gastrointestinal tract) is possible with a proctoscope. The position most frequently used for this procedure is the knee-chest position. The warmed and lubricated instrument is passed with the obturator in place to its full length. The obturator is removed, and the proctoscope is removed slowly while the examiner observes for ulcers, inflammation, strictures, or the cause of a palpable mass. Biopsy may be performed through the tube.

Sigmoidoscopy. Visual examination of the upper portion of the rectum that cannot be felt with the examining finger is possible with a sigmoidoscope; it allows direct visualization of the lower 24 cm of the gastrointestinal tract. This examination is particularly important since one-half of all carcinomas occur in the rectum and colon. The early detection of polyps and malignant lesions may result in early and successful treatment of an otherwise fatal disease.

Careful explanation of the procedure and gentle manipulation of the client's tissue allow the examination to take place with little discomfort to the client.

The procedure is effective for the identification of proctitis, polyps, and carcinoma. Sigmoidoscopy is

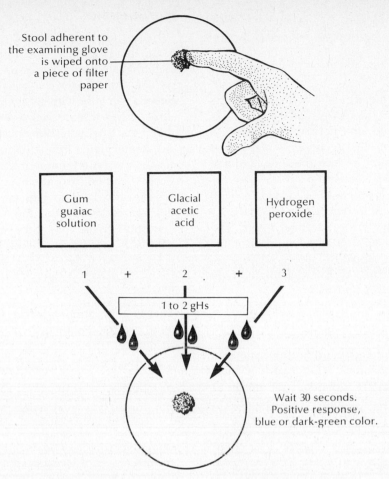

Stool adherent to the examining glove is wiped onto a piece of filter paper

Gum guaiac solution

Glacial acetic acid

Hydrogen peroxide

1 + 2 + 3

1 to 2 gHs

Wait 30 seconds. Positive response, blue or dark-green color.

Fig. 18-4. Procedure for the guaiac assessment for occult blood. (Adapted from Dunphy, J. E., and Botsford, T. W.: Physical examination of the surgical patient; an introduction to clinical surgery, ed. 4, Philadelphia, 1975, W. B. Saunders Co.)

also helpful in the identification of diarrhea of colonic origin. The mucous membrane may be inspected, and scrapings may be taken for microscopic examination.

PATHOLOGY
Pilonidal cyst or sinus

Pilonidal sinus is generally first diagnosed between the ages of 15 and 30, even though it is a congenital lesion. It is located superficial to the coccyx or lower sacrum. The opening may look like a dimple, with another very small opening in the midline. In other cases a cyst is observed and may be palpated; in more advanced conditions a sinus tract may be palpated. The area may become erythematous, and a tuft of hair may be observed. The ingrowth of the hairs is probably the cause of infection, cyst, and fistula formation.

Pruritus ani

Excoriated, thickened, and pigmented skin may result from chronic inflammation of pruritus ani. The itching and burning of the rectal area are most often traceable to pinworms in children and to fungal infections in adults. Diabetic clients are particularly vulnerable to fungal infections. A dull, grayish pink color of the perianal skin is a characteristic of fungal infections. The radiating folds of skin may appear enlarged, and the skin may be cracked or fissured. Pruritus ani characterized by dry and brittle skin is thought to be related to psychosomatic disease.

Rectal tenesmus

Rectal tenesmus is the painful straining at stool associated with spasm of anal and rectal muscles; the client complains of a distressing feeling of urgency. The client is questioned concerning the nature of the stool. A hard, dry stool is indicative of constipation. A bloody, diarrheal stool might be indicative of ulcerative colitis. Rectal fissure may be the cause of tenesmus with normally constituted stools.

Tenesmus may also be a symptom experienced by the client with a perirectal inflammation, such as prostatitis.

The client who complains of constant rectal pain is examined carefully for thrombosed rectal hemorrhoids.

Fecal impaction

Fecal impaction is the accumulation and dehydration of fecal material in the rectum. When motility of the rectum is inhibited, the normal progression of feces does not occur and more water is reabsorbed through the bowel wall. The feces become hard and difficult to pass and may lead to complete obstruction. Fecal impaction is observed in individuals with chronic constipation and in individuals who have retained barium following gastrointestinal x-rays. The client complains of a sense of rectal fullness or urgency. Frequent small, liquid-to-loose stools may occur in incomplete obstruction. The dehydrated fecal mass is easily felt on palpation.

Anal fissure

A thin tear of the superficial anal mucosa, generally weeping, may be identified by asking the client to perform Valsalva's maneuver. The fissure is most commonly (more than 90%) found in the posterior midline of the anal mucosa and less frequently in the anterior midline.

Anal fissure is generally the result of the trauma associated with the passage of a large, hard stool. The client may complain of local pain, itching, or bleeding. Pain generally accompanies the passage of stool and blood may be observed on the stool or on the toilet tissue. The inspection findings may include a sentinel skin-tag or ulcer through which the muscles of the internal sphincter may be visible at the base. Because the examination is painful to the patient, making it difficult to relax the anal muscles, local anesthesia may be necessary.

Fistula in ano

A tract from an anal fissure or infection that terminates in the perianal skin or other tissue is termed an anorectal fistula; it usually has its origin from local crypt abscesses. The fistula is a chronically inflamed tube made up of fibrous tissue surrounding granulation tissue and may frequently be palpated. The external opening is generally visible as a red elevation of granulation tissue. Local compression may result in the expression of serosanguinous or purulent drainage. Palpation (bidigital) is best accomplished with a finger in the anorectal cavity compressing the tissue against the thumb on the skin surface. The fistulous tract feels like an indurated cord.

The site from which drainage from an anal infection occurs can be identified by relating the location of the external opening of the fissure to the anus (Table 18-2 and Fig. 18-5).

Hemorrhoids

Hemorrhoids are dilated congested veins of the hemorrhoidal group. The swelling is associated with increased hydrostatic pressure in the portal venous system. The pressure associated with hemorrhoids correlates highly with pregnancy, straining at stool, chronic liver disease, and sudden increases in intra-abdominal pressure. Bowel habits also play a role in that hemorrhoids frequently occur with diarrhea or incomplete bowel emptying. Local factors such as abscess or tumor may also contribute to venous stasis.

Hemorrhoidal skin tags are ragged, flaccid, skin sacs located around the anus. These skin tags cover connective tissue sacs and are the locus of resolved external hemorrhoids. Clients describe these tags as

Table 18-2. Location of fissure site related to the external opening

	External opening	Location in the anus
Goodsell's rule	Posterior to a line between the ischial tuberosities	Posterior
	Radial from the drainage site	Anterior
Salmon's law	Posterior to the anus or more than 2.5 cm anterior or lateral	Posterior
	Anterior or less than 2.5 cm lateral	Anterior

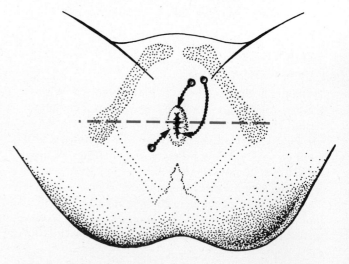

Fig. 18-5. Salmon's law. Fissure location related to the aperture of the fistula. (Adapted from Dunphy, J. E., and Botsford, T. W.: Physical examination of the surgical patient; an introduction to clinical surgery, ed. 4, Philadelphia, 1975, W. B. Saunders Co.)

painless. Internal hemorrhoids occur proximal to the pectinate line, whereas external hemorrhoids are those that are seen distal to this boundary. External hemorrhoids are covered by skin or anal squamous tissue.

External hemorrhoids are often accompanied by pain, particularly if the skin is stretched by a sudden increase in mass; since the mass is located near the sphincter muscles, spasm is not uncommon. External hemorrhoids often cause itching and bleeding on defecation. These dilated veins may not be apparent at rest, but may appear as bluish, swollen areas at the anal verge when thrombosed. A thrombosed hemorrhoid is one in which blood has clotted, both within and outside the vein.

Internal hemorrhoids generally do not contribute to pain sensation unless they are complicated by thrombosis, infection, or erosion of overlying mucosal surfaces. Discomfort is increased if the hemorrhoids prolapse through the anal opening. Bleeding may occur from the internal hemorrhoids with or without defecation. Proctoscopy is generally necessary for their identification.

Rectal polyps

Rectal polyps, which feel like soft nodules, are encountered frequently. They may be pedunculated (on a stalk) or sessile (irregularly moundlike, growing from a relatively broad base, and closely adherent to the mucosal wall). Because of their soft consistency they may be difficult or impossible to identify by palpation. Proctoscopy is usually necessary for identification, and a biopsy is performed to identify malignant lesions.

A pedunculated rectal polyp occasionally prolapses through the anal ring.

Rectal prolapse

Internal hemorrhoids are the type most commonly identified because of mucosal tissue prolapsing through the anal ring. The pink-colored mucosa is described as appearing like a doughnut or rosette. In the older client, however, protruding mucosa may herald eversion or prolapse of the rectum. Incomplete prolapse involves only mucosa, whereas complete rectal prolapse involves the sphincters.

The prolapse of tissue through the anal ring is described by the client as occurring on exercise or while straining at stool. Frequently, the client describes being able to push the mass back in with digital pressure. Inspection reveals a red, bulging, mucosal mass protruding through the anal ring.

Anal incontinence

The loss of the voluntary ability to control defecation is called incontinence. The loss may range from the involuntary passage of flatus to complete loss of sphincter tone. The loss of fecal gases or liquids may also occur in the presence of a normal sphincter in hyperdynamic bowel states.

Abscesses or masses

Abscesses of the lower gastrointestinal tract that may be identified by physical examination (Fig. 18-6) include:

1. *Perirectal abscess.* This abscess may be palpated as a tender mass adjacent to the anal canal. The increased temperature of the mass may be helpful in the identification of the inflammatory process.
2. *Ischiorectal abscess.* This abscess may be palpated as a tender mass protruding into the lateral wall of the anal canal.

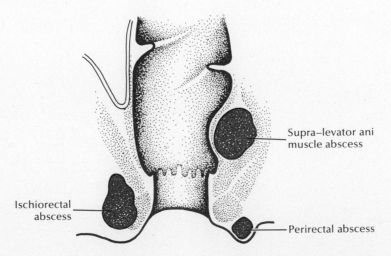

Fig. 18-6. Common sites of abscess formation of the lower gastrointestinal tract. (Adapted from Dunphy, J. E., and Botsford, T. W.: Physical examination of the surgical patient; an introduction to clinical surgery, ed. 4, Philadelphia, 1975, W. B. Saunders Co.)

3. *Supra–levator ani muscle abscess.* This abscess may be felt by the examining finger as a tender mass in the lateral rectal wall.

The presence of a mass in the rectum deserves special attention since nearly half of those discovered are malignant. The client frequently denies pain or other symptoms. Early lesions are felt as small elevations or nodules with a firm base. Ulceration of the center of the lesion results in a crater that may be palpated. An ulcerated carcinoma may be identified through palpation by its firm, nodular, rolled edge. The lesion of carcinoma is described by including annular or tubular shape, degree of fixation, and distance from the anus. The consistency of the malignant mass is often stony and hard, and the contour is irregular. Extension of metastatic carcinoma from the peritoneum to the pelvic floor is described as a rectal shell. It is palpated as a hard, nodular ridge.

SUMMARY

I. Inspection of perianal skin and perineum
   A. Pilonidal sinus
   B. Pruritus ani
   C. Fissure
   D. Fistula in ano
   E. Hemorrhoids
   F. Prolapse
II. Palpation
   A. Sphincter tone
   B. Prostate evaluation
      1. Size
      2. Shape
      3. Consistency
   C. Seminal vesicles
   D. Polyp
   E. Abscess
   F. Tumor
      1. Nature of mass
      2. Rectal shelf
III. Inspection of stool
   A. Pus
   B. Blood
   C. Guaiac test for occult blood

BIBLIOGRAPHY

Brooks, F. P., editor: Gastrointestinal pathophysiology, New York, 1974, Oxford University Press, Inc.

Deyhle, P., and Demlingi, L.: Colonscopy: technic, results and indications, Endoscopy 3:143, 1971.

Dunphy, J., and Botsford, T.: Physical examination of the surgical patient; an introduction to clinical surgery, Philadelphia, 1975, W. B. Saunders Co.

Dworken, H. J.: The alimentary tract, Philadelphia, 1974, W. B. Saunders Co.

Earnest, D. L.: Diseases of the anus. In Schleisenger, M. H., and Fordtran, J. S., editors: Gastrointestinal disease, Philadelphia, 1973, W. B. Saunders Co.

Ganchrow, M. I., Bowman, E., and Clark, J. F.: Thrombosed hemorrhoids: a clinicopathologic study, Dis. Colon Rectum 14:331, 1971.

Graham-Stewart, C. W.: The etiology and treatment of fissure in ano, Int. Abstr. Surg. 115:511, 1962.

Mazier, W. P.: The treatment and care of anal fistulas: a study of 1000 patients, Dis. Colon Rectum 14:134, 1971.

Ostrow, J. D., and others: Sensitivity and reproducibility of chemical tests for fecal occult blood with an emphasis on false positive reactions, Am. J. Dig. Dis. 18:930, 1973.

19 Assessment of the male genitalia and assessment of the inguinal area for hernias

Male genitalia

The examination of the genital organs of any client is usually perceived by both the client and the practitioner as being different from the examination of other body parts. Culturally, male gynecologists have been accepted and sometimes even preferred by female clients. This chapter discusses the approach of the female practitioner to the examination of the male client's genital system.

First, the female practitioner should feel emotionally comfortable with the examination. If she does not, she should routinely refer this part of the physical examination to a male practitioner. Next, if she is comfortable with the examination, she must accept the possibility of the male client's reluctance to having his genitalia examined by a woman. Cajoling a client into an uncomfortable procedure may destroy further rapport; his wishes in the situation should be respected. In most clinical settings, there is a male practitioner present who would be available for a few minutes to examine the male genitalia. Our experience has been that most male clients are agreeable to examination by a woman; if there is discomfort, it is usually on the part of the examiner. It is therefore recommended that the beginning female examiner critically analyze her own feelings, fears, and beliefs; attempt male genital examination under supervision and with several cooperative clients; and then reexamine her feelings.

The examination should be preceded by a thorough history of the urinary system and a history of sexual functioning. As with the female client, questioning about sexual activity or performance while the genitalia are being handled may be perceived by the client as evaluative or provocative.

ANATOMY

The following is a review of the anatomy of the male genitalia (Fig. 19-1).

The shaft of the penis is formed by three columns of erectile tissue bound together by heavy fibrous tissue to form a cylinder. The dorsolateral columns are called the corpora cavernosa; the ventromedial column is called the corpus spongiosum, and this column contains the urethra. Distally the penis terminates in a cone-shaped entity called the glans penis. The glans penis is formed by an extension and expansion of the corpus spongiosum penis, which fits over the blunt ends of the corpora cavernosa penis The corona is the prominence formed where the glans joins the shaft. The urethra traverses the corpus spongiosum, and the external urethral orifice is a slit-like opening located slightly ventrally on the tip of the glans.

The skin of the penis is thin, hairless, dark, and only loosely connected to the internal parts of the organ. At the area of the corona, the skin forms a free fold, called the prepuce or foreskin. When allowed to remain, this flap covers the glans to a variable extent. Often the prepuce is surgically removed in circumcision (Fig. 19-2).

The scrotum is a deeply pigmented cutaneous pouch, containing the testes and parts of the spermatic cords (Fig. 19-3). The sac is formed by an outer layer of thin, rugous skin overlying a tight muscle layer. The left side of the scrotum is often lower than the right side because the left spermatic cord is usually longer. Internally the scrotum is divided into halves by a septum; each half contains a testis and its epididymis and part of the spermatic cord. The testes are ovoid and are suspended vertically, slightly for-

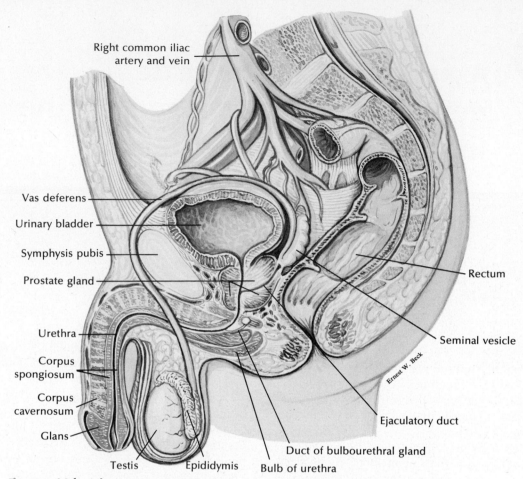

Right common iliac
artery and vein

Vas deferens

Urinary bladder

Symphysis pubis

Prostate gland

Rectum

Urethra

Seminal vesicle

Corpus
spongiosum

Corpus
cavernosum

Ernest W. Beck

Glans

Ejaculatory duct

Duct of bulbourethral gland

Testis   Epididymis   Bulb of urethra

Fig. 19-1. Male pelvic organs. (From Anthony, C. P., and Thibodeau, G. A.: Anatomy and physiology, ed. 10, St. Louis, 1979, The C. V. Mosby Co.)

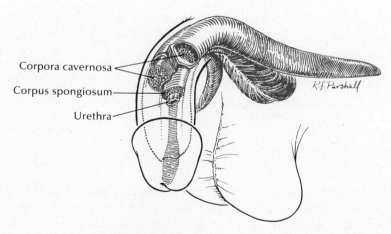

Corpora cavernosa

Corpus spongiosum

Urethra

R.f. Parshall

Fig. 19-2. Circumcised penis.

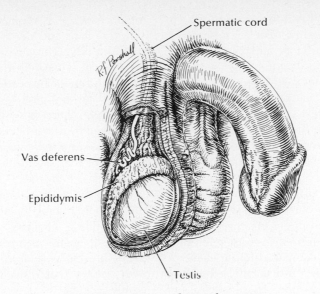

Fig. **19-3.** Scrotum and scrotal contents.

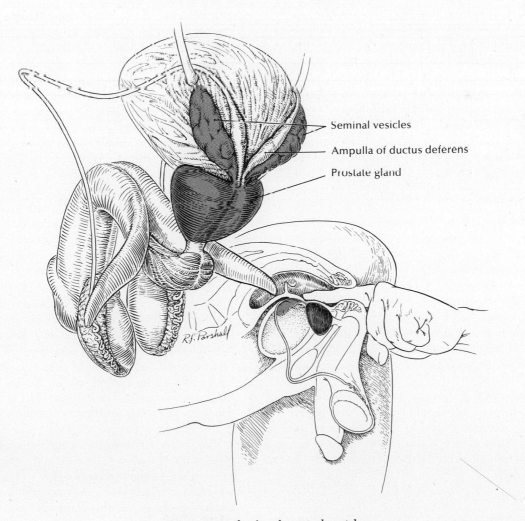

Fig. **19-4.** Prostate gland and seminal vesicles.

ward; they lean slightly laterally in the scrotum. The mediolateral surfaces are flattened. Each is approximately 4 to 5 cm long, 3 cm wide, and 2 cm thick.

The epididymis is a comma-shaped structure that is curved over the posterolateral surface and upper end of the testis; it creates a visual bulge on the posterolateral surface of the testis. The ductus deferens (or vas deferens) begins at the tail of the epididymis, ascends the spermatic cord, travels through the inguinal canal, and eventually descends on the fundus of the bladder (Fig. 19-1).

The prostate, a slightly conical gland, lies under the bladder, surrounds the urethra, and measures approximately 4 cm at its base or uppermost part, 3 cm vertically, and 2 cm in its anteroposterior diameter. The prostate gland has been compared to the chestnut in size and shape. It has three lobes, left and right lateral lobes and a median lobe. These lobes are not well demarcated from each other. The median lobe is the part of the prostate that projects inward from the upper, posterior area toward the urethra. It is the enlargement of this lobe that causes urinary obstruction in benign prostatic hypertrophy.

The posterior surface of the prostate is in close contact with the rectal wall and is the only portion of the gland accessible to examination. Its posterior surface is slightly convex; a shallow median furrow divides all except the upper portions of the posterior surface into right and left lateral lobes.

The seminal vesicles are a pair of convoluted pouches, 5 to 10 cm long, which lie along the lower posterior surface of the bladder, anterior to the rectum (Fig. 19-4).

EXAMINATION

The techniques of inspection and palpation are used to examine the male genitalia. After the inguinal and genital areas are exposed, the skin, hair, and gross appearance of the penis and scrotum are inspected. Examination of the skin, nodes, and hair distribution are discussed elsewhere in this text. The size of the penis and the secondary sex characteristics are assessed in relationship to the client's age and general development. If inflammation or lesions are observed or suspected, gloves are used for the examination.

The onset of the appearance of adult sexual characteristics is extremely variable. Pubic hair appears and the testes enlarge between the ages of 12 and 16 years. Penile enlargement and the onset of seminal emission normally occurs between the ages of 13 and 17 years.

Penis

The penis is observed for lesions. nodules, swelling, inflammation, and discharge. If the client is un-

circumcised, he is requested to retract the prepuce from the glans and the glans and foreskin are examined carefully. The client is also asked to compress the glans anteroposteriorly. This opens the distal end of the urethra for inspection. If any discharge is present, a smear and culture for gonorrhea are obtained (see Chapter 20 on assessment of the female genitalia and procedures for smears and cultures). If the client has reported a discharge, he is requested to milk the penis from the base to the urethra; if a discharge is present, it is cultured.

Among the more common penile lesions are syphilitic chancre, condylomata acuminata, and cancer. The syphilitic chancre is the primary lesion of syphilis. It begins as a single papule that eventually erodes into an oval or round red ulcer with an indurated base that discharges serous material. It is usually painless.

Condylomata acuminata are wart-appearing growths. They are caused by a venereal infection and may be seen occurring singly or in multiple, cauliflowerlike patches.

Carcinoma of the penis occurs most frequently on the glans and on the inner lip of the prepuce. It may appear dry and scaly, ulcerated, or nodular. It is usually painless.

The urethral meatus should be positioned rather centrally on the glans. When the distal urethral ostium occurs on the ventral corona or at a more proximal and ventral site on the penis or perineum, the condition is called hypospadias (Fig. 19-5). A similar malpositioning of the urethral meatus in the dorsal area is called epispadias.

When hypospadias or epispadias is noted, the location of the urethral meatus should be described as precisely as possible. Hypospadias can be classified as being glandular, penile, penoscrotal, or perineal. Epispadias can be classified as being glandular, penile, or complete. Glandular refers to a location somewhere between the normal position and the junction of the glans with the body of the penis. Penile refers to a location on the penile shaft. Penoscrotal hypospadias indicates a positioning of the meatus along the anterior margin of the scrotum. Hypospadias is described as perineal when the urethral orifice is on the perineum. In the latter condition, the scrotum is bifid. Epispadias is described as complete when the urethral orifice is located anterior to and off of the penis.

The prepuce should be easily retractable from the glans and returnable to its original position. Phimosis exists when retraction cannot occur (Fig. 19-6). This condition presents problems with cleanliness and prevents observation of the glans and interior surfaces of the prepuce. If the foreskin has been partially retracted but has impinged on the penis, so that it

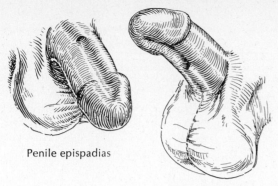

Penile epispadias

Penile hypospadias

Fig. 19-5. Malpositioning of the urethral meatus.

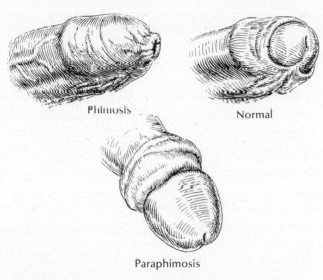

Phimosis

Normal

Paraphimosis

Fig. 19-6. Phimosis, normal retraction of the prepuce, and paraphimosis.

cannot be returned to its usual position, the condition is called paraphimosis.

The penile shaft should be carefully palpated. Occasionally, hard, nontender subcutaneous plaques are palpated on the dorsomedial surface. The client with this condition, called Peyronie's disease, may report penile bending with erection and painful intercourse.

Scrotum

The client is instructed to hold the penis out of the way, and the examiner observes the general size, superficial appearance, and symmetry of the scrotum. The scrotum may normally appear asymmetrical because the left testis is generally lower than the right testis. Also, the tone of the dartos muscle determines the size of the scrotum; it contracts when the area is cold and relaxes when the area is warm. In advanced age, the dartos muscle is somewhat atonic and the scrotum may appear pendulous.

When the scrotal skin is being observed, its rugated surface should be spread. Also, the examiner

should remember to inspect the posterior and posterolateral as well as anterior and anterolateral skin areas. A common abnormality, occurring as a single lesion or as multiple lesions, is that of sebaceous cysts. These are firm, yellow to white, nontender cutaneous lesions measuring up to 1 cm in diameter.

The scrotum may become edematous, and palpation may produce pitting. This may occur in any condition that causes edema in the lower trunk, for example, cardiovascular disease.

The contents of each half of the scrotal sac are palpated. Both testes should be present in the scrotum at birth; if not present, their location should be determined by retracing their course of descent back into the abdomen.

Both testes are palpated simultaneously between the thumb and the first two fingers. Their consistency, size, shape, and response to pressure are determined. They should be smooth, homogenous in consistency, regular, equal in size, freely movable, and slightly sensitive to compression.

Next, each epididymis is palpated. The epididymides are located in the posterolateral area of the testes in 93% of males. In approximately 7% of males they are in the anterolateral or anterior areas. They are palpated, and their size, shape, consistency, and tenderness are noted. Then each of the spermatic cords is palpated by bilaterally grasping each between the thumb and the forefinger. The vas deferentia feel like smooth cords and are movable; the arteries, veins, lymph vessels, and nerves feel like indefinite threads along the side of the vas.

If swelling, irregularity, or nodularity is noted in the scrotum, attempts are made to transilluminate it by darkening the room and placing a lit flashlight behind the scrotal contents. Transillumination is a red glow. Serous fluid will transilluminate; tissue and blood will not. The more commonly occurring abnormalities of the scrotum are described and illustrated in Table 19-1.

All scrotal masses should be described by their placement, size, shape, consistency, tenderness, and whether they transilluminate.

Prostate gland

With an ambulatory client it is most satisfactory to execute the rectal and prostate examination with the client standing, hips flexed, toes pointed toward each other, and upper body resting on the examining table. This position flattens the buttocks, deters gluteal contraction, and makes the anus and rectum more accessible to evaluation. A debilitated client may be examined in the left lateral or lithotomy position. In the left lateral position he is reminded to flex his right knee and hip and to have his buttocks close to the edge of the examining table. The gen-

Table 19-1. Description of scrotal abnormalities

Abnormality	Illustration	Definition/causation	Basis for diagnosis
Hydrocele		An accumulation of serous fluid between the visceral and parietal layers of the tunica vaginalis	Transilluminates; fingers can get above the mass
Scrotal hernia		A hernia within the scrotum	Bowel sounds auscultated; does not transilluminate; fingers cannot get above the mass
Varicocele		Abnormal dilatation and tortuosity of the veins of the pampiniform plexus; often described as a "bag of worms" in the scrotum*	Complaints of a dragging sensation or dull pain in the scrotal area; feels like a soft bag of worms; collapses when the scrotum is elevated and increases when the scrotum is dependent; more commonly present on the left side; usually appears at puberty
Spermatocele		An epididymal cyst resulting from a partial obstruction of the spermatic tubules*	Transilluminates; round mass, feels like a third testis; painless
Epididymal mass or nodularity		May be due to benign or malignant neoplasms, syphilis, or tuberculosis	Nodules are not tender; in tuberculosis lesions, vas deferens often feels beaded

Table 19-1. Description of scrotal abnormalities—cont'd

Abnormality	Illustration	Definition/causation	Basis for diagnosis
Epididymitis		An inflammation of the epididymis, usually due to *Escherichia coli*, *Neisseria gonorrhea*, or *Mycobacterium tuberculosis* organisms*	Spermatic cord often thickened and indurated; pain relieved by elevation
Torsion of the spermatic cord		Axial rotation or volvulus of the spermatic cord, resulting in infarction of the testicle	Elevated mass; pain not relieved by further elevation; more common in childhood or adolescence; history of extreme pain and tenderness of the testis, followed by hyperemic swelling and hydrocele
Testicular tumor		Multiple causes	Usually not painful; hydroceles may develop secondary to tumor—if a testis cannot be palpated, fluid may need to be aspirated so that the testis can be accurately evaluated.

*Betesh, S., editor: Diseases of the urinary tract and male genital organs, Geneva, 1974, Council for Internal Organizations for Medical Sciences, pp. 86-90.

eral procedure for the anal and rectal examination is described in Chapter 17 on assessment of the abdomen and rectosigmoid region. The general rectal examination is performed first; then the prostate gland and seminal vesicles are palpated (Fig. 19-4). The pad of the index finger is used for palpation. The prostate gland is located on the anterior rectal wall but should not be protruding into the rectal lumen.

Prostatic enlargement is protrusion of the prostate gland into the rectal lumen and is commonly described in grades:

Grade I: Encroaches less than 1 cm into the rectal lumen.

Grade II: Encroaches 1 to 2 cm into the rectal lumen.

Grade III: Encroaches 2 to 3 cm into the rectal lumen.

Grade IV: Encroaches more than 3 cm into the rectal lumen.

The gland should be approximately 3 cm in length,

symmetrical, movable, and of a rubbery consistency. Its median sulcus normally can be felt. The proximal portions of the seminal vesicles can sometimes be palpated as corrugated structures above the lateral to the midpoint of the gland. Normally they are too soft to be palpated. The examiner should attempt to examine all available surfaces of the prostate gland and seminal vesicles. Significant abnormalities of the prostate gland or seminal vesicles include protrusion into the rectal lumen; hard, nodular areas; bogginess; tenderness; and asymmetry.

The examiner should mentally consider the following questions about these structures:

Surface: Smooth or nodular?

Consistency: Rubbery, hard, boggy, soft, or fluctuant?

Shape: Rounded or flat?

Size: Normal, enlarged, or atrophied?

Sensitivity: Tender or not?

Movability: Movable or fixed?

A hard, single or multiple lesion on a firm and

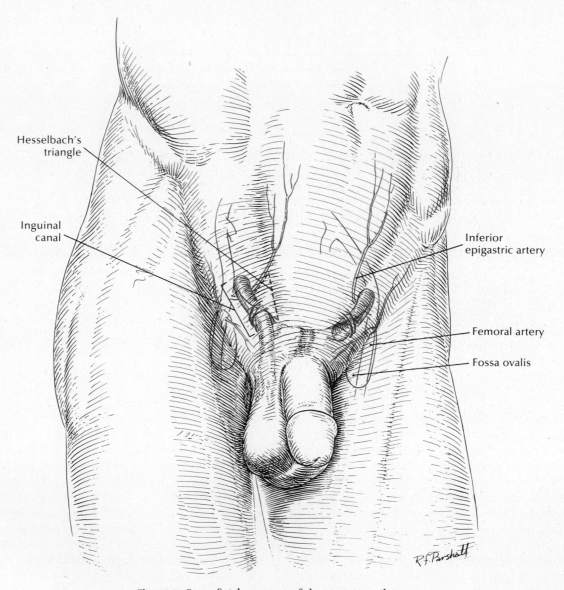

Hesselbach's
triangle

Inguinal
canal

Inferior
epigastric artery

Femoral artery

Fossa ovalis

R.F.Parshall

Fig. 19-7. Superficial anatomy of the anterior pelvic area.

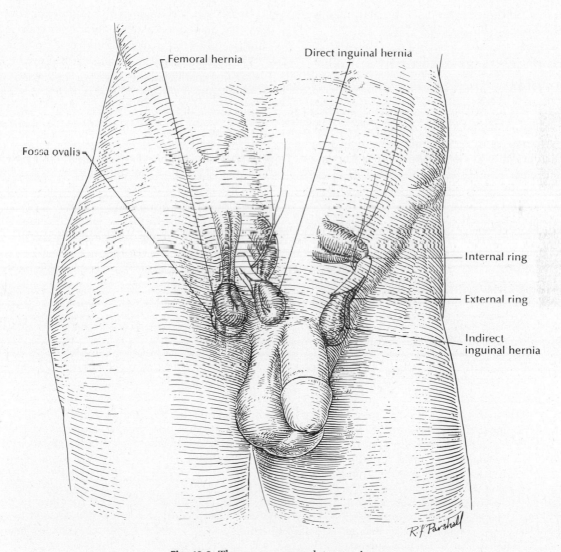

Fig. 19-8. Three common pelvic area hernias.

fixed prostate gland may be carcinoma or tuberculosis. The initial lesion of carcinoma is frequently on the posterior lobe and can be easily identified during the rectal examination. A soft, symmetrical, boggy, nontender prostate gland may indicate benign prostatic hypertrophy, a condition very common in men over 50 years of age. In the later stages of this condition, the median sulcus may be obliterated. A boggy, fluctuant, or tender prostate gland may indicate acute or chronic prostatitis. The prostate gland can be massaged centrally from its lateral edges to force secretions into the urethra. Secretion at the urethral opening can be examined and cultured.

Inguinal area: assessment for hernias

If a client has an inguinal or groin area hernia, he (or she) will probably complain of a swelling or bulging in that area, especially during abdominal straining. All clients should be screened for inguinal and femoral hernias, even if they do not complain of groin swelling, as part of the routine physical examination.

No special equipment is needed for the examination.

ANATOMY

The following is a review of the anatomy of the inguinal area (Fig. 19-7).

The inguinal (Poupart's) ligament extends from the anterosuperior spine of the ilium to the pubic tubercle. The inguinal canal is a flattened tunnel between two layers of abdominal muscle, measuring approximately 4 to 6 cm in the adult. Its internal ring is located 1 to 2 cm above the midpoint of the inguinal ligament. The spermatic cord traverses through this internal ring, passes through the canal, exits the canal at its external (subcutaneous) ring, and then moves up and over the inguinal ligament and into the scrotum.

Hesselbach's triangle is the region superior to the inguinal canal, medial to the inferior epigastric artery, and lateral to the margin of the rectus muscle.

The femoral canal is a potential space just inferior to the inguinal ligament and 3 cm medial and parallel to the femoral artery. If the examiner's right hand is placed on the client's right anterior thigh with the index finger over the femoral artery, the femoral canal will be under the ring finger.

The three main types of pelvic area hernias are shown in Fig. 19-8. In the *indirect inguinal hernia*, the hernial sac enters the internal inguinal canal and its tip is located somewhere in the inguinal canal or beyond the canal. In males, indirect inguinal hernias may descend into the scrotum. The *direct inguinal hernia* emerges directly from behind and through the external inguinal ring. The *femoral hernia* emerges through the femoral ring, the femoral canal, and the fossa ovalis.

Table 19-2. Comparison of inguinal and femoral hernias

| | Inguinal hernia | | Femoral hernia |
	Indirect	Direct	
Course	Sac emerges through the internal inguinal ring, lateral to the inferior epigastric artery; can remain in the canal, exit the external ring, or pass into the scrotum	Sac emerges directly from behind and through the external inguinal ring; located in the region of Hesselbach's triangle	Sac emerges through the femoral ring, the femoral canal, and the fossa ovalis; observed lateral to the femoral vein
Incidence	More common in infants under 1 year and in males 16 to 20 years; more common in males than in females at a ratio of approximately 4:1; 60% of all hernias	Most often observed in men over 40 years of age; rarer than the indirect hernia	Less common than inguinal hernias; seldom seen in children; more common in women; 4% of all hernias
Cause	Congenital or acquired	Congenital weakness exacerbated by (1) lifting, (2) atrophy of abdominal muscles, (3) ascites, (4) chronic cough, or (5) obesity	Acquired; may be caused by (1) stooping frequently, (2) increased abdominal pressure, or (3) loss of muscle substance
Clinical symptoms and signs	Soft swelling in the region of the internal inguinal ring—swelling increases when client stands or strains, is sometimes reduced when client reclines; pain during straining	Abdominal bulge in the area of Hesselbach's triangle, usually in the area of the internal ring; usually painless; easily reduced when client reclines; rarely enters scrotum	Right side more commonly affected; pain may be severe; strangulation frequent; sac may extend into the scrotum, into the labium, or along the saphenous vein

EXAMINATION

Inspection and palpation are the techniques used. Whenever possible, the examination for hernias is performed with the client standing. However, if the client is debilitated or especially tense, the examination may be performed while the client is lying down on a flat surface.

First, the areas of inguinal and femoral hernias are exposed and observed with the client at rest and while the client holds his breath and exerts abdominal pressure with the diaphragm. Straining is preferred to coughing because a more sustained pressure is elicited. Sometimes the impulse of coughing can be confused with the impulse of a hernia. Often, small hernias in women and children are more easily observed than felt because of the fatty tissue in the area.

The examiner palpates for a direct inguinal hernia by placing two fingers over each external inguinal ring and instructing the client to bear down. The presence of a hernia will produce a palpable bulge in the area.

To determine the presence of an indirect inguinal hernia, the client is asked to flex the ipsilateral knee slightly while the examiner attempts to direct his index or little finger into the path of the inguinal canal. When the finger has traversed as far as possible, the client is asked to strain. A hernia will be felt as a mass of tissue meeting the finger and then withdrawing. The left index or little finger, hand with palm side out, is used to examine the client's left side. The right hand in turn is used for the client's right side. In women, the canal is narrow and the

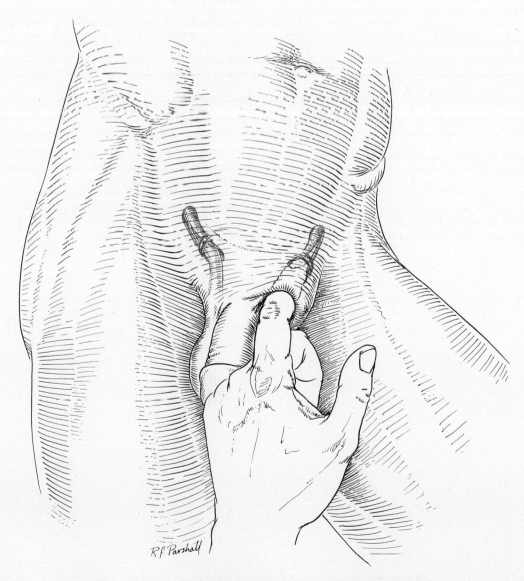

Fig. 19-9. Examination of a male client for indirect inguinal hernia.

finger cannot be inserted far, if at all. In men, the finger invaginates scrotal skin into the inguinal canal (Fig. 19-9).

In both men and women, each fossa ovalis area is palpated while the client is straining. The femoral hernia will be felt as a soft tumor at the fossa, below the inguinal ligament and lateral to the pubic tubercle.

Occasionally, the client may complain of the symptoms of hernia but none can be palpated. In such cases a load test is suggested. The client lifts a heavy object while the inguinal area is being observed. A previously unobserved bulge may become prominent.

SUMMARY

I. Male genitalia
   A. General inspection
      1. Skin
      2. Hair
         a. Distribution
         b. Parasites
      3. Inguinal area
         a. Swelling
         b. Inflammation
   B. Inspection of the penis
      1. Size relative to age and general development
      2. Discharge
      3. Skin
      4. Urethral meatus
      5. Prepuce
   C. Palpation of the penis
   D. Palpation of the inguinal nodes
   E. Inspection of the scrotum
      1. Skin
      2. Symmetry
      3. Size
   F. Palpation of the scrotum
      1. Testes
      2. Epididymides
      3. Spermatic cords
   G. Transillumination (if any swellings or masses are present)
   H. Observation and palpation of the rectal area
      1. General rectal examination
      2. Prostate gland
      3. Seminal vesicles
II. Inguinal area: assessment for hernias (direct, inguinal, and femoral)
   A. Inspection
   B. Palpation

BIBLIOGRAPHY

Badenoch, A. W.: Manual of urology, ed. 2, London, 1974, William Heinemann Medical Books, Ltd.

Bodner, H.: Diagnostic and therapeutic aids in urology, Springfield, Ill., 1974, Charles C Thomas, Publishers.

Brandes, D., editor: Male accesory sex organs, New York, 1974, Academic Press, Inc.

Btesh, S., editor: Disease of the urinary tract and male genital organs, Geneva, Switzerland, 1974, Council for International Organizations for Medical Sciences.

Calman, C. H.: An atlas of hernia repair, St. Louis, 1966, The C. V. Mosby Co.

Johnson, D. E., editor: Testicular tumors, Flushing, N.Y., 1972, Medical Examination Publishing Co., Inc.

Maingot, R., editor: Abdominal operation, ed. 6, New York, 1974, Appleton-Century-Crofts.

Ravitch, M. M.: Repairs of hernias, Chicago, 1969, Year Book Medical Publishers, Inc.

Scott, R., editor: Current controversies in urologic management, Philadelphia, 1972, W. B. Saunders Co.

20 Assessment of the female genitalia and procedures for smears and cultures

Female genitalia

Most female clients perceive the examination of their reproductive organs as being different from the examination of other body parts. Past admonitions of "do not touch" and "keep it covered" have created a population of anatomically unaware and sometimes inappropriately "modest" women who are often unnecessarily difficult to examine. Most practitioners believe that a great amount of information about a female client can be obtained by examining the genital area and performing screening tests; but because of their experience with the fearful and tense reactions of many clients, practitioners have sometimes routinely omitted the examination of the genital organs or have referred their clients to gynecological specialists for screening examinations.

One cause of the female client's tenseness during an examination of the genital area may be fear of discovery. During the history the practitioner investigates areas of anatomical and physiological function and dysfunction. The review of systems on all clients should include a sexual history. If this portion of the history is accomplished skillfully and if the client has been cooperative, she should not be apprehensive about the possible discovery of sexual "secrets."

Other causes of tenseness during the pelvic examination include fear of discovery of disease and the memory of previous, uncomfortable pelvic examinations.

Also, many clients are not knowledgeable regarding the anatomy of the pelvic area. The practitioner should determine the client's need for basic information regarding the structure of the genital organs and provide this instruction before the pelvic examination, along with a demonstration of the instruments and an explanation of the procedure. If a relatively

short amount of time were taken to inform and orient all female clients at the time of their first examination, practitioners and clients would reap the benefits of enhanced mutual cooperation.

Teaching the client a relaxation technique will often make an examination shorter or even possible. One relaxation technique that has been successful is the following: the client is instructed to place her hands on her chest at about the level of the diaphragm, breathe deeply and slowly through her mouth, concentrate on the rhythm of breathing, and relax all body muscles with each exhalation. The tense client is apt to hold her breath and tighten. Even the coached client may forget and hold her breath; a gentle reminder, advising her to keep breathing, usually enables the client to maintain relaxation. This technique is particularly helpful in the adolescent or virginal client, whose introitus may be especially tight.

Another relaxation or, more specifically, distraction technique that has been used by some practitioners is the placement of a sign or mobile above the examining table. Clients appreciate having something to look at, and their attention is constructively diverted from the activities of the examiner.

For most clients it is distressing to attempt to converse while in a lithotomy position. Most clients appreciate an explanation and reassurance from the examiner but prefer not to have to respond to questions until they are again upright and at eye level with the examiner. Questioning a client during the pelvic examination is apt to make her tense.

Environmental conditions are also important in enhancing cooperation during the examination of the genital area. The environment and the client should be warm. The examining area should be private and safe from unexpected intrusion.

ANATOMY AND PHYSIOLOGY
External genitalia

The external female genitalia are termed the vulva or pudendum (Fig. 20-1). The symphysis pubis is covered by a pad of fat called the mons pubis or mons veneris. In the postpubertal female the mons is covered by a patch of coarse, curly hair that extends to the lower abdomen. The abdominal portion of the female escutcheon is flat and forms the base of an inverted triangle of hair.

The labia majora are two bilobate folds of adipose tissue extending from the mons to the perineum. After puberty, their outer surfaces are covered with hair and their inner surfaces are smooth and hairless. The labia minora are two folds of skin that are thinner and darker in color than the labia majora. The labia minora lie within the labia majora and extend from the clitoris to the fourchette. Anteriorly, each labium minus divides into a medial and a lateral part. The lateral parts join posteriorly to form the prepuce of the clitoris, and the medial parts join anterior to the clitoris to form the frenulum of the clitoris. The clitoris is composed of erectile tissue and is homolo-

gous to the corpora cavernosa of the penis. Its body is normally about 2.5 cm in total length; the length of its visible portion is 2 cm or less.

The vestibule is the boat-shaped anatomical region between the labia minora. It contains the urethral and vaginal orifices. The urethral orifice is located approximately 2.5 cm posterior to the clitoris and is visualized as an irregular, vertical slit. The vaginal orifice, or introitus, lies immediately behind the urethral orifice and can be observed as a thin vertical slit or as a large orifice with irregular skin edges, depending on the condition of the hymen. The hymen is a membranous, annular, or crescentic fold at the vaginal opening. When unperforated, it is usually a continuous membrane but on occasion may be cribriform. After perforation small rounded fragments of hymen attach to the introital margins; these are called hymenal caruncles.

The ducts of two pairs of glands open on the vulva. Skene's glands are multiple, tiny organs located in the paraurethral area. Their ducts, numbering approximately 6 to 31, lie inside and just outside of the urethral orifice and are usually not visible. These ducts open laterally and slightly posterior to the urethral orifice in approximately 5 and 7 o'clock positions; the urethral orifice is the center of the clock.

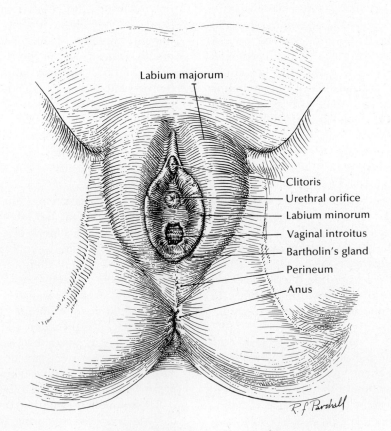

Labium majorum

Clitoris
Urethral orifice
Labium minorum
Vaginal introitus
Bartholin's gland
Perineum
Anus

Fig. 20-1. External female genitalia.

Bartholin's glands are small, ovoid organs located lateral and slightly posterior to the vaginal orifice, partially behind the bulb of the vestibule. Their ducts are approximately 2 cm long and open in the groove between the labia minora and the hymen. These ducts are also usually not visible.

The perineum consists of the tissues between the introitus and the anus.

The pelvic floor consists of a group of muscles attached to points on the bony pelvis (Fig. 20-2). These muscles form a suspended sling that assists in holding the pelvic contents in place. The muscles are pierced by the urethral, vaginal, and rectal orifices and function both passively as a pelvic support and actively in voluntary contraction of the vaginal and anal orifices.

Internal genitalia

Fig. 20-3 illustrates the internal genitalia.

The vagina is a pink, transversely rugated, collapsed tube that in the adult is approximately 9 cm long posteriorly and 6 to 7 cm long anteriorly. It inclines posteriorly at approximately a 45-degree angle with the vertical plane of the body. The vagina is highly dilatable, especially in its superior portion and anteroposterior dimension. When collapsed, it is

H shaped in transverse section. Superiorly and usually anteriorly, the vagina is pierced by the uterine cervix. The recess between the portion of the vagina adjacent to the cervix and the cervix is called the vaginal fornix. Although it is actually continuous, the fornix is anatomically divided into anterior, posterior, and lateral fornices.

The uterus is an inverted, pear-shaped, muscular organ that is flattened anteroposteriorly. It is usually found inclined forward 45 degrees from the vertical plane of the erect body and is approximately 5.5 to 8 cm long, 3.5 to 4 cm wide, and 2 to 2.5 cm thick. The uterus of the parous client may be normally enlarged an additional 2 to 3 cm in any of the three dimensions. The uterus is divided into two main parts: the body and the cervix. The body in turn is composed of three parts: the fundus, the prominence above the insertion of the fallopian tubes; the body, or main portion, of the uterus; and the isthmus, the constricted lower portion of the uterus, which is adjacent to the cervix. The cervix extends from the isthmus and into the vagina.

The uterine cavity communicates with the vagina via an ostium, the cervical os. The os is a small, depressed, circular opening in the nulliparous client. In women who have borne children the os is en-

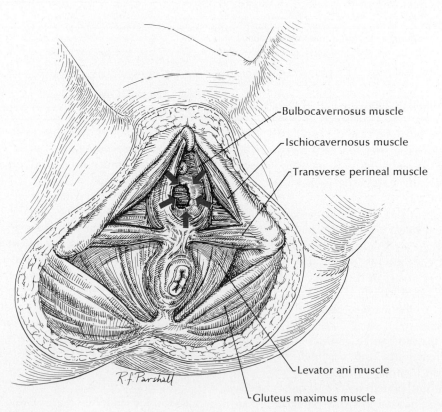

R.f. Parshall

Bulbocavernosus muscle

Ischiocavernosus muscle

Transverse perineal muscle

Levator ani muscle

Gluteus maximus muscle

Fig. 20-2. Muscles of the pelvic floor. Arrows illustrate the direction of contraction of the bulbocavernosus muscle.

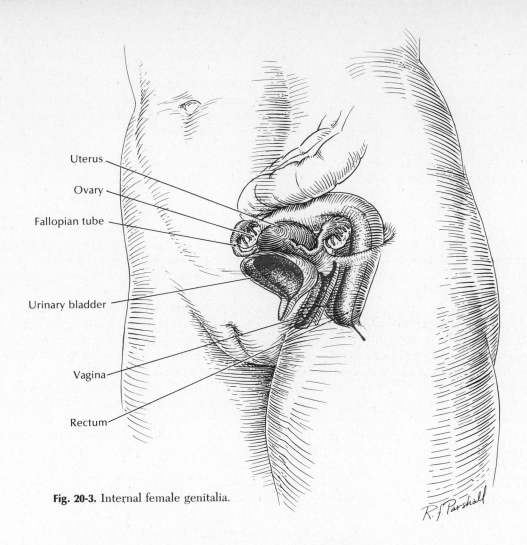

Uterus

Ovary

Fallopian tube

Urinary bladder

Vagina

Rectum

R. f. Parshall

Fig. 20-3. Internal female genitalia.

larged and irregularly shaped. The position of the uterus is not fixed; it is a relatively movable organ. The uterus may be anteverted, anteflexed, retroverted, or retroflexed in position; or it may be in midposition. In the normal adult with an empty bladder the uterus is usually anteverted and slightly anteflexed in position.

The ovaries are a pair of oval organs; each is approximately 3 cm long, 2 cm wide, and 1 cm thick. They are usually located near the lateral pelvic wall, at the level of the anterosuperior iliac spine. The two uterine tubes insert in the upper portion of the uterus, are supported loosely by the broad ligament, and run laterally to the ovaries. Each tube is approximately 10 cm long.

The uterus, ovaries, and tubes are supported by four pairs of ligaments: the cardinal, uterosacral, round, and broad ligaments (Fig. 20-4).

The rectouterine pouch, or Douglas' cul-de-sac, is a deep recess formed by the peritoneum as it passes over the intestinal surface of the rectum. It is the lowest point in the abdominal cavity.

EXAMINATION
Preparation

Clients should be advised not to douche during the 24 hours preceding the pelvic examination and reminded to empty their bladders immediately before the examination.

Some clients have difficulty assuming the lithotomy position, especially in moving their buttocks sufficiently downward to the edge of the table. The practitioner can assist the client by asking the client to raise her buttocks (while the client is lying on the table with heels in the stirrups) and by guiding the client's buttocks downward from a position at the client's side or from a position at the foot of the table. Clients usually feel more comfortable wearing shoes when their feet are in the stirrups, rather than supporting their weight with bare heels against the hard, cold stirrups.

Materials needed for the examination should be assembled and readily available before the client is put in the lithotomy position. Materials needed for the examination minimally include:

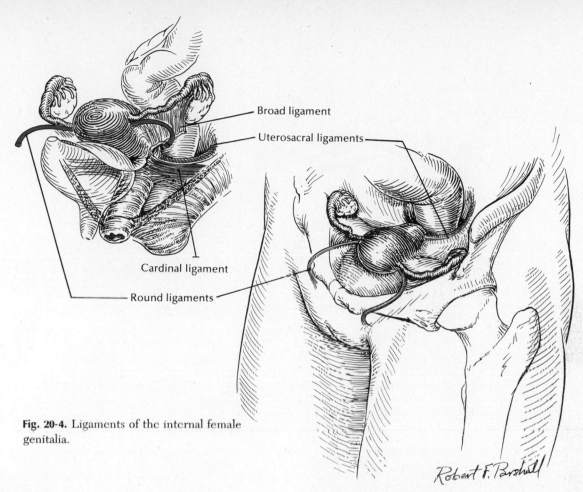

Fig. 20-4. Ligaments of the internal female genitalia.

- Broad ligament
- Uterosacral ligaments
- Cardinal ligament
- Round ligaments

Rubber gloves
Speculums of various sizes
Culture plates for gonorrhea screening
Glass slides
Glass cover slides
Ayre spatula
Sterile cotton swabs
Lubricant on a piece of paper or gauze
Cotton balls
Sponge forceps
Cytology fixative
Source of light

Components of the examination

The regional examination of the female genital system consists of (1) the abdominal examination, (2) inspection of the external genitalia, (3) palpation of the external genitalia, (4) the speculum examination, (5) the obtaining of specimens, (6) the bimanual vaginal examination, and (7) the rectovaginal examination.

The abdominal examination is discussed in Chapter 17 on assessment of the abdomen and rectosigmoid region. The examination of the female genital system should be preceded by a thorough examination of the abdomen.

It is recommended that the examiner wear two gloves for the genital area examination. This will allow for a thorough external examination and complete spreading of the labia and also will protect subsequent clients from the possible transfer of infection.

Inspection of the external genitalia. First, the skin and hair distribution are observed. Hair distribution should be approximately shaped as an inverse triangle. Some abdominal hair is normal and may be hereditary. Male hair distribution patterns in females are abnormal. Growth of hair commences approximately 1 year before menarche. The total skin area is inspected for lesions and parasites. The gloved fingers should be used to spread the hair and labia so that all skin surfaces can be adequately visualized. The area of the clitoris particularly is a common site for chancres of syphilis in the younger client and for cancerous lesions in the older client.

The labia are flat in childhood and atrophic in old age. Estrogen influences fat deposition, which causes a round, full appearance of the labia. The labia majora of the nulliparous client will be in close approximation, covering the labia minora and the vestibule area. After a vaginal delivery, the labia may be slightly shriveled and gaping in appearance.

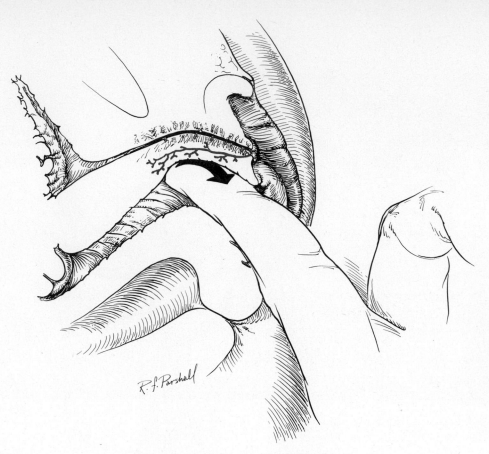

R. J. Parshall

Fig. 20-5. Palpation of Skene's glands.

The skin of the vulvar area is of a slightly darker pigment than the skin of the rest of the body. The mucous membranes are normally dark pink in color and moist in appearance.

Common abnormalities of the skin and labia include parasites, skin lesions of all types, areas of leukoplakia, varicosities, hyperpigmentation, erythema, depigmentation, and swelling. Leukoplakia appears as white, adherent patches on the skin; it may be likened to spots of dried white paint.

The clitoris is examined for size; the visible portion of the clitoris should not exceed 2 cm in length and 1 cm in width.

The urethral orifice normally appears slitlike or stellate and is of the same color as the membranes surrounding it. The openings of the paraurethral (Skene's) glands are not usually visible. Erythema or a polyp located in this area or a discharge from the urethra or gland ducts is abnormal.

The examiner next observes the area of the Bartholin's glands and their ducts for swelling, erythema, duct enlargement, or discharge. The presence of any of these conditions is abnormal.

The perineum is inspected for evidence of an episiotomy and its healing. The anus is also inspected at this time (see Chapter 17 on assessment of the abdomen and rectosigmoid region).

Palpation of the external genitalia. Any areas of observed abnormality are palpated to determine the size, shape, consistency, and tenderness of the mass or lesion. The labia are palpated. They should feel soft, and the texture should be homogenous.

The index finger and the middle finger are inserted into the vagina. First, the urethra and area of Skene's duct openings are gently milked from about the level of 4 cm in on the anterior vaginal wall down to the orifice (Fig. 20-5). This procedure should not normally cause pain or discharge. If a discharge is present, a specimen is inoculated onto a Thayer-Martin culture plate. Then the area of Bartholin's glands and their ducts are palpated for swelling or tenderness (Fig. 20-6). Normally Bartholin's glands are not palpable.

While the examiner's fingers are in the vagina, several maneuvers are performed to assess the integrity of the pelvic musculature. First, the perineal area is palpated between the fingers inside the vagina and the thumb of that same hand. In the nulliparous client the perineum is felt as a firm, muscular body. After an episiotomy has healed, the perineum feels

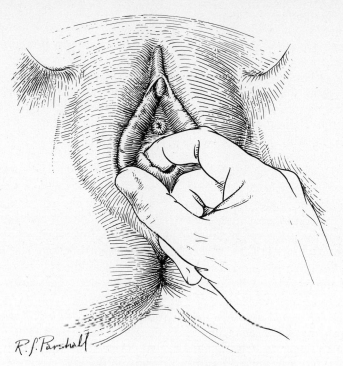

Fig. 20-6. Palpation of Bartholin's glands.

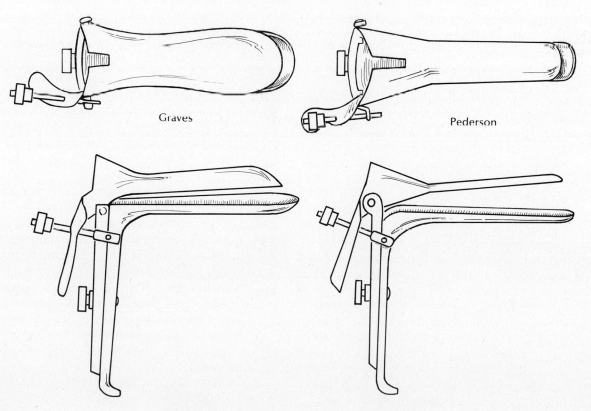

Graves

Pederson

Fig. 20-7. Graves speculum and Pederson speculum.

thinner and more rigid because of scarring. If this area is very thin and if the palpating fingers can almost approximate, the client should be questioned again about bowel or sexual problems.

The client is then asked to constrict her vaginal orifice around the examiner's fingers while they are still placed in the vagina. Again, a nulliparous client will demonstrate a high degree of tone and a multiparous client, less tone. A client whose vaginal orifice has poor tone will probably admit to some dissatisfaction expressed by her sexual partner.

In the third maneuver the index and middle fingers remain in the vagina; they are spread laterally, and the client is asked to push down against them. The presence of urinary stress incontinence, cystocele, rectocele, enterocele, or uterine prolapse can be observed if present.

Cystocele is the prolapse into the vagina of the anterior vaginal wall and the bladder. Clinically, a pouching would be seen on the anterior wall as the client strains.

Rectocele is the prolapse into the vagina of the posterior vaginal wall and the rectum. Clinically, a pouching would be seen on the posterior wall as the client strains.

Enterocele is a hernia of the pouch of Douglas into the vagina. Clinically, a bulge would be seen emerging from the posterior fornix. If this is observed, the client should be additionally examined by assessing the effect of straining (1) during the speculum examination with the speculum inserted, half opened, three-fourths of its length into the vagina; and (2) during the bimanual examination with the intravaginal fingers in the posterior fornix.

There are three degrees of *uterine prolapse*. In first-degree prolapse, the cervix appears at the introitus when the client strains. In second-degree prolapse, the cervix is outside of the introitus when the client strains. In third-degree prolapse, the whole uterus is outside the introitus and the vagina is essentially turned inside out when the client strains.

Speculum examination. The examiner will have obtained clues regarding the most appropriate type and size of speculum to use in the speculum examination through the history and inspection of the external genitalia. There are two basic types of speculums, the Graves speculum and the Pederson speculum (Fig. 20-7). The Graves speculum is one of the most commonly used in the examination of the adult female client. It is available in lengths varying from 3½ to 5 inches and in widths from ¾ to 1½ inches. The Pederson speculum is both narrower and flatter than the Graves speculum and is used with virgins, nulliparous clients, or clients whose vaginal orifices have contracted postmenopausally.

A metal speculum needs to be warmed before insertion. An effective way to do this is by running warm water over it. Lubricant is bacteriostatic and also distorts cells on Papanicolaou (Pap) smears; thus, it cannot be used if a culture or smear is to be obtained. The warm water also assists in lubricating both the metal and plastic speculums and may be used if cultures and smears are to be taken.

The index finger and middle finger are placed 1 inch into the vagina. The fingers are then spread, and pressure is exerted toward the posterior vaginal wall. The client is advised that she will feel intravaginal pressure. The speculum is held in the opposite hand with the blades between the index and middle fingers. The client is asked to bear down. This maneuver helps to additionally open the vaginal orifice and to relax perineal muscles (Fig. 20-8).

The speculum blades are inserted obliquely, taking advantage of the H configuration of the relaxed vagina (Fig. 20-8, *B*). They are inserted at a plane parallel to the examining table until the end of the speculum has reached the tips of the fingers in the vagina.

The speculum is then rotated to a transverse position, and the plane is altered in adaptation to the plane of the vagina, approximately one of a 45-degree angle with the examining table (Fig. 20-8, *C*). The intravaginal fingers are simultaneously withdrawn, and the speculum is inserted until it touches the end of the vagina. The lever of the speculum is then depressed; this opens the blades and allows visualization. Hopefully, the cervix is seen between the blades (Fig. 20-8, *D*). Sometimes, however, especially for the beginning examiner, it is not. In such cases the speculum is either anterior (usually the situation) or posterior to the cervix. If this occurs, the speculum is withdrawn halfway and reinserted in a different plane. After the entire cervix is in view of the examiner, the depressed lever is fixed in an open position.

The appearance of the normal cervix has already been described. The cervix is observed for color, position, size, projection into the vaginal vault, shape, general symmetry, surface characteristics, shape and and patency of the os, and discharge:

1. *Color:* The color of the cervix is normally pale after menopause and cyanotic in pregnancy. Cyanosis can occur with any condition that causes systemic hypoxia or regional venous congestion. Hyperemia may be an indication of inflammation. An additional cause of pallor is anemia.
2. *Position:* A cervix projecting more deeply than 3 cm into the vaginal vault may indicate uterine prolapse. A cervix situated on a lateral vaginal wall may indicate tumor or adhesion of a superior structure.
3. *Size:* A cervix larger than 4 cm in diameter is

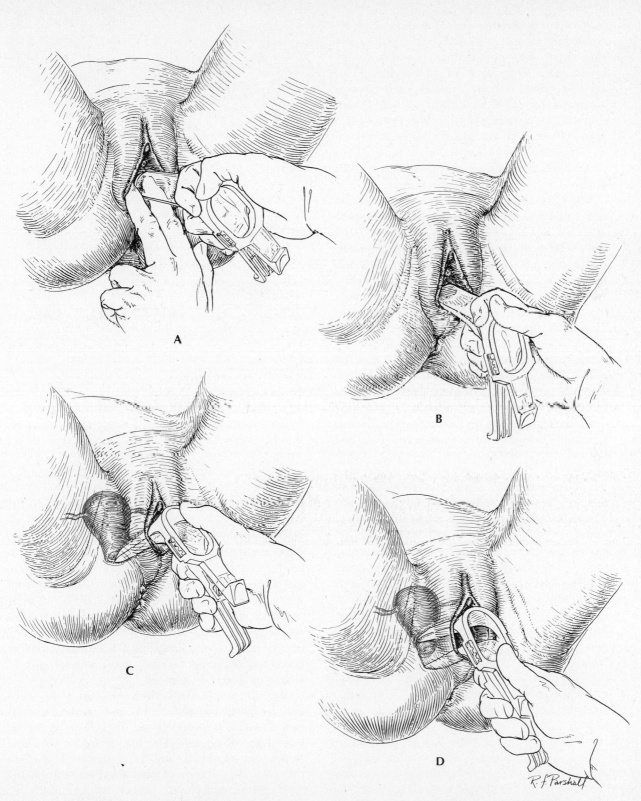

Fig. 20-8. Procedure for vaginal examination. **A,** Opening of the introitus. **B,** Oblique insertion of the speculum. **C,** Final insertion of the speculum. **D,** Opening of the speculum blades.

hypertrophied, and the presence of inflammation or tumor should be considered.

4. *Surface characteristics:* Lesions and polyps are commonly seen on the cervix and require more than visual assessment to determine if pathology exists. Any irregularity or nodularity of the cervical surface should be considered possibly abnormal (Fig. 20-9). One relatively benign condition is the presence of nabothian cysts, which appear as smooth, round, small (less than 1 cm in diameter) yellow lesions. Nabothian cysts are caused by obstruction of the cervical gland ducts.

When the squamocolumnar junction is on the ectocervix, the columnar epithelium will appear as a red, relatively symmetrical circle around the os. This condition may be a normal variation of the placement of the squamocolumnar junction or may be caused by the separation by speculum blades of a cervix whose external os has been altered and enlarged by childbirth. This condition is termed eversion or ectropion. Erosions appear similar to eversions. However, erosions are usually irregular, rough, and friable. Erosions frequently indicate pathology and require further assessment and treatment. Because of the occasional presence of the squamocolumnar junction on the ectocervix, the differential assessment of normal cervix from abnormal cervix using inspection alone is impossible.

Diffuse punctile hemorrhages, colloquially termed "strawberry spots," are occasionally observed in association with trichomonal infections.

5. *Discharge:* The character of the normal cervical mucus varies in the menstrual cycle. It is always odorless and nonirritating. Its color and consistency may vary from clear to white and from thin to thick and stringy. Colored or purulent discharges exuding from the os or present in the area of the cervix are probably abnormal.

6. *Shape of the os:* The cervical os of the nulliparous client is small and evenly round. The cervical os of a parous client shows the effects of the stretching and laceration of childbirth and is irregular in shape.

After the cervix is inspected, a Pap smear, culture for gonorrhea, and hanging drop specimen may be obtained if indicated. The procedures for these are described at the end of this chapter. The vagina is then inspected. This is done during speculum insertion, while the speculum is open, and during its removal. The color and condition of the vaginal mucosa and the color, odor, consistency, and appearance of

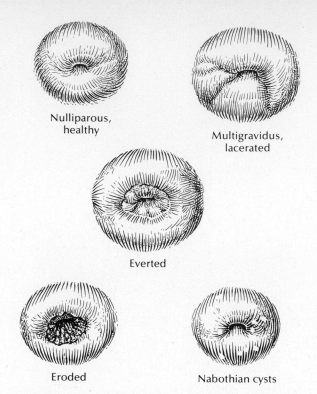

Fig. 20-9. Common appearances and lesions of the cervix.

vaginal secretions are noted. Pallor, cyanosis, and hyperemia may be present for the same reasons as described for the cervix. Leukoplakia may also occur on vaginal mucosa.

As with cervical discharge, vaginal discharge is normally odorless, nonirritating, thin or mucoid, and clear or cloudy. Also, the presence of some whitish, creamy material is normal. Any other vaginal discharge should be described according to its color, odor, consistency, amount, and appearance. Three basic types of vaginal infections produce observable discharge: monilial infections, characterized by thick, white, curdy, exudates that appear as adherent patches and free discharge; trichomonal infections, characterized by a profuse watery, gray or green, frothy, odorous discharge; and bacterial infections, characterized by an odorous, gray, homogenous discharge of moderate amount.

After the inspection of the vaginal area, the speculum is slowly withdrawn. As it is withdrawn, the nut, or catch, is loosened and the lever is again controlled by the thumb. The blades are slowly closed as they are removed, and the speculum is carefully rotated so that all areas of vaginal tissue are inspected. As the blades are closed, caution is taken to prevent pinching of tissue or the catching of hairs in the blades.

The speculum is inspected for odors and is either discarded or placed in a soaking solution.

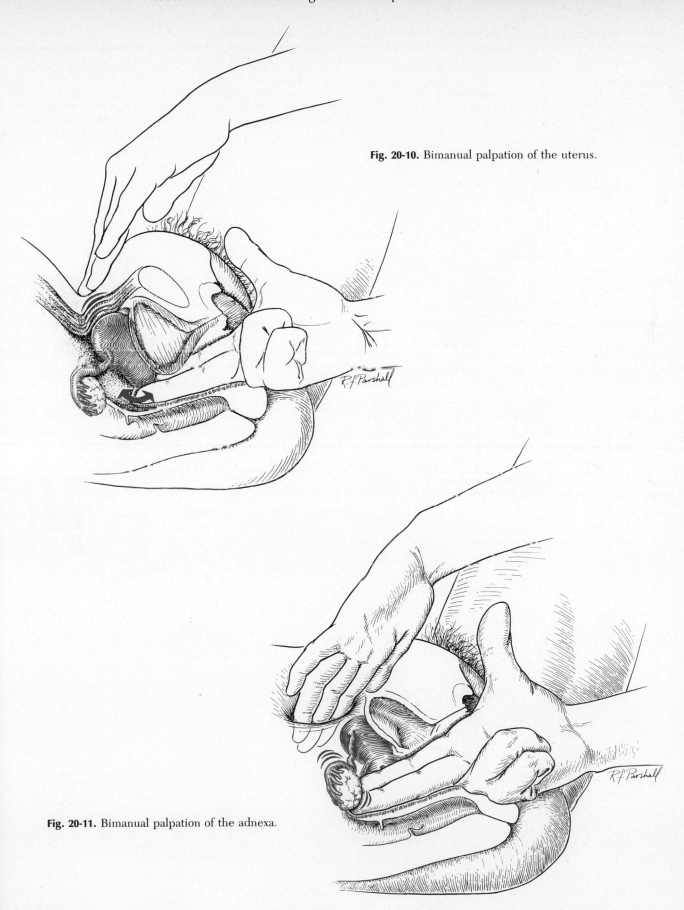

Fig. 20-10. Bimanual palpation of the uterus.

Fig. 20-11. Bimanual palpation of the adnexa.

Table 20-1. Findings in bimanual vaginal and rectovaginal examination

Position of uterus	Bimanual		
	Illustration	Position of the cervix	Body and fundus
Anteverted		Anterior vaginal wall	Palpable by one hand on the abdomen and the fingers of the other in the vagina
Midposition		The apex of the vagina	May not be palpable
Retroverted		Posterior vaginal wall	Not palpable

Anterior and posterior portion of uterus	Rectovaginal		
	Illustration	**Cervix**	**Body and fundus**
Palpable as the uterus is rotated even more anteriorly		Palpable through the rectovaginal septum	Not palpable by fingers in the rectum
May not be palpable		Posterior portion felt through the rectovaginal septum	May not be palpable
Posterior portion may be palpable by fingers in the posterior fornix		May not be palpable by fingers in the rectum	Body easily palpable by fingers in the rectum; fundus may not be palpable

Continued.

Table 20-1. Findings in bimanual vaginal and rectovaginal examination—cont'd

| Position of uterus | Bimanual | | |
	Illustration	Position of the cervix	Body and fundus
Anteflexed		Anterior vaginal wall or apex	Easily palpable; angulation of the isthmus may be felt in the anterior fornix
Retroflexed		Anterior or posterior vaginal wall or apex	Not palpable

Bimanual vaginal examination. The purpose of the bimanual examination is the palpation of the pelvic contents between the examiner's two hands (Figs. 20-10 and 20-11). Examiners vary in their preference of the placement of the dominant, more sensitive hand. The beginning examiner should attempt alternating hands for examinations and then decide on a routine that is most workable for him.

The client remains in the lithotomy position. The vaginal examining hand assumes the obstetrical position: index and middle fingers extended and together, thumb abducted, and fourth and little fingers folded on the palm of the hand. The vaginal examining fingers are lubricated. The labia are spread with the thumb and index finger of the opposite hand. The lubricated fingers are inserted into the vagina with the palmar surface of the hand directed toward the anterior vaginal wall. The examiner should always palpate with the palmar surface of the fingers rather than with the less sensitive tips or backs. The other hand is placed on the abdomen. This hand will be used to press the abdominal and pelvic contacts toward the intravaginal hand. Movement of both hands should be slow and firm. In order for the examiner to palpate adequately, the client must be relaxed. If the client becomes tense, the procedure is stopped, and the client is helped to relax; however, the examiner's hands remain in position.

The cervix is located and assessed for size, contour, surface characteristics, consistency, position, patency of the os, and mobility. The palmar surfaces of both fingers are used to completely palpate the cervix and the fornices. A finger is gently placed into the external os to assess its patency. It is determined on which vaginal wall the cervix is placed and if the cervix is approximately midline. The fingers are placed in the lateral fornices, and the cervix is wagged, or moved back and forth, between the fin-

| Anterior and posterior portion of uterus | Rectovaginal | | |
	Illustration	Cervix	Body and fundus
Easily palpable	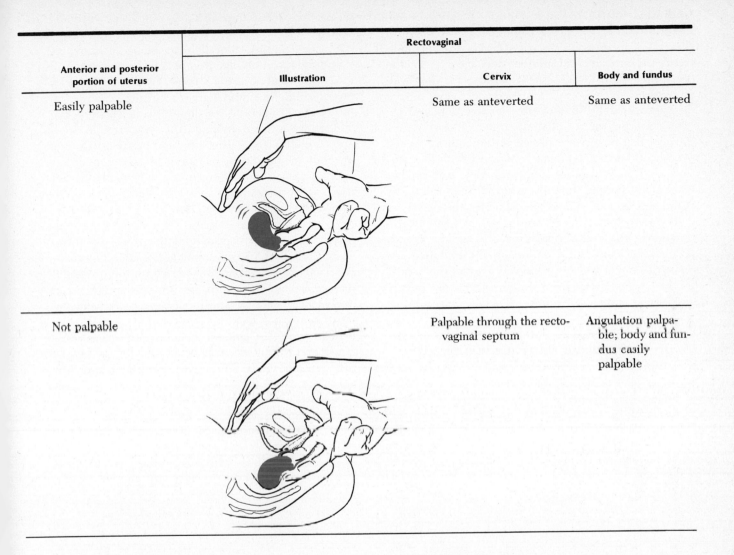	Same as anteverted	Same as anteverted
Not palpable		Palpable through the rectovaginal septum	Angulation palpable; body and fundus easily palpable

gers for approximately 1 to 2 cm in each direction. The cervix and uterus should be freely movable and should move without tenderness. An immobile or tender cervix and uterus are abnormal.

The surface of the cervix is normally smooth. Nabothian cysts, tumors, or lesions will make it feel nodular or irregular. The consistency of the cervix is firm and slightly resilient and feels analogous to the tip of the nose. The cervix softens in pregnancy and hardens with tumors. The cervix is normally located on the anterior wall in the midline or on the posterior wall. A laterally displaced cervix may indicate tumor or adhesion. The external os in the nonpregnant client should admit a finger for about a quarter inch. It should be open and firm. A stenosed external os is abnormal.

The size, shape, surface characteristics, consistency, position, mobility, and tenderness of the uterine body and fundus are assessed. First it is use-

ful to determine the position of the uterus because techniques used to assess the uterine body and fundus will vary with the uterine position in the client (Table 20-1). The uterus is in one of the three basic positions: anteversion, midposition, or retroversion. Version in this context indicates deflection, specifically the relationship of the long axis of the uterus to the long axis of the body. If the axis of the uterus is deflected anteriorly, the uterus is said to be anteverted; if the uterus is deflected posteriorly, the uterus is said to be retroverted; and if the long axis of the uterus is roughly parallel to that of the total body, the uterus is in midposition. When the long axis of the uterus is not straight but is bent upon itself, the uterus is said to be flexed. Thus, the anteverted or retroverted uterus can be flexed or bend upon itself to produce two additional variations of position: anteflexion and retroflexion.

The position of the cervix provides the examiner

with clues of the uterine position. A cervix on the anterior wall may indicate an antepositioned or retroflexed uterus; a centrally located cervix probably indicates a uterus in midposition; and a cervix on the posterior vaginal wall usually indicates a uterus in retroposition.

Approximately 85% of uteri are in anteposition; therefore, palpation is first attempted anteriorly. The intravaginal fingers are placed in the anterior fornix. The hand on the abdomen is placed flat on the midline and in a position approximately halfway between the symphysis pubis and the umbilicus. This hand acts as a resistance against which the pelvic organs are palpated by the intravaginal fingers. The fingers in the anterior fornix gently lift the tissues against the hand on the abdomen. If the uterus is in anteposition, it will be palpated between the hands. If the uterus is not palpated anteriorly, the fingers are placed in the posterior fornix and again raised forward toward the hand on the abdomen. If the uterus is in retroversion, only the isthmus will be felt between the hands and the corpus may be felt with the backs of the intravaginal fingers. A retroverted

uterus is felt best during the rectovaginal examination.

If the uterus is identified as being in anteposition or midposition, an attempt is made to palpate all its anterior and posterior surfaces by maneuvering its position and by "walking up" its surface with the intravaginal fingers. After the uterus is palpated, the adnexal areas are examined. The structures in these areas are of a size, consistency, and position that they may not be specifically palpated. If the examiner has appropriately examined the area and no masses larger than the normal-size ovaries are identified, it is assumed that no masses are present.

Each of the adnexal areas, left and right, are palpated. The index and middle finger of the intravaginal hand are placed in one of the lateral fornices; the hand on the abdomen is placed on the ipsilateral iliac crest; and the hands are brought together and moved in an inferior and medial direction, allowing the tissues lying between the two hands to slip between them. The hand on the abdomen acts as resistance, and the intravaginal hand palpates the organs between the hands. Frequently, no specific organ is

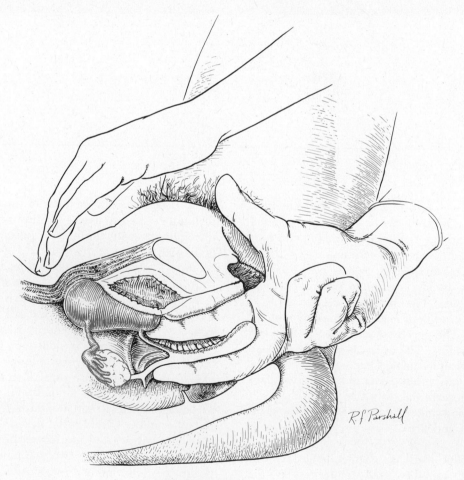

Fig. 20-12. Rectovaginal palpation.

palpated in this maneuver. If normal ovaries are palpated, they are smooth, firm, slightly flattened, ovoid, and no larger than 4 to 6 cm in their largest dimension. Ovaries of prepubertal girls or postmenopausal women are normally smaller than 4 cm in their largest dimension. The ovaries are sensitive to touch but are not tender. They are highly movable and will easily slip between the palpating hands.

Normal fallopian tubes are not palpable. One clue to an ectopic pregnancy is the presence of arterial pulses in the adnexal areas.

Cordlike structures that are sometimes palpable are round ligaments.

Rectovaginal examination. After the completion of the vaginal examination, the hands are withdrawn, the secretions are washed off of the gloved fingers,

and the index and middle fingers are relubricated. The index finger is placed into the vagina and the middle finger is placed into the rectum. The intravaginal finger remains on the cervix, identifying it, lest it be mistaken for a mass by the intrarectal finger.

The uterine position is confirmed by the rectal examination. If the uterus is retroverted, its body and fundus are now palpated. In addition, the adnexal areas are reassessed. The procedure is the same as that described with the vaginal examination (Fig. 20-12).

The area of the rectovaginal septum and cul-de-sac are palpated. The rectovaginal septum should be palpated as a firm, thin, smooth, pliable structure. The posterior cul-de-sac is a potential space. The normal pelvic organs are palpated through it. Often,

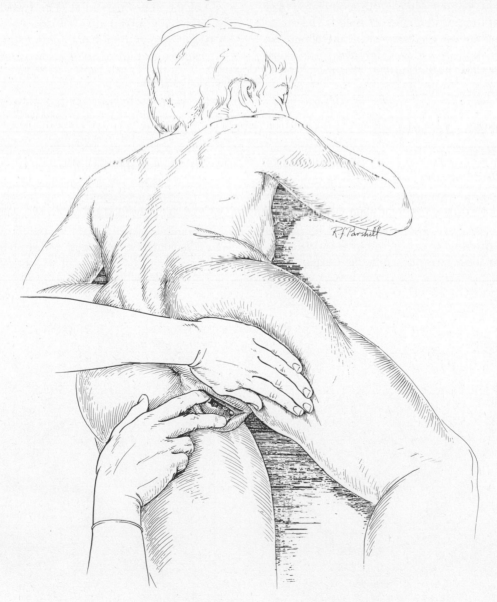

Fig. 20-13. Left lateral position for genital examination.

abnormal masses and normal ovaries are discovered in the cul-de-sac.

Uterosacral ligaments may be palpable.

The rectal examination is completed (see Chapter 18 on assessment of the anus and rectosigmoid region), and the client is helped up.

Examination of clients who are unable to assume the lithotomy position

The lithotomy position is the optimal one for a pelvic examination. However, it may be difficult for a very ill or debilitated client to assume and maintain a lithotomy position. An alternative position for the female genital examination is a left lateral or Sims's position (Fig. 20-13). The client's buttocks should be as close to the edge of the examining table as safety allows. The left leg is positioned on top of or over the right leg and bent and abducted. The examiner stands behind and at the side of the client. All of the examination procedures described previously in this chapter can be performed with the client in this position.

Procedures for smears and cultures

CERVICAL PAPANICOLAOU SMEAR

The client is in the lithotomy position, and the speculum has been inserted. All materials listed earlier in the chapter are assembled. If a cervical mucous plug is present, it can be removed with a cotton ball held with forceps. There are many varia-

tions among laboratories regarding the areas from which cell samples are to be obtained, the mixing of cells from two or more areas, and the fixing of cells. One procedure is described here. However, variations are acceptable and the practitioner should consult with the cytopathologist reading the smears for locally recommended procedures.

Endocervical smear

Fig. 20-14 illustrates the procedure for an endocervical smear:

1. A sterile applicator is inserted approximately 0.5 cm into the cervical os. It is rotated 360 degrees and left in 10 to 20 seconds to ensure saturation.

2. The endocervical smear is spread on the portion of the slide marked *E*. The swab is rotated so that all sampled areas are smeared on the slide. The smear should not contain thick areas that would be difficult to visualize microscopically.

Cervical smear

Fig. 20-15 illustrates the procedure for a cervical smear:

1. The larger humped end of the Ayre spatula is inserted into the cervical os, so that the cervix fits comfortably into the groove created by the two humps. With moderate pressure, the spatula is rotated 360 degrees, scraping the entire cervical surface and the squamocolumnar junction.

2. The material from both sides of the spatula is spread on the portion of the slide marked *C*.

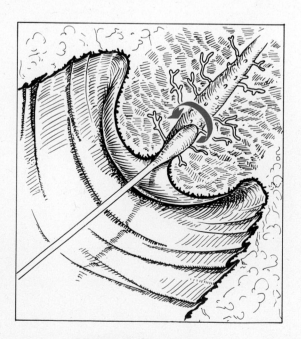

Fig. 20-14. Endocervical smear.

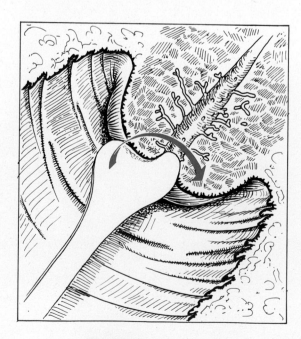

Fig. 20-15. Cervical smear.

Vaginal pool smear

1. With the paddle or handle end of the Ayre spatula, the area of the posterior fornix is scraped.
2. The material on the spatula is spread in the area marked V.
3. The slide is fixed immediately by spraying or immersion into a fixative solution.

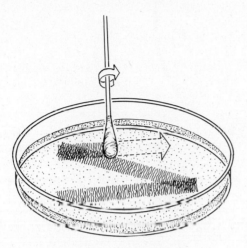

Fig. 20-16. Inoculation of the Thayer-Martin culture.

GONORRHEAL CULTURE

The female client is in the lithotomy position. The male client can be seated when a urethral specimen is to be taken. If a rectal culture is also to be taken, the male client may assume the Sims's position or bend over an examining table with buttocks exposed, feet spread, and toes pointing inward. An oropharyngeal culture is sometimes indicated.

Endocervical culture

1. A specimen from the endocervical canal is obtained with a sterile cotton applicator. The technique is the same as that described for the Pap smear.
2. The Thayer-Martin culture plate is inoculated. With the medium at room temperature, the swab is rolled in a large **Z** pattern on the culture plate; the swab is simultaneously rotated as it is creating the **Z**, so that all swab surfaces will be inoculated (Fig. 20-16).
3. The culture plate is incubated within 15 minutes of its inoculation in a warm, anaerobic environment. The culture plate is placed medium side up in a candle jar; the candle is lit; the cover of

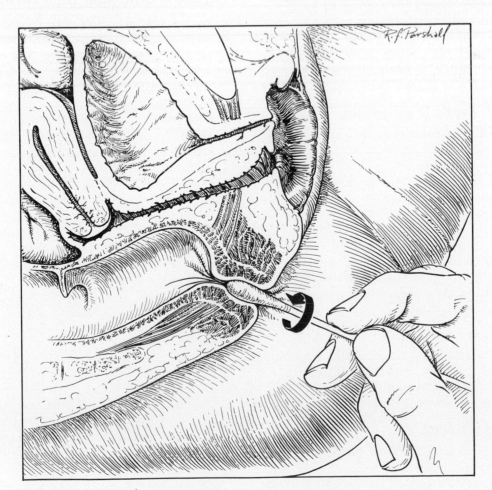

Fig. 20-17. Anal smear.

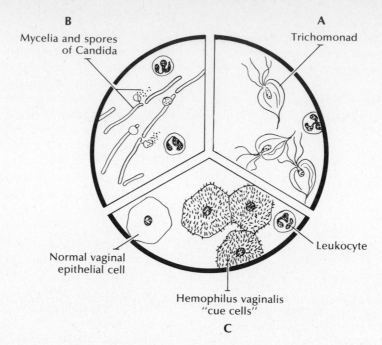

B
Mycelia and spores
of Candida

A
Trichomonad

Leukocyte

Normal vaginal
epithelial cell

Hemophilus vaginalis
"cue cells"

C

Fig. 20-18. Microscopic appearance of vaginal microorganisms. **A,** Trichomonads. **B,** Mycelia and spores. **C,** Epithelial cells stippled by *Hemophilus vaginalis* bacteria.

the jar is tightly secured; and the jar is left in a warm area until specimens can be placed in an incubator. In some clinic situations, the inoculation is immediately cross-streaked with a sterile wire loop. Usually, however, this is done in the laboratory, not in the examining room.

Anal culture: female or male client

Fig. 20-17 illustrates the procedure for an anal culture:
1. A sterile cotton-tipped applicator is inserted into the anal canal. The applicator is rotated 360 degrees and moved from side to side. It is left in for a total of 10 to 30 seconds to allow for absorption of secretion and organisms. If the swab contains feces, it is discarded and another specimen taken.
2. The culture plate is inoculated and incubated as described previously, using a separate culture plate.

Urethral culture: male client

1. A urethral culture is obtained. A sterile bacteriological loop is inserted into the urethra for 1 to 2 cm, and the mucosa is gently scraped.
2. The culture medium is inoculated and incubated.

Oropharyngeal culture

1. A specimen of secretion from the oropharynx is obtained with a sterile swab.
2. The medium is inoculated and incubated as described for endocervical specimens.

SMEARS FOR VAGINAL INFECTIONS

1. A specimen of vaginal secretions is obtained directly from the vagina or from material in the inferior speculum blade. For *Trichomonas vaginalis*, the secretions are mixed with a drop of normal saline solution on a glass slide. For *Candida albicans*, the secretions are mixed with a drop of 10% potassium hydroxide solution on a slide. For *Hemophilus vaginalis*, the secretions are not mixed with any solution.
2. A cover glass is placed on the slide.
3. The slide is immediately observed under a microscope (Fig. 20-18). If positive for *T. vaginalis*, trichomonads will be seen. These are single-cell flagellates about the size of a white blood cell. If positive *C. albicans*, mycelia and spores are seen. If positive for *H. vaginalis*, characteristic "cue cells" are seen.

SUMMARY

I. External genitalia
  A. Inspection
    1. Hair distribution
    2. Skin
    3. Labia
    4. Clitoris
    5. Urethral orifice
    6. Bartholin's glands
    7. Perineum
  B. Palpation
    1. Skene's glands
    2. Bartholin's glands

II. Muscular integrity
  A. Strength of the bulbocavernosus muscle, that is, general vaginal tone
  B. Observation for bladder, rectal, uterine, and intestinal prolapse
III. Speculum examination
  A. Inspection of the cervix
  B. Gonorrhea culture
  C. Pap smear
  D. Inspection of vaginal mucosa
IV. Bimanual vaginal palpation
  A. Cervix
  B. Uterus
  C. Cul-de-sac area
  D. Adnexal area
    1. Ovaries
    2. Fallopian tubes
V. Rectovaginal palpation
  A. Uterus
  B. Adnexal area
  C. Cul-de-sac area
  D. Rectovaginal septum
  E. Rectum

BIBLIOGRAPHY

Barr, W.: Clinical gynecology, Edinburgh, 1972, Churchill Livingstone.

Burghardt, E.: Early histological diagnosis of cervical cancer, Philadelphia, 1973, W. B. Saunders Co.

Frankfort, E.: Vaginal politics, New York, 1972, Quadrangle Books.

Garrey, M. M., and others: Obstetrics illustrated, ed. 12, Edinburgh, 1974, Churchill Livingstone.

Greenhill, J. P.: Office gynecology, Chicago, 1971, Year Book Medical Publishers, Inc.

Greenhill, J. P., and Friedman, E. A.: Biological principles and modern practices of obstetrics, Philadelphia, 1974, W. B. Saunders Co.

Howkins, J., and Bourne, G.: Shaw's textbook of gynecology, Edinburgh, 1971, Churchill Livingstone.

Hughes, E. C., editor: Obstetric-gynecologic terminology, Philadelphia, 1972, W. B. Saunders Co.

Kistner, R. W.: Gynecology; principles and practice, ed. 2, Chicago, 1971, Year Book Medical Publishers, Inc.

Novak, E. R., Jones, G. S., and Jones, H. W., Jr.: Textbook of gynecology, ed. 9, Baltimore, 1975, The Williams and Wilkins Co.

U.S. Department of Health, Education, and Welfare: Criteria and techniques for the diagnosis of gonorrhea, Atlanta, 1974, U.S. Public Health Service.

Wilson, R. J., and Carrington, E. R.: Obstetrics and gynecology, ed. 6, St. Louis, 1979, The C. V. Mosby Co.

21 Health assessment of the prenatal client

In this chapter the physical changes that occur in normal pregnancy are presented, as well as the adaptation of the health history and the physical examination for the pregnant client. The student practitioner should either know or review the performance of the female genital examination presented in Chapter 20 because it is a component of the assessment of the prenatal patient. That assessment procedure will not be repeated here except as the examination or findings may change in pregnancy.

PHYSICAL CHANGES IN PREGNANCY
Hormonal changes

All of the physiological changes of pregnancy are directly or indirectly initiated by the hormones produced by the fetal chorionic tissues and placenta. In early pregnancy, the fetal trophoblast produces large amounts of human chorionic gonadotropic hormone (HCG) that provides the basis for biological pregnancy testing. HCG is present in detectable amounts by immunological tests 8 to 10 days after conception.

Large amounts of estrogens and progesterone are produced during pregnancy. Estriol, an estrogen, is produced in large amounts during middle and late pregnancy and is the basis for biological tests of placental and fetal well-being because a well-functioning placenta, a healthy fetus, and intact fetal circulation are prerequisites for the continuous production of this hormone. The estrogens and progesterone maintain the decidua of pregnancy and cause the growth and hyperemia of the uterus, other pelvic organs, and the breasts.

The thyroid gland is enlarged in over 50% of prenatal patients as a result of hyperplasia of glandular tissue, new follicle formation, and increased vascularity. The basal metabolic rate is increased largely because of increased growth and oxygen consumption by the pregnant uterus, the fetus, and the placenta.

Changes in the uterus, cervix, and vagina

Changes in the uterus include the development of the decidua, hypertrophy of muscle cells, increased vascularity, formation of the lower uterine segment, and softening of the cervix. The overall size of the uterus increases five to six times, the weight increases about 20 times, and the capacity increases from approximately 2 to 5,000 ml.

Hormones supply the initial stimulus for uterine hypertrophy. During the first 6 to 8 weeks of pregnancy, the uterus will increase in size whether the pregnancy is uterine or extrauterine. In early pregnancy, the uterus is a pelvic organ and only internally palpable. At about 10 to 12 weeks' gestation, the growing uterus is double its nonpregnant size and reaches the top of the symphysis, where it is palpable abdominally. The uterine fundus is about half-way between the symphysis and umbilicus at about 16 weeks and is at the umbilicus at about 20 to 22 weeks' gestation. After the twentieth week, the average upward growth of the uterus is about 3.75 cm per month. At approximately 36 weeks' gestation, the uterus reaches the xiphisternum. In the last month of pregnancy, the fundus of the uterus may drop several centimeters if the fetal head descends deeply into the pelvis.

The position of the uterus changes during gestation. In early gestation an exaggerated anteflexion is common. As the uterus ascends into the abdomen, a slight dextrorotation develops. The uterus changes from a flattened pear shape to a globular shape in early pregnancy. This globular shape continues until approximately 20 to 24 weeks, when a definite ovoid shape develops and continues until delivery.

In about the sixth to eighth week of gestation, the uterine isthmus becomes softened and easily compressible, to the extent that the cervix, upon palpation, seems almost detached from the uterine fundus.

At about the eighth week of gestation, the entire uterus softens in consistency.

During pregnancy the uterus contracts intermittently. These painless contractions, called Braxton-Hicks contractions, begin in early pregnancy, and are first noted by the client and examiner at about 24 weeks' gestation. They can be stimulated by palpation of the uterus. If a contraction occurs during abdominal examination, the examiner should wait until the contraction ends to continue palpation and subsequently palpate more gently.

Three major changes occur in the cervix: (1) hypertrophy of the glands in the cervical canal, (2) softening of the cervix, and (3) bluish discoloration. These changes begin early in pregnancy—at about the sixth week of gestation. Because of changes in the cervical epithelium, commonly a portion of the squamous epithelium is replaced by an outward extension of the columnar epithelium, producing an observable cervical ectropion or eversion of the cervical canal. This condition usually persists throughout pregnancy but disappears soon after.

The increase in pelvic vascularity causes a bluish discoloration of the cervix, vagina, and vulva at about 6 to 8 weeks. In addition, the vaginal mucosa thickens, the connective tissue becomes less dense, and the muscular areas hypertrophy. These changes are reflected in palpatory findings of softening and relaxation. The hypertrophied glands secrete more mucus, and the total vaginal discharge is increased and is more acid in reaction.

Changes in the breasts

Breast changes begin at about the eighth week of pregnancy with the enlargement of the breasts. Shortly afterward, the nipples become larger and more erectile, the areolae become more darkly pigmented, and the sebaceous glands (Montgomery's tubercles) in the areolae hypertrophy. Sometimes an irregular secondary areola develops, extending from the primary areola. Hypertrophy of the breasts often causes a slight tenderness. In women with well-developed axillary breast tissue, the hypertrophy may produce symptomatic lumps in the armpits. Colostrum can be expressed from the breasts at about the twenty-fourth week of pregnancy. The colostrum appears clear and yellowish at first but it becomes cloudy later.

Stretching of the skin on the breasts may produce striae and increased vascular supply may visibly engorge superficial breast veins.

Abdominal changes

The muscles of the abdominal wall stretch to accommodate the growing uterus, and the umbilicus becomes flattened or protrudes. The rapid stretching of abdominal skin may cause the formation of striae gravidarum, which appear pink or red during pregnancy and become silvery white after delivery. In the third trimester of pregnancy, the rectus abdominis muscles are under considerable stress, and their tone is diminished. A wide, permanent separation of these muscles, called diastasis recti abdominis, may occur. This condition allows abdominal contents to protrude in the midline of the abdomen.

In pregnancy, peristaltic activity is reduced, resulting in decreased bowel sounds. Smooth muscle relaxation or atony contributes to a variety of changes in gastrointestinal function. These include a high incidence of pregnancy-associated nausea and vomiting, heartburn, and constipation. In addition, the increased regional blood flow to the pelvis and venous pressure contribute to hemorrhoids—a source of discomfort in late pregnancy. Nausea and vomiting should not persist beyond the third month, but heartburn, constipation, and hemorrhoids are more characteristic and troublesome in late pregnancy.

Less frequently noted gastrointestinal symptoms include ptyalism or excessive salivation, and pica, a craving for substances of little or no food value. Pica is often an expression of the folkways of some cultural groups and is a common concern when it interferes with good nutrition.

The enlarging uterus displaces the colon laterally, upward, and posteriorly. This changes the anatomical situation of the appendix, and signs of appendicitis during pregnancy are not localized in McBurney's area of the right lower quadrant.

Skin, mucous membrane, and hair changes

The melanocytes in all portions of the skin are extremely active in pregnancy. There is a tendency toward generalized darkening of all skin, especially in skin hyperpigmented in the nonpregnant state. In some women a brownish black pigmented streak may appear in the midline of the abdomen. This line of pigmentation is called the linea nigra. Some women develop a dark, pigmented configuration on the face that has been characteristically called the "mask of pregnancy," or chloasma. Scars and moles may also darken during pregnancy from the influence of melanocyte-stimulating hormone (MSH). Palmar erythema and spider nevi on the face and upper trunk may accompany pregnancy.

Many women observe hypertrophy of gums or epulis resulting from hormones and increased vascularity.

The hair of pregnant women may straighten and change in oiliness. Some women experience hair loss, especially in frontal and parietal areas. Occasionally, increases in facial and abdominal hair resulting from increased androgen and corticotropic hormone are noted.

Cardiovascular system changes

Many changes—too numerous to adequately discuss here—occur in the maternal circulatory system during pregnancy. Several of those changes that alter physical examination findings are mentioned.

Blood volume is increased up to 45% and cardiac output is increased up to 30% in pregnancy as compared to the prepregnant state. Blood volume and cardiac output changes contribute to auscultatory changes common in pregnancy. There is accentuation of the heart sounds, and a low-grade systolic murmur (usually Grade II) is often noted.

As pregnancy advances, the heart is displaced upward and laterally. The point of maximal impulse (PMI) is displaced to a point 1 to 1.5 cm lateral to that of the nonpregnant client. The pulse rate increases up to about 10 beats per minute more than prepregnant rates and palpitations may be noticed during pregnancy. The blood pressure is unchanged or sometimes decreases in the second trimester.

There is a progesterone-induced generalized relaxation of the smooth muscle, arteriolar dilatation, and increased capacity of the vascular compartment. Systolic blood pressure remains the same or slightly lower during midpregnancy. There is no change in venous pressure in the upper body, but venous pressure increases in the lower extremities when the woman is supine, sitting, or standing. This predisposes the woman to varicosities of the legs and vulva, to edema, and to faintness from hypotensive effects. Hypotensive tendencies are aggravated by a supine position, and approximately 10% to 20% of gravida develop the supine hypotensive syndrome, manifested by dizziness, diaphoresis, nausea, and hypotension when they are lying on their backs.

Respiratory system changes

During pregnancy, tidal volume increases and there is a slight increase in respiratory rate. Alveolar ventilation is increased and a more efficient exchange of lung gases occurs in the alveoli. Oxygen consumption rises by almost 20% and plasma carbon dioxide content is decreased.

As the uterus enlarges, the thoracic cage and diaphragm are pushed upward and the thorax is widened at the base. A change in respiration from abdominal to costal may be noted on physical examination. Also, dyspnea is a common complaint, especially in the last trimester, and deep respirations and sighing may be more frequent.

The tissue of the respiratory tract and nasopharynx manifest hyperemia and edema. This may contribute to engorgement of the turbinates, nasal stuffiness, and mouth breathing. Some women note increased nasal and sinus secretion and nosebleeds. Vocal cord edema may cause voice changes. Increased vascularity of the tympanic membranes and blockage of the eustachian tubes may contribute to decreased hearing, a sense of fullness in the ears, or earaches.

Musculoskeletal system changes

The pelvic joints exhibit slight relaxation in pregnancy resulting from some unknown mechanism. This relaxation is maximum from about the seventh month onward. Because the gravid uterus has caused the pregnant client's weight to be thrust forward, the muscles of the spine are used to achieve a temporary new balance. The pregnant woman throws her shoulders back and straightens her head and neck. The lower vertebral column is hyperextended.

The musculoskeletal changes are often reflected in postural and gait changes, lower backache, and fatigue. Often the pregnant woman's gait is described as waddling.

PRENATAL HEALTH HISTORY

The health history is important in pregnancy because information derived from the history assists the practitioner in differentiating the patient who is essentially normal and who will be expected to deliver a full-term, healthy baby from the high-risk expectant mother whose pregnancy is likely to negatively affect her own health or who may not deliver a full-term or healthy baby. High-risk clients are given special care in most health care systems. The early identification and referral of the high-risk patient enable the special program to achieve maximal benefit for the mother and baby.

The health history for the obstetrical client follows the same basic protocol as that presented for all adults in Chapter 3. However, in prenatal care, the following areas of history-taking should receive special and complete attention:

   I.   Age
  II.   Race
 III.   Marital status
  IV.   Parity
        A four-number code is often used to summarize parity information. The first digit in the code is used to denote the number of full-term births; the second, the number of preterm births; the third, the number of abortions; and the fourth, the number of living children. Thus, for example, the parity of 2-1-1-3 indicates that the client has three living children, two of whom were delivered after full-term gestation and one of whom was premature, and has had one abortion.
   V.   Past obstetrical history, including:
        A.   Date of delivery

B. Duration of gestation

C. Significant problems

D. Manner in which labor started, specifically whether labor was spontaneous or induced; if induced, the reason for induction should be noted. Abortion should be described as being spontaneous (S) or induced (I).

E. Length of labor

F. Complications of labor

G. Presentation of infant at delivery

H. Type of delivery—vaginal or cesarean; if cesarean, the reason

I. Type of anesthesia used at delivery

J. Condition of infant(s) at birth and birth weight

K. Postpartum problems, especially infections, hemorrhage, or thrombophlebitis

L. Problems of the infant, especially jaundice, respiratory distress, infection, or congenital anomalies

M. Type of infant feeding

N. Current health of infant

VI. Present obstetrical history

A. Last normal menstrual period (LNMP)

An important task during the prenatal history is the estimation of the expected date of confinement (EDC). Because the exact date of conception is unknown for the majority of prenatal patients, the EDC is calculated according to the first day of the last normal menstrual period (LNMP). The EDC is determinated by counting backwards 3 calendar months from the LNMP and adding 7 days (Nägele's rule). The year, of course, may change. For example, if the LNMP were 10-15-80, the EDC would be 7-22-81. If the patient has a history of irregular menses, the EDC would be more accurately estimated by physical examination than by using the LNMP. Critical features that aid in determination or validation of the EDC are the date of quickening, when the mother first notices fetal movement (at about 18 weeks), and the time at which the fetal heart tones can be auscultated (at about 20 weeks' gestation). Because of the variation that characterizes these events, ultrasonic measurement of fetal size and growth is being used more frequently to "date" pregnancy and assess fetal growth, along with measurement of the progressive enlargement of the uterus

B. Symptoms of pregnancy

C. Feelings about pregnancy, especially determination if pregnancy was planned or unplanned

D. Bleeding since last normal menstrual period

E. Date when fetal movements were first felt

F. Fetal exposure to infections, x-ray, and drugs

VII. Current or past medical and gynecological history

A. Urinary or venereal infections

B. Bacterial or viral infections during pregnancy

C. Diabetes

D. Hypertension

E. Heart disease

F. Endocrine disorders

G. Anemia

H. Genital tract history, especially:

1. Anomaly

2. Cervical incompetence

3. Myomas

4. Contracted pelvis

5. Ovarian mass

6. Vaginal infections

7. Surgery

8. Abnormal Pap test results

9. Use of hormones (for example, birth control pills)

10. Menstrual history and functioning

11. Endometriosis

I. Medication history

J. Habitual use of alcohol, tobacco, or mood-altering drugs

VIII. Family history

Features of the family history that have special significance in pregnancy include diabetes, renal or hematological disorders, hypertension, multiple pregnancy, and congenital defects or retardation. It is important to learn if the primigravida's mother had preeclampsia or high blood pressure with her pregnancies, especially if she convulsed. A woman with a family history of hypertension during pregnancy is three times more likely to develop hypertension with her pregnancy (24% incidence) than most other primigravida (7% to 8% incidence of preeclampsia, or pregnancy-induced hypertension).

IX. Emotional-psychological status

Pregnancy is an important developmental event in the life of a woman. Development involves the achievement-relevant tasks, and the developmental tasks of pregnancy are incorporation, differentiation, and, eventually, separation from the fetus. These tasks roughly coincide with the three trimesters of pregnancy.

During the first trimester, the gravida is involved with the process of accepting the fetus as a fact and a part of her body. Most women initially experience some ambivalence about their pregnancy with a resultant increase in anxiety. Many body changes occur that cause increased somatic awareness and inward focus. Relationships with key persons, especially the baby's father and the gravida's mother, become especially important. Unresolved feelings and conflicts undergo reexamination. Feelings of dependency and vulnerability occur and can be additional causes of anxiety.

In the second trimester, the fetus develops a separate identity. The gravida has had some time to become accustomed to her bodily changes and often feels better because the nausea has ceased. The baby's movements are an important event, confirming the presence of the fetus and reminding the woman of the independence of the fetal movements from her control She begins to daydream about the baby and their future. Worries about the possibility of producing an abnormal baby are common.

In the last trimester of pregnancy, the gravida prepares her separation from the fetus and entrance into a new relationship with the newborn. This time is occupied with preparatory activities such as attending parents' classes and buying clothing and equipment for the newborn. Concerns about labor and delivery and physical discomforts of late pregnancy contribute to the woman's readiness for separation from the fetus and movement to the tasks of parenthood.

X. Social-economic status

PRENATAL RISK FACTORS

The following is a list of factors that have been associated with increased morbidity and mortality of mothers and infants:

Maternal characteristics
Age: less than 18 or over 35
Poverty
Unmarried
Family disorganization
Conflict about pregnancy
Height less than 5 feet
20% overweight or underweight
Inadequate diet
Nonwhite race

Reproductive history
More than one previous abortion
Gravity over 8
Stillbirth
Neonatal death
Infant less than 2,500 g
Infant over 4,000 g
Infant with isoimmunization or ABO incompatibility
Infant with major congenital perinatal disease
Preeclampsia or eclampsia
Antepartal hemorrhage
Cesarean section
Difficult midforceps delivery
Genital tract anomaly
Myomas
Ovarian masses

Medical problems
Hypertension
Renal disease
Diabetes mellitus
Heart disease
Sickle cell disease
Anemia
Pulmonary disease
Endocrine disorder

Present pregnancy
Bleeding after 20 weeks gestation
Premature rupture of membranes
Anemia
No prenatal care
Preeclampsia or eclampsia
Hydramnios
Multiple pregnancy
Low or excessive weight gain
Hypertension (blood pressure greater than 140/90, or a 30 mm Hg systolic increase, or a 15 mm Hg diastolic increase)
Abnormal fasting blood sugar
Rh-negative sensitized
Exposure to teratogens
Viral infections
Syphilis
Bacterial infections
Protozoan infections
Postmaturity
Abnormal presentation

PHYSICAL ASSESSMENT DURING PREGNANCY
General physical examination

A complete physical examination should be made on the first prenatal visit because (1) the examination may reveal problems that need special or immediate attention, and (2) initial data serve as a baseline against which changes later in pregnancy can be compared. The initial, general physical examination of the prenatal patient is the same as that for other patients, except for special emphasis on the diagnosis of pregnancy, the assessment of the adequacy of the pelvis, and the assessment of the growth and well-being of the fetus.

A number of nonreproductive system signs may be normally altered in pregnancy. Such alterations of physical findings include:

Respiratory system
Change in breathing from abdominal to costal
Shortening and widening at the base of the thoracic cage
Elevation of the diaphragm
Increase in respiratory rate

Cardiovascular system
Displacement of the point of maximal impulse laterally 1 to 1.5 cm
Grade II systolic murmur
Increase in pulse rate
Slight fall in blood pressure in the second trimester

Musculoskeletal system
Slight instability of pelvis
Alteration of standing posture and gait to accommodate for gravid uterus

Abdominal region
Contour changes because of gravid uterus
Striae gravidarum
Decrease in muscle tone
Linea nigra
Reduced peristaltic activity

Skin and mucous membranes
Chloasma
Linea nigra
Palmar erythema
Spider nevi on face and upper trunk
Striae gravidarum on breasts and abdomen
Gum hypertrophy

Breasts
Enlargement
Large, erect nipples
Darkening of areolar pigment
Development of a secondary areola
Hypertrophy of sebaceous glands in the areola
Formation of colostrum
Tenderness on palpation
Striae gravidarum
Engorgement of superficial veins

Diagnosis of pregnancy

The diagnosis of pregnancy is made from the history of subjective symptoms noticed by the woman together with objective signs noted by the examiner. In addition, laboratory tests are especially helpful in confirming early pregnancy.

Traditionally, the signs and symptoms of pregnancy have been categorized as presumptive symptoms, probable signs, and positive signs.

Presumptive symptoms are those concerns that the prenatal client identifies in the present illness and chief complaint portions of the history and several additional general physical signs. They are the subjective data that led the client to seek confirmation of pregnancy. Presumptive symptoms include: (1) absence of menses 10 or more days after the expected date of onset, (2) morning nausea or appetite change, (3) frequent urination, (4) soreness or a tingling sensation in the breasts, (5) Braxton–Hicks' contractions, (6) quickening, (7) abdominal enlargement, and (8) bluish discoloration of the vagina.

The following are probable signs of pregnancy: (1) progressive enlargement of the uterus, (2) softening of the uterine isthmus (Hegar's sign), (3) asymmetrical, soft enlargement of one uterine cornu (Piskacek's sign), (4) bluish or cyanotic color of the cervix and upper vagina (Chadwick's sign), (5) softening of the cervix (Goodell's sign), (6) internal ballottement, (7) palpation of fetal parts, and (8) positive test results for HCG in urine or serum. These signs are termed "probable" because clinical conditions other than pregnancy can cause any of these signs. However, if they occur together, a strong case can be made for the presence of a pregnancy.

In pregnancy, uterine enlargement can be noted on pelvic examination about 6 to 8 weeks after the last normal menses. The uterus first enlarges in the pelvis and by 12 weeks' gestation it can be palpated ab-dominally just above the symphysis pubis. In addition to enlarging, the uterus becomes globular and then ovoid in shape.

The uterus softens in pregnancy because of increased vascularity. The isthmus of the uterus is the first part to soften. At about 6 to 8 weeks' gestation, the softened isthmus produces a dramatic palpatory finding. On palpation, the enlarged, globular uterus feels almost detached from the still not completely softened cervix because the isthmus feels so indistinct (Fig. 21-1). This phenomenon is called Hegar's sign. By 7 or 8 weeks the cervix and uterus can be easily flexed at their junction (McDonald's sign).

Cyanosis of the cervix is noted on speculum examination as early as 6 to 8 weeks' gestation and results from the increased vascularity in the area.

Often uterine enlargement does not progress symmetrically. Rather, the area of placental development enlarges more rapidly. This produces a palpatory asymmetrical enlargement of one uterine cornu, called Piskacek's sign (Fig. 21-2).

Immunological tests for the presence of HCG are commonly used to assist in the diagnosis of pregnancy. These tests depend on an antigen-antibody reaction between HCG and an antiserum obtained from rabbits immunized against this antigen. These tests are available for use by both health professional and women themselves and are very sensitive. Most commercial tests use standardized anti-HCG rabbit serum and standardized latex particles coated with HCG. Anti-HCG serum is mixed first with a sample of the client's urine, then HCG particles are added. The lack of agglutination is a positive test because urine containing HCG had neutralized the HCG antibodies. If the urine sample contains no HCG, agglutination would occur, indicating a negative test for pregnancy.

Pregnancy tests based on the presence of HCG in the urine can be reliably made in the period from 2 weeks after the first missed menses through 16 weeks' gestation. During this period of time, the production of HCG is at its peak.

The positive signs of pregnancy are those that prove the presence of a fetus. These signs are: (1) documentation of a fetal heart beat by auscultation, electrocardiogram, or Doppler instrument; (2) palpation of active fetal movements; and (3) the radiological or ultrasonographical demonstration of fetal parts. Ultrasonographical techniques can demonstrate the presence of a gestational sac as early as the sixth week of gestation. Doppler instruments can detect a fetal heartbeat as early as 10 to 12 weeks.

Currently, clinical diagnosis of pregnancy is more dependent on the probable signs than the presumptive symptoms and positive signs of pregnancy. How-

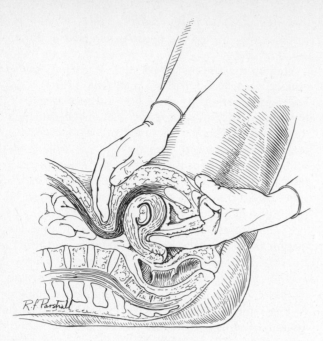

Fig. 21-1. Hegar's sign, softening of the lower uterine segment.

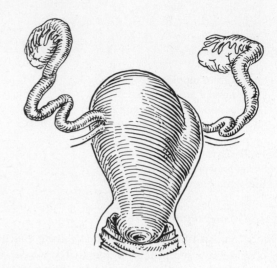

Fig. 21-2. Piskacek's sign, asymmetrical enlargement of the uterine fundus.

Table 21-1. The physical signs of pregnancy

Approximate gestation (weeks since last menses)	Sign	Approximate gestation (weeks since last menses)	Sign
2	Amenorrhea	16-20	Fetal movements noted by mother ("quickening")
4-6	Softening of the cervix (Goodell's sign)		Pigment changes may occur
5-6	Softening of the cervicouterine junction (Ladin's sign)	20	Uterine fundus at the lower border of the umbilicus
6	Gestational sac may be noted by ultrasonography		Fetal heartbeat auscultated with fetoscope
6-8	Compressibility of the lower uterine segment (Hegar's sign)	24	Fetus palpable
	Dilatation of breast veins	24-26	Mother begins to notice Braxton-Hicks contractions
	Pulsation of uterine arteries in lateral fornices (Oslander's sign)		Uterus changes from globular to ovoid shape
7-8	Flexing of fundus of cervix (McDonald's sign)	28	Fetus easily palpable, very mobile, and may be found in any lie, presentation, or position
	Asymmetrical softening and enlarging of the uterus (Piskacek's sign)		The uterus is approximately one-half of the distance from the umbilicus to the xiphoid
	Uterus changes from pear to globular shape	32	The fetus usually lies longitudinally with a vertex presentation
8-12	Bluish coloration of the vagina and cervix (Chadwick's sign)		The uterine fundus is approximately two-thirds of the distance between the umbilicus and the xiphoid
10-12	Detection of fetal heartbeats with a Doppler instrument	34	The uterine fundus is just below the xiphoid
12	Uterus palpable just above the symphysis pubis	36-40	The vertex presentation may engage in the pelvis
16	Ballottement of the fetus possible by abdominal and vaginal examination		
	Uterus palpable halfway between the symphysis and umbilicus		

ever, with new developments in immunological blood testing, radioimmunoassay, and more available ultrasonographical technology, the methods of pregnancy diagnosis may change.

The radioimmunoassay test that is specific for the B subunit of the HCG molecule at very low concentrations is also considered a positive test for pregnancy. With this test there is no cross-reaction with luteinizing hormone as with other immunological tests and, thus, it is more accurate for HCG itself.

The timetable for physical signs of pregnancy is presented in Table 21-1.

PRENATAL EXAMINATIONS

Subsequent to the initial assessment, the prenatal client is examined at regular intervals. Reexamination schedules vary for clients, but the schedule includes examination approximately every 3 to 4 weeks during the first 28 weeks of pregnancy and every 1 to 2 weeks during the final 12 weeks.

At each prenatal revisit, the following assessments are usually made:

1. Weight
2. Blood pressure
3. Urine screening for glucose and protein
4. Determination of the presence of edema
5. Abdominal assessment
   a. Determination of fundal height
   b. Determination of fetal presentation and position
   c. Measurement of fetal heart rate

Weight gain

Optimal weight gain during pregnancy based on the lowest rate of complications and low birth weight infants is 24.0 to 27.5 pounds (a wider range is 20 to 30 pounds). High prepregnancy weight correlates significantly with an increased risk of preeclampsia. Women with low prepregnancy weight who gain little weight during pregnancy are more likely to have low birth weight babies (that is, babies weighing 2,500 g or less). Sudden weight gain, especially in the third trimester, usually means fluid retention and is evaluated in conjunction with maternal blood pressure. Apart from this transient cause of weight gain many women tend to add to their body fat stores during pregnancy and this weight gain may not be entirely lost after delivery. The gain in weight should occur gradually, averaging 1½ to 2 pounds per month during the first 24 weeks and ½ to 1 pound a week during the remainder of pregnancy.

Blood pressure

Mean systolic blood pressure and mean diastolic blood pressure are essentially unchanged during pregnancy except, as indicated, for a mild and transient decrease during the middle trimester. Hypertension, however, contributes significantly to prenatal morbidity and mortality and pregnancy-induced hypertension is a disease peculiar to pregnancy. This disorder typically develops after the twenty-fourth week of pregnancy and is characterized by:

1. A systolic blood pressure of at least 140 mm Hg or a rise of 30 mm Hg or more above the usual level in two readings 6 hours apart
2. A diastolic pressure of 90 mm Hg or more or a rise of 15 mm Hg above the usual level in two readings 6 hours apart
3. Proteinuria
4. Edema of the face or hands

Researchers have described what has come to be known as the roll-over test to detect gravidas who are likely to develop hypertension in late pregnancy. Such women have an increased vascular reactivity and have lost their resistance to vasopressor substances that characterize normal pregnancy. This sensitivity or vascular reactivity is exhibited by an increase of 20 mm Hg in diastolic pressure when a woman of 28 to 32 weeks' gestation turns from her side to her back. This increase is termed a positive roll test, and such a woman requires closer monitoring of her blood pressure during the latter portion of her pregnancy because she is much more likely to develop the classical signs and symptoms of preeclampsia.

Assessment of edema and the extremities

Ankle swelling and edema of the lower extremities occur in two-thirds of women in late pregnancy. Women notice this swelling later in the day after standing for a period of time. Sodium and water retention caused by steroid hormones, an increased hydrophilic property of intracellular connective tissue, and increased venous pressure in the lower extremities during pregnancy contribute to this edema. Assessment includes palpation of the ankles and pretibial areas to determine the extent of the edema and observation for hand, face, or generalized edema. Generalized edema may be manifested by pitting in the sacral area or by the appearance of a depression on the gravid abdomen from the rim of the fetoscope after it has been pressed against the abdomen to auscultate the fetal heart rate.

In addition to assessment for edema formation, examination of the legs includes inspection for varicose veins and dorsiflexion of the foot with the legs extended to check for Homan's sign and thrombophlebitis. In the presence of an elevated or a borderline elevated blood pressure, deep tendon reflexes are assessed. Hyperreflexia and clonus, combined with other signs, can indicate preeclampsia.

Leg cramps during pregnancy may accompany extension of the foot and sudden shortening of leg muscles. This may be caused by an elevation of serum phosphorus with a diet that includes a large quantity of milk.

A variety of discomforts and sensations in the legs is attributed to compression of nerves from pressure of the enlarging uterus. This includes numbness in the lateral femoral area resulting from compression of that nerve beneath the inguinal ligament. Medial thigh sensation may result from the compression of the obturator nerve against the side walls of the pelvis. Periodic numbness of the fingers is reported to occur in at least 5% of gravidas. This is apparently caused by a brachial plexus traction syndrome from drooping shoulders. This drooping is associated with the increased weight of breasts as pregnancy advances. Skilled movement of fingers may be impaired by compression of the median nerve in the arm and hand caused by physiological changes in fascia, tendons, and connective tissue during pregnancy. This is known as carpal tunnel syndrome and is characterized by a paroxysm of pain, numbness, tingling, or burning in the sides of the hands and fingers—particularly the thumb, second, and third fingers, and the side of the fifth finger.

Abdominal examination

As pregnancy progresses, the uterus enlarges steadily. The height of the fundus serves as a rough guide to fetal gestation and overall fetal growth. Fig. 21-3 displays the expected fundal height at various gestational ages. At the twelfth week of pregnancy, the fundus is palpable just above the symphysis. At 16 weeks, the fundus is approximately halfway between the symphysis and umbilicus. At the twentieth gestational week, the fundus usually reaches the lower border of the umbilicus. After the twentieth week, the uterus increases in height at approximately 3.75 cm per month or around 1 cm per week until weeks 34 to 36, when the fundus almost reaches the xiphoid. Then, in approximately 65% of gravidas, the fetal head drops further into the pelvis with lightening. If this occurs, the fundal measurement at 36 may be greater than that later in pregnancy.

Unless the fetal head drops into the pelvis, the fundal height between weeks 37 to 40 will stay the same. During this period the fetus is increasing in size, but the amount of amniotic fluid decreases.

The routine procedure for abdominal reevaluation during pregnancy is (1) inspection, (2) palpation and measurement, and (3) auscultation.

In addition to the observations the practitioner makes when observing the abdomen, for example, skin and scars, for the pregnant client, the examiner observes the size and configuration of the enlarging uterus.

Normally, the uterine size should relate to the estimated gestational age. Any discrepancy between observed size and estimated gestational age should be further explored. A uterus larger than expected may indicate incorrect gestational age estimation or multiple pregnancy. A smaller than expected uterus may indicate a poorly growing fetus or gestational miscalculation.

Abdominal assessment

Observation of the abdomen may provide the first clues to the presentation and position of the fetus. Asymmetrical appearance or distention in width versus longitudinal enlargement may suggest a transverse or oblique lie of the fetus that can be verified by palpation. After about week 28 fetal movements may be seen.

The uterus is palpated to determine the top, or height, of the fundus. The examiner stands at the right side of the supine client. The ulnar surface of the examiner's left hand is placed approximately 3 to 4 cm above where the fundal apex is expected to be located in the midline of the abdomen. This hand

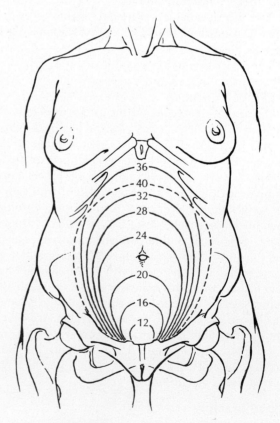

Fig. 21-3. Approximate levels of the uterine fundus at various gestational points. Numbers indicate weeks of gestation.

palpates downward in small progressive steps until the examiner can differentiate between the softness of the abdomen generally and the firm round fundal edge (Fig. 21-4). The use of only the palmar surface of the middle finger of the examining hand can assist in locating the precise level of fundal height.

When the fundal edge is located, its distance from the symphysis is estimated. When the fundus is below the umbilicus, the measurement in centimeters above the symphysis or below the umbilicus can be estimated or measured with a tape.

When the fundus is above the umbilicus, measurement with a measuring tape is recommended. The examiner places the zero point of the tape at the top of the symphysis and measures the distance to the top of the fundus (Fig. 21-5). Various methods exist for estimating fundal height. Methods that avoid the measurement of the fundal curve and abdominal adipose tissue are more accurate estimations of actual fundal growth. The practitioner should choose one method and use it consistently. This measurement is approximate and estimates of fundal height measurement may vary 1 to 2 cm among examiners. However, measurement is more reliable than visual estimation beyond 20 weeks and, if it is practiced consistently by one examiner, should provide an excellent picture of fetal growth with each visit.

The examiner next palpates the abdomen to determine fetal lie, presentation, position, attitude, and size.

The lie is the relationship of the long axis of the fetus to the long axis of the uterus. The lie can be longitudinal, oblique, or transverse (Fig. 21-6).

The presentation of the fetus is that fetal part that is most dependent. The presentation can be vertex, brow, face, shoulder, or breech (Fig. 21-7).

The position is the relationship of a specified part of the fetal presentation, the denominator, to a particular part of the maternal pelvis (Fig. 21-8). The denominator in a vertex presentation is the occiput (O); in a breech presentation, it is the sacrum (S); and in a face presentation, it is the mentum (M), that is, the chin. The position is standardly abbreviated according to the left or right of the pelvis, the denominator, and the pelvic portion as follows:

Side of pelvis	Denominator	Pelvic portion
L = left	O = occiput	A = anterior
R = right	S = sacrum	P = posterior
	M = mentum	L = lateral

For example, if the occiput were closest to the left, anterior portion of the pelvis, the fetal position would be LOA.

The fetal attitude is the relationship of the fetal head and limbs to its body (Fig. 21-9). The fetus may be fully flexed, poorly flexed, or extended. When the fetus is fully flexed, the spine is flexed, the head is flexed on the chest, and the arms and legs are crossed over the chest and abdomen.

Engagement is said to have occurred when both the biparietal and suboccipitobregmatic diameters of the fetal head have passed into the inlet of the pelvis (Fig. 21-10). When this has occurred, the fetal head can be felt at the level of the ischial spines on vaginal palpation.

Determination of fetal lie, presentation, position,

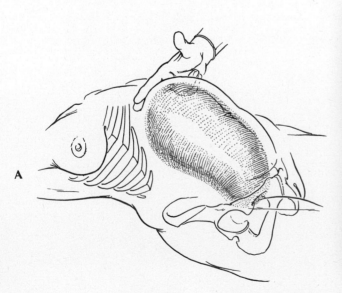

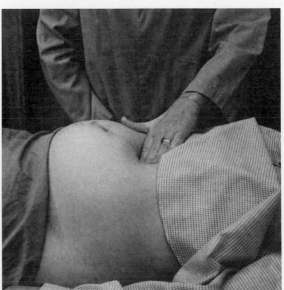

Fig. 21-4. Palpation to determine the height of the uterine fundus.

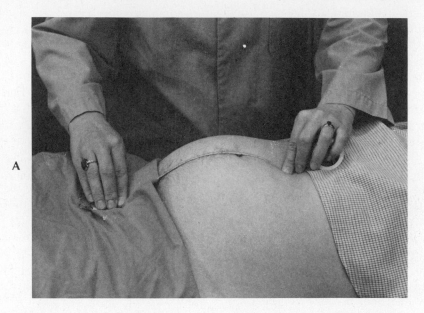

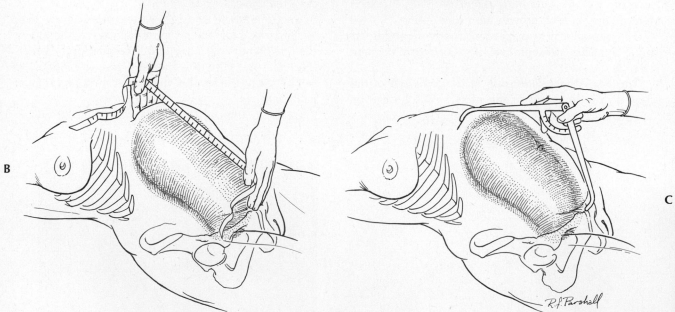

Fig. 21-5. Various methods of measuring the height of the fundus. **A,** Measurement accounting for some of the fundal curve. **B,** Measurement avoiding the fundal curve. **C,** Measurement using obstetrical calipers. This method also avoids measuring the fundal curve.

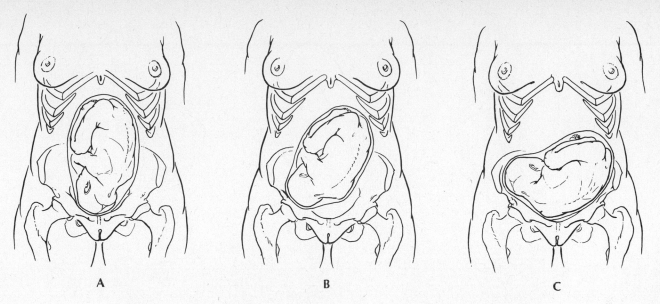

Fig. 21-6. Examples of fetal lie. **A,** Longitudinal lie. **B,** Oblique lie. **C,** Transverse lie.

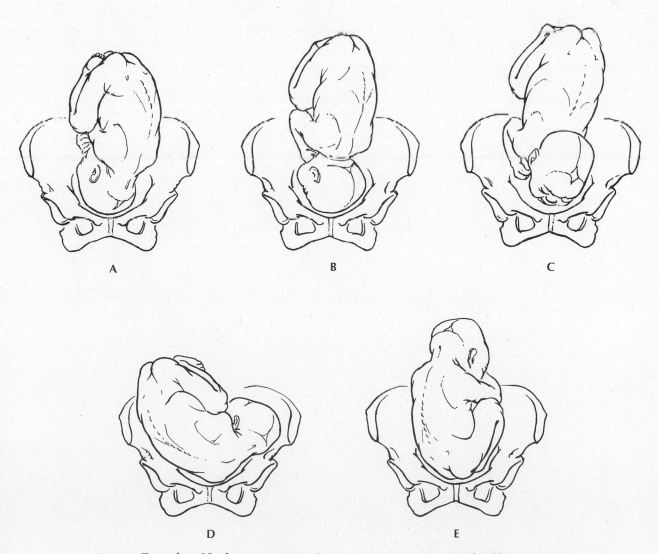

Fig. 21-7. Examples of fetal presentation. **A,** Vertex. **B,** Brow. **C,** Face. **D,** Shoulder. **E,** Breech.

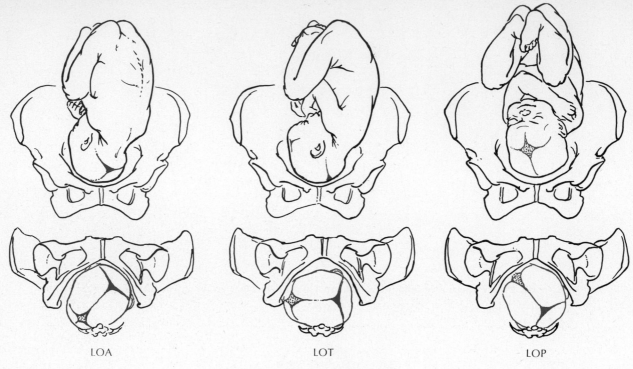

LOA   LOT   LOP

Fig. 21-8. Examples of fetal position.

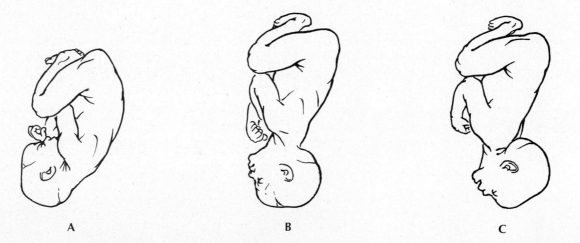

A   B   C

Fig. 21-9. Fetal attitude. **A,** Fully flexed. **B,** Poorly flexed. **C,** Extended.

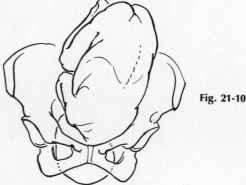

Fig. 21-10. Engagement.

attitude, and size is accomplished by abdominal palpation. The abdomen is systematically palpated using Leopold's maneuvers:

1. Fundal palpation
2. Lateral palpation
3. Pawlik palpation
4. Deep pelvic palpation

Leopold's maneuvers are usually not especially productive until 26 to 28 weeks' gestation, when the fetus is large enough for its parts to be differentiated through abdominal and uterine structures.

For this examination the client is supine. Elevation of the client's knees may assist in decreasing tension of the abdominal muscles and making the examination more comfortable for the client.

FUNDAL PALPATION

The examiner stands at the client's right side, facing her head, and places the palmar surface of both hands on the uterine fundus to determine what part of the fetus is occupying the fundus (Fig. 21-11). Leopold's first maneuver, the method of determining the location of the top of the fundus has already been described. Usually the buttocks of the fetus will be in

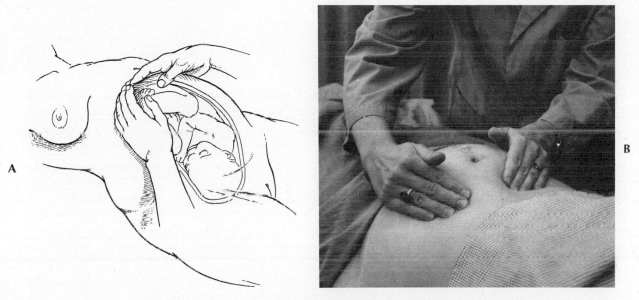

Fig. 21-11. Palpation to determine the contents of the uterine fundus.

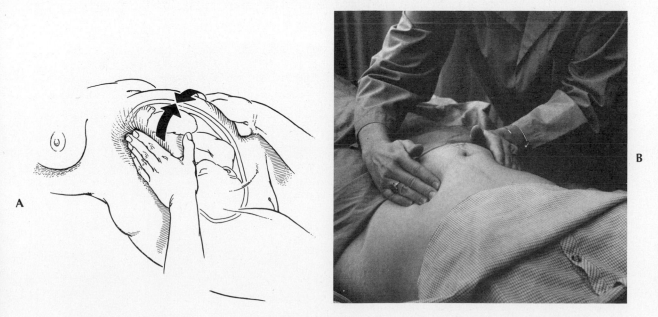

Fig. 21-12. Palpation of lateral uterine fundus to determine the position of the back and extremities of the fetus.

the fundus and felt as a soft, irregular, and slightly movable mass. The lower limbs are felt adjacent to the buttocks. If the head is in the fundus, it is felt as smooth, round, hard, and ballotable. The groove of the neck is felt between the trunk and the upper limbs. The head is freely movable in contrast to the buttocks, which can only move sideways and with the trunk.

LATERAL PALPATION

For Leopold's second maneuver (Fig. 21-12), the examiner, while still facing the patient's head, moves both hands to either side of the uterus to determine which side the fetal back is on. The examiner supports the fetus with one hand while the other hand palpates the fetus. The examiner then reverses the procedure to palpate each side of the uterus. The fetal back is felt as a continuous, smooth, firm object, whereas the fetal limbs, or small parts, are felt as small, irregular, sometimes moving objects. On each side, the examiner palpates the flank to the midline, making special note of the edge of the fetal back as a landmark in determining the fetal position.

PAWLIK PALPATION

This procedure is done with the right hand only to determine what fetal part lies over the pelvic inlet. The right hand is placed over the symphysis so that the fingers are on the left side of the uterus and the thumb is on the right side (Fig. 21-13). The hand

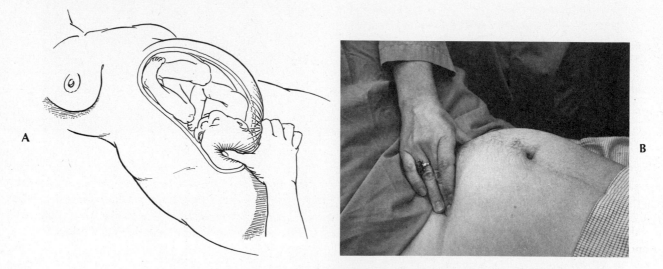

Fig. 21-13. Pawlik palpation to determine fetal presenting part.

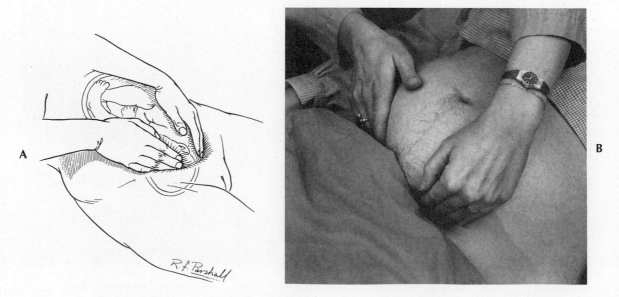

Fig. 21-14. Deep pelvic palpation to determine the attitude and descent of the fetus.

should be approximately around the fetal presenting part, usually the head. The presenting part is gently palpated to determine its form and consistency, and grasped and gently moved sideways to determine its movability. This palpation confirms impressions about the presenting part and determines if the presenting part (if the fetal head) might be engaged. If the fetal head is movable above the symphysis, it is not engaged. If the head is not movable, it may be engaged. Engagement can only be confirmed by pelvic examination to determine if the biparietal diameter of the fetal head is level with the ischial spines.

DEEP PELVIC PALPATION

The examiner changes position (Fig. 21-14). The examiner remains on the right side of the client but is turned so that she or he is facing the woman's feet. A hand is placed on each side of the uterus near the pelvic brim. The client is asked to take a deep breath and to exhale slowly. As she does, the examining fingers are allowed to sink deeply above the pubic bones to palpate the presenting part and to determine which side the cephalic prominence is on. If the presenting part is the head, the location of the cephalic prominence, that is, the forehead, assists in determining the fetus' position and attitude. If the head is flexed, the occiput lies deeper in the pelvis, is flatter, and is less defined than the forehead, which is more prominent and on the same side as the small parts. If the head is not well flexed, the cephalic and occipital prominences will be palpated at the same level, and the occipital portion may feel more prominent and is on the same side as the back.

Throughout these maneuvers the examiner assesses the congruence of the size of the fetus with the gestational age.

In summary to this section on abdominal assessment, a series of questions the examiner mentally asks about each client are listed with an indication of the procedures that assist in answering the questions.

Question	Methods of obtaining evidence to answer the question
What is the fetal lie?	Abdominal inspection
	Lateral abdominal palpation
What is the fetal presentation?	Fundal palpation
	Pawlik palpation
	Deep pelvic palpation
What is the fetal position?	Lateral palpation
	Deep pelvic palpation
What is the fetal attitude?	Deep pelvic palpation
Is the fetal growth congruent with gestational age?	Fundal height measurement
	All of Leopold's maneuvers

Auscultation

The fetal heart rate is an indicator of the health status of the fetus and is monitored throughout pregnancy. Auscultation of the fetal heart rate is accomplished by use of a special stethoscope, or fetoscope, or a Doppler instrument. With the Doppler instrument, the fetal heart rate can be monitored after about 10 weeks gestation. Using a fetoscope, the examiner can first hear the fetal heart rate between the sixteenth and twentieth weeks of gestation.

The use of the fetoscope is demonstrated in Fig. 21-15. The fetal heart rate is rapid and soft. The use of a fetoscope avoids noises produced by fingers on the stethoscope and makes use of the benefits of both air and bone conduction. The bell of an ordinary stethoscope can be used but is less effective than a fetoscope in listening to fetal heartbeats, especially around 20 weeks.

The fetal heart rate is normally between 120 and 160 beats per minute, and the heartbeats resemble a watch tick heard through a pillow. They are best heard through the fetal back. When the fetus is large enough for its position to be determined, the bell of the fetoscope or the Doppler head is placed at the back of the fetal thorax. When the fetus is under 20 weeks' gestation, the heart rate is often best heard at the midline, just above the pubic hairline.

The fetal heart rate is counted for at least 15 seconds and is recorded in number of beats per minute. The fetal heart rate is normally much faster than the maternal heart rate and thus can usually be well differentiated from it. Moreover, the fetal and maternal heart rates are not synchronous, and the maternal rate can be differentiated by palpating the mother's pulse while auscultating the abdomen.

Blood rushing through the placenta can be heard as a uterine souffle. The uterine souffle is a soft, blow-

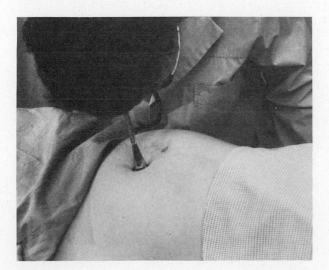

Fig. 21-15. Use of the fetoscope to auscultate the fetal heartbeat.

ing sound that is synchronous with the maternal pulse. The intensity of the souffle has been interpreted as an indicator of uterine blood flow and placental function. A loud uterine souffle has been associated with high urinary estriol levels, and soft or absent souffle with lower estriol levels. Thus, a soft or absent uterine souffle may indicate poor uterine blood flow and placental function, particularly in late pregnancy.

Examination of the bony pelvis

The purpose of the examination of the bony pelvis is to determine if the pelvic cavity is of adequate size to allow for the passage of a full-term infant. This examination is performed on the initial prenatal evaluation and need not be repeated if the pelvis is of adequate size. However, if findings indicate that the pelvis is of borderline adequacy or if the examination could not be done on the initial visit because of client tenseness and subsequent muscular contraction, the examination should be repeated between 32 to 36 weeks' gestation. In the third trimester of pregnancy, there is a relaxation of pelvis joints and ligaments, and the client is more accustomed to examination. Thus, the examination of the bony pelvis can be more thoroughly and accurately accomplished then.

The examination of the bony pelvis is done not so much to diagnose the type of pelvis but to determine its configuration and size. Because the examiner does not have direct access to the bony structures and because the bones are covered with variable amounts of soft tissue, estimates are approximate. Precise bony pelvis measurements can be determined using x-rays. However, x-rays are not needed or indicated for the vast majority of prenatal patients.

The assessment of the bony pelvis needs to be put in the perspective of the capacity needed to accommodate a full-term fetus. When the head of a full-term fetus is well flexed, the two largest presenting diameters are the biparietal and the suboccipitobregmatic, each measuring approximately 9.5 cm (Fig. 21-16).

The pelvis consists of four bones: the two innominate bones, the sacrum, and the coccyx. Each innominate bone consists of three bones that fuse after puberty. These three bones are the ilium, the ischium, and the os pubis (Fig. 21-17). The innominate bones form the anterior and lateral portions of the pelvis.

The sacrum and coccyx form the posterior portion of the pelvis. The sacrum is composed of five fused vertebrae. Its upper anterior portion is termed the sacral promontory, which forms the posterior margin of the pelvic brim. The coccyx is composed of three to five fused vertebrae and articulates with the sacrum.

The pelvis is divided by the brim into two parts: the false pelvis and the true pelvis. The false pelvis is that part above the brim and is of no obstetrical interest.

The true pelvis is that portion of the pelvis that includes the brim and the area below. The true pelvis is divided into three parts: the inlet or brim, the midpelvis or cavity, and the outlet. The inlet is formed anteriorly by the upper margins of the pubic bones, laterally by the iliopectineal lines, and posteriorly by the anterior, upper margin of the sacrum, the sacral promontory. The cavity is formed anteriorly by the posterior aspect of the symphysis pubis, laterally by the inner surfaces of the ischial and iliac bones, and posteriorly by the anterior surface of the sacrum. The outlet is diamond-shaped and is formed anteriorly by the inferior rami of the pubic and ischial bones, laterally by the ischial tuberosities, and posteriorly by

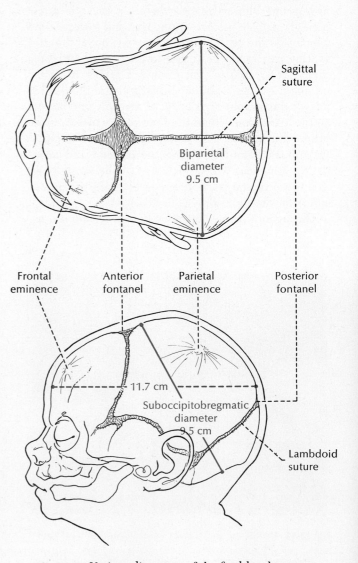

Fig. 21-16. Various diameters of the fetal head at term.

the inferior edge of the sacrum, if the coccyx is movable.

Each of the pelvis portions can be imagined as a series of planes: the plane of the brim, or pelvic inlet; the planes of the midpelvis; and the plane of the outlet. These planes are illustrated in Fig. 21-18.

The plane of the inlet in an average female pelvis measures approximately 11 to 13 cm in the anteroposterior diameter and 13 to 14 cm in the transverse diameter. The anteroposterior diameter of the inlet measured from the middle of the sacral promontory to the superior, posterior margin of the symphysis pubis is called the true conjugate and is an important obstetrical measurement. However, it cannot be assessed directly, except by radiographic methods. An estimate of the true conjugate is made by measuring the diagonal conjugate, which is the distance between the inferior border of the symphysis pubis

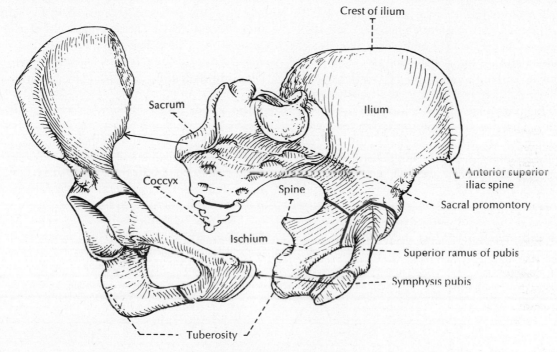

Fig. 21-17. Bones of the pelvis.

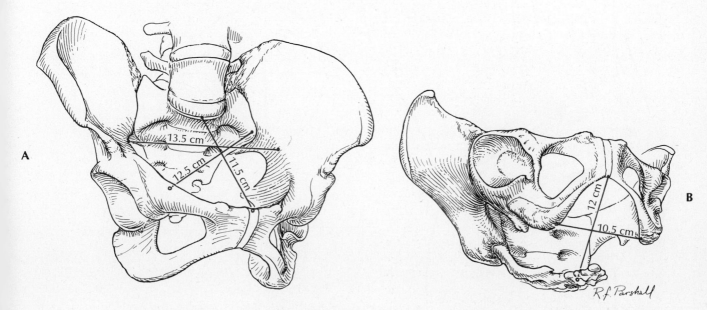

Fig. 21-18. Planes of the pelvic inlet and midpelvis. (Measurements are averages within normal limits.)

and the sacral promontory. The diagonal conjugate is about 1 to 2 cm longer than the true conjugate, depending on the height and inclination of the symphysis. The clinical measurement of the diagonal conjugate, the most valuable single measurement of pelvic adequacy, will be discussed later in this section.

The midpelvis contains the planes of greatest at least pelvic dimensions. The plane of least pelvic dimensions is bounded by the junction of the fourth and fifth sacral vertebrae, the apex of the symphysis, and the ischial spines. The average dimensions of this plane are 12 cm (anteroposterior diameter) and 10.5 cm (transverse diameter). The transverse diameter is the distance between the ischial spines.

The pelvic outlet is composed of two triangular planes, having a common base in the most inferior portion of the transverse diameter between the ischial tuberosities. The obstetrical anteroposterior diameter of the outlet is the distance between the inferior edge of the symphysis pubis and the edge of the sacrum, if the coccyx is movable. This measurement is usually 11.5 cm.

The transverse diameter of the outlet is the distance between the inner surfaces of the ischial tuberosities and usually measures about 11.0 cm (Fig. 21-19).

Although there is a characteristic shape of the adult female pelvis that is different from the characteristically male pelvis, a female client may have any one of four types of human pelvises, or a mixture of these types. In addition, the pelvis shape may have been distorted congenitally or by disease.

The four basic pelvic types as classified by Caldwell and Moloy (1939) are (1) gynecoid, (2) android, (3) anthropoid, and (4) platypelloid.

The typical female pelvis is the gynecoid pelvis, which is found in approximately 40% to 50% of adult females. This pelvis is characterized by a rounded inlet, except for a slight projection of the sacral promontory; a deep posterior half, made possible by a wide sacrosciatic notch and concave sacrum, and a wide anterior half made possible by a wide, subpubic angle.

The android pelvis is found in approximately 15% to 20% of adult females. This pelvic type is roughly wedge- or heart-shaped with the transverse diameter of the inlet approximately equal to the anteroposterior diameter, but with the widest transverse diameter located closer to the sacrum. Other characteristics of the android pelvis include:
1. Narrow subpubic arch
2. Convergent side walls
3. Large encroaching spines

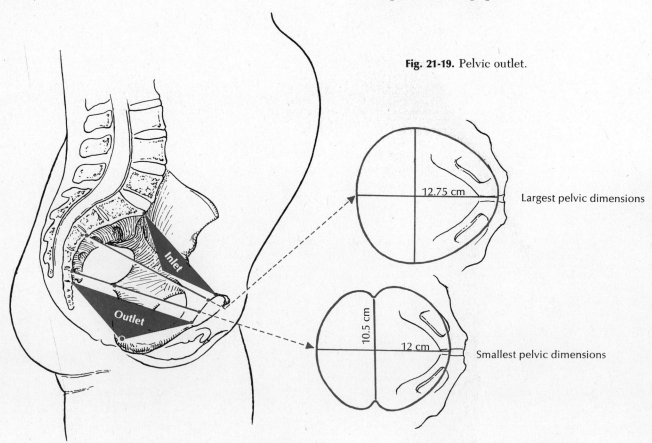

Fig. 21-19. Pelvic outlet.

4. Short sacrosciatic notch and sacrospinous ligament
5. Short interspinous diameter
6. Straight sacrum
7. Short intertuberous diameter

The anthropoid pelvis has an elongated anteroposterior diameter and is found in approximately 25% to 35% of women. It is characterized by:

1. Narrow subpubic arch
2. Prominent ischial spines
3. Wide sacrosciatic notch and long sacrospinous ligaments
4. Deeply curved sacrum

The platypelloid pelvis had a flattened anteroposterior dimension with a relative widening of the transverse diameter. This pelvic type is seen in approximately 5% of women. The platypelloid pelvis is characterized by:

1. Wide subpubic arch
2. Flat ischial spines
3. Wide sacrosciatic notch and long sacrospinous ligaments
4. Straight sacrum

The various dimensions of the four basic pelvic types are compared and contrasted in Fig. 21-20. Pure pelvic types are unusual; most pelvises are admixtures

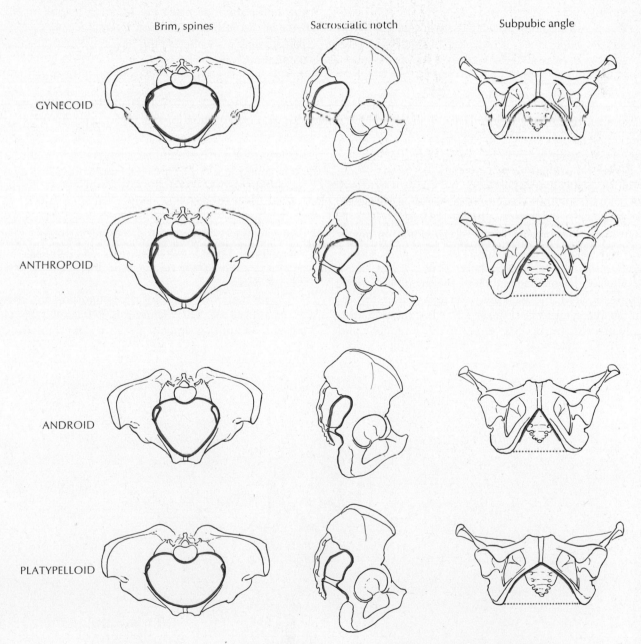

Brim, spines   Sacrosciatic notch   Subpubic angle

GYNECOID

ANTHROPOID

ANDROID

PLATYPELLOID

Fig. 21-20. Comparisons and contrasts of various portions of the four basic pelvic types.

of two pelvic types, with the characteristics of one type predominating.

The examination of the bony pelvis can be uncomfortable for the client. It should be done after the internal examination of the soft pelvic organs. The preparation of the client should include the explanation of the procedure, the client's emptying of her bladder, and instructions to the client for relaxation.

A routine standard procedure is recommended for the bony pelvis examination, beginning with the examination of the anterior pelvis, proceeding to lateral examination on one side, comparing the initially examined side with the opposite side, and concluding with the examination of the posterior and inferior portions.

The following bony pelvis parts and landmarks are especially important in examining the pelvis:

1. Subpubic arch
2. Symphysis pubis
3. Side walls
4. Ischial spines
5. Sacrosciatic notch
6. Sacrum
7. Coccyx
8. Sacral promontory
9. Ischial tuberosities

The width of the subpubic arch is palpated and its angle is estimated. Normally both examining fingers should fit comfortably in the arch, which optimally forms an angle measuring slightly more than a right angle (that is, a 90 degree angle) (Fig. 21-21).

The length and inclination of the symphysis pubis are estimated by sweeping the examining fingers under the symphysis (Fig. 21-22). Also, the examiner palpates the retropubic curve of the forepelvis and envisions its configuration. Measurement difficulties created by a large amount of soft tissue in the area and reliability with slope measurements preclude a precise estimation of the length and inclination of the symphysis. The examiner essentially screens for an unusually long or steeply inclined symphysis pubis and for an angular rather than a rounded forepelvis.

Next, the right or left lateral pelvic area is examined. First, the side walls are palpated to determine if they are straight, convergent, or divergent. The splay of the side walls can be assessed by following a line from the point of origin of the widest transverse diameter of the inlet downward to the inner aspect of the tuberosity. Another method for assessing the side walls is to place the examing fingers on the base of the ischial spine as a landmark and then to palpate above and below the landmark to determine inclination.

The ischial spine and sacrospinous ligament are examined. The spine is assessed as being blunt, prominent, or encroaching. The sacrosciatic notch is outlined with palpating fingers, if possible, and its width is determined in centimeters or finger breadths. Often the examiner cannot trace the entire notch, and the sacrospinous ligament is useful in estimating the width of the notch (Fig. 21-23).

The other side of the pelvis is then examined in the manner previously described to determine overall pelvic symmetry. The examiner should attempt to do this part of the examination with the palm of the hand up, rather than rotating the hand so that the palm is down.

The interspinous diameter is an important obstetrical measurement. This diameter is estimated by moving the examining fingers in a straight line from

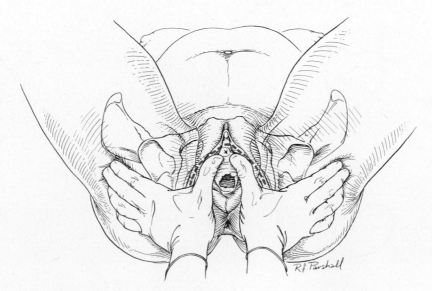

Fig. 21-21. Method of estimating the angle of the subpubic arch.

one spine across to the other (Fig. 21-24). The hand may need to be pronated for this estimation. The estimate is calculated in centimeters. The usual measurement is 10.5 cm. Special calipers are available to measure the interspinous diameter, but these are not often used in clinical practice.

Next the sacrum and coccyx are examined. The fingers are swept down the sacrum, noting whether it is straight, curved, or hollow, and if its inclination is forward or backward. The coccyx is examined

gently because it may be tender on movement. The coccyx is gently pressed backward to determine if it is movable or fixed. Its tilt is noted as anterior or posterior.

The diagonal conjugate is assessed last because this assessment can be especially uncomfortable for the client. A moderate amount of constant pressure is needed to depress the perineum adequately. Pressure is better exerted by the body than by the hand and forearm. It is recommended that the examiner place the foot (the one on the same side as the examining hand) on a stool and the elbow of the examining arm on the thigh or hip. The needed pressure is then applied and controlled by the trunk of the examiner's body. For this examination, the fingers and wrist should form a straight line with the forearm.

The examiner locates the sacrum with the examining fingers and, with the middle finger, walks up the sacrum until the promontory is reached or until the examiner can no longer reach the sacrum. The point where the patient's symphysis touches the examiner's hand is marked with the thumb of the opposite hand and the distance is measured in centimeters by a ruler (Fig. 21-25). In obstetric examining rooms, a ruler is often fixed to the wall for this measurement.

Often, the examiner will not reach the sacral promontory. The examiner should become familiar with the "reach" of his or her examining fingers and record the findings as greater than ($>$) the centimeters of this reach. Normally the diagonal conjugate is greater than 12.5 cm.

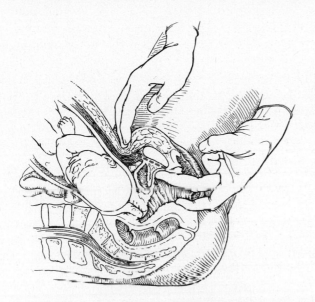

Fig. 21-22. Estimation of the length and inclination of the symphysis pubis.

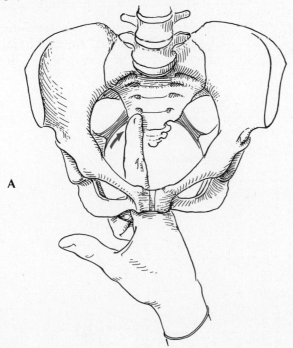
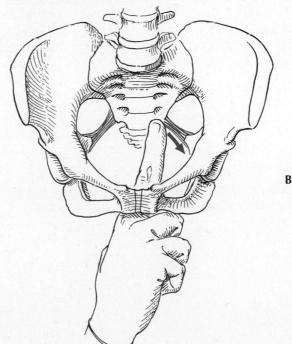

Fig. 21-23. Measurement of the width of the sacrosciatic notch.

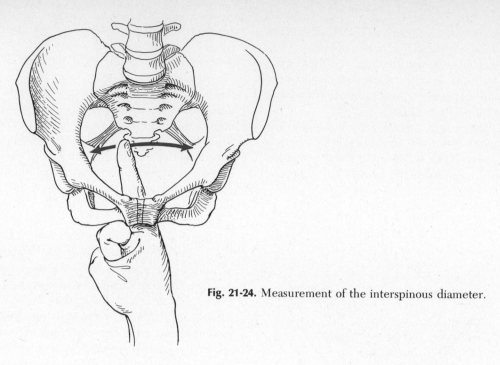

Fig. 21-24. Measurement of the interspinous diameter.

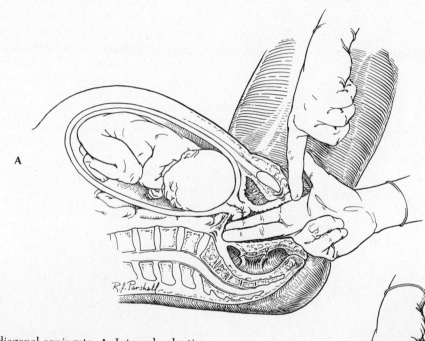

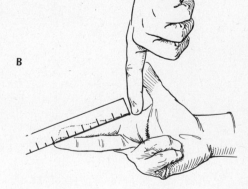

Fig. 21-25. Measurement of the diagonal conjugate. **A,** Internal palpation. **B,** Use of a ruler to specify estimation in centimeters.

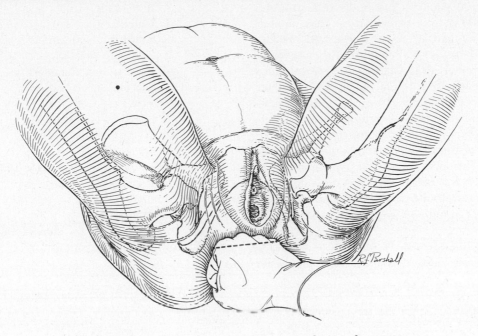

Fig. 21-26. Use of a fist to estimate the intertuberous diameter.

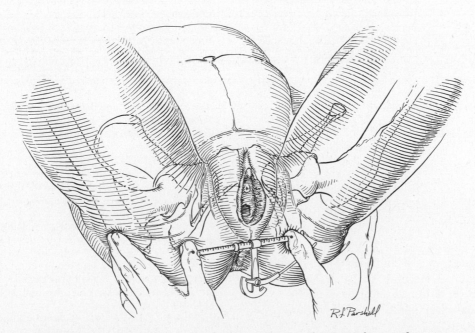

Fig. 21-27. Use of the Thom's pelvimeter to measure the intertuberous diameter.

The examining hand is withdrawn from the vagina and the intertuberous diameter is measured. Using both thumbs, the examiner externally traces the descending rami down to the tuberosities. The examiner then makes a fist and attempts to insert the fist between the tuberosities to measure the transverse diameter of an outlet (Fig. 21-26). The intertuberous diameter is usually 10 to 11 cm. Again, the examiner knows the span of his or her own fist and estimates the intertuberous diameter accordingly.

An instrument called the Thom's pelvimeter can be used to measure the intertuberous diameter (Fig. 21-27). This instrument has two arches that are held against the tuberosities by the examiner's thumbs. The precise intertuberous diameter can be determined by calibrations on the instrument's midportion.

In summary, the areas of bony pelvic examination and the assessment descriptors for these areas are noted:

Sequence of areas of bony pelvis examination	Assessment descriptors
1. Subpubic arch	Less than 90°; more than 90°
2. Side walls	Parallel; convergent; divergent
3. Ischial spines	Size: small; average; large
	Prominence: blunt; prominent; encroaching
4. Sacrosciatic notch Sacrospinous ligament	Estimated width or length in centimeters or fingerbreadths (FB) Usual length 3 to 4 cm
5. Opposite pelvic side	Symmetrical; asymmetrical
6. Interspinous diameter	Estimated length in centimeters Usual length 10.5 cm
7. Sacrum	Concave; straight; convex
8. Coccyx	Position: straight; projects anteriorly; projects posteriorly Movability: movable; fixed
9. Diagonal conjugate	Actual length or length greater than the measurement the examiner can reach Usual length 12.5 cm
10. Intertuberous diameter	Actual length in centimeters if Thom's pelvimeter is used, or an estimated length using a closed fist Usual length 10 to 11 cm

SUMMARY

I. First visit
   A. Complete physical examination, including the female genital examination (see Chapter 23, "Integration of the Physical Assessment")
   B. Abdominal assessment (prenatal portion)
      1. Palpation
         a. Fundal height
         b. Fetal position, using Leopold's maneuvers
      2. Auscultation—fetal heart rate

   C. Bony pelvis assessment
      1. Subpubic arch
      2. Side walls
      3. Ischial spine
      4. Sacrospinous ligament
      5. Opposite side
      6. Interspinous diameter
      7. Sacrum
      8. Coccyx
      9. Diagonal conjugate
      10. Intertuberous diameter
II. Repeat visits
   A. Regional examinations as indicated by history and current condition
   B. Weight
   C. Blood pressure
   D. Urine screening for glucose and protein
   E. Abdominal assessment
      1. Palpation
         a. Fundal height
         b. Fetal position, using Leopold's maneuvers
      2. Auscultation—fetal heart rate

BIBLIOGRAPHY

American College of Obstetricians and Gynecologists: Standards for ambulatory care, Chicago, 1974, The College.

Bailey, R. E.: Mayes' midwifery, London, 1976, Cossell & Collier Macmillan.

Caldwell, W. E., Moloy, H. C., and Swenson, P. C.: The use of the roentgen ray in obstetrics; anatomical variations in the female pelvis and their classification according to morphology, Am. J. Roentgenol. 41:505, 1939.

Gant, N. F., and others: A clinical test for predicting the development of acute hypertension in pregnancy, Am. J. Obstet. Gynecol. 120:1, 1974.

Greenhill, J. P., and Friedman, E. A.: Biological principles and modern practice of obstetrics, Philadelphia, 1974, W. B. Saunders Co.

Hickman, M. A.: An introduction to midwifery, Oxford, 1978, Blackwell Scientific Publications, Ltd.

Martin, L. L.: Health care of women, Philadelphia, 1978, J. B. Lippincott Co.

Page, E. W., Willee, C. A., and Villee, D. B.: Human reproduction: the core content of obstetrics, gynecology, and perinatal medicine, ed. 2, Philadelphia, 1976, W. B. Saunders Co.

Oxhorn, H., and Foote, W.: Human labor and birth, New York, 1975, Appleton-Century-Crofts.

Romney, S. L., and others: Gynecology and obstetrics: the health care of women, New York, 1975, McGraw-Hill Book Co.

Spellacy, W. N.: Management of the high risk pregnancy, Baltimore, 1976, University Park Press.

Walker, J., MacGillivray, I., and Macnaughton, M. C.: Combined textbook of obstetrics and gynecology, ed. 9, Edinburgh, 1976, Churchill Livingstone.

Willson, R. J., and Carrington, E. R.: Obstetrics and gynecology, ed. 6, St. Louis, 1979, The C. V. Mosby Co.

22 Musculoskeletal assessment

The skeletal system is made up of 206 bones and the joints by which they articulate. Bone, cartilage, and connective and hematopoietic (myeloid) tissues make up this system. These structures (1) provide support for the body, (2) allow movement as those muscles attached to the bones shorten in contraction (thereby pulling the bones), and (3) provide for the formation of red blood cells.

The musculoskeletal system is comprised of more than 600 voluntary or striated muscles and constitutes the principal organ of movement as well as a repository for metabolites. The muscle mass accounts for as much as 40% of the weight of the adult man.

It is the partial contracture of skeletal muscle that makes all of the characteristic postures of human beings possible, including the upright position that distinguishes the anthropoid.

Seven types of joint motion have been defined. These movements are flexion, extension, abduction, adduction, internal rotation, external rotation, and circumduction (Figs. 22-1 to 22-4).

Flexion is the bending of the joint so as to approximate the bones it connects, thereby decreasing the joint angle. *Extension* is the straightening of a limb so that the joint angle is increased, the placement of the distal segment of a limb in such a position that its axis is continuous with that of the proximal segment, or the pulling or dragging force exerted on a limb in a direction away from the body.

Abduction is the movement of a limb away from the midline of the body or one of its parts. *Adduction* is the movement of a limb toward the central axis of the body or beyond it.

Internal rotation is the turning of the body part inward toward the central axis of the body. *External rotation* is the turning of the body part away from the midline.

Circumduction is the movement of a body part in a circular pattern. This is not a singular motion but a combination of the other motions.

Muscles are categorized according to the type of joint movement produced by their contraction. Muscles, thus, are flexors, extensors, adductors, abduc-

tors, internal rotators, external rotators, or circumflexors. Muscles shorten on contraction and in so doing exert pull on the bones to which they are attached to move them closer together. Most muscles attach to two bones that articulate at an intervening joint. Generally, one bone moves while the other is held stable. This is due to simultaneous shortening of other muscles. The body of the muscle that produces movement of an extremity generally lies proximal to the bone that is moved.

Thus, the joint, with its synovial membrane, capsule, ligaments, and the muscles that cross it, is considered to be the functional unit of the musculoskeletal system. This discussion of musculoskeletal assessment assumes that the practitioner has an understanding of the anatomy and physiology of the joints involved.

The examination of neuromuscular coordination begins as the practitioner first meets and observes the client, and it continues as the client advances into the room, sits, rises from a sitting position, climbs onto the examining table, lies down, and rolls over. The practitioner should note the speed, coordination, and strength of motion. He should particularly note clumsy, awkward, or involuntary movements, as well as tremor or fasciculation. An estimate of muscle strength may be gained from the handshake of the patient. During the interview the flamboyance or paucity of gesture may provide valuable clues to the client's personality and general mobility.

The chief complaint of the client may indicate the direction for emphasis of the physical assessment. The individual with a chief problem of bodily deformity, paralysis, weakness, or pain associated with movement causes the examiner to focus attention on the bones, joints, and muscles as the possible sites of disorder.

EQUIPMENT FOR THE MUSCULOSKELETAL ASSESSMENT

The structure and function of the body's equipment for movement are explored essentially through the techniques of inspection and palpation, assess-

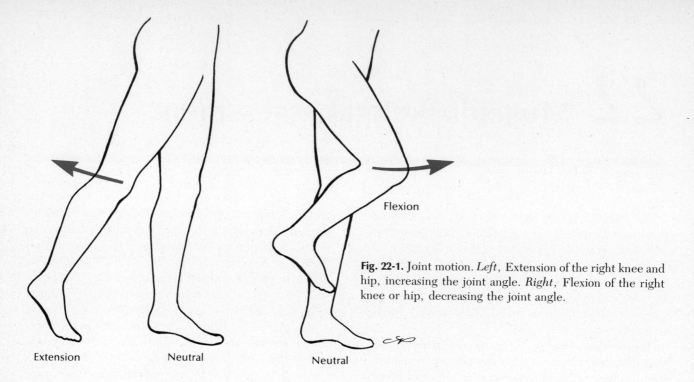

Flexion

Neutral

Extension   Neutral

Fig. 22-1. Joint motion. *Left,* Extension of the right knee and hip, increasing the joint angle. *Right,* Flexion of the right knee or hip, decreasing the joint angle.

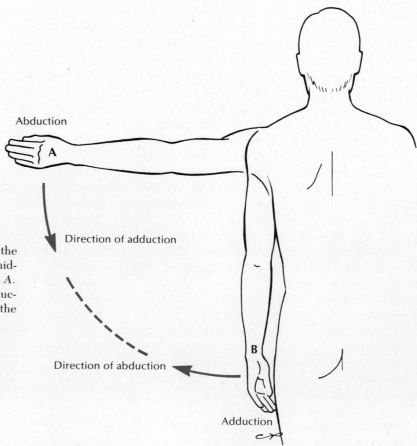

Abduction

Direction of adduction

Fig. 22-2. Joint motion. Abduction is the movement of a limb away from the midline of the body, as seen in position *A*. Position *B* illustrates an arm in adduction, the movement of a limb toward the central axis of the body.

Direction of abduction

Adduction

Fig. 22-3. Joint motion. Internal rotation is the turning of a body part inward toward the midline, as seen in position *A*. Position *B* illustrates external rotation, the turning of a body part away from the midline.

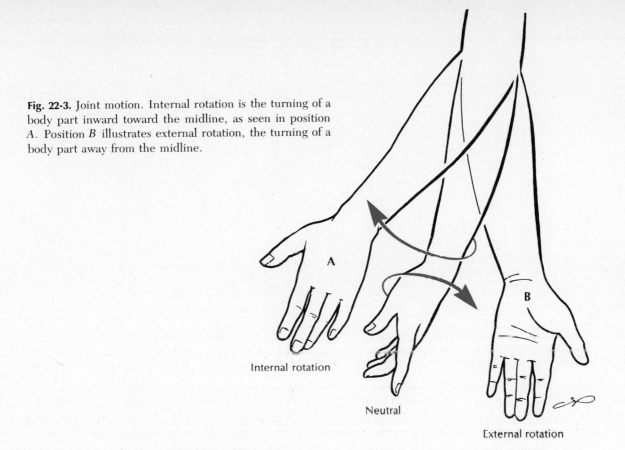

Internal rotation

Neutral

External rotation

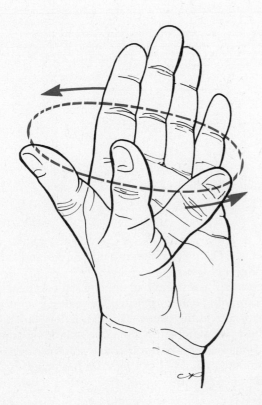

Fig. 22-4. Joint motion. Circumduction is the movement of a body part in a circular pattern.

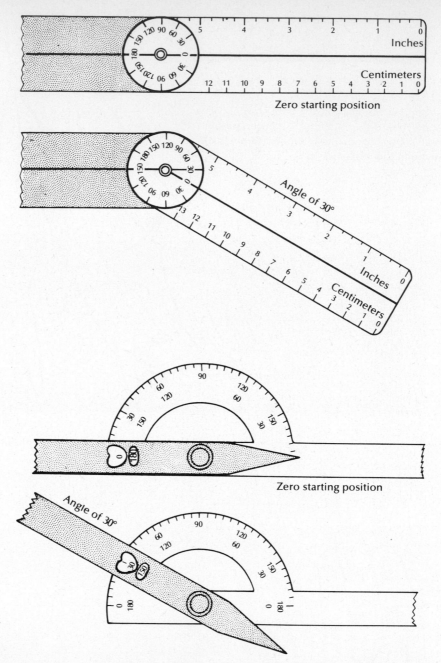

Fig. 22-5. Goniometers used to measure joint motion. The extended anatomical position is accepted as zero degrees. (From Joint motion; method of measuring and recording, Chicago, 1965, American Academy of Orthopaedic Surgeons.)

ment of the ranges of active and passive motion, and tests for muscle strength. A cloth or metal tape measure that will not stretch and a goniometer—a protractor with movable arms that is used to measure the range of joint motion—are necessary to this examination (Fig. 22-5).

THE ASSESSMENT

As in previously described assessments, the cephalocaudal (head to toe) organization for examination is

used in the examination of the bones, joints, and muscles. This organization provides order and aids in avoiding omissions.

Thorough assessment of the musculoskeletal system can only be accomplished through the appropriate exposure of the client. The ambulatory individual can best be examined in shorts or swimming trunks. In this manner the extremities and spine are available for examination. Modesty may be protected for the female client by allowing her to wear a brassiere or

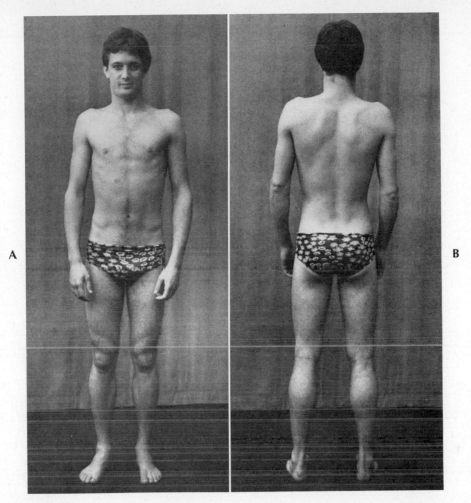

Fig. 22-6 A, B. The body is inspected, both **A,** anterior and, **B,** posterior surfaces, for symmetry of contour and size, gross deformities, swelling, ecchymosis, or other discoloration.

some other abbreviated form of chest cover. Although every effort is made to protect the modesty of the client, an accurate examination cannot be made on a fully clothed client.

For each examination the client should be in the position that provides the greatest stability of joints.

Muscles and joints are examined in symmetrical pairs, that is, first one and then the other for equivalence in size, contour, and strength. The contralateral, matching muscle pairs should be uniformly positioned while they are examined. They are examined both at rest and in a state of contraction.

INSPECTION

General inspection of the musculoskeletal system includes a visual scanning for symmetry, contour, size, and involuntary movement of the two sides of the body, gross deformities, areas of swelling or edema, and ecchymoses or other discoloration.

The posture, or stance, and body alignment are viewed from both in front of and behind the client.

The structural relationship of the feet to the legs and the hips to the pelvis are noted, as are those of the upper extremities, shoulder girdle, and upper trunk.

The shape of the spine is assessed, and its structural apposition to the shoulder girdle, thorax, and pelvis are ascertained.

A deformity is an abnormality in appearance. *Varus* and *valgus* are terms used to describe an angular deviation from the normal structure of an extremity. The reference point is the midline of the body. A varus deformity of the leg (bowlegs) is the lateral deviation of the leg from the midline (Fig. 22-7). A valgus deformity (knock-knees) is one wherein the deviation of the deformity is toward the midline (Fig. 22-8).

Scoliosis is a deformity of the spine seen as a lateral deviation (Fig. 22-9). This angling of the spine produces a downward slant of the thoracic cage on the affected side and an upward tilt of the pelvis on the contralateral side. A rotary deformity of the rib

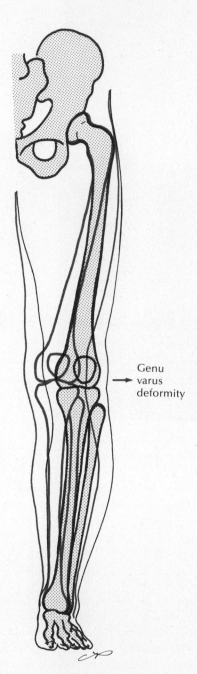

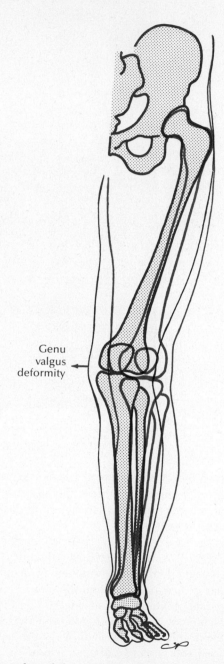

Genu
varus
deformity

Genu
valgus
deformity

Fig. 22-7. Varus deformity of the leg: lateral deviation from the midline (bowleg). This condition was called valgus deformity in earlier times. Red outline figure shows normal position; black, the deformity.

Fig. 22-8. Valgus deformity of the leg: deviation of the leg toward the midline (knock-knee). This condition was called varus deformity in earlier times. Red outline figure shows normal position; black, the deformity.

Fig. 22-9. Deformity of the spine. Scoliosis is the lateral deviation of the spine. Red outline figure shows the normal position; black, the deformity.

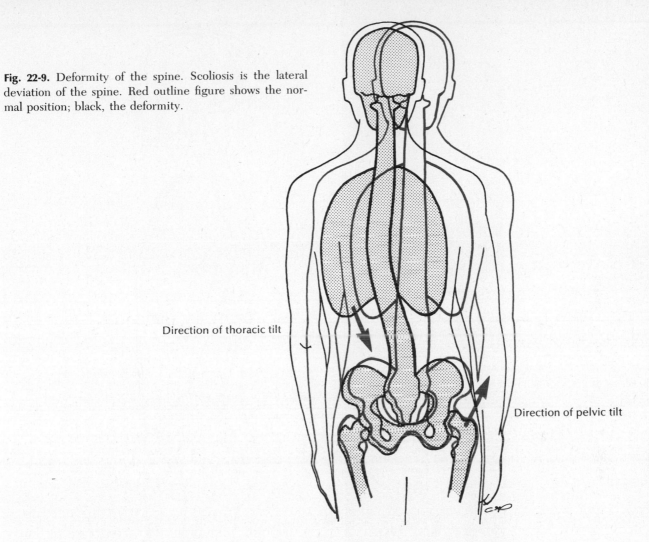

Direction of thoracic tilt

Direction of pelvic tilt

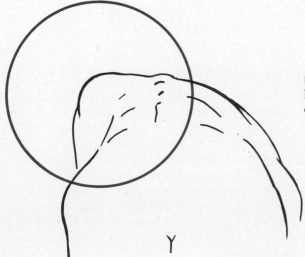

Fig. 22-10. The rotary deformity of scoliosis produces a hump or "razor back" deformity. This deviation is best demonstrated by asking the client to bend at the waist.

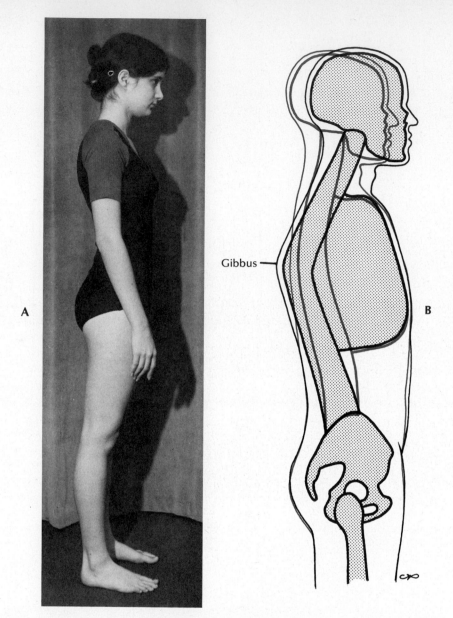

Gibbus

Fig. 22-11. A, Normal curvature of the spine. **B,** Deformity of the spine. Kyphosis is flexion of the spine. When the angle of the defect is sharp, the apex is called a gibbus. Red outline figure shows the normal position; black, the deformity.

cage occurs as well. The ribs protrude posteriorly on the convex side of the spine. A hump or "razor back" may be observed. The protrusion may be made more obvious by asking the client to bend over to touch his toes. The deformity is best observed from behind (Fig. 22-10).

Kyphosis is a flexion deformity (Fig. 22-11, *B*). When the angle of the defect is sharp, the apex is called a gibbus.

Lordosis (swayback) is an extension deviation of the spine commonly found in the lumbar area (Fig. 22-12).

Measurement of the extremities

The musculoskeletal examination frequently includes the measurement of the extremities for length and circumference. Measurements of length are made when there is a question of symmetry between two limbs or when the limbs are in normal range for length. The measurements are made with the client lying relaxed on a hard surface (examining table) with the pelvis level and the hips and knees fully extended and with both hips equally adducted. Frequently, apparent discrepancies in limb size are due to position.

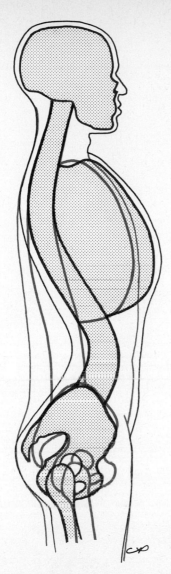

Fig. 22-12. Deformity of the spine. Lordosis (swayback) is extension of the spine. It is most commonly found in the lumbar area. Red outline figure shows the normal position; black, the deformity.

The length of the upper extremity is the distance from the tip of the acromion process to the tip of the middle finger; the shoulder is adducted and the other joints are at neutral zero (anatomical position—limb in extension). The length of the lower extremity is the distance from the lower edge of the anterosuperior iliac spine to the tibial malleolus (Table 22-1).

Measurement of muscle mass

The muscles are examined for gross hypertrophy or atrophy. Only in the markedly obese client are changes in muscle mass difficult to assess. The difference in the firm, hypertrophic muscle of the athlete and the limp, atrophic muscle of the paralytic are obvious both on inspection and to the palpating

Table 22-1. Anatomical guideposts for measuring extremities

Area	From	To
Entire upper extremity	Tip of acromion process	Tip of middle finger
Upper arm	Tip of acromion process	Tip of olecranon process
Forearm	Tip of olecranon process	Styloid process of ulna
Entire lower extremity	Lower edge of anterosuperior iliac spine	Tibial malleolus
Thigh	Lower edge of anterosuperior iliac spine	Medial aspect of knee joint
Lower leg	Medial aspect of knee	Tibial malleolus

finger. Although muscle size is largely a function of the use or disuse of the muscle fibers, changes in the size of muscles may be indicative of disease. Malnutrition and lipodystrophy tend to reduce muscle size as well as markedly weaken the strength of contraction. Lack of neural input due to lesions of the spinal cord or peripheral motor neuron may lead to a reduction in muscle size of as much as 75% of the normal volume; this may occur over as short a time as 3 months. Measurements taken of limbs at their maximum circumference may provide a baseline for comparison when swelling or atrophy are suspected or in subsequent routine examination. The limbs should be in the same position and the muscles in the same state of tension each time measurements are performed. Several corresponding points may be measured above and below the patella and olecranon process. Some clinics routinely measure at 10 cm below and at points 10 and 20 cm above the midpatella in order to provide uniformity. At any rate, a small diagram showing the points measured (Fig. 22-13) will obviate ambiguity. Differences in symmetry or of limb size at different times of less than 1 cm are not significant (Fig. 22-14).

PALPATION

Palpation is utilized in the examination of the musculoskeletal system to detect swelling, localized temperature changes, and marked changes in shape.

The consistency of the muscle on palpation is noted.

Muscle tone or tonus is the tension that is present in the resting muscle. This is the slight resistance that is felt when the relaxed limb is passively moved.

While palpating the muscle, the examiner should be alert to fasciculations, which are involuntary contractions or twitchings of groups of muscle fibers.

The client should be requested to tell the examiner

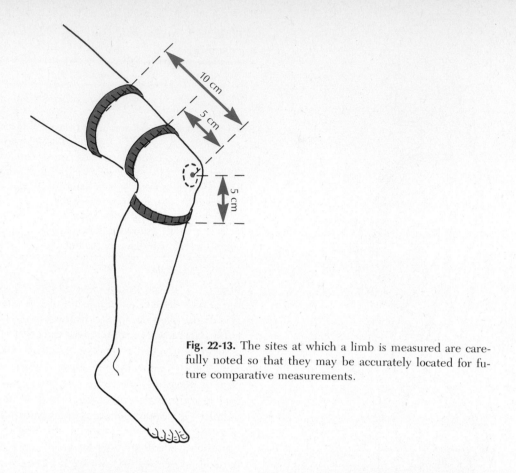

Fig. 22-13. The sites at which a limb is measured are carefully noted so that they may be accurately located for future comparative measurements.

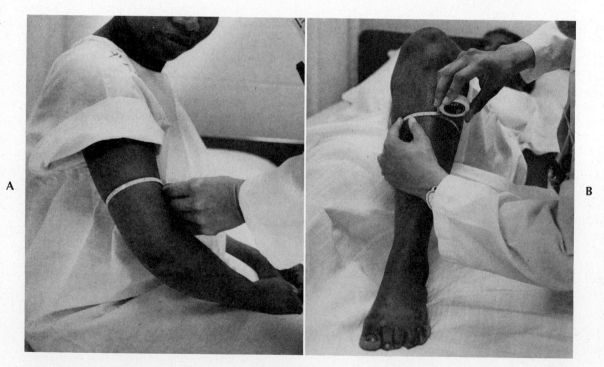

Fig. 22-14. A, Measurement of upper midarm circumference. **B,** Measurement of midgastrocnemius circumference.

of any sensation he has while the muscles and tendons are being felt. The client's descriptions of pain or tenderness on palpation are recorded.

Tendon stretch reflexes, described in Chapter 21 on neurological assessment, are generally altered in muscle disease, especially if the peripheral nerves are involved. For instance, the tendon reflexes are diminished in muscular dystrophy and polymyositis in proportion to the loss of muscle strength. A lengthened reflex cycle is characteristic of hypothyroidism, whereas a shortened period is indicative of the hypermetabolic state.

TESTING OF MUSCULOSKELETAL FUNCTION

Muscle strength is assessed throughout the full range of motion for each muscle or group of muscles. The usual method of testing is manual and subjective. Resistance is applied to the muscles; the client is placed in the position that best allows movement through the full range. The muscle contractions are graded according to the examiner's judgment of the client's responses.

The following criteria for recording the grading of muscle strength has been frequently used:

Functional level	Lovett scale	Grade	Percentage of normal
No evidence of contractility	Zero (0)	0	0
Evidence of slight contractility	Trace (T)	1	10
Complete range of motion with gravity eliminated	Poor (P)	2	25
Complete range of motion with gravity	Fair (F)	3	50
Complete range of motion against gravity with some resistance	Good (G)	4	75
Complete range of motion against gravity with full resistance	Normal (N)	5	100

Some examiners prefer simple descriptive words, such as *paralysis*, *severe weakness*, *moderate weakness*, *minimal weakness*, and *normal*. Disability is considered to exist if the muscle strength is less than grade 3; external support may be required to make the involved part functional, and activity of the part cannot be achieved in a gravity field.

There is an expectation that muscle strength will be greater in the dominant arm and leg. Movements should be coordinated and painless.

Screening test for muscle strength

Although muscle weakness in adults is generally mild and transitory, it may be the outcome of musculoskeletal, neurological, metabolic, or infectious problems. Therefore, an evaluation is necessary. A simple screening test has been suggested that can be performed in less than 5 minutes and allows the examiner to find nearly any muscle or reflex abnormality. The test allows for a systematic testing of muscle groups from head to toe. As he walks into the examining room and undresses, the client is carefully observed for cues to neurological and motion deficit. He is carefully observed to ascertain that the chief complaint is verifiable by physical evidence. The following procedure may then be used:

1. The examiner assesses the ocular musculature by asking the client to close his eyes tightly as the examiner attempts to open the lids. The client is instructed to look up, down, right, and left as the examiner checks for lid lag and appropriate tracking of the eyes.
2. The examiner assesses the facial musculature by asking the client to blow out his cheeks while the examiner assesses the pressure against the fingers held against the resultant cheek bulge. The client is then asked to put his tongue into the cheek, and the tension created in this bulge is tested. The client is then asked to stick out his tongue and to move it to the right and left.
3. The examiner assesses the neck musculature by asking the client to extend his head backward while standing erect as the examiner attempts to break the extension (Fig. 22-15). The client is then asked to bend his chin toward his chest forcefully as far as he is able while the examiner attempts to bend the chin upward.
4. The examiner tests the deltoid muscles by asking the client to hold his arms upward while the examiner tries to push them down. The client is asked to extend his arms while the examiner attempts to press them down.
5. The examiner tests the biceps by asking the client to fully extend his arms and then to try to flex them while the examiner attempts to pull them into extension (Fig. 22-16).
6. The examiner tests the triceps by asking the client to flex his arms and then to extend them while the examiner attempts to push them into a flexed position (Fig. 22-17).
7. The examiner assesses the wrist and finger musculature by asking the client to extend his hand and then to try to resist the examiner with the hand up, alternately with the fingers out or together, in an attempt to flex the wrist (Fig. 22-18). The handshake provides a measure of the strength of the grasp (Fig. 22-19).

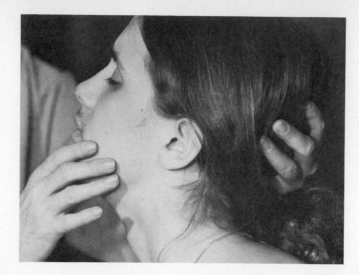

Fig. 22-15. Assessment of the neck musculature. The client flexes his head backward while the examiner attempts to break the extension.

Fig. 22-16. Assessment of biceps strength. The client flexes his arm while the examiner attempts to pull the arm into extension.

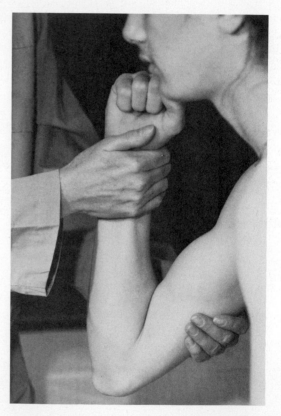

Finger strength may be assessed by trying to move the fingers together as the client attempts to spread them (Fig. 22-20).

8. The examiner assesses hip strength by asking the client to assume the supine position and then to raise the extended leg while the examiner attempts to hold it down.

9. The examiner assesses the hamstring, gluteal, abductor, and adductor muscles of the leg by asking the client to sit and perform alternate leg crossing (Fig. 22-21).

10. The examiner assesses quadriceps muscle

strength by asking the client to extend the leg stiffly as the examiner tries to bend it (Fig. 22-22).

11. The examiner assesses the hamstring muscles by asking the client to bend his knees as the examiner tries to straighten them (Fig. 22-23).

12. The examiner assesses the ankle and foot musculature by asking the client to exert upward foot pressure and then big toe pressure against the examiner's hands.

13. The client is asked to walk naturally for a short distance in order to observe gait (if the exam-

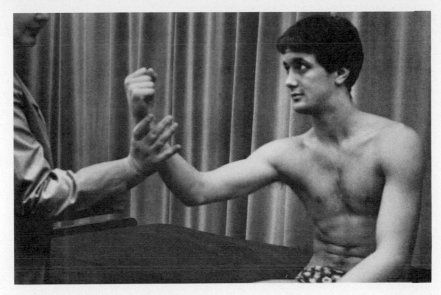

Fig. 22-17. Assessment of triceps strength. The client attempts to extend his arm while the examiner attempts to push the arm into a flexed position.

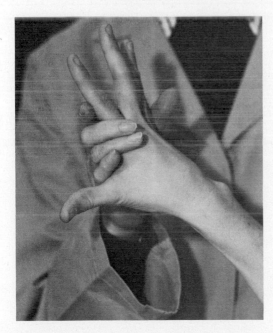

Fig. 22-18. Assessment of wrist strength. The client pushes against the examiner's hand in an attempt to flex the wrist.

iner has not already done so). Then the client is asked to take a few steps on his toes and a few steps on his heels.

Muscle fasciculations are checked for in the face, neck, torso, and extremities. A sharp tap to the muscle mass may induce this visible twitching.

Screening assessment of neurological adequacy

Neurological adequacy can be assessed by examining the pupillary reflex and the fundus. Pyramidal tract function is evaluated through the use of deep tendon reflex tests, including Babinski's sign.

Cerebellar tract function may be elicited by asking the client to stand erect with his eyes closed and then checking Romberg's sign. The client is then asked to touch his finger to his nose and to rapidly rotate his hands inward and outward. Sensory perception is assessed by checking for pain, vibration, and temperature responses. (Neural function tests are described in Chapter 23 on neurological assessment.) The screening test is the only one performed unless the examiner suspects a musculoskeletal problem. A more extensive discussion of range of motion and joint examination, which may be helpful in a more inclusive examination, follows.

Measurement of the range of joint motion

A standardized method for measuring and recording joint motion has been published by the American Academy of Orthopaedic Surgeons (1965). The range of motion is described in degrees of deviation from a defined neutral zero point for each joint. The position of neutral zero is that of the extended extremity or anatomical position.

Goniometry and arthrometry are the terms used to describe the measurement of joint motion. The practitioner should learn to use the goniometer to measure the range of motion and to communicate the findings to other health team professionals.

The two arms of the goniometer are a protractor and a pointer that are joined at the zero point of the protractor (Fig. 22-5). The hinge should provide sufficient friction that the instrument remains in position when picked up for reading after being set

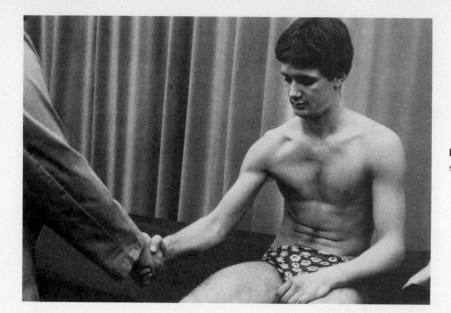

Fig. 22-19. The handshake provides a measure of the strength of the hand grasp.

Fig. 22-20. Finger strength is assessed as the examiner resists the client's attempts to spread them.

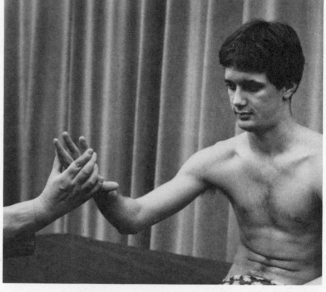

against the joint. The scale should be easily read from a distance of 18 inches. Some goniometers have full-circle scales, whereas others have half-circle scales. The length of the arms is generally about 6 inches so that it can be easily carried.

Motion is described as active when the client moves the joint and passive when the examiner provides the motion. Active joint motion that is smooth and painless through its complete range generally indicates the absence of any advanced lesion.

Active motion. Less muscle tension and joint compression are produced by the voluntary movement of the joints through their range of motion than when the joints are moved against resistance as in the

strength tests. Therefore, the range of active motion should be assessed before muscle strength since the more marked contraction may induce pain in the client, which may skew the test results.

Should the range of active motion of a given joint be less than the range of passive motion, further investigation should focus on true weakness, joint stability, pain, malingering, or hysterical weakness as possible causes.

Passive motion. The examiner moves the relaxed joint through the limits of its movement. When the range of motion is limited, the examiner explores further to determine whether there (1) is an excess of fluid within the joint, (2) are loose bodies in the joint,

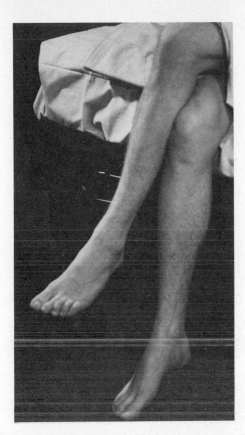

Fig. 22-21. Alternate leg crossing for assessment of hamstring, gluteal, abductor, and adductor muscle strength.

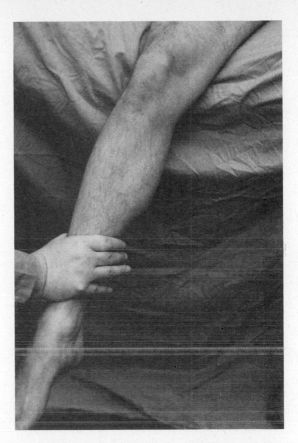

Fig. 22-22. Assessment of quadriceps muscle strength. The client attempts to straighten the leg while the examiner attempts to flex it.

or (3) is joint surface irregularity or contracture of the muscles, ligaments, or capsule. Moving the joint through the range of its motion may also reveal hyper mobility of the joint. In this case, further examination is directed toward differentiating among (1) a connective tissue disruption such as the relaxation of the ligaments that occurs in Marfan's syndrome, (2) a ligamentous tear, and (3) an intraarticular fracture. An example of how this information might aid in diagnosis would be seen in a joint that could be flexed to a smaller angle with passive movement than with active flexion. Such a finding would probably indicate a problem related to the musculature rather than a problem within the joint causing a block in the flexion.

Testing by functional group

The movement of the neck and the trunk are examined in functional groups in order to determine muscle strength and the range of joint motion. The full range of motion is not assessed as part of the screening examination unless the history or other parts of the physical examination indicate that muscular or neural dysfunction is a possible problem for the client.

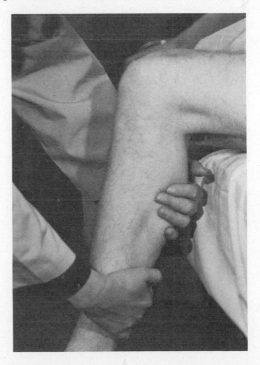

Fig. 22-23. Assessment of hamstring muscle strength. The client flexes his knees while the examiner tries to straighten them.

Text continued on p. 496.

Table 22-2. Testing for muscle strength and range of joint motion

NECK

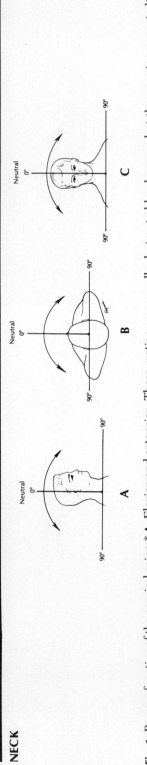

Fig. 1. Range of motion of the cervical spine.* **A,** Flexion and extension. These motions are usually designated by degrees, but the examiner may indicate the distance the chin lacks from touching the chest. **B.** Rotation. This is estimated in degrees from the neutral position or in percentages of motion, as compared to individuals of similar age and physical build. **C,** Lateral bend. This motion is also measured in degrees but can be indicated by the number of inches the ear lacks from reaching the shoulder.

Movement	Muscles	Motor nerves	Positions for testing	Instructions and tests for muscle strength

Flexion	Prime mover: sternocleido-mastoid (Fig. 2†)
	
	Accessory muscles
	  Scalenus anterior
	  Scalenus medius
	  Scalenus posterior
	  Rectus capitis anterior
	  Longus capitis
	  Longus colli
	  Infrahyoid group
		Spinal accessory nerve (cranial XI)
		Cervical 2, 3
			Standing, sitting, supine	"Bend your head to touch your chin to your chest." Resistance is applied to the forehead. Pressure is exerted over the tip of the xiphoid process to obviate the tendency to contract the abdominal muscles to raise the chest (Fig. 3).

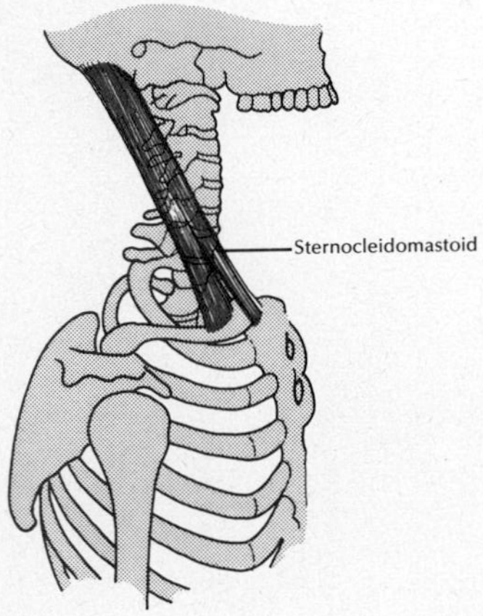

Fig. 3

Sternocleidomastoid

Fig. 2

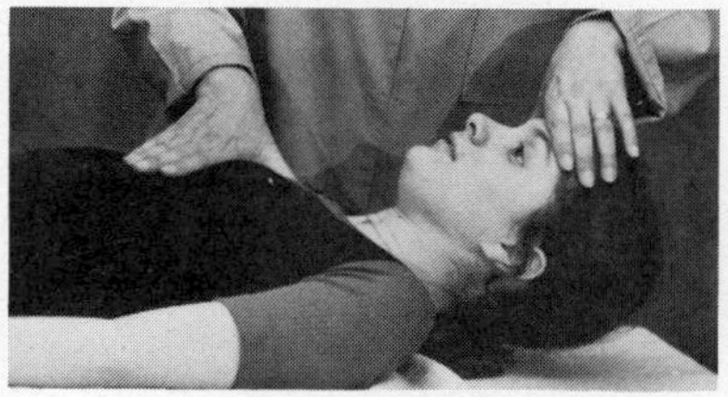

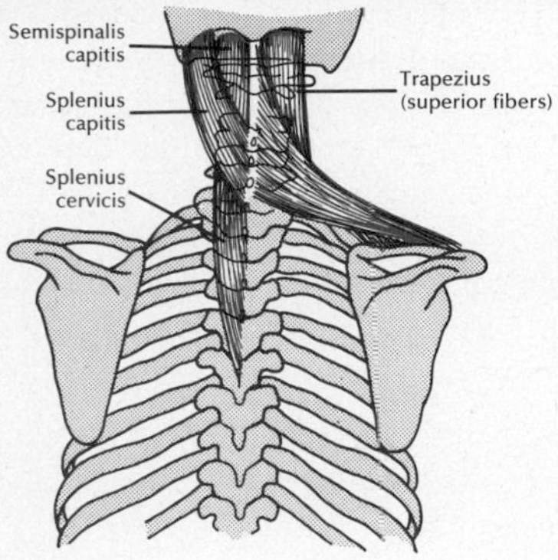

Fig. 4

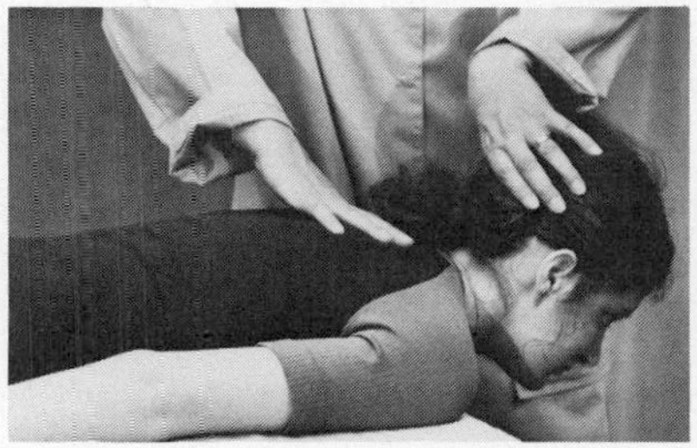

Labels: Trapezius (superior fibers); Semispinalis capitis; Splenius capitis; Splenius cervicis

Fig. 5

Motion	Position	Instructions	Prime movers	Nerves
Extension	Standing, sitting, prone	"Bend your head back as far as possible." "Lift your head up as far as you can." Resistance is applied to the occipital prominence (Fig. 5).	Prime movers (Fig. 4†) Trapezius (superior fibers)	Spinal accessory nerve (cranial XI) Cervical 3, 4
			Semispinalis capitis	Dorsal rami of spinal nerves
			Semispinalis cervicis	Dorsal rami of spinal nerves
			Splenius capitis	Dorsal rami of middle and lower cervical nerves
			Splenius cervicis	Dorsal rami of middle and lower cervical nerves
			Spinalis capitis	Adjacent spinal nerves
			Spinalis cervicis	Adjacent spinal nerves
			Longissimus capitis	Adjacent spinal nerves
			Longissimus cervicis	Adjacent spinal nerves
			Accessory muscles Levator scapulae Multifidi Obliquus capitis Rectus capitis posterior	
Rotation				
Anterolateral	Standing, sitting, supine	"Bend your head forward and turn your head as far as you can to the right [left]." "Bend your head so that your ear is close to your chest." Resistance is applied to the right (left) temple.	Prime mover: sternocleido-mastoid (Fig. 2)	Spinal accessory nerve (cranial XI) Cervical 2, 3
			Accessory muscles Scalenus anterior Scalenus medius Scalenus posterior Rectus capitis anterior Longus capitis Longus colli Infrahyoid group	
Posterolateral	Standing, sitting, prone	"Bend your head back and turn your head to the right [left]." Resistance is applied to the right (left) occiput.	Prime movers (Fig. 4) Trapezius (superior fibers)	Spinal accessory nerve (cranial XI) Cervical 3, 4
			Semispinalis capitis	Dorsal rami of spinal nerves
			Semispinalis cervicis	Dorsal rami of spinal nerves
			Splenius capitis	Dorsal rami of middle and lower cranial nerves

Continued.

*From Joint motion; method of measuring and recording, Chicago, 1965. American Academy of Orthopaedic Surgeons.
†Adapted from Daniels, L., and Worthingham, C.: Muscle testing; techniques of manual examination, ed. 3, Philadelphia, 1972, W. B. Saunders Co.
‡From Francis, C. C., and Farrell, G. L.: Integrated anatomy and physiology, St. Louis, 1957, The C. V. Mosby Co.
§From Anthony, C. P., and Kolthoff, N. J.: Textbook of anatomy and physiology, ed. 9, St. Louis, 1975, The C. V. Mosby Co.
‖From Mann, R. A.: DuVries' surgery of the foot, ed. 4, St. Louis, 1978, The C. V. Mosby Co.

Table 22-2. Testing for muscle strength and range of joint motion—cont'd

Movement	Muscles	Motor nerves	Positions for testing	Instructions and tests for muscle strength
Posterolateral—cont'd	Splenius cervicis	Dorsal rami of middle and lower cranial nerves		
	Spinalis capitis	Adjacent spinal nerves		
	Spinalis cervicis	Adjacent spinal nerves		
	Longissimus capitis	Adjacent spinal nerves		
	Longissimus cervicis	Adjacent spinal nerves		
	Accessory muscles			
	Levator scapulae			
	Multifidi			
	Obliquus capitis			
	Rectus capitis posterior			
Lateral bend	Prime mover: sternocleido-mastoid (Fig. 2)	Spinal accessory nerve (cranial XI) Cervical 2, 3	Standing, sitting, supine	"Bend your head so that your right [left] ear touches your shoulder. Don't bring your shoulder up to meet your ear." Resistance is applied to the right (left) temporal bone.
	Accessory muscles			
	Scalenus anterior			
	Scalenus medius			
	Scalenus posterior			
	Rectus capitis anterior			
	Longus capitis			
	Longus colli			
	Infrahyoid group			

TRUNK

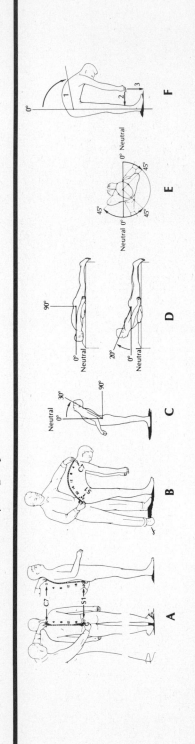

A B C D E F

Fig. 6. Range of motion of the spine. * **A** and **B**, Steel tape measure method. This is perhaps the most accurate clinical method of measuring true motion of the spine in flexion. The flexible steel or plastic tape adjusts very accurately to the thoracic and lumbar contours of the spine. **A,** With the client standing, the 1-inch marker of the tape is held over the spinous process C7 and the distal tape over the spinous process S1. **B,** As the client bends forward, if the lumbar curve reverses and the spinous processes spread, this will be indicated by lengthening of the measured distance from C7 to S1. In the normal healthy adult there is an average increase of 4 inches in forward flexion. If the client bends forward with his back straight (as in rheumatoid spondylitis), the tape will not record motion. The examiner can record motion of the thoracic spine per se by measuring from the spinous process C7 to the spinous process T12. Likewise, motion of the lumbar spine can be measured from T12 to S1. Usually, if the total spine lengthening in flexion is 4 inches, the examiner will find that 1 inch occurs in the dorsal spine and 3 inches occur in the lumbar spine. **C,** Client standing (extension). **D,** Client lying prone (extension). **E,** Rotation of spine. **F,** Client bending forward (flexion). *1,* Degrees of inclination of trunk (note reversal of lumbar curve); *2,* level of fingertips to leg; *3,* distance between fingertips and floor.

Movement	Muscles	Motor nerves	Positions for testing	Instructions and tests for muscle strength
Flexion	Prime mover: rectus abdominis (Fig. 7) Accessory muscles Obliquus internus abdominis Obliquus externus abdominis	Intercostal nerves (thoracic 6-12, lumbar 1)	Standing Supine (knees not bent)	"Bend over; touch your toes" (Fig. 8). "Try to sit up without using your hands." Legs are stabilized (Fig. 9). Two important signs may be elicited in assessing abdominal muscle strength: 1. Beevor's sign, upward movement of the umbilicus on contraction of the abdominal muscles, is associated with comparative weakness of the lower abdominal muscles in relation to the upper abdominal muscles. 2. Hyperextension of the lumbar spine when the client tries to rise to a sitting position occurs when strong hip flexors are contracted in the presence of weak abdominal muscles.

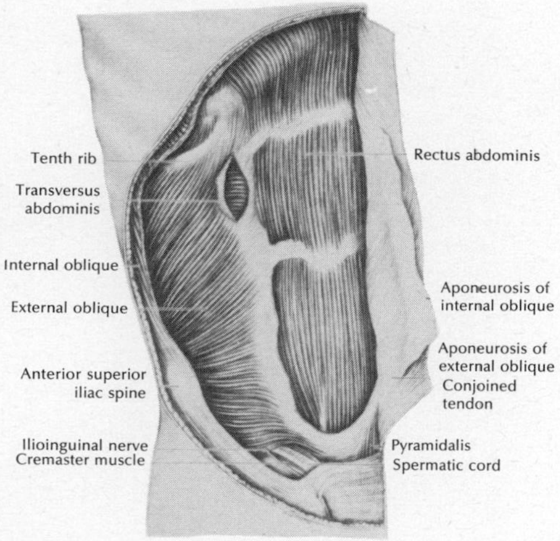

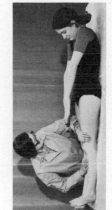

Fig. 7

Labels: Tenth rib, Transversus abdominis, Internal oblique, External oblique, Anterior superior iliac spine, Ilioinguinal nerve, Cremaster muscle, Rectus abdominis, Aponeurosis of internal oblique, Aponeurosis of external oblique, Conjoined tendon, Pyramidalis, Spermatic cord

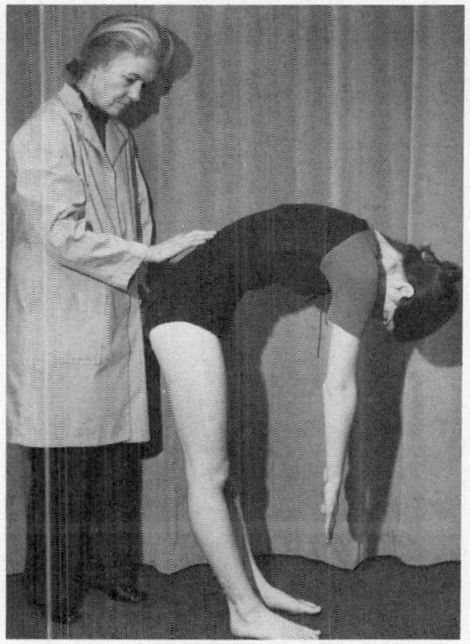

Fig. 8

Fig. 9

Continued.

Table 22-2. Testing for muscle strength and range of joint motion—cont'd

Movement	Muscles	Motor nerves	Positions for testing	Instructions and tests for muscle strength
Extension	Prime movers (Fig. 10†) Longissimus thoracis Iliocostalis thoracis Spinalis thoracis Iliocostalis lumborum Quadratus lumborum Accessory muscles Rotators Multifidi Semispinalis	Adjacent spinal nerves Adjacent spinal nerves Adjacent spinal nerves Adjacent spinal nerves Thoracic 12, lumbar 1	Standing Prone	"Bend your head and shoulders back as far as you can." "Lift your head and shoulders up from the table without using your hands." Pelvis is stabilized. Resistance is applied between the scapulae (Fig. 11).
Rotation	Prime movers (Fig. 12†) Obliquus externus abdominis Obliquus internus abdominis Accessory muscles Rectus abdominis Latissimus dorsi Semispinalis Multifidi Rotators	Intercostal nerves (thoracic 8-12) Intercostal nerves (thoracic 8-12)	Sitting (hips flexed) Supine (hands behind head, legs stabilized)	"Twist your right [left] shoulder to the opposite knee." "Turn your right [left] shoulder to the opposite knee" (Fig. 13). Resistance may be applied against the right (left) anterior shoulder.

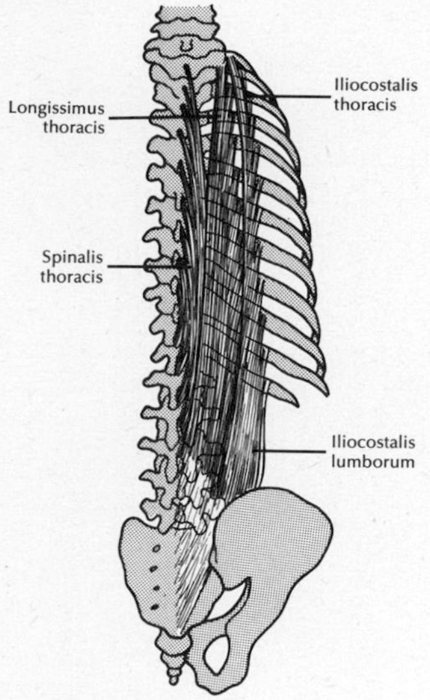

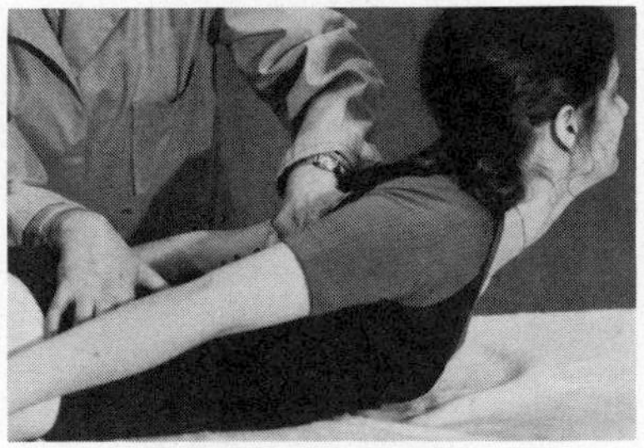

Fig. 11

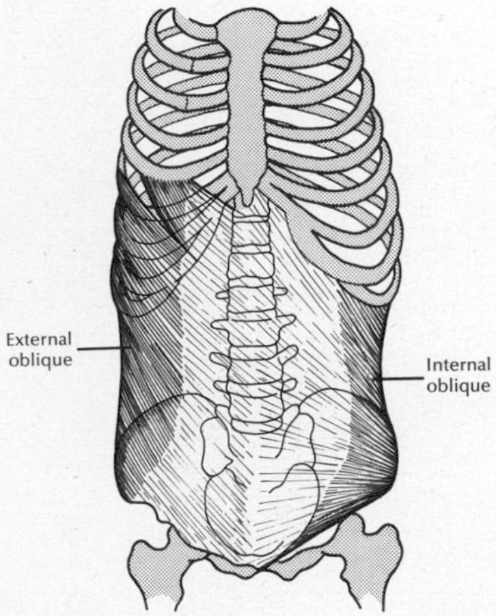

Fig. 13

Iliocostalis thoracis

Iliocostalis lumborum

Longissimus thoracis

Spinalis thoracis

Fig. 10

Internal oblique

External oblique

Fig. 12

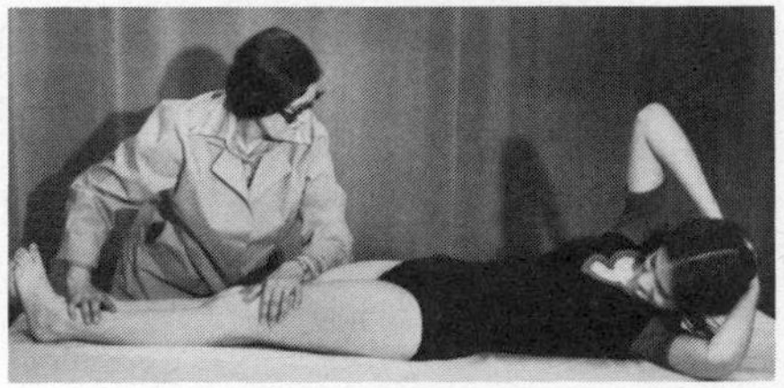

Elevation

Prime movers (Fig. 14f)
Quadratus lumborum
Iliocostalis lumborum
Accessory muscles
   Obliquus internus abdominis
   Obliquus externus abdominis
   Latissimus dorsi
   Abductor muscles of hip

Fig. 14

Thoracic 12; lumbar 1, 2
Adjacent spinal nerves

Supine (legs together)

"Try to lift your right [left] hip toward your shoulder." Resistance is applied by the examiner holding the ankle (Fig. 15).

Fig. 15

Standing

"Thrust your right [left] hip forward and up."

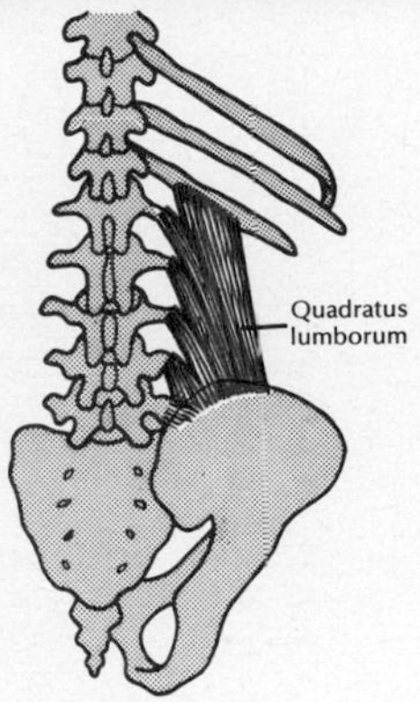

SHOULDER

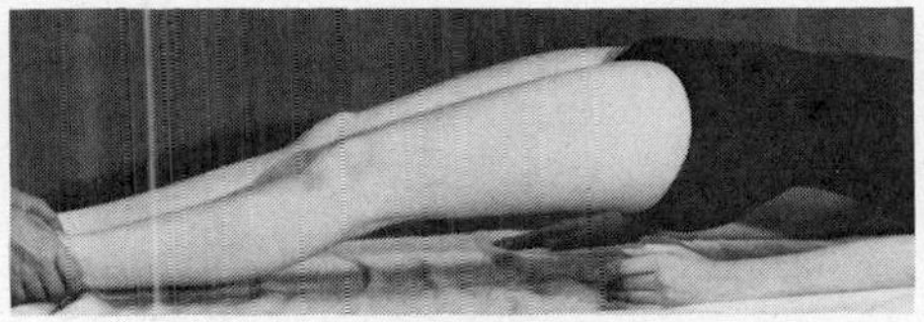

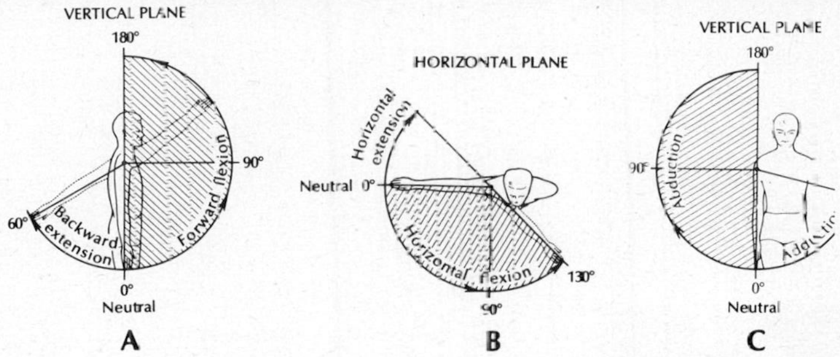

Fig. 16. Range of motion of the arm at the shoulder.* **A,** Forward flexion (or forward elevation) and backward extension. *Forward flexion* is the forward upward motion of the arm in the anterior saggital plane of the body from zero to 180 degrees. The opposite motion to the zero position may be termed "depression" of the arm. *Backward extension* is the upward motion of the arm in the posterior saggital plane of the body from zero to approximately 60 degrees. **B,** Horizontal flexion and horizontal extension. *Horizontal flexion* is the motion of the arm in the horizontal plane anterior to the coronal plane across the body. This motion is measured from zero to approximately 130 or 135 degrees. *Horizontal extension* is the horizontal motion of the arm in the horizontal plane posterior to the coronal plane of the body. **C,** Abduction and adduction. *Abduction* is the upward motion of the arm away from the side of the body in the corneal plane from zero to 180 degrees. *Adduction* is the opposite motion of the arm toward the midline of the body or beyond it in an upward plane.

Continued.

Table 22-2. Testing for muscle strength and range of joint motion—cont'd

Movement	Muscles	Motor nerves	Positions for testing	Instructions and tests for muscle strength
Forward flexion	Prime movers (Fig. 17†) Deltoid (anterior fibers) Coracobrachialis Accessory muscles Deltoideus (middle fibers) Pectoralis major (clavicular fibers) Biceps brachii	Axillary nerve (cervical 5, 6) Musculocutaneous nerve (cervical 6, 7)	Standing, sitting, supine	"Move your arms forward and up." Resistance is applied at the level of the interior angle of the scapula on the upper side of the arm (Fig. 18).
Backward extension	Prime movers (Fig. 19†) Latissimus dorsi Teres major Deltoideus Accessory muscles Teres minor Triceps brachii (long head)	Thoracodorsal nerve (cervical 6, 7, 8) Lowest subscapular nerve (cervical 5, 6) Axillary nerve (cervical 5, 6)	Standing, sitting, prone	"Move your arms downward and back." "Clasp your arms behind your back." Resistance is applied to the posterior aspect of the arm proximal to the elbow (Fig. 20).

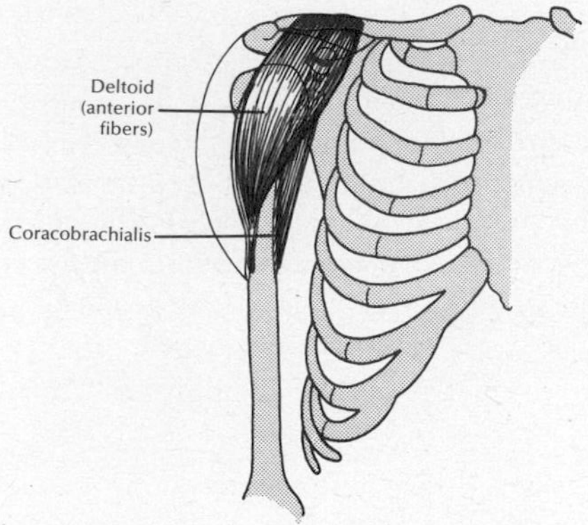

Deltoid (anterior fibers)

Coracobrachialis

Fig. 17

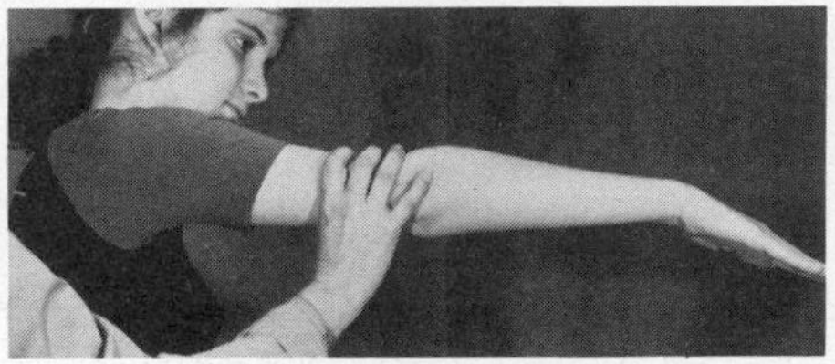

Fig. 18

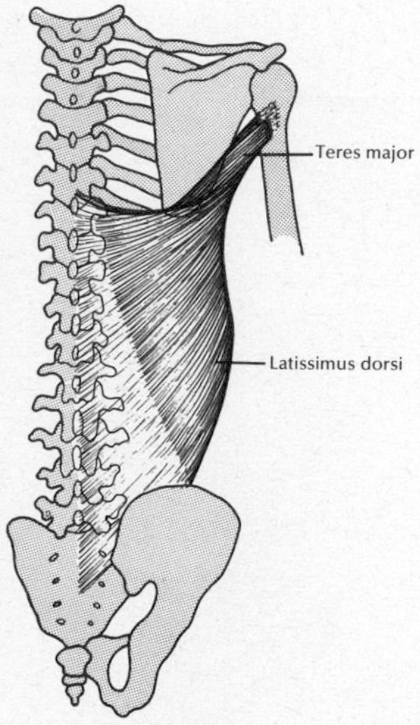

Teres major

Latissimus dorsi

Fig. 19

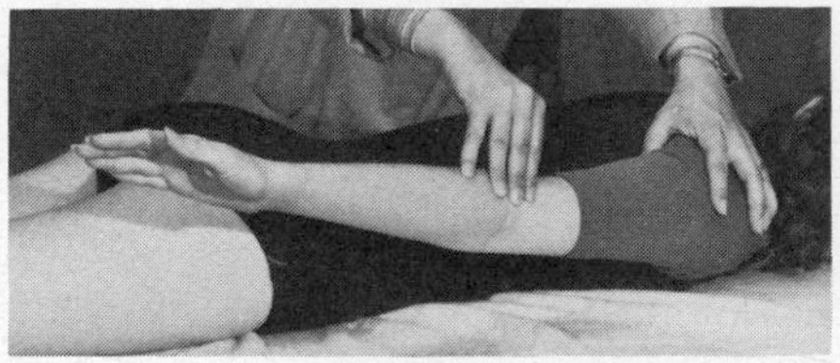

Fig. 20

Abduction

Prime movers (Fig. 21†)
Deltoideus (middle fibers)
Supraspinatus
Accessory muscles
Deltoideus (anterior and posterior fibers)
Serratus anterior

Axillary nerve (cervical 5, 6)
Suprascapular nerve (cervical 5)

Standing, sitting (scapula stabilized)

"Lift your arm straight out and to your side, away from your body."
Resistance is applied to the superior aspect of the arm proximal to the elbow (Fig. 22).

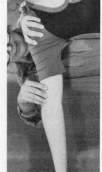
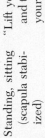

Fig. 21

Supraspinatus

Deltoid (middle fibers)

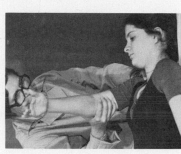

Fig. 22

Horizontal adduction

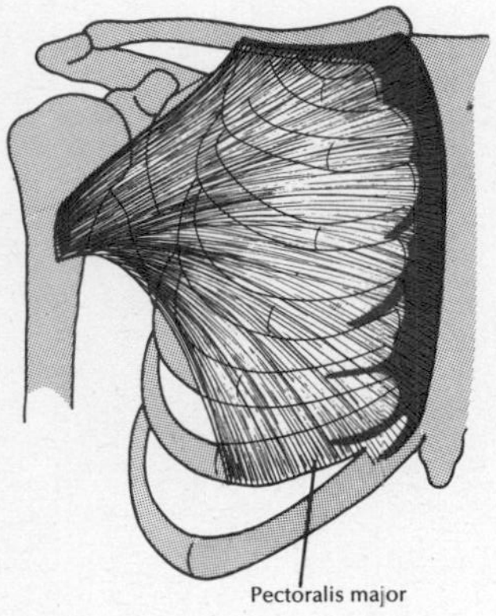

Prime mover: pectoralis major (Fig. 23†)

Accessory muscle: deltoid (anterior fibers)

Medial and internal pectoral nerves (cervical 5, 6, 7, 8; thoracic 1)

Standing, sitting, supine (arm abducted)

"Bring your straight arm over your chest."
Resistance is applied on the medial side of arm proximal to the elbow (Fig. 24).

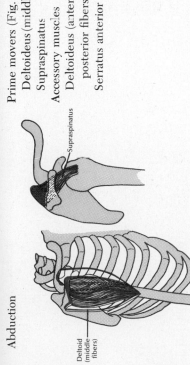

Pectoralis major

Fig. 23

Fig. 24

Continued.

Table 22-2. Testing for muscle strength and range of joint motion—cont'd

Movement	Muscles	Motor nerves	Positions for testing	Instructions and tests for muscle strength
Horizontal abduction	Prime mover: deltoideus (posterior fibers) (Fig. 25†) Accessory muscles Teres minor Infraspinatus	Axillary nerve (cervical 5, 6)	Standing, sitting, prone (scapula stabilized, arm adducted)	"Keeping your arm at shoulder height, move it backward as far as you can." Resistance is applied on the posterior surface of the arm proximal to the elbow (Fig. 26).

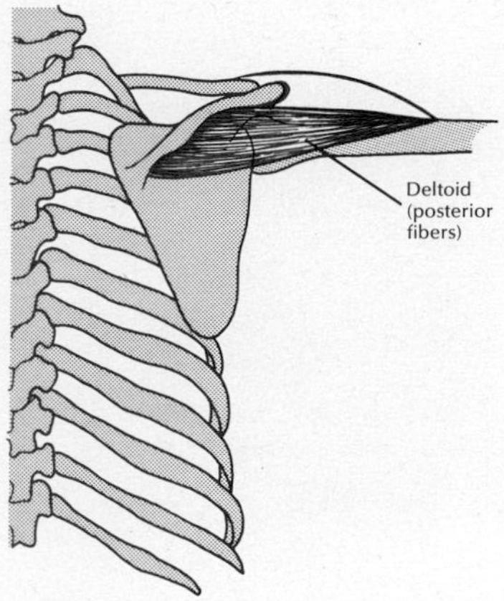

Fig. 26

Deltoid (posterior fibers)

Fig. 25

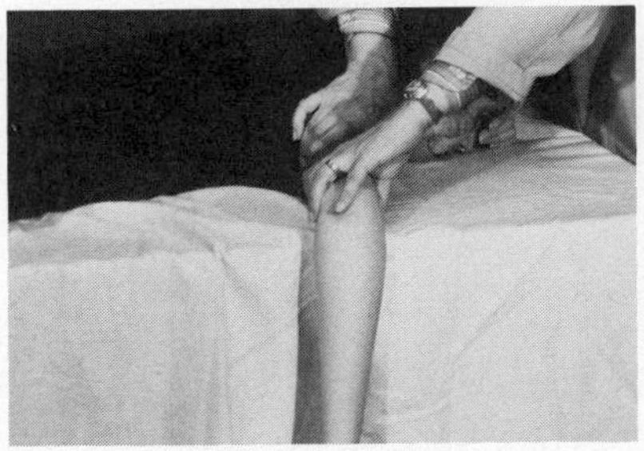

SHOULDER—cont'd

Neutral 0°

Inward rotation (internal)

Outward rotation (external)

90°

90°

A

Outward rotation (external)

0° Neutral

Inward rotation (internal)

90°

90°

B

C

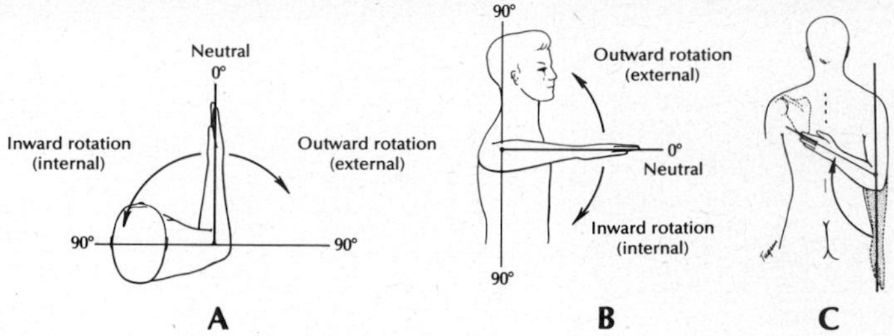

Fig. 27. Rotation of the shoulder.* **A,** Rotation with arm at side of body. Inward and outward rotation is recorded in degrees of motion from the neutral starting point. **B,** Rotation in abduction. Rotation in this position is less than with the arm at the side of the body. It is recorded in degrees of motion from the zero starting point. **C,** Internal rotation posteriorly. A clinical method of estimating function is the distance the fingertips reach in relation to the scapula or the base of the neck.

Movement	Muscles	Motor nerves	Positions for testing	Instructions and tests for muscle strength
Rotation **Internal**	Prime movers (Fig. 28†) Subscapularis	Upper and lower subscapular nerves (cervical 5, 6)	Standing, sitting, prone (scapula stabilized)	"Rotate your shoulder inward, swing your arm backward with your palm upward, and point your fingers toward the ceiling." Resistance is applied to the volar surface of the wrist (Fig. 29).
	Pectoralis major	Medial and lateral pectoral nerves (cervical 5, 6, 7, 8; thoracic 1)		
	Latissimus dorsi Teres major	Thoracodorsal nerve (cervical 6, 7, 8) Lowest subscapular nerve (cervical 5, 6)		
	Accessory muscle: deltoideus (anterior fibers)			
External	Prime movers (Fig. 30†) Infraspinatus	Suprascapular nerve (cervical 5, 6)	Standing, sitting, prone (scapula stabilized)	"Rotate your shoulder outward with your palm facing you posteriorly; bring your arm upward as if throwing a ball behind you." Resistance is applied to the dorsum of the wrist (Fig. 31).
	Teres minor	Axillary nerve (cervical 5)		
	Accessory muscle: deltoideus			

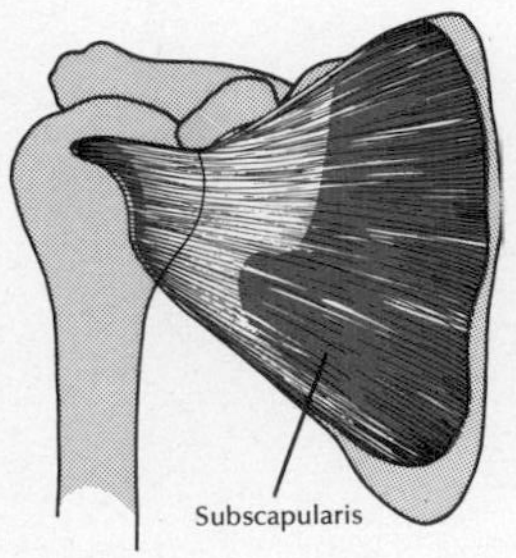

Subscapularis

Fig. 28

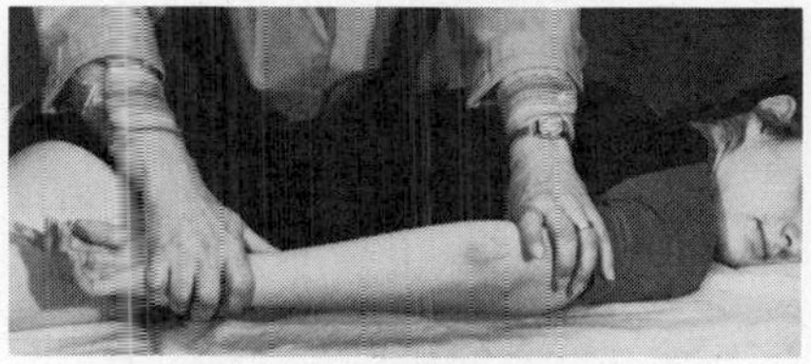

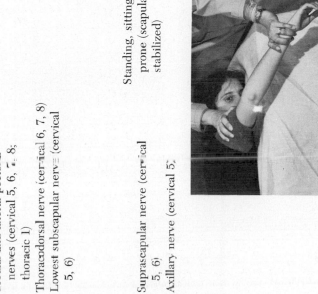

Fig. 29

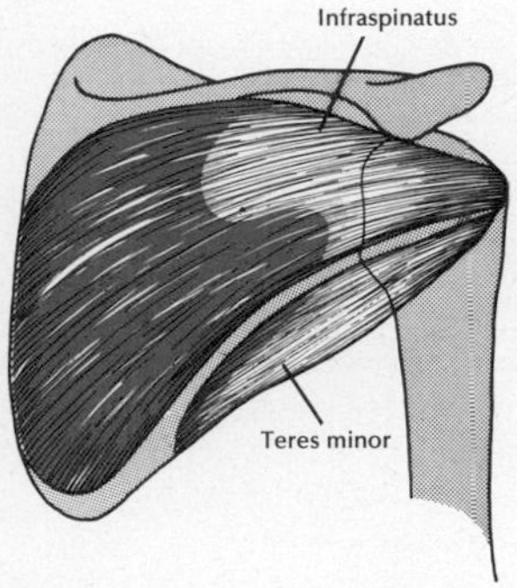

Infraspinatus

Teres minor

Fig. 30

Fig. 31

Continued.

Table 22-2. Testing for muscle strength and range of joint motion—cont'd

SHOULDER—cont'd

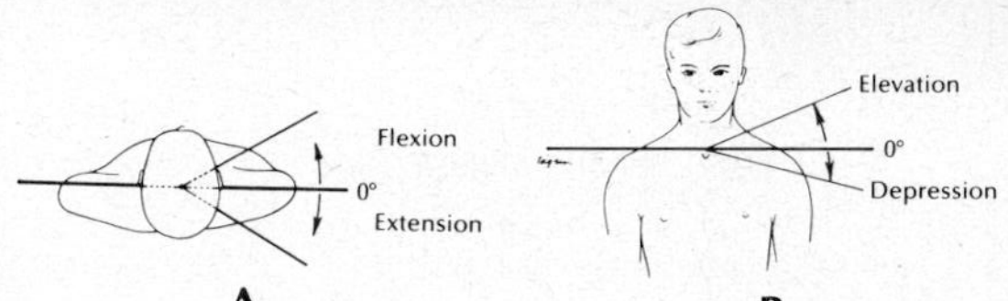

Fig. 32. Range of motion of the shoulder girdle.* **A,** Flexion and extension. Forward flexion and backward extension of the shoulder girdle are measured in degrees from the neutral starting position. This is primary motion of the scapula and the clavicle. **B,** Elevation and depression. Upward motion of the shoulder girdle in elevation is measured in degrees. The opposite downward motion may be described as "depression" of the shoulder. Rotatory motion in the shoulder girdle is possible but cannot be accurately measured. It can be estimated in percentage of motion as compared to individuals of similar age and physique.

Movement	Muscles	Motor nerves	Positions for testing	Instructions and tests for muscle strength
Scapular abduction and upward rotation	Prime mover: serratus anterior (Fig. 33†)	Long thoracic nerve (cervical 5, 6, 7)	Standing, sitting	"Push your arm upward and forward as if pushing open a door." Resistance is applied with a hand at the wrist and elbow, making pressure toward the chest (Fig. 34).

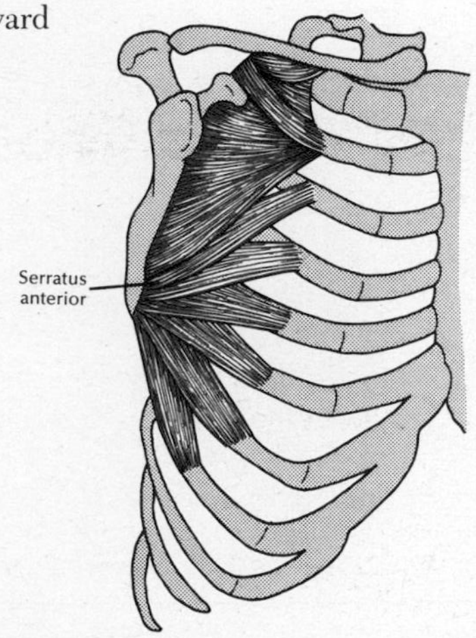

Fig. 33

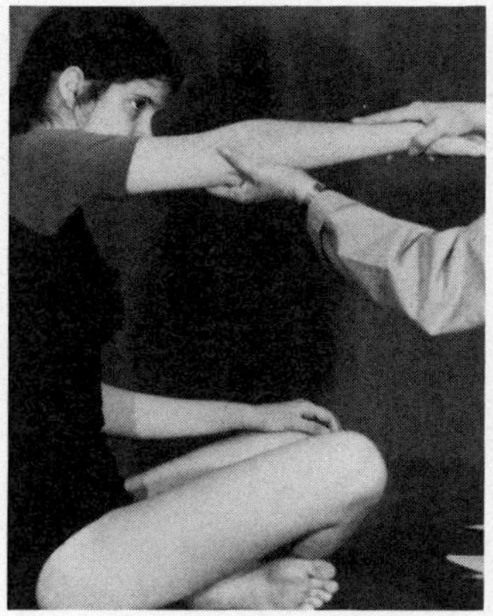

Fig. 34

Scapular adduction

Prime movers (Fig. 35†)
Trapezius (middle fibers)

Rhomboideus major

Rhomboideus minor

Accessory muscle: trapezius (upper and lower fibers)

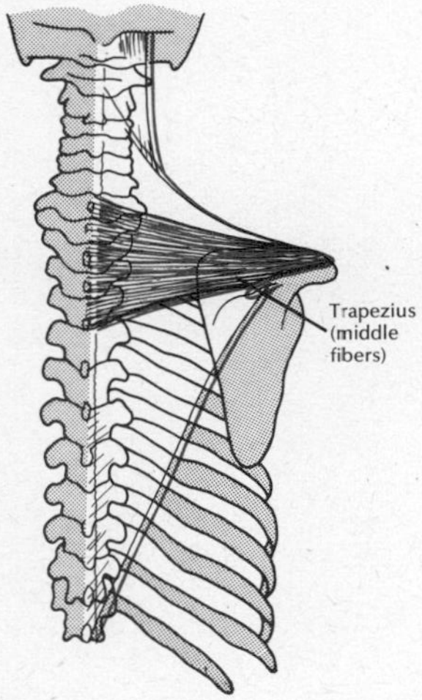

Spinal accessory nerve (cranial XI)
Cervical 3, 4
Dorsal scapular nerve (cervical 5)
Dorsal scapular nerve (cervical 5)

Standing, sitting, prone

"Try to bring you shoulder blades together in back."
Resistance is applied over the posterior shoulder (Fig. 36).

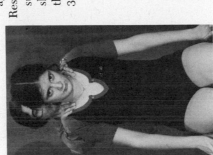

Fig. 36

Trapezius (middle fibers)

Fig. 35

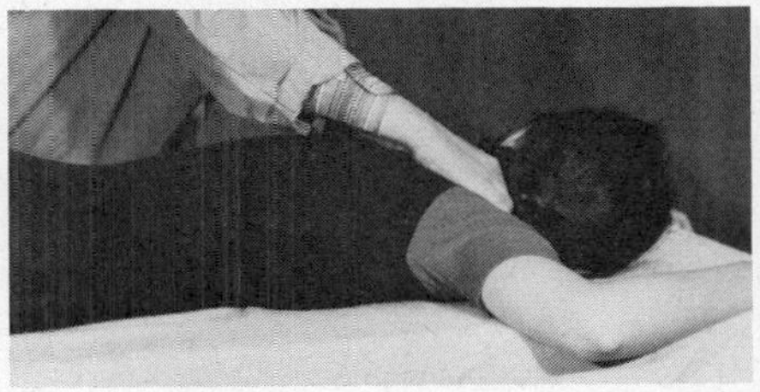

Scapular elevation

Prime movers (Fig. 37†)
Trapezius (superior fibers)
Levator scapulae
Accessory muscles
Rhomboideus major
Rhomboideus minor

Spinal accessory nerve (cranial XI)
Cervical 3, 4

Standing, sitting, lying

"Shrug your shoulders."
"Hunch your shoulders against my hand."
Resistance is applied to the superior aspect of the shoulder centered over the trapezius muscle (Fig. 38).

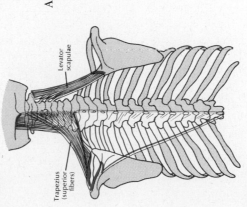

Fig. 38

Levator scapulae

Trapezius (superior fibers)

Fig. 37

Continued.

Table 22-2. Testing for muscle strength and range of joint motion—cont'd

Movement	Muscles	Motor nerve	Positions for testing	Instructions and tests for muscle strength
Scapular depression and adduction	Prime mover: trapezius (inferior fibers) (Fig. 39†)	Spinal accessory nerve (cranial XI) Cervical 3, 4	Standing, sitting, prone	"Lift your arm and bring your shoulder blade down and close against your back chest wall. Bring the shoulder blade down against the chest." Upward pressure is applied against the deltoid muscle (Fig. 40).
Adduction and downward rotation	Prime movers (Fig. 41†) Rhomboideus major Rhomboideus minor	Dorsal scapular nerve (cervical 5) Dorsal scapular nerve (cervical 5)	Standing, sitting, prone (arm adducted over back in medial rotation)	"Lift up your arm. Concentrate on your elbow." Resistance is applied over the scapula (Fig. 42).

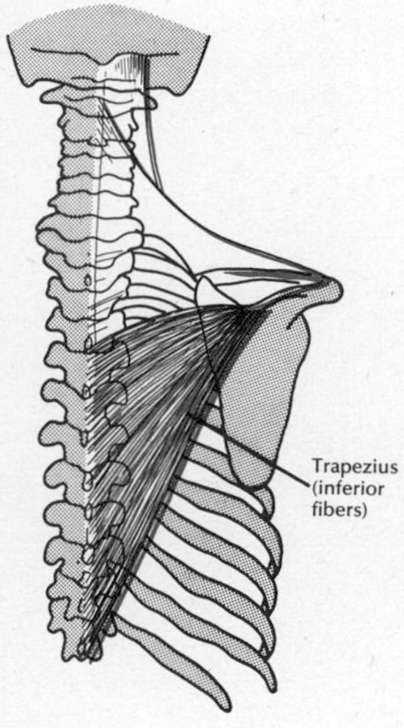

Fig. 39

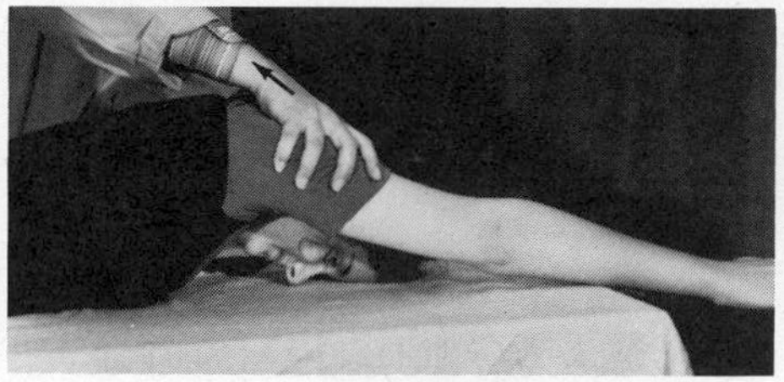

Fig. 40

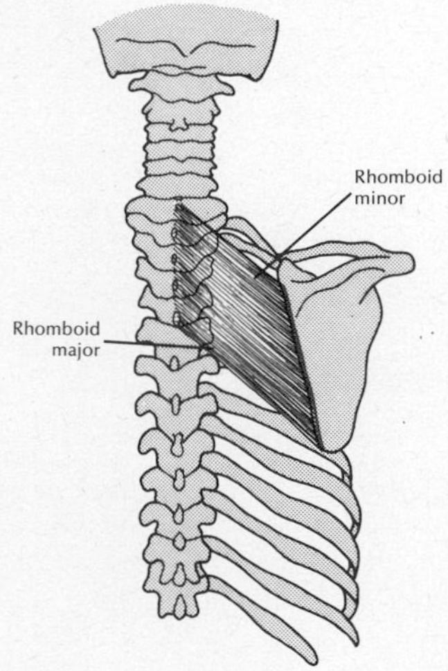

Fig. 41

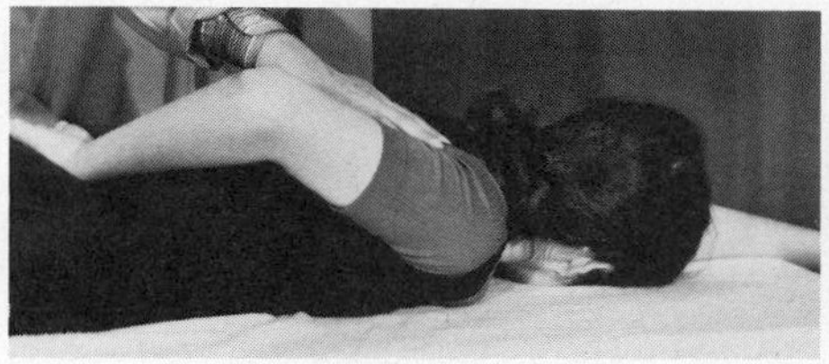

Fig. 42

ELBOW

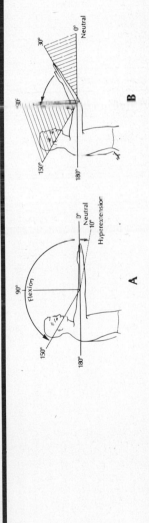

Fig. 43. Range of motion of the elbow.* **A,** Flexion and hyperextension. *Flexion:* zero to 150 degrees. *Extension:* 150 degrees to zero (from the angle of greatest flexion to the zero position). *Hyperextension:* measured in degrees beyond the zero starting point. This motion is not present in all individuals. When it is present, it may vary from 5 to 15 degrees. **B,** Measurement of limited motion. (The unshaded area indicates the range of limited motion.) Limited motion may be expressed in the following ways: (1) the elbow flexes from 30 to 90 degrees (30° → 90°); (2) the elbow has a flexion deformity of 30 degrees with further flexion to 90 degrees.

Movement	Muscles	Motor nerves	Positions for testing	Instructions and tests for muscle strength
Flexion	Prime movers (Fig. 44§) Biceps brachii	Musculocutaneous nerve (cervical 5, 6)	Standing, sitting, supine (arm extended)	"Move your right [left] hand to your right [left] shoulder."
	Brachialis	Musculocutaneous nerve (cervical 5, 6)		"Make a fist; try to bring your fist to your shoulder."
	Brachioradialis	Radial nerve (cervical 5, 6)		Resistance is applied to the lower arm (Fig. 45).
	Accessory muscles: flexor muscles of forearm			

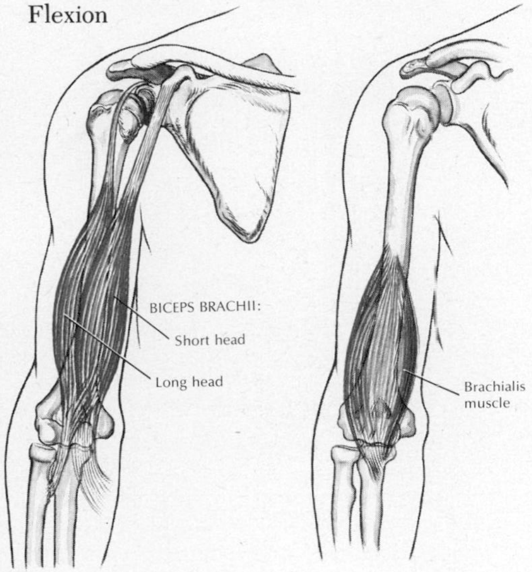

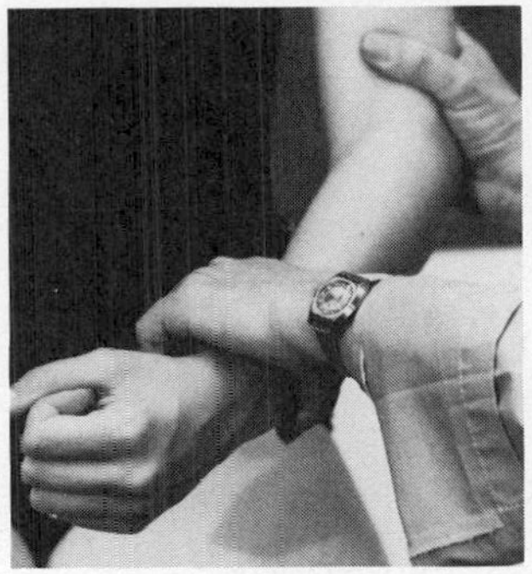

Fig. 45

Fig. 44

Continued.

Table 22-2. Testing for muscle strength and range of joint motion—cont'd

Movement	Muscles	Motor nerves	Positions for testing	Instructions and tests for muscle strength
Extension	Prime mover: triceps brachii (Fig. 46§) Accessory muscles Anconeus Extensor muscles of fore-arm	Radial nerve (cervical 7, 8)	Standing, sitting, supine (arm flexed)	"Straighten out your right [left] arm." Resistance is applied to the dorsal surface of the arm (Fig. 47).

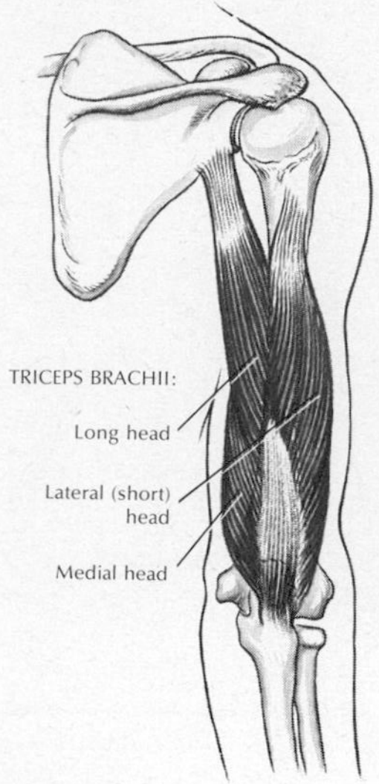

TRICEPS BRACHII:
Long head
Lateral (short) head
Medial head

Fig. 46

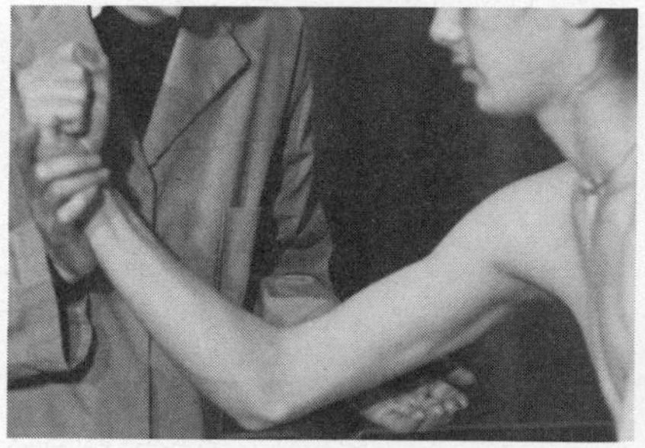

Fig. 47

FOREARM

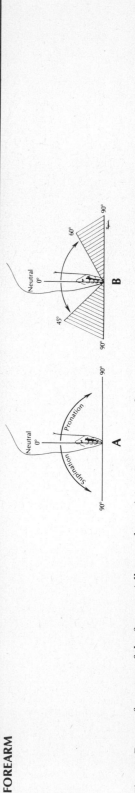

A, Pronation and supination.

Neutral 0° Supination Pronation 90° 90°

B

Neutral 0° 45° 60° 90° 90°

Fig. 48. Range of motion of the forearm (elbow and wrist).* **A,** Pronation and supination. *Pronation:* zero to 80 or 90 degrees. *Supination:* zero to 80 or 90 degrees. *Total forearm motion:* 160 to 180 degrees. Individuals may vary in the range of supination and pronation. Some individuals may reach the 90-degree arc, whereas others may have only 70 degrees plus. **B,** Limited motion. *Supination:* 45 degrees (0 → 45°). *Pronation:* 60 degrees (0 → 60°). *Total joint motion:* 105 degrees.

Movement	Muscles	Motor nerves	Positions for testing	Instructions and tests for muscle strength
Pronation	Prime movers (Fig. 49§) Pronator teres Pronator quadratus Accessory muscle: flexor carpi radialis	Median nerve (cervical 6, 7) Median nerve (cervical 8, thoracic 1)	Standing, sitting, supine (elbow flexed, hands extended, palms up)	"Rotate your right [left] hand inward so that your palm is downward." Resistance is applied at the base of the thumb on the volar surface (Fig. 50).
Supination	Prime movers (Fig. 51†) Biceps brachii Supinator Accessory muscle: brachio-radialis	Musculocutaneous nerve (cervical 5, 6) Radial nerve (cervical 6)	Standing, sitting, supine	"Rotate your right [left] hand outward so that the palm is upward." Resistance is applied on the base of the thumb or over the surface of the hand on the dorsal surface (Fig. 52).

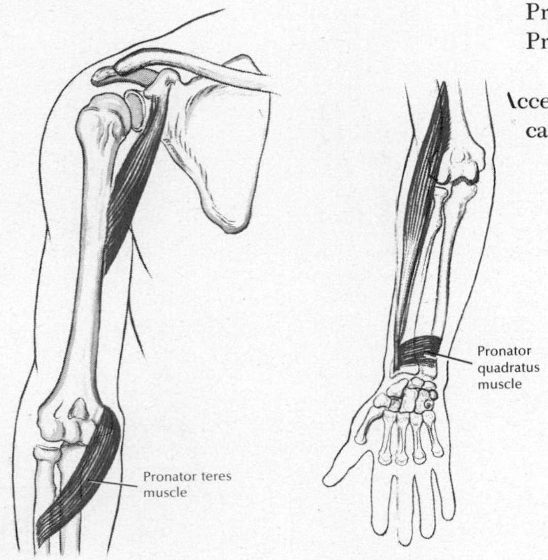

Pronator quadratus muscle

Pronator teres muscle

Fig. 49

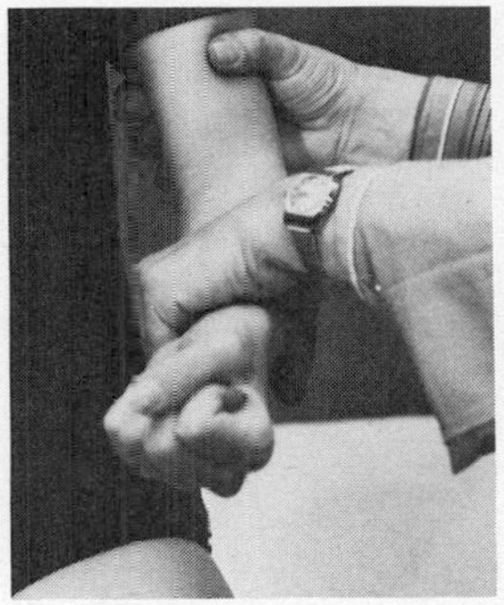

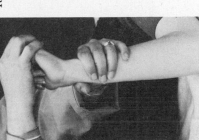

Fig. 50

Biceps brachii

Supinator

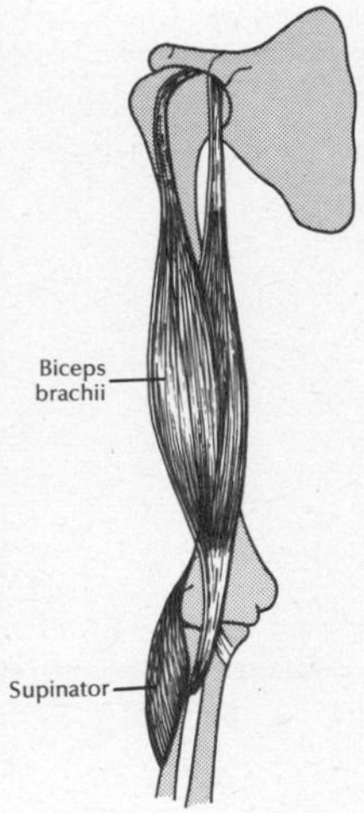

Fig. 51

Fig. 52

Continued.

Table 22-2. Testing for muscle strength and range of joint motion—cont'd

WRIST

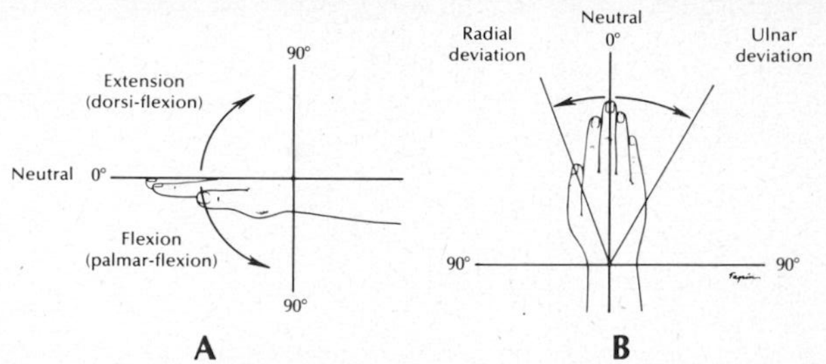

Fig. 53. Range of motion of the wrist.* **A,** Flexion and extension. *Flexion* (palmar flexion): zero to ±80 degrees. *Extension* (dorsiflexion): zero to ±70 degrees. **B,** Radial and ulnar deviation. *Radial deviation:* zero to 20 degrees. *Ulnar deviation:* zero to 30 degrees. Ulnar deviation is usually measured with the wrist in pronation. When measured in supination, ulnar deviation will be somewhat increased.

Movement	Muscles	Motor nerves	Positions for testing	Instructions and tests for muscle strength
Flexion	Prime movers (Fig. 54§) Flexor carpi radialis Flexor carpi ulnaris Accessory muscle: palmaris longus	Medial nerve (cervical 6, 7) Ulnar nerve (cervical 8, thoracic 1)	Standing, sitting, supine (unextended)	"Bend your right [left] hand down toward you." Resistance is applied to the volar surface of the hand (Fig. 55).

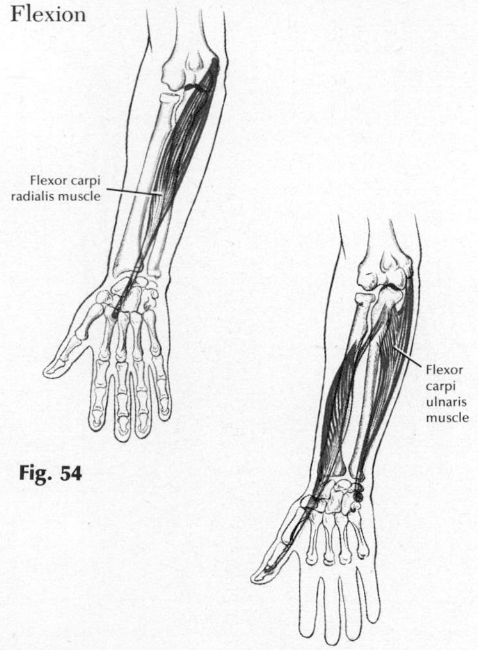

Fig. 54.

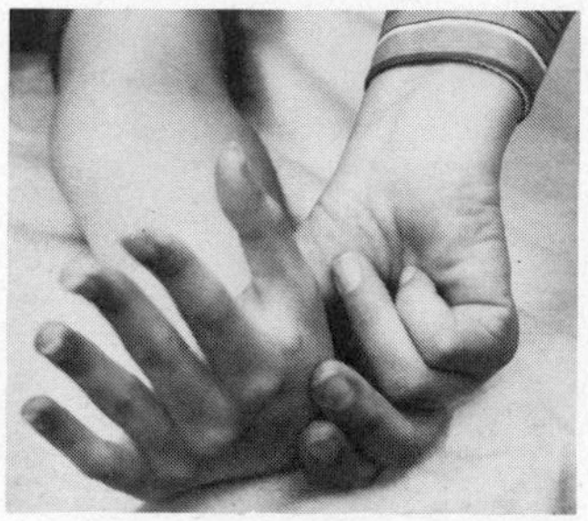

Fig. 55

Extension

Prime movers (Fig. 56†)

Extensor carpi radialis longus — Radial nerve (cervical 6 7)

Extensor carpi radialis brevis — Radial nerve (cervical 6 7)

Extensor carpi ulnaris — Radial nerve (cervical 6 7, 8)

Standing, sitting, supine (wrist flexed)

"Bend your right [left] hand back on itself." Resistance is applied on the dorsal surface of the hand (Fig. 57).

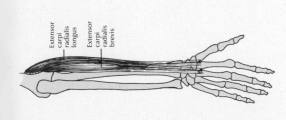

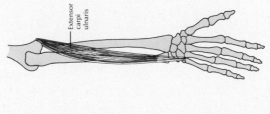

Fig. 56

Fig. 57

Continued.

Table 22-2. Testing for muscle strength and range of joint motion—cont'd

THUMB

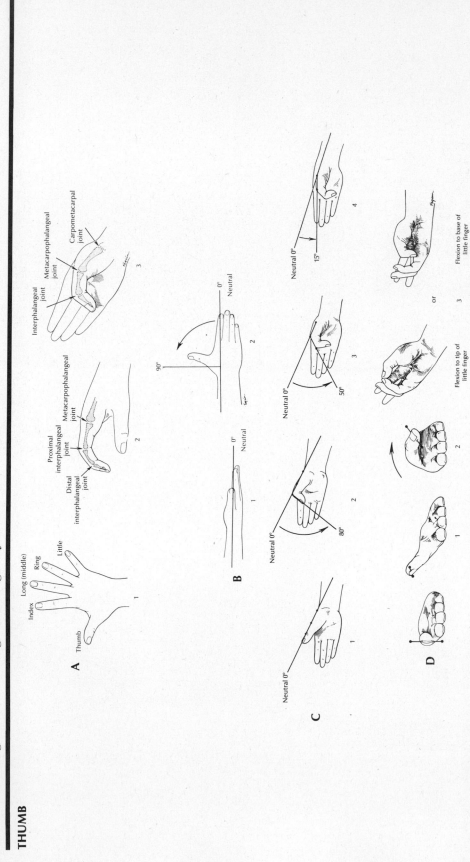

Fig. 58. Hand and range of motion of the thumb.* **A,** Hand. *1,* Nomenclature: in order to avoid mistaken identity, the fingers and thumb are referred to by name rather than by number. Anatomical nomenclature is used for joints of the fingers and thumbs. *2,* Joints of the fingers and thumbs. *3,* Joints of the thumb. **B,** Abduction. *1,* Zero starting position: the extended thumb alongside the index finger, which is in line with the radius. *Abduction* is the angle created between the metacarpal bones of the thumb and index finger. This motion may take place in two planes. *2,* Abduction parallel to the plane of the palm (extension). **C,** Flexion. *1,* Zero starting position: the extended thumb. *2,* Flexion of the interphalangeal joint: zero to ±80 degrees. *3,* Flexion of the metacarpophalangeal joint: zero to ±50 degrees. *4,* Flexion of the carpometacarpal joint: zero to ±15 degrees. **D,** Opposition. Zero starting position *(far left):* the extended thumb in line with the index fingers. *Opposition* is a composite motion consisting of three elements: *1,* abduction, *2,* rotation, and *3,* flexion. This motion is usually considered complete when the tip, or pulp, of the thumb touches the tip of the fifth finger. Some surgeons, however, consider the arc of opposition complete when the tip of the thumb touches the base of the fifth finger. Both methods are illustrated.

Movement	Muscles	Motor nerves	Positions for testing	Instructions and tests for muscle strength
Flexion of joints Metacarpophalangeal Interphalangeal	Prime movers (Fig. 59†) Flexor pollicis brevis Flexor pollicis longus	Median nerve (cervical 6, 7) Ulnar nerve (cervical 8, thoracic 1)	Standing, sitting, supine (thumb extended)	"Bend your right [left] thumb to touch your palm." Resistance is applied to the thenar eminence—the dorsal surface of the distal phalanx (Fig. 60).
Extension of joints Metacarpophalangeal Interphalangeal	Prime movers (Fig. 61†) Extensor pollicis brevis Extensor pollicis longus	Radial nerve (cervical 6, 7) Radial nerve (cervical 6, 7, 8)	Standing, sitting, supine (thumb flexed)	"Straighten out your thumb as if thumbing a ride." "Thumb your nose." Resistance is applied to the dorsal surface of the distal phalanx (Fig. 62).

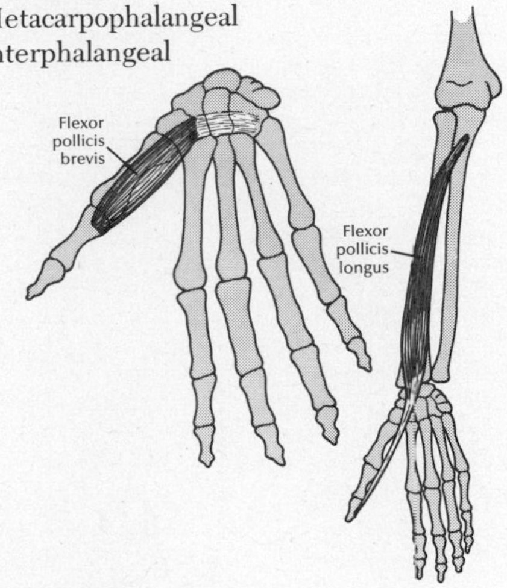

Fig. 59

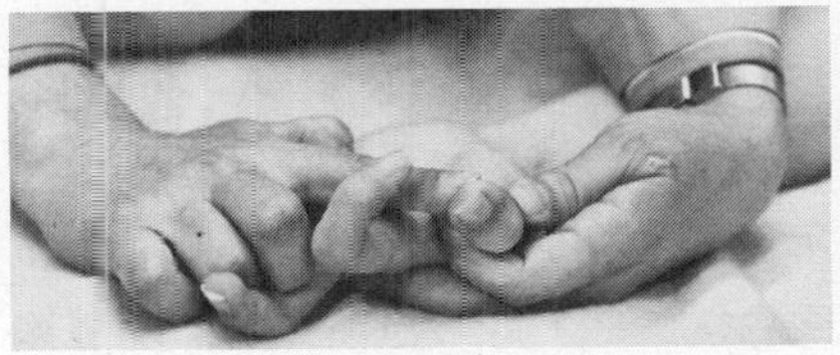

Flexor pollicis longus

Flexor pollicis brevis

Fig. 60

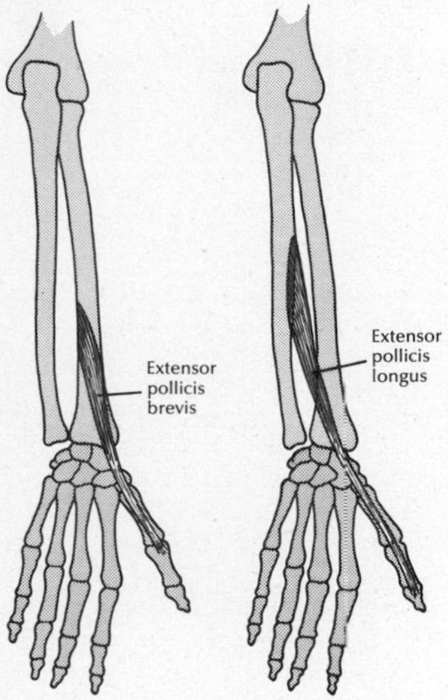

Fig. 61

Extensor pollicis longus

Extensor pollicis brevis

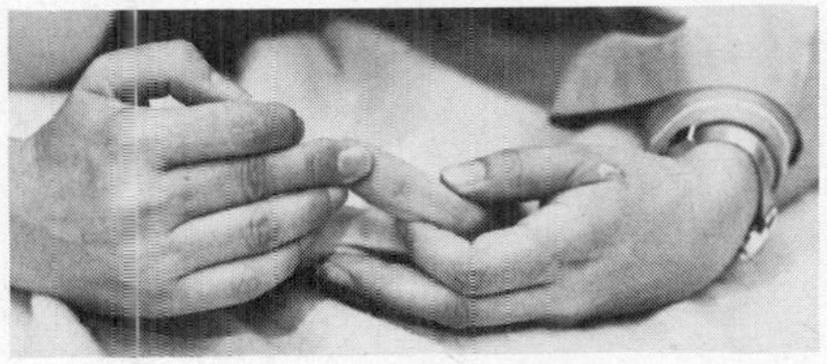

Fig. 62

Continued.

Table 22-2. Testing for muscle strength and range of joint motion—cont'd

Movement	Muscles	Motor nerves	Positions for testing	Instructions and tests for muscle strength
Abduction	Prime movers (Fig. 63†) Abductor pollicis longus Abductor pollicis brevis Accessory muscle: palmaris longus	Radial nerve (cervical 6, 7) Median nerve (cervical 6, 7)	Standing, sitting, supine (arms extended, may have hands in clapping position)	"Raise your right [left] thumb to the ceiling." Resistance is applied to the dorsal surface of the thumb (Fig. 64).
Adduction	Prime movers (Fig. 65†) Adductor pollicis oblique Adductor pollicis transverse	Ulnar nerve (cervical 8, thoracic 1) Ulnar nerve (cervical 8, thoracic 1)	Standing, sitting, supine	"Bring your thumb down against the index finger." Resistance is applied against the terminal phalanx.

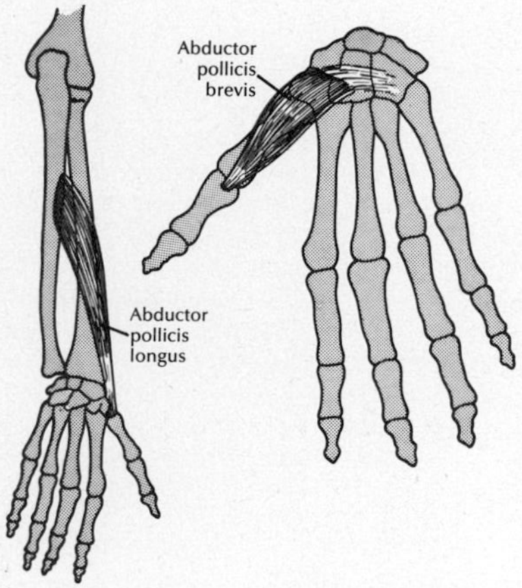

Fig. 64

Abductor pollicis brevis

Abductor pollicis longus

Fig. 63

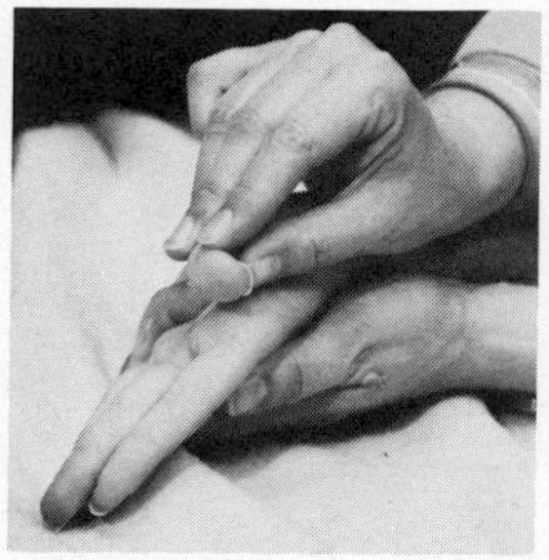

Adductor pollicis

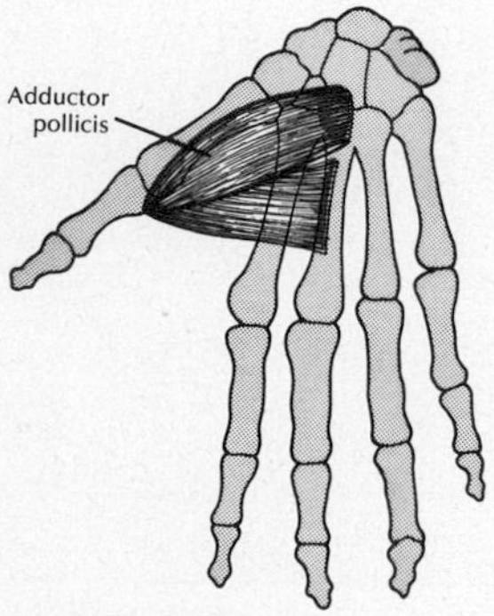

Fig. 65

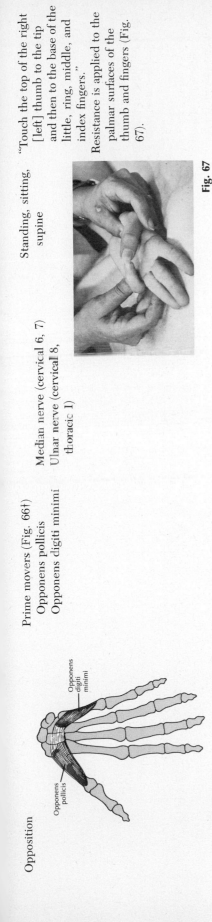

Opposition	
Prime movers (Fig. 66†)	Median nerve (cervical 6, 7)	Standing, sitting, supine	"Touch the top of the right [left] thumb to the tip and then to the base of the little, ring, middle, and index fingers."
Opponens pollicis	Ulnar nerve (cervical 8, thoracic 1)		Resistance is applied to the palmar surfaces of the thumb and fingers (Fig. 67).
Opponens digiti minimi			

Fig. 66

Fig. 67

FINGERS

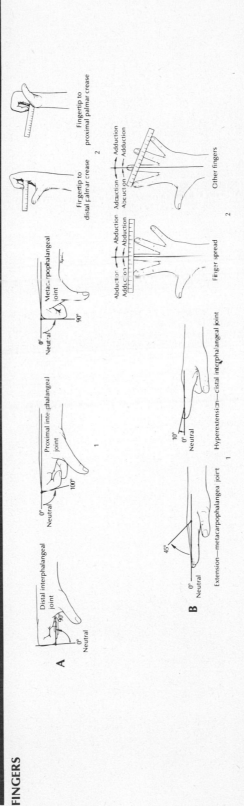

Fig. 68. Range of motion of the fingers.* **A,** Flexion. *1,* This motion can be estimated in degrees or in centimeters. Flexion is a natural motion in all joints of the fingers. *2,* Composite motion of flexion. This motion can be estimated by a ruler as the distance from the tip of the finger (indicate midpoint of pad and nail edge) to the distal palmar crease (*left*) (this measures flexion of the middle and distal joints) and the proximal palmar crease (*right*) (this measures the distal, middle, and proximal joints of the fingers). **B,** Extension, abduction, and adduction. *1,* Extension and hyperextension. Extension is a natural motion at the metacarpophalangeal joint, but an unnatural one in the proximal interphalangeal joint and in the distal interphalangeal joint. *2,* Abduction and adduction. These motions take place in the plane of the palm away from and to the long or middle finger of the hand. This can be indicated in centimeters or inches. The spread of fingers can be measured from the tip of the index finger to the tip of the little finger (*right*). Individual fingers spread from tip to tip of indicated fingers (*left*).

Table 22-2. Testing for muscle strength and range of joint motion—cont'd

Movement	Muscles	Motor nerves	Positions for testing	Instructions and tests for muscle strength
Flexion of joints Metacarpophalangeal	Prime movers (Fig. 69†) Lumbricales Dorsal interossei Palmar interossei Accessory muscles Flexor digiti minimi brevis Flexor digitorum superficialis Flexor digitorum profundus	Ulnar nerve (cervical 8) Ulnar nerve (cervical 8) Ulnar nerve (cervical 8, thoracic 1)	Standing, sitting, supine	"Bend your fingers at the first [proximal] joint." Resistance is applied to the palmar surface of the proximal phalanges (Fig. 70).
Proximal interphalangeal	Prime mover: flexor digitorum superficialis	Median nerve (cervical 7, 8; thoracic 1)	Standing, sitting, supine	"Bend your fingers at the middle joint." "Crook your fingers." Resistance is applied to the palmar surface of the middle phalanges.
Distal interphalangeal	Prime mover: flexor digitorum profundus	Ulnar nerve (cervical 8, thoracic 1)	Standing, sitting, supine	"Bend your distal finger joint." "Crook your finger." Resistance is applied to the pad of the finger (Fig. 71).

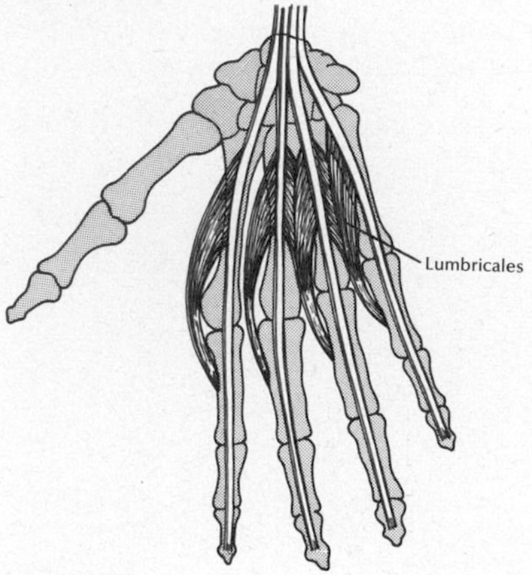

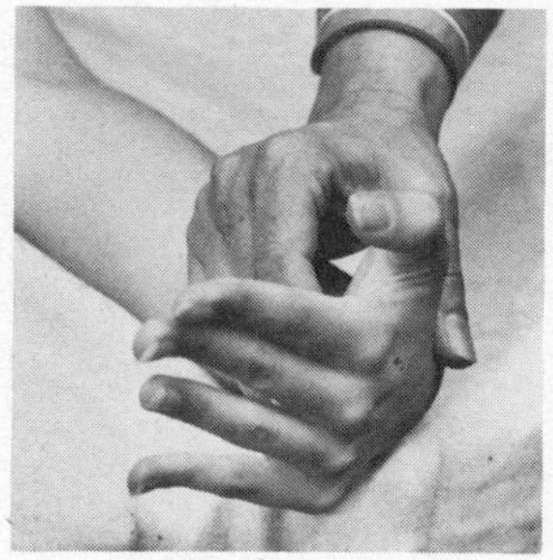

Fig. 70

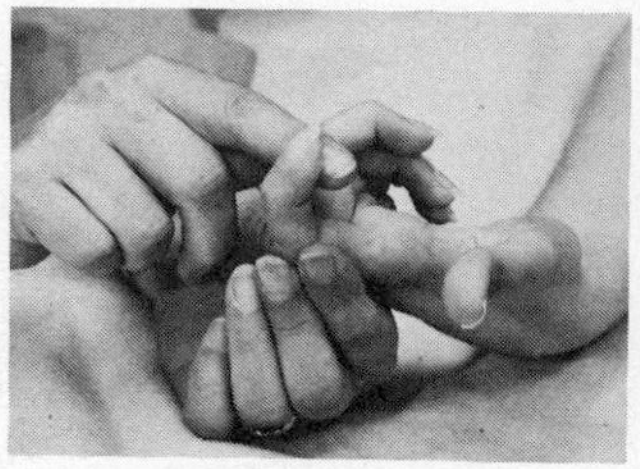

Fig. 71

Lumbricales

Fig. 69

Extension of metacarpophalangeal joints

Prime movers (Fig. 72†)
Extensor digitorum communis — Radial nerve (cervical 6, 7, 8)
Extensor indicis proprius — Radial nerve (cervical 6, 7, 8)
Extensor digiti minimi — Radial nerve (cervical 7)

Standing, sitting, supine (fingers flexed)

"Straighten out your fingers." Resistance is applied to the dorsal surface of the proximal and distal phalanges (Fig. 57).

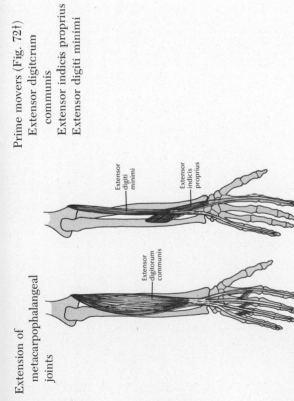

Extensor digiti minimi
Extensor indicis proprius
Extensor digitorum communis

Fig. 72

Abduction

Prime movers (Fig. 73†)
Interossei dorsales — Ulnar nerve (cervical 8, thoracic 1)
Abductor digiti minimi — Ulnar nerve (cervical 8)

Standing, sitting, supine (fingers together)

"Spread your fingers as far apart as possible." Pressure is exerted against the outside surfaces of the fingers being tested to resist spread of the fingers (Fig. 74).

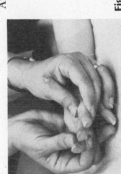

Fig. 74

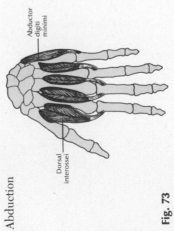

Abductor digiti minimi
Dorsal interossei

Fig. 73

Adduction

Prime movers: interossei palmares (Fig. 75†) — Ulnar nerve (cervical 8, thoracic 1)

Standing, sitting, supine (fingers apart)

"Put your fingers together. Press them hard against each other." An attempt is made to pull them apart (Fig. 76).

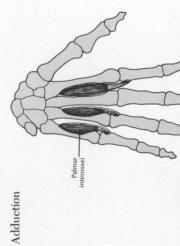

Fig. 76

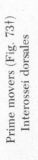

Palmar interossei

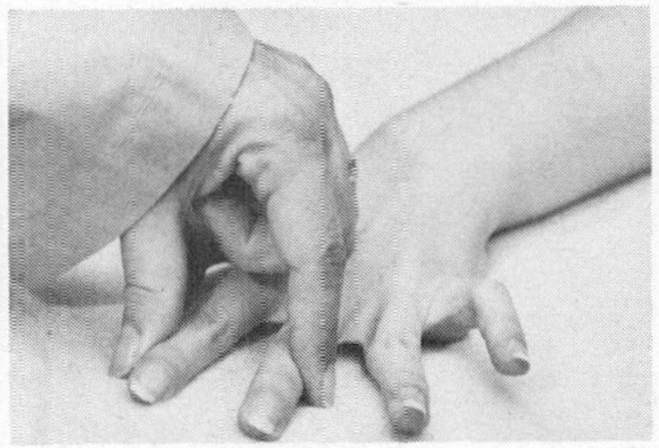

Fig. 75

Continued.

Table 22-2. Testing for muscle strength and range of joint motion—cont'd

HIP

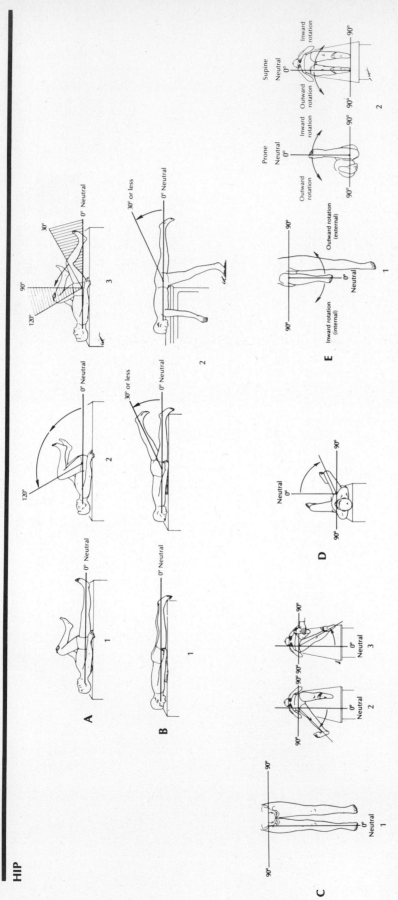

Fig. 77. Range of motion of the hip.* **A,** Flexion. *1,* Zero starting position of the right hip: client is supine on a firm, flat surface with the opposite hip held in full flexion. This flattens the lumbar spine and demonstrates a flexion deformity of the hip if present. *2,* Flexion. The motion is recorded from zero to 110 or 120 degrees. The examiner should place one hand on the iliac crest to note the point at which the pelvis begins to rotate. *3,* Limited motion in flexion. Limited motion is noted as in the elbow and knee: the hip flexes from 30 to 90 degrees (30° → 90°); the hip has a flexion deformity of 30 degrees with further flexion to 90 degrees. **B,** Extension. *1,* Zero starting position: client is prone on a firm, level surface. *2,* The upward motion of the hip is measured in degrees from the zero starting position. Two methods are commonly used. *Left,* With the client prone and a small pillow under the abdomen, the leg is extended with the knee straight or flexed. *Right,* With the opposite extremity flexed over the end of the examining table, the hip is extended. This method is a more accurate method of measuring extension. There is an anatomical question whether extension is present in the hip at all. Extension as seen from examination is that deviation of the extremity past the zero position and reflects some back motion. **C,** Abduction and adduction. *1,* Zero starting position: client is supine with the legs extended at right angles to a transverse line across the anterosuperior spine of the pelvis. *2,* Abduction. The outward motion of the extremity is measured in degrees from the zero starting position. *3,* Adduction. In measuring adduction the examiner should elevate the opposite extremity a few degrees to allow the leg to pass under it. **D,** Abduction in flexion. Abduction can be measured in degrees at any level of flexion. Usually, this is carried out in 90 degrees of flexion. **E,** Rotation. *1,* Rotation in flexion. Zero starting position: client is supine with the hip and knee flexed 90 degrees each and the thigh perpendicular to the transverse line across the anterosuperior spine of the pelvis. *Inward (internal) rotation* is measured by rotating the leg away from the midline of the trunk with the thigh as the axis of rotation, thus producing inward rotation of the hip. *Outward (external) rotation* is measured by rotating the leg toward the midline of the trunk with the thigh as the axis of rotation, thus producing outward rotation of the hip. *2,* Rotation in extension. Zero starting position: with client prone *(left),* the knee is flexed to 90 degrees and is perpendicular to the transverse line across the anterosuperior spine of the pelvis. *Inward rotation* is measured by rotating the leg outward. *Outward rotation* is measured by rotating the leg inward. Rotation in extension can also be measured with the client supine *(right).*

Movement	Muscles	Motor nerves	Positions for testing	Instructions and tests for muscle strength
Flexion	Prime movers (Fig. 78†) Psoas major Iliacus Accessory muscles Sartorius Rectus femoris Tensor fasciae latae Pectineus Adductor brevis Adductor longus Adductor magnus (oblique fibers)	Femoral nerve (lumbar 2, 3) Femoral nerve (lumbar 2, 3)	Supine Sitting	"Draw your knees up to your chest." "Bend your right [left] knee up to your chest." Resistance is applied to the anterior surface of the leg proximal to the knee (Fig. 79).
Extension	Prime movers (Fig. 80§) Gluteus maximus Semitendinosus Semimembranosus Biceps femoris (long head)	Inferior gluteal nerve (lumbar 5, sacral 1, 2) Sciatic nerve (lumbar 4, 5; sacral 1, 2) Sciatic nerve (lumbar 5; sacral 1, 2) Sciatic nerve (sacral 1, 2, 3)	Prone	"Lift your right [left] leg toward the ceiling." Resistance is applied to the dorsal surface of the leg proximal to the knee (Fig. 81).

Fig. 79

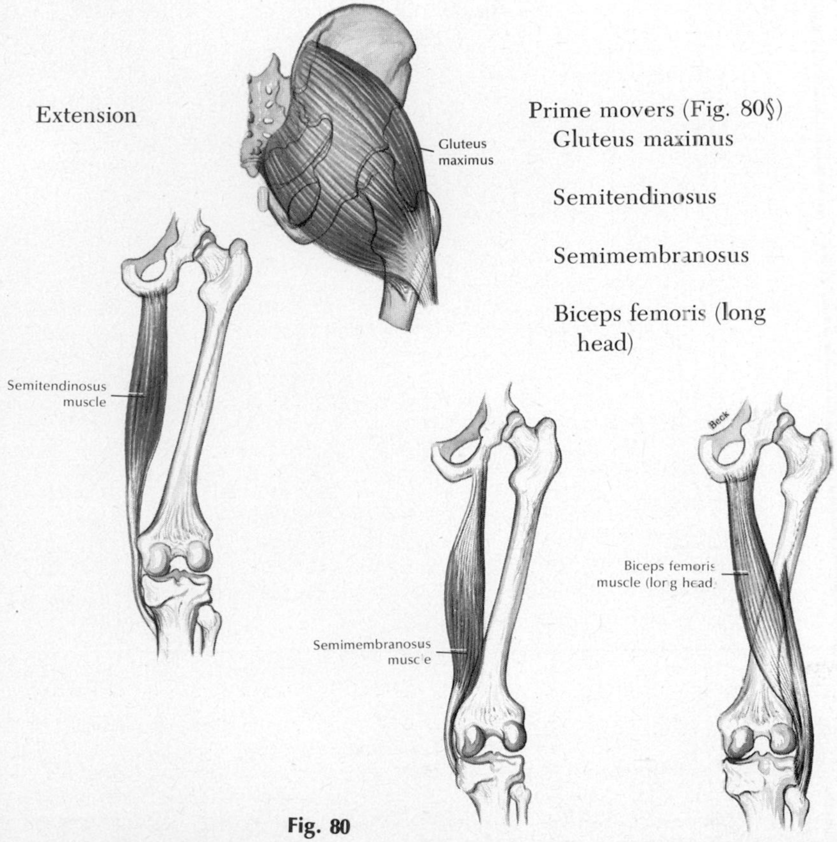

Fig. 81

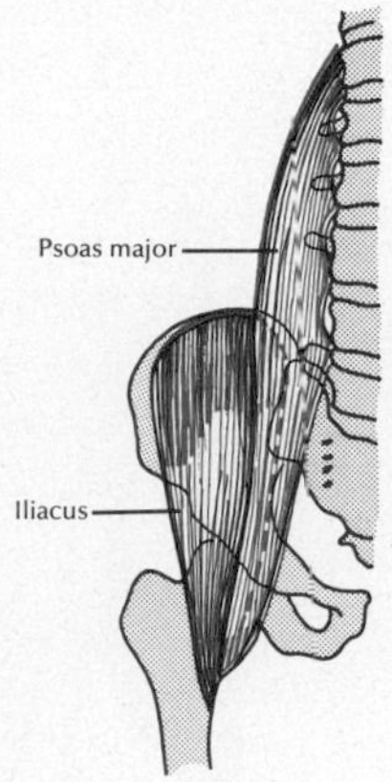

Psoas major

Iliacus

Fig. 78

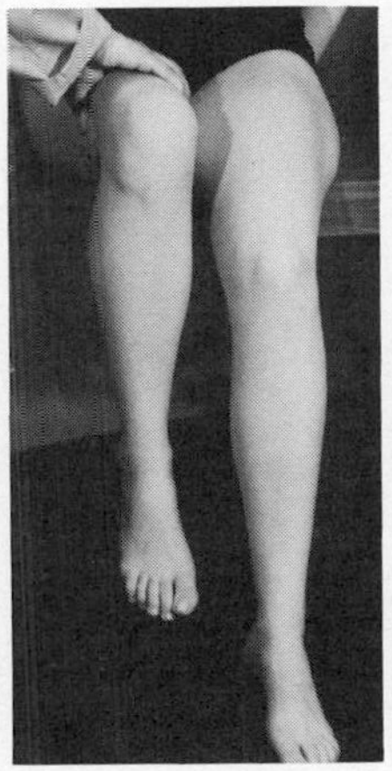

Gluteus maximus

Semitendinosus muscle

Biceps femoris muscle (long head)

Semimembranosus muscle

Fig. 80

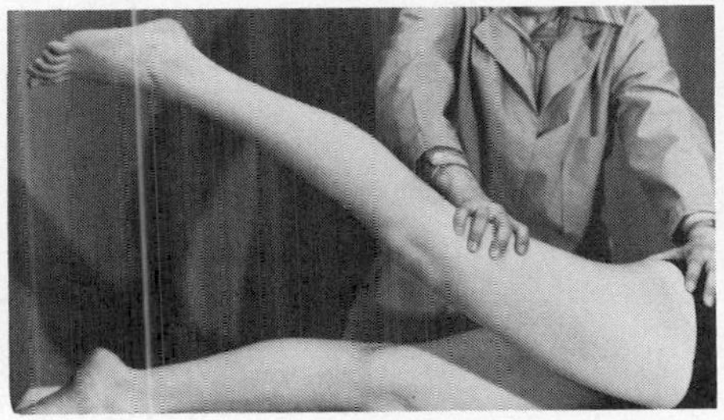

Continued.

Table 22-2. Testing for muscle strength and range of joint motion—cont'd

Movement	Muscles	Motor nerves	Positions for testing	Instructions and tests for muscle strength
Abduction	Prime mover: gluteus medius (Fig. 82§) Accessory muscles Gluteus minimus Tensor fasciae latae Gluteus maximus (upper fibers)	Superior gluteal nerve (lumbar 4, 5; sacral 1)	Lateral lie	"Move your upper leg toward the ceiling." Resistance is applied to the lateral surface of the upper leg (Fig. 83).
Adduction	Prime movers (Fig. 84§) Adductor magnus Adductor brevis Adductor longus Pectineus Gracilis	Obturator nerve (lumbar 3, 4) Obturator nerve (lumbar 3, 4) Obturator nerve (lumbar 3, 4) Obturator nerve (lumbar 2, 3, 4) Obturator nerve (lumbar 3, 4)	Lateral lie, legs apart	"Try to bring your legs together." Resistance is applied to the medial surface of the thighs proximal to the knees (Fig. 85).

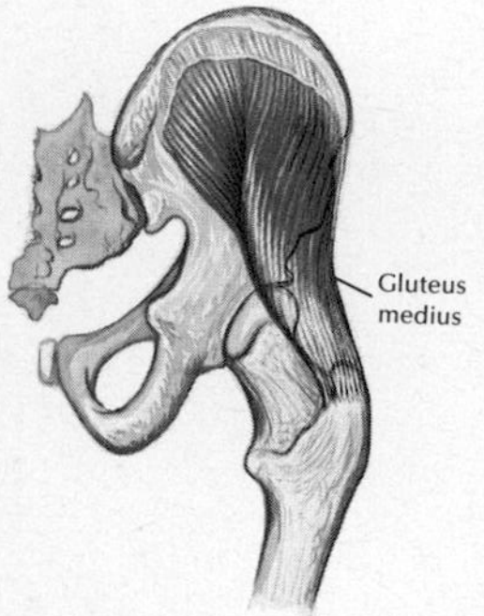

Fig. 82

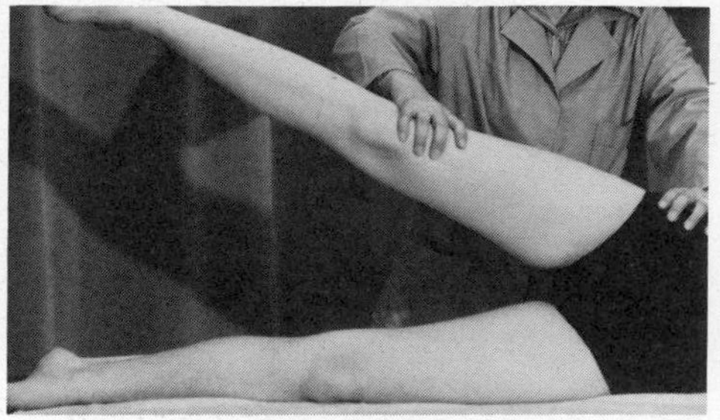

Fig. 83

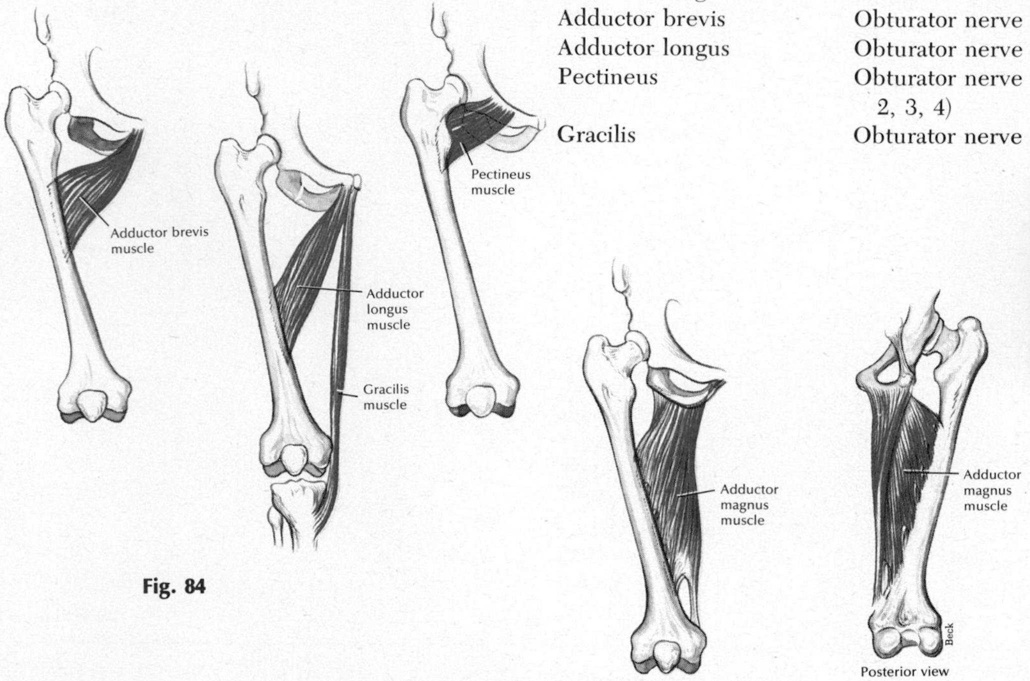

Fig. 84

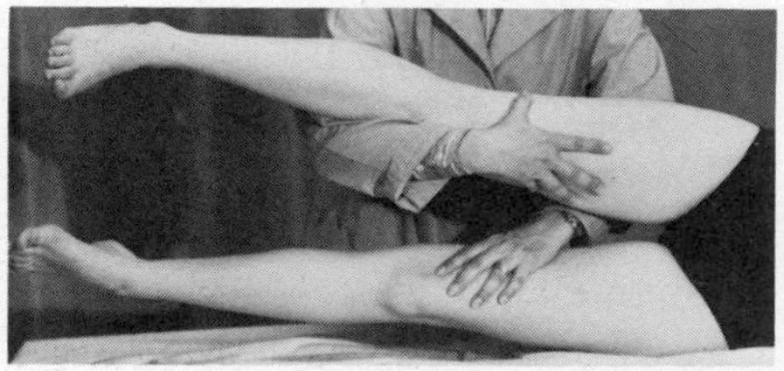

Fig. 85

Rotation (knees extended)

Internal

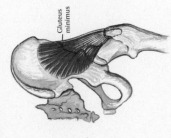

Fig. 86

Prime movers (Fig. 86§)

Gluteus minimus — Superior gluteal nerve (lumbar 4, 5; sacral 1)

Tensor fasciae latae — Superior gluteal nerve (lumbar 4, 5; sacral 1)

Accessory muscles
Gluteus medius (anterior fibers)
Semitendinosus
Semimembranosus

Sitting (legs about a foot apart at ankle)

"Pivot your right hip inward—your foot will move away from your body." Resistance is applied toward the midline at the lateral surface of the ankle (Fig. 87).

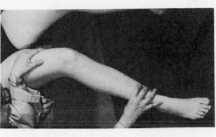

Fig. 87

External

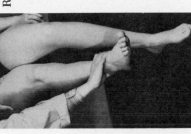

Fig. 88

Prime movers (Fig. 88†)

Obturator externus — Obturator nerve (lumbar 3, 4)

Obturator internus — Obturator nerve (lumbar 5; sacral 2, 3)

Quadratus femoris — Obturator nerve (lumbar 5; sacral 1)

Piriformis — Obturator nerve (sacral 1, 2)

Gemellus superior — Obturator nerve (lumbar 5; sacral 1, 2, 3)

Gemellus inferior — Obturator nerve (lumbar 5; sacral 1)

Gluteus maximus — Obturator nerve (lumbar 5; sacral 1)

Accessory muscles
Sartorius
Biceps femoris (long head) — Obturator nerve (lumbar 5; sacral 1, 2)

Sitting

"Rotate your hip outward; your foot will turn in." Resistance is applied to the medial aspect of the ankle (Fig. 89).

Fig. 89

Continued.

Table 22-2. Testing for muscle strength and range of joint motion—cont'd

Movement	Muscles	Motor nerves	Positions for testing	Instructions and tests for muscle strength
Rotation (knees flexed)	Prime mover: sartorius Accessory muscles External rotators of hip Flexors of hip, knee	Femoral nerve (lumbar 2, 3, 4)	Supine (knees flexed)	"Rotate your knees outward. Bend them toward the table. Bring them as close as you can to the table." Resistance is applied to the lateral aspects of the knees.
Abduction	Prime mover: tensor fasciae latae Accessory muscles Gluteus medius Gluteus minimus	Superior gluteal nerve (lumbar 4, 5; sacral 1)	Supine	"Bend your knees out." Resistance is applied to the upper outer aspect of each leg.

KNEE

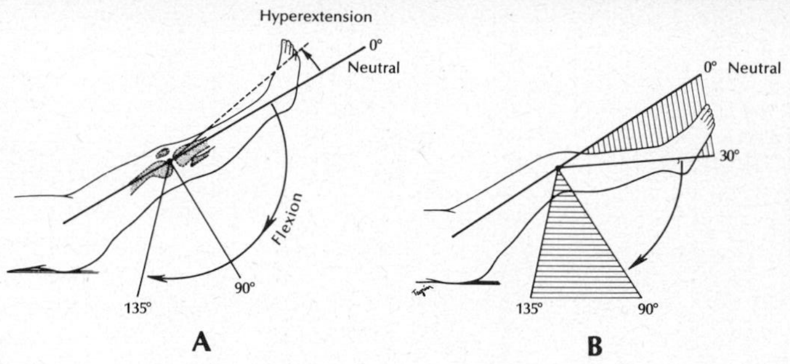

Fig. 90. Range of motion of the knee.* **A,** Flexion. Zero starting position: the extended straight knee with client either supine or prone. *Flexion* is measured in degrees from the zero starting point. *Hyperextension* is measured in degrees opposite to flexion at the zero starting point. **B,** Measurement of limited motion of the knee. The terminology for recording limited motion of the knee is similar to that of the elbow and hip: (1) the knee flexes from 30 to 90 degrees ($30° \rightarrow 90°$); (2) the knee has a flexion deformity of 30 degrees with further flexion to 90 degrees.

Movement	Muscles	Motor nerves	Positions for testing	Instructions and tests for muscle strength
Flexion	Prime movers (Fig. 91§)		Prone	"Bend your right [left] leg. Try to touch your heel to the back of your leg." Resistance is applied to the dorsal aspect of the ankle (Fig. 92).
	Biceps femoris (long head)	Sciatic nerve (sacral 1, 2, 3)		
	Biceps femoris (short head)	Sciatic nerve (lumbar 4, 5; sacral 1, 2)		
	Semitendinosus	Sciatic nerve (lumbar 4, 5; sacral 1, 2, 3)		
	Semimembranosus	Sciatic nerve (lumbar 4, 5; sacral 1, 2, 3)		
	Accessory muscles			
	Popliteus			
	Sartorius			
	Gracilis			
	Gastrocnemius			

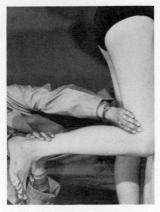

Fig. 92

Continued.

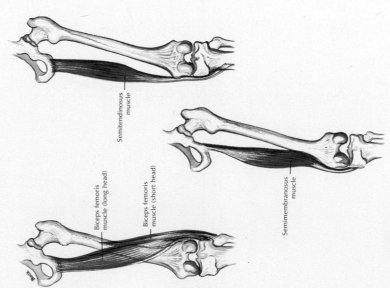

Biceps femoris muscle (long head)

Biceps femoris muscle (short head)

Semitendinosus muscle

Semimembranosus muscle

Fig. 91

Table 22-2. Testing for muscle strength and range of joint motion—cont'd

Movement	Muscles	Motor nerves	Positions for testing	Instructions and tests for muscle strength
Extension	Prime movers (Fig. 93§) Rectus femoris Vastus intermedius Vastus medialis Vastus lateralis	Femoral nerve (lumbar 2, 3, 4) Femoral nerve (lumbar 2, 3, 4) Femoral nerve (lumbar 2, 3, 4) Femoral nerve (lumbar 2, 3, 4)	Sitting	"Straighten out your right [left] leg." Resistance is applied against the anterior aspect of the ankle.

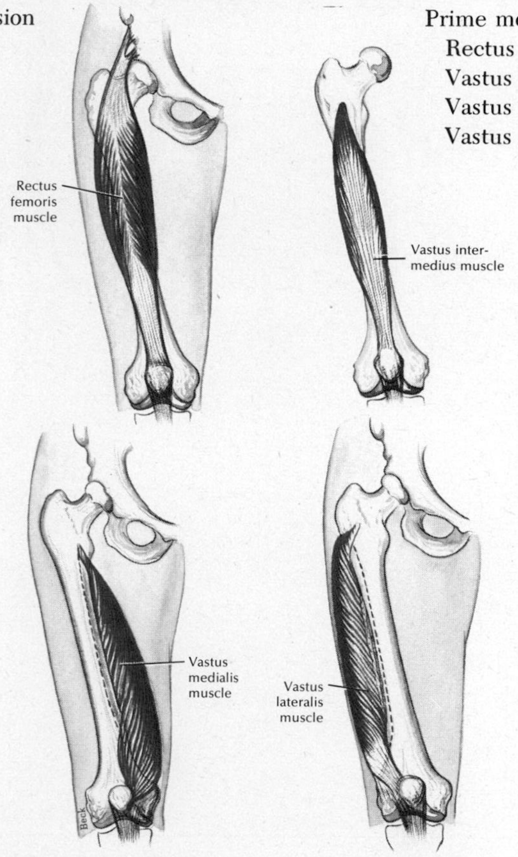

Fig. 93

ANKLE

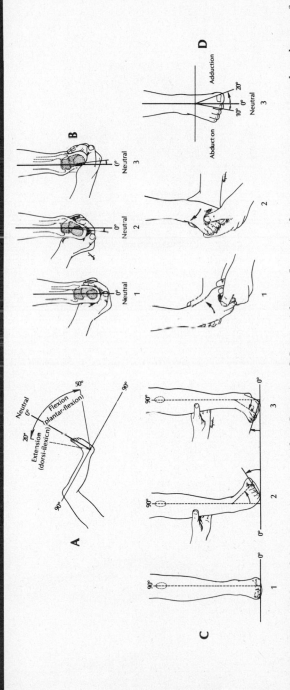

Fig. 94. Range of motion of the ankle and foot.* **A,** Extension (dorsiflexion) and flexion (plantar flexion). These motions are measured in degrees from the right-angle neutral position or in percentages of motion as compared to the opposite ankle. **B,** Motions of the hind part of the foot (passive motion). *1,* Zero starting position: the heel is in line with the midline of the tibia. *2,* Inversion. The heel is grasped firmly in the cup of the examiner's hand. Passive motion is estimated in degrees or percentages of motion by turning the heel inward. *3,* Eversion. This motion is estimated by turning the heel outward. **C,** Motions of the fore part of the foot (active motion). *1,* Zero starting position: the foot is in line with the tibia in the long axis from the ankle to the knee. The axis of the foot is the second toe. *2,* Active inversion. The foot is directed medially. This motion includes supination, adduction, and some degree of plantar flexion. This motion can be estimated in degrees or expressed in percentages as compared to the opposite foot. *3,* Active eversion. The sole of the foot is turned to face laterally. This motion includes pronation, abduction, and dorsiflexion. NOTE: Problems exist when the foot motions are divided into forefoot and hindfoot descriptions. Care must be made to record motions pertaining to that part of the foot described or to the whole foot, as the case may be. **D,** Motions of the fore part of the foot (passive motion). *1,* Inversion. The examiner carries the foot passively through the motions of active inversion. The heel must be held firmly by the examiner's hand, with the other hand turning the foot inward. *2,* Eversion. The examiner passively turns the foot outward in pronation, abduction, and slight dorsiflexion. *3,* Adduction and abduction. These passive motions are obtained by grasping the heel and moving the fore part of the foot inward or outward. This motion must take place in the plane of the sole of the foot.

Continued.

Table 22-2. Testing for muscle strength and range of joint motion—cont'd

Movement	Muscles	Motor nerves	Positions for testing	Instruction and tests for muscle strength
Dorsiflexion	Prime mover: tibialis anterior (Fig. 95†)	Deep peroneal nerve (lumbar 4, 5; sacral 1)	Sitting, supine	"Bend your toes toward your knees." Resistance is applied to the dorsal aspect of the foot.
Internal rotation and dorsiflexion	Prime mover: tibialis posterior (Fig. 95)	Deep peroneal nerve (lumbar 5; sacral 1)	Sitting, supine	"Rotate your right [left] foot toward the left [right] foot. Turn it as far as you can." Resistance is applied to the medial aspect of the foot at the first metatarsal joint.
Plantar flexion	Prime movers (Fig. 96†) Gastrocnemius Soleus Accessory muscles Tibialis posterior Peroneus longus Peroneus brevis Flexor hallucis longus Flexor digitorum longus Plantaris	Tibial nerve (sacral 1, 2) Tibial nerve (sacral 1, 2)	Sitting, supine	"Point your toes away from you [downward] as far as you can." Resistance is applied to the ball of the foot (Fig. 97).

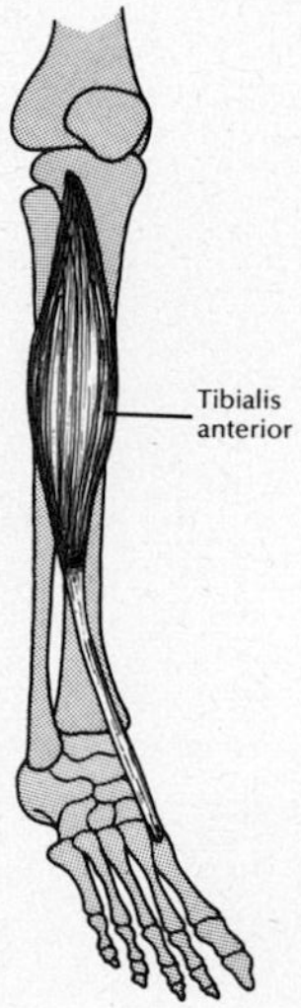

Tibialis anterior

Fig. 95

Gastrocnemius

Soleus

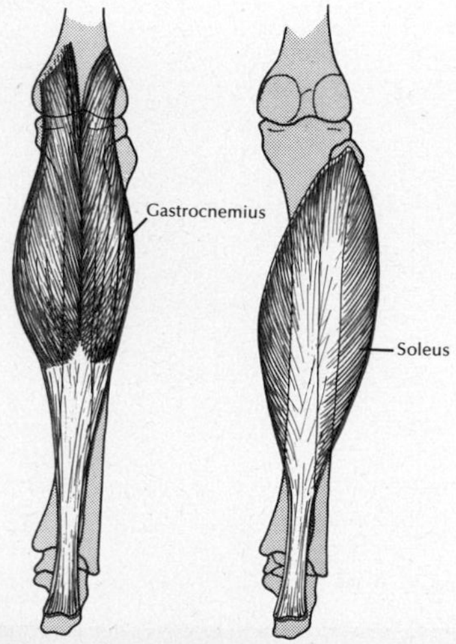

Fig. 96

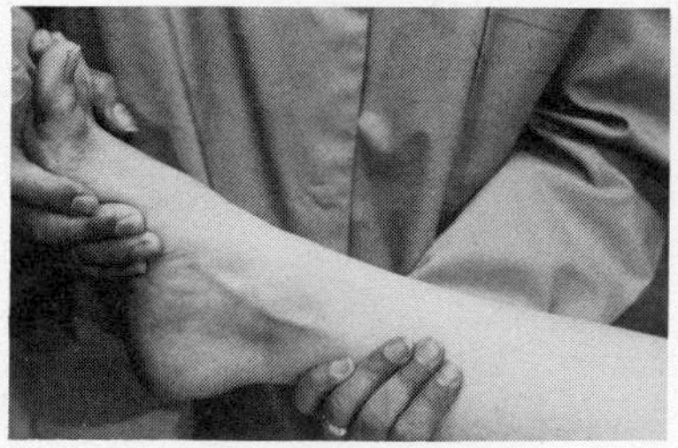

Fig. 97

FOOT

Movement	Muscles	Motor nerves	Positions for testing	Instructions and tests for muscle strength
Inversion	Prime mover: tibialis posterior (Fig. 98†) Accessory muscles Flexor digitorum longus Flexor hallucis longus Gastrocnemius (medial head)	Tibial nerve (lumbar 5, sacral 1)	Sitting, supine	"Point your toes; then rotate them inward." Resistance is applied against the medial aspect of the first metatarsal bone (Fig. 99).
Eversion	Prime movers (Fig. 100†) Peroneus longus Peroneus brevis Accessory muscles Extensor digitorum longus Peroneus tertius	Superficial peroneal nerve (lumbar 4, 5; sacral 1) Superficial peroneal nerve (lumbar 4, 5; sacral 1)	Sitting, supine	"Point your toes and rotate them outward." Resistance is applied against the lateral aspect of the fifth metatarsal bone.

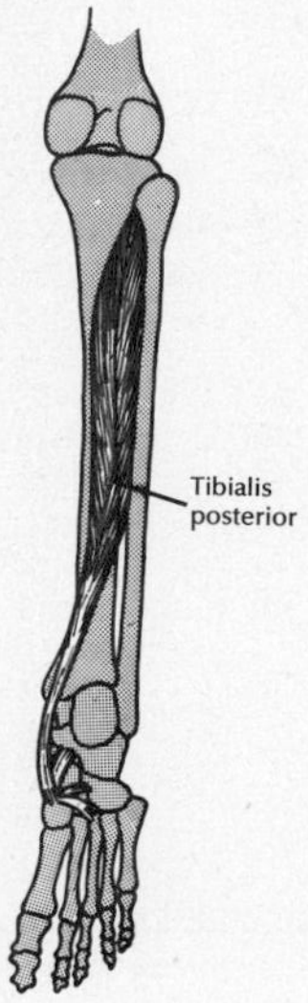

Fig. 99

Tibialis posterior

Fig. 98

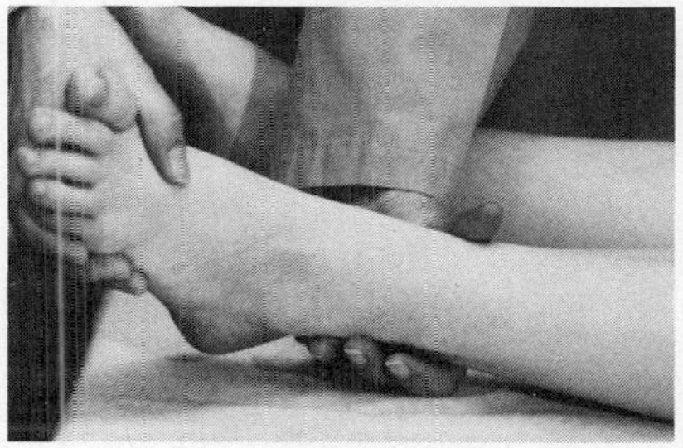

Peroneus brevis

Peroneus longus

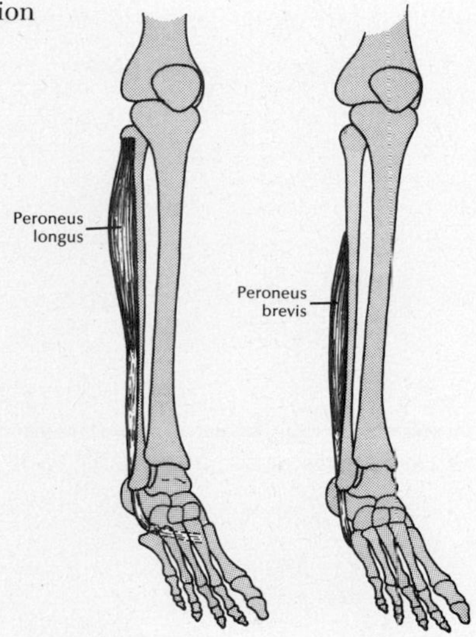

Fig. 100

Continued.

Table 22-2. Testing for muscle strength and range of joint motion—cont'd

GREAT TOE

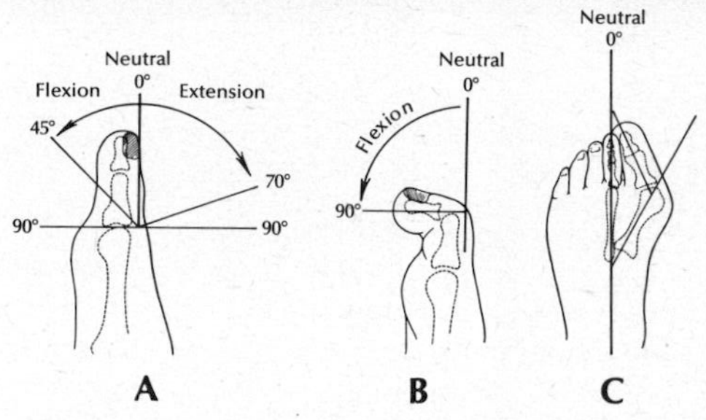

Fig. 101. Range of motion of the great toe.* **A,** Flexion and extension of the great toe. Zero starting position: the extended great toe is in line with the first metatarsal bone. **B,** Flexion and extension are present at the metatarsophalangeal joint, and flexion only is present at the interphalangeal joint. **C,** The degree of deformity of the great toe in this instance, hallux valgus, may be measured in degrees of abduction of the metatarsal bone and in degrees of adduction of the proximal and distal phalanges.

Movement	Muscles	Motor nerves	Positions for testing	Instructions and tests for muscle strength
Flexion of joints Metatarsophalangeal	Prime mover: flexor hallucis brevis (Fig. 102) Accessory muscle: flexor hallucis longus	Medial plantar nerve (lumbar 4, 5; sacral 1)	Sitting, supine	"Bend your right [left] big toe down." "Curl your toe." Resistance is applied to the plantar side of the toe (Fig. 103).

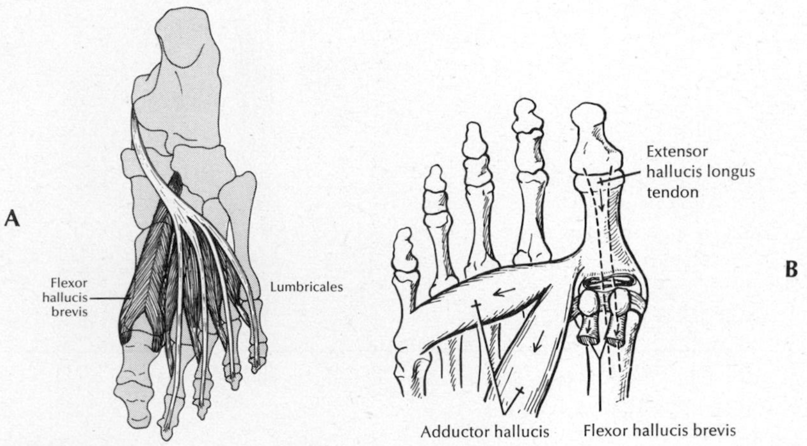

Fig. 102

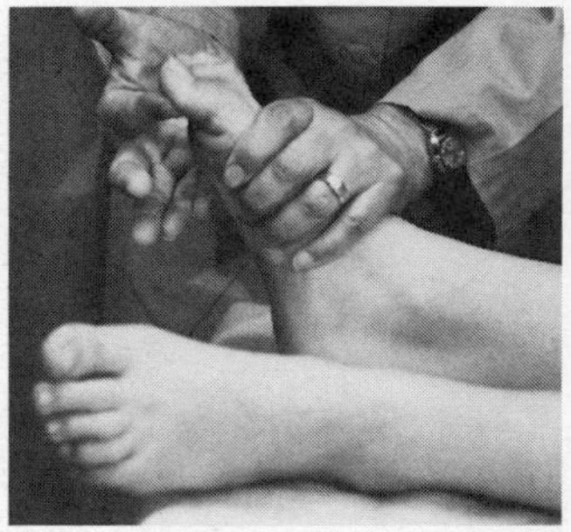

Fig. 103

Interphalangeal

Prime mover: flexor hallucis longus (Fig. 104†)

Tibial nerve (lumbar 5; sacral 1, 2)

Sitting, supine

"Bend your right [left] big toe down." "Curl your toe." Resistance is applied to the plantar surface of the distal phalanges.

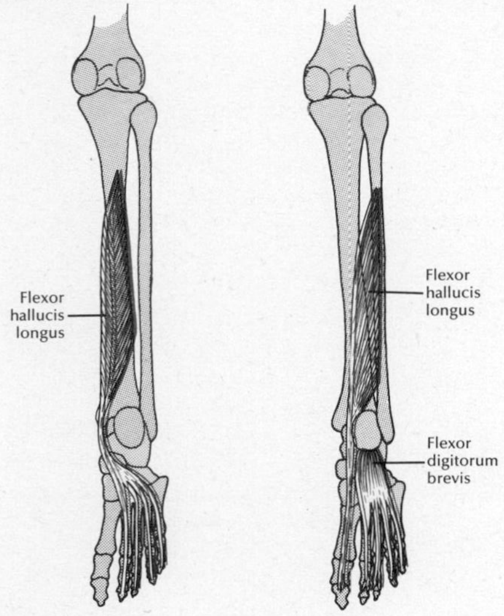

Flexor hallucis longus

Flexor hallucis longus

Flexor digitorum brevis

Fig. 104

Extension of metatarsophalangeal joint

Prime movers (Fig. 105†) Extensor digitorum longus Extensor digitorum brevis

Deep peroneal nerve (lumbar 4, 5; sacral 1) Deep peroneal nerve (lumbar 5; sacral 1)

Sitting, supine

"Bend your big toe upward." Resistance is applied to the dorsum of the toe (Fig. 106).

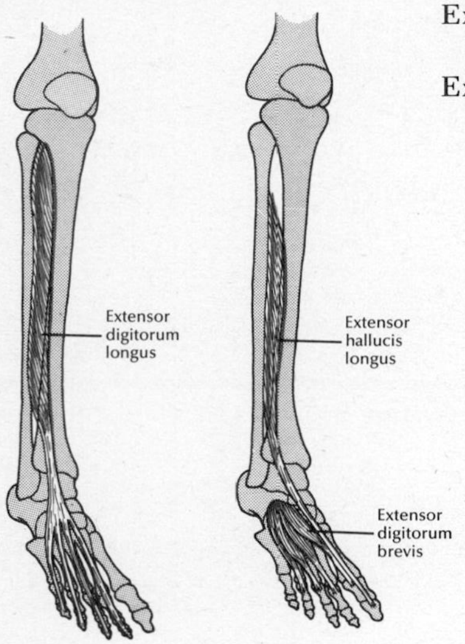

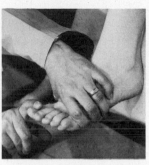

Fig. 106

Extensor digitorum longus

Extensor hallucis longus

Extensor digitorum brevis

Fig. 105

Continued.

Table 22-2. Testing for muscle strength and range of joint motion—cont'd

LATERAL FOUR TOES

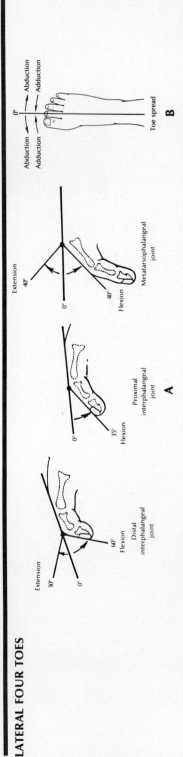

Fig. 107. Range of motion of the lateral four toes.* **A,** Second to fifth toes. Motion in flexion is present in the distal, middle, and proximal joints of the toes. Extension is present at the metatarsophalangeal joint. These motions can be simply expressed in degrees. **B,** Abduction and adduction (toe spread). This can be measured in relation to the second toe, which is the midline axis of the foot.

Movement	Muscles	Motor nerves	Positions for testing	Instructions and tests for muscle strength
Flexion of toe joints Metatarsophalangeal	Prime mover: lumbricales (Fig. 102) Accessory muscles Interossei dorsales and plantares Flexor digiti quinti brevis Flexor digotorum longus Flexor digitorum brevis	Medial plantar nerve (lumbar 4, 5) Lateral plantar nerve (sacral 1, 2)	Sitting, supine	"Bend all your toes down-ward." Resistance is applied to the plantar surface of the proximal phalanges.
Proximal interphalangeal	Prime mover: flexor digitorum brevis (Fig. 104)	Medial plantar nerve (lumbar 4, 5)	Sitting, supine	"Bend your toes down-ward." Resistance is applied to the plantar surface of the medial phalanges.

Distal interphalangeal

Prime mover: flexor digitorum longus (Fig. 104)

Tibial nerve (lumbar 5, sacral 1)

Sitting, supine

"Bend your toes downward." Pressure is applied to the plantar surface of the distal phalanges (Fig. 108).

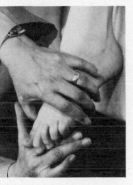

Fig. 108

Extension of metatarsophalangeal joint

Prime movers (Fig. 105):
Extensor digitorum longus
Extensor digitorum brevis

Deep peroneal nerve (lumbar 4, 5, sacral 1)
Deep peroneal nerve (lumbar 5, sacral 1)

Sitting, supine

"Straighten out your toes. Point your toes upward." Resistance is applied to the dorsum of the proximal phalanges.

Recording of data

The following chart provides a listing of clinically testable muscles. Although the methodical recording of data for each muscle is painstaking, it serves as a baseline for subsequent changes and does indicate that the muscle was actually tested.

Special tests of musculoskeletal function

Although the following tests are described separately, they may be incorporated into the systematic evaluation of the client, which progresses in a cephalocaudal direction.

Range of motion	Tone	Fasciculation	Strength				Range of motion	Tone	Fasciculation	Strength
				Face:						
				Neck:	Flexor	Sternocleidomastoid				
					Extensor group					
				Trunk:	Flexor	Rectus abdominis				
					Rotators Right oblique internal abductor Left oblique internal abductor Left oblique external abductor Right oblique external abductor					
					Extensors	Thoracic group Lumbar group				
					Pelvic elevator	Quadratus lumbar				
				Scapula:	Abductor	Serratus anterior				
					Elevator	Trapezius (superior)				
					Depressor	Trapezius (inferior)				
					Adductors	Trapezius (middle) Rhomboid major and minor				
				Shoulder:	Flexor	Deltoid (anterior)				
					Extensors	Latissimus dorsi Teres major				
					Abductor (to 90°)	Deltoid (middle)				
					Horizontal abductor	Deltoid (posterior)				
					Horizontal adductor	Pectoralis major				
					Rotators Lateral rotator group Medial rotator group					
				Elbow:	Flexors	Biceps brachii Brachialis				
					Extensor	Triceps brachii				
				Forearm:	Extensors Supinator group					
					Pronator group					

*Adapted from Daniels, L., and Worthingham, C.: Muscle testing; techniques of manual examination, ed. 3, Philadelphia, 1972, W. B. Saunders Co.

Range of motion	Tone	Fasciculation	Strength				Range of motion	Tone	Fasciculation	Strength
				Wrist:	Flexors	Flex. carpi radialis Flex. carpi ulnaris				
					Extensors	Ext. carpi rad. longus and brevis Ext. carpi ulnaris				
				Fingers:	MP flexors	Lumbricales				
					IP flexors (first)	Flex. digit. superficialis				
					IP flexors (second)	Flex. digit. profundus				
					MP extensors	Ext. digit. communis				
					Adductors	Interossei palmares Interossei dorsales				
					Abductors	Abductor digiti minimi Opponens digiti minimi				
				Thumb:	MP flexor	Flex. poll. brevis				
					IP flexor	Flex. poll. longus				
					MP extensor	Ext. poll. brevis				
					IP extensor	Ext. poll. longus				
					Abductors	Abd. poll. brevis Abd. poll. longus				
					Adductors	Adductor pollicis Opponens pollicis				
				Hip:	Flexor	Iliopsoas				
					Extensor	Gluteus maximus				
					Abductor	Gluteus medius				
					Adductor group					

					Rotators
					  Lateral rotator group
					  Medial rotator group					

				Knee:	Flexors	Biceps femoris Inner hamstrings				
					Extensor	Quadriceps femoris				
				Ankle:	Plantar flexors	Gastrocnemius Soleus				
				Foot:	Invertors	Tibialis anterior Tibialis posterior				
					Evertors	Peroneus brevis Peroneus longus				
				Toes:	MP flexors	Lumbricales				

Continued.

Range of motion	Tone	Fasciculation	Strength				Range of motion	Tone	Fasciculation	Strength
				Toes—cont'd	IP flexors (first)	Flex. digit. brevis				
					IP flexors (second)	Flex. digit. longus				
					MP extensors	Ext. digit. longus Ext. digit. brevis				
				Hallux:	MP flexor	Flex. hall. brevis				
					IP flexor	Flex. hall. longus				
					MP extensor	Ext. hall. brevis				
					IP extensor	Ext. hall. longus				

Gait:

DISTINCTION BETWEEN UPPER AND LOWER MOTOR NEURON INVOLVEMENT

A concept of clinical importance in the examination of the musculoskeletal system is the distinction between upper and lower motor neuron involvement. The cells of the upper motor neurons are in the cortex and terminate in the brainstem (corticobulbar) tract or cross over in the anterior gray horn of the medulla and end in the spinal cord (corticospinal tract). The corticobulbar fibers terminate in cranial nerve nuclei.

The corticospinal axons passing through the medullary pyramids are known as the pyramidal tracts. The lower motor neurons include the cranial nerve nuclei and their axons as well as anterior horn cells of the cord and their axons.

Lesions of the upper motor neuron produce a spasticity or hypertonicity of the affected muscles, and muscle strength is diminished. Tendon stretch reflexes are brisk and Babinski's sign is present if the lesion is in the corticospinal tract. Atrophy occurs only with disuse of the muscles. By contrast, lesions of the lower motor neurons produce flaccidity or loss of muscle tone. The hypotonus leads to atrophy. Fasciculations are seen. Tendon reflexes are depressed or absent.

The distinctions between the two types of nerve involvement can often be made by palpation of the muscle and tests for muscle strength.

MUSCLE WEAKNESS

The client who has difficulty in getting up from the sitting position, who is able to rise only by pushing off with his hands and arms or by pulling himself up by grasping some nearby furniture, may have a problem involving the hip girdle musculature. Further tests would be needed to ascertain the presence of muscular dystrophy, myasthenia gravis, parkinsonism, or polymyositis. Myasthenia gravis may be more strongly suspected if the following are true: (1) The client is instructed to sit back and relax for a few minutes, after which he can rise easily; (2) the client is a woman in her 20s or a man in his 50s or 60s; (3) muscle atrophy is not present; and (4) the client has a ptosis or extraocular muscle weakness resulting in diplopia.

The presence of myasthenia gravis may be conclusively determined in the client with ptosis by the use of the Tensilon test, which is performed in the following manner. The examiner injects edrophonium (Tensilon) chloride, 2 mg, while watching the client's eyelids. If there is no change after a minute, the examiner injects another 8 mg. In 90% of clients who have myasthenia gravis the ptosis is markedly improved as muscle strength increases following the injection.

The client who has polymyositis may have pain, muscle atrophy, or a rash, particularly around the eyelids, as well as a low-grade fever.

Parkinsonism may be the underlying cause when the aging client has difficulty rising from a chair. This impression may be substantiated if the client says stiffness is one of his problems. The examiner should be alert in this case for signs of flexion posture, slow and intermittent movement, frequent tremor, masked facies, or movement of several joint units at one time because these signs are also characteristic of Parkinson's disease.

Viral, upper respiratory tract infections may be suspected in the individual who has a mild elevation in

Table 22-3. Topographical patterns of muscle palsy

Muscle weakness of paralysis	Signs	Possible etiology
Ocular	Diplopia Ptosis Strabismus	Myasthenia gravis Thyroid disease Ocular dystrophy and botulism
Bifacial	Inability to smile Inability to expose teeth Inability to close eyes	Myasthenia gravis Facioscapulohumeral dystrophy Guillain-Barré syndrome
Bulbar	Dysphonia Dysarthria Dysphagia Hanging jaw facial weakness (may or may not be present)	Myasthenia gravis Myotonic dystrophy Botulism Diphtheria Poliomyelitis Early polymyositis
Cervical	Inability to lift head from pillow (hanging head syndrome) Weakness of posterior neck muscles	Polymyositis Dermatomyositis Progressive muscular dystrophy
Bibrachial	Weakness, atrophy, and fasciculations of hands, arms, and shoulders (hanging arm syndrome)	Amyotrophic lateral sclerosis
Bicrural	Lower leg weakness Floppy feet Inability to walk on heels and toes	Diabetic polyneuropathy
Limb-girdle	Inability to raise arms Inability to rise from sitting position Difficulty in climbing stairs without use of arms Waddling gait	Polymyositis Dermatomyositis Progressive muscular dystrophy
Distal limb	Foot drop with steppage gain Weakness of all leg muscles Wrist drop—weakness of handgrips ("claw hand") (later sign)	Familial polyneuropathy
Generalized or universal	Limb and cranial muscle weakness (acute in onset and periodic) Slow onset and progressive paralysis Atrophy Fasciculations of limb and trunk muscles No sensory loss Paralysis developing over several days Mild degree of generalized weakness	Electrolyte imbalance Hypokalemia Hypocalcemia Hypomagnesemia Motor system disease Guillian-Barré syndrome Glycogen storage diseases Vitamin D deficiency
Single muscles or groups of muscles	Inability to contract affected muscles	Tyrotoxic myopathy (almost always neuropathic)

temperature and whose chief complaint revealed that he had no symptoms only a day or so before but now feels weak, almost unable to move.

If the initial examination fails to demonstrate muscular or neural disease, the possibility of fatigue should be entertained.

The client who complains of intermittent bouts of muscle weakness should be investigated for ischemic attacks, disorders of glucose metabolism (diabetes), anemia, and serum electrolyte disturbances, particularly of potassium or calcium ion concentrations.

Transient ischemic attacks (TIAs) may cause a focal episode of motor dysfunction related to vascular disease, such as arteriosclerosis or essential hypertension. It is particularly important to listen for bruits over the neck vessels in the elderly client with muscle weakness, since these bruits might strengthen the impressions of vascular disease.

Clinical correlation of signs of muscle weakness and disease entities have shown that each neuromuscular disease has a general predilection for a particular group of muscles. A given pattern of weakness, then, suggests the possibility of a certain disease and excludes others. An example lies in the adage that peripheral muscle involvement in the extremities is of muscular origin, whereas distal disease is of neuropathic origin. Further explanation of the correlation of assessment data with underlying disease processes appears in Table 22-3.

Hypokalemia

Since the ratio of the concentrations of potassium ion of the intracellular milieu to the extracellular fluid determines the rate of cell firing, a deficit of this ion is accompanied by disorders of structure and function in muscular and neural tissues. Both skeletal and smooth muscles are affected by hypokalemia. The client complains of varying degrees of weakness and lassitude. Extreme hypokalemia may be accompanied by muscular paralysis. Some other signs that will help to confirm the cause of muscle weakness as due to hypokalemia are abnormalities in motor and secretory activities of the gastrointestinal tract, changes in electrocardiograms, and dilute urine. Some of the conditions known to be correlated with a deficiency of this ion are diarrhea, excessive losses in the urine due to the use of chlorothiazide or mercurial diuretics or steroid hormones; Cushing's syndrome; and primary aldosteronism.

Age-related muscle weakness

Wasting of muscles and a decrease in muscle strength have been traditionally attributed to the aging process. Histologically, the muscle tissue shows increased amounts of collagen initially, followed by fibrosis of connective tissue.

INVOLUNTARY CONTRACTION OF SKELETAL MUSCLES
Fasciculations

Fasciculations are the visible, spontaneous contraction of a number of muscle fibers supplied by a single motor nerve filament. Visible dimpling or twitching may be seen, although there is usually insufficient power generated to move the joint.

Twitching. Fasciculations during muscular contraction occur in conditions of irritability that result in poorly coordinated contraction of small and large motor units. Benign fasciculation occurs in the nor-

mal individual and is characterized by normal muscle strength and size. Rarely, myokymia, a rippling appearance of the muscle occasioned by numerous fasciculations, is noted in a normal individual.

Fascicular twitches that occur during rest in a client with exaggerated muscular weakness and atrophy are characteristic of a peripheral motor neuron disorder. Generalized fascicular twitching occurring in a progressive, wavelike pattern over an entire muscle and progressing to complete paralysis is characteristic of certain types of poisoning (organic phosphate) and of poliomyelitis.

Cramps, spasm (Table 22-4)

Muscular spasm may occur at rest or with movement and may occur in the normal individual with metabolic and electrolyte alterations. Cramping is commonly noted following excessive sweating and with hyponatremia, hypocalcemia, hypomagnesemia, and hyperuricemia. Diseases that magnify these alterations are correlated with the presence of muscle spasm. A continuous spasm that is heightened by attempts to move the affected muscles is seen in tetanus and following the bite of the black widow spider.

Paravertebral muscle spasm is often responsible for low back pain.

Tetany. Hypocalcemia, as well as hypomagnesemia, may cause the involuntary spasms of skeletal muscle that resemble cramping. The clacium deficit causes depolarization of the distal segments of the motor nerve; furthermore, there is a change within the muscle fibers themselves since nerve section or block does not prevent these tetanic contractions. Tetanic cramps can be elicited by percussing the motor nerve leading to a muscle group at frequencies of 15 to 20 per second. *Chvostek's sign* is the spasm of the facial muscles produced by tapping over the facial nerve near its foramen of exit. The instability of the neuromuscular unit is heightened by hyperventilation (alkalosis) and hypoxia (ischemia). *Trousseau's sign* is the production of tetany of the carpal muscles following occlusion of the blood supply to the arms by a tourniquet. The client may also describe tingling and prickling paresthesia due to the stimulation of sensory nerve fibers. Electromyographic tracings show fast-frequency doublets and triplets of motor unit potentials. Tetany in its mildest form affects the distal musculature in the form of carpopedal spasm but may involve all the muscles of the body except those of the eye.

Muscle cramp. Muscle cramp frequently occurs after a day of vigorous exercise. As the feet cool, a sudden movement may trigger a strong contraction of the foot and leg. The musculature is visible, and the muscle feels hard on palpation. The spasm will cease

Table 22-4. Tremor classification

Etiology	Type and rate of movement	Description
Anxiety	Fine, rapid, 10 to 12 per second	Irregular, variable Increased by attempts to move part; decreased by relaxation of part
Parkinsonism	Fine, regular, or coarse, 2 to 5 per second	Occurs at rest May be inhibited by movement Involves flexion of finger and thumb "pill rolling" Accompanied by rigidity, "cogwheel" phenomena, bradykinesia
Cerebellar tremor	Variable rate	Evident only on movement (most prominent on finger-to-nose test) Dysmetria (seen when client is asked to pat rapidly—pats are of unequal force and do not all arrive at same point)
Essential or senile	Coarse, 3 to 7 per second	Involves the jaw, sometimes the tongue, and sometimes the entire head
Metabolic		Disappears on complete relaxation or in response to alcohol Variable Client is obviously ill; if illness is due to hepatic failure, client will have other signs, such as palpable liver, spider nevi

in response to stretch of the fibers. In the case of the gastrocnemius muscle, the stretch can be achieved by dorsiflexion of the foot. Occasionally massage is helpful in relaxing the spasm. Fasciculations may frequently be observed before and after the cramp and are further evidence of the hyperexcitability of the neuromuscular unit. Electromyogram recordings show high-frequency action potentials during the cramp. These muscle spasms have greater frequency when the client is dehydrated or sweating and in the pregnant client.

The cause of the pain associated with muscle cramp has not been determined but is thought by some to be due to the increased metabolic needs of the hyperactive muscles and to the collection of the metabolic waste products such as lactic acid within the muscle.

MUSCLE ENZYME LEVELS

Destructive diseases of striated muscle fibers result in the loss of enzymes from the intracellular compartment of the muscle. The enzymes enter the blood and can be measured. The usual laboratory analysis of serum enzymes includes alkaline phosphatase, lactic dehydrogenase (LDH), serum glutamic oxaloacetic transaminase (SGOT), and creatine phosphokinase (CPK). Enzymes are found in all tissues. Since high concentrations of these enzymes are found in the heart and liver, elevated serum level values may be due to myocardial infarction or hepatitis. However, CPK, though present in the heart and brain, is most concentrated in the striated muscle. The level may rise from a normal level of 0 to 65 inter-

national units (IU) to more than 1,000 IU in clients with destructive lesions of the striated muscles.

MYALGIA

"I hurt all over" is frequently the chief complaint for the diffuse muscle pain that accompanies many types of systemic infection, for example, influenza, measles, rheumatic fever, brucellosis, dengue fever, or salmonellosis. Soreness and aching are other descriptive terms for this type of involvement. Little is known of the cause. Fibromyositis (myogelosis) is the term used to describe the inflammation of the fibrous tissue in muscle, fascia, and nerves. The client may complain of pain and tenderness in a muscle after exposure to cold, dampness, or minor trauma.

Firm, tender zones occasionally several centimeters in diameter are found on palpation. Palpation, active contraction, or passive stretching increases the pain. Intense pain localized to a smaller group of muscles may be due to epidemic myalgia, also called pleurodynia, "painful neck," or "devil's grip." Intense pain at the beginning of neurological involvement has been seen in poliomyelitis and herpes zoster.

The pain of poliomyelitis is described as marked during the initial involvement of the nerve, whereas the later sensation of the paralyzed muscle is said to be one of aching. The segmental pattern of the intense pain of herpes zoster is caused by the inflammation of spinal nerves and dorsal root ganglia that occurs 3 to 4 days prior to the skin eruption.

The initial symptoms of rheumatoid arthritis may

be diffuse muscular soreness and aching, which may antedate the joint involvement by weeks or months. The muscles are tender, and the client describes the pain as occurring not at the time of activity but hours later. An increased sedimentation rate or a positive latex fixation test may support the conclusion of rheumatoid involvement.

ELECTROMYOGRAPHY

The electromyogram is the graph generated from the electrical potential of individual muscles. The test is accomplished by inserting needles directly into the muscle being studied and recording the potential with the muscle at rest, with slight voluntary contractions, and at maximal flexion. Whereas the heart can be sampled from a number of surface electrode positions, the skeletal muscles are variable in size, widely separated, and numerous. Therefore, no small number of leads can give an adequate picture of their activity. Furthermore, surface electrodes yield only a summation of the underlying activity. To ascertain the bursts of individual muscle units, sterile needle electrodes must be used to register the activity.

Thus, the electromyogram must be done for one muscle at a time. Information obtained from the tracing is useful in determining neural adequacy of the muscle and the presence of intrinsic muscle disease.

MUSCLE BIOPSY

Muscle biopsy was first used by Cachenne in 1868. Currently the use of muscle biopsy is believed to be indicated for five clinical problems: (1) atrophy of the muscle that is progressive (when doubt exists as to whether the disease is myogenic or neurogenic); (2) localized inflammatory disease of the muscle wherein biopsy may contribute to isolating the causative agent, thus allowing institution of the appropriate therapeutic regimen; (3) certain metabolic diseases wherein the histological or biological data, or both, thus provided may help to identify the disease; (4) fever associated with many visceral and cutaneous lesions wherein biopsy of the muscle may reveal further connective tissue and vascular involvement to support the conclusions of a generalized involvement; and (5) trauma wherein the biopsy may further define the degree of nerve and muscle injury.

ASSESSMENT OF GAIT

Gait is evaluated in both phases—the stance and the swing—for rhythm and smoothness. *Stance* is considered to consist of three processes: (1) heel strike—the heel contacts the floor or ground; (2) mid-stance—body weight is transferred from the heel to the ball of the foot; and (3) push-off—the heel leaves the ground (see General assessment).

The *swing* phase also consists of three processes: (1) acceleration; (2) swing through—the lifted foot travels ahead of the weight-bearing foot; and (3) deceleration—the foot slows in preparation for the heel strike.

The description of the observation of the client's gait should include: *phase* (conformity); *cadence* (symmetry, regular rhythm); *stride length* (symmetry, length of swing); *trunk posture* (related to phases); *pelvic posture* (related to phases); and *arm swing* (symmetry, length of swing).

If pain is present, it should be described in relationship to the phases of gait.

EXAMINATION OF BONES AND JOINTS
Bones

Bones are examined for deformity or tumors. Bones are also examined for integrity by testing resistance to a deforming force. Palpation of the bone is performed to assess the presence of pain or tenderness. Tenderness of a bone may indicate tumor, inflammation, or the aftermath of a trauma. Frequently, traumatic injuries are associated with damage to both bone and nerve. Paralysis of the ulnar and median nerves in the hand is frequently the result of a hand injury and may result in a clawlike posture of the hand.

Joints

Pain, swelling, partial or complete loss of mobility, stiffness, weakness, and fatigue are the signs and symptoms most frequently associated with disorders of the joints. Joint disease may be indicated by skin that feels warm, is red, has lesions, or is ulcerated. In the condition of psoriatic arthritis the lesions and the nails have been shown to be involved in about 50% of cases. Pitting is the most commonly recognized change. There may be isolated pitting of a single nail or the pitting may be *uniformly* distributed across all the nails.

Pain. *Pain* is the symptom that most frequently causes the client to seek help and understanding the character of the pain may be helpful in determining its cause in the physical assessment of the involved joints. The client should be encouraged to try to recall those events occurring prior to the onset of pain because most individuals tend to forget minor injuries or unusual physical activity in the weeks before the pain began. The client is unlikely to correlate symptoms and signs of infection in the months before with his current joint pain. The nature of the onset of pain is also important because rheumatoid symptoms are known to begin gradually, whereas gouty attacks are characterized by sudden onset that frequently wakes the client from sleep.

The client frequently has difficulty in localizing the pain associated with joint disease. His description may involve large areas of the body, that is, "my neck" (while moving his hand from his head to the thoracic vertebra), "my back," or "all down my arm." This difficulty in localizing the pain may be related to whether the pain is deep or superficial and whether a nerve is involved.

The locations or distribution of the pain may also provide valuable information. Rheumatoid involvement is known to be migratory, that is, involving first one joint, which improves, then another. On the other hand most infectious arthritis is confined to one joint. The joint involvement in rheumatoid arthritis tends to be symmetrical, whereas that of gout, psoriatic arthritis, and Reiter's syndrome tends to occur initially in one or two joints but becomes polyarticular in later stages. Spondylitis is first detected in the spine and then spreads to peripheral joints (centrifugal spread), whereas rheumatoid arthritis starts peripherally in the hands and feet and then involves the large joints of the hips, shoulders, and spine in the later stages of the disease (centripetal spread).

The time that pain occurs may also be diagnostic. The individual with osteoarthritis generally reports that the pain is made worse by increased use of the affected joint and, thus, frequently has pain later in the day or when tired. The individual with rheumatoid arthritis generally reports stiffness and pain that occurs early in the morning and some improvement when he forces himself to exercise the part.

Questions directed to a description of referred pain may prove helpful. Spinal nerve root involvement is frequently felt in peripheral tissues. For instance, lumbosacral nerve root irritation (sciatica) may be experienced as pain in the thigh or the knee on the involved side. The area of referred pain corresponds with the segmental innervation of the structures. The description of this type of pain may include words associated with paresthesias, that is, "prickling," "like an electric shock," "pins and needles," and "numbing." Pain of muscle origin may be described by such words as "pulled" or "charleyhorse." Joint pain descriptions may be noted along a spectrum from dull, aching, or stiff to excruciating and intolerable.

A knowledge of those measures known to alleviate the pain may also be valuable diagnostically. Some of these have already been discussed, for example, exercise for rheumatoid arthritis and rest for osteoarthritis.

Limitation of range of motion. The client may voluntarily limit the motion of a joint in response to pain. Spasm of the muscles involved in the movement of a joint may limit its motion. Mechanical obstruction to movement may accompany bony overgrowth as well as scar tissue. Limitation of motion in a joint is accompanied by weakness and atrophy of the muscles that are involved.

Deformity. Deformities of the joint include absorption of tissues, flexion contracture, and bony overgrowth. Absorption may produce a flail joint such that the bones making the joint move erratically. Deformities result from scarring phenomena following inflammation and infection.

Swelling. The amount of swelling of the joint may range from difficult to detect to visually evident fluid within the joint, that is, visible or palpable as a bulging of the joint capsule. Pressure on the sac at one point causes the fluid within to shift and may lead to bulging at another site. The sac may feel from soft to tense and the involvement may be symmetrical or unilateral. Frequently the swelling is fusiform. Redness, warmth, swelling, and pain in a joint are the classical descriptors of an inflammatory process. The inflammation may be within the joint itself or in the soft tissue surrounding it. Swelling may also result from intraarticular effusion, synovial thickening, or bony overgrowth. The swelling may also result from the deposition of fat in the region adjacent to the joint.

The synovial membrane is not palpable in normal joints. The palpation of a "boggy" or "doughy" consistency generally indicates a thickened or otherwise abnormal synovial membrane.

Heberden's or Bouchard's nodules of the fingers or bony spurs, particularly the knees, are typical of osteoarthritis.

Crepitation. Crepitation (crackling or grating sounds) produced by motion of the joint is caused by irregularities of the articulating surfaces. The coarseness of surface may involve the cartilage or the bony capsule.

A systematic assessment of individual joints may be made during the performance of the head to toe physical examination or all of the joints may be examined at a preselected time during the examination. As with all bilateral structures, the paired joints should be compared.

The joints that are given special consideration are the temporomandibular, sternoclavicular, manubriosternal, shoulder, elbow, wrist, hip, knee, and ankle.

TEMPOROMANDIBULAR JOINT

The temporomandibular joint is the articulation between the mandible and the temporal bone (Fig. 22-24). The joint is divided into two cavities by a fibrocartilaginous disc. Swelling is observed as a tumescence over the joint but must be considerable in order for it to be visible. Palpation is accomplished

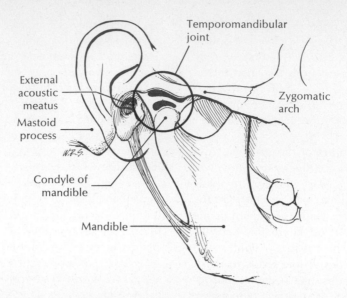

Fig. 22-24. The temporomandibular joint. A fibrocartilaginous disc divides the articulation point into two synovial cavities. Note the proximity to external acoustic meatus.

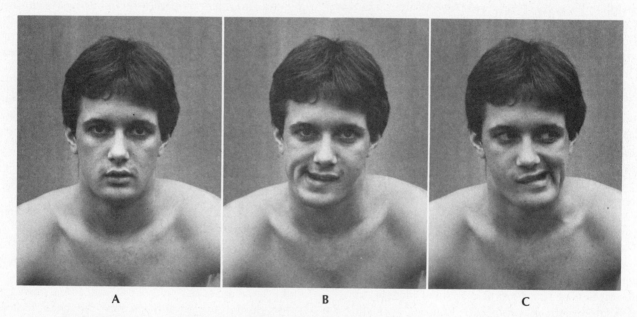

A   **B**   **C**

Fig. 22-25. Lateral motion is determined by asking the client to move the lower jaw from side to side. The distance measured is the distance the midline of the lower lip deviates in each direction. The midline of the stationary upper lip may be used as the baseline.

by placing the fingertips anterior to the external meatus of the ear. In the normal joint, there is a depression over the joint. Swelling may make this indentation difficult to feel. The jaw is palpated while it is moved through its range of motion: opening and closure of the mouth, protrusion (jutting of the jaw), retrusion (tucking in of chin), and side-to-side sliding of the mandible. The normal range of distance between the upper and lower incisors is 3 to 6 cm. Lateral motion of the jaw may be measured by asking the client to protrude the jaw and move it from side to

side. The distance is measured by the distance that the midline of the lower lip deviates in each direction. The normal range of motion is 1 to 2 cm (Fig. 22-25). "Clicks" may be heard on movement and may be regarded as normal.

STERNOCLAVICULAR JOINT

The sternoclavicular joint is located at the juncture of the clavicle and the manubrium of the sternum. The joint is divided into two synovial cavities by a disc of cartilage and fibrous material. The joint

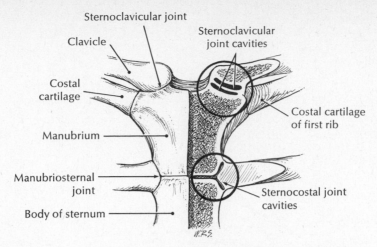

Fig. 22-26. The sternoclavicular joint is divided into two synovial cavities. Movement of the shoulder girdle may cause pain when these joints are diseased. The manubriosternal joint examination is largely by inspection and palpation since these joints move minimally.

is reinforced by a fibrous capsule and ligaments (Fig. 22-26). The obtuse angle formed by the junction of the manubrium and body of the sternum is called the angle of Louis and has been used as a landmark for counting the ribs. Observation of this joint is readily accomplished because there is little tissue overlying it. Swelling, redness, bony overgrowth, and dislocation are not difficult to see. Swelling of the joint appears as a smooth, round bulge. While this joint is often overlooked, it is often involved following surgery of the neck. Palpation is done with the fingertips. Movements of the shoulder are dependent on the normal function of this joint. Inflammation of the sternoclavicular joint may result in pain on movement of the shoulder girdle.

MANUBRIOSTERNAL JOINT

The hyaline cartilage–lined joint covers the articular surface of the second rib and those of the manubrium and body of the sternum (Fig. 22-26). Little tissue overlies this joint. Observation is thus a more accurate method of examination. Observation is the only technique of examination because movement of the joint is minimal.

SHOULDER JOINT (GLENOHUMORAL)

The shoulder joint is a ball-and-socket joint that is the articulation of the humerus and the glenoid fossa of the scapula (Fig. 22-27). Protection of the joint is afforded by muscles and ligaments. A fibrous capsule surrounds the joint completely. Overlying these structures is the subacromial bursa. The portion of the bursa that lies beneath the deltoid is called the subdeltoid bursa. The clavicle and the acromion process of the scapula are articulated by the acromioclavicular joint. Inspection may reveal anterior dislo-

cation of the shoulder as flattening of the lateral aspect of the shoulder. Swelling of the joint as a result of fluid collection may be observed only when the amount of fluid is moderate to large. Visible swelling is generally observed over the anterior aspect of the shoulder. Palpation should include the joint and bursal sites. In the event that neoplasia or infection are suspected, the axilla is palpated for lymph nodes. Special attention is also given to the tendons of the teres minor and infraspinatus muscles (called the rotator cuff). These tendons are palpated for swelling, nodes, tears, and pain. The client is instructed to adduct the arm by bringing it over the chest. The examiner, standing in front of the client, puts his thumb on the anterior surface of the joint and the tips of the fingers on the posterior aspect. The client is asked to move the humerus backward about 20 degrees. Moving behind the client and with the fingertips over the head of the humerus, the examiner asks the client to move his arm behind his body (internal rotation) with the hand between the scapulae.

ELBOW JOINT

The elbow is the articulation of the humerus, radius, and ulna (Fig. 22-28). The three articulating surfaces are enclosed in a single synovial cavity. The synovial membrane is generally only palpable on the posterior aspect of the joint. Radial and ulnar ligaments provide protection to the joint. The olecranon bursa is the largest bursa of the elbow, although several smaller bursae are present. Swelling and redness are easily observed over the posterior aspect of the elbow. Palpation is accomplished with the tips of the fingers while applying pressure on the opposite side of the joint with the thumb of the dominant hand and while supporting the arm with the other. The

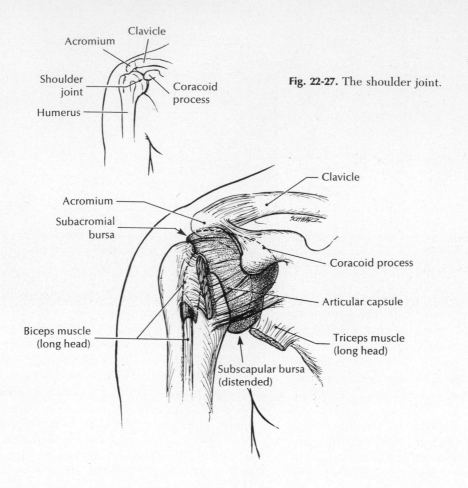

Fig. 22-27. The shoulder joint.

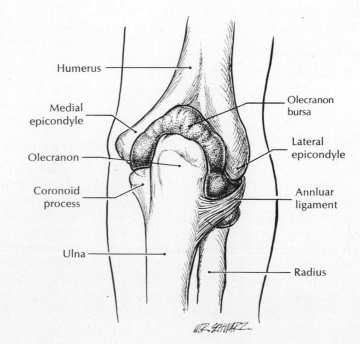

Fig. 22-28. The elbow joint, posterior view.

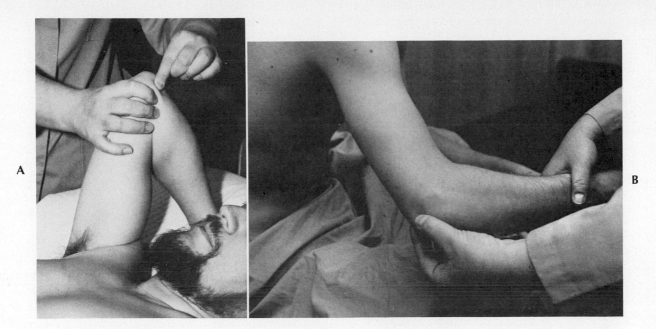

Fig. 22-29. A, Examination of the extensor surface of the elbow joint in the supine position. **B,** Examination of the extensor surface of the elbow joint in the sitting position.

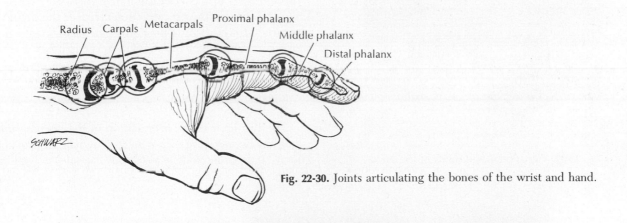

Radius   Carpals   Metacarpals   Proximal phalanx   Middle phalanx   Distal phalanx

Fig. 22-30. Joints articulating the bones of the wrist and hand.

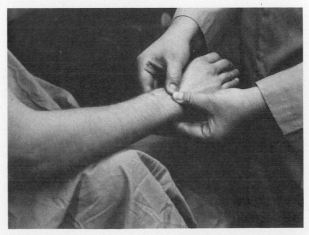

Fig. 22-31. Examination of the wrist.

client's arm is flexed 70 degrees. Joint swelling is most often palpable in the medial groove (Fig. 22-29).

WRIST JOINT

The wrist joint contains the points of articulation between the distal radius and the proximal portions of the following carpal bones; scaphoid or navicular, lunate, and triangular (Fig. 22-30). An articular disc divides the radius from the ulnar bone and also separates the radius from the wrist joint. The wrist joint is protected by a fibrous capsule as well as ligaments. The joint is lined by synovial membrane.

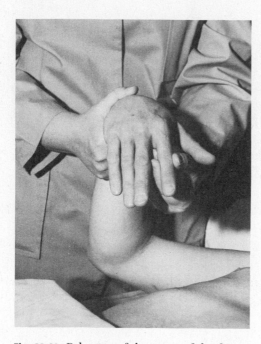

Fig. 22-32. Palpation of the joints of the finger.

Swelling of the wrist joint is most frequently observed on the dorsal surface distal to the ulnar tip. Two hands for palpation are used such that the thumb and index fingers are opposed on either side of the wrist. Enough pressure is applied to outline bony and soft tissue structures (Fig. 22-31).

CARPAL, METACARPAL, AND PHALANGEAL JOINTS

The joints between the carpal, metacarpal, and phalangeal bones are also examined by observation and palpation. Swelling is easily observed over the dorsal surface of the hand because there is little tissue over the joints. The thumb and index fingers are used to palpate the entire perimeter of each of these joints (Fig. 22-32).

Carpal tunnel syndrome. Thickening of the flexor tendon sheath of the median nerve may lead to feelings of numbness and paresthesia. The thickness of the sheath may be observed on the palmar surface of the wrist. In addition, tests may elicit these altered sensory phenomena. In the first of these tests, the client is asked to maintain palmar flexion for 1 minute. The experience of numbness and paresthesia over the palmar surface of the hand and the first three fingers and part of the fourth is called Phalen's sign. The symptoms resolve quickly after the hand is returned to the resting position. The second test consists of tapping over the median nerve (palmar aspect of wrist). The client's sensation of tingling or prickling is known as Tinel's sign.

HIP JOINT

The hip joint is the articulation of the acetabulum and the femur (Fig. 22-33). It is a ball-and-socket joint. It is protected by a fibrous capsule as well as

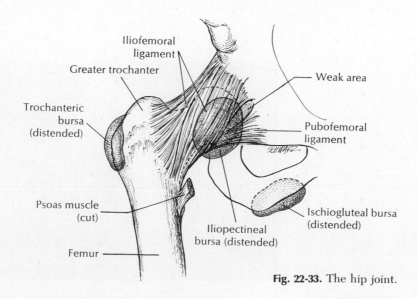

Fig. 22-33. The hip joint.

ligaments. Three bursae reduce friction in the hip: (1) the trochanteric, between the posterolateral greater trochanter and the gluteus maximus; (2) the ileopectineal, between the anterior surface of the joint and the iliopsoas muscle; and (3) the ischiogluteal, situated over the ischial tuberosity. Inspection of the hip joint includes an assessment of gait. Antalgic limp is characteristic of disease that produces pain in a hip joint. Antalgic limp is seen as a body tilt toward the involved diseased hip such that the weight of the body is directly over the hip. This decreases the need for abductor muscle movement and thus may decrease muscle spasm. If the abductor muscles are weak, that is, unable to support the pelvis, the unaffected hip may move downward such that the weight is borne on that side. This is called Trendelenberg's limp.

The synovial cavity of the hip is generally not palpated, even when it is distended. The bursae are not palpable unless they are swollen. Swelling and tenderness are the diagnostic findings of pathology of these structures.

KNEE JOINT

The knee joint is the articulation of the femur, tibia, and patella (Fig. 22-34). The lining of the joint is a fibrous membrane. Synovial membrane covers the articular surface of the femur and tibia with folds to the patella. The medial and lateral menisci are fibrocartilaginous discs whose outside edges (horns) are attached to the tibia and continuous with the articular capsule. The medial convexity of the femur rotates with the inner portion of the meniscus attached to it. A spiral distortion of the menisci occurs on rotation, making them susceptible to rupture. The surfaces of the menisci have no synovial membrane. They are thought to aid in the spread of synovial fluid and this may account for their existence. An anterior pouch in the knee joint that separates the patella and quadriceps tendon and muscle from the femur is called the suprapatellar pouch.

The bursae of the knee are numerous. On the anterior knee the prepatellar bursa lies immediately in front of the patella. The superficial infrapatellar bursa lies anterior to the patellar ligament, while the deep infrapatellar bursa is behind the ligament. Those of the posterior knee include the two gastrocnemius bursae, one of which separates the lateral head of the gastrocnemius muscle from the articular capsule and the other of which separates the medial head of the gastrocnemius from the articular capsule. In addition, there is a large bursa separating the medial head of the gastrocnemius muscle from the semimembranosus muscle.

Inspection of the knee should be made with the patient walking (to observe gait), sitting, supine with knees extended. The examiner should be familiar with the normal contour of the knee, because loss of the contour may occur with swelling. The client may voluntarily maintain the knee at 15 to 20 degrees of flexion because the knee joint is at maximum capacity at this angle and, thus, pain is reduced. Swelling as a result of synovitis is most apparent at the suprapatellar pouch. Swelling as a result of meniscal cysts is observed at the lateral or the medial joint surface. Popliteal swelling is more obvious when the knee is extended. Swelling of the knee observed on the anterior aspect of the knee is called "housemaid's knee."

Palpation of the knee may be performed with the client in the sitting or supine position, whichever affords more comfort for the client. Palpation of the suprapatellar pouch (Fig. 22-35) is accomplished with the thumb and fingers of one hand while the other hand is used to push the contents of the articular cavity upward. To do this the thumb is placed on the lateral surface of the joint posterior to the patella with the fingers on the other lateral surface such that the arch formed by thumb and fingers is below the patella. An inward and upward pressure thus applied moves fluid upward into the suprapatellar bursa. The examining hand is placed about 10 cm above the patella and moves gradually to the patella.

A second procedure for the palpation of the knee (Fig. 22-36) involves applying downward pressure over the suprapatellar pouch in order to localize the synovial fluid in the lower portion of the articular cavity. The other hand is used to palpate the lateral and medial joint surfaces with the fingers while steadying with the thumb. In instances when considerable fluid is in the suprapatellar pouch, ballottement of the patella may be possible (Fig. 22-37). Ballottement is accomplished by applying downward pressure with one hand while the patella is pushed backward against the femur with a finger of the opposite hand. The popliteal region may be examined with the client in the prone position or standing. Swelling of the joint in the popliteal region is called a "Baker's cyst" and is generally an extension of the articular cavity.

Sprains or tears of the ligaments are the most common injuries of the knee. Two sets of ligaments play a role in movement of the knee. They are the anterior and posterior cruciate ligaments and medial and lateral collateral ligaments. The anterior cruciate ligament limits extension and rotation, while the posterior stabilizes the femur against forward dislocation. The collateral ligaments prevent lateral dislocation of

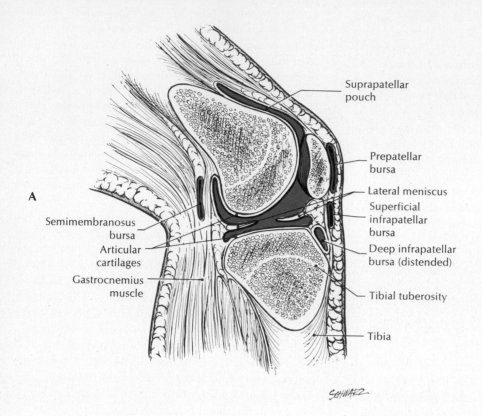

Suprapatellar pouch

Prepatellar bursa

Lateral meniscus

Superficial infrapatellar bursa

Deep infrapatellar bursa (distended)

Tibial tuberosity

Tibia

A

Semimembranosus bursa

Articular cartilages

Gastrocnemius muscle

SCHWARZ

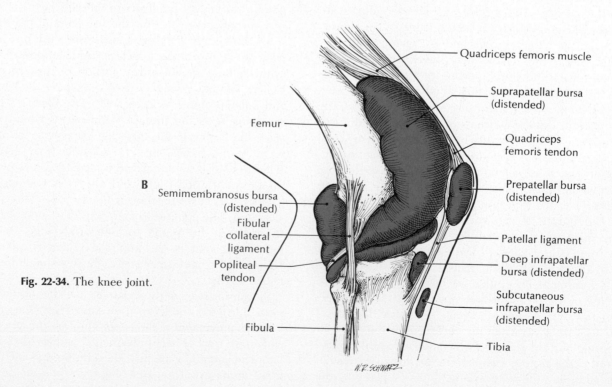

Quadriceps femoris muscle

Suprapatellar bursa (distended)

Quadriceps femoris tendon

Prepatellar bursa (distended)

Patellar ligament

Deep infrapatellar bursa (distended)

Subcutaneous infrapatellar bursa (distended)

Tibia

Femur

B

Semimembranosus bursa (distended)

Fibular collateral ligament

Popliteal tendon

Fibula

W.R.SCHWARZ

Fig. 22-34. The knee joint.

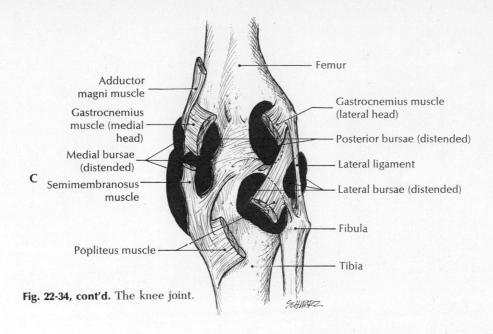

Femur

Adductor
magni muscle

Gastrocnemius
muscle (medial
head)

Medial bursae
(distended)

C

Semimembranosus
muscle

Popliteus muscle

Gastrocnemius muscle
(lateral head)

Posterior bursae (distended)

Lateral ligament

Lateral bursae (distended)

Fibula

Tibia

Fig. 22-34, cont'd. The knee joint.

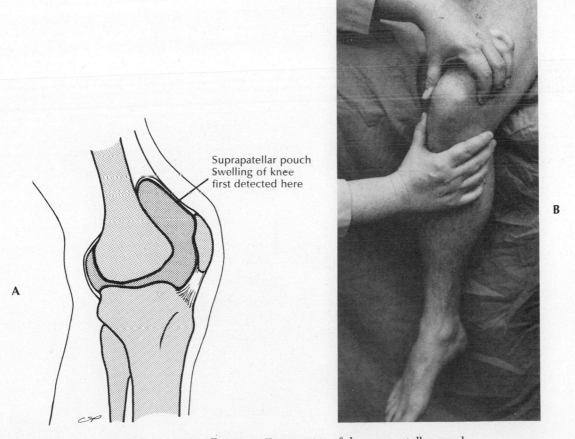

Suprapatellar pouch
Swelling of knee
first detected here

A

B

Fig. 22-35. A, Knee effusion. **B,** Examination of the suprapatellar pouch.

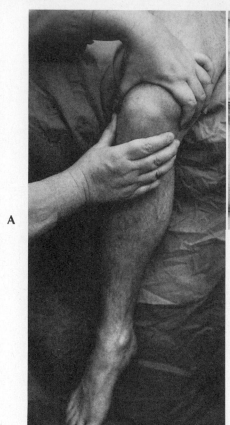

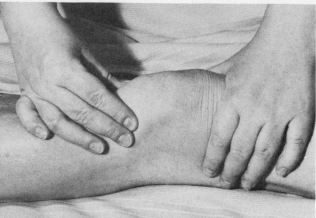

Fig. 22-36. Examination of the lateral aspects of the knee. A, Sitting. B, Supine.

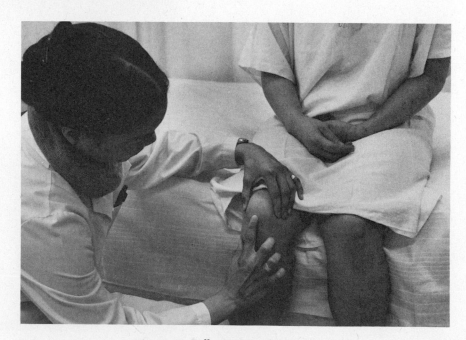

Fig. 22-37. Ballottement of the patella.

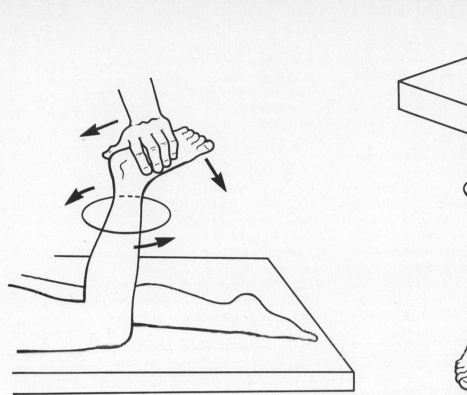

Fig. 22-38. Elicitation of Apley's sign.

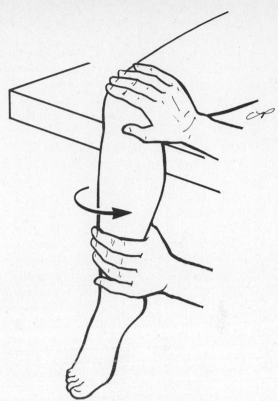

Fig. 22-39. Elicitation of McMurray's sign.

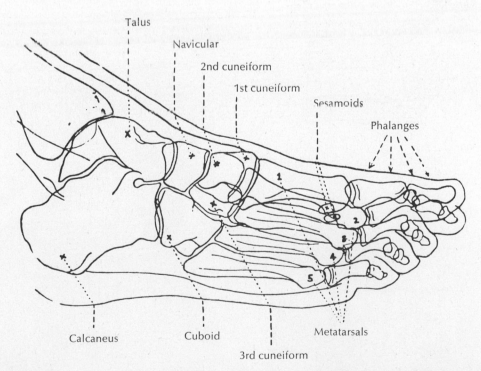

Talus

Navicular

2nd cuneiform

1st cuneiform

Sesamoids

Phalanges

Calcaneus

Cuboid

3rd cuneiform

Metatarsals

Fig. 22-40. Bones of the ankle and foot. (From Mann, R. A.: DuVries' surgery of the foot, ed. 4, St. Louis, 1978, The C. V. Mosby Co.)

the knee. Abnormal movements of the knee may indicate dislocation. The tears may be palpated in the assessment of the knee.

Indications of pathology of menisci include (1) pain or tenderness on the lateral surfaces of the knee joint; (2) popping, snapping, or grating sounds with movement; and (3) inability to fully extend the knee. The medial meniscus is more often injured than the lateral.

Tests for a foreign body in the knee

APLEY'S SIGN. An attempt is made to elicit Apley's sign (Fig. 22-38) in the client who is suspected of having a loose object in the knee joint or who has given a history of knee joint locking. The client assumes the prone position with the suspected knee flexed to 90 degrees. The tibia is firmly opposed to the femur by exerting downward pressure on the foot. The leg is rotated externally and internally. Locking of the knee (positive sign) or the sound of clicks may indicate that a loose body, such as torn cartilage, is trapped in the articulation. Clicks or popping sounds are generated as the object escapes.

MCMURRAY'S SIGN. An attempt is made to elicit McMurray's sign (Fig. 22-39) in the individual who says he "feels something in the knee joint" or complains that "sometimes it just won't bend." The test may be performed with the client in the sitting position and while obtaining as much flexion of the suspected knee as possible. The leg is internally rotated while it is slowly being extended with one hand. The other hand is used to provide resistance at the medial aspect of the knee. Extension of the knee may not be possible (positive sign) if a loose body impedes its movement. The procedure may be repeated employing external rotation and resistance applied to the lateral aspect of the knee.

ANKLE AND FOOT JOINTS

The ankle joint is the articulation between the tibia, fibula, and the talus (Fig. 22-40). The capsule is lined with synovia. The ankle joint is protected by ligaments on the medial and lateral surfaces but not on the anterior or posterior surfaces.

Talocalcaneal joint. The joint between the talus and calcaneous bones is called the talocalcaneal or subtalar joint. The forward extension of the joint cavity is the articulation of the talus and the navicular bones. Articular capsules lined with synovial membrane separate the remainder of the tarsal, metatarsal, and phalangeal bones of the foot.

Inspection of the ankle and foot is made with the client standing, walking, and sitting (not bearing weight). Swelling is best observed over the dorsal aspect of the foot because there is less tissue over the

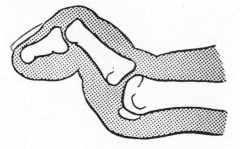

Fig. 22-41. Hammered great toe. (From Mann, R. A.: DuVries's surgery of the foot, ed. 4, St. Louis, 1978, The C. V. Mosby Co.)

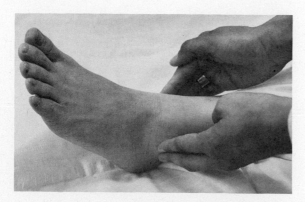

Fig. 22-42. Examination of the ankle joint.

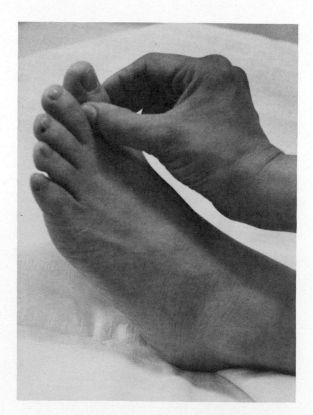

Fig. 22-43. Examination of the joint of the toe.

bone. Hallux valgus is lateral deformity of the great toe such that it may lie above or below the second toe. The metatarsophalangeal joint is distorted in such a way that the first metatarsal bone is angled medially. A callus or bursal distention generally occurs at the joint. Hammer toe is a result of hyperextension of the metatarsophalangeal joint and flexion of the proximal phalangeal joint (Fig. 22-41).

Palpation of the ankle and foot is best accomplished with the fingertips of one hand while holding the foot behind the ankle with the other (Fig. 22-42). The metatarsal and phalangeal joints are palpated with the fingers on the anterior surface and the thumb on the sole surface (Fig. 22-43).

Results of examination of these joints may be conveniently summarized on a diagram by circling the joint involved (Fig. 22-44) and briefly noting any pathology.

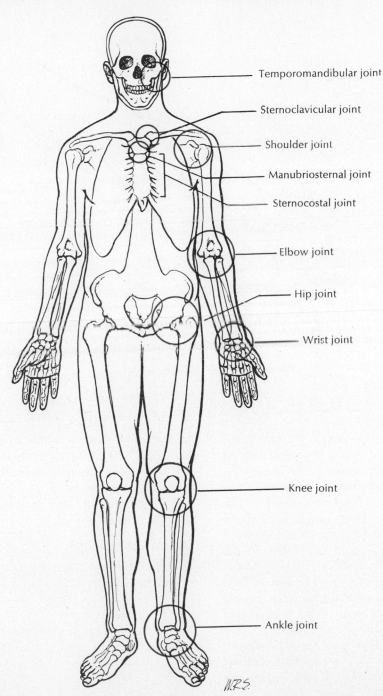

Fig. 22-44. Results of the examination of joints may be summarized by circling the joint involved and briefly noting the pathology.

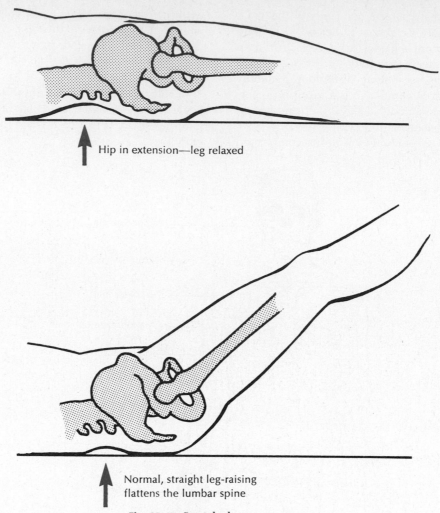

Hip in extension—leg relaxed

Normal, straight leg-raising
flattens the lumbar spine

Fig. 22-45. Straight leg-raising test.

Straight leg-raising test. The straight leg-raising test (Fig. 22-45) is useful in defining herniated lumbar disc as the cause of sciatic nerve pain. The test is indicated for those individuals who complain of low back pain or of pain that radiates down the leg. The test is performed with the client lying on his back on a firm surface. The leg and thigh should be as relaxed as possible. The extended leg is raised behind the heel maintaining the heel and the foot in dorsiflexion until the client complains of pain. The foot is then dorsiflexed. Pain induced in this manner is caused by pressure on the dorsal roots of the lumbosacral nerves and is characteristic of herniated disc. The other leg is treated similarly and results are compared. In the normal person, the leg may be flexed to 90 degrees without pain. Nerve root irritation is suggested by pain in lumbar, hip, or posterior leg or muscle spasm.

In flexion of the hip in the normal individual the lumbar spine flattens in the lumbar region. For the individual with an immobile hip continued flexion of the lumbar spine is seen when the leg is raised. Extending the leg stretches the ligaments and extensor muscles of the hip. Pain may indicate pathology in these structures.

SUMMARY

I. Muscle
   A. Inspection
      1. Size—swelling
      2. Shape
      3. Involuntary movement
   B. Palpation
      1. Tenderness
      2. Masses
      3. Heat
   C. Range of motion against resistance—screening examination

1. Position
   a. Head extension and flexion
   b. Arm extension and flexion
   c. Wrist extension and flexion
   d. Finger extension and flexion
   e. Leg extension and flexion
   f. Ankle extension and flexion
2. Standing
   a. Back posture—flexion and rotation
3. Walk on toes, heels, hop

II. Joints
   A. Inspection
      1. Size—swelling
      2. Shape—contractures
      3. Redness
   B. Palpation
      1. Effusion
      2. Heat
      3. Masses
   C. Auscultation—crepitation
   D. Range of motion

BIBLIOGRAPHY

Adams, R.: Diseases of the muscle, New York, 1975, Harper and Row, Publishers.

Beetham, W., and others: Physical examination of the joints, Philadelphia, 1965, W. B. Saunders Co.

Daniels, L., and Worthingham, C.: Muscle testing; techniques of manual examination, ed. 3, Philadelphia, 1972, W. B. Saunders Co.

Enneking, W. F., and Sherrard, M. G.: Physical diagnosis of the musculoskeletal system, Gainesville, Fla., 1969, Storter Printing Co., Inc.

Goodgold, J., and Eberstein, A.: Electrodiagnosis of neuromuscular diseases, Baltimore, 1972, The Williams & Wilkins Co.

Inman, V. T.: DuVries surgery of the foot, St. Louis, 1973, The C. V. Mosby Co.

Joint motion; method of measuring and recording, Chicago, 1965, American Academy of Orthopaedic Surgeons.

Knapp, M. E.: Electromyography, Postgrad. Med. 47:213, 1970.

Layzer, R. B., and Rowland, L. P.: Cramps, N. Engl. J. Med. 285:31, 1971.

McCarty, D. J.: Arthritis, ed. 9, Philadelphia, 1979, Lea & Febiger.

Moosa, A.: Paediatric electrodiagnosis, Arch. Dis. Child 46(6):149, 1972.

Polley, H. F., and Hunder, G. G.: Physical examination of the joints, Philadelphia, 1978, W. B. Saunders Co.

Rosse, C., and Clawson, D.: Introduction to the musculoskeletal system, New York, 1970, Harper and Row, Publishers.

Walton, J. N.: Disorders of voluntary muscle, ed. 3, Baltimore, 1974, The Williams and Wilkins Co.

Yates, D. A.: The electrodiagnosis of muscle disorders, Proc. R. Soc. Med. 65:617, 1972.

23 Neurological assessment

The neural system provides integration for all the functions of the body, but it also derives its homeostatic balance from the appropriate functioning of the peripheral organs. The cells of the central nervous system, for example, depend on an adequate supply of glucose for their metabolic processes, and this supply can be maintained only when those tissues that play a role in intermediary metabolism function well. This balance makes neurological assessment a part of all the components of the history and the physical examination.

The neurological system controls cognitive and voluntary behavioral processes as well as the subconscious and involuntary bodily functions of the organism. The major functions of the nervous system are reception (sensory), integration, and adaptation. That is, the normal nervous system receives stimuli from the environment, compares the adaptive processes necessary to adjustment to the environment with the functions the body is currently employing, and effects changes as necessary to assure homeokinesis or survival.

Equipment needed for neurological assessment includes vials of coffee, vanilla, tobacco, and oil of cloves for olfactory assessment, and vials of glucose solution (sweet), salt solution, vinegar or lemon juice (sour), and quinine (bitter) for taste assessment. Test tubes of water are used for assessment of hot and cold temperature perception. Also necessary are an ophthalmoscope, a Snellen chart for visual acuity, a Rosenbaum pocket-vision screener, a tuning fork, a reflex hammer, a tongue blade, an applicator, and a wisp of cotton.

The mental status examination is an integral part of the neurological examination. In the context of the total assessment of health, however, this appraisal occurs much earlier in the examination. Most examiners make assessments of mental status while obtaining the client's history and do special tests immediately afterward.

CRANIAL NERVE FUNCTION
CN I: olfactory nerve

The olfactory nerve is sensory in function and makes possible the sense of smell, or olfaction.

The peripheral neurons of the olfactory nerve are bipolar neurons. The ciliated, distal neurons penetrate the nasal mucosa in the roof of the nose, the upper septum, and the medial wall of the superior nasal concha. Unless the individual sniffs or inspires deeply, most of the inspired air does not contact the olfactory epithelium; during normal respiration inspired air does not rise this high in the nares. Deep inspiration or sniffing causes a sudden rush of air into the upper nose, as well as initiating swirling or turbulence of air around the olfactory mucosa. The central, unmyelinated axons are grouped in 15 to 20 bundles that pass through the cribriform plate of the ethmoid bone to synapse within the olfactory bulb. The second-order neurons course posteriorly from the bulb to the olfactory trigone, where they divide into medial and lateral striae. The medial striae terminate in the cortex of the medial subcallosal gyrus and the inferior portion of the cingulate gyrus. The lateral striae terminate in the uncus, the anterior portion of the hippocampal gyrus, and amygdaloid

---

Physical examination

The remainder of the neurological physical examination may be performed as five areas of investigation:

1. Assessment of cranial nerve function
2. Assessment of proprioception and cerebellar function
3. Musculoskeletal assessment (see Chapter 22)
4. Assessment of sensory function
5. Assessment of reflexes

nucleus. Testing of the sense of smell is a test of the integrity of the entire system. When the same odor is smelled continuously, the olfactory cells are thought to be fatigued because a decreased awareness of odor is reported on long exposures.

CLINICAL EXAMINATION

The client is asked to close his eyes (if the substance can be identified visually), occlude one nostril, and attempt to identify familiar substances with the open one, sniffing or inhaling deeply. The substances should be mildly aromatic (volatile oils and liquids) and unambiguous, such as coffee, cigarettes, soap, peanut butter, toothpaste, oranges, vanilla, chocolate, and oils of wintergreen, lemon, lime, almond, and cloves. It has been shown that the most easily identified substances are coffee, oil of almond, chocolate, and oil of lime. Strongly aromatic compounds should be avoided in determining olfactory function because the vapors may prevent the perception of weaker substances. Substances that stimulate either gustatory receptors or trigeminal branches of the nasal mucosa should also be avoided, including chloroform, oil of peppermint, camphor, ammonia, alcohol, and formaldehyde.

The substances are housed in test tubes that are kept closed until the examiner is prepared to present them to the client.

The client is asked whether he smells anything; then he attempts to identify the substance. The process is repeated for each nostril in order to determine symmetry (Fig. 23-1).

Both the number of substances used as stimuli and the number of correct responses should be recorded, along with differences in sensitivity from one nostril to the other.

If the client has difficulty identifying substances, he should be asked whether he is able to smell anything at all. In addition, the examiner should determine whether the nasal passages are patent.

Anosmia is the loss of the sense of smell or the inability to discriminate vapors. Diminution of the ability to smell is termed hyposmia. The client is not always aware of a deficit in olfaction. A pathophysiological condition of the nasal mucosa or olfactory bulb or tract can interfere with the sensation of smell.

The individual with an impaired sense of smell also has difficulty in identifying flavors. Since the tongue has receptors for only sweet, salt, sour, and bitter, these must be regarded as the true tastes and will be retained in hyposmia and anosmia. However,

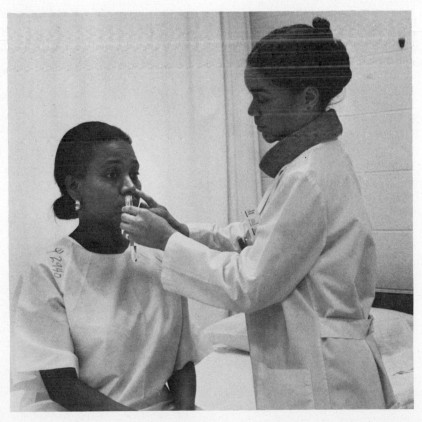

Fig. 23-1. Testing for ability to smell. The client is asked to sniff as the test tube containing the test substance is placed beneath the nostril. The examiner holds the other nostril closed.

flavor perception is a synthesis of odor, taste, and perceptions from stimulation of end organs in the mouth and pharynx. The individual with CN I involvement may complain only of loss of the sense of taste. The examiner should note that olfactory acuity is thought to be more acute prior to eating than after a meal.

The mucosal surfaces are examined when the client has difficulty in smelling, since an inflammation of the mucous membranes (viral, bacterial) decreases the sense of smell. Allergic rhinitis and excessive cigarette smoking are common causes of anosomia or hyposmia.

Lesions of the sinuses may result in distortion or hallucinations of smell but do not result in a loss of olfactory sensation. Unilateral loss of smell may be an early indication of a neoplasm involving the olfactory bulb or tract. Total anosmia may follow head trauma, especially fractures involving the cribriform plate. Parosmia is a perversion of the sense of smell that sometimes accompanies trauma or tumors of the uncus. Olfactory hallucinations that are offensive are known as cacosmia.

CN II: optic nerve

The optic nerve is described in Chapter 11 on eye assessment (note the sections on examination of visual acuity, visual fields, and the pupils—tests of pupillary constriction). Fig. 23-2 illustrates an examination for unilateral protrusion of an eye.

CN III: oculomotor nerve, CN IV: trochlear nerve, CN VI: abducens nerve

The oculomotor, trochlear, and abducens nerves are also described in Chapter 11 (note the sections on neuromuscular and extraocular muscle function—tests of eye movement).

DOLL'S HEAD MANEUVER (VESTIBULAR OCULOGYRIC REFLEX)

Rapid turning of the head to one side results in ocular deviation to the contralateral side. In deep coma or other conditions resulting in paralysis of the oculomotor nerves or muscles, conjugate gaze to the contralateral side may be diminished or lost.

CN V: trigeminal nerve

The trigeminal nerve is motor to the muscles of mastication and sensory to the face and to the mucosa of the nose and mouth in perceiving touch, temperature, and pain.

The nuclei of the trigeminal nerve are located in the midportion of the pons. The bulk of the cell bodies of the sensory portion of the trigeminal nerve lie in the gasserian ganglion, with the remainder in the mesencephalic nucleus. The sensory fibers to the gasserian ganglion are contained in one of the three proximal divisions of the nerve: ophthalmic, maxillary, or mandibular (Fig. 23-3). Peripheral nerve endings of the ophthalmic branch are sensory to the cornea, conjunctiva, upper lid, forehead, bridge of the nose, and scalp as far posteriorly as the vertex. The maxillary division of CN V conducts sensation from the skin of the lateral aspect of the nose, cheek, upper teeth, and jaw, as well as the mucosa of the lower nasal cavity, nasopharynx, hard palate, and uvula. The mandibular division contains the motor fibers that innervate the masseter, temporal, pterygoid, and digastric muscles. This division is also sensory to the skin of the lower jaw, pinna of the ear,

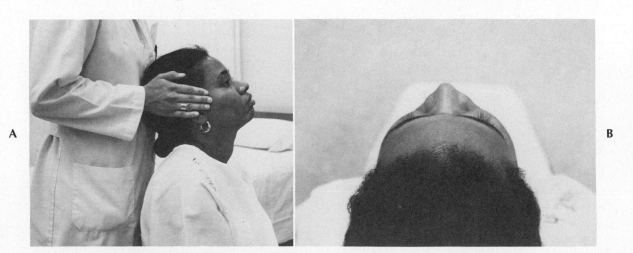

A   B

Fig. 23-2. An examination for unilateral protrusion of an eye. The examiner stands behind the client and slowly extends the neck. The eyelashes should be sighted simultaneously for both eyes if they are similar in size and position.

anterior portion of the external auditory canal, side of tongue, lower gums, lower teeth, floor of the mouth, and buccal surface of the cheek.

Afferent fibers from the gasserian ganglion enter the lateral portion of the pons and bifurcate into ascending and descending branches. The ascending branches pass to the main sensory nucleus responsible for the sensation of touch and to the mesencephalic nucleus that serves proprioception from the muscles of mastication and the periodontal membrane. The descending branch provides sensations of pain and temperature. The motor nucleus is located in the midcentral pons.

The muscles of mastication are evaluated by asking the client to bite down with as much force as possible. The masseter muscles (Fig. 23-4) are evaluated by palpation, as are the temporal muscles (Fig. 23-5). Resistance is applied with downward pressure on the chin.

The pterygoid muscles may be examined by asking the client to press his jaw laterally against the examiner's hand with the mouth slightly open.

Atrophy of the muscle is recorded. Deviation of the jaw to one side indicates that the muscles of the side to which it is pulled are stronger than those of the opposite side. The individual is able to move the jaw to the unparalyzed side but not to the paralyzed side.

The client may be asked to bite on a tongue blade; the position of the upper and lower incisors are compared to measure any deviation. An idea of the extent of weakness of the muscle might be gained by asking the client to move his jaw toward the weak side. Muscle tone and strength are also assessed, with the muscles observed for fasciculations.

The usual tests of sensation (see sensory assessment) are employed on both sides of the face, taking care that each division of the nerve is tested. Both skin and mucous membranes are examined. A wooden applicator may be used to touch various areas of the mucosa inside the mouth to test sensitivity to touch. The trigeminal nerve contains the afferent fiber for the corneal reflex (see Chapter 11 on eye assessment) and both the afferent and efferent fibers for the jaw closure reflex (described later in this chapter).

MOTOR PATHOPHYSIOLOGY

Myasthenia gravis. The weakness and ready fatigability of muscles that occur in myasthenia gravis may involve the muscles of mastication, making chewing difficult or impossible.

Amyotrophic lateral sclerosis. Degeneration of the motor nucleus of the trigeminal nerve may occur in amyotrophic lateral sclerosis, resulting in weakness

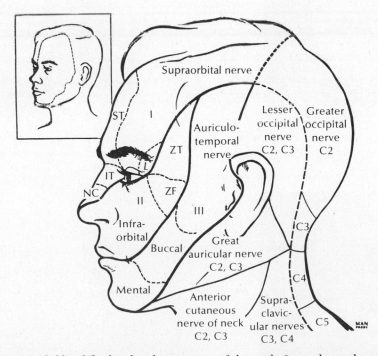

Fig. 23-3. Cutaneous fields of the head and upper part of the neck. Inset shows the area of sensory loss in the face following resection of the trigeminal nerve. The cutaneous fields of the three branches of the trigeminal nerve are identified as *I,* ophthalmic; *II,* maxillary; and *III,* mandibular. (From Haymaker, W., and Woodhall, B.: Peripheral nerve injuries, ed. 2, Philadelphia, 1959, W. B. Saunders Co.)

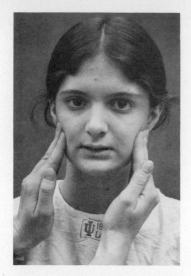

Fig. 23-4. Palpation of the masseter muscles for size, strength, and symmetry to test CN V.

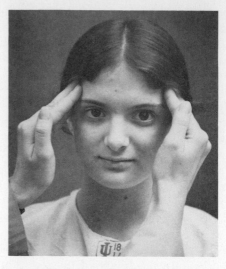

Fig. 23-5. Palpation of the temporal muscles for size, shape, and symmetry to test CN V.

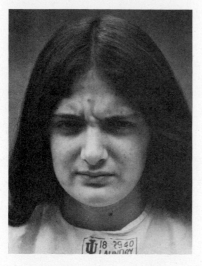

Fig. 23-6. Test of CN VII. Client's ability to frown is inspected as a function of the facial muscles.

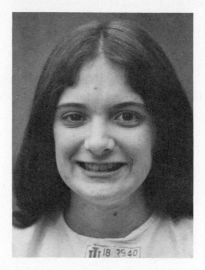

Fig. 23-7. Test of CN VII. Client's ability to expose the teeth is inspected as a function of the facial muscles and platysma muscle of the neck.

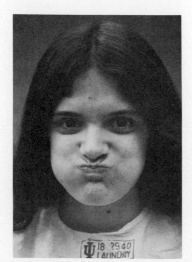

Fig. 23-8. Test of CN VII. Client's ability to puff out the cheeks is inspected as a function of the facial muscles.

and atrophy of the muscles of mastication. The client may be unable to chew or close his mouth.

Tetanus. Rigidly spastic muscles are frequently observed in tetanus infections. Spasm of the muscles of mastication is called lockjaw.

SENSORY PATHOPHYSIOLOGY

Neuritis. Painful neuritis is caused by infection, vitamin deficiencies, and chemical irritants. When pain is severe, there is radiation over the three branches of the trigeminal nerve.

Trigeminal neuralgia (tic douloureux). Trigeminal neuralgia is characterized by excruciating pain of the lips, gums, or chin. The regions of pain may map out one of the divisions of the trigeminal nerve. These zones are supraorbital, infraorbital, and inferior to the labial fold midway to the angle of the jaw. Sharp pain may be elicited by applying pressure at the point where the trigeminal nerve emerges from the bone. Cold may also precipitate the pain. The condition generally occurs in elderly people. Clinical examination does not reveal impairment of sensory or motor function.

Herpes zoster (shingles). The gasserian ganglia, just as any ganglion of the body, may be affected by the herpes virus. A characteristic papulovesicular rash generally involving the ophthalmic division may be observed. The vesicles are located over the forehead, eyelid, and cornea. These lesions may later ulcerate and keratinize. A neuralgia may remain after the rash has disappeared, and sensation may be lost from the involved area.

CN VII: facial nerve

The facial nerve is a motor to the facial muscles and sensory to taste sensation of the anterior two-thirds of the tongue. It also conducts exteroceptive sensation from the eardrum area and proprioceptive information from the muscles it supplies. Visceral sensation from the salivary glands and mucosa of the mouth and pharynx is also conducted by CN VII. The facial nerve also carries parasympathetic fibers that stimulate secretion of the salivary glands, the lacrimal glands, and the mucosa of the nose, palate, and nasopharynx. The reticular formation of the pons is the location of the motor nucleus of the facial nerve.

Taste sensation is mediated by the taste buds of the tongue, and the sensation is conducted via the lingual nerve; the neurons of the lingual nerve have their cell bodies in the geniculate ganglion. Gustatory sensation is then conducted via the sensory portion of the intermediate nerve to the solitary tract of the pons.

The muscles controlled by the motor component of the facial nerve play a role in all the voluntary and involuntary movements of the face, except for move-

ments of the jaw. The client's face is inspected for indications of facial muscle weakness, such as drooping of one side of the mouth, flattening of the nasolabial fold, and laxity of the lower eyelid.

The client is asked to perform the following facial movements: elevate his eyebrows, wrinkle his forehead by looking upward, frown (Fig. 23-6), smile or show his teeth (in this test, in addition to the facial muscles, the platysma muscle of the neck is noted) (Fig. 23-7), puff out his cheeks against the pressure of the examiners fingers (Fig. 23-8), or whistle. The examiner evaluates the movements for muscle strength and symmetry. The client is told to close his eyes, first lightly and then tightly, while the examiner tries to open them. The platysma muscle is checked by asking the client to open his mouth slightly and to "jut out" his jaw.

In infants the facial muscles are evaluated during crying, evaluating tone and noting any atrophy and fasciculations.

MOTOR PATHOPHYSIOLOGY

Motor weakness of CN VII is defined by the location of the particular lesion. Corticobulbar or upper motor neuron lesions are those that involve the motor cortex. The motor neurons supply the face or the axons of those neurons that form the corticobulbar tracts coursing through the internal capsule, cerebral peduncle, or pons. Corticobulbar paralysis is rarely complete and is contralateral to the lesion. The nuclear center of the brain that controls the upper part of the face receives both contralateral and ipsilateral fibers. The lower portion of the face, however, receives only contralateral fibers.

Chvostek's sign is produced by tapping the facial nerve. A positive response is a brisk contraction of the facial muscles that are innervated distal to the point of contact with the nerve. This may be elicited with a finger or a reflex hammer. The sign is seen in hypocalcemia, as in hypoparathyroidism.

Peripheral nerve facial palsy of acute onset and unknown cause is called *Bell's palsy*. Evidence of this lower motor neuron disorder is seen when only one eye closes as the client attempts to close both eyes. Observation of a flat nasolabial fold may add to this suspicion. When the client attempts to raise his eyebrows, the eyebrow on the affected side will not raise and the forehead does not wrinkle. Other lower motor neuron weakness may result in partial or complete paralysis of an entire side of the face or a flat facial expression. The client may exhibit epiphora (overflow of tears), be unable to hold fluids because of a sagging mouth, or be unable to pronounce such labials as *b*, *m*, or *w*.

Upper motor neuron paralysis (hemiparesis) is rarely complete and is a possibility if the nasolabial folds appear flat when the client closes his eyes. In this case, both eyebrows raise and the forehead wrinkles. In upper motor neuron pathology, involuntary contractions of the facial muscle such as smiling may show normal strength, whereas voluntary contractions such as retracting the corner of the mouth may prove to be weak or absent. There may also be paralysis of eyelid closure (widening of palpebral fissure) or weakness of lid closure.

Taste sensation for the anterior two-thirds of the tongue is mediated through the sensory component of the facial nerve (CN VII) and is the only aspect of sensation that is tested. To test taste sensation, solutions of the following substances are applied with an applicator or pipette to the appropriate region of the lateral aspect of the tongue: sweet, salty, sour (vinegar, lemon juice), and bitter (quinine) (Figs. 23-9 and 23-10). A different applicator is used for each substance, and the client is allowed a sip of water inbetween testing to avoid mixing tastes. In addition, the tongue should remain protruded throughout each test to avoid spreading the test substance over the tongue. The client is given a card with the words "salty," "sweet," "sour," and "bitter" and asked to point to the one that best describes the solution on the tongue. Each substance is used twice. Both sides of the tongue must be assessed. The number of tests and the number of correct responses are recorded.

The facial nerve also innervates the submandibular, submaxillary (sublingual), and lacrimal glands. However, the functions of salivation and lacrimation are generally not tested as a part of the routine physical examination.

SENSORY PATHOPHYSIOLOGY: AGEUSIA

Ageusia is the loss of taste or the lack of ability to discriminate sweet, sour, salty, and bitter tastes. The nature of the loss of taste sensation may aid in making a diagnosis. For example:

1. Unilateral loss of taste may be caused by lesions of the solitary tract and its nucleus.
2. Bilateral ageusia may be caused by pathophysiological phenomena occurring near the midline of the pons.
3. Hallucinations or perversions of taste may be caused by lesions of the uncus.

CN VIII: acoustic nerve

The acoustic nerve has two divisions: the vestibular and the cochlear.

VESTIBULAR DIVISION

Neurons of the vestibular division of CN VIII are bipolar. The cell bodies are located in the vestibular

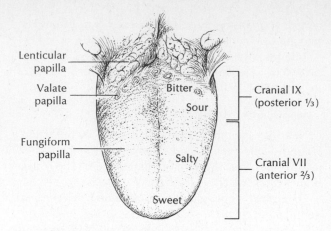

Fig. 23-9. Localization of taste buds of tongue.

ganglion. Peripheral fibers terminate in the neuroepithelium of the semicircular canals, utricle, and saccule, while the central portion terminates in the medulla in the vestibular nucleus. Axons from the cell bodies located in the vestibular nucleus terminate in the spinal cord (vestibulospinal tract) to produce reflex movements of the trunk and limbs, also contributing to the medial longitudinal fasciculus to produce conjugate eye movements in response to head movements. Fibers also terminate in the cerebellum, providing changes in muscle tone.

Tests for vestibular functions are *not routine* in the physical examination. The three types of stimuli used are caloric, rotational, and electrical. These stimuli produce changes in the flow of endolymph in the vestibular structures.

Bárány's test *(caloric).* The client is placed in a sitting position with the head tilted 60 degrees in extension (backward). The ear is irrigated with 5 to 10 ml of ice water (32° to 50° F) or 100 to 200 ml of cold water (68° F). The response of an individual with normal vestibular apparatus tested in the right ear is nausea, dizziness, and nystagmus. Horizontal nystagmus with the slow component to the right is normal. The slow phase is in the direction of endolymph flow. In addition, the client is tested for past pointing by asking the client to touch his index finger to that of the examiner. Past pointing and falling to the right occur in normal subjects. There will be no response in persons who have no vestibular function. The individual who has hyperirritability of the vestibular system may show vestibular responses to less strong stimuli, such as turning the head from side to side; the symptoms of vertigo and nausea will be stronger and vomiting may occur.

Nylen-Bárány test. This is a test for positional nystagmus. With client's head hanging 45 degrees backward over the head of the examining table and 45 degrees to one side, the examiner observes for nys-

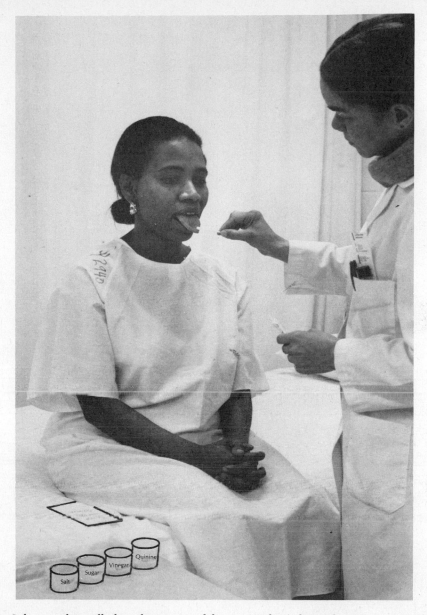

Fig. 23-10. Solutions that will elicit the taste modalities are salty (saline solution), sweet (sugar), sour (vinegar or lemon juice), and bitter (quinine). The solutions are applied one at a time to the appropriate sensory area of the tongue.

tagmus. The head is then turned in the opposite direction, and the observation is repeated.

Bárány chair rotation test. The client is rotated 10 times in 20 seconds and stopped suddenly. The examiner observes for nystagmus and postural deviation and checks for past pointing. Nystagmus, past pointing, and postural deviation are in the direction of the movement of the chair in the normal subject. Vertigo, the hallucination of continued movement, is in the opposite direction.

Electronystagmography. With this process, nystagmus may also be recorded from differences in electrical potential.

Vertigo is the most common symptom of vestibular disease. Any of the responses to the vestibular function tests, such as nausea, dizziness, or nystagmus, may be present in labyrinth disease. Nystagmus may be horizontal, vertical, or rotary. Etiology of disease of the semicircular canals may include inflammation, hemorrhage, edema, and pressure alterations. Vertigo may also result from disorders of the cortex or other central nervous system structures.

Labyrinthitis and hemorrhage into the labyrinth have been termed *Meniere's disease*, even though this term is more correctly applied to the presence of excessive endolymph or edema.

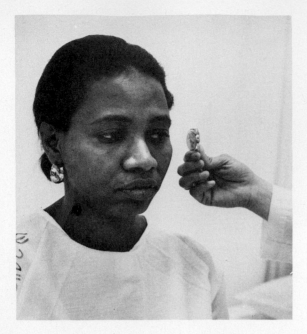

Fig. 23-11. Gross test of hearing to assess cochlear function. The ticking watch is moved away from the ear until the client no longer hears it.

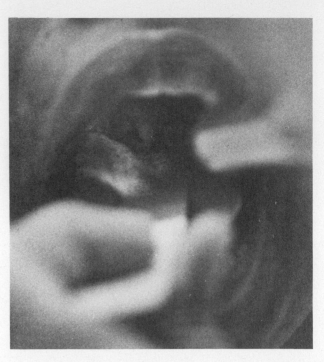

Fig. 23-12. Test of glossopharyngeal and vagal nerve function. Uvula is observed in midline.

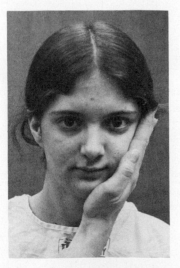

Fig. 23-13. Assessment of the symmetry, size, and strength of the sternocleidomastoid muscle in test of CN XI. The client is asked to turn the head to one side to push the chin against the resistance of the examiner's hand. The contralateral sternocleidomastoid muscle will stand out as it contracts. The muscle is palpated to assess tension.

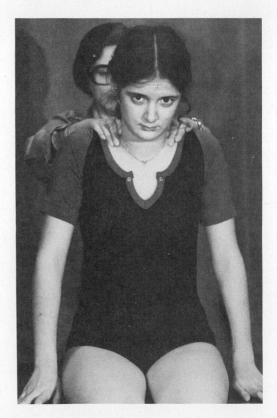

Fig. 23-14. Assessment of the symmetry, size, and shape of the trapezius muscles in test of CN XI. The client shrugs the shoulders against the resistance of the examiner's hand.

COCHLEAR DIVISION

Tests for cochlear function (Fig. 23-11) are described in Chapter 10 on ears, nose, and throat assessment (note testing of auditory function—audiogram, Weber, and Rinne tests).

CN IX: glossopharyngeal nerve,
CN X: vagus nerve

The glossopharyngeal and vagus nerves are closely related both anatomically and physiologically. These nerve are tested clinically as a unit.

The glossopharyngeal nerve contains sensory and motor fibers. The sensory fibers arise from the posterior third of the tongue, middle ear, and eustachian tube and have their cell bodies in the petrosal ganglia and terminate in the solitary tract in the medulla. From the solitary tract, fibers connect with the cells of the superior salivary nucleus. Motor fibers arise from the upper portion of the ambiguous nucleus in the medulla to innervate the stylopharyngeus muscle.

The glossopharyngeal nerve is sensory for taste for the posterior third of the tongue and conveys general sensation from the tonsillar and pharyngeal mucosa. It also has afferent sensory fibers for the carotid sinus and body. Testing for taste sensation is conducted for the posterior tongue at the time of examination of the anterior tongue (see CN VII: facial nerve).

The vagus nerve is sensory for the walls of the gastrointestinal viscera (to the transverse colon) and for the heart, lungs, and aortic bodies. The vagus is a motor nerve to the palate, pharynx, larynx, and the thoracic and abdominal visceral organs.

Testing of vagal function can be difficult. The clinical examination focuses on the musculature of the palate, pharynx, and larynx. The soft palate is inspected for symmetry. The uvula is identified and any deviation from the midline is recorded (Fig. 23-12). Unilateral weakness is characterized by the drooping of the affected side and the absence of the arch on that side.

The client is asked to say, "Ah." The palate should rise symmetrically. The palatal reflex is elicited by stroking the mucous membrane of the soft palate with an applicator. The side touched retracts upward.

The gag reflex is obtained by touching the posterior wall of the pharynx with an applicator or a tongue blade. The response includes elevation of the palate and contraction of the pharyngeal muscles.

Swallowing is evaluated by giving the client a small quantity of water to drink and observing him while he swallows it. Retrograde passage of water through the nose while drinking indicates a weakness of the soft palate wherein the nasopharynx is not closed off during the swallow.

In the presence of a lesion of the vagus nerve, the uvula and soft palate deviate to the unaffected side since the muscles on the intact side are unopposed.

The client who is hoarse or who complains of a problem with vocalization is examined by indirect laryngoscopy. A laryngeal mirror and headlight allow visualization of the vocal cords.

CN XI: spinal accessory nerve

Cell bodies of the spinal accessory nerve are located in the gray matter of the first five cervical cord segments and give off axons to the sternocleidomastoid and trapezius muscles, providing these muscles with motor innervation.

To test the spinal accessory nerve, the symmetry, size, and strength of these muscles are evaluated.

For assessment of the sternocleidomastoid muscle, the client is asked to turn his head to one side and push the chin in the same direction against the resistance of the examiner's hand. The contralateral sternocleidomastoid muscle will stand out and may be inspected and palpated (Fig. 23-13).

For assessment of the trapezius muscles, the client is asked to shrug his shoulders while the examiner exerts downward pressure against the muscles. As the muscles contract, they may be evaluated for strength and symmetry (Fig. 23-14).

The trapezius muscles may be further tested by asking the client to raise his arms to a vertical position. Weakness of the trapezius muscles makes this position difficult to achieve.

Neck trauma is the most frequent cause of dysfunction of the spinal accessory nerve. Radical neck dissection is often followed by symptoms of CN XI damage.

Torticollis is a condition of intermittent or constant contraction of the sternocleidomastoid muscle wherein the head is flexed forward and the chin is rotated away from the affected side.

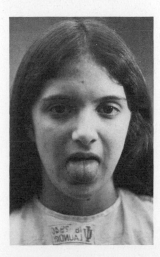

Fig. 23-15. Assessment for symmetry, size, shape, and fasciculations of the muscles of the protruded tongue in test of CN XII.

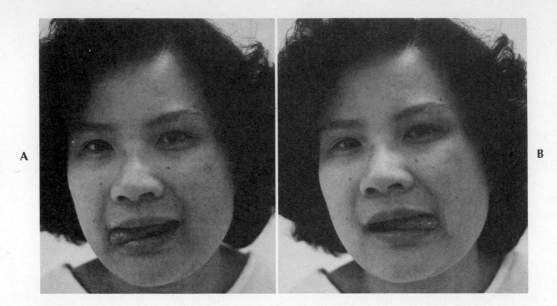

Fig. 23-16. The client moves the tongue from side to side, progressively increasing the speed of motion.

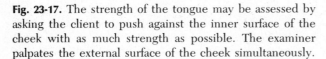

Fig. 23-17. The strength of the tongue may be assessed by asking the client to push against the inner surface of the cheek with as much strength as possible. The examiner palpates the external surface of the cheek simultaneously.

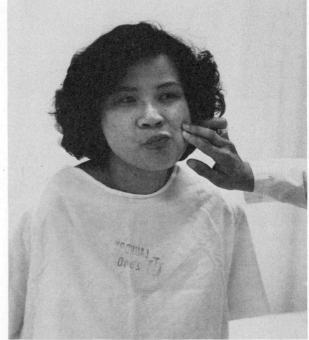

CN XII: hypoglossal nerve

The nucleus of the hypoglossal nerve is in the medulla and provides motor fibers to both the extrinsic and the intrinsic muscles of the tongue, making possible articulation of lingual speech sounds and swallowing.

The tongue is inspected for size (atrophy), symmetry, and fasciculations. Deviation to the affected side is characteristic of unilateral peripheral nerve damage because of the dominance of the genioglossus muscle on the nonaffected side. The posterior fibers of this muscle push the tongue toward the opposite side.

The client is asked to stick out his tongue as far as he can. The examiner notes the ability of the client to stick the tongue straight out, the strength of the movement, and how far out the client sticks the tongue (Fig. 23-15). The client also moves the tongue rapidly in and out and from side to side (Fig. 23-16). Upper motor neuron disease may result in slowness

Table 23-1. The cranial nerves

Nerve	Function	Clinical test	Cells of origin	Major components	Afferent	Efferent
I Olfactory	Smell	Odor applied to one nostril	Olfactory epithelium	Olfactory filaments	Visceral special Smell	
II Optic	Vision	Visual acuity: Snellen chart Visual fields: confrontation, tangent screen, perimeter	Retinal ganglion cells	Optic nerves Optic chiasm Optic tracts	Somatic special Vision	
III Oculomotor	Upward, downward, medial eye movement Lid elevation	Eye movement Lid movement	Nucleus 3	Oculomotor nerve		Somatic Extraocular muscles Levator palpebrae Superior rectus Inferior rectus Inferior oblique
	Pupil constriction	Pupillary response to light and accommodation	Edinger-Westphal nucleus	Oculomotor nerve Ciliary ganglion Ciliary nerves		Visceral general Intrinsic eye muscles, iris, ciliary muscle
IV Trochlear	Downward, medial eye movement	Eye movement	Nucleus 4	Trochlear nerve		Somatic Superior oblique muscle
V Trigeminal	Sensory Face Scalp Nasal mucosa Buccal mucosa	Corneal reflex Sensation Face Anterior scalp Nasal mucosa Buccal mucosa	Gasserian ganglion	Ophthalmic nerve Maxillary nerve Mandibular nerve	Somatic general Sensory Anterior half of scalp Face Buccal mucosa Dura, anterior, and middle fossa Proprioception Muscles of mastication	
	Jaw muscles		Mesencephalic Nucleus 5	Motor root		
	Motor Masseter muscle Temporal muscle Diagastric muscle	Muscle strength of masseter and temporal muscles; muscles palpated with jaw clenched	Motor nucleus 5	Motor root		Visceral special Muscles for mastication
VI Abducens	Lateral eye movement	Eye movement	Nucleus 6	Abducens nerve		Somatic Lateral rectus

Continued.

Table 23-1. The cranial nerves—cont'd

Nerve	Function	Clinical test	Cells of origin	Major components	Afferent	Efferent
VII Facial	Sensory					
	External ear	Sensation	Geniculate ganglion	Intermediate nerve Ramus of vagus nerve	Somatic general	
	Taste: anterior two-thirds of tongue	Taste: sweet, salty, sour	Geniculate ganglion	Intermediate nerve Chorda tympani nerve Lingual nerve	Visceral special	
	Deep facial	Sensation, deep facial		Intermediate nerve	Visceral general	
	Motor					
	Facial movement Scalp muscle Auricular muscle Stylohyoid muscle Digastric posterior belly	Corneal reflex Facial movement: client frowns, wrinkles forehead, shows teeth	Motor nucleus 7	Temporofacial branch Cervicofacial branch		Visceral special
	Salivation: submaxillary glands, sublingual glands		Superior salivary nucleus	Intermediate nerve Chorda tympani nerve Lingual nerve Submaxillary ganglion		Visceral general
	Lacrimation: lacrimal glands Mucous membrane Nasopharynx		Superior salivary nucleus	Intermediate nerve Petrossal nerve Sphenopalatine ganglion		Visceral general
VIII Acoustic	Vestibular		Vestibular ganglion	Vestibular nerve	Somatic special	
	Hearing	Audiometry	Spiral ganglion of cochlea	Cochlear nerve	Somatic special	
IX Glossopharyngeal	Sensory					
	External ear (part)		Superior ganglion	Ramus of vagus nerve	Somatic general	
	Taste: posterior third of tongue	Taste: sweet, salty, sour	Petrosal ganglion		Visceral special	
	Carotid: reflexes, baroreceptors and chemoreceptors, sinus, body			Carotid sinus nerve	Visceral special	
	Motor					
	Pharynx: gag reflex, swallowing, pharyngeal muscles	Gag test: give drink; watch swallow	Petrosal ganglion Ambiguous nucleus	Pharyngeal branch Lingual branch Pharyngeal plexus		Visceral special Visceral special
	Parotid gland: salivation		Inferior salivatory nucleus	Tympanic nerve Petrosal nerve		Visceral general

Nerve	Component	Function	Assessment	Nucleus / Ganglion	Pathway	Modality
X Vagus	Sensory	External ear (part)		Jugular ganglion		Somatic general
		Pharynx		Nodose ganglion		Visceral general
		Thoracic and abdominal viscera				
		Aortic arch			Carotid sinus nerve	Visceral special
		Chemoreceptors				
		Baroreceptors				
	Motor	Swallowing, gag reflex	Give drink; watch swallow	Ambiguous nucleus	Pharyngeal plexus	Visceral special
		Phonation	Observe speech		Laryngeal nerves	Visceral special
		Cardiac slowing		Dorsal motor nucleus 10		Visceral general
		Bronchoconstriction				Visceral general
		Gastric secretion				Visceral general
		Peristalsis				Visceral general
XI Accessory	Motor	Swallowing: pharyngeal muscles	Give drink; watch swallow	Ambiguous nucleus	Cranial root	Visceral special
		Turning of head: sternocleidomastoid muscles	Client turns head against resistance	Ventral horn C2; Ventral root branch	Spinal root	Visceral special
		Elevation of shoulders: trapezius muscles	Client shrugs shoulders against resistance	Ventral horn C3, 4; Ventral root branch		Visceral special
XII Hypoglossal	Motor	Muscles that move tongue: hypoglossus, genioglossus, styloglossus	Client sticks out tongue, moves tongue from side to side; Observe speech	Nucleus 12	Hypoglossal nerve	Somatic

of alternate movements. In another test, the client curls the tongue upward as to touch the nose and downward as to lick the chin surface. The client may also be tested for muscle strength by asking him to push out the cheek with his tongue while the examiner pushes against it from the outside (Fig. 23-17).

The examiner tests lingual speech sounds by giving the client a phrase for repetition that includes a number of words containing *l, t, d,* or *n.*

SUMMARY

Table 23-1 is a summary of the cranial nerves, including their functions, assessment, makeup, and components.

PROPRIOCEPTION AND CEREBELLAR FUNCTION

The proprioceptive system of the nervous system maintains posture, balance, and other acts of coordination. The neural structures that are involved in proprioception are the posterior columns (gracilis and cuneatus) of the spinal cord, the cerebellum, and the vestibular apparatus. The posterior columns carry stimuli from the proprioceptors in muscle tendons and joints. The posterior columns also carry fibers for touch sensation and two-point discrimination. Deficit of function of the posterior column results in impairment of muscle and position sense. Clients with such an impairment are often observed to be watching their own arm and leg movements so as to know the position of the limbs from these visual cues.

The cerebellum functions primarily in the integration of muscle contractions for the maintenance of posture. Loss of cerebellar function results in dyssynergia (impairment of muscle coordination or of the ability to perform movements smoothly), intention tremor, or hypotonia.

Abnormalities of muscle tone, gait, speech, and nystagmus in lateral gaze may also indicate cerebellar dysfunction. Disturbances in the timing of movements may also be evident.

The vestibular system is concerned with righting movements. Vestibular disease is characterized by vertigo, nausea, and vomiting. A subjective phenomenon, vertigo is the illusion of movement of the individual or his environment. Nausea and vomiting frequently accompany vertigo. Nystagmus is also frequently associated with vertigo and may be vertical, horizontal, or rotary.

Ataxia is the impairment of position sense. Ataxia is more severe if visual images are excluded in posterior column disease but not in cerebellar dysfunction.

The client with a *cerebellar gait* walks with a wide base; the trunk and head are held rigidly; the legs bend at the hips; arm movements are not coordinated with the stride; the client lurches and reels, frequently falling.

The client with *cerebellar speech* has slow, hesitant, or dysarthric verbalization.

Jerking movements are noted in the client with a *cerebellar sitting posture* as the client attempts to maintain balance.

The client with proprioceptive or cerebellar dysfunction may experience difficulty with the following tests of posture maintenance or coordination.

The client is asked to pat his knees with the palms of the hands followed by the backs of the hands at an ever increasing rate. The client with cerebellar disease has difficulty with rapid patting as well as supination-pronation alterations. The problem involves both smooth control of muscles and the starting and stop-

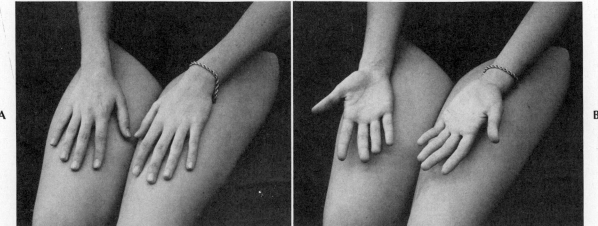

A   B

Fig. 23-18. Test for dysdiadochokinesia—pronation and supination of the hands, with progressively more rapid movement.

ping of motion (Fig. 23-18). Clumsiness of movement and irregular timing are characteristic of affected individuals.

A test for dysdiadochokinesia, the ability to stop a movement and replace it by a movement in the opposite direction, is the pronation and supination test. The arms may be outstretched or flexed at the elbow. The movements are performed as rapidly as possible (Fig. 23-18). Any movement may be tested that involves the alternated action of agonists and antangonists.

Accuracy of movement direction may be tested by asking the client to touch his nose with the index finger of first one hand and then the other with the eyes closed (Fig. 23-19). The client is then asked to repeat this activity several times while gradually increasing the speed of performance.

The client may be asked to touch his nose and then the examiner's finger at a distance of about 18 inches (Figs. 23-20 and 23-21). This maneuver is also repeated with increasing speed. The finger-to-finger test involves asking the client to spread the arms broadly and then to bring them together in the midline. It is done slowly and then rapidly with the eyes

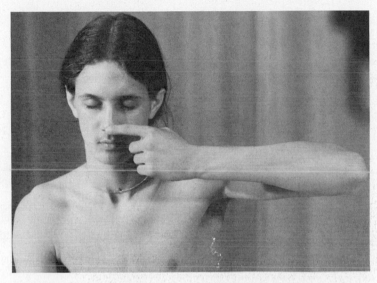

Fig. 23-19. Test of the proprioceptive system. The client is asked to alternately touch his nose with the tip of the index finger of each hand, repeating the motion with increasing speed.

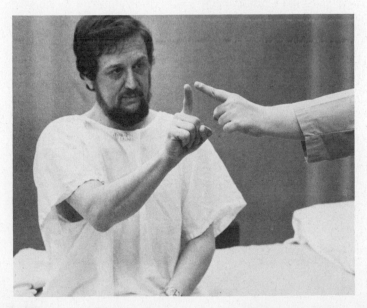

Fig. 23-20. Test of the proprioceptive system. The client is asked to touch the examiner's finger, which is placed about 18 inches from the client's eye.

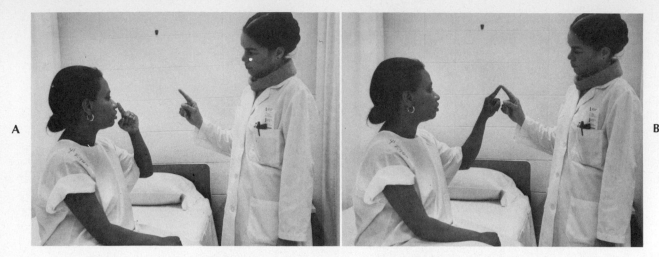

Fig. 23-21. Test of the proprioceptive system. **A,** The client is asked to touch her nose with an index finger and then **B,** to touch the examiner's index finger at a distance of about 18 inches, repeating the motion with increasing speed.

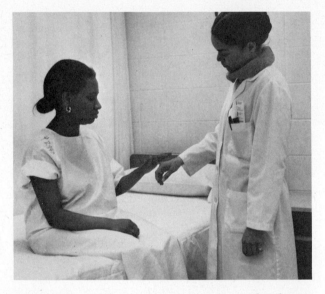

Fig. 23-22. Test of the proprioceptive system. The client is asked to pat the examiner's hand, progressively increasing the speed of motion.

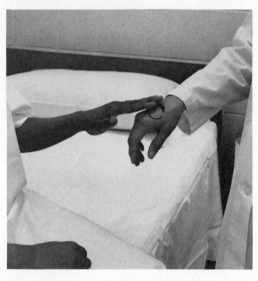

Fig. 23-23. Test of the proprioceptive system. The client is asked to make a polishing (circular) motion on the volar surface of the examiner's hand, progressively increasing the speed of motion.

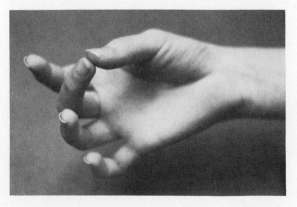

Fig. 23-24. Test of the proprioceptive system. The client is asked to touch each finger of one hand to the thumb of the same hand as rapidly as possible.

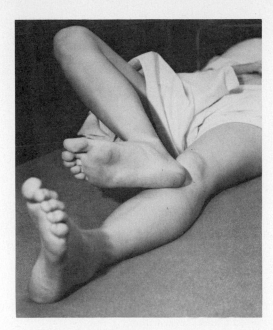

Fig. 23-25. Test of the proprioceptive system. The client is asked to run the heel of each foot down the opposite shin.

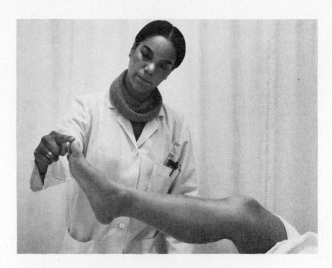

Fig. 23-26. Test of the proprioceptive system. The client is asked to touch the examiner's finger with his large toe.

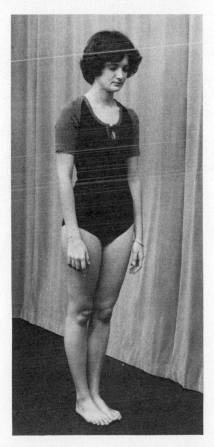

Fig. 23-27. Test of the proprioceptive system. Romberg test—individual should be able to stand with eyes closed and feet together without swaying for approximately 5 seconds.

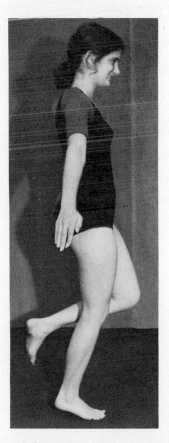

Fig. 23-28. Test of the proprioceptive system. The client who has demonstrated Romberg's sign is asked to hop in place on one foot and then the other.

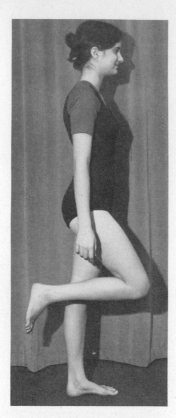

Fig. 23-29. Test of the proprioceptive system. The client is asked to stand on one foot and then the other. The normal individual is able to do this for about 5 seconds with the eyes closed.

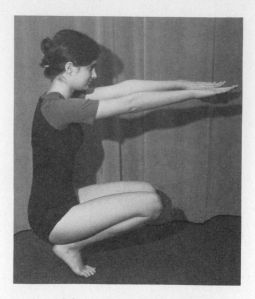

Fig. 23-30. Test of the proprioceptive system. The client is asked to do a knee bend without support.

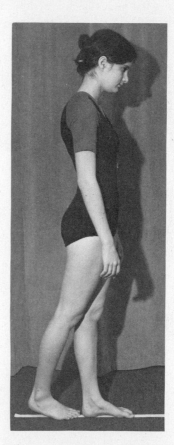

Fig. 23-31. Test of the proprioceptive system. The client is asked to walk a straight line placing heel to toe.

open and then closed. The client is asked to pat and then use a polishing motion on the examiner's hand, progressively increasing the speed (Figs. 23-22 and 23-23).

In a test for rapid, skilled movement, the client touches each finger of one hand to the thumb of the same hand as rapidly as possible (Fig. 23-24).

The client is also asked to run the heel of each foot down the opposite shin (Fig. 23-25).

The client may be asked to draw a figure eight in the air while lying on his back.

While lying on his back, the client is asked to touch the ball of each foot to the examiner's hand. The client is also asked to touch the examiner's finger with his large toe (Fig. 23-26).

In the Romberg test, the client is asked to stand with his feet together, first with his eyes closed and then with them open, and is evaluated for swaying movement (Fig. 23-27). Slight swaying is normal. The examiner stands close enough to the client to prevent falling. The client who demonstrates Romberg's sign is asked to hop in place on one foot and then the other (Fig. 23-28).

Gait is assessed as the client walks with his eyes closed and then with them open.

The client is asked to stand on one foot and then the other. The normal client is able to do this for about 5 seconds with his eyes closed (Fig. 23-29).

The client who is reasonably steady may be asked to do a knee bend from a standing position without support (Fig. 23-30).

Table 23-2. Proprioceptive dysfunction: signs and symptoms

Cerebellar dysfunction

Ataxia not made worse in darkness or with eyes closed	Dysmetria
	Dysdiadochokinesia
	Scanning speech
Clumsiness	Hypotonia
Poor coordination	Asthenia
Decomposition of movement	Tremor
	Nystagmus

Posterior column dysfunction

Ataxia made worse in darkness or with eyes closed	Astereognosis
	Loss of two-point discrimination
Positive Romberg's sign	
Inability to recognize limb position	Loss of vibratory sensation

Vestibular dysfunction

Nystagmus	Nausea
	Vomiting
	Ataxia

The client is asked to walk a straight line, placing the heel of the leading foot against the toe of the other foot (Fig. 23-31).

The client is asked to pull against the resistance of the examiner's hands, and the client's hands are released without warning. The client with cerebellar disease may have difficulty in starting and stopping movement. Thus, there may be excessive after-movement or rebound, so that the client hits himself.

DEFINITIONS

decomposition of movement Movements smoothly coordinated in the normal individual are performed in several parts.

dysdiadochokinesia Disturbance in the ability to stop one movement and follow it by the opposite action, such as supination and pronation of hands.

dysmetria Disturbance in the ability to stop a movement.

These definitions may be helpful in recording signs observed in cerebellar or proprioceptive dysfunction (Table 23-2).

SENSORY FUNCTION

The equipment needed for sensory testing includes a cotton wisp or soft brush, a safety pin, test tubes for cold and warm water, a tuning fork, and calipers or a compass with dull points.

Although it is not necessary to evaluate sensation over the entire skin surface, stimuli should be applied strategically so that the dermatomes and major peripheral nerves are tested. A minimal number of test sites would include areas on the forehead, cheek, hand, lower arm, abdomen, foot, and lower leg.

As a general rule, the more distal area of the limb is checked first. In the screening examination the nerve may be assumed to be intact if sensation is normal at its most peripheral extent. If evidence of dysfunction is found, the site of the dysfunction must be localized and mapped. This means determining the boundaries of the loss of sensation. A lucid method of recording would include a sketch of the region involved and a description of the sensory change.

The intensity of the stimulus is kept to a minimal level on initial application. Gradual increases in magnitude may be made until the client is aware of the stimulus.

Variation in sensitivity of skin areas is seen in the normal client, so that a stronger stimulus is required over the back, the buttocks, and areas where the skin is heavily cornified. Symmetry of sensation is established by checking first one spot and then its mirror-image area.

The client's eyes should be closed during evaluation of sensory modalities. The visual cuing that occurs when the client is able to see the examiner apply the stimulus may lead to false positive responses in the client who is highly sensitive to suggestion.

Spurious results to sensory testing are risked when either the client or the examiner is fatigued. Inattention to instruction or lack of motivation may lead to an impression of sensory loss.

The examiner should avoid predictable patterns in applying the stimulus. That is, the examiner should vary testing sites and timing so that the client cannot predict the response he is expected to give.

DEFINITIONS

anesthesia Absence of touch sensation.

hyperesthesia Greater than normal sensation to touch stimuli.

hypoesthesia Less than normal sensation to touch stimuli.

paresthesia Abnormal or perverted sensation; may include burning, itching, pain, or the feel of an electric shock.

The above definitions may be helpful in recording sensory dysfunction.

Light touch sensation

Light touch and deep touch are mediated by different nerve endings. Sensory fibers for simple touch enter the spinal cord and travel upward before crossing to enter the anterior spinothalamic tract to the thalamus. Light touch is the sensory system that is least often obtunded. Both anterior spinothalamic tracts must suffer destruction before transmission of light touch is lost.

Light touch is tested by touching the skin with a wisp of cotton (Fig. 23-32) or a soft brush (Fig. 23-33). Pressure is applied in such a way that sensation is stimulated but not enough to perceptibly depress

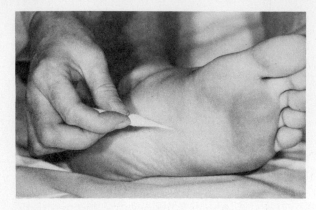

Fig. 23-32. Test of sensation of light touch using a wisp of cotton applied firmly enough to stimulate the sensory nerve endings but not so much that the skin is indented.

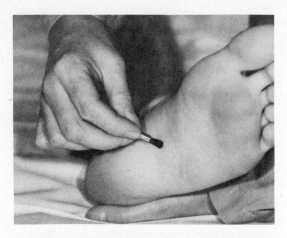

Fig. 23-33. Test of light touch sensation using a soft brush.

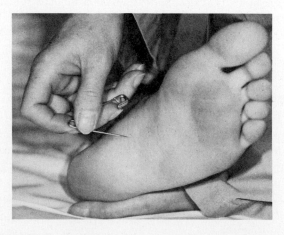

Fig. 23-34. Evaluation for superficial pain using the sharp point of a safety pin.

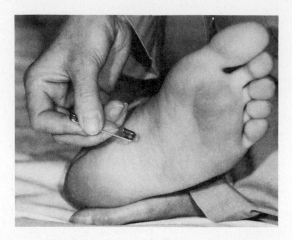

Fig. 23-35. Alternate use of the dull end of the pin for evaluation of pain.

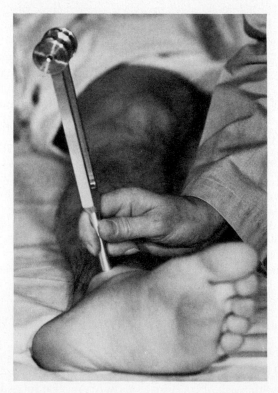

Fig. 23-36. Test of sensitivity to vibration. The base of the vibrating tuning fork is applied to bony prominences such as the sternum, elbow, or ankle.

the skin. The client is instructed to say, "Yes" or "Now" when he feels his skin being touched. The hair of the skin should be avoided when testing for touch sensation in the skin. The follicles are innervated with sensory fibers that are stimulated by movement of the hair. Instances of distortion of sensation or anesthesia are recorded.

Tactile localization (point localization). The client is asked to point to the spot where he was touched.

Pain sensation

Pain and temperature fibers both travel in the dorsolateral fasciculus for a short distance, after which they cross and continue to the thalamus in the lateral spinothalamic tract.

Superficial pain. The evaluation of the sensory perception of superficial pain and pressure may be conducted through the use of the sharp and dull points of a safety pin (Figs. 23-34 and 23-35): however, recent studies have indicated a risk of infection with safety pins and some examiners are using the hub (dull) and point (sharp) of a hypodermic needle. The client is asked to say, "Sharp," "Dull," or "Can't tell," when he feels the pin touch his skin. At least 2 seconds should be allowed between successive tests to avoid summation effects (several successive stimuli perceived as one). Pain sensation may be lost in the presence of lesions of the tegmentum of the brain stem.

Deep pressure. Deep pressure is tested over the eyeball, Achilles tendon, forearm, and calf muscles.

Temperature sensation

In the screening examination, temperature assessment need not be done when pain sensation is found to be within normal limits. When it is performed, the stimuli are tubes filled with warm and cold water that are rolled against the skin sites to be tested. The examiner tests the stimuli on his own skin in order to avoid burning the client and to provide a comparison. The client is asked to say, "Hot," "Cold," or "Can't tell." The tubes are applied to a sufficient number of areas to ascertain that all dermatomes are included.

Vibration sensation

The normal client is able to distinguish vibration when the base of a vibrating tuning fork is applied to a bony prominence such as the sternum, elbow, or ankle. The client perceives the vibration as a buzzing or tingling sensation.

The greatest sensitivity to vibration is seen when the tuning fork is vibrating between 200 and 400 cycles per second. A large tuning fork is suggested since the decay of vibration occurs more slowly in the larger instrument.

After the client closes his eyes, the vibrating tuning fork may be applied to the clavicles, spinous pro-cesses, elbows, finger joints, knees, ankles, and toes (Fig. 23-36). The client is asked to say, "Yes" or "Now," (1) when he first feels the vibrations and (2) when the vibrations stop. The examiner must emphasize to the client the importance of signifying the cessation of the feeling of vibration. The examiner may damp the vibrations of the tuning fork in order to move along more rapidly.

Vibratory sensation is diminished in the older client (after 65 years of age), particularly in the extremities.

Tactile discrimination

Tactile discrimination requires cortical integration. Three types of tactile discrimination that are tested clinically include: (1) stereognosis, (2) two-point discrimination, and (3) extinction. Afferent fibers for vibration, proprioception, and stereognosis are found to take one of three courses after entering the spinal cord: they (1) synapse immediately with motor cells to form a reflex arc, (2) run superiorly in the dorsal column to the cerebellum, or (3) travel in dorsal columns to the medulla and cross-run to the thalamus.

Stereognosis. Stereognosis is the act of recognizing objects on the basis of touching and manipulating them. This is a function of the parietal lobes of the cerebral cortex. Objects used to test stereognosis should be universally familiar items, such as a key or coin (Fig. 23-37).

Two-point discrimination. Two-point discrimination is defined as the ability to sense whether one or two areas of the skin are being stimulated by pressure. This may be done with pins. One pin is held in each hand and both are applied to the skin simultaneously. The client is asked if he feels one or two pinpricks. This determination may also be accomplished using calipers or a compass with dull points (Fig. 23-38).

In the adult client there is considerable variability of perceptual ability over the different parts of the body. The following are minimum distances between the two points of the calipers at which the normal adult is capable of sensing simultaneous stimulation:

Tongue: 1 mm
Fingertips: 2.8 mm
Toes: 3 to 8 mm
Palms of hand: 8 to 12 mm
Chest, forearms: 40 mm
Back: 40 to 70 mm
Upper arms, thighs: 75 mm

Extinction. The normal client, when touched in corresponding areas on both sides of the body, perceives touch in both areas. The failure to perceive touch on one side is called the extinction phenomenon. Impairment of the extinction phenomenon is frequently noted in lesions of the sensory cortex.

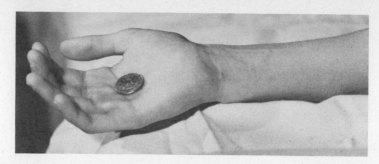

Fig. 23-37. Test for stereognosis. The normal client can discriminate a familiar object (coin, key) by touching and manipulating it.

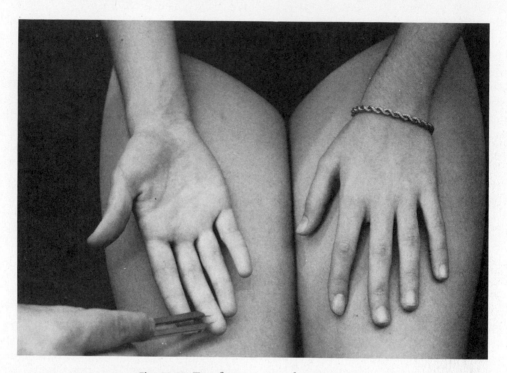

Fig. 23-38. Test for two-point discrimination.

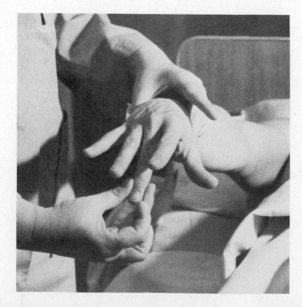

Fig. 23-39. Test of kinesthetic sensation. The normal client can discriminate the position of his body parts. With the client's eyes closed, the examiner changes the position of a finger. The client describes how the position was changed.

Table 23-3. Patterns of sensory loss

Pathological involvement	Common etiology	Characteristics
Peripheral nerve	Metabolic disorders, such as diabetes or nutritional deficiencies	Peripheral structures more frequently involved—"glove and stocking" involvement—may involve all sensory modalities
Specific peripheral nerve or root	Trauma Vascular occlusion	May map area of sensory loss specific to area innervated by the nerve and distal to the pathological lesion
Dorsal root		Loss of sensation in the segmented distribution (dermatome)
Spinal cord—hemisection (Brown-Séquard syndrome)	Trauma Medullary lesion Extramedullary lesion	Loss of pain and temperature perception on contralateral side, one or two segments below the lesion Loss of position sense, two-point discrimination, and vibratory sensation on ipsilateral side below the lesion
Brain stem	Trauma Neoplasm Vascular occlusion	Loss of pain and temperature sensation on contralateral side of body, ipsilateral side of face
Thalamus	Trauma Neoplasm Vascular occlusion	Loss of sensory modalities on contralateral side of body
Cortex—lesions of post-cortical cortex	Trauma Neoplasm Vascular occlusion	Loss of discriminatory sensation on contralateral side of body Loss of position sense, two-point discrimination, or stereognosis

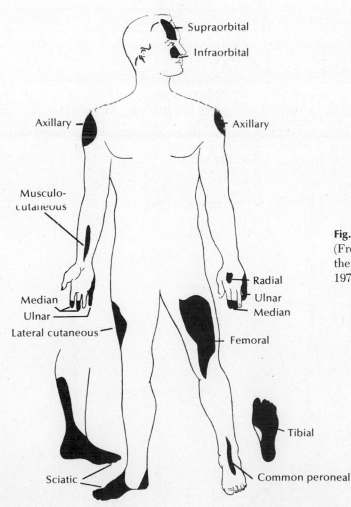

Fig. 23-40. Areas of sensory loss from peripheral nerve lesions. (From Prior, J. A., and Silberstein, J. S.: Physical diagnosis; the history and examination of the patient, ed. 4, St. Louis, 1973, The C. V. Mosby Co.)

Kinesthetic sensation (position awareness)

Kinesthetic sensation is that facilitated by proprioceptive receptors in the muscles, tendons, and joints. Perception of the position, orientation, and motion of limbs and body parts is obtained from kinesthetic sensations.

With the client's eyes closed and the joint in a neutral position, the examiner changes the position of one finger of the client's hand. It is important that the joint be held at the lateral aspect. The client is asked to describe how the position of the finger was changed. The finger is always moved to a neutral position before it is moved again (Fig. 23-39). This procedure may be done for any joint.

Graphesthesia

The normal client can discern the identity of letters or numbers inscribed on the palm of the hand, back, or other areas with a blunt object.

Patterns of sensory loss

Loss of discriminatory sensation may indicate a lesion of the posterior columns or sensory cortex. Bilateral sensory loss in both lower extremities sug-

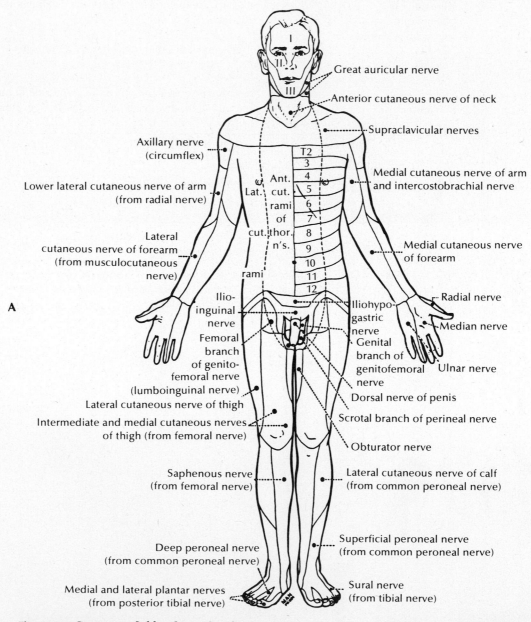

Fig. 23-41. Cutaneous fields of peripheral nerves from the anterior **(A)** and posterior **(B)** aspects. (From Haymaker, W., and Woodhall, B.: Peripheral nerve injuries, ed. 2, Philadelphia, 1959, W. B. Saunders Co.)

gests a peripheral neuropathy, such as diabetic neuropathy. Often the pattern of sensory loss is useful in establishing a diagnosis. Some common patterns of sensory deficit are described in Table 23-3.

Sensory loss resulting from disease in a single peripheral nerve may be mapped over the skin surface distribution of that nerve. The nerves most commonly involved in disease include the medial, radial, ulnar, sciatic, femoral, and peroneal nerves. The examiner should be knowledgeable of the sensory, motor, and reflex distribution of these and other major nerves (Fig. 23-40). Body surface projections of the major nerves are seen in Fig. 23-41.

Pathophysiological conditions involving the dorsal root may result in sensory loss distributed over the dermatome for that root (Fig. 23-42). Clear description of sensory loss for a given segment may be difficult to obtain since a good deal of sensory overlap occurs between the distribution of one root and another.

Both nerve and root sensory loss may result from disease involving a plexus. This phenomenon is frequently observed for the brachial plexus. Superior brachial plexus lesions involve C5 and C6, resulting in sensory loss in the shoulder and in the lateral arm and forearm. In addition, there may be weakness of

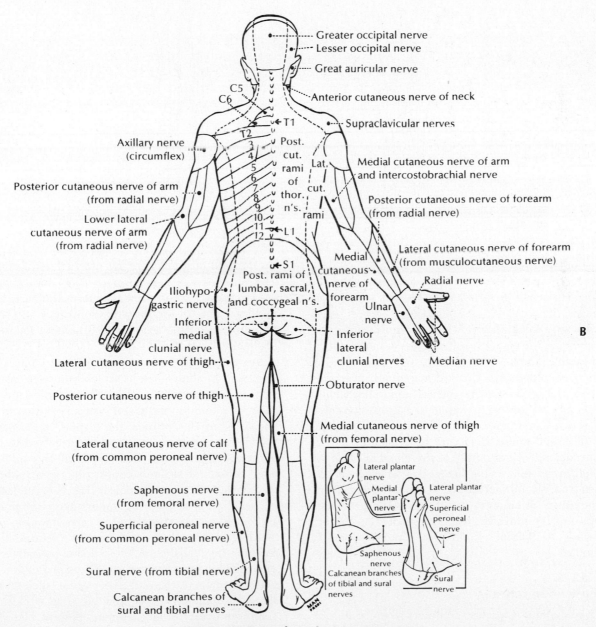

Fig. 23-41, cont'd. For legend see opposite page.

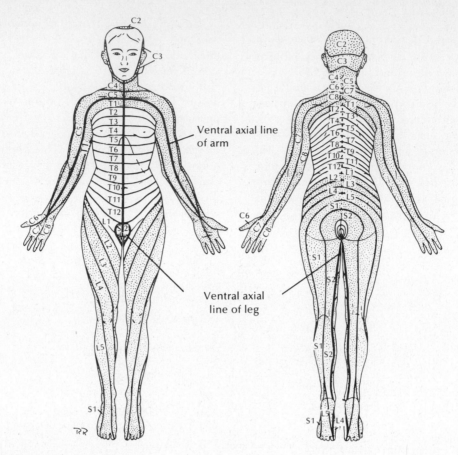

Fig. 23-42. Distribution of spinal dermatomes. (From Keegan, J. J., and Garrett, F. D.: Anat. Rec. **102**:411, 1948.)

the shoulder muscles. Inferior brachial plexus lesions involve C8 and T1, resulting in sensory loss of the medial surface of the arm and in weakness of the arm muscles.

Pathophysiological conditions of the thalamocortical fibers on the cortex result in a loss of those cortical integrating functions (kinesthesis, two-point discrimination, stereognosis). Cortical mapping of the brain is seen in Fig. 23-43; the cortical integrating center for peripheral sensory phenomena is in the postcentral gyrus. Gross perceptions of vibration, pain, temperature, and crude touch may be retained.

The degree of awareness of the client is often recorded in relation to the manner in which he reacts to external stimuli according to the following: alert, cooperative, orientation intact, responds to spoken words and commands, responds to tactile stimuli, responds to painful stimuli, does not respond to stimuli.

REFLEXES
Deep tendon reflex

The skeletal muscles contract when they are stretched by contraction of the antagonistic muscle,

by the pull of gravity, or by external manipulation. The muscles will also contract when their tendons are stretched. These principles form the basis for an understanding of the deep tendon reflex (DTR). Afferent fibers for the reflex arise from both the muscle itself and the tendon.

Muscle spindles or fusiform capsules have been identified in abundance in skeletal muscles, particularly in antigravity muscles. The spindles are capsules surrounding two to ten specialized muscle cells known as intrafusal fibers; these spindles are parallel with surrounding muscles and are attached to them by connective tissue. Both ends of the intrafusal fiber consist of striated contractile tissue, whereas the central portion, the nuclear bag, is expanded and nucleated. These bags are innervated, but primary afferent fibers are stimulated to carry impulses when the bag is stretched or otherwise deformed. On reaching the spinal cord, these action potentials activate the alpha motor neurons. The alpha motor neurons terminate at the end-plates of the skeletal muscle and stimulate their contraction (Fig. 23-44).

Afferent nerve fibers (gamma afferent fibers) encased in a fibrous capsule are called Golgi tendon

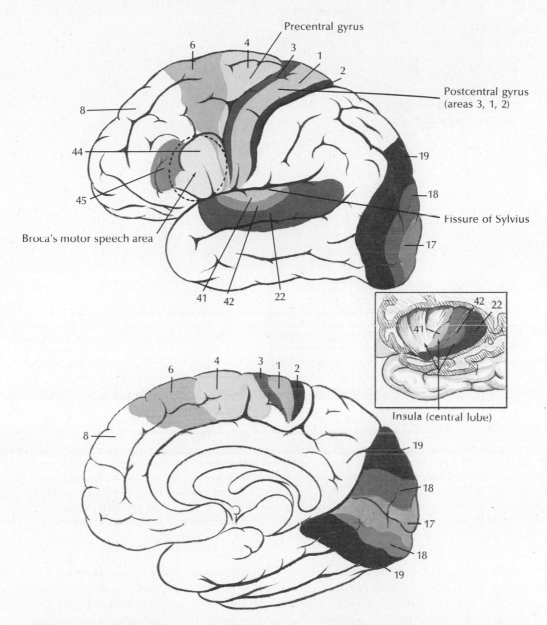

Fig. 23-43. Map of the human cortex. Identity of each numbered area is determined by structural differences in the neurons that compose it. Some areas whose functions are best understood are the following: areas *3*, *1*, and *2*, somatic sensory areas; area *4*, primary motor area; area *6*, secondary motor area; area *17*, primary visual area; areas *18* and *19*, secondary visual areas; areas *41* and *42*, primary auditory areas; area *22*, secondary auditory area. Area *44* and the posterior part of area *45* constitute the approximate location of Broca's motor speech area. (From Anthony, C. P., and Kolthoff, N. J., Textbook of anatomy and physiology, ed. 9, St. Louis, 1975, The C. V. Mosby Co. Modified from Brodmann, K.: Feinere Anatomie des Grosshirns. In Handbuch der Neurologie, Berlin, 1910, Springer-Verlag.)

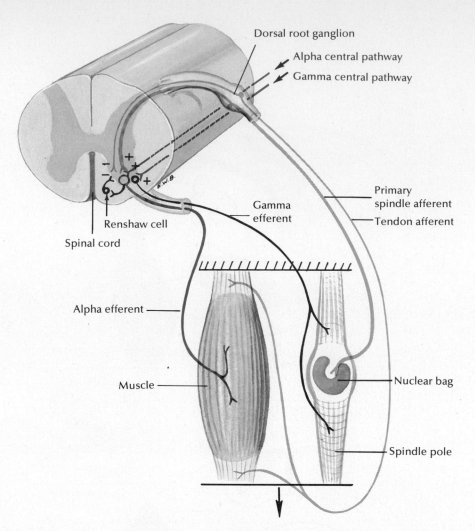

Fig. 23-44. Neural basis for the stretch reflex. Afferent fibers from muscle spindle and tendon organs and efferent fibers to muscle and spindle (gamma fibers) are shown. Excitation is indicated by plus signs, inhibition by minus signs. The Renshaw cell is an interneuron that provides recurrent inhibition to the active motoneuron pool. Muscle is rigidly fixed at the upper end and subject to stretch in the direction of the arrow at the lower end. (From Schottelius, B. A., and Schottelius, D. D.: Textbook of physiology, ed. 18, St. Louis, 1978, The C. V. Mosby Co.)

organs or tendon end-organs and are found in the tendons of skeletal muscles. Stretching of the muscle deforms and activates these afferent nerves, which end on and inhibit the alpha motor neurons. The threshold for activation of the Golgi organs is significantly greater than that of the muscle spindles, and these organs are thought to modulate excessive stretching through inhibition of the muscle spindle (autoinhibition).

Another cell that may inhibit reflex contraction of a muscle is the Renshaw cell, an interneuron between axons of motor nerves. The full nature of this inhibition is not understood.

Golgi efferent nerves terminate in the muscle spindles and may regulate their sensitivity.

Fig. 23-45 illustrates the tendon reflex, using pa-

tellar tendon reflex as an example. The patellar tendon of the quadriceps muscle, an extensor muscle of the upper leg, is attached to the tibia. Deforming this tendon with a reflex hammer causes the muscle to be stretched, activating the muscle spindles, and thereby the primary afferent nerve, in terminating on the alpha motor nerve in the cord segment (L3 and L4). The action potential thus stimulates the alpha efferent fibers, resulting in shortening of the quadriceps muscle, which pulls up the tibia to extend the leg. Dysfunction of the tendon reflex, then, could be attributed to lesions of the afferent or efferent arc of the nerve or to lesions of the muscle, tendon, or spinal segment involved.

Assessment of the DTRs allows the examiner to obtain information about the function of the reflex arcs

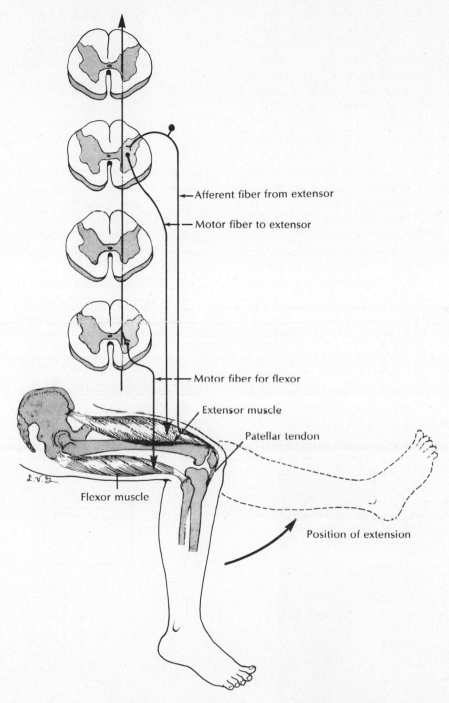

Afferent fiber from extensor

Motor fiber to extensor

Motor fiber for flexor

Extensor muscle

Patellar tendon

Flexor muscle

Position of extension

Fig. 23-45. Tendon reflex (knee jerk or patellar tendon reflex). Note that the patellar tendon of the extensor muscle is attached to the tibia below the knee. (From Schottelius, B. A., and Schottelius, D. D.: Textbook of physiology, ed. 18, St. Louis, 1978, The C. V. Mosby Co.)

and spinal cord segments without implicating other cord segments or higher neural structures.

Reflexes may be altered in pathophysiological changes involving the sensory pathways from the tendons and muscles or the motor component, that is, the corticospinal or corticobulbar pathways (upper motor neuron), or the anterior horn cells or their axons (lower motor neuron).

The best muscle contraction is obtained in testing deep muscle tendons when the muscle is slightly stretched before the tendon is stretched (tapped with the reflex hammer).

Augmentation of the reflex may be obtained by isometrically tensing muscles not directly involved in the reflex arc being tested. For example, the client may be asked to clench the fists or to lock the fingers together and pull one hand against the other (Jendrassik's maneuver) (Fig. 23-46) as the examiner attempts to elicit reflexes in the lower extremity. To reinforce the reflex arcs of the upper extremities, the client may be asked to clench the jaws or to set the quadriceps.

Elicitation of reflexes

Three categories of reflexes are described: (1) DTRs, elicited by deforming (tapping) a tendon (synonyms are muscle stretch reflexes, muscle jerks,

and tendon jerks); (2) superficial or cutaneous reflexes, obtained by stimulating the skin; and (3) pathological reflexes, which are usually present only in disease.

Reflexes may be graded for the record as follows:

4$^+$ or + + + +	Brisk, hyperactive, clonus, often associated with disease
3$^+$ or + + +	More brisk than normal, not necessarily indicative of disease
2$^+$ or + +	Normal
1$^+$ or +	Low normal, slightly diminished response
0	No response

The symmetry of the reflex from one side of the body to the other is also recorded. Differences in response on one side of the body may be helpful in locating the site of the lesions.

A succinct method of recording the reflex findings is the stick figure representation (Fig. 23-47). This lends itself well to expression of both amplitude and symmetry.

Jaw closure reflex. The maxillary reflex, or jaw jerk, is elicited by tapping; the examiner's thumb is placed on the midline of the client's chin but below the lip, with the mouth slightly open. The normal response is an elevation of the mandible (closure of the mouth). The reflex may be difficult to demonstrate.

Arm reflexes. Reflexes that are frequently elicited in the arms are the pectoralis, biceps, triceps, and brachioradialis reflexes and finger flexion.

PECTORALIS REFLEX. This test is not done in the screening examination. The client's arm is held in a position about 6 inches from the body. The exam-

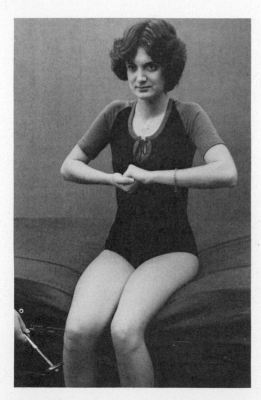

Fig. 23-46. Augmentation maneuver for deep tendon reflexes.

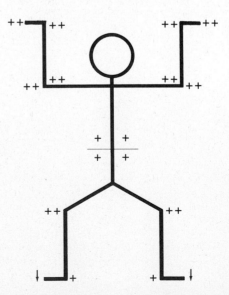

Fig. 23-47. Stick figure drawing for recording reflexes. These are the reflexes usually tested in the screening examination; "++" values shown here are normal.

iner's thumb is placed over the tendon while the hand encircles the shoulder. The thumb is struck with the reflex hammer (Fig. 23-48) in such a way that the blow is transmitted to the tendon. The normal response is adduction of the arm.

BICEPS REFLEX (Fig. 23-49). The client's arm is flexed at the elbow. The examiner's thumb is placed over the biceps tendon. The thumb is struck with the reflex hammer with a slight downward thrust in order to augment the tendon stretch. The normal response is flexion of the arm at the elbow.

TRICEPS REFLEX (Fig. 23-50). The client's arm is flexed at the elbow. The triceps tendon is tapped with the reflex hammer. The normal response is extension of the arm or straightening.

BRACHIORADIALIS REFLEX (Fig. 23-51). The client's arm is placed in a relaxed position. The styloid process (body prominence on the thumb side of the wrist) or the radius is dealt a blow with the percussion hammer after palpation for the tendon (best elicited 3 to 5 cm above the wrist). The normal re-

sponse is flexion of the arm at the elbow (pronation, supination) and at the forearm. The fingers of the hand may also flex (Fig. 23-52).

Finger flexor reflex (finger-thumb reflex). The client's arm is placed so that the wrist is relaxed and pronated. The fingers are slightly flexed at the metacarpophalangeal joint but relaxed. A tap is delivered to fingertips. Flexion of the fingers is accompanied by flexion of the distal phalanx of the thumb.

Lower limb reflexes. Reflexes commonly elicited in the lower limb are the patellar, Achilles tendon, and plantar reflexes.

PATELLAR REFLEX (Fig. 23-53). The tendon is located directly inferior to the patella, or kneecap. With the legs of the client hanging freely over the side of the bed or chair or with the client in a supine position, the tendon is dealt a blow with the percussion hammer. The normal response is extension or kicking out of the leg as the quadriceps muscle contracts.

ACHILLES TENDON REFLEX (Fig. 23-54). The client's foot is held in the hand in a slightly dorsiflexed

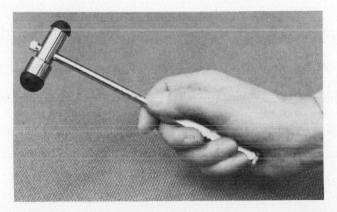

Fig. 23-48. The percussion hammer is held between the thumb and index finger.

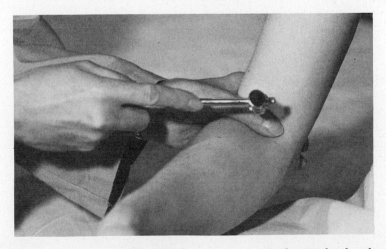

Fig. 23-49. Elicitation of the biceps reflex. A downward blow is struck over the thumb, which is situated over the biceps tendon. The normal response is flexion of the arm at the elbow.

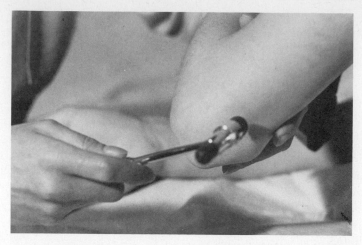

Fig. 23-50. Elicitation of the triceps reflex. With the arm flexed at the elbow, the triceps tendon is tapped with the percussion hammer. The normal response is straightening or extension of the arm.

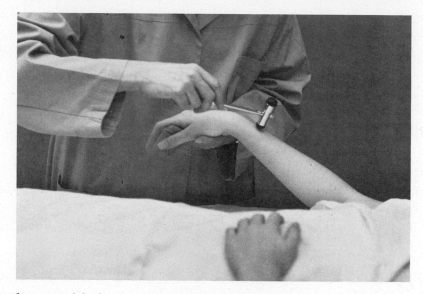

Fig. 23-51. Elicitation of the brachioradialis reflex. The styloid process is dealt a blow with the percussion hammer. The normal response is flexion of the arm at the elbow and slight flexion of the fingers.

position. The Achilles tendon is delivered a blow with the percussion hammer. The normal response is plantar flexion of the foot.

PLANTAR REFLEX (Fig. 23-55). Plantar reflexes are superficial reflexes. A key, pin, half a tongue blade, an applicator stick, or the handle portion of the reflex hammer may be used to elicit the reflex. The stimulus is applied to the lateral border of the client's sole, starting at the heel and continuing to the ball of the foot and then proceeding at a right angle over the ball of the foot toward the great toe. The normal response (negative Babinski's reflex) is flexion of all of the toes (Fig. 23-56).

Before the child can walk, fanning and extension of the toes are the normal response.

Babinski's reflex is dorsiflexion of the great toe and fanning of the other toes (Fig. 23-57). Lesions of the pyramidal tract or motor nerves may be present in the client when Babinski's reflex is found.

If the examiner has difficulty in obtaining the plantar response, a similar reflex may be elicited by stimulating the lateral aspect of the dorsum of the foot. *Chaddock's sign* is the positive response (dorsiflexion of the great toe and fanning of the other toes) to this stimulus.

Other tests for eliciting the plantar response are

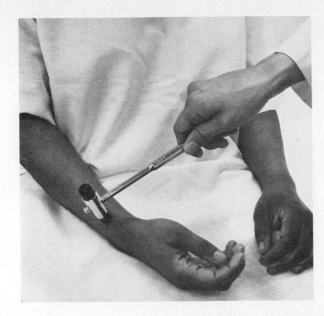

Fig. 23-52. Elicitation of the brachioradialis reflex in the sitting position. The normal response is flexion of the arm at the elbow and slight flexion of the fingers.

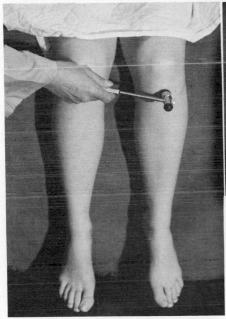

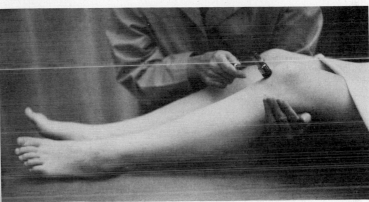

Fig. 23-53. Elicitation of the patellar reflex. With the legs handing freely over the side of the bed **(A)** or with the client in a supine position **(B)**, a blow with the percussion hammer is dealt directly to the patellar tendon, inferior to the patella. The normal response is extension or kicking out of the leg.

Gordon's reflex (elicited by squeezing the calf muscles), *Oppenheim's reflex* (elicited by moving the thumb and index finger simultaneously and firmly over the tibial surface in a caudal direction) (Fig. 23-58), and *Schäffer's reflex* (elicited by squeezing the Achilles tendon).

Abdominal reflexes. See Chapter 17 on assessment of the abdomen and rectosigmoid region.

Cremasteric reflex. The client's inner thigh is stimulated with a sharp object, such as a key or the stick end of an applicator, or with cold or hot water. The expected response is retraction (elevation) of the testis on the same side, as the cremaster muscle contracts.

Gluteal reflex. The client's buttocks are spread, and the perianal area is stimulated. The normal response is contraction of the anal sphincter.

Reflexes elicited in disease states

WARTENBERG'S REFLEX. The examiner grasps the flexed fingers of the client with his own flexed fingers. Both individuals pull against the other; in doing so, the normal client will extend the thumbs. The individual with upper motor neuron disease will adduct and flex the thumb.

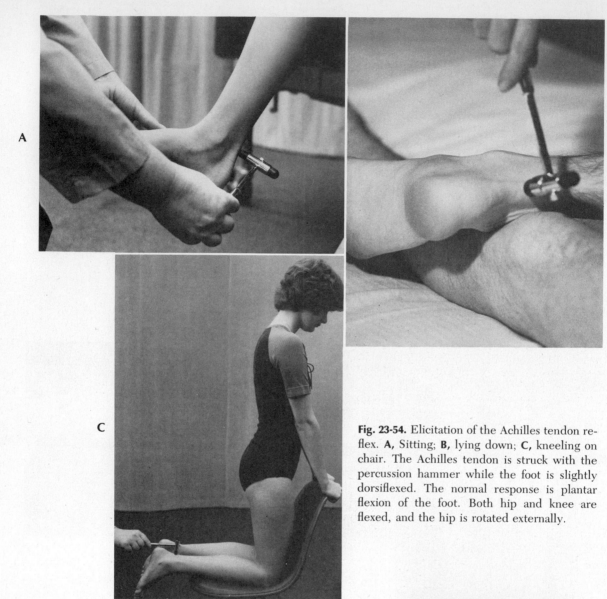

Fig. 23-54. Elicitation of the Achilles tendon reflex. **A**, Sitting; **B**, lying down; **C**, kneeling on chair. The Achilles tendon is struck with the percussion hammer while the foot is slightly dorsiflexed. The normal response is plantar flexion of the foot. Both hip and knee are flexed, and the hip is rotated externally.

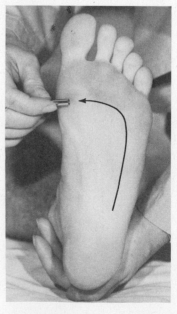

Fig. 23-55. Elicitation of the plantar reflex. A hard object is applied to the lateral surface of the sole, starting at the heel and going over the ball of the foot, ending beneath the great toe. Extension or dorsiflexion of the great toe and fanning of the others is a positive Babinski's reflex.

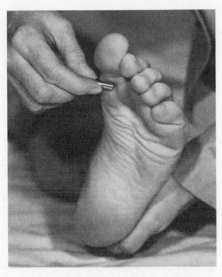

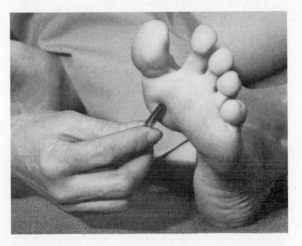

Fig. 23-56. Normal response (negative Babinski's reflex) to plantar stimulation: flexion of all the toes.

Fig. 23-57. Elicitation of a positive Babinski's reflex: dorsiflexion of the great toe and fanning of the other toes.

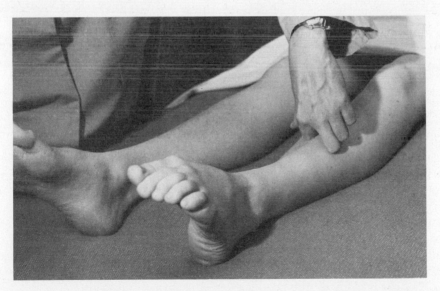

Fig. 23-58. Elicitation of Oppenheim's reflex. Plantar flexion of the toes is obtained by running the index finger and thumb firmly down the tibial surface in a caudal direction.

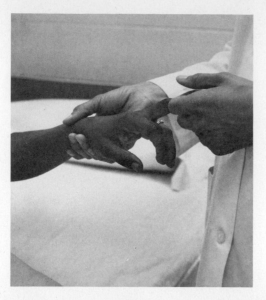

Fig. 23-59. Preparation for elicitation of finger flexion reflex by Hoffman's method: the middle finger is extended to stretch the flexor tendons. The examiner then depresses the distal phalanx and allows it to flip up sharply. Flexion of the thumb or the other fingers may be indicative of pyramidal tract lesion.

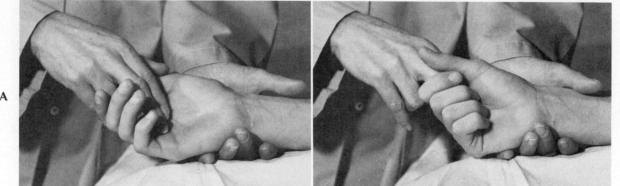

Fig. 23-60. Elicitation of the grasp reflex. **A,** The examiner places the index and middle finger in the client's palm and gently withdraws them. **B,** A positive response consists of the client grasping the examiner's fingers.

FINGER FLEXOR REFLEX. In *Trommer's method,* the metacarpophalangeal joint of the middle finger is extended (to stretch the flexor tendons). The palmar side of the distal phalanx is flicked by the examiner.

In *Hoffmann's method,* (Fig. 23-59) the examiner depresses the distal phalanx and allows it to flip up sharply. A positive response is recorded if flexion of the thumb and other finger is observed. This reflex is normally not elicited. Hoffmann's sign is the name given to the reflex when it is elicited. The presence of a pyramidal lesion may be suspected.

GRASP REFLEX (Fig. 23-60). The examiner places the index and middle finger in the client's palm, entering between the thumb and the index finger. The examiner's fingers are gently withdrawn, pulling the fingers across the skin of the client's palm. A positive response consists of the client grasping the examiner's fingers. Present in individuals with widespread brain damage, the grasp reflex is normal in infants less than 4 months of age.

Loss of reflexes

With loss of or diminution of reflexes on the same side, the examiner might suspect corticospinal lesions.

The reappearance of primitive reflexes such as Babinski's is also indicative of corticospinal pathology.

Loss of sensation from a segment (dermatome) coupled with loss of reflexes suggests lesions in the sensory arc. Tabes dorsalis (neurosyphilis) produces this form of disorder.

INDICATIONS OF DISEASE
Early indications of interruptions of the corticospinal tract

The examiner may elicit the *pronation sign* by asking the client to extend his arms at the level of the shoulders with the palms upward (Fig. 23-61). The arm on the affected side will drift downward and pronate.

The examiner may elicit *Barré's sign* by asking

Table 23-4. Deep tendon reflex and muscle changes in upper and lower motor neuron lesions

Lesion	Common etiology	Characteristics
Upper motor neuron lesion (corticospinal tract)	Cerebrovascular occlusion	Brisk reflexes
	Neoplasm—cerebral hemispheres	Contralateral arm and leg muscles spasticity—more marked in the flexors in arm and leg extensions
	Amyotrophic lateral sclerosis	Muscle weakness—disuse atrophy of those muscles that oppose the spastic muscles
	Deficiency diseases, pernicious anemia	Hyperreflexia
	Trauma	Babinski's sign present; clonus frequently seen
Lower motor neuron lesion (anterior horn cell, somatic motor part of cranial nerves)	Poliomyelitis	Hyporeflexia
		Diminution or absence of deep tendon reflexes
	Amyotrophic lateral sclerosis	Muscle atrophy
	Neoplasm	
		Muscle weakness, fasciculation, and fibrillation of muscle
	Trauma	Babinski's sign—diminished or absent

Table 23-5. Reflexes commonly tested in the physical examination

Reflexes	Segmental level
Deep tendon	
Jaw	Pons
Biceps	Cervical 5, 6
Triceps	Cervical 6, 7, 8
Brachioradialis	Cervical 5, 6
Patellar	Lumbar 2, 3, 4
Achilles	Sacral 1, 2
Superficial	
Corneal	Pons
Palatal	Medulla
Pharyngeal	Medulla
Abdominal (upper)	Thoracic 7, 8, 9
Abdominal (lower)	Thoracic 12, lumbar 1
Cremasteric	Lumbar 1, 2, 3
Gluteal	Lumbar 4, 5
Plantar	Lumbar 4, 5; sacral 1, 2

the client to flex his knees 90 degrees while in the prone position (Fig. 23-62). The affected leg will move downward.

Fine movements of the hands, such as picking up coins or pencils, are done slowly when there are lesions of the corticospinal tract. The ability to touch the thumb to the fingers is performed less rapidly.

Cortical lesions

Disturbance in the ability to discriminate objects or symbols by means of the senses, assuming the individual previously had this skill, is termed agnosia. *Visual agnosia*, caused by lesions of the occipital cortex, is the inability to recognize objects. *Auditory agnosia*, caused by lesions below the sylvian fissure, is the inability to recognize familiar sounds. *Tactile agnosia*, caused by lesions of the parietal lobe, is the inability to recognize objects by feeling them.

A disturbance in the recognition of body parts is termed autotopagnosia.

Lack of insight of an individual to his disease is termed anosognosia.

Lesions of the cerebral hemisphere dominant for language

Aphasia, the inability to comprehend or use language symbols, is caused by a disorder of the cortical areas necessary to speech or by neural connections in the cerebral hemisphere dominant for speech; aphasia encompasses dysarthria and dysphonia. *Nonfluent aphasia* is the inability to produce words in either spoken or written form. The client with *fluent aphasia* has the ability to produce words but frequently chooses inappropriate words (*paraphasia*) or makes errors in content, occasionally creating words.

Lesions of the cerebral hemisphere not dominant for language

A disturbance in the ability to perform a purposeful act when comprehension is intact is termed apraxia. For example, given a fork, the client may be unable to use it to eat; the client may be unable to dress or button his shirt. *Constructional apraxia* is the inability to draw or construct forms of two or three dimensions.

Signs of meningeal irritation

Meningeal irritation is most commonly due to infection or to intracranial hemorrhages. The following

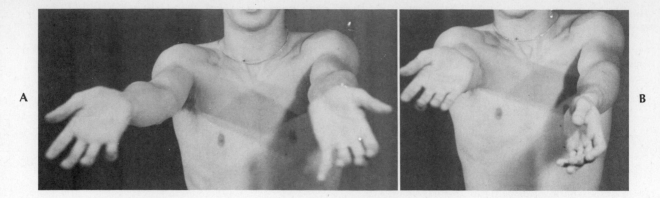

Fig. 23-61. Elicitation of the pronation sign. **A,** The client is asked to extend his arms at shoulder height with the palms upward. **B,** Frequently in disease of the corticospinal tract, the affected arm will drift downward and pronate.

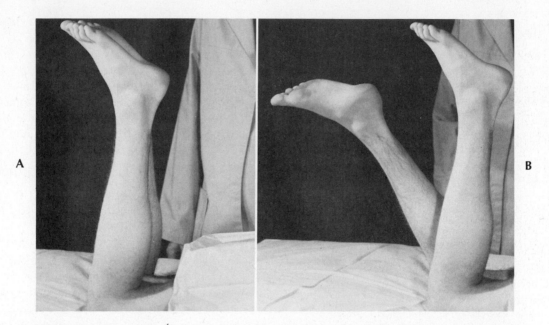

Fig. 23-62. Elicitation of Barré's sign. **A,** The client is asked to lie on his abdomen, flexing the legs at a 90-degree angle. **B,** Frequently in disease of the corticospinal tract, the affected leg will drift downward.

signs indicate the need for laboratory work to confirm the diagnosis.

Nuchal rigidity (stiff neck) is a common sign of meningitis and may be demonstrated through the use of cervical flexing.

Brudzinski's sign (Fig. 23-63) is elicited with the client supine. The head is lifted toward the sternum. The individual with meningeal irritation will resist the movement and may flex the hips and knees. The movement is commonly accompanied by pain.

Kernig's sign is the inability to extend the lower leg when that leg is flexed at the hip, or there may be resistance or pain during the process. Knee extension is usually possible to approximately 135 degrees.

Lasègue's sign (straight leg) is elicited by lifting the leg, supporting it under the heel, in order to maintain extension. A positive sign is pain, resistance, or a decreased angle of flexion of the hip.

Neurological (equivocal) or "soft" signs

Neurological (equivocal) or "soft" signs may be of neurological significance but involve only slight dysfunctions that are present occasionally or inconsistently. The following signs are recorded when observed: short attention span; minimal or lack of coordination; clumsiness; frequent falling, disturbances of gait, or failure to maintain balance; hyperkinesis, both voluntary and involuntary; uneven per-

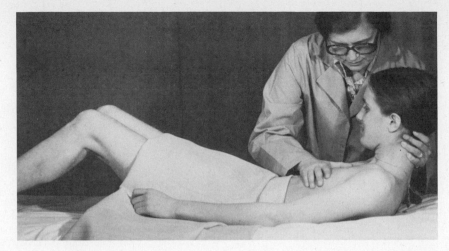

Fig. 23-63. Elicitation of Brudzinski's sign. With meningeal irritation, pain is elicited when the head is flexed.

ceptual development; incomplete laterality, for example, left handed but right footed, with no side clearly dominant; language disturbances; articulation disorders; dyslexia; motor outflow (motor movements involving more muscles than intended); and mirroring movements of the extremities, for example, when one hand performs a function, the other is also in motion.

Levels of consciousness

The levels of consciousness (responsiveness) are generally described according to the behavior exhibited by the individual. Table 8-4 includes a useful categorization of the levels of consciousness.

SUMMARY

I. Mental status examination (see Chapter 8)
  A. Description of appearance and behavior
  B. Level of consciousness
    1. Time
    2. Place
    3. Person
  C. Cognitive function
    1. Memory
      a. Immediate
      b. Recent
      c. Remote
    2. Calculation
    3. Abstract reasoning
    4. Language skills—facility
  D. Emotional status
  E. Thought content
  F. Observation for agnosia, apraxia, and aphasia
II. Assessment of the cranial nerves
  A. CN I: olfactory—normal smell
  B. CN II: optic—with assessment of the eye
    1. Visual acuity
    2. Color vision

  C. CN III: oculomotor—all performed with assessment of the eye
    CN IV: trochlear
    CN VI: abducens—all performed
    1. Extraocular movement
    2. Nystagmus
    3. Elevation of eyelids
    4. Pupil size
      a. Consensus
      b. Accommodation
  D. CN V: trigeminal
    1. Sensory in ophthalmic, maxillary, mandibular divisions
      a. Pressure, pain
      b. Vibration
      c. Temperature
      d. Corneal reflex
    2. Motor—muscles of mastication
  E. CN VII: facial
    1. Motor—muscles of facial expression
    2. Sensory—anterior two-thirds of tongue (test posterior one-third at same time)
  F. CN VIII: auditory and vestibular
    1. Auditory—done with assessment of the ear
      a. General
      b. Weber
      c. Rinné
    2. Vestibular—not generally done
  G. CN IX: glossopharyngeal
    CN X: vagus
    1. Uvular position and movement
    2. Gag reflex
    3. Swallowing
  H. CN XI: spinal accessor—movement of sternocleidomastoid and trapezius

1. Turn head to side against resistance
2. Shrug shoulders against resistance
I. CN XII: hypoglossal
   1. Stick out tongue
   2. Move tongue from side to side against resistance
III. Cerebellar function
   A. Pronation, supination
   B. Finger to nose
   C. Finger to examiner's finger
   D. Each finger to thumb
   E. Heel down shin
   F. Romberg test
IV. Motor function—dont in musculoskeletal examination
   A. Muscle size
   B. Muscle tone
   C. Involuntary movements
   D. Muscle strength
V. Sensory function
   A. Pressure, pain, and vibration in all dermatomes
   B. Temperature if pressure, pain, and vibration abnormal
   C. Discrimination
      1. Stereognosis
      2. Two-point discrimination
VI. Reflex assessment
   A. Deep tendon reflexes (DTRs)
      1. Jaw closure
      2. Biceps
      3. Triceps
      4. Brachioradialis
      5. Patellar
      6. Achilles
   B. Superficial reflexes
      1. Plantar (Babinski's)
      2. Abdominal—done in abdominal examination
      3. Cremasteric
      4. Gluteal—not generally done in screening

BIBLIOGRAPHY

Alpers, B. J., and Mancall, E. L.: Essentials of the neurological examination, Philadelphia, 1971, F. A. Davis Co.

DeJong, R. N.: The neurologic examination: incorporating the fundamentals of neuroanatomy and neurophysiology, ed. 4, New York, 1979, Harper & Row, Publishers.

DeMyer, W.: Technique of the neurologic examination, ed. 2, New York, 1974, McGraw-Hill Book Co.

Haymaker, W.: Bing's local diagnosis in neurological diseases, ed. 15, St. Louis, 1969, The C. V. Mosby Co.

Haymaker, W., and Woodhall, B.: Peripheral nerve injuries, principles of diagnosis, ed. 2, Philadelphia, 1953, W. B. Saunders Co.

Mayo Clinic: Clinical examinations in neurology, ed. 4, Philadelphia, 1976, W. B. Saunders Co.

Plum, F., and Posner, J. B.: The diagnosis of stupor and coma, ed. 2, Philadelphia, 1972, F. A. Davis Co.

Schneider, F. A.: The sense of smell in man: its physiological basis, N. Engl. J. Med. **277**:299, 1967.

Simpson, J. F., and Magee, K. R.: Clinical evaluation of the nervous system, Boston, 1973, Little, Brown and Co.

Sumner, D.: On testing the sense of smell, Lancet **2**:895, 1962.

Wartenberg, R.: The examination of reflexes; a simplification, Chicago, 1945, Year Book Medical Publishers, Inc.

24 Assessment of the pediatric client

MURIEL MOSS, R.N., M.A.
JOANNA SCHLEUTERMANN, R.N., M.P.H.

Pediatric care is, to a large extent, health care aimed at promoting the health of the child and preventing illness and disability through early identification of problems.

The examination of the child is ideally carried out over an extended period of time in a planned sequential pattern. The dynamic changes that occur in the normal growth and development of the child require the practitioner to carefully assess the increments in growth; the changes in physiological function; and the development of cognitive, social, and motor skills of the child during each examination.

It is by comparing the individual child's current growth achievements and parameters of health with that found in previous examinations and with other normal healthy children that the health of the child is determined. The child should be seen more frequently during infancy, when the growth changes are most rapid and dramatic, and then at less frequent intervals throughout the childhood years.

The examination of the child also gives consideration to the environment in which the child lives and to the parental concerns in child rearing. The adults responsible for the child's care often have concerns about the development of the child and about their own ability to manage. They need respect, support, and guidance that encourages them to express the concerns they may have and to discuss their needs and the needs of the child. The mother is usually the person most familiar with the child and his care and is the one most likely to detect changes, both normal and abnormal, that go unnoticed by others, including the health practitioner. The practitioner should also be alert to any signs of stress between the mother and child. A mother who is concerned, anxious, or angry about a child's behavior or physical condition may be showing evidence of stress that can interfere with the mother-child relationship and ultimately with the development of the child. There-

fore, consideration is given to the needs of the mother or other adults caring for the child as well as to those of the child himself.

The attitude of the practitioner should always demonstrate respect for both the child and the parent, a willingness to listen to the problems, and a concerned interest in finding adequate solutions. Both the child and the parent will be sensitive to the attitudes of the practitioner and will respond according to the impressions they receive.

In essence, the examiner needs to be sensitive to the child as a growing, developing human being who is ever changing.

This chapter includes a discussion of the approaches to the child and the parent and some of the techniques used in obtaining health information and in assessing the health of the child. In addition, some of the physical differences between the child and the adult are discussed.

It is not possible to include a survey of all the components of child development that are assessed. The reader is referred to standard pediatric texts and Chapter 4, "Developmental Assessment," for assistance in understanding the parameters of normal development and health of children.

THE PEDIATRIC HISTORY

The pediatric history provides the opportunity to interview both the child and the parent in order to gather information about the child's health, development, relationships with others, and care. It also provides the opportunity for the child to become acquainted with the practitioner before he is examined. The pediatric history is an adaptation of the model used for an adult history. It also incorporates areas uniquely pertinent to the child, such as the history of the mother's health during the pregnancy and the history of birth and the neonatal period.

The informant for the history may be a parent, a

relative, a caretaker, or the child himself. The interviewer should identify the informant and indicate the reliability of the information obtained. It is common for the child, even the young child, to participate in the interview and to volunteer useful information. The information gained from the child should be indicated as such in the history.

Chief complaint

The chief complaint (CC) statement gives the reason for making the visit and should be in the words of the informant. Children are seen most frequently for health care, and the CC statement may indicate a visit for routine health care rather than for the treatment of a health problem. An example would be "It is time for his checkup." The chief complaint may be recorded in the words of the adult or the older child when the child is young.

Present illness

The present illness (PI) section incorporates the same categories of information obtained in the adult health history and includes a statement about the usual health, a description of the chronological story, any relevant family history, negative information, and a disability assessment. The following is an example of a history of the present illness of a child brought to the examiner for health care:

This 7-year-old, white female, who is a student in the second grade of the Urban Elementary School, was brought to the clinic by her mother for an annual physical examination. She has been in good health except for occasional colds, approximately four colds, since her visit 1 year ago in July. The child, Debbie, stated that she enjoys school but thinks her teacher "is too hard sometimes." Her mother indicated that all school reports are good and that Debbie has many friends in school and the neighborhood and has recently started "sleeping over" with one or two of her girl friends. The only problem that the mother expressed was in regard to dental care. Debbie has two small cavities, which were found on her first visit to the dentist 2 months ago and the mother is questioning the value of having "baby teeth filled." Debbie has complained of a toothache on only one occasion, just prior to the visit to the dentist. The pain was relieved by giving aspirin, 5 grains.

The PI description in this example is that of a child in good health who is functioning well. The negative information concerning the dental caries gives information that the dental caries are not interfering with the child's ability to function but that further consideration is necessary to prevent a more serious problem for the child. An attempt should be made to learn the reason for deciding not to continue dental care. The mother may be seeking assurance that she is right in not making a plan for dental care or she may be seeking information that the experience will not be difficult for the child and should be planned. Whatever the outcome, information and support need to be given to help the child and the parent reach a more appropriate decision.

Past history

The past history of infants, young children, and any child with a possible developmental deficiency should include the following information:

1. The health of the mother during the pregnancy with this child, including the mother's feelings about the pregnancy, the amount of prenatal care, and any history of complications (excessive weight gain, hypertension, vaginal bleeding, nausea and vomiting, urinary problems, infections such as rubella or venereal disease), and any medications or drugs prescribed or used
2. The birth history, including the date, the hospital where the child was born, the duration of the pregnancy, the parity of the mother, the birth weight, the nature and duration of the labor, the type of delivery, the use of any sedation or anesthesia, the state of the infant at birth, and the use of any special procedures
3. The postnatal history, including information about skin color, bleeding, seizures, fever, congenital anomalies or birth injuries, difficulty in sucking, rashes, or poor weight gain during the first days and weeks after birth
4. A developmental history, including the age at which the child attained specific developmental achievements (holding the head erect, rolling over, sitting alone, pulling up, walking with help, walking alone, saying first words, using sentences, urinary continence during the day, urinary continence during the night, control of feces), a comparison of this child's development with that of siblings, any periods of decreased or increased growth, the school grade attained, and the quality of school work
5. A history of hospitalizations, serious illnesses, or injuries and dates of occurrence
6. A history of communicable diseases (measles, mumps, pertussis, chickenpox, rheumatic fever), the age at which the disease occurred, the severity, and any complications
7. A history of immunizations, including booster inoculations and dates
8. A history of allergies to food and drugs and any history of hay fever, asthma, or eczema

Family history

The family history of the child includes questions about familial illnesses or anomalies; the health and age of the grandparents, as well as that of the parents; the age, sex, and health of siblings; and the age at death and the cause of death of immediate members of the family, including a history of stillbirths, miscarriages, and abortions.

Nutritional history

Nutritional assessment of the child is one of the most important aspects of health care. Because infant nutrition is different from infant feeding, there are distinct implications about the taking of a nutritional history. Nutrition refers to "the nature and nurturing properties of the material being assimilated as food," whereas feeding is the transferral of food to the infant's intestine (Filer, 1977). Because most health professionals focus on infant feeding when they take a history, the child's caretaker is frequently left to make the decisions about the child's nutrition. And too often the only statement made in the nutritional history is that the infant, child, or adolescent, eats well or poorly.

One of the first questions to ask the mother of a new infant is whether she is breast-feeding or using a formula. This inquiry is to be made in a manner that does not tell the mother that she is right or wrong in the choice she has made, but is to be supportive of her decision. However, if one were providing health care counseling to the pregnant woman, the practitioner would make sure that the prospective mother has sufficient and accurate information about the dietary, immunological, and psychological advantages of breast-feeding. Determining the method of feeding the infant is insufficient.

If the mother is breast-feeding, the interviewer needs to explore the mother's care of her breasts, her program of daily exercise and rest, her daily dietary intake, and whether she is supplementing the baby's diet. In the latter case, it is necessary to determine the nature of the supplement, for example, formula, cereal, and/or other solid foods, and how frequently and how much the infant consumes. Also, the mother's self-confidence needs to be promoted. It is useful to explore her ideas and feelings about the sensuous nature of the breast-feeding relationship with her infant and any effects it has on the marital relationship she shares with her husband. Identifying her beliefs about breast size, adequacy of the richness and the amount of her milk, and her opinion of whether it satisfies her baby or not is important. Specifying who in her family and peer group support or undermine her choice to breast-feed is helpful. It is necessary to assess whether her reasons for breast-feeding are realistic.

Inquiries are made to see if the mother is planning to introduce solid foods and whether she knows it is

---

Examples of medicants, foods, and sundries that are excreted in breast milk and may affect infants*

Analgesics
  Codeine in habituated doses
  Heroin in habituated doses
  Meperidine in habituated doses
  Morphine in habituated doses
  Propoxyphene in IV
  Sodium salicylate in high doses
Antihistamines
Antimicrobials
  Ampicillin
  Chloramphenicol
  Penicillin
  Sulfonamides
  Tetracyclines
Depressants
  Barbiturates
    Long-acting, hypnotic doses
    Short-acting, hypnotic doses
  Others
    Alcohol
    Bromides, hypnotic doses
    Chloral hydrate
    Diazepam
    Reserpine
Diuretics
  Hydrochlorothiazide, chlorothiazide
Hormonal compounds
  Iodides
  Oral contraceptives
  Pregnane beta-diol
  Propylthiouracil
  Thyroid
Anthraquinone derivatives
  Cascara
  Danthron
Social drugs (legal)
  Caffeine
  Tobacco
Social drugs (illegal)
  Abuse drugs: stimulants, depressants, narcotics, psychedelics in high doses
Miscellaneous
  Anticoagulants, oral
  DDT
  Ergotrate maleate
  Fluorides
  Foods: white navy beans, corn, egg white, chocolate, unripe fruit, pickles, peanuts, cottonseed, and wheat

---

*Data from Levin, R.: In Herfindal, E. T., and Hirschman, J., editors: Clinical pharmacy and therapeutics, Baltimore, 1975, The Williams & Wilkins Co.

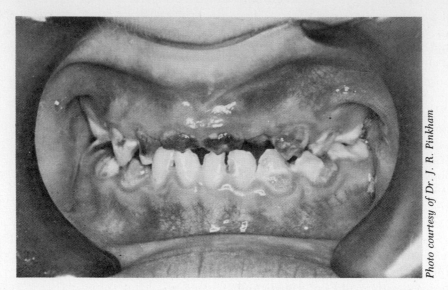

Photo courtesy of Dr. J. R. Pinkham

Fig. 24-1. Mouth of 2-year-old boy with "nursing bottle syndrome," demonstrating extensive carious destruction of the maxillary anterior primary teeth. The mandibular teeth are affected to a lesser extent, probably because of the position of the tongue in relation to the nursing nipple and the protective bathing action of saliva from submandibular and sublingual salivary glands. (From Fomon, S.: Infant nutrition, ed. 3, Philadelphia, 1974, W. B. Saunders Co.)

not recommended by many physicians or needed before 6 months of age. Dry infant cereal, as a source of iron, can be used as a supplement when the child is 4 to 6 months of age. It should be continued until the child is at least 18 months of age (Committee on Nutrition, 1976). Breast-feeding is only rarely associated with iron deficiency. Intestinal blood loss is rare in breast-fed infants in comparison to infants fed fresh cow milk. Also, the absorption of the small amount of iron present in human milk is quite good, the average being 49% (Fomon, 1974).

The practitioner will need to inquire whether the mother is using any medications, including birth control pills. In addition, specifying the name, amount, frequency taken, purpose, and effectiveness is useful in assessing whether it may be harmful to the infant and whether it is necessary for the mother's health. The box on p. 561 provides a list of drugs that are known to be excreted in human milk and to have side effects in breast-fed infants.

Last, the mother's plan for weaning should be investigated. Some health professionals recommend that any weaning before 9 months of age be to the bottle; formula rather than whole milk is used. It is thought that the child may associate formula with the cup and not make as smooth a transition when the time comes to be weaned to the cup and to whole milk. Others believe that the infant should be breast-fed as long as possible, for example, 12 months, and then weaned directly to the cup when whole milk is introduced.

If the infant is formula-fed, the preceding questions are easily and appropriately adapted. The mother is instructed to choose an iron and zinc–fortified formula. The early use of iron-fortified formula helps to store iron and prevent iron deficiency between the ages of 6 and 18 months, when the risk is greatest. Two servings a day (3 to 6 tablespoons each serving) will provide a sufficient supplement of iron for most infants and is to be used throughout the second year of life as iron requirements remain high. If the child is preterm, iron supplementation begins at age 2 months instead of 4 months (Committee on Nutrition, 1976). Weaning from the bottle by 12 months is strongly advised by pedodontists to prevent dental caries and malocclusions. Inquiries are made about putting the baby to bed with a bottle of milk or fruit juice in his mouth. She is advised not to do this because of the danger of dental caries and destruction of the maxillary anterior teeth, commonly referred to as "baby bottle syndrome" (Fig. 24-1). If the child shows signs of dental caries between 6 and 18 months of age he should be referred for dental care.

In order for the practitioner to complete a nutritional assessment, data that reflect caloric intake, liquid and solid intake, and the pattern of output must be obtained. In the breast-fed infant, it is necessary to determine how long the child nurses, whether he sucks well, whether he empties a breast, whether he suckles at both breasts each feeding, how often he feeds, and whether he seems satisfied. In the formula-fed infant, inquiries are made about the

Table 24-1. Calories, ounces of formula, number of feedings in 24 hours, and the quantity of feedings for children age birth to 5 months*

Age	Calories per day	Ounces of formula per day	Number of feedings in 24 hours	Quantity per feedings (ounces)
Birth–10 days	250-350	12-25	6-10	2-3
1 month	300-350	15-25	5-6	3-4½
2 months	400-580	20-24	5-6	3½-6
3 months	480-650	24-32†	4-5	4-7
4 months	560-700	28-35	4-5	5-8
5 months	630-750	31-37	4-5	6-8

*Data from Pediatric Series, 1975.
†When the intake of milk formula reaches 650 to 700 calories or 32 ounces a day, other foods should be added to the diet.

Table 24-2. Guidelines for vitamin, iron, and zinc supplementation and the introduction of solid foods in breast-fed or formula-fed infants*

Age (months)	Food
Birth	Vitamin D supplement for breast-fed infants if sunshine is inadequate
	Fluoride drops for any infant living in a community where the water contains less than 1 mg/L fluoride
	Iron and zinc supplement for noniron- and nonzinc-fortified formula-fed infants
	or
	Iron- and zinc-fortified formula for formula-fed infants
2	Iron supplement for preterm infant using iron-fortified dry cereal or iron drops
4	Iron-fortified dry cereal or iron drops to supplement full-term infants
6	Strained fruits, strained vegetables, diluted fruit juices
7-9	Mashed fruits and vegetables, mashed, cooked egg yolk, soft finger foods, toast, zwieback
12	Cooked egg white
	Multivitamin supplement as milk intake decreases and solid foods are increased

*Data on vitamin supplementation from Fomon, 1974; zinc and iron supplementation from Filer, 1977; introduction of solid foods from personal clinical experiences. These guidelines would need to be adjusted if the child had a malabsorptive disorder or was being fed a nonmilk formula.

type of formula, whether it contains iron and/or zinc, how it is prepared, how frequently the child feeds, and how much he consumes. If the child receives solid foods, it is helpful to determine when they were first introduced, in what order and combination they were started, any dermatological or gastrointestinal reactions, how frequently they are fed, how much is consumed, and how they are prepared or altered to encourage feeding. Table 24-1 describes general guidelines for formula-fed infants. Table 24-2 provides guidelines for supplementation in breast-fed or formula-fed infants.

Another important question is how the foods are given, that is, by spoon or in the bottle. Mothers need to be advised that spoon feeding solid foods is a valuable step in assisting their child's development, especially in the manipulation of food in his mouth, swallowing, chewing, and feeding himself. They are to be cautioned about the dangers of aspiration when the nipple is opened for thicker foods and is then used for thinner formula. Also, nipple widening can discourage an infant from vigorous sucking as he tries to avoid getting too much milk into his mouth. When infants are receiving water, it is necessary to know whether sugar has been added, the amount, the type, gastrointestinal effect, how often it is fed, and the amount consumed. Food preferences of the mother and family, in addition to the child, are helpful in assessing the likelihood of the infant being exposed to a varied and balanced diet. Likewise, the effects of culture, religion, and ethnicity on the types of foods available, the methods of preparation, and the use of food as a reward are important concerns. Need for attention, overprotection from parents, and insecurity are to be evaluated as they relate to food intake. The causes of obesity are many and complex, but obesity is rarely an isolated problem and often begins in early childhood as mothers frequently measure their child's growth by the amount of weight gained. Knowledge of the family's budget is vital to assessing the mother's ability to provide the foods the health professional may be recommending for her infant's nutrition. Whether the mother is utilizing iron drops or vitamin supplements with her child is assessed. Information obtained includes the type, when they were started, the amount, and the length of time they have been used. In the older child, food preferences and snack foods become more evident. These food habits need to be explored in terms of their nutritional value, effect of weight gain, any dermatological reactions, and potential for chronic disease in adulthood—for example, foods that serve as an energy booster, are a source of empty calories, are antagonists to acne, or increase cholesterol or high blood pressure.

Urinary output is an important factor in nutritional assessment. "Most commercially prepared formulas, as well as cow milk with added carbohydrate and water, will yield renal solute loads that are considerably less than that resulting from whole cow milk, though greater than the renal solute load presented by human milk" (Fomon, 1974). Urinary output may be increased if water is being used as a supplement and may falsely be interpreted as reflecting sufficient milk intake. The mother is to be counseled to observe and report about the urinary stream, the color,

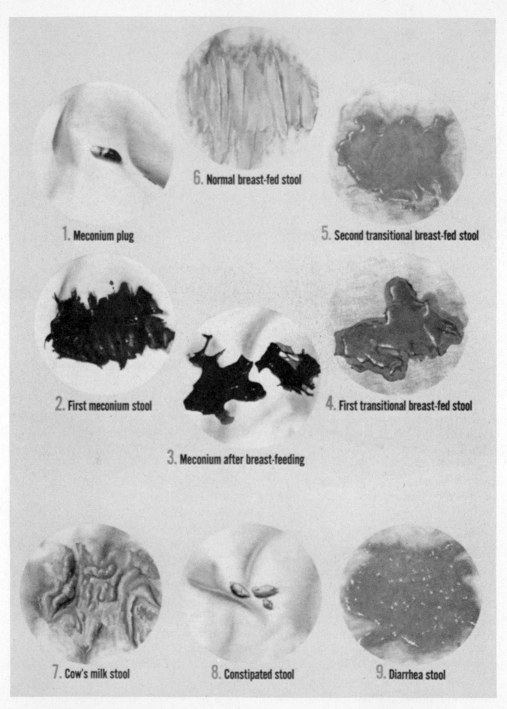

1. Meconium plug

6. Normal breast-fed stool

5. Second transitional breast-fed stool

2. First meconium stool

3. Meconium after breast-feeding

4. First transitional breast-fed stool

7. Cow's milk stool

8. Constipated stool

9. Diarrhea stool

Fig. 24-2. Normal stool cycle of breast-fed and formula-fed infants. (Modified from *Nursing Education Aids*, Clinical Educational Aid, courtesy Ross Laboratories, Columbus, Ohio.)

odor, and presence of blood, frequency of urination, and degree of wetness, that is, whether the diaper is wringing wet or barely wet.

Gastrointestinal output varies in relationship to the source of nutrition. A breast-fed infant has a very distinctive stool. Question the mother to determine if the stool is soft, yellow, and with the consistency and form of scrambled eggs. It may be infrequent once the child adapts to regular feedings and the mature milk is produced. As many as 5 to 6 days may go by between stool passages. Before this time, the infant usually passes a stool after each feeding and even spots a diaper periodically throughout the day. A formula-fed infant's stool is firmer, deeper in color, and follows a more frequent and regular pattern of excretion. Fig. 24-2 illustrates the normal stool cycle of a breast-fed infant compared to a formula-fed infant. As solid foods are introduced the mother will notice color, texture, frequency, and odor changes.

When a child experiences diarrhea, the loss of water in the stool can be a critical factor in his ability to recover, particularly if he is not eating well. A breast-fed infant has protection against the enteroviral infections that are the most common etiological agents in infant diarrhea. The stool may indicate to the practitioner blood loss, malabsorption, or other disorders of the gastrointestinal system, such as allergy to cow's milk, anemia, cystic fibrosis, or celiac diseases.

Of course nutritional assessment would be incomplete without the mother's interpretation of her child's growth, weight gain, and appetite. A comparison of this infant to other siblings of the same age can give insight into familial patterns and parent expectations. A sample of an interview form to assess the nutritional status of a child is provided here.

Sample interview form to assess nutritional status of child*

Date of evaluation _____

Name _____

Address _____

Birth date _____ Birth weight _____ Birth order _____

Sex: ☐ Male ☐ Female   Multiple birth: ☐ Yes ☐ No

Who prepares the meals? _____ Who is responsible for feeding the child? _____

Does the home have a working stove? ☐ Yes ☐ No Oven? ☐ Yes ☐ No

Does the home have a refrigerator? ☐ Yes ☐ No

Home location? ☐ Urban ☐ Suburban ☐ Rural nonfarm ☐ Farm ☐ Other

Does the family do any of the following to obtain part of its food supply? ☐ Have a vegetable garden
  ☐ Keep a cow ☐ Raise chickens ☐ Fish

Feeding during first year

	Duration (months)				
	0	**1**	**1-3**	**3-6**	**6-12**
Breast					
Iron-fortified formula					
Other formula					
Other milk—specify					

	Duration (months)				
Dietary supplements	**1**	**1-6**	**6-12**	**12-24**	**Now**	**Brand name if known**
Vitamins						
Vitamins with iron						
Vitamins with fluoride						
Vitamins with fluoride and iron						

Regularity of administration (specify) _____

*From U.S. Department of Health, Education and Welfare: Screening children for nutritional status, Washington, D.C., 1971, U.S. Government Printing Office.

Continued.

Sample interview form to assess nutritional status of child—cont'd

Immunizations
- ☐ DPT primary series
- ☐ DPT, DT, or tetanus booster
- ☐ Smallpox vaccine
- ☐ Oral polio vaccine
- ☐ Measles vaccine
- ☐ German measles (rubella) vaccine
- ☐ Mumps vaccine

Walked alone at _____ months

Serious illnesses:

Hospitalizations (give age, time hospitalized, and nature of illness):

☐ Ill now? If ill, indicate nature of illness: _____

FOOD INTAKE
Form A—24-hour recall

Name _____

Date and time of interview _____

Length of interview _____

Date of recall _____

Day of the week of recall: 1-M 2-T 3-W 4-Th 5-F 6-Sat 7-Sun

"I would like you to tell me about everything your child ate and drank from the time he got up in the morning until the time he went to bed at night and what he ate during the night. Be sure to mention everything he ate or drank at home, at school, and away from home. Include snacks and drinks of all kinds and everything else he put in his mouth and swallowed. I also need to know where he ate the food, but now let us begin."

What time did he get up yesterday? _____

Was it the usual time? _____

What was the first time he ate or had anything to drink yesterday morning? (list on the form that follows)

Where did he eat? (list on the form that follows)

Now tell me what he had to eat and how much?

(Occasionally the interviewer will need to ask:)

    When did he eat again? or, is there anything else?

    Did he have anything to eat or drink during the night?

Was intake unusual in any way? ☐ Yes ☐ No

    (If answer is yes) Why? _____

        In what way? _____

What time did he go to bed last night? _____

Does he take vitamin and/or mineral supplements? ☐ Yes ☐ No

    (If answer is yes) How many per day? _____

        Per week? _____

    What kind? (Insert brand name if known)

    Multivitamins _____

    Ascorbic acid _____

    Vitamins A and D _____

    Iron _____

    Other _____

Sample interview form to assess nutritional status of child—cont'd

Suggested form for recording food intake

Time	Where eaten*	Food	Type and/or preparation	Amount	Food code†	Amount code†

*Code
  H—Home
  R—Restaurant, drug store, or lunch counter
  CL—Carried lunch from home
  CC—Child care center
  OH—Other home (of a friend, babysitter, or relative)
  S—School
  FD—Food dispenser
†Do not write in these spaces

Form B—Dietary questionnaire

Name _____ Date _____

1. Does the child eat at regular times each day? _____
2. How many days a week does he eat—
    a morning meal? _____ a lunch or mid-day meal? _____ an evening meal? _____
    during the night* _____
3. How many days a week does he have snacks—
    in mid-morning? _____ in mid-afternoon? _____ in the evening? _____ during the night* _____
4. Which meals does he usually eat with your family? ☐ None ☐ Breakfast ☐ Noon meal ☐ Evening meal
5. How many times per week does he eat at school or child care center or day camp?
    Breakfast _____ Lunch _____ Between meals _____
6. Would you describe his appetite as ☐ Good? ☐ Fair? ☐ Poor?
7. At what time of day is he most hungry? ☐ Morning ☐ Noon ☐ Evening
8. What foods does he dislike? _____
_____
9. Is he on a special diet now? ☐ Yes ☐ No
    If *Yes*, why is he on a diet? (check)
      ☐ For weight reduction (own prescription)
      ☐ For weight reduction (doctor's prescription)
      ☐ For gaining weight
      ☐ For allergy, specify _____
      ☐ For other reason, specify _____
    If *No*, has he been on a special diet within the past year? ☐ Yes ☐ No
      If *Yes*, for what reason? _____
10. Does he eat anything which is not usually considered food? ☐ Yes ☐ No
    If *Yes*, what? _____ How often? _____
11. Can he feed himself? ☐ Yes ☐ No
    If *Yes*, with his fingers? _____ with a spoon? _____
12. Can he use a cup or glass by himself? ☐ Yes ☐ No

_____

*Include formula feeding for young children.

Continued.

Sample interview form to assess nutritional status of child—cont'd

13. Does he drink from a bottle with a nipple? ☐ Yes ☐ No
    If *Yes*, how often? _____ At what time of day or night? _____
    _____

14. How many times *per week* does he eat the following foods (at any meal or between meals)?
    Circle the appropriate number:

Bacon	0 1 2 3 4 5 6 7	>7, specify _____
Tongue	0 1 2 3 4 5 6 7	>7, specify _____
Sausage	0 1 2 3 4 5 6 7	>7, specify _____
Luncheon meat	0 1 2 3 4 5 6 7	>7, specify _____
Hot dogs	0 1 2 3 4 5 6 7	>7, specify _____
Liver—chicken	0 1 2 3 4 5 6 7	>7, specify _____
Liver—other	0 1 2 3 4 5 6 7	>7, specify _____
Poultry	0 1 2 3 4 5 6 7	>7, specify _____
Salt pork	0 1 2 3 4 5 6 7	>7, specify _____
Pork or ham	0 1 2 3 4 5 6 7	>7, specify _____
Bones (neck or other)	0 1 2 3 4 5 6 7	>7, specify _____
Meat in mixtures (stew, tamales, casseroles, etc.)	0 1 2 3 4 5 6 7	>7, specify _____
Beef or veal	0 1 2 3 4 5 6 7	>7, specify _____
Other meat	0 1 2 3 4 5 6 7	>7, specify _____
Fish	0 1 2 3 4 5 6 7	>7, specify _____

15. How many times *per week* does he eat the following foods (at any meal or between meals)?
    Circle the appropriate number:

Fruit juice	0 1 2 3 4 5 6 7	>7, specify _____
Fruit	0 1 2 3 4 5 6 7	>7, specify _____
Cereal-dry	0 1 2 3 4 5 6 7	>7, specify _____
Cereal-cooked or instant	0 1 2 3 4 5 6 7	>7, specify _____
Cereal-infant	0 1 2 3 4 5 6 7	>7, specify _____
Eggs	0 1 2 3 4 5 6 7	>7, specify _____
Pancakes or waffles	0 1 2 3 4 5 6 7	>7, specify _____
Cheese	0 1 2 3 4 5 6 7	>7, specify _____
Potato	0 1 2 3 4 5 6 7	>7, specify _____
Other cooked vegetables	0 1 2 3 4 5 6 7	>7, specify _____
Raw vegetables	0 1 2 3 4 5 6 7	>7, specify _____
Dried beans or peas	0 1 2 3 4 5 6 7	>7, specify _____
Macaroni, spaghetti, rice, or noodles	0 1 2 3 4 5 6 7	>7, specify _____
Ice cream, milk pudding, custard or cream soup	0 1 2 3 4 5 6 7	>7, specify _____
Peanut butter or nuts	0 1 2 3 4 5 6 7	>7, specify _____
Sweet rolls or doughnuts	0 1 2 3 4 5 6 7	>7, specify _____
Crackers or pretzels	0 1 2 3 4 5 6 7	>7, specify _____
Cookies	0 1 2 3 4 5 6 7	>7, specify _____
Pie, cake or brownies	0 1 2 3 4 5 6 7	>7, specify _____
Potato chips or corn chips	0 1 2 3 4 5 6 7	>7, specify _____
Candy	0 1 2 3 4 5 6 7	>7, specify _____
Soft drinks, popsicles or Koolaid	0 1 2 3 4 5 6 7	>7, specify _____
Instant Breakfast	0 1 2 3 4 5 6 7	>7, specify _____

16. How many servings *per day* does he eat of the following foods?
    Circle the appropriate number:

Bread (including sandwich), toast, rolls, muffins (1 slice or 1 piece is 1 serving)	0 1 2 3 4 5 6 7	>7, specify _____
Milk (including on cereal or other foods) (8 ounces is 1 serving)	0 1 2 3 4 5 6 7	>7, specify _____
Sugar, jam, jelly, syrup (1 teaspoon is 1 serving)	0 1 2 3 4 5 6 7	>7, specify _____

Sample interview form to assess nutritional status of child—cont'd

17. What specific kinds of the following foods does he eat most often?

Fruit juices _____

Fruit _____

Vegetables _____

Cheese _____

Cooked or instant cereal _____

Dry cereal _____

Milk _____

SUGGESTIONS FOR INTERVIEWERS

Information will usually be obtained from the person responsible for feeding the child. Older children may be able to give more reliable information regarding their own intakes than will the responsible adult. The interviewer should judge this in each individual case.

How questions are asked is important. Avoid questions that suggest the correct answers—e.g., Did you have a dark-green or deep-yellow vegetable today? Avoid expressing approval or disapproval of the foods reported. If you feel there are omissions, ask additional questions: What did he drink with his lunch? What did he have on his toast?

Check carefully for the following information to help complete the 24-hour recall intake form:

A. *Additions to foods already recorded, such as:*
   1. Fats: Butter, margarine, honey-butter, peanut butter, mayonnaise, lard, meat drippings, cheese spreads, and others.
      - Used on toast, bread, rolls, buns, cookies, crackers, sandwiches.
      - Used on vegetables.
      - Used on potatoes, rice, noodles, etc.
      - Used on other foods.
   2. Sugars: Jam, jelly, honey, syrup, sweetening, etc.
      - Used on breads, sandwiches, vegetables, fruit, cereal, coffee, tea, other foods.
   3. Other spreads: Catsup, mustard, etc.
   4. Milk: Cream, half and half, skim milk, etc.
      - Used on cereal, coffee, tea, desserts, other foods.
   5. Gravies: Used on bread, biscuits, meat, potatoes, rice, noodles, other foods.
   6. Salad dressings: Used on vegetables, salads, sandwiches, other foods.
   7. Chocolate or other flavoring to milk, e.g., Quik, Bosco.

B. *Food preparation*
   1. Preparation of eggs, e.g., fried, scrambled, boiled, poached.
   2. Preparation of meat, poultry, fish, e.g., fried, boiled, stewed, roasted, baked, broiled.
   3. Preparation of mixed dishes—major ingredients used, e.g., tuna fish and noodles, macaroni and cheese.
   4. Special preparation of food—strained, chopped, etc.

C. *Special additional detail about food items*
   1. Kinds of milk (whole, partially skim, skim, powdered, chocolate, etc.)
   2. Kinds of carbonated beverages (regular, low-calorie).
   3. Kinds of fruits (canned, frozen, fresh, dried, cooked with sugar added).
   4. Kinds of fruit juices, fruit drinks, or juice substitutes.

By carrying a few standardized props it will be possible to obtain more accurate recording of amounts: a teaspoon and tablespoon; several sizes of glasses and bowls (including a 4-oz. and an 8-oz. measure); something to indicate thickness of meat—a ruler or a standard form such as a model of a slice of bread.

Habits and care

The history of habits and care includes a description of the following items:

1. Eating patterns
2. Sleeping habits, including the number of hours and any disturbances, restlessness, or nightmares
3. Play interests and the amount of exercise
4. Urinary and bowel continence and the care given to the child in developing independence and control
5. Medications and drugs given to the child
6. Parental concerns and management of any specific behavior, such as masturbation, thumbsucking, temper tantrums, or bedwetting

Social history

The social history gives information about the child's pattern of health care; his place of birth; his placement and progress in school; his relationships with family members, peers, and the important people outside the home; the socioeconomic status of the family; and the marital status of the parents.

Review of systems

The review of systems is essentially the same as that carried out in the adult history (see Chapter 3) except for age-appropriate modifications. The following are examples of modifications:

General (additional questions)
Recent and significant gain or loss of weight or *failure to gain weight appropriate for age*.
Changes in behavior such as increased crying, irritability, or nervousness. (These questions are usually found under the review of the CNS in the adult history. However, behavior changes in children may represent the first symptoms of a problem in any physical system.)

Skin (additional questions)
Birthmarks

Eyes (additional questions)
Strabismus

Mouth and throat (additional questions)
Age of eruption of teeth
Cleft lip or cleft palate
Number of teeth at 1 year

Neck and nodes (additional questions)
Limitation of movement

Breasts (deletions and additional questions)
Questions about breast development should be addressed to the preadolescent and the adolescent boy or girl.
Questions about individual concerns regarding breast development such as comparisons made with peers or the unequal development of the breasts.
Delete the questions about self-examination until the breasts begin to develop.

Respiratory and cardiovascular systems (additional questions)
Reduced exercise tolerance—does child play as actively as other children or does he curtail strenuous exercise?

Genital system (deletions and additional questions)
Male
Questions about the development of the secondary sex characteristics should be addressed to the preadolescent and adolescent male:
  Increase in size of testes
  Appearance of pubic hair
  Appearance of hair on face and body
  Appearance of axillary hair
Questions about individual concerns regarding sexual development should be asked.
Delete the question about impotence until late adolescence when a determination has been made that the young man is sexually active.

Female
Questions about development of the secondary sex characteristics should be addressed to the preadolescent and the adolescent female:
  Appearance of pubic hair
  Appearance of axillary hair
  Onset of menses
Questions about individual concerns regarding sexual development should be asked.
Delete the questions about menses until menarche has occurred.
Delete the questions about obstetrical history unless it is determined that the girl is sexually active.
Delete the question about Pap tests until onset of menses.

Both sexes
Questions about sexual activity and venereal disease should be delayed until adolescence. An explanation should be given as to why questions need to be asked.

Extremities and musculoskeletal system (additional questions)
Postural deformities or changes
Changes in gait

Central nervous system
Additional information about this system will be obtained in the developmental history and social history.

THE PHYSICAL EXAMINATION

The importance of a physical examination is the opportunity to obtain objective information. Diagnostic clues obtained can become extremely valuable, especially when the child is unable to communicate or when the parents are poor historians.

The physical examination of the infant or child varies according to the primary purpose of the visit. There are three types of examinations that might be performed. The first is the screening of a healthy child. This examination is usually complete but does not go into any great depth in a particular organ system. The second is the evaluation of a chief complaint and a more intensive examination of a particular area may be in order. The third is the follow-up examination of a complaint or disease that has been under treatment, and the focus is usually on one or two organ systems. Sometimes these three types of examinations are combined, particularly when it is the child's first visit and he is in need of a screening examination as well as a careful evaluation of a chief complaint.

Performance of the physical examination of the infant or child also varies according to the age, development, and behavior of the child and the type of setting in which the care is being provided. If consideration is not given to the child's age and development, it is likely that the examination will be incomplete. For example, the practitioner must have a fine appreciation for the physical differences and developmental milestones according to age. If the child is overly fearful or fatigued, the practitioner would do well to be selective in his examination. If a complete examination is warranted, then the practitioner needs to be quick and efficient in his or her examination technique. The type of setting in which the care is delivered can affect which examination services are rendered. The agency's philosophy of care, their type of staffing, and their source of funding may have direct influence on patient care.

When carrying out a pediatric examination, the examiner should keep in mind that each visit for health care is a learning experience for the child and his parent(s). The experience may result in increased confidence in themselves and others, or they may experience feelings of failure and distrust in the people who care for them. Thus it is most productive to provide opportunities to develop positive relationships during the visits for routine health care. It also is important to remember that any separation of the child from the parent may be anxiety-provoking to both and may increase their level of fear and distrust. Therefore it is important to encourage the parents to participate as much as comfortably possible for them in order to support their child. The older child may be able to participate more freely without the parent present all the time. Most parents will recognize the child's need to develop independence and encourage him to participate by himself.

It is important to prepare the child and parent for any new or painful procedures. Some procedures do not hurt but feel uncomfortable because of new and strange sensations. A special kind of appreciation for the feelings of children and parents will result in greater cooperation on their part. The practitioner should always be forthright with a child, no matter how young. Even if the child is too young to understand what is being said, the parent is listening too and can learn from the practitioner's behavior. One must always talk to the family in a warm, honest, and reassuring way. Regardless of whether the child can understand, the tone of voice is to be kind and determined. The tone of the practitioner's voice often sets the stage for the child's reactions.

The performance of the physical examination of a child needs to be organized and systematic. There are, however, differences between an adult and a pediatric examination. The practitioner performs distressing parts of the examination at the end, especially if it is believed that the child will be unable to cope and continue with the examination, for example, ear, nose, and throat examination. The order of the examination may be altered to accommodate the individual child's behavior, for example, listening to the heart and lungs early in the examination before crying starts or becomes more vigorous. A good idea is to start the examination of a child with a body part that is least likely to interfere with his developing a sense of trust and confidence, for example, inspection of the hands and feet. Finally, the practitioner should take the time to wash the hands before examining the child. The first reason is to warm them before touching the child. The second reason is to let the mother know that the practitioner is concerned about being clean before seeing her child. Third, it assists in reducing the spread of infection.

Approach to the child

Little difficulty is encountered in the performance of the physical examination of the infant in the first 6 months of life, since the infant has little fear of strangers. The infant often enjoys having his clothing removed and is easily distracted by the parent or the examiner with repetitive vocal sounds and smiles. However, the examination of the ears and mouth may cause distress and should be the last part of the examination. It is wise to take advantage of the opportunities that are offered. If the infant is quiet or sleepy, it is best to start with the auscultation of the chest; if the infant is playful and active, it is easier to start with the extremities and wait for a quieter moment to examine the chest.

During the last half of the first year of life, the infant experiences an increasing fear of strangers; thus, it is often profitable to conduct the entire examination while the infant is held on the parent's lap. Even under the best of circumstances, it may not be possible to create a situation that is ideal; the infant may remain resistant throughout the examination. This requires the examiner to be efficient in carrying out the examination in the least amount of time and with the use of minimal restraint of the infant. The parent often experiences discomfort or embarrassment because of the infant's behavior and needs reassurance that the infant is behaving normally. The situation is

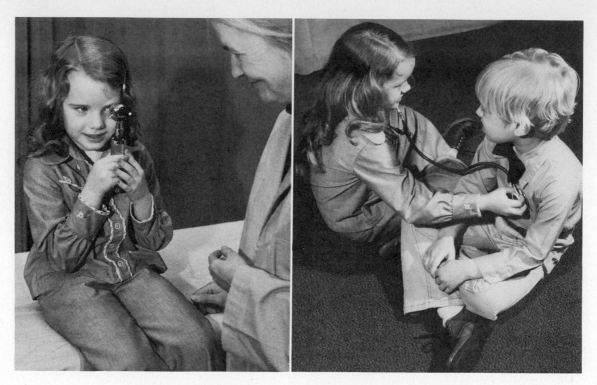

Fig. 24-3. The child enjoys trying out the examiner's equipment.

ideal for helping the parent understand normal development and the needs of the infant at this age.

The child from 1 to 3 years of age is a challenge to even the most experienced examiner. The child is learning to use his body and to manipulate and experiment with all aspects of the environment. Any restraint in the pursuit of his desired activities may be seen by the child as an interference, resulting in unhappiness or frustration for the child. The child at this age is getting lots of pleasure from recently acquired skills such as walking and talking and enjoys his new ability to manipulate objects such as doors and wastebaskets. At the same time, he is still unsure of strangers and needs the parent's presence in order to feel safe. The 2- or 3-year-old child may be charming and cooperative or difficult to examine; whichever the case, the examiner is required to make many modifications in the organization of the examination. The child may be examined in a standing position or on the parent's lap. He usually does not like to have all of his clothing removed at one time but will often cooperate if only one article of clothing is removed at a time as the examination is carried out. The child also needs the opportunity to handle and use the examining instruments. He may enjoy doing this but may also reject the offer if it is too fear-provoking. Despite the difficulties in examining the child of this age, the ability of the child to relate more positively at each subsequent visit can be rewarding and profitable for the examiner.

The child at 3 or 4 years of age is usually able to understand and cooperate during the examination. He is anxious to please and is usually a delightful participant. He has better control of his feelings and his behavior than the younger child but may still lose control if his fear is great. He should receive recognition for his efforts to participate, so that his self-image is enhanced. This child especially enjoys trying out the examiner's equipment and will very likely demonstrate his new learning in future play activities; this is a way to incorporate the role of the examiner and master his fears (Fig. 24-3).

When examining the school-aged child or adolescent, the practitioner needs to provide an opportunity for the child to discuss his feelings and to ask questions about the physical examination. The school-aged child is often curious and interested in what is being done and why. The adolescent needs time to explore any questions he may have about his bodily functions and anatomical features. Often during this talk, a girl expresses concern about engaging in sexual activity, and a sexually active boy may be concerned that he has a penile discharge. These two problems are unlikely to be discussed openly in front of parents. And so, for part of his health visit, it is desirable to see the adolescent alone. Sometimes shyness and modesty pervade when it is necessary to undress in front of a stranger. If the child is distressed about removing his clothing, it is usually best to leave the boy's shorts or the girl's tee-shirt or bra on until it becomes necessary to examine those parts of the body. Allowing the child time to redress before proceeding with the remainder of the examination is supportive and indicates respect for their modesty. Often, in the case of the adolescent, the practitioner will choose not to conduct an examination on the first visit. This occurs when the adolescent seems extraordinarily anxious or hostile or has no immediate medical reason to be examined.

Safety in child restraint and handling

Because of the nature of the health visit, there are occasions when the physical examination involves an uncooperative child. The practitioner will benefit by displaying patience, kindness, determination, and efficiency in carrying out this task. The practitioner may reassure the parent that the child's behavior is the result of fear and that it is normal for the child to want to cry or to get away from the source of fear. The practitioner conveys to the parent the reason the examination cannot be delayed, as in the case of confirming a diagnosis or ruling out a hidden condition, for example, otoscopic examination to confirm or rule out otitis media.

The practitioner may need to utilize one or more of a variety of safe child-restraint methods. Clinical experience and knowledge of the child's behavior during previous visits will aid the practitioner in the choice of a safe restraint method. A frightened and thrashing child is a danger to himself, his parents, and the professional. It is likely that the child will use the same behavioral methods to resist the examiner that he uses at home to "manage" his parents. The child who has been allowed to scream and kick at home is likely to try the same methods with the examiner. If he has not, he may still try these behaviors at least once to test the examiner and his parents in a new situation. It must be demonstrated to the child that unreasonable behavior will gain him neither frustration nor affection from his parents and neither anger nor cessation of the examination from the practitioner.

The principles that form the basis for child restraint are effective restraint, safety, and self-control. The first two are obvious. The last means the practitioner maximizes an area in which the child can exercise control during the restraint procedure.

Once a child gains mobility and especially when he begins to ambulate, he may resist any attempt to place him in a prone position. He often fights to get to a sitting or to a standing position. If the examination or procedure can be made with the child sitting in his parent's lap, this is preferred; it is one way to help the child gain control over himself in a fearful situation.

Another way to give him a sense of control is to bargain with him. In exchange for not moving, he can scream as loud as he wishes. This is an outlet he can regulate himself, that is, volume and duration.

In the youngest of infants, up to 3 months, when the Moro reflex is still quite prominent, the child, when startled, will cry, quiver his lower lip, shake his body, extend his arms and legs, and flex his thumbs and forefingers. This reflex can be interrupted and the child restored to comfort by placing him in a prone position on a padded table, a person's lap, or against a person's chest. This is a helpful hint to pass on to the parent. Bodily contact with a large surface area stimulates the child to hug the source and gain security.

Another fundamental method of relatively passive control is distraction. This method is most helpful with the infant up to 6 months old but works with any age, including adults. A kind but firm tone of voice that remains consistent in tonal quality is used. This can be reassuring to the child and aids in setting limits. For the older child, the practitioner should try to empathize and tell the child that it is alright to cry as long as he does not move.

For the 4- to 9-month-old, hand occupation is a good strategy—simply place an object in each hand. An object commonly used is a tongue blade. The child usually will grasp it and play, allowing the examiner to complete auscultating the heart, lungs, and abdomen. One note of concern is to watch that a young child with quick hand movements may poke the blade into his eye. Also, the tongue blade is checked for smooth edges because the infant may well put it in his mouth. A set of keys made from nontoxic materials is a safe alternative to the tongue blade. It is an interesting item to rattle, to finger, and to put into the mouth and it can be washed. The infant 9 or more months old can be occupied with some of the very items used in screening the child's development, that is, blocks and rattles. There are two precautions when selecting an object as a distractor. A noisemaker should not be chosen. A child often perseveres in an activity and it can really prove a distractor—to the parent and to the professional—as the visit progresses. Second, the object should always be too large to be accidentally swallowed by the child.

A third method of child restraint is the "hug." Usually, the adult involved is the parent. But if the parent prefers not to assist in the restraint of his child, this decision should be supported and a staff person should be requested to assist. The adult is to sit in a chair that will not move too easily along the floor. He holds the child in his arms so that the child is in a semisitting position, with his head resting in the bend of the adult's arm. This same arm wraps around the child with the hand of the adult firmly grasping the child's elbow joint. The adult's free arm then comes over the body of the child approximately at his hip level, firmly grasping the child's knee joint that is farthest away from the adult's body. The principles used in this restraint method include simulating a hug, where a child comes in bodily contact with a person he trusts or at least feels the warmth of a person's body against his own. The second principle is to immobilize only those joints where movement would interfere with the practitioner. A child normally swings his arms at the practitioner or at the object in the practitioner's hand, such as a syringe or otoscope.

A fourth method, called the straddle, can be used with a heftier, long-legged, or older child. In this instance, the child sits on the adult's lap or stands in such a way that his legs are between the adult's legs. The adult holds his own legs together firmly so that the child can remain sitting or standing but cannot kick. Again, the adult's arms wrap around the child, with a firm grasp at the child's elbows. In this position, the child can be facing the adult pressing his head against the adult's chest. The child could also choose to face the practitioner and lean back against the adult's chest. In both the hug and straddle positions, the adult holding the child is advised to lean forward as the child tries to move away from the examiner. This will help to steady the child and keep the practitioner from overreaching his stance.

The next restraint position is done with the child lying down on a padded table and requires two persons. The child can recline in a prone or a supine position. The adult stands near the child's head. The arms of the child are fully extended upward and lay close to the sides of his head. The adult firmly grasps the elbow joints. Since the child can see and hear the adult, he may be soothed and distracted. The practitioner faces the child and applies his upper body weight across the child's hip area. In this fashion, the child cannot raise his hips off the table, but he can move his lower legs. Using this method, the practitioner has both hands free to perform an examination or procedure. This technique can be adapted when the examiner needs access to the lower instead of the upper parts of the child's body.

The last method described here is called swaddling or mummifying. In this technique, a cloth or sheet is used to wrap the child's arms, legs, and body so as to totally contain them. This method is seldom used.

Frequently, the practitioner needs to evaluate whether the mother holds and turns over her child safely. For example, during breast-feeding or bottle-feeding, the safest way to hold a child is in a semi-sitting position with his head resting in the bend of the mother's elbow. Her arm extends around him and gently grasps his elbow joint. This leaves the free hand to hold his legs, to caress him, to push away the breast if it is obstructing his breathing, or to hold a bottle of formula to his mouth.

In order to safely turn the child over, the mother should be instructed to use her left hand to grasp hold of the child's right shoulder. She needs to place her hand palm side down on the anterior surface of the shoulder and chest. The adult's right arm reaches under the child's right leg and grasps the left leg. In one smooth motion, the child is then picked up and turned from a face-up to a face-down position. The head is turned to the side, if the child cannot do this for himself. This maneuver also can be adapted to return the child to a supine position.

In all the positions described, it is assumed that the examiner and/or adult is right-handed and that the examiner is approaching the child from the right side. Left-handed persons will need to reverse, and in some instances also to adjust, these positions in relation to the child.

Measurements

The measurements of the temperature, pulse rate, respiratory rate, blood pressure, height, and weight are part of the physical examination of the child. In addition, the measurements of the head circumference and chest circumference are noted for the child under 2 years of age. The comparison of the physical measurements of a child with those of other healthy children over a period of time makes it possible to determine if the child is progressing within the normal parameters of health or if there are significant deviations.

TEMPERATURE

The three body areas commonly used for obtaining temperature measurements—the mouth, the axilla, and the rectum—are discussed in Chapter 7 on general assessment. In pediatric care, there are advantages and disadvantages associated with each method, and the practitioner needs to decide which site is appropriate, depending on the child's ability to cooperate and his health status.

An axillary temperature reading can be performed on any child if a proper and safe method is used. The child can be held safely in the restraint method called the "hug." Taking an axillary temperature reduces the risk of injury that may occur with the oral or the rectal method, and it also reduces the risk of spreading infection. The axillary method requires a clean glass thermometer that has been shaken down below 97° F. It takes 3 to 11 minutes to obtain an accurate measurement because there is less proximity to the blood supply and because it may be difficult to avoid air contact, which produces cooling.

A rectal temperature is often the method used during the first few years of a child's life. The main drawback is the danger of perforation of the rectum in the young infant and the increased discomfort for the young child, who experiences this as an intrusive procedure. It should not be used with children who cannot tolerate this kind of stimulus to the central nervous system, as is the case with some children who have epilepsy. A safe restraint method for taking a rectal temperature of a young infant is to lay the child face down on the mother's lap or on a padded table. The adult should place the left forearm firmly across the child's hip area, so that the child cannot raise the buttocks off the adult's lap or the table. The practitioner uses the left thumb and forefinger to separate the buttocks, then the right hand is free to gently insert the lubricated thermometer. The infant's rectum is quite short; therefore the thermometer should be inserted only a short distance. Three considerations that may be used to determine sufficient entry include: noting that the column of mercury is rising steadily, inserting no more than ½ inch, and observing a decrease in the child's effort to push against the thermometer. It is normal for the child to push against the thermometer as the rectal sphincter muscles contract in response to the stimulus. The practitioner waits until the sphincter relaxes before continuing to insert. The thermometer is held firmly enough to keep the child from pushing it out. Care must be taken to hold the thermometer firmly but not to push it in further. Also, the child must be held securely to prevent jerking and pushing the thermometer further into the rectum. It takes at least 1 minute to get a rectal temperature reading.

Obtaining an oral temperature reading is usually reserved for children who are 5 to 6 years of age and older. The child must be able to understand not to bite on the glass thermometer and to keep his mouth closed during the procedure. Sometimes, the child's health condition interferes with being able to use this method, for example, mouth breathing or limited intellectual functioning. The elongated bulb thermometer is used and placed well under the child's tongue for 2 to 3 minutes.

A temperature up to 100° F (37.8° C) may be considered normal in a child, as a child's temperature is usually higher than an adult's. Apprehension and physical activity are two factors that may affect the child's body temperature in addition to illness. Fever is a sign of illness, not the illness itself. Fever serves as a measure of the child's ability to cope with illness, an aid in differential diagnosis, and help in assessing the effectiveness of treatment. The absence of fever can be just as significant as its presence. Likewise, a fever in a child under 3 months of age is unusual and should be diagnosed by a competent health care professional.

The treatment of a fever is usually done only if it is interrupting the child's sleep, causing fatigue to the child or his parents, or contributing to a state of dehydration. Fever over 102.2° F is usually treated with an age/weight appropriate dose of acetaminophen. The child may also be sponge-bathed or wet-toweled if he remains febrile, despite medications, fluids, and rest. Great care is to be exercised in these procedures, monitoring the child's body temperature to prevent hypothermal shock.

Causes of fever are many and varied. In brief, fever of 1 week's duration is probably the result of an acute infection, whereas fever that persists into a second week suggests a chronic bacterial infection. After 2 weeks, the practitioner is cautioned to consider two other major causes of fever—the autoimmune disorders and neoplasms. Acute rheumatoid arthritis and, in older children, lupus erythematosus are possible. An acute lymphatic leukemia is a neoplasm to be considered in children. Other possible causes, by major groups of diseases, include hypersensitization, central nervous sytem disorders, and dehydration. Short-term fevers of recurrent nature may be of psychophysiological origin. Prolonged excitement and tension in a child other than when he is engaged in a physical activity may be a factor in fever episodes. A fever may be found in a school-aged child who is experiencing fear and tension in the school setting (Kempe, 1978).

PULSE AND RESPIRATION

Apprehension, crying, and physical activity, as well as the examination procedure itself, can alter a child's heart and respiratory rates. Thus, it is desirable to take these measurements while the child is at rest, either sleeping or lying quietly. If the child has been active, the measurement is delayed until the child has relaxed about 5 to 10 minutes.

The child's pulse is to be examined for rate, rhythm, quality, and amplitude, just as in an adult. Auscultation of the heart—measuring the apical pulse—is the most easily obtained pulse in a young infant. The average heart rate of the infant at birth is 140 beats per minutes. At 2 years of age the child's heart has adjusted downward to 110. At 10 years the rate is 85, and by the time the child reaches age 18, his pulse may be observed to have lowered to 82. A child, usually an adolescent, who engages in exercise regularly, such as swimming laps, may exhibit a much slower rate, that is, in the 60s. Table 24-3 lists the average heart rates for children from birth to 18

Table 24-3. Average heart rate for infants and children at rest*

Age	Average rate
Birth	140
1st mo	130
1-6 mo	130
6-12 mo	115
1-2 yr	110
2-4 yr	105
6-10 yr	95
10-14 yr	85
14-18 yr	82

*Data from Lowrey, G. H.: Growth and development of children, Chicago, 1978, Year Book Medical Publications, Inc.

years. Heart rhythm in children is not always regular. Often it reflects the phasic action of the heart in relation to the respiratory cycle. This is called sinus arrhythmia and it is considered normal in children.

Palpation of the brachial and the femoral pulses is an essential step in the examination of the young infant. Irregularities often are the first signs of serious heart dysfunction. The amplitude and time of appearance of the femoral pulse are expected to equal those of the brachial pulse. Absence or weakness of the femoral pulse alerts the examiner to the possibility of coarctation of the aorta in the young infant. Table 24-4 compares some differences in amplitude, quality, and site and how they may relate to the differential diagnosis of heart disorders in children.

The respiratory rate may be obtained by inspection and/or auscultation. The average range of normal respirations is 30 to 80 per minute in the newborn period as compared to 20 to 30 in the 2-year-old. By 10 years of age the rate has adjusted to 17 to 22, and by age 20 it averages 15 to 20 respirations per minute. Table 24-5 exhibits variations in respiration with age.

BLOOD PRESSURE

It was once thought that young infants and children rarely exhibited hypotension except in instances of excess blood loss. Chronic hypertension in children was virtually never reported. Now, of course, we know that blood pressure disorders do prevail in children and can be detected early with regular and periodic screening. The American Academy of Pediatrics has supported regular blood pressure monitoring of children and Early Periodic Screening and Development Testing (EPSDT) requires screening annually of children aged 3 years and older.

The levels of blood pressure gradually increase during childhood. The average systolic pressure of the individual at 1 day of age is 78; at 1 year of age it reaches 96. By 3 years of age, it has increased to 99

Table 24-4. Amplitude, quality of the heart rate, and site, as they relate to differential diagnosis of heart dysfunction in young infants and children*

Amplitude, quality, site	Cardiac dysfunction
Narrow, thready	Congestive heart failure Severe aortic stenosis
Bounding	Patent ductus arteriosus Aortic regurgitation
Pulsation in suprasternal notch	Aortic insufficiency Patent ductus arteriosus Coarctation of the aorta
Palpable thrill in suprasternal notch	Aortic stenosis Valvular pulmonary stenosis Coarctation of the aorta, occasionally patent ductus arteriosus

*Data from Kempe, C. H., and others: Current pediatric diagnosis and treatment, ed. 5, Los Altos, Calif., 1978, Lange Medical Publications.

Table 24-5. Variations in respiration with age*

Age	Rate/minute
Premature	40-90
Newborn	30-80
1 yr	20-40
2 yr	20-30
3 yr	20-30
5 yr	20-25
10 yr	17-22
15 yr	15-20
20 yr	15-20

*Data from Lowrey, G. H.: Growth and development of children, Chicago, 1978, Year Book Medical Publications, Inc.

and by 10 years of age it is 110. At the age of 18 the systolic pressure has climbed to 120. Diastolic pressure also increases over time. It is noted to rise from 42 on day 1 to 65 by age 3; it is 60 by age 10 and at 18 years of age is again elevated to 65. Table 24-6 shows the range of systolic and diastolic pressure for children aged 1 day to 16 years.

The most common method of obtaining a blood pressure in children in still auscultation using a mercury or aneroid sphygmomanometer set. The Doppler method is being used with various age ranges, but it still is not available in many clinical settings because of its formidable price. For the child who is not able to understand or cooperate with the examiner or when Korotkoff sounds are inaudible, the flush method is to be used. This method is described in detail in Chapter 7 on general assessment.

Regardless of the method used, when it involves

Table 24-6. Normal blood pressure for various ages*

Age	Systolic (mm Hg)	Diastolic (mm Hg)
1 day	78	42
1 mo	86	54
6 mo	90	60
1 yr	96	65
2 yr	99	65
4 yr	99	65
6 yr	100	60
8 yr	105	60
10 yr	110	60
12 yr	115	60
14 yr	118	60
16 yr	120	65

*The figures under 1 year were obtained by the Doppler method. From 1 year on, the figures were obtained by auscultation using the first sound to indicate diastolic pressure. Data from Lowrey, G. H.: Growth and development of children, Chicago, 1978, Year Book Medical Publications, Inc.

Table 24-7. Arbitrary standards for defining hypotension in neonates*

Length of term	Systolic pressure
Full-term infant	Less than 55
Preterm infant	Less than 50
Any other infant	Less than 40

*Data from Haddock, N.: Blood pressure monitoring in neonates, Matern.-Child Nurs. J. 5:131, 1980.

using a blood pressure cuff, much care and attention are to be paid that the cuff fits correctly. It is to be comfortable and to fit between one-half and two-thirds of the length of the extremity being used. It cannot be emphasized enough that if the cuff is too narrow, the blood pressure will read artificially high, and if the cuff is too wide, the reading will be artificially low. Cuffs are available for neonates, toddlers, 1- to 4-year-olds, 4- to 8-year-olds, and adults and in an extra-large width for use with obese persons. The blood pressure is often neglected in children because of lack of correct equipment and lack of any sign of illness.

As in adults, hypertension in children can also be a silent disease. Hypertension does not occur frequently in the newborn period. If it is observed in the neonate, the examiner should be alert to look for an artificial elevation caused by use of the wrong size cuff; to note whether the child was agitated or crying, because these factors elevate blood pressure; and to be aware that hypertension may be secondary to umbilical artery catheterization. The practitioner

needs to be alert for renal disease or congenital renal abnormalities. In addition to renal disorders, there are several cardiovascular conditions associated with hypertension, for example, coarctation of the aorta, patent ductus arteriosus, and Marfan's syndrome. Other conditions, such as lead poisoning, encephalitis, burns, and acute bacterial endocarditis, may also account for an increase in blood pressure in the older child. Of course, one also has to consider the hypertensive effects of emotional tension and diet.

Blood pressure is also used to screen for hypotension. In the newborn, hypotension may be the result of hypovolemia from obstetrical bleeding. After the first 12 hours, it may be from decreased cardiac output as seen in congenital heart disease, coarctation of the aorta, septic shock, internal bleeding, air block with increased intrathoracic pressure, or drugs that have crossed the placental barrier. Arbitrary standards for defining hypotension as reported by Haddock (1980) are noted in Table 24-7.

ANTHROPOMETRIC PARAMETERS

Measurement of a child's growth is a screening procedure rather than a diagnostic one. And, as such, it is one of the most frequently performed in pediatric primary care. The seven parameters that may be measured are length or height, weight, head circumference, chest circumference, body proportion (including volume and tissue thickness), bone ossification, and secondary sex characteristics. Before detailing the reasons and method for obtaining these measurements in children, a discussion about growth of children seems warranted.

Breckenridge and Vincent (1966) presented seven laws governing the regulation of growth that still hold true today.

1. Growth is both quantitative and qualitative.
2. Growth is a continuous and orderly process.
3. The rate of growth is not even.
4. Different areas of the body grow at different rates.
5. The rate and pattern of growth can be modified by conditions within or outside of the body.
6. Each child grows in his unique way.
7. Growth is complex in nature and all its aspects are closely related.

In view of these laws, it is easy to understand why the task of measuring a child's growth can be a difficult one. The value of the measurements obtained is determined by their accuracy, reliability, recording, interpretation, and follow-up (Hamill and Moore, 1976).

Although anthropometric studies are screening procedures, the role of the practitioner is to make an assessment of the child's growth. He has four goals in mind: (1) to confirm the child is within normal limits, (2) to determine any sign of pathology, (3) to note the effects of any planned intervention, and (4) to identify a plan to continue or to alter the child's rate and pattern of growth. In this process, he has indeed made a diagnosis about the child's state of health as it relates to his overall growth. He will expand this assessment to draw conclusions about its fit to other sources of data, such as social and nutritional history, knowledge of the family's physical characteristics, and observations of the child himself. He may even need to view photographs of the family and of the child with his classmates.

In order to determine whether the child is within normal limits, serial measurements are obtained. They are compared with previous measurements of the child and with measurements of other children of the same age, sex, and ethnic background. Measurements are made at regular intervals as well as during episodes of illness and are plotted on a standardized growth curve, that is, one that plots a series of consecutive measurements so that the total amount of growth, over time, can be observed. It is necessary for the practitioner to be well informed about the relative strengths and weaknesses of different growth charts.

The first growth grid for average height and weight of American children is credited to Bowditch in 1870. Early research was limited to school-aged population groups. In 1921, Woodbury provided the first physical growth reference data for children under 6. As new data were generated new growth charts became available. Height-weight-age relationships were being combined with other anthropometric measures, that is, head and chest circumference and skinfold thickness. It did not take long for confusion to develop about how the charts were constructed, the nature of the sampling, and other aspects of the research methodology. Of the various charts that were tested in practice, the Stuart-Meredith charts remained the most popular until 1971, when a conference on the assessment and recording of measurements of growth in children concluded that the measurements no longer represented the children in the United States.

Two new growth curves were generated by the National Center for Health Statistics (NCHS) Task Force (Fig. 24-4). The age intervals are birth to 36 months, 2 years to prepuberty, and 2 to 18 years. Separate sets of reference data are provided for each sex. These new data now assist the examiner in determining where the child ranks relative to all "contemporary" children in the United States who are the same age and sex (Hamill and Moore, 1976). Less ambiguity about the meaning of the percentile is be-

coming evident. For example, if a child's height and weight are plotted to be at the fifth percentile, it means that the child weighs less and is shorter than 95 of every 100 children in the United States who are the same age and sex. The examiner can also determine that a child whose growth is plotted in the central percentiles is within normal limits. Standardized reference data for the nation make the comparison of measurements easier now that the reference data are the same. It is anticipated that the NCHS growth charts will survive the test of time.

The validity and reliability of growth standards are dependent on the socioeconomic and cultural descriptors of test standard subjects and the individual being measured, the consistent use of one standard to plot individual measurements, the utilization of referent data to form a baseline of comparison, and the accuracy of the method of measurement. The last place for invalid and unreliable measurement rests with the person who does the actual measuring. The four pitfalls in measurement are positioning, instrument, preparation of the subject, and anatomical referent. These will be discussed further as each anthropometric measurement is described.

Length or height. When a child is under the age of 6, the recumbent position is used (Chinn and Leitch, 1974). This measurement is called length and can be obtained most easily by using a measuring board on a pediatric examining table (Fig. 24-5). The child is laid within the confines of the measuring board. His head rests firmly against the fixed end of the board. The child is well aligned, with extremities extended, and the opposite end of the measuring device is pulled out until it reaches the bottom of the child's heels. This location is then observed on the attached ruler and the number of centimeters is recorded as the child's length.

If it is necessary to rely on a tape measure, the child needs to be placed on a flat surface. The table cannot be molded or equipped with a mattress pad. The flat surface is covered with a piece of paper. The child is placed in a supine position. If he is too young to lie still, an adult may gently restrain him by raising the child's arms above and next to the sides of his head. The examiner needs to ensure that the body is properly aligned and that the extremities are fully extended, with the heels perpendicular to the table. The practitioner moves quickly in this procedure and marks the paper at the top of the child's head and at the bottom of his heels. The child is then removed from the table. The distance between the two marks is measured and recorded as the child's length. This last method depends on accuracy in positioning and the use of a flat surface. One other factor influencing accuracy in measuring length is the

Text continued on p. 591.

BOYS FROM BIRTH TO 36 MONTHS

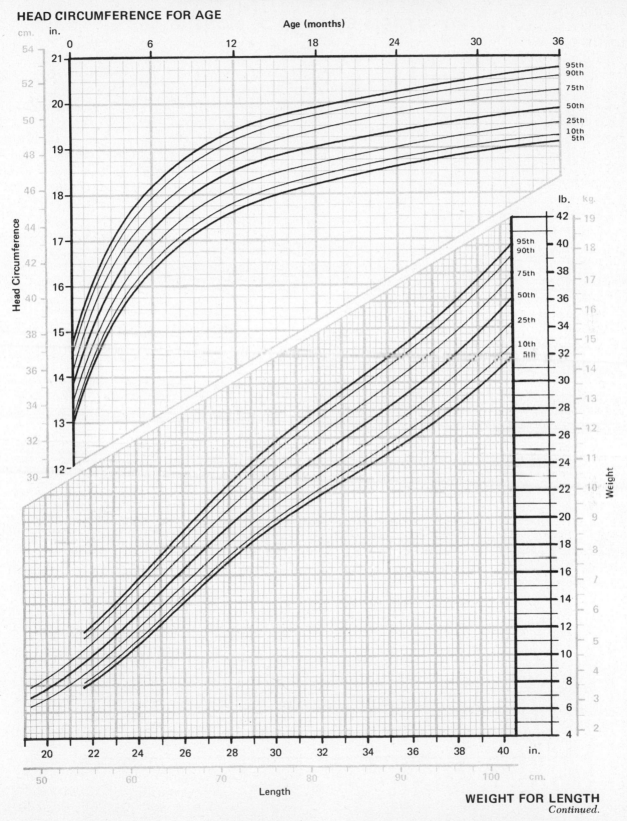

HEAD CIRCUMFERENCE FOR AGE

WEIGHT FOR LENGTH
Continued.

Fig. 24-4. National Health Center statistics growth charts for various ages and both sexes.

BOYS FROM BIRTH TO 36 MONTHS

WEIGHT FOR AGE

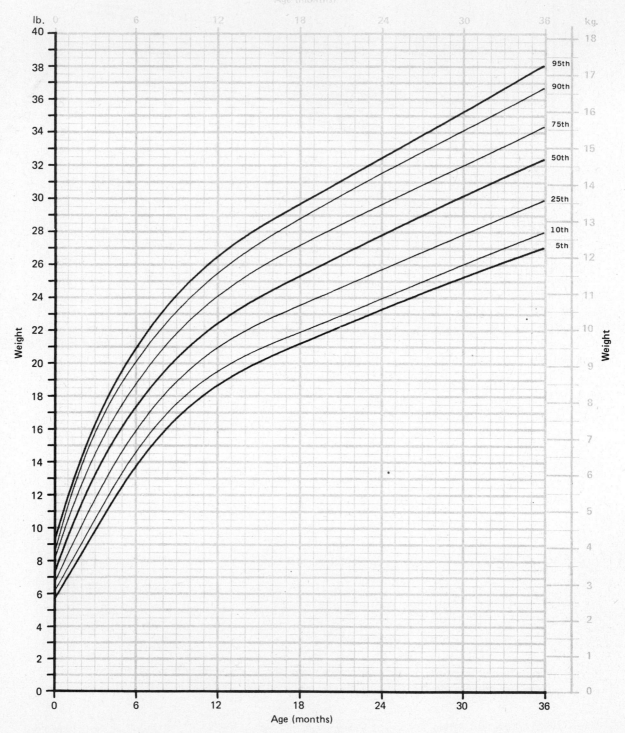

BOYS FROM BIRTH TO 36 MONTHS
LENGTH FOR AGE

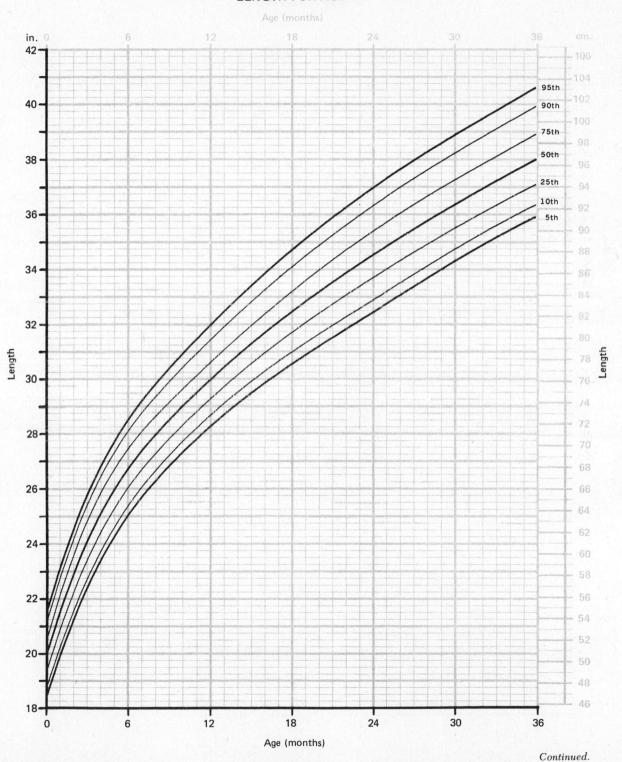

Continued.

BOYS FROM 2 TO 18 YEARS

WEIGHT FOR AGE

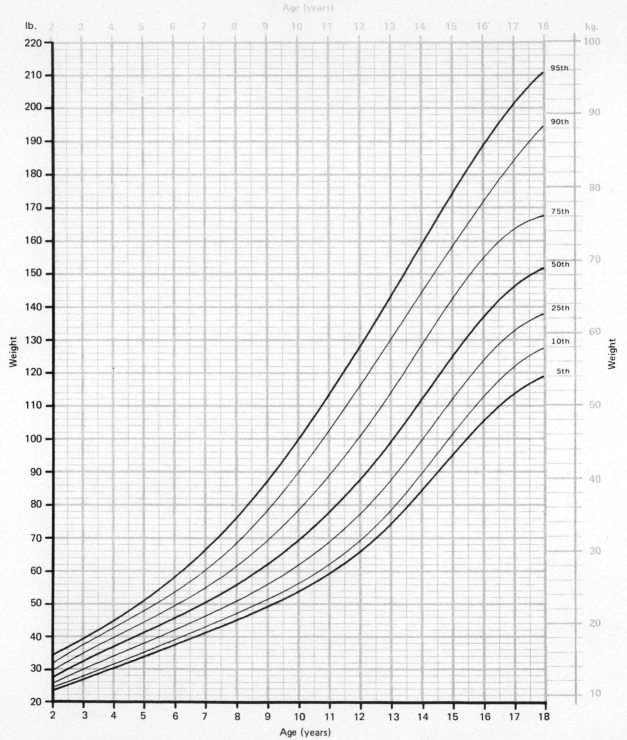

PRE-PUBERTAL BOYS FROM 2 TO 11½ YEARS

WEIGHT FOR STATURE

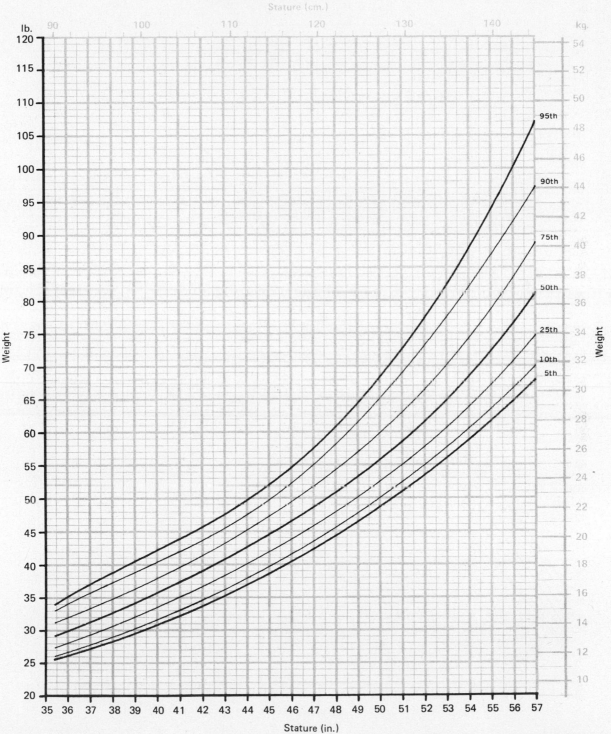

Continued.

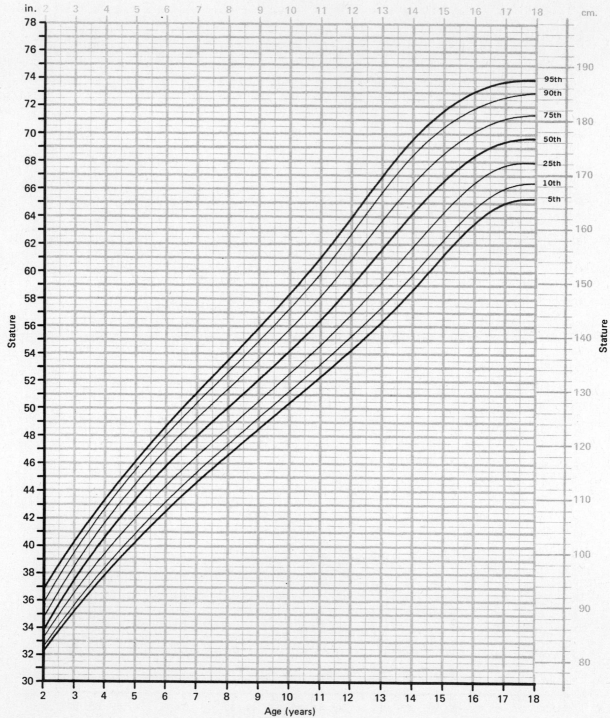

BOYS FROM 2 TO 18 YEARS

STATURE FOR AGE

Age (years)

Stature

Age (years)

GIRLS FROM BIRTH TO 36 MONTHS

HEAD CIRCUMFERENCE FOR AGE

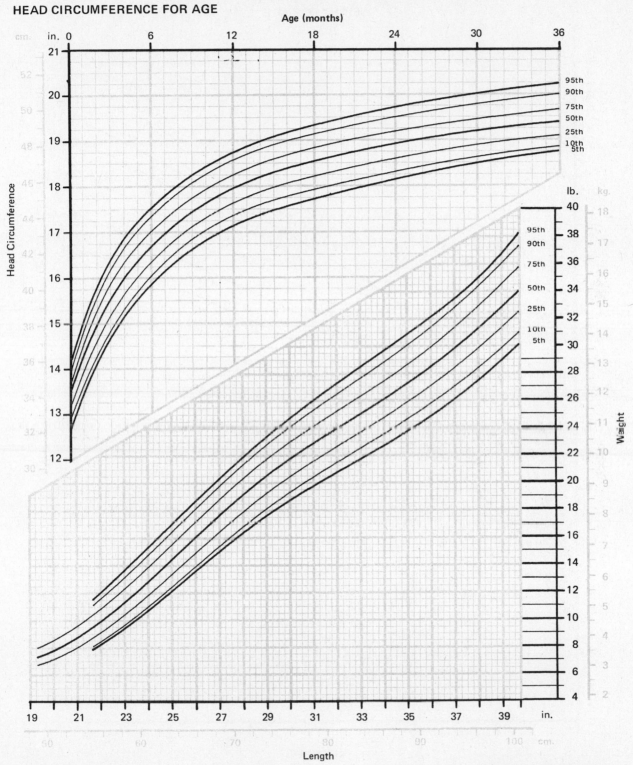

WEIGHT FOR LENGTH
Continued.

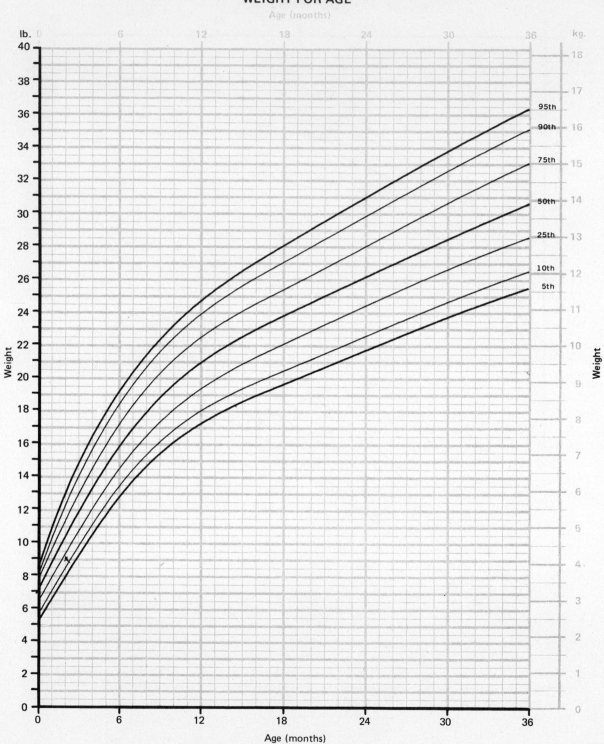

GIRLS FROM BIRTH TO 36 MONTHS
WEIGHT FOR AGE

GIRLS FROM BIRTH TO 36 MONTHS

LENGTH FOR AGE

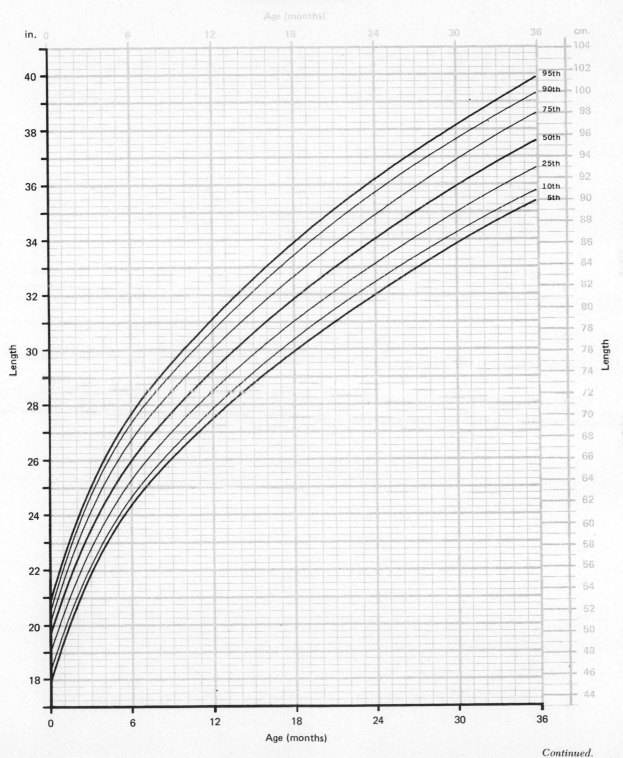

Continued.

GIRLS FROM 2 TO 18 YEARS
WEIGHT FOR AGE

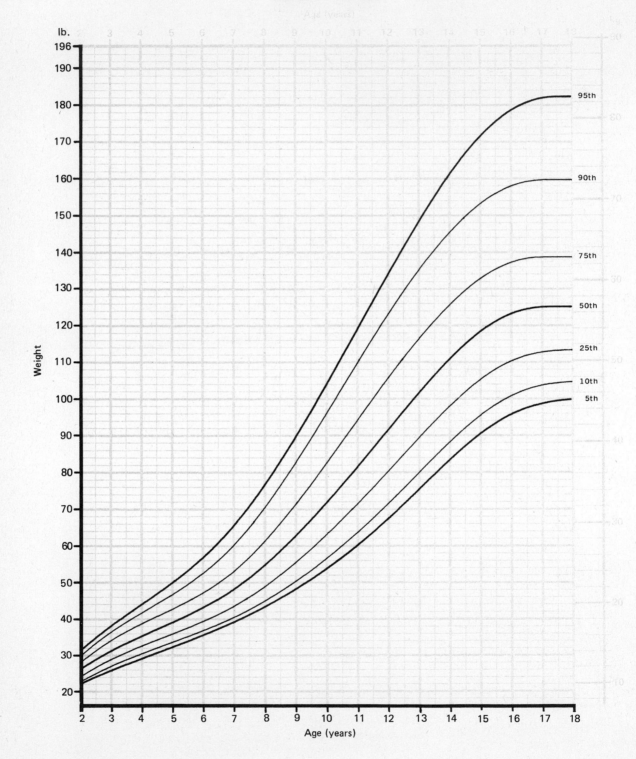

PRE-PUBERTAL GIRLS FROM 2 TO 10 YEARS
WEIGHT FOR STATURE

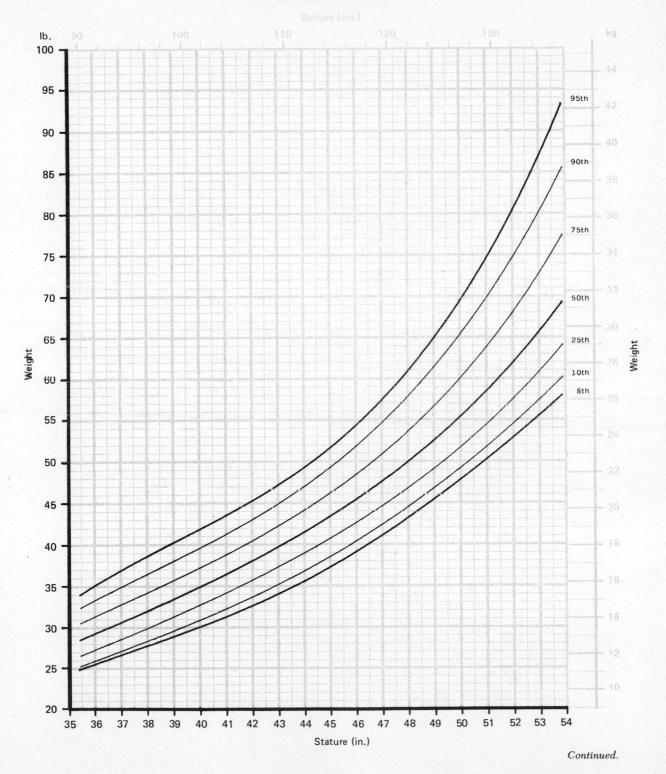

Continued.

GIRLS FROM 2 TO 18 YEARS
STATURE FOR AGE

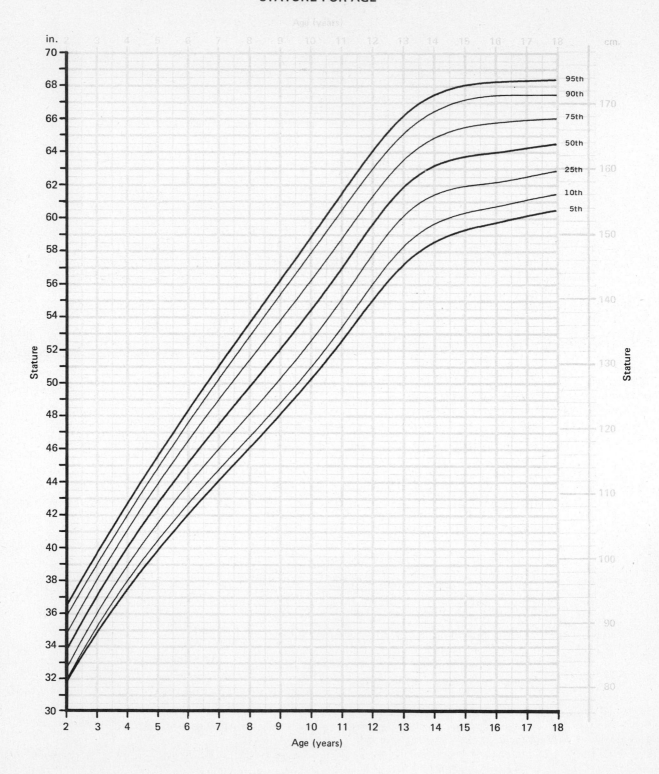

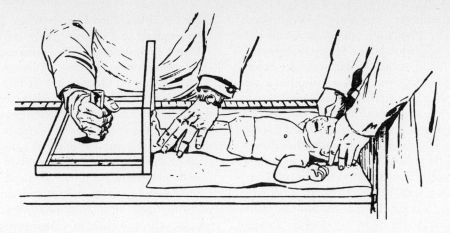

Fig. 24-5. Pediatric device to measure length of infant. (From the U.S. Department of Health, Education, and Welfare, Public Health Service, Center for Disease Control, Atlanta, Georgia.)

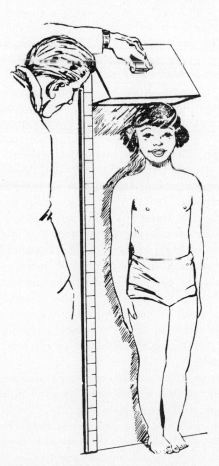

Fig. 24-6. Pediatric device to measure height in children over 6 years of age. (From U.S. Department of Health, Education, and Welfare, Public Health Service, Center for Disease Control, Atlanta, Georgia.)

use of both heels of the child's feet. When measurement is taken from only one heel, the child's squirming may cause inaccuracy. Also, the examiner may fail to observe that one of the child's extremities is shorter than the other.

When height is measured, the child remains in a standing position with his shoes off. He is instructed to stand on his toes and to stretch his fingers "to the sky." This stretch exercise assists the body in regaining its full skeletal length after being used so many hours to hold up the body's weight. When the child relaxes from his stretch, the examiner quickly places the child's heels against the wall. With care that the child's extremities are correctly aligned, a mark is made at the top of his head. In light of many current hair fashions, it may be necessary to flatten the hair before making this mark. The distance between the mark on the wall and the floor can be measured with a tape measure or with a device similar to the one illustrated in Fig. 24-6.

Although the length or height seems troublesome to obtain, it is an important parameter of growth. Height is not influenced by as many factors as weight. A child does not lose height. The significant feature about height is that it is a parameter usually affected last by serious illness. Often these effects are irreversible. This means that a child may not be able to grow to his full height potential even with treatment. Therefore, observation that a child is not growing in height warrants immediate attention and follow-up either to explain a normal slowing of growth or to cite cause for impaired growth and to determine a plan of treatment.

Weight. When measuring the child's weight, the important concern is that the child be consistently weighed with his clothes removed or at least down to his underwear. A younger child should be weighed without his diapers. The child can sit or lie on the infant scale, as is appropriate for his development. An older child can stand on an upright scale. In either case, *before* the child is placed on the scale, the scale should be checked to be certain it is balanced. Each time a child is weighed, the weights are returned to the starting position and the balance observed to rest in the middle. If the balance is skewed in either direction, the scale needs to be adjusted. There are times when a child, through fear or fatigue, is uncooperative, but a weight needs to be obtained. This can be accomplished by having the mother hold her undressed child and weighing them together on an upright scale. The mother is then reweighed by herself on the same scale. The mother's weight is then subtracted from the combined weight to obtain the child's weight.

In both the measurement of length or height and weight, the person doing the measurement should note any deviation from the normal routine of measurement on the patient's record, for example, measuring a child under 3 in an upright position. It is possible to find a discrepancy of ½ to 1½ inches between a recumbent and an upright position. This difference may seem small, but it would then be possible to see the child's recorded length at one visit, when a height was measured, fall one or even two percentiles below that of the last visit, when a length was measured. Of course the child did not lose any length. But at first glance, he appears to be dropping off his cumulative growth curve. This kind of erroneous data has serious implications for children and their parents. They may find themselves undergoing extensive histories and laboratory or radiographic studies to determine if some hormonal problem exists. Therefore, in all cases of suspected growth problems, the first step in management is to verify the measurements.

Head circumference. The head circumference is measured during each examination between birth and 2 years of age. A nonstretchable cloth tape measure is passed over the most prominent part of the occiput and just above the supraorbital ridges. This measurement is repeated three times, once at each temple and at the midforehead, and the largest reading is recorded. The average head circumference at birth is 35 cm (14 inches) and by age 2 has increased to 49 cm (19.2 inches). Table 24-8 lists head circumferences of children of various ages. The head circumference is an important measure to obtain because it is related to intracranial volume and allows an estimation of the rate of growth of the brain. Sequential measurements (Table 24-8) are plotted on the appropriate NCHS growth chart. Any discrepancy or deviation should be checked. The conditions of microcephaly and hydrocephaly are considered.

Chest circumference. The measurement of the circumference of the chest at delivery and in early infancy has become significant in that it may indicate birth injury, congenital anomalies, or system dysfunction, for example, cardiac enlargement. Otherwise, measuring the chest circumference on a regular basis after the first 9 months of life is unnecessary. Exceptions to this might include observed body disproportion or malformation of the thoracic cage. The chest circumference of the child is measured by placing a nonstretchable cloth tape measure at the level of the nipple, with the child in a supine position. Measurement is made midway between inspiration and expiration. Table 24-9 lists chest circumferences for various ages.

Head and chest circumferences are both made with a flexible tape measure, preferably not a paper one. Even though paper tapes are disposable, when they are used improperly or with a moving child they can produce paper cuts of the forehead, eyelid, cornea, or skin on the back or chest. In clinical practice, this means the examiner never pulls a paper tape out from under a child's back or head.

Tissue thickness. Volume and thickness of tissue can be measured in several ways. The circumference of the upper arm or calf of the leg is determined. This measurement is best accomplished by measuring down from a consistent anatomical reference, for example, 4 inches below the acromion process or 7 inches below the hip. Likewise, a measurement by radiography can be obtained. It is seldom necessary to use this measurement in children unless they are laying fat or muscle poorly, as with the under- or overnourished child or the child suspected of having a muscle-wasting disease. Skinfold measurements using calibrated calipers are described in Chapter 5 on nutritional assessment. Again, this is seldom performed in children unless serial measurements are desired in order to assess a normal or moderately obese child's laying down of fat in relation to his caloric intake.

Body proportions can be observed at different ages of the child to note differences expected relative to head, trunk, and extremities (Fig. 24-7).

Bone growth can be measured in three ways: by height, by use of calipers to measure prominent bony diameters, or by actual measurement of long bones via radiography. The usual bone ossification centers studied in children are the wrist and hand; the knee and foot are also helpful before age 2 (Kempe, 1978). These studies are costly and can be intrusive to the child as well as worrisome to the parent. They are necessary if growth patterns are suspicious, but only after exhausting other sources of data, for example, history of nutrition, pica, or the physical characteristics of the family.

Secondary sex characteristics are measured by inspection and noting the time of onset, via the history. In females, the primary foci of development are axillary and pubic hair, breast enlargement, and onset of the menarche. In males, the characteristics include facial, axillary, and genital hair; testicular enlargement; penile enlargement; rugae of the scrotal sac; and onset of seminal emission. Because sexual maturation is closely associated with bone age, girls'

height is seen to be related to the onset of the menarche. Generally, in the year preceding menarche, the girl adds her maximum increment in height. This is, in part, a function of changes in hormones and their effect on epiphyseal growth. Oral contraceptives, certain antibiotics, and thyroid medications are not recommended for use in the prepubertal female. If they are needed, caution should be exercised by regularly monitoring their effects on the child's growth. Although girls with early menarche have a more rapid growth, the period of growth is shorter and so their cumulative growth is less than girls who

Table 24-8. Average head circumference of American children*

| Age | Mean average | |
	Inches	Centimeters
Birth	13.8	35
1 mo	14.9	37.6
2 mo	15.5	39.7
3 mo	15.9	40.4
6 mo	17.0	43.4
9 mo	17.8	45.0
12 mo	18.3	46.5
18 mo	19.0	48.4
2 yr	19.2	49.0
3 yr	19.6	50.0
4 yr	19.8	50.5
5 yr	20.0	50.8
6 yr	20.2	51.2
7 yr	20.5	51.6
8 yr	20.6	52.0
10 yr	20.9	53.0
12 yr	21.0	53.2
14 yr	21.5	54.0
16 yr	21.9	55.0
18 yr	22.1	55.4
20 yr	22.2	55.6

*Data from Lowrey, G. H.: Growth and development of children, Chicago, 1978, Year Book Medical Publishers, Inc.

Table 24-9. Average chest circumference of American children*

| Age | Chest circumference | |
	Inches	Centimeters
Birth	13.7	35
3 mo	16.2	40
6 mo	17.3	44
1 yr	18.3	47
18 mo	18.9	48
2 yr	19.5	50
3 yr	20.4	52
4 yr	21.1	53
5 yr	22.0	55
6 yr	22.5	56
7 yr	23.0	57
8 yr	24.0	59
9 yr	24.5	60
10 yr	25.1	61
12 yr	27.0	66
14 yr	29.0	72
16 yr†	31.0	77
18 yr†	33.0	82
20 yr†	34.5	86

*Data from Lowrey, G. H.: Growth and development of children, Chicago, 1978, Year Book Medical Publishers, Inc.
†Males only.

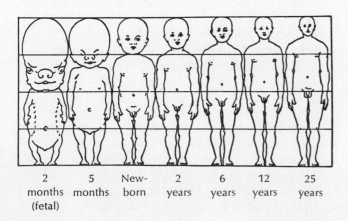

2 months (fetal)   5 months   New-born   2 years   6 years   12 years   25 years

Fig. 24-7. Relative proportions of head, trunk, and extremities at different ages. (From Stratz; modified by Robbins and others: Growth, Yale University Press, 1928.)

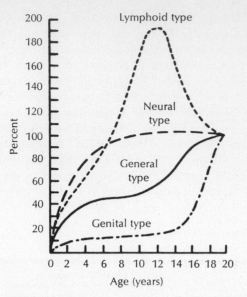

Fig. 24-8. Graph showing major types of postnatal growth of various parts and organs of the body. **Lymphoid type:** Thymus, lymph nodes, intestinal lymphoid masses. **Neural type:** Brain and its parts, dura, spinal cord, optic apparatus, many head dimensions. **General type:** Body as a whole, external dimensions (with exception of head and neck), respiratory and digestive organs, kidneys, aorta and pulmonary trunks, spleen, musculature as a whole, skeleton as a whole, blood volume. **Genital type:** Testis, ovary, epididymis, uterine tube, prostate, prostatic urethra, seminal vesicles. (Modified from Scammon, R. E.; redrawn and reproduced, with permission, from Holt, McIntosh, and Barnett: Pediatrics, ed. 13, Appleton-Century-Crofts, 1962.)

mature later. However, "late" maturers tend to be shorter as a result of little or no growth before closure of the epiphyses (Kempe, 1978).

Growth curves of the body as a whole and of the three types of tissue—lymphoid, neural, and genital—are illustrated in Fig. 24-8. These curves demonstrate the age ranges when children are expected to exhibit growth spurts.

Areas of assessment
SKIN

The examination of the skin provides valuable information about the general health of the child as well as evidence of specific skin problems. The skin of the entire body should be noted at each examination. The normal condition of the skin changes with age, and it is helpful to become familiar with those changes seen in children.

The skin of the newborn is soft, smooth, and appears almost transparent. The superficial vessels are prominent, giving the skin its red color. A mild degree of jaundice is present after the second or third day in normal infants; if the jaundice is severe or

occurs in the first 24 hours, however, the examiner should consider the presence of a serious problem. Small papular patches, called nevus flammeus, may be present over the occiput, forehead, and upper eyelids in the newborn period and usually disappear by the end of the first year of life. The nose and cheeks are frequently covered by small white papules caused by plugging of the sebaceous glands during the neonatal period. Both sweat and sebaceous glands are present in the newborn but do not function until the second month of life. Some desquamation is common during the first weeks and varies in individual babies. Mongolian spots, which are blue, irregularly shaped flat areas, are found in the sacral and buttocks area of some infants, usually those who have more darkly pigmented skin. These usually disappear by the end of the first or second year but occasionally persist for a longer time. There is a considerable amount of fine hair, called lanugo, over the body of the newborn, which is lost during the first weeks of life. The nails of the full-term newborn are well formed and firm in contrast to those of the premature infant, which are imperfectly formed.

During the first year of life there is a continuing increase in the proportion of subcutaneous fat, and raw areas resulting from skin rubbing against skin are more prevalent in young obese infants. This is called intertrigo. During the second year of life there is a decrease in the proportion of subcutaneous fat, and intertrigo is less common.

After the first year of life the normal child shows little changes in the skin until the onset of puberty, when there is considerable development of both sweat and sebaceous glands. Associated with the development of the sebaceous glands is acne vulgaris, which is so common in its mildest forms that it is sometimes considered as a normal physiological change. Early evidence of acne is the occasional comedo or blackhead on the nose and chin. At age 13 or 14, papules and small pustules may begin to appear, and by age 16 many children will have recovered completely. There are also changes in the amount and distribution of hair. Hair growth becomes heavier; the appearance of pubic, axillary, and most of the more prominent body hair is influenced by sexual development during adolescence.

LYMPH NODES

Lymph nodes in children have the same distribution as that found in adults, but the nodes are usually more prominent until the time of puberty. The amount of lymphoid tissue is considerable at birth and increases steadily until after puberty. It is common to find shotty, discrete, movable, small, nontender nodes in the occipital, postauricular, anterior and posterior cervical, parotid, submaxillary, sublingual, axillary, epitrochlear, and inguinal areas in the normal healthy child. Lymph nodes are examined during the examination of each part of the body.

HEAD AND NECK

The shape of the newborn infant's head is often asymmetrical as a result of the molding that occurs during the passage through the birth canal, and it may be a few days or weeks before the normal shape is restored. The newborn has a skull that molds easily because the bones are soft and pliable. Trauma may result in caput succedaneum or cephalohematoma. *Caput succedaneum* is an edematous swelling of the superficial tissues of the scalp that is manifested by a generalized soft swelling not bounded by suture lines. *Cephalohematoma* occurs as a result of bleeding into the periosteum and results in swelling that does not cross the suture line. These problems are temporary and are usually resolved in a matter of days or weeks. Flattening of the head is often seen in normal children but can also be indicative of problems such as mental retardation or rickets.

The sutures of the skull are palpated and can usually be felt as ridges until the age of 6 months. The fontanels are palpated during each examination of the infant and young child to determine the size, shape, and presence of any tenseness or bulging. Normally, the posterior fontanel closes by 2 months of age and the anterior fontanel closes by the end of the second year (Fig. 24-9). Tenseness or bulging of the fontanels is most easily detected when the child is in a sitting position and should be assessed when the child is quiet. Bulging of the fontanels is evidence of intracranial pressure. The fontanels may be depressed when the infant is dehydrated or malnourished. Early closure or delayed closure of the fontanels should be noted. Early closure may result from microcephaly and delayed closure from prolonged intracranial pressure.

The importance of measuring the head circumference of the child up to 2 years of age has already been discussed.

Transillumination of the skull is a useful procedure in the initial examination of the infant and for any infant with an abnormal head size. Transillumination is carried out in a completely darkened room with an ordinary flashlight equipped with a rubber adaptor. The light is placed against the infant's head. If the cerebrum is absent or greatly thinned, as from increased intracranial pressure, the entire cranium lights up. Often, defects transilluminate in a more limited way. Auscultation of the skull may reveal bruits, which are commonly found in normal children up to 4 years of age. After the age of 4, bruits are

evidence of problems such as aneurysms or increased intracranial pressure.

The young infant's scalp is inspected for evidence of crusting, which often results from a seborrheic dermatitis.

The shape of the face is inspected. A facial paralysis is most easily observed when the child cries or smiles and the asymmetry is increased. An abnormal or unusual facies may indicate a chromosomal abnormality such as Down's syndrome.

The frontal and maxillary sinuses should be percussed by the direct method and palpated in the child over 2 or 3 years of age. Until that age the sinuses are too small and poorly developed for percussion or palpation (Fig. 24-10).

The submaxillary and sublingual glands are palpated in the same way as in the adult examination. Local swelling of the parotid gland is most easily determined by observing the child in the sitting position with the head raised and the neck extended and by noting any swelling below the angle of the jaw. The swollen parotid gland may be felt by palpating downward from the zygomatic arch. Unilateral or bilateral swelling of the parotid gland is usually indicative of mumps.

The neck is examined with the child lying flat on his back. The size of the neck is noted. The neck of the infant normally is short; it lengthens at about 3 or 4 years of age. The lymph nodes are palpated, as are the thyroid gland and trachea. The sternocleidomastoid muscle is carefully palpated. A mass on the lower third of the muscle may indicate a congenital torticollis. Finally, the mobility of the neck is determined by lifting the child's head and turning it from side to side. Any resistance to flexion may be indicative of meningeal irritation.

EYES

The examination of the eyes is most easily accomplished when the child is able to cooperate. The school-age child is able to participate, and the examination is carried out as described in Chapter 11 on assessment of the eyes. The infant and young child are much more of a challenge to the examiner.

Visual function at birth is limited but improves as the structures develop. Vision may be grossly tested in the very young infant by noting the pupillary response to light; this is one of the most primitive visual functions and is normally found in the newborn infant. The blink reflex is also present in normal newborns and young infants. The infant will blink his eyes when a bright light is introduced. At 5 or 6 weeks of age the child should be able to fixate and give some evidence of following a bright toy or light. At 3 or 4 months of age the infant begins to reach for objects at

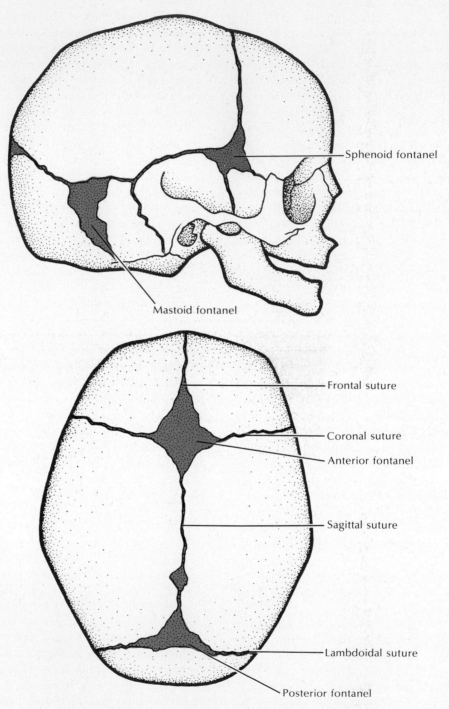

Fig. 24-9. Skull bones of the infant, showing fontanels and sutures.

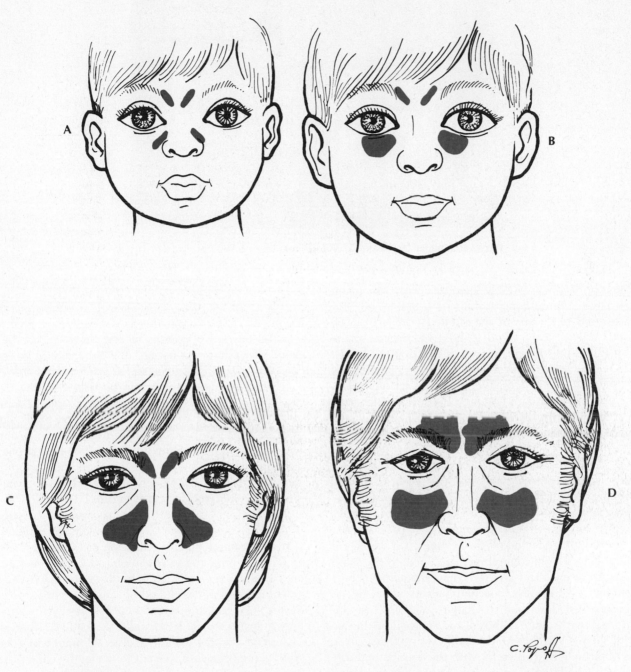

Fig. 24-10. Development of the frontal and maxillary sinuses. **A,** Early infancy. **B,** Early childhood. **C,** Adolescence. **D,** Adulthood.

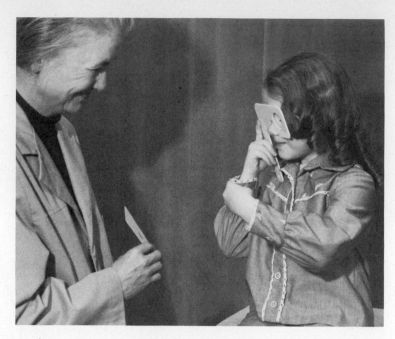

Fig. 24-11. Preparing the child for participation in testing of visual acuity.

different distances. At 6 to 7 months of age, the infant can have a funduscopic examination performed. For children 3 to 6 years of age Snellen's *E* chart can be used. The child is asked to hold his fingers in the same direction as the fingers of the *E* (Fig. 24-11). The young child is normally far-sighted and does not achieve visual acuity of 20/20 until the age of 7 years.

Tests for strabismus (squint, cross-eye), which is an imbalance of the extraocular muscles, are of importance because strabismus can lead to amblyopia exanopsia (lazy eye), a functional loss of vision in one eye that occurs when there is a disconjugate fixation. Early recognition is essential for restoration of binocular vision as the prognosis for a successful outcome for the child over 6 years of age is poor. An easy method for detecting strabismus is the observation of a bright light reflected off the corneas. The reflection of the light should come from approximately the same part of the eye, and any deviation should be noted. Another test to assess muscle imbalance is the cover-uncover test described in Chapter 10. This test can be used with older children and in some instances with younger children. A modification of the cover test that may be successful with the younger child is accomplished by the examiner placing the palm of the hand on top of the child's head and extending the thumb down over one eye without touching it (Fig. 24-12). As the vision of the one eye is obstructed by the examiner's thumb, the other eye is observed for movement. Then the examiner lifts the thumb and the recently covered eye is observed for movement. A slight jerking movement of the eye as it is

uncovered is indicative of strabismus. The test is repeated for the other eye. Transient strabismus is frequently seen during the first months of life; if it persists beyond 6 months of age, however, or becomes fixed at an earlier age, the child should be referred to an ophthalmologist.

Extraocular movements can be tested during the first weeks of life, as soon as the child is able to demonstrate following movement. The visual fields can also be at least partially examined in infants and young children by having the child sit on the parent's lap with the head in the midline and one eye covered. As the light or bright object is brought into the visual field, the child will look at it or reach for it.

Inspection of the outermost structures of the eyes is done in the same way as in the adult examination. The ophthalmoscopic examination of the eyes is dependent on the ability of the child to cooperate and on the examiner's efficiency in observing as much as possible in a limited period of time. Attempts to restrain the child and force the eyes to remain open prove unsuccessful. If possible, the child's attention should be directed toward an object or light while the examiner approaches without touching the child. The appearance of the red reflex alone is important information for ruling out opacities of the cornea and lens and cataracts.

EARS

Examination of the ears is often difficult but is important because the immature structure of the young child's ears makes them more prone to infection.

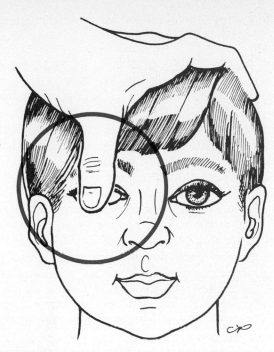

Fig. 24-12. Modification of the cover test for testing young children for strabismus.

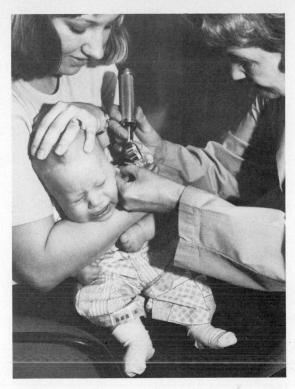

Fig. 24-13. Examination of the child's ear may be facilitated if he is held by the parent. Note that the pinna is pulled downward.

The external ear and the posterior mastoid areas are inspected and palpated for any obvious deformities. The position and size of the ears are noted. Normally the top of the ear is on a horizontal line with the inner and outer canthus of the eye.

Next, the otoscope is used. This examination becomes more difficult as the child grows older, and it is usually helpful to spend some time preparing the child by letting him see the light and by inserting the speculum gently for only a few seconds and then removing it to assure him that discomfort will be minimal. When it is necessary to use restraint, the child should be held firmly by the parent. Before the otoscope is inserted, the meatus is inspected for evidence of a foreign body or external otitis. In infancy and early childhood the auditory canal is directed upward, and the pinna should be pulled downward to aid in visualization. The otoscope is held so that the hand holding it rests firmly on the head, and the top of the speculum is inserted only ¼ or ½ inch into the canal to avoid any unnecessary discomfort (Fig. 24-13). Before the drum is examined, the canal should be carefully examined for evidence of furuncles or redness.

If the canal is filled with cerumen, it may occasionally be necessary to remove the cerumen by irrigation or curettage. If the wax is hard, it should first be softened with several drops of a mild liquid detergent, and after 10 minutes the ear should be gently irrigated with lukewarm water. Some examiners use a few drops of mineral oil to soften the wax. The irrigation procedure is unpleasant, may cause vomiting, and is not done unless necessary. It is never done if a perforation of the tympanic membrane is suspected. It is inadvisable to clean the wax out with a curette unless the examiner is skillful. The procedure may cause pain and bleeding and result in increased crying, which only increases the redness of the membrane. Often the cerumen that is not dry but is fairly soft will move during the period of the examination. Visualization of the membrane then becomes possible without any special procedures to remove the cerumen. It is important to avoid discomfort so that the child will not become conditioned to expect pain with future ear examinations.

The hearing is estimated. In the infant it can be tested by asking an assistant to stand behind the child and make a noise, such as a hand slap, several inches away from the ear while the examiner observes the child for an eye blink. In the young child, hearing can be grossly tested with the whispered voice. The examiner stands behind the child and whispers the child's name. The child will usually turn if he hears his name.

NOSE

Any unusual shape of the nose is noted, as well as flaring of the nostrils and the character and amount of discharge.

Examination of the septum, turbinates, and vestibule is accomplished by pushing the tip of the nose upward with the thumb of the left hand and shining a light into the naris. A speculum is usually not necessary; it might cause the child to be apprehensive.

MOUTH AND OROPHARYNX

This area is usually examined last, since this examination is often the most fear-provoking to the child. However, it is helpful to some children to do this examination first. The child who is anticipating discomfort may be relieved to have it accomplished and can then cooperate with the rest of the examination. This approach requires the examiner to have knowledge about the individual child's behavior and responses.

The procedures are the same as in the adult examination; however, there are differences from adults in the findings. The number of deciduous and permanent teeth and the pattern of eruption are determined by the age and development of the child. There are 20 deciduous teeth, and their eruption is completed by the age of 2½ years. The first permanent molar and lower incisor erupt at 6 years of age. The tonsils are normally larger in children than in adults and usually extend beyond the palatine arch until the age of 11 or 12 years.

CHEST

The examination of the chest begins with an inspection of the general shape and circumference. In infancy the chest is almost round; the anteroposterior diameter is as great as the transverse diameter. The circumference is normally the same as or slightly less than the head circumference until the age of 2 years, as discussed earlier in this chapter. Respiratory activity is abdominal and does not become primarily thoracic until the age of 7 years. Little intercostal motion is seen in infants and young children. Therefore, if intercostal motion is seen in the young child, lung disease may be suspected.

Palpation may be carried out and tactile fremitus evaluated, while the child is crying.

Percussion of the chest may be done directly or by the indirect method; the chest is normally more resonant than in the adult.

Auscultation with the bell stethoscope is most satisfactory, because of the small size of the child's chest (Fig. 24-14). Breath sounds will seem much louder because of the thinness of the chest wall and are almost all bronchovesicular.

HEART

The examination of the cardiovascular system as described in Chapter 16, applies to the examination of the child. However, there are some cardiac findings of normal children that are not considered normal in adults.

The pulse rate found in children of different ages is discussed earlier in this chapter. The palpation of pulses in all the extremities is a part of the cardiovascular examination; and the pulses in the lower extremities, especially the femoral pulses, are of special importance in children. Their absence or diminution may indicate coarctation of the aorta.

During infancy the heart is more nearly horizontal and has a larger diameter in comparison with the total diameter of the chest than it does in the adult (Fig. 24-15). The apex is one or two intercostal spaces above that considered normal for the adult. Therefore, the apical impulse in young children is normally felt in the fourth intercostal space just to the left of the midclavicular line. This location changes gradually and by 7 years of age the apical impulse is normally found in the fifth intercostal space at the midclavicular line.

Sinus arrhythmia is a normal finding in infants and children. The degree of arrhythmia is less in the young infant and greatest in the adolescent.

The heart sounds are louder because of the thinness of the chest wall. They are also of a higher pitch and shorter duration than those of the normal adult. A splitting of the second heart sound can be heard in the second left intercostal space in most infants and children. The split normally widens with inspiration. A third heart sound is present in about one-third of all children and is best heard at the apex.

Many children have murmurs without heart disease, and the significance of a murmur may be difficult to determine. Innocent murmurs are characteristically systolic in timing, are grade 1 or 2 in intensity, and are not transmitted to other areas. They are loudest in the recumbent position and disappear when the child sits up or exercises. It is not always possible to determine whether the murmur is innocent or pathological by auscultation alone, although murmurs of grade 3 or louder are usually indicative of heart disease. A venous hum is commonly found in children. It is a continuous, low-pitched sound originating in the internal jugular vein and is heard either above or below the clavicles. It is accentuated in the upright position and disappears when the child is lying down. As it is not pathologically significant, it should be differentiated from a murmur.

ABDOMEN

The examination of the abdomen may be done first, since it requires few instruments and may be less frightening to the child. However, if the child is upset, it may be done later. When the child is re-

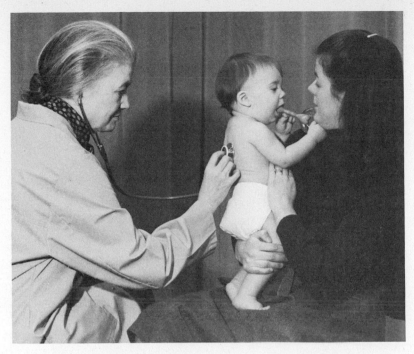

Fig. 24-14. Auscultation of breath sounds is most easily accomplished when the child is comfortable.

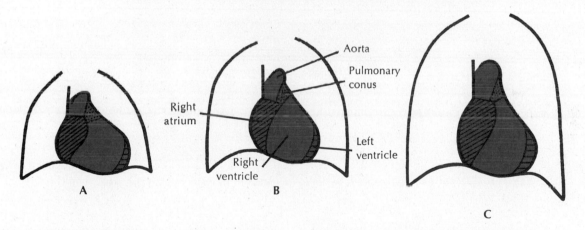

Fig. 24-15. Position of the heart at different ages. **A,** Early infancy. **B,** Early childhood. **C,** Adulthood.

laxed, the abdomen is somewhat easier to examine than in the adult, because of the less well developed abdominal wall. To win the child's cooperation, several approaches may be helpful: a bottle may be offered to the infant; the young child may be more comfortable and relaxed if examined while sitting on the parent's lap. Each examiner will find the approaches that are most productive for him (Fig. 24-16).

The order of the abdominal examination procedures for the young child may be changed to avoid introducing the stethoscope and using percussion until after the child has experienced procedures that appear less threatening. First, the abdomen is inspected. The abdomen is larger than the chest in children under 4 years of age and appears "pot bellied" in both supine and sitting positions. The child up to 13 years of age will have a "pot belly" in the standing position. This normal shape needs to be differentiated from the real distention that is caused by enlargement of organs or the presence of tumors, cysts, or ascites. A depressed abdomen may result from dehydration of malnutrition. Respirations are largely abdominal in children up to 7 years of age. Any splinting or loss of movement may be indicative of peritonitis, appendicitis, or other acute problems.

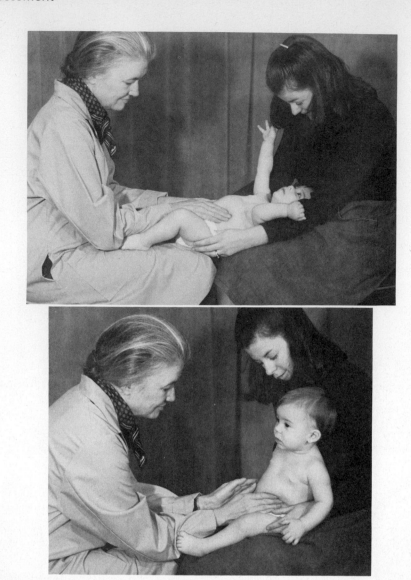

Fig. 24-16. Modification in approach to the examination of the abdomen of the young child.

The umbilicus is normally closed, but umbilical hernias are common in white children up to 2 years of age and for longer periods in black children. The abdomen is also observed for peristaltic waves and dilated veins.

Palpation is carried out in the same way as in the examination of the adult except for the modifications in approach and in the positions of the child. Light palpation enables the examiner to determine the tenseness of the abdominal muscles, the presence of superficial masses, and the presence of tenderness. The child is often not able to pinpoint the area of tenderness, and only by watching the facial expressions can the examiner determine the point of maximal tenderness. The liver is generally palpable 1 to 2 cm below the right costal margin during the first year of life. If it extends more than 2 cm below the costal margin, further investigation is warranted. The spleen is normally palpable 1 to 2 cm below the left costal margin in the first weeks of life. Any increase in size should be noted, and any evidence of tenderness may be an indication of serious blood dyscrasias or other problems. Tissue turgor is also determined by grasping a few inches of skin and subcutaneous tissue over the abdomen, pulling it up, and then quickly releasing it. If the creases formed do not disappear immediately, dehydration is present. Deep palpation is done in all four quadrants by single-handed or bimanual methods. The inguinal and femoral regions are palpated for hernias, lymph nodes, and femoral pulses.

Auscultation of the abdomen is carried out in the same manner as described in the examination of the adult.

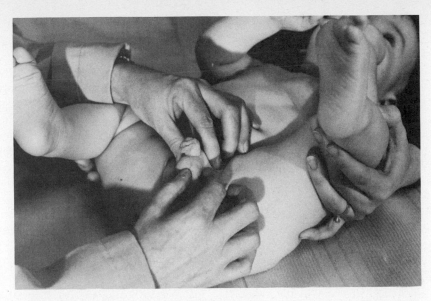

Fig. 24-17. Palpation of the scrotum to determine if the testes are descended.

Finally, percussion may be useful in obtaining the boundaries of the liver spleen, and any tumors

GENITALIA

The examination of the genitalia of both male and female children is usually carried out by inspection and palpation.

Male genitalia. In the male child there are two primary areas to be examined; the penis and the scrotum. The foreskin of the penis is examined first. The foreskin of the uncircumcised infant is normally tight for the first 2 or 3 months of life and does not retract easily. If the tightness persists beyond this period, it is called a phimosis and should be observed to determine if there is any interference with urination. Any retraction of the foreskin should be done carefully, since the delicate membranes attached to the foreskin may be easily torn and result in adhesions. Next, the meatus is examined to determine its position and the presence of any ulceration. The meatus is normally located at the tip of the shaft. An abnormal location of the meatus on the ventral surface is called a hypospadias; an abnormal location on the dorsal surface is called an epispadias.

The scrotum is inspected for evidence of enlargement. An enlarged scrotum may be indicative of a hernia or hydrocele. The scrotum is also palpated to determine if the testes are descended (Fig. 24-17). The examiner's index finger is used to block the inguinal canal and is gently pushed toward the scrotum. The finger and thumb of the opposite hand are used to palpate the scrotum and grasp the testes as it is pushed downward into the scrotum. If the testes cannot be easily palpated in an older boy, he should

sit in a chair with his legs apart, his heels on the seat of the chair, and his arms around his knees. This procedure interrupts the cremasteric reflex and creates pressure by flexing abdomen and thigh. The testes are felt as a soft mass about 1 cm in diameter and are normally descended if they can be palpated in the scrotum even if retraction into the inguinal canal occurs immediately.

Female genitalia. The female child is examined early in infancy for structural intactness. This examination procedure must be done with great care. Both the child and the parents may not understand what is going to be done and may fear the procedure. With proper preparation of the child and a gentle technique, the gynecological examination can prove a valuable tool. The examination can be performed with emotional and physical support measures, with analgesia, or if required with anesthesia. A small infant can be examined in a dorsal lithotomy position, while lying in the mother's lap. An older child may lie on an examining table, using the Teg lithotomy blocks instead of stirrups. The child's fear can be allayed, and her tense abdomen relaxed, by gaining her participation in the examination. The child can hold a speculum, help to separate the labia, or help palpate her abdomen.

In the pediatric client, inspection and palpation consist of identifying structural defect or absence, such as the presence of masses, the appearance of the labia, the presence of a vagina, the size of the clitoris, the structure of the mons veneris, the presence of pubic hair, the presence of a urethral orifice in the expected location, and the presence of masses in the groin. A manual rectal examination will rule out masses in the adnexa and allow for palpation of the cervix and estimation of the ratio of fundus to cervix. Extrapelvic sex areas to be considered in any gynecological assessment include height, weight, general body contours, and the presence or absence of secondary sex characteristics.

The last step in examining a young child is visualization of the vagina and cervix. This procedure requires instruments that have been adapted to the small size of the child and still allow for visualization of the upper vagina and cervix.

Although the order of the examination of the adolescent remains the same as in the younger child, the climate is usually one of suspicion and conflict as well as fear. The practitioner needs to address the history to both the client and the adolescent's parents. Most often the gynecological examination is best performed without the parent present in the room. The gynecological examination procedure is the same as in an adult and is discussed in Chapter 17, "Assessment of Female Genitalia." The bimanual rectal pelvic examination is done to rule out masses in the adnexa and in the vagina. The Huffman vaginal speculum or the small-sized Pederson speculum is thought to be the most useful and comfortable instrument in visualizing the vagina and the cervix of the sexually inactive adolescent. The examiner is also to be alert to breast development, changes in the pigmentation, texture and integrity of the skin, and the development and pattern of pubic hair.

MUSCULOSKELETAL SYSTEM

Much of the examination is done while watching the child or while playing with the child. The younger child or infant is not able to understand directions, and much of the examination is done by helping the child passively go through range-of-motion movements. An older child will be able to follow directions, and a routine musculoskeletal examination can be completed.

The skeleton of the infant and young child is made up largely of cartilaginous tissues, which accounts for the relative softness and malleability of the bones. It is also the reason that many defects identified early in life can be corrected with more ease than in later years.

The common orthopedic problems of childhood are age-related. This occurs, in part, because of certain environmental factors, such as constrained uterine position, birth trauma, improper diet and caloric intake, inadequate footgear, poor foot hygiene, age-inappropriate athletics, poor body mechanics, and lack of regular exercise. In addition, one must acknowledge the role that disease conditions, like arthritis, and deformities, like scoliosis, play in musculoskeletal dysfunction. Table 24-10 is a composite of the common orthopedic problems seen in various age groups.

In the neonate, the four major areas in which orthopedic problems are encountered are the head, hip, leg, and foot. An asymmetrical deformity of the head and neck, in which the child tilts his head toward the affected side, is called congenital muscular torticollis. It is more common in females than males; and if not present at birth, it may present itself by the second or third week. The mother's chief concern is that the child does not seem to turn his head equally well in both directions. Physical examination requires palpation of the sternocleidomastoid muscle. The finding usually is a hard, nontender, fusiform swelling. It is likely to enlarge gradually for 2 to 4 weeks. Then it regresses slowly, disappearing in 2 to 6 months. An x-ray of the cervical spine may be warranted to rule out cervical anomalies. An x-ray of the neck region may be necessary to differentiate torticollis from a tumor of the muscle. Generally, torticollis will treat itself. In mild cases, passive stretching exercises or using a mobile in the crib to attract the child to turn his head toward the unaffected side may help. Having the mother, who is formula-feeding hold the child so that he must turn his head to reach the nipple, having the mother who is breast-feeding, hold the child when he is sucking for comfort so that he must turn his head toward the unaffected side, and/or rolling up a towel and positioning his head during nap or nightime sleeping periods can be recommended. In severe cases surgery is required to shorten the opposite muscle and help regain facial symmetry and head alignment.

Asymmetry of the mandible often accompanies torticollis. However not all asymmetry will disappear. Sometimes, when the constraint of the fetus in utero has been significant, molding of the head or jaw remains. Except for showing the parent ways to style the child's hair to help round out his facial appearance or head shape, there is little to be done.

Four deformities of the feet noted in the neonate are varus, valgus, equinus, and calcaneus. There are also combinations of these deformities. Table 24-11 points out the position of the heel, forefoot, and/or toes in these deformities. Foot deformities usually are a result of constraint of the fetus' position in utero. It may help the examiner to try and determine the position of comfort for the neonate. The newborn may be folded into what was believed to be his uterine position. There should be no resistance to this manipulation. Often, the examiner can gain much insight into the origin of the orthopedic problem at hand. An example of this phenomenon is when the examiner notes a unilateral varus and a unilateral

Table 24-10. Orthopedic disorders common to various age groups of children

Neonate	Preschooler	School age child	Young adult
Oligohydramnios	Postural/orthopedic abnor-	Idiopathic adolescent	Disabling low back pain
Compressed face	malities of the foot	scoliosis	Osteoarthritis
Limb deformities	Abnormalities of the toenail	Other types of scoliosis	Athletic injuries
Thoracic compression	Disorders of skin	Kyphosis	Jogging-related injuries
Lung hypoplasia	Deviations in gait	Lordosis	
Prolonged breech position	Poor foot hygiene	Alignment problems of	
Dislocation of hip	Inadequate footgear	lower extremity	
Deformations of knee		Juvenile arthritis	
Hyperextension of knee		Athletic injuries	
Dislocation of knee		Unstable knee	
Foot deformities		Upper extremity, elbow	
Calcaneovalgus		clean	
Metatarsus adductus		Epiphyseal injuries	
Equinovarus			
Overlapping toes			
Craniofacies			
Compressed face			
Molding of calvarum			
Mandibular asymmetry			
Torticollis			
Dislocated hip(s)			
Postural scoliosis			

Table 24-11. Four primary deformities of the foot in relation to the position of the heel, forefoot, and/or toes*

Primary deformity	Heel	Forefoot	Toes
Varus	Inverted	Adducted inverted (sole in)	
Valgus	Everted	Abducted everted (sole out)	
Equinus	Plantar flexed		At level lower than heel
Calcaneus	Dorsiflexed		At level higher than heel
Combinations:			
Equinovarus	Plantar flexed inverted	Adducted inverted (sole in)	At level lower than heel
Equinovalgus	Plantar flexed everted	Abducted everted (sole out)	At level lower than heel
Calcaneovarus	Dorsiflexed inverted	Adducted inverted (sole in)	At level higher than heel
Calcaneovalgus	Dorsiflexed everted	Abducted everted (sole out)	At level higher than heel

*Data from Swanger, R.: Common problems of toddlers and preschoolers, lecture, 1972.

valgus, commonly known as windblown feet. By folding the child into his position of comfort, the practitioner soon is able to visualize that both feet were tucked in and facing one direction in utero.

One of the most problematical foot deformities to deal with is talipes equinovarus, or clubfoot. This is more common in males. It occurs as often as once in every 1,000 births. This deformity can include such a severe degree of plantar flexion, heel inversion, and forefoot adduction that the foot appears to be backward, that is, with the toes facing the rear. X-rays will illustrate the actual anatomical deformity. In this condition, the child's foot is usually fixed and resists fully the examiner's attempts to manipulate it into a neutral position. Treatment usually includes plaster casting, exercises, and operative procedures.

The second most common foot disorder is metatarsus varus, or what is sometimes referred to as one-third of a clubfoot. The child displays forefoot adduction and inversion. In this deformity, the child's foot can be manipulated with some resistance into a normal, neutral position. This disorder is often accompanied by internal tibial torsion. Plaster casts, exercises, Denis-Browne bar, using reversed shoes, or attaching shoes at the heels may be done (Fig. 24-18).

Problems encountered with the leg are usually alignment difficulties. Tibial torsion may be internal or external. Internal is more common and may be associated with bowing of the legs or clubfoot. External torsion of the tibia is sometimes seen with genu valgum (knock-knees) and flat feet. An x-ray will confirm the diagnosis. Treatment ranges from none to casting, use of the Denis-Browne splint, and/or Thomas heels and wedges. Occasionally, corrective surgery is performed in the older child.

The second leg deformity seen by the practitioner in pediatric primary care is genu varum, or bowlegs. An x-ray will confirm an outward bowing of the femur and the tibia, and a flaring at the knee. Treatment is usually limited to exercises of the feet or positioning to encourage abduction. Sometimes Thomas heels and wedges are applied.

Genu valgum, or knock-knees, refers to the distance between the medial malleoli. This condition is usually found with flat feet. Providing support to the arch of the foot so that the hips, legs, and ankles can be kept in proper alignment is the treatment used. If the distance between malleoli is less than 2½ to 3 inches, the prognosis is good.

When the examiner is concerned over the alignment of the lower extremities, one of the more helpful procedures is to try to draw a straight line from the anterior superior spine of the ilium, through the middle of the patella, to the second toe. If any deviation from this line is noted, the examiner then determines whether it is limited to a specific bone and whether bowing, torsion, or rotation is part of the presenting picture. Manual manipulation of the extremities at each joint can help to differentiate if the lack of alignment is from muscle torque or skeletal deformity.

Congenital dislocation of the hip means that the femoral head is displaced and out of the acetabular socket. It is more common in females and affects the left hip three times more frequently than the right. In 25% of all cases, it is bilateral. The examiner may note asymmetry of skin folds of the thigh, gluteal folds (Fig. 24-19) and popliteal creases. When the examiner places the hip in a 90-degree flexed position and with passive manipulation attempts to abduct the affected hip, the movement will be lim-

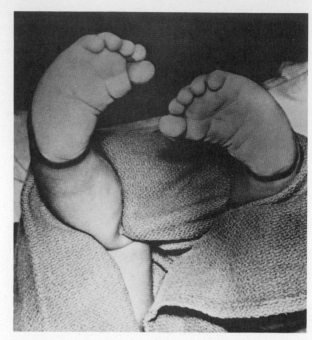

Fig. 24-18. Marked metatarsus varus. (Mead Johnson & Co., Evansville, Ind., 1971.)

ited. When the infant lies with his knees flexed at right angles, the shortening of the femur is seen. This is called Galeazzi's sign. The Ortolani test may be performed. Starting with both hips in a neutral position, the practitioner examines one hip at a time, using the other hip to stabilize the pelvis. The examiner applies abduction, traction, and inward pressure over the greater trochanter with his index and middle fingers. A reducible dislocation results in the examiner *feeling* a click in the hip, not necessarily hearing it. Proceeding with Barlow's test, the examiner adducts the hip, uses the length of the fingers to apply pressure along the axis of the femur, and produces outward pressure with the thumb. This maneuver slips the reduced hip posteriorly over the acetabulum's edge. Both these procedures assume the hip to be dislocated posteriorly (Asher, 1977). Dislocated hips can resolve spontaneously. However, there is no way to know which ones will, thus all are treated. Splinting of the hip may consist of casting or skin or skeletal traction followed by hip spica casting. Delay in identification of a dislocated hip and immediate referral can cost the child an additional 10 weeks of treatment for every month lost.

In most instances, the foot bones of school-aged children are developed sufficiently so that they are unable to give the maximum response to treatment. Shapiro and Rhee (1970) demonstrated that a screening of 8,995 preschool and kindergarten children revealed 37% to have postural and orthopedic problems, 16% skin abnormalities, 15% gait deviations,

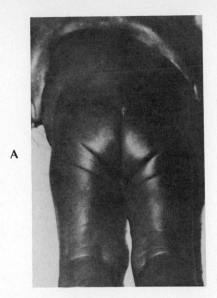
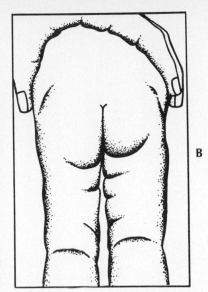

Fig. 24-19. Examination of the hips. **A,** Normal gluteal folds. **B,** Abnormal gluteal folds. (Courtesy Mead Johnson & Co., Evansville, Ind., 1972.)

and 4% nail abnormalities. Of these children 997 were referred for treatment and 838 for further study. Four hundred nine children received treatment at the time of the publication. Additionally, the study pointed out the need for improved foot hygiene and the use of adequate footgear.

In the school-aged child, as young as 5 to 6 years of age, girls are to be screened for scoliosis. This procedure is outlined in detail in Chapter 18. It is late to identify scoliosis in the 10 to 13 or older age range, as the thoracic cage is having to deal with increased body weight and breast development. The best results in treating idiopathic adolescent scoliosis occur when treatment begins with curves that are less than 20 to 25 degrees. While viewing the entire body from the front, side, and rear, the examiner notes scapular asymmetry and unilateral prominence, waist and hip asymmetry or fullness, shoulder level, and asymmetry in distance between the arms and the torso. An extensive history and complete x-ray examination are performed. Nonsurgical corrective techniques include exercise, Milwaukee brace, body casts, and traction. Surgical procedures focus on spinal fusion.

Juvenile rheumatoid arthritis is a chronic and disabling disease of young children. The time of onset and the number of joints involved are categorized into different syndromes, which have varying patterns and prognoses. Juvenile arthritis impairs growth in children. The long bones of the hands and feet may not grow, the jaw may not develop, sexual development can be delayed, and erosion of the joint cartilage and bone may occur, with joint contractures becoming evident. The older the child, the more similar his symptoms are to the adult with rheumatoid arthritis. But the young child frequently presents with a maze of signs and symptoms that must be sorted out. These may include fever, rash, joint symptoms, endocarditis, pericarditis, palpable spleen, limited joint movement, and lymphadenopathy.

Athletic injuries are fast becoming a new field of health care. Hard-hitting sports like tackle football require repeated blows to the body; or putting all the body weight on one joint, as with running; or stressing a joint such as the elbow, as in tennis. Often the sport is inappropriate for the individual child's build and stage of development. Stress fractures of the fibula, heel cord injuries, epiphyseal fractures, sprains and bursitis of the elbow, and damage to the articular cartilage of the knee are just a few of the athletic-related injuries a child may sustain. Rest, reduction of inflammation, and relief of fluid buildup are the usual treatment methods. Radiography is needed to confirm suspicion of stress fractures. Surgery may be necessary to reduce a fracture or to apply a fixation device. Growth disturbance can occur when the epiphyseal center is displaced. This is not always seen on roentgenogram, if the child is very young and the epiphyses are not yet highly visible. It is important that children who sustain athletic injuries with a possibility of growth disturbance be checked regularly to prevent, identify, and/or treat any deformity that may result.

NEUROLOGICAL SYSTEM

The formal neurological examination of the infant or child must be adapted to the age of the individual,

Table 24-12. Normal findings in the neurological examination of various age groups of children.

	Age			
	Premature (weeks gestation)	Full-term	4 Months	6-18 Months
Posture	Lax and floppy	Firm, rounded		
	Fetal position is open	Fetal position is closed		
Tone	Hypotonia inversely proportional to gestational age	Predominance of flexor tone in extremities		
Motor	Jerky and asymmetric movements, floppy head	Symmetrical movement of extremities, poor control of head	Follows objects with eyes, waves hands at dangling objects, kicks both feet simultaneously	Maturing prehensile function, transfers objects from hand to hand, opposition of thumb and forefinger; sits, propels self, crawls reciprocally, pulls self up, cruises walks with, then without support, toddles with wide based gait
Reflexes Infant	Extensor toe	Extensor toe	Uses either hand to remove cloth from face	Steady gait develops
	Marked Moro by 32 wks	Moro	Head control when prone or supine, raises chest from table when prone, pulled to sit and rights neck, pushes symmetrically with his feet when supported, Moro disappearing, incurvation gone, sucking/rooting disappears, righting fuses into voluntary movement, primary walk disappears	Triceps
	Incurvation by 24	Incurvation		Crossed adduction
	Sucking by 28	Sucking		Moro gone, tonic neck not reproducible, parachute response appears, Landau
	Rooting by 24	Rooting		
	Palmar and plantar by 24	Palmar and plantar		
	Vertical righting by 34	Neck and vertical righting		
	Primary walking by 34	Primary walking		
		Primary stepping		
		Placing		
		Quadriceps		
		Ankle		
		Abdominal		
		Cremasteric		
Deep				
Superficial				
Cranial nerves I—Olfactory		Grimaces; likes sugar, dislikes salt		
II—Optic		Pupillary reflex	Follows objects	Retrieves objects
III—Oculomotor		Doll's eye phenomena	Nystagmus decreasing	Follows light
IV—Trochlear		Can not assess rooting, sucking		Accommodation
V—Trigeminal				
VI—Abducens				
VII—Facial				
VIII—Acoustic		Auditory induced Moro		
IX—Glossopharyngeal		swallow, cry, motility of palate		
X—Vagus		Gag		
XI—Accessory		Head control		
XII—Hypoglossal		Sucking		
Sensation Pain				
Touch				
Vibratory		Can not assess yet		12-18 mos can assess

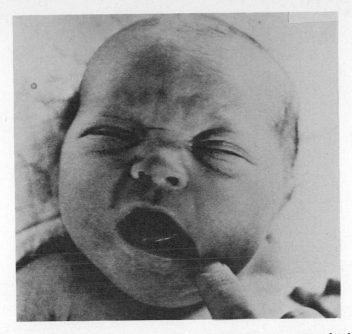

Fig. 24-20. Eliciting the rooting reflex in a full-term infant. (Courtesy Mead Johnson & Co., Evansville, Ind., 1965.)

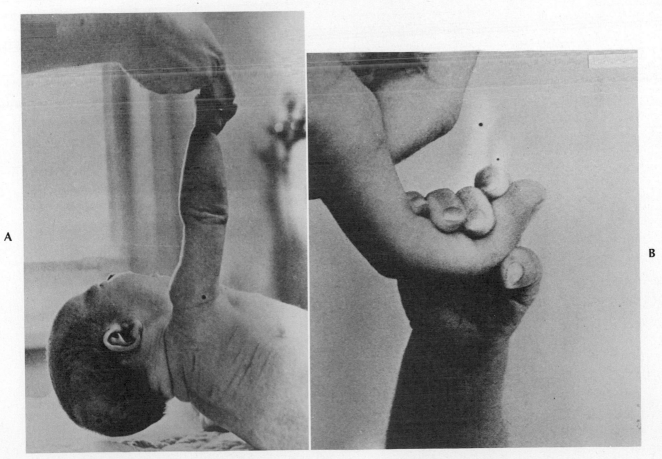

A   B

Fig. 24-21. Eliciting the grasp reflex of the hand of a full-term infant. (Courtesy Mead Johnson & Co., Evansville, Ind., 1965.)

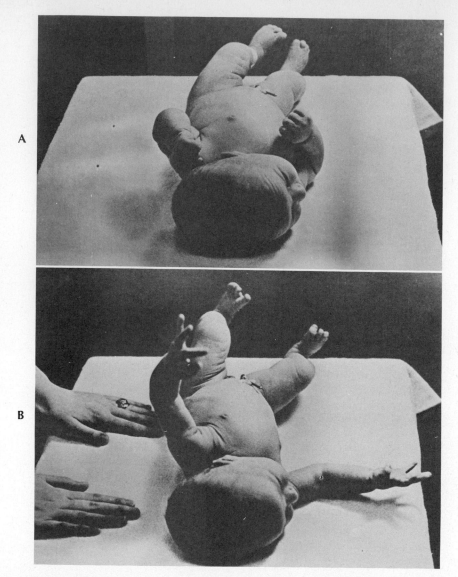

A

B

Fig. 24-22. Eliciting the Moro reflex in a full-term infant. (Courtesy Mead Johnson & Co., Evansville, Ind., 1965.)

but at all times a complete examination consists of an assessment of the cranial nerves and special senses, the motor system, coordination and cerebellar function, sensation, and both superficial and deep reflexes. In children under 2 years of age, the neurological assessment is closely related to the increasing myelinization and maturation of the neural system. In this age group, the degree of maturation can only be estimated rather than quantified.

In the newborn, infant, and child over 2 years, the primary mode of examination is one of observation and inspection. This is usually reinforced by palpation and passive manipulation, although other modes may be used, such as, auscultation. Usually these methods are not necessary in the daily practice of the primary care practitioner. Observation of the

child in his natural state and then with purposeful stimulation is often the most valuable tool of the examiner. This is the best opportunity to determine how the child's overall function and behavior meet age-related norms. Seven areas can be observed: symmetry of spontaneous movements, appearance, positioning, posture, movement of extremities, seizure activity, and responsiveness of the infant to his parents and environment.

Because the neurological system affects every other system, it is necessary to integrate the neurological examination. For example, changes in the pigmentation of the skin, lesions of the skin, masses in the abdomen, abnormal size and shape of the head, gaps and protrusions in the spinal column, and limited range of motion can all reflect a disease, lesion, or

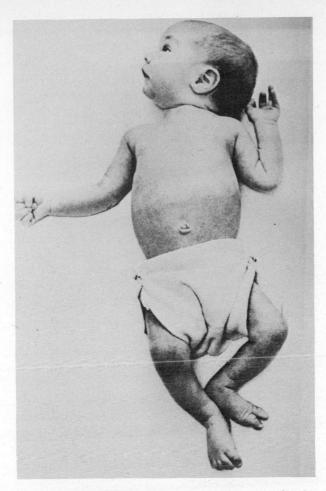

Fig. 24-23. Tonic neck reflex displayed by full-term infant when his head was gently turned to the right side. (Courtesy Mead Johnson & Co., Evansville, Ind., 1965.)

injury to the nervous system. In addition, because a child is going through an intense period of development that is in part related to the increasing myelinization and maturation of the neural system, a meticulous look at the child's developmental progress is required. The quality, pitch, loudness, and duration of a child's cry; drowsiness; irritability; and social, adaptive, language, and motor skills are all measures of how well his neurological system is functioning. Table 24-12 lists some of the normal findings the examiner expects in children of various age groups.

The automatic infant reflexes that are normal at birth and disappear around 4 months of age, as voluntary control begins to develop, include the Moro reflex, the palmar grasp reflex, and the rooting reflex. Absence of these reflexes may indicate a severe problem of the central nervous system. Persistence of these reflexes may be equally serious. The *Moro reflex* is elicited by placing the infant in a supine position and surprising him with a loud noise or by allowing the head to suddenly drop a few inches. The infant will respond with an overall grasping movement;

the arms extend and then flex, and the knees and hips flex. The *palmar grasp reflex* is obtained by the examiner's placing one of his fingers in contact with the plamar surface of the infant's fingers. The infant will automatically grasp the fingers tightly. The *rooting reflex* is obtained by touching the infant's cheeks. The infant will turn his head toward the stimulus as if searching for it.

The tonic neck reflex appears at 1 month of age and disappears at 4 to 6 months of age. It is elicited by placing the infant in the supine position and turning the head to the left or right. The arm on the side toward which the head is turned will extend, and the other arm will flex.

Babinski's reflex is normally present in the newborn and disappears by the age of 12 to 24 months. Figs. 24-20 through 24-23 illustrate several of the reflexes found in a full-term infant.

Children two years of age or older can be examined with many of the same methods used with an adult. Only the conversation, directions, and developmental tasks are altered to be more suitable to the interests

Text continued on p. 620.

Table 24-13. Health surveillance chart: birth to 21 years*

Age	History	Approach to client	Order of examination	Physical examination
1 mo	Prenatal course of mother, delivery Family Genetic diseases General health Respiratory Digestive Eating Elimination Urinary Behavior/misc. Sleep, crying Problems/concerns Mother's perception of child	Examine while quiet on mother's lap Examine while sitting on mother's lap Examine while lying on mother's lap Examine on table	General observation and examination of skin are done first for all children Chest Head and neck Eyes (more apt to remain open in sitting position or when held over mother's shoulder) Abdomen Extremities Genitalia and rectum Spine Reflexes Ears Nose Oral cavity	Complete, including for cyanosis Pulses Murmur Genitalia Congenital anomalies Reflexes Skin Mother-child interaction
2-3 mo	General health Respiratory Digestive Eating Elimination Urinary Sensory/motor development Behavior/misc. Sleeping Crying Happiness Feeding Problems/concerns			Murmurs Ortolani's sign Cyanosis Denver Developmental Screening Test (DDST)
4-5 mo	General health Respiratory Digestive Eating Elimination Urinary Sensory/motor development Language development Behavior/misc. Current living situation Parent-child interaction Problems/concerns			Complete (tibial torsion) Cyanosis Hips DDST

*Adapted in part from Farrand, L.: Health surveillance chart, 1978, unpublished communication. Used with permission.

Auditory-visual	Laboratory	Developmental landmarks	Nutrition	Anticipatory guidance	Immunization/other
Vision 　Corneal light reflex Pupillary response to light	Phenylketonuria (PKU) test	Eyes follow midline Regards face While prone lifts head off table	Method 　Acceptability 　Schedule 　Supplement 　　Breast milk—vitamins A and D 　　Evaporated milk —vitamin C and iron	Car seat Sneezing, hiccups, bowel patterns, sleeping and breathing patterns Night bottle Colic "Spoiling" Accidents/safety Siblings Temperature taking	
Vision 　Red reflex 　Corneal light reflex 　Observe response to direction of light Hearing	Vocalizes Smiles responsively Holds head and chest up to make 90° angle with table		Feeding schedule	Solid foods Immunization Thumbsucking Accidents/car seat Sleeping without rocking, holding Coping with frustrations Sibling rivalry Determining illness Encourage vocalization	Diphtheria-pertussis-tetanus/oral poliovirus vaccine no. 1
Strabismus		Holds head erect and steady when held in sitting position Squeals Grasps rattle Eyes follow object for 180°	Solids—plain, strained Rice cereal (iron fortified) Starting foods (fruit then yellow vegetables, then green vegetables)	Feeding schedule to fit in with family Attitude of father Respiratory infections Teething Role of iron in diet	DPT/OPV #2

Continued.

Table 24-13. Health surveillance chart: birth to 21 years—cont'd

Age	History	Approach to clinet	Order of examination	Physical examination
6-7 mo	General health Respiratory Digestive Eating Elimination Urinary Sensory/motor development Behavior/misc. Sleeping Exposure to lead Problems/concerns	Examine on mother's lap; child can be distracted with toy, bottle, or examiner's voice Examine on table	General observation Chest Head and neck Eyes Abdomen Ears Nose Oral cavity Extremities Reflexes Genitalia and rectum Spine	Complete observation Strabismus Fundi Skin DDST
9-10 mo	General Health Respiratory Digestive Eating Elimination Urinary Sensory/motor development Behavior/misc. Relationship with peers/siblings Exposure to lead Problems/concerns			Complete EOM Mother-child interaction DDST
12-15 mo	Same as for 9-10 mo			Complete Pulses Tibial torsion EOM DDST Bloodpressure (BP) (and each visit hereafter)

Auditory-visual	Laboratory	Developmental landmarks	Nutrition	Anticipatory guidance	Immunization/other

Vision
  Corneal light reflex (strabismus; extraocular movements [EOM]
  Fundi
Hearing
  Differentiates sounds
Should look toward source of speech
	Hematocrit (Hct)
	Hemaglobin (Hgb)
		No head lag if pulled to sitting position	Add vegetables, fruit—plain/strained with desserts
			Avoid mixed dinners
			Use natural juices
				Feeding
				Accidents/lead poisoning
				Night crying
				Fear of strangers
				Separation anxiety
				Use of teething ring/ice for teething
					DPT/OPV #3

	Lead Hgb Electrophoresis	Looks after object that has fallen Transfers block from one hand to other Feeds crackers to self Sits alone for 5 sec after support is released	Add strained meats Avoid mixed dinners Use spoon/cup Finger foods	Normal to display unpleasant behavior Discipline Use of cup Eats with fingers Fear of strangers Accidents Ipecac prescription Need for affection Pica Shoes Use of books Explore feelings of parenting	Tuberculosis screening (TBC)
Vision Amblyopia may develop	Urinalysis (U/A)	Cruises—walks around holding on to furniture Stands alone 2-3 sec if outside support is removed Bangs together two objects (one held in each hand) Imitates vocalization heard within preceeding minute Plays pat-a-cake	Nutritious snacks	Negativism Likelihood of respiratory infections Push/pull toys "Getting into things" Weaning from bottle Proper dose of vitamins Control of drugs and poisons Safety	Mumps-measles-rubella (MMR)—15 mo (TBC before MMR)

Continued.

Table 24-13. Health surveillance chart: birth to 21 years—cont'd

Age	History	Approach to client	Order of examination	Physical examination
15-19 mo	General health Respiratory Digestive Eating Elimination Urinary Sensory/motor development Speech Behavior/misc. Current living situation Parent-child interaction Pica Relationship to peers/siblings Problems/concerns	Examination modified to take advantage of opportunities Examine while standing and walking Examine while standing or on mother's lap Examine on mother's lap or on the examining table; child may need restraint—examination should be carried out as as quickly and efficiently as possible	General observation Extremities Spine Chest Head and neck Eyes Abdomen Reflexes Genitalia and rectum Ears Nose Oral cavity	Complete DDST
23-25 mo (2 yr)	General health Respiratory Digestive Eating Elimination Urinary Sensory/motor development Toilet training Speech Behavior/misc. Current living situation Social adjustment Problems/concerns			Complete DDST
3 yr	Same as for 2 yr			Complete BP Initial dental examination DDST

Auditory-visual	Laboratory	Developmental landmarks	Nutrition	Anticipatory guidance	Immunization/other
Vision Convergence well established	U/A Lead	Puts one block on another Mimics household chores such as dusting Feeds self with spoon Indicates wants	Limit milk 2-3 cups daily Monitor quality of snack foods	Reaction towards peers/siblings Toilet training readiness Speech development Discipline/limit setting Toys: play dough, tricycle, picture books Sexual play is normal	DPT/OPV #4
EOM Squint Lead	U/A Lead	Kicks ball with foot and without support Scribbles spontaneously—purposeful marking of more than one stroke on paper Balances four blocks on top of one another Points correctly to one body part Dumps small objects out of bottles after demonstration Does simple tasks in house Uses phrases	Cease night bottles	Need for peer companionship Immaturity—inability to share or take turns Play: color and shape games Brush teeth, twice daily	
Test vision (20/40) Ocular adjustment	Lead Hct Urine culture (female)	Jumps in place Pedals tricycle Dumps small objects out of bottle without demonstration Uses plurals Washes and dries hands	Decreased appetite	Sex education Nursery schools qualifications of good one Obedience and discipline Toilet training, bedwetting Fear of darkness, animals, and so on	TBC

Continued.

Table 24-13. Health surveillance chart: birth to 21 years—cont'd

Age	History	Approach to client	Order of examination	Physical examination
4 yr	Same as for 2 yr	Enjoys conversation and responds to questions Needs simple explanations of what examiner is doing; enjoys opportunity to handle equipment Examine while standing and walking Examine on table; usually tolerates if mother remains nearby	General observation Extremities Spine Complete the rest of the examination, leaving the ears, nose, and oral cavity until last	School readiness
5 yr	Same as for 2 yr (omit toilet training) Kindergarten—mother's readiness Problems/concerns			Complete BP Dental examination
6 yr	Same as for 2 yr Peer adjustment			
7 yr		Usually more comfortable with mother present Modest and often shy but cooperative Needs to have equipment and procedures of examination explained	Same order as the adult examination; genitalia and rectum examined last	

Auditory-visual	Laboratory	Developmental landmarks	Nutrition	Anticipatory guidance	Immunization/other
Test vision (20/30) Audiogram	Lead	Builds bridge of three blocks after demonstration Copies cross and circle Identifies longer of two lines Knows first and last names Understands what to do when "tired" Plays with other children in games of interaction, such as tag Dresses with supervision	Food overindulgence common	Readiness for kindergarten Use of money Dental care Safety (leading causes of injury: burns, drowning, auto accident)	
Vision E chart Color blindness Audiogram	Hct U/A Lead Urine culture (female)	Hops two or more times Catches ball thrown 3 feet Dresses without supervision Tolerates separation from mother without anxiety	Readiness for school Span of attention and how to increase it Sleep problems Bedwetting		DPT/OPV
Same as for 5 yr Vision acuity approaches 20/20 Audiogram	Lead	Bicycle riding Copies a square Draws a man with six parts Defines six simple words, such as ball, lake, and horse Names materials of which things (spoon, door) are made	Suggest nutritious snacks, such as fruit and nuts	School readiness or performance Allowance	
	Hct			Able to brush own teeth Safety Responsible for money Obedience/discipline Need for praise Sex education Sleep (11-12 hr) Swimming	

Continued.

Table 24-13. Health surveillance chart: birth to 21 years—cont'd

Age	History	Approach to client	Order of examination	Physical examination
8 yr				
10 yr		May not need to have parent present Modest but wants to participate Needs to be informed about methods and procedures of examination	Same order as the adult examination; genitalia and rectum examined last.	
12 yr				Genital development BP
13-15 yr	General health Peer relationships Menarche or seminal emission Problems/concerns			Complete BP
16-21 yr	General health Peer relationship Pap smear Problem/concerns			BP

and knowledge level of a child. In a child of this age, more specific examination is possible, including auditory testing, funduscopic examination, and stereogenesis testing. Assessment can be expanded to observe the quantity and quality of spontaneous voluntary motor activity, the ease in performing voluntary movements, lateral dominance, spontaneous drawing, articulation of sounds, and language acquisition. Also, the examiner notes the child's auditory discrimination, memory, and reading, speech, and calculation skills. Lastly, the child can be tested for awareness of his body parts, spatial orientation and emotional lability.

In a child of any age, if the examiner suspects meningeal irritation during an illness episode, he is to note the presence of paradoxical irritability, Kernig's, and/or Brudzinski's signs. In paradoxical irritability, the child is not easily comforted when held by his parent, contrary to his usual behavior. To elicit Kernig's sign, the examiner has the child lie on the table, face up, with the thigh bent at the knee. The examiner then attempts to extend the hip by raising the knee. If pain and resistance are encountered the maneuver is positive for meningeal irritation. Brudzinski's sign is obtained by having the child lie supine on a table, and the examiner proceeds to gently bend the neck. If the child's knees flex spontaneously, this sign is positive.

Babinski's reflex is normally present in the newborn and disappears by the age of 12 to 24 months.

The overall development of motor skills, communication skills, and behavior is evaluated by obtaining a developmental history and by observing the child's behavior. Comparison of the child's development with the expected development for his age may be accomplished by utilizing developmental charts that

Auditory-visual	Laboratory	Developmental landmarks	Nutrition	Anticipatory guidance	Immunization/ other
Vision test Audiogram	Urine culture (female)		Smoking Drugs	Peer relationships increasingly more important	
Vision test	Hct			Same as for 7-8 yr Prepare child for puberty and body changes	
Vision test	Hct U/A Rubella serology (nonvac- cinated fe- male)			Smoking Drug abuse Hygiene, skin care Breast self-examina- tion Sleep (10 hr)	TBC (Rubella vac- cine if not immunized or titer negative and not pregnant)
Vision test	U/A		Need for calories Adequate calcium intake	Venereal disease (VD) Drugs Pap smear Accidents/injuries Sports Adequate rest/sleep Sexuality	Diphtheria tetanus (DT)
Vision test	Hct		Need for calories Adequate calcium intake	VD Drugs Pap smear Accidents/injuries Sports	

provide information about the range of ages in which specific developmental abilities are expected to occur.

SUMMARY

The organization of the examination and the approach to the child need to be modified at different ages and stages of development. The following brief Table 24-13 describes some of the adaptations that can be made when examining children. It also lists the recommended times to elicit specific aspects of the history, to perform selected parts of the physical examination, to order laboratory studies, to consider topics for anticipatory guidance, and to plan for the administration of immunizations.

BIBLIOGRAPHY

American Academy of Pediatrics: Standards of child health care, ed. 3, Evanston, Illinois, 1977.

Asher, M.: Orthopedic screening, Pediatr. Clin. North Am. 24(4):713, 1977.

Barich, D.: Approach to the physical examination of the pediatric client. Personal notes of lecture given in Cleveland, Ohio, 1971.

Block, S.: Juvenile rheumatoid arthritis, Nurs. Dig. Summer, 1976, p. 50.

Breckenridge, M., and Vincent, L.: What are some of the laws that govern growth? In Haimowitz, M., and Haimowitz, N. editors: Human development, ed. 2, New York, 1966, Thomas Crowell Co.

Capraro, V.: Gynecologic examination in children and adolescents, Pediatr. Clin. North Am. 19(3):511, 1972.

Chinn, P., and Leitch, C.: Child health maintenance, a guide to clinical assessment, St. Louis, 1974, The C. V. Mosby Co.

Clarren, S., and Smith, D.: Congenital deformities, Pediatr. Clin. North Am. 24(4):665, 1977.

Collins, H. R.: Epiphyseal injuries in athletes, Cleve. Clin. Q. 42(4):285, 1975.

Committee on Nutrition: Iron supplementation for infants, Pediatrics 58(5):765, 1976.

DeHaven, K.: Elbow problems in the adolescent athlete, Cleve. Clin. Q. 42(4):297, 1975.

Filer, L. J., editor: Infant nutrition, a foundation for lasting health? Part One, Bloomfield, New Jersey, 1977, Health Learning Systems, Inc.

Fomon, S.: Infant nutrition, ed. 3, Philadelphia, 1974, W. B. Saunders Co.

Haddock, N.: Blood pressure monitoring in neonates, Matern.-Child Nurs. J. **5:**131, 1980.

Hamill, P. and Moore, W., editors: Growth charting in the U.S., Pediatr. Nurs. Currents **23**(5):17, 1976.

Hoole, A., editor: Patient care guidelines for family nurse practitioners, Boston, 1976, Little, Brown & Co.

Jones, K.: The unstable knee of the young athlete, J. Arkansas Medic. Soc. **72**(11):461, 1976.

Kempe, C. H., and others: Current pediatric diagnosis and treatment, ed. 5, Los Altos, California, 1978, Lange Medical Publications.

Levin, R.: Teratogenicity and drug excretion in breast milk (maternogenicity). In Herfindal, E. T., and Hirschman, J., editors: Clinical pharmacy and therapeutics, Baltimore, 1975, The Williams & Wilkins Co.

Lowrey, G. H.: Growth and development of children, Chicago, 1978, Year Book Medical Publishers, Inc.

Mayo Clinic and Foundation: Clinical examinations in neurology, ed. 4, Philadelphia, 1976, W. B. Saunders Co.

Nichols, G. A.: Taking adult temperatures; rectal measurement, Am. J. Nurs. **72:**1092, 1972.

Nichols, G. A., and Kucha, D. H.: Taking adult temperatures, oral measurements, Am. J. Nurs. **72:**1090, 1972.

Owen, G.: The assessment and recording of measurements of growth of children, Pediatrics **51**(3):461, 1973.

Reid, U. V.: Screening for adolescent idiopathic scoliosis, Can. Nurse, November, 1975, p. 13.

Swanger, R.: Common problems of toddlers and preschoolers. Personal notes of lecture, 1972.

Tibbits, C.: Adolescent idiopathic scoliosis, Nurse Pract. March-April, 1980, p. 11.

U.S. Department of Health, Education and Welfare: Screening children for nutritional status, Washington, D.C., 1971, U.S. Government Printing Office.

U.S. Department of Health, Education and Welfare: Comparison of body weights and lengths or heights of groups of children, Atlanta, Georgia, 1974, Center for Disease Control.

Valadian, I., and Porter, D.: Assessing physical growth and development, Boston, 1977, Little, Brown & Co.

25 Assessment of the aging client

THE INTERVIEW AND HEALTH HISTORY

The social use of the age 65 as the demarcation point between middle age and old age had its origin in Bismarck's laws. This is the time designated for retirement from work and for the eligibility for funds and services designated for the aged. Gerontologists have classified old age into two groups:

1. *Early old age or later maturity:* 65 to 74
2. *Advanced old age:* 75 and older

Although the use of specific years has been useful for governmental and social agency purposes, it has served to prejudice the public as well as health personnel, so that all the changes attributable to the aged, both ill and well, are expected to be present in each aged client.

The life expectancy has not changed significantly in the United States over the past 20 years. The following figures reflect the life expectancy of children born in 1970:

Race	Men	Women
White	67.5	74.9
Black	60.1	67.5

Both black and white women outlive their respective male counterparts, so that women make up more than 55% of the elderly population. There are five times as many widows as widowers over age 65. The total number of elderly persons in the United States was estimated to be 20 million in 1970; this figure represents 10% of the total population. It is believed that at least 60% of all hospitalized people are elderly.

The number of elderly individuals in the United States is increasing. Medicare and other health care insurance plans have enabled older persons to obtain more health care. However, the majority of health care provided older persons is curative rather than preventive.

Two general thoughts should be borne in mind by the practitioner in examining the older individual. On the one hand, advancing years are not necessarily equated with disease. Thus, the practitioner should not expect all older clients to be ill. On the other hand, when one problem is identified, others must be suspected, since multiple disease is the primary characteristic of health problems in the elderly. In addition, the differentiation of the client's major problem may be complicated by decreases of acuity in the sensory processes, so that clearly defined symptoms may not be reported.

Although a representative of the U.S. Census Bureau has declared that the majority of the elderly in the United States are poor, uneducated, and generally unemployed, it is important to remember that many clients are educated and gainfully employed. A 1975 study showed that only 2% of white people had no formal schooling and 19% had 1 to 7 years. Among black persons, 12% had no schooling and 50% had 1 to 7 years.

The usual age for retirement in the United States is 62 years (and even younger in dangerous occupations), but it has been shown that 42% of individuals between 70 and 74 years of age and 19% of those between 75 and 79 years of age are still working for pay. Often, however, forced retirement means retirement from a valued job to a less satisfying form of work, such as caretaker or watchman, which this society values little and therefore allots to the elderly.

For those not working, retirement may be fraught with financial worries, particularly if the client has been stretching his income to the limit during his working years or for other reasons has been unable to establish any savings. Thus, one of the problems of the elderly in the United States (except those 70 or older) is earning money to meet the costs of living without jeopardizing their qualifications for Social Security benefits. Most of the cost-of-living estimates indicate that governmental support to the elderly is not sufficient for total support. Few states have enacted legislation that will allow the elderly the option of seeking work without risking the loss of Social Security payments. The elderly constitute 13% of the nation's poor.

Although the more affluent may not experience the problems related to the curtailment of monetary supply, they may experience an even more universal feeling. This is the feeling of loss or demoralization associated with aging. This society has devalued the elderly by making them ineligible for many highly valued activities that are reserved for younger members. The aging person is considered appropriate for menial, boring, and low-paying jobs. In addition, the elderly are frequently rejected in a real or imagined sense by younger relatives and acquaintances.

The presence of emotional illness has been estimated to be as high as 20% in the otherwise well population over 65 years of age and 40% in those with physical illness. Thus, particularly in assessment of the elderly, consideration must be given to both the psychological and the social, as well as the physical, aspects of the client's development. One must also bear in mind that a problem associated with one of these functional areas may well lead to a disturbance in one or both of the other two.

Taking the health history

Although the objective of obtaining as much relevant information about the client and his problems as possible is valid for the elderly as well as for other age groups, techniques for obtaining more information may need to be adapted to compensate for aging changes. In addition, in interpreting the relationship to problems, the examiner may need to weigh the information regarding symptoms that are unique to these clients. For instance, it has been shown that the elderly complain less of pain than do younger adults with a similar disease. For example, some aging clients may sense biliary colic as a dull ache. Since the aged complain less of pain in general, the complaint of pain may be less characteristic of a symptom complex.

It may be necessary to devote a good deal more time and patience in order to get an adequate history from the aging client. Difficulties in obtaining information may relate to sensory loss, since sensory losses in both reception and perception are particularly prevalent in the aging client.

The loss of auditory acuity is the most common sensory loss among aging individuals and may seriously impede history taking. It has been reported that nearly one-third of the population 65 years of age or older has substantial bilateral hearing loss. This loss is often associated with personality changes that may further complicate the history-taking process. Hearing loss has been shown to be associated with suspiciousness and irritability. Communication techniques that are used with the partially deaf client should include a commonly accepted vocabulary and simple, direct questions. The examiner should face the client so that the client can clearly see the lips and eyes. In cases of extreme hearing loss, electronic amplifying equipment or even an old-fashioned speaking tube may be used. Since shouting obscures the consonants and only amplifies vowels, this process should be avoided with the client who has hearing loss. In instances where the client is totally deaf, it may be necessary to communicate entirely in writing. When the interview has to be conducted in writing, only the most pertinent questions should be asked, since this process is quite exhausting for the majority of such clients. It may be wiser to identify only that a symptom exists at the first interview and to establish other clues, such as how long and how much, at a subsequent interview.

Vision perception diminishes from the middle years onward. One of the changes that can be seen during the interview is a change in pupil size. The reduction in pupil size limits the amount of light that reaches the retina. The client may appear to have slow adaptation and a degree of blindness. These changes may be compensated by increasing the illumination without glare and by utilizing color contrast. The client's ability to follow directions may be markedly increased by using color contrast in the furniture and walls of the room. "Sit on the yellow chair" may be an easier task than "Sit on the middle chair." If written interview forms are utilized, a high-wattage lamp, placed so that the light is reflected onto the page and not the client's eyes, may improve the responses that the client can make. Since light-dark adaptation occurs more slowly, the level of general illumination in examining rooms should be the same level of brightness. Differences in intensity of lighting should be avoided. Floor and table lamps should not be used; these frequently appear as spots of bright light surrounded by dark or dim spaces and are confusing to the individual with slow visual adaptation.

As previously mentioned, a sensory loss that makes the history taking of the elderly client difficult is the apparent decrease in the perception of pain. In the laboratory the aging client perceives and responds to cutaneous and visual pain-producing stimuli to a lesser degree than the healthy young adult. A more intense stimulus is required to evoke a response in the older client. Further evidence of sensory loss with aging is the lessening of hypersensitivity reactions. Thus, the aging client may not report symptoms attested to by younger individuals in the early stages of some illnesses.

Laboratory testing has shown that there is a loss of tactile perception that accompanies aging. Thus, "I don't know why I fell" may mean that the client did not feel the object under the sole of his foot that caused him to trip. Furthermore, his loss of visual acuity may have made the object difficult to see.

One of the common fallacies of thinking that must be avoided by the examiner of aging clients is that general intelligence declines as a function of advancing years. Although some of the older correlation studies would seem to support this conclusion, more recent, controlled studies deny this phenomenon. Studies performed on individuals at various time intervals in their lives (using them as their own controls) have shown an increase in intelligence test scores that continued to 55 or 60 years of age. Furthermore, there is little evidence to support the fact that a decline of intelligence occurs even after age 60 unless systemic or neurological disorders are superimposed. Impaired oxygen delivery to central nervous system (CNS) structures, such as that which accompanies decreased cerebral blood perfusion, is cited as the major cause of intellectual deterioration. Thus, the examiner should interact with the aging client with respect for both the intelligence and the experience the client's years have granted him.

Although the general intelligence has been shown to remain intact, there may be an uneven decline in some of those intellectual skills thought to comprise intelligence. Problem-solving skills involving numerical manipulation, analogies, block design, and number series suffer loss starting in early adult years. However, this may be a disuse phenomenon; if so, it should be less likely to be found in individuals using these skills in their careers, such as engineers, who would constantly challenge their mathematical skills. Vocabulary skills and inventories of available information show little change from early adulthood through the aging years. For some aged clients memory appears to be less efficient for recent events than for those of the distant past. This failure to relate events in the immediate past has also been correlated with the physical health of the client; the older person in good health has much less of a deficit.

As with any individual, learning that involves the unlearning of previously held information is the most difficult type of learning for the older client. By virtue of his greater number of learning years, the client may have a good deal to unlearn during the acquisition of most new information. Thus, difficulties for the aging person in learning new tasks may be understood.

When disorders of memory or learning ability are apparent, the examiner should be alert to the necessity of repeating questions, instructions, and explanations. Directions should be given in simple phrases and in words familiar to the older client.

Should the client be confused or intellectually impaired, it may be necessary to obtain the history from a relative or an individual who has spent a good deal of time with the client. The testimony of persons who have been with the client at home may be particularly valuable in answering questions concerning changes in behavior or symptoms that the client may have identified prior to this assessment. Such a question might be "Has he complained of 'stomach' pain to you?"

Previous medical records should be sought to provide evidence concerning the duration of current symptoms and signs since particularly recent symptoms may not be remembered.

Although the family history is important, the hereditary diseases deserve less attention in the elderly client since genetic diseases are usually diagnosed at an earlier age. An exception to this might be diabetes mellitus. One of the major values of the family history is that it may yield clues concerning the support systems of the client.

Pharmaceutical history

It is particularly important to assess the medicines prescribed for the older client and those nonprescription medicines he is ingesting at his own discretion. In addition to a careful drug history taken at the initial interview, a periodic review of drug intake is important to the care of the elderly client.

Many of the drugs frequently prescribed for common medical problems pose a greater danger to the aged client than to the younger adult. Mucosal irritation and bleeding of the gastrointestinal tract caused by aspirin, digitalis intoxication, bizarre or hypersensitive reactions to barbiturates, bleeding phenomena as a result of heparin, potassium depletion resulting from diuretics, and extrapyramidal symptoms resulting from phenothiazine and phenylbutazone toxicity are known to have a higher incidence in older adults. The changes in reaction to drugs may be caused by diminished CNS function, altered metabolism, and a reduction in elimination of drugs as a result of the functional decline of both the liver and the kidney.

Frequently, iatrogenic illness is not identified, because practitioners do not recognize symptoms as drug induced since they are a part of the stereotype of old age: slowed reaction time, confusion, disorientation, loss of memory, tremors, loss of appetite, noncompliant behavior, or anxiety.

Chronic laxative abuse is frequently seen in the elderly and may explain symptoms of potassium deficiency or general malnourishment. Tranquilizers and sleeping medications are also recognized as being frequently used by the elderly.

Just as important as the drugs that are being used are those that have been ordered by a physician and not taken. Some clients do not fill prescriptions. Others stop taking medicine because they feel better. The examiner may ask to see the containers of all drugs that are currently being taken and advise the client to bring all of his medicine with him on future visits so that the examiner may see them first-hand. This will allow the practitioner to count the pills remaining and to calculate whether they are being taken as prescribed. This may also obviate confusion from descriptions such as, "It is a little yellow one with a mark in the middle."

PHYSICAL APPRAISAL

The approach to the physical examination in the elderly is essentially identical to that performed on a client of any age. The client should be allowed to establish his own pace. The examiner may need to allow more time for response to requests such as a change of position. The examiner should note evidence of muscle weakness or lack of coordination in order to give assistance to the client when he needs help in moving or turning.

Patience is the most helpful asset in dealing with the elderly. Valuable information may be lost because the practitioner did not wait to see the full range of response to a test. A hurried and annoyed manner of dealing with the elderly client may cause him to retreat or make minimal attempts to comply with procedures.

The following review of examinations includes only those parameters that may differ in the aged client as compared to the younger adult.

General inspection

The elderly client may measure 1.5 cm or more shorter than when he was young. This change is attributed to the thinning of cartilages between bones.

Longitudinal studies have shown a steady loss in weight in men past age 65. However, the majority of women show a tendency toward progressive weight gain. With weight loss, contours appear sharper and hollows are deeper, especially the orbits and axillae. Muscles appear more prominent.

Because cartilage continues to be laid down in old age, the ears and nose of the elderly client may be larger and appear more prominent in relation to the face.

Wrinkling and relaxation (sagging) of the skin are recognized as signs of the aging process, as is the loss of pigmentation and thinning of the hair.

Histological changes correlated with aging

A gradual loss of cells has been documented in the aging individual. The cells that decline with age are the postmitotic cells, those that are incapable of reproduction. The cells most affected are neurons and muscle cells. Cells also accumulate pigment in storage granules of the cytoplasm with aging.

Decreased and distorted mitochondria, chromosomal fragmentation, and collagen changes have also been observed in the elderly client. An increase in collagen and cross-linking of collagen fibers is common in aging tissues. The increased density of the extracellular matrix may impair diffusion. Elastin fragments and calcifies with aging. Both of these connective tissue changes lead to a reduction in elasticity of body tissue.

Areas of assessment
METABOLISM

The physiology of the healthy aged individual is essentially the same as that of the younger adult. However, the response to stressful stimuli occurs at a slower rate in the older person, such as the slower return of normal pH in the person challenged with an oral dose of sodium bicarbonate.

The metabolic rate declines with age, and the thyroid gland has been shown to undergo a reduction in cell size and function. The rate of thyroxin metabolism also declines with age. Glucose clearance time—the reflection of insulin secretion in response to stimulation of the beta cells—is lengthened in the aged. One estimate is that one-half of the elderly population has at least minimal diabetes; that is, the response to glucose stimulation of the beta cells to produce insulin is impaired. It has been suggested that impaired glucose clearance may be related to elevated levels of insulin antagonists in the elderly client.

EYES

The lacrimal glands decrease in tear production with aging, so that the eyes may appear dry and lusterless. Other eye changes may include arcus senilis, scleral discolorations, and diminution of pupil size. Arcus senilis is the accumulation of a lipid substance on the cornea. It characteristically appears as a grayish arc or complete circle almost at the edge of the cornea. It may be seen as a dotlike accumulation even in those individuals in their 20s or 30s. As more of the lipid is deposited, the cornea may be completely infiltrated, thickened, and even raised in appearance. The iris may frequently have pale brown discolorations. This condition occurs earlier in persons with hyperlipidemia.

Loss of elasticity and transparency of the lens causes vision changes, requiring many aging individuals to wear corrective lenses. Normal changes in the eye may predicate changes in the eyeglasses every 3 to 5 years. The examiner should assess visual acuity with the client wearing his glasses and determine how long the client has had them.

Peripheral vision is diminished in the aged. In addition, the cornea tends to cloud with age. There is a decrease in the rate of dark adaptation. Sclerotic changes in the iris result in a small and somewhat fixed pupil. An elevation in the threshold for visible light perception has been noted, along with a loss of visual acuity in dim lighting. The elderly are also less able to perceive purple colors.

Glaucoma and cataracts are other problems frequently associated with aging. Surgical removal of the cataract followed by ocular correction will obviate the loss of vision.

The ophthalmoscopic examination reveals mildly narrowed vessels, granular pigment in the macula, drusen in the posterior pole, and a loss of bright macular and foveal reflexes.

EARS

Hearing loss in the elderly is most frequently the result of presbycusis or otosclerosis. *Presbycusis* is the loss in perception of auditory stimuli that accompanies degenerative changes of the neural structures of the inner ear or the auditory nerve, or both. The first symptom is the loss of high-frequency tones. Threshold increases for auditory perception at all frequencies for pure tone.

Otosclerosis is a common condition of the otic capsule in which abnormally excessive bone cells are deposited. This generally results in fixation of the footplate of the stapes in the oval window; occasionally, however, the otosclerotic process may affect the cochlea, resulting in a neural deafness.

NOSE

The sense of smell is markedly diminished in the older adult because of a decrease of olfactory nerve fibers and atrophy of the remaining fibers.

MOUTH

Atrophy of the papillae of the lateral edges of the tongue is common in persons past age 45. One of the indications of loss of taste perception is that the elderly need to be exposed to three times the concentration of sugar needed by younger clients to sense sweetness.

Most clients of age 65 or greater are edentulous. If teeth are still present, they are generally diseased. Salivary glands are known to atrophy as well, so that the mucosal surfaces of the mouth are drier.

BREASTS

The amount of fat in the breasts increases in most women, whereas glandular tissues atrophy. As a rule, the general size remains the same. However, the breasts change in consistency and shape and are often described as pendulous (elongated) or flaccid. Because of the diminution of connective tissue, the presence of breast lesions is detected earlier than in the

Table 25-1. Visual changes in the elderly

Visual function	Changes with aging
Lens transparency	Decreased
Acuity	Decreased
Accommodation to far object	Improved
Accommodation to near object	Decreased
Astigmatism	Corneal shape more spherical
Adaptation (light to dark)	Reduced
Color vision	Decreased; pastels discriminated less readily; color blindness worse
Flicker adaptation	Decreased
Peripheral vision	Decreased
Pupillary response	Decreased response to light changes; pupil smaller
Intraocular fluid reabsorption	Decreased; glaucoma more likely

younger adult. The detection of a lump in the elderly woman is of greater significance because cystic mastitis is not common past the menopausal years.

RESPIRATORY SYSTEM

There is an advancing kyphosis with aging associated with changes in cartilage, osteoporosis, and vertebral collapse. There may be calcification of the vertebral cartilages, resulting in reduced mobility of the ribs and partial contraction of the intercostal muscles. Thus, the chest wall is less compliant and the strength of muscle contraction is diminished.

The intraalveolar septi degenerate with aging, resulting in coalesced or large alveoli and widening of the alveolar ducts and bronchioles. Loss of compliance of the lung also occurs.

Tracheal deviation in the elderly may be the result of upper dorsal scoliosis. Changes in calcium metabolism may result in an increase in the anteroposterior diameter of the chest.

Maximum breathing capacity, forced vital capacity, vital capacity, and inspiratory reserve volume are known to decline with age, while functional residual capacity increases. The breaths taken by the elderly client are not as deep as those taken by the younger client, and the older client may complain of discomfort if asked to breathe more deeply. Furthermore, there is a loss of diffusion capacity, or the passage of oxygen from the environment into the pulmonary capillaries and of carbon dioxide from the pulmonary capillaries to the external side of the alveolus. For identical pulmonary blood flow rates, the client of 80 years of age gets one-third as much oxygen into his cardiovascular system as a 20-year-old.

As with the younger adult, nocturnal dyspnea and orthopnea may suggest a cardiovascular origin. The elderly client with cardiac disease more frequently presents a chief complaint of fatigue than of shortness of breath. The elderly client with known respiratory disease who has marked fatigue that has been present for only a short time is frequently found to be suffering an acute respiratory system infectious process. Cough is the most frequent symptom of pulmonary congestion.

The elderly client's complaints of chest pain may sound less severe than those described by the younger individual for both pleural and cardiac problems.

CARDIOVASCULAR SYSTEM

The resting heart rate and stroke volume at maximum load decline in the elderly, along with the cardiac output. The heart rate returns to the resting state more slowly following a challenge in the elderly. The heart also becomes less distensible as collagen increases.

Areas of fibrosis and lipofuchsin deposits in the myocardial cells have been noted. Sclerosis of the coronary vessels occurs as a result of fibrosis of the media and elastocalcinosis. The ECG reveals a decrease in the amplitude of the QRS complex as well as lengthening of the P-R, QRS, and Q-T intervals.

The effective strength of blood vessels is decreased as connective tissue replaces smooth muscle cells, and fibroconnective tissue deposits have been observed. Elasticity is also decreased as elastic fibers fragment. The proximal arteries tend to thin and dilate as aging progresses, whereas the peripheral arterial walls become thicker and dilate less readily. The occurrence of varicose veins is more frequent in elderly clients. Baroreceptor sensitivity is known to be blunted with age.

The older individual's response to maximal exercise is not as great as that of the younger adult for either cardiac output or heart rate. Both contraction and relaxation rates of cardiac muscle are prolonged. The older person develops a greater increase in systolic blood pressure than does a young adult performing the same amount of physical work. Cardiac valves stiffen and hypertrophy with age.

Kyphoscoliosis, frequently seen in the aging individual, may cause a downward dislocation of the cardiac apex, so that its location loses diagnostic significance.

The National High Blood Pressure Coordinating Committee (September, 1979) reaffirmed the validity of the indirect method of blood pressure recording in the elderly in spite of sclerotic changes of the vessel wall and indicated systolic measurements 160 mm Hg and diastolic 95 mm Hg as the pressures at which drug treatment should begin. The committee estimated that more than 40% of the individuals over age 65 are hypertensive.

Dizziness, blackouts, or syncope seen in the elderly may be the result of marked aortic stenosis but may also result from impairment of carotid flow. Fainting also occurs when cardiac output is not increased in response to exertion and also with marked vasodilatation of skeletal muscle beds.

Many elderly clients have ectopic heartbeats, which may be innocuous, but those that are not must be identified.

Data from phonocardiographic studies show that murmurs are present in 60% or more of aging clients. The most common is a soft systolic ejection murmur heard at the base of the heart as a result of sclerotic changes at the bases of the cusps of the aortic valve.

Whereas in the younger individual there are often typical symptoms related to heart attack, such as heavy, squeezing pressure on the sternum radiating to the neck, back, or arm, the descriptions given by the elderly client may be indefinite. This may be the result of changes in perception or the sensory nerve endings and fibers being altered in such a way that the intensity of signals reaching the brain is diminished. This decrease in reporting of pain sensation has a higher incidence in the client with diabetes mellitus. These individuals frequently report no experience of pain at the time of myocardial infarction.

Although there is an overall increase in incidence of heart disease with advancing age, there are no heart diseases that are peculiar to old age.

Tricuspid stenosis is generally found in marked rheumatic heart disease and therefore is seldom seen in the elderly, since the victims generally succumb in middle age. Thus, the practitioner need devote less attention to ruling out this phenomenon.

Pulses. The artery is felt more readily in the elderly because of a loss of adjacent connective tissue and increased hardness of the arteries due to arteriosclerosis and atherosclerosis. The vessels may be more tortuous as well, because vessels become longer with age and are anchored at fixed points; thus lengthening results in folding or kinking. The increased rigidity is the result of a deposit of fatty material (arteriosclerotic plaque) in the intimal part of the artery and of calcification of the middle layer.

ABDOMEN

Examination of the abdominal structures may be accomplished more easily in the nonobese client than in the fat or heavily muscled client. Since there is a general loss of fibroconnective tissue as well as muscle wasting in the elderly, the abdominal wall of the elderly client will be slacker and thinner, making palpation simpler and ostensibly more accurate than in the younger client.

Abdominal wall rigidity is not as common a sign

of peritoneal irritation in the elderly client as it is in the younger individual.

In an acute abdominal emergency, the elderly client generally complains less of discomfort than would the younger person with a similar condition.

Gastrointestinal function. Salivation and gastric acid secretion have been shown to decline with advancing age. Decreases in the production of both hydrochloric acid and pepsin as well as in digestive enzymes of the pancreas (amylase, lipase, trypsin) have been measured and may explain the elderly client's complaints of anorexia and difficulty in digesting meals.

Constipation is also a frequent complaint. However, although a decline in the motility of the gastrointestinal tract has been proved to occur with advancing years, it has been shown that 90% of individuals over 60 years of age have at least one bowel movement a day.

GENITOURINARY SYSTEM

Because of the decreased cardiac output, blood flow to the kidney and glomerular filtration rate are markedly diminished in the aged, leading to a loss of kidney function.

The two most common signs of genitourinary dysfunction in the elderly are nocturnal frequency of micturition and incontinence of urine.

In addition to the frequency of urination, the volume passed during each episode should be investigated. Small amounts of urine passed frequently may be the result of a mucosal irritation caused by inflammation or trauma. Large volumes of urine passed frequently may be the result of chronic renal failure or poorly regulated diabetes mellitus. The client should be questioned as to the exact amount of fluid he ingests. In addition, he should be asked if he is taking a diuretic and, if so, the time he takes it.

In the elderly male client frequency of micturition accompanied by problems in initiating and ending the stream is generally the result of prostatic enlargement with urinary retention.

Relaxation of the perineal muscles in the elderly female client leads to stress incontinence.

REPRODUCTIVE STATUS

Female client. Since the cells of the reproductive tract and the breasts are estrogen-dependent, both for growth and for function, the decline of estrogen production starting at menopause is responsible for many changes observed in these tissues in elderly female clients.

The uterus is diminished in size because of a loss of myometrial fibers; the uterine mucosa is normally thin and atrophic and is rarely secretory. The cervix is also decreased in size, and the cervical mucus is less than during the reproductive years. When the mucus is examined, it is seen to be thick and cellular. The fern test is negative. The vagina of the elderly client is observed to be narrower and shorter because of an increase in the amount of the submucosal connective tissue. The vaginal epithelium atrophies, and the surface appears thin and pale. Because of the fragility of the mucosa, special attention should be devoted to observing for erosion, ulcerations, and adhesions. Furthermore, as estrogen deficiency becomes marked, the glycogen content and acidity of the vaginal mucus decline, allowing pathogenic organisms to replace the normally protective Döderlein's bacilli. Thus, the examiner should be alert to the presence of vaginitis. Dyspareunia is a common symptom of the loss of vaginal epithelium and associated changes in mucus.

It is considered inadvisable to routinely administer

Table 25-2. Changes noted in the four phases of intercourse in the aging female client

Phase	Alteration
Excitement	Delay in production of vaginal secretion and lubrication
Plateau	Reduction in expansion, both length and width, of vagina
	Uterus does not elevate into false pelvis as much as in younger women
	Labia majora flaccid—do not elevate and flatten against perineum
	Labia minor does not undergo sex color change from pink to burgundy or become congested
	Clitoral size decreases after 60 years of age
Orgasmic	Shorter than in younger women
Resolution	Occurs more rapidly

Table 25-3. Changes noted in the four phases of intercourse in the aging male client

Phase	Alteration
Excitement	Slower increment in excitement; sex flush less in duration and intensity; involuntary spasms diminished; longer time required to obtain erection; less testicular elevation and scrotal sac vasocongestion in erection
Plateau	Longer duration; increase in penile diameter since less preejaculatory fluid emission
Orgasmic	Shorter duration; fewer contractions in expulsion of semen bolus
Resolution (refractory)	Lasts 12 to 24 hours as compared to 2 minutes in the youthful client; loss of erection (return of penis to flaccid state) may take a few seconds as compared to minutes or hours in the youthful client

estrogen to postmenopausal women to prevent the atrophic and functional changes of the reproductive tissues. Estrogen and progesterone are administered on the basis of the client's need as determined by blood assay. The practitioner must assess the client who is medicated with estrogen to determine the effect of the hormone and the presence of side effects. The client should be examined for the presence of uterine bleeding, mastalgia, weight gain, fluid retention, hypertension, and neoplasm, all of which have been implicated in long-term estrogen therapy.

Male client. Although the decline of testosterone production in the male client occurs at a later time in life than that of estrogen in the female client, clinically observable signs and symptoms do accompany the decline in production of this reproductive hormone.

The client may report a decline in sexual energy. During the act of intercourse, physiological reactions are less intense and reactions are slowed.

There is a gradual decline in strength of the muscles associated with the act of intercourse. The testes decrease in size and are less firm on palpation. Histologically, there is an increase in connective tissue in the tubules, so that they are thickened. The result of this degenerative change is a decrease in production of spermatozoa. The prostate gland is increased in size, and secretion is impaired. The seminal fluid is reduced in amount and viscosity.

These changes do not necessarily mean a decrease in libido or a loss in the sense of satisfaction from the sex act. A frequency of intercourse of one or two times per week in most men over 60 has been reported.

MUSCULOSKELETAL SYSTEM

Although muscle mass is known to decline progressively with age, loss of strength is not necessarily the result. The practitioner may use the opportunity afforded by the examination session to determine if the aging client is exercising all of his muscles. The client is queried concerning his planned exercise or calisthenics, movements during recreation, and the amount of activity experienced through his work. If the client is a housewife, it is important to find out just how much physical activity is actually involved in her particular housecleaning; the number of rooms and floors in her home (determining the extent of stair climbing) plus the thoroughness with which cleaning is done provide a wide range of exercise commitment. Remedial exercise may be advised if deficits are identified.

Osteoarthritic changes in the joints are almost universally observed in the elderly. The changes are of such a general nature that some roentgenologists claim to be able to estimate the age of individuals past 40 years of age through examination of roentgenograms of the cervical spine. Proliferative changes in the spine cause protrusion and lipping of the vertebrae. These bony overgrowths are called osteophytes. Osteoarthritic bony overgrowths involving the distal finger joints are termed Heberden's nodes. Bouchard's nodes are overgrowths involving the proximal joints.

A nodular thickening of the palmar fascia may be associated with the contraction deformity of the lateral fingers, so that full extension is impossible. A higher incidence of this contraction, called Dupuytren's contraction, is observed more in clients with diabetes than those without. The overall occurrence in the elderly population is 10%.

Kyphosis in the elderly client may be the first indication of osteoporosis, a type of pathophysiological condition characterized by increased mobilization of calcium from the bones. The client may complain of aches and pains along the vertebrae; this may also signal the presence of osteoporosis. Bone loss in women is approximately 25%, while the decrement in men is 12%.

SKIN

Skin changes are not necessarily associated with a specific period in the individual's life. Aging changes of the skin are influenced by many factors, such as heredity, enzymatic changes in the connective and epithelial tissues, endocrine alterations, and inadequate nutrition as a result of vascular changes. Excessive exposure to the sun and extremes of weather are known to accelerate the changes characteristic of aging.

The appearance of senile white skin has been described as wrinkled, dry, and inelastic. In many cases the skin takes on a yellowish hue and resembles parchment. Aging changes in black skin occur at a later age than in white skin.

Pruritus, or itching, is a common symptom of aging skin. The itching may be related to the drying of the aging skin, but the examiner must be alert to other symptoms and signs of systemic disease also associated with pruritus, such as liver disease, diabetes, kidney disease, and thyroid disorders.

A decrease in connective tissue, which becomes more marked with aging, is evident in examination of the skin. The skin appears thinner, particularly over the backs of the hands. Because of the loss of elastic fibers, the skin, when pinched between the examiner's thumb and finger, takes a good deal longer to return to its natural shape. Sebaceous and sweat glands are less active. Thus, the client may complain of "dry skin," particularly over the extremities where circulation is less effective. In addition, hair growth often becomes scanty or absent as the peripheral circulation is compromised. This is particularly evident over the dorsum of the feet and lower legs. Along with the general thinning of the hair that is characteristic of the aging phenomenon, the elderly suffer a loss of scalp hair. In women the hairs appear finer or sparser, or both. There is also a general thinning of pubic and axillary hair, while the hairs of the nostrils, ears, and eyebrows are coarser and bristlelike. Nails grow more slowly in the elderly.

In examination of the skin, the examiner should be particularly alert to the presence of ecchymoses, since the presence of a bruise may indicate a recent injury. The client may have forgotten the injury or may have been unaware of it because of the decrease in sensory perception.

Small, scarlet structures scattered over the skin, called senile telangiectasia, are noted to increase in number from the middle years onward.

Pigment may be deposited as melanotic freckles (lentigines), although overall the skin may be paler. Cells lose their capacity to spread out melanin. Vitiligo, areas of skin lacking pigment (melanocytes), may be localized or generalized in distribution; there is some tendency for this hypopigmentation to increase with age.

The presence of warts or hyperkeratosis consisting of raised pale, brown, or black epidermal overgrowth may be noted. These senile warts are generally located with their long axis following those of the client's skin creases. These are normal overgrowths and are not removed unless the client desires them excised for cosmetic reasons.

Cutaneous tags called acrochordons are a common skin change seen in the elderly. The lesions are soft, flesh colored, and pedunculated and vary in size from a pinhead to a pea. They are most commonly noted on the vertical and lateral surfaces of the neck and in the axillary area. The lesions have no clinical significance and can be ignored, unless the client frequently injures them with clothing or jewelry or if they are disturbing from a cosmetic point of view.

NEURAL SYSTEM

After age 50, brain cells decrease in number at a rate of about 1% per year. However, because of the immense number of reserve cells involved, no clinical signs may be observed.

A decrease in the number of interconnections between dendrites has been observed. Intracellular deposits of lipofuchsin are seen in storage granules, and senile plaques and neurofibrillary tangles are increasingly apparent with aging.

Autopsies of individuals who were assessed as hav-

ing normal behavior have shown extensive disease of neural structures. This finding has led to the conclusion that compensation to neurological disease is possible. It has been postulated that alternate tissues may be available for many functions. Thus, physical diagnostic procedures may not be sufficient to unmask all of the pathology that exists.

Conduction velocity in some nerves is known to decline with age. The startle response takes twice as long in some aged clients.

Position sense is impaired in many elderly clients. Since the tactile sense is known to be blunted, more intense clues may be used to test this sensory modality. The assessment of these sensory abilities is particularly important in effectively advising modifications of the client's living quarters to increase sensory input and to avoid serious accidents. Some suggestions to the client that may be helpful are (1) the use of very marked textural differences and (2) the use of color contrasts.

The aged need stronger signals (greater amplitude) to detect vibration; this is probably the result of decline of CNS function.

Although the response to deep tendon reflex testing is decreased or absent in some elderly clients, all of these reflexes may be elicited in the healthy elderly adult.

BIBLIOGRAPHY

Agate, J. N.: The practice of geriatric medicine, ed. 2, London, 1970, William Heinemann Medical Books Ltd.

Brocklehurst, J. C.: Textbook of geriatric medicine and gerontology, Edinburgh, 1973, Churchill Livingstone.

Buckley, E. C. III, and Dorsey, F. C.: The effect of aging on serum immunoglobulin concentrations, J. Immunol. **105:**964, 1970.

Busse, E. W., and Pfeiffer, E., editors: Behavior and adaptation in late life, Boston, 1969, Little, Brown and Co.

Butler, R. N., and Lewis, M.: Aging and mental health, ed. 2, St. Louis, 1977, The C. V. Mosby Co.

Caird, F. I., and Judge, T. G.: Assessment of the elderly patient, London, 1974, Pitman Publishing Ltd.

Hershey, D.: Life span and factors affecting it, Springfield, Ill., 1974, Charles C Thomas, Publisher.

Jones, H. E.: Trends in mental abilities, 1958, Institute of Child Welfare, University of California.

Owens, W. J.: Age and mental abilities; a second adult follow-up, J. Educ. Psychol. **67:**311, 1966.

National High Blood Pressure Coordinating Committee, Washington, D.C., September, 1979, U.S. Government Printing Office.

Post, F.: The clinical psychiatry of late life, Oxford, 1965, Pergamon Press Ltd.

Reichel, W., editor: Clinical aspects of aging, Baltimore, 1978, The Williams & Wilkins Co.

Rossman, I.: Clinical geriatrics, ed. 2, Philadelphia, 1979, J. B. Lippincott Co.

Shanas, E.: Health status of older people, Am. J. Public Health **64:**261, 1974.

Steinberg, F. U.: Cowdry's the care of the geriatric patient, ed. 5, St. Louis, 1976, The C. V. Mosby Co.

26 Integration of the physical assessment

This chapter contains a discussion of two issues relating to the complete physical assessment: the performance of an integrated, screening physical examination and the recording of the physical examination.

PERFORMANCE OF THE SCREENING PHYSICAL EXAMINATION

After practicing and acquiring proficiency in the performance of regional examinations, the student is recommended to develop a procedure for the performance of an integrated physical examination. In actual practice, the examiner will need to perform complete regional examinations, such as in acute care settings, as well as complete screening examinations, such as in health maintenance or screening situations.

In developing a personal routine for a complete examination, the student should consider factors of efficiency and client comfort. If procedures are performed systematically and efficiently, time is conserved and the examiner is less likely to forget a procedure or a part of the body than if the examination were performed haphazardly.

Clients who are ill or debilitated lose energy quickly. Developing a system of examination that requires the fewest number of position changes of clients will enhance acceptability and decrease the number of examinations that need to be deferred because of client intolerance.

The manner in which the examiner conducts the physical examination can enhance or destroy rapport developed during the history-taking interview. A disorganized examiner who leaves the room to obtain missing equipment, who runs around the bed several times in a short period, or who has the client changing positions frequently may lose the client's confidence.

The outline presented here is a suggested procedure for the performance of the physical examination. It is intended to be a guide for the beginning practitioner and is intended for use in practice sessions. In actual client care situations this outline may require adaption because of the client's age or disability or because of the examination protocols and priorities of the care agency.

The suggested procedure is organized in such a way as to avoid excessive movement of the client or examiner. Examination of body systems is integrated into the examination of body regions.

Outline for examination

I. *Client* is sitting on the bed or examination table, head and shoulders uncovered. *Examiner* is facing client (Fig. 26-1)
   A. Observe generally.
   B. Observe and palpate upper extremities.
      1. Examine skin (color, temperature, vascularity, lesions, hydration, turgor, texture, edema, masses), muscle mass, and skeletal configuration.
      2. Examine nails (color and condition).
   C. Assess pulses (apical and brachial).
   D. Measure blood pressure (both arms).
   E. Measure respiration.
   F. Examine head.
      1. Ask about deformities.
      2. Observe scalp and face.
      3. Palpate head and face.
      4. Palpate sinus area.
   G. Examine eyes.
      1. Measure visual acuity (cranial nerve [CN] II).
      2. Assess visual fields (CN II).
      3. Determine alignment of eyes (perform cover test and light reflex).
      4. Test extraocular movements (CN III, CN IV, CN VI).
      5. Observe eyebrows, eyelids, conjunctiva, cornea, sclera, iris, and lens.
      6. Palpate lacrimal organs.

7. Inspect pupillary responses.
8. Perform ophthalmoscopic examination of lens, media, and retina (CN II).
H. Examine ears.
   1. Inspect auricle.
   2. Palpate auricle.
   3. Perform otoscopic examination.
   4. Determine auditory acuity (CN VIII).
   5. Perform Weber and Rinne tests.
I. Examine nose.
   1. Determine patency of each nostril.
   2. Test for olfaction (CN I).
   3. Determine position of septum.
   4. Inspect mucosa, septum, and turbinates with nasal speculum.
J. Examine mouth and pharynx.
   1. Inspect lips, total buccal mucosa, teeth, gums, tongue, sublingual area, roof of the mouth, tonsillar area, and pharynx.
   2. Test glossopharyngeal nerve (CN IX) and vagus nerve (CN X) ("ah" and gag reflex).
   3. Test hypoglossal nerve (CN XII) (tongue movement).
   4. Test taste (CN VII).
K. Complete examination of cranial nerves and face.
   1. Test trigeminal nerve (CN V) (jaw clenching, lateral jaw movements, corneal reflex, pain, and light touch to face).

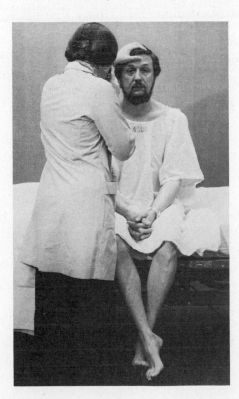

Fig. 26-1. Client seated, examiner facing client.

2. Test facial nerve (CN VII) (client raises eyebrows, shows teeth, puffs cheeks, keeps eyes closed against resistance).
3. Test spinal accessory nerve (CN XII) (trapezius and sternocleidomastoid muscles).
L. Palpate temporomandibular joint.
M. Observe range of motion of the head and neck.
N. Palpate nodes (preauricular, posterior auricular, occipital, tonsillar, submaxillary, submental, anterior cervical, posterior cervical, supraclavicular, and infraclavicular nodes).
O. Palpate carotid arteries.
P. Palpate thyroid gland.
Q. Palpate for position of trachea.
R. Auscultate carotid arteries and thyroid gland.

II. *Client* is sitting on the bed or examining table, total chest uncovered if male, breasts covered if female (Fig. 26-2). *Examiner* is standing behind client.
A. Examine back.
   1. Inspect spine.
   2. Palpate spine.
   3. Inspect skin and thoracic configuration.
   4. Palpate muscles and bones.
   5. Palpate costovertebral area, asking client about tenderness.
B. Examine lungs (apices and lateral and posterior areas). *Note:* Apical, posterior, and lateral lung regions can usually be examined from a position behind client.
   1. Observe respiration and total thorax.
   2. Palpate for thoracic expansion and tactile fremitus.
   3. Percuss systematically.
   4. Determine diaphragmatic excursion.
   5. Auscultate systematically.
   6. Auscultate for vocal fremitus.

III. *Client* is sitting on the bed or examining table, uncovered to the waist. *Examiner* is facing client (Fig. 26-3).
A. Examine breasts.
   1. Observe breasts with client's arms and hands at the side; above the head; and pressed into the hips, eliciting pectoral contraction.
   2. Observe breasts with client leaning forward.
   3. Ask client about lesions; if present, palpate them.
   4. If large breasts, perform a bimanual examination.

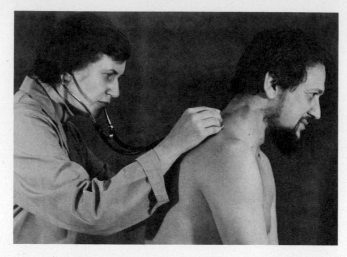

Fig. 26-2. Client seated, examiner behind client.

B. Palpate axillary nodes.
C. Examine lungs (anterior areas).
   1. Inspect configuration and skin.
   2. Palpate for tactile fremitus.
   3. Percuss lungs systematically.
   4. Auscultate lungs systematically.
D. Examine heart.
   1. Inspect precordium.
   2. Palpate precordium.
   3. Auscultate precordium.
   4. Observe external jugular vein and internal jugular pulsations.

IV. *Client* is supine. *Examiner* is at the right side of client (Fig. 26-4).
A. Examine breasts.
   1. Palpate breasts systematically.
   2. Attempt to express secretion from the nipples.
B. Examine heart.
   1. Inspect precordium.
   2. Palpate precordium.
   3. Auscultate precordium.
   4. Observe jugular venous pulses and pressures.
C. Measure blood pressure (both arms).
D. Examine abdomen.
   1. Inspect abdomen.
   2. Auscultate bowel sounds, aorta, renal arteries, and femoral arteries.
   3. Percuss liver and spleen systematically.
   4. Palpate liver, spleen, inguinal and femoral node and hernia areas, and femoral pulses systematically.
   5. Test abdominal reflexes.
E. Examine genitalia of male client.
   1. Inspect penis, uretheral opening, and scrotum.
   2. Palpate scrotal contents.

F. Examine lower extremities.
   1. Inspect skin, hair distribution, muscle mass, and skeletal configuration.
   2. Palpate for temperature, texture, edema, popliteal pulses, posterior tibial pulses, and dorsal pedal pulses.
   3. Test range of motion.
   4. Test strength.
   5. Test sensation (pain, light touch, and vibration).
   6. Test position sense.

V. *Client* is sitting on the bed or examining table. *Examiner* is standing in front of client (Fig. 26-5).
A. Assess neural system.
   1. Elicit deep tendon reflexes (biceps, triceps, brachioradialis, patellar, and Achilles reflexes).
   2. Test for Babinski's reflex.
   3. Test for coordination of upper and lower extremities.
B. Test upper extremities for strength, range of motion sensation, vibration, and position.

VI. *Female client* is in lithotomy position, genital area uncovered. *Examiner* is sitting, facing the genital area.
A. Examine genitalia.
   1. Inspect genitalia.
   2. Palpate external genital area.
   3. Perform speculum examination.
   4. Take smears and cultures.
   5. Perform bimanual vaginal examination.
B. Examine rectum: perform bimanual rectovaginal examination.

VII. *Client* is standing. *Examiner* is standing next to client (Fig. 26-6).
A. Examine spine.

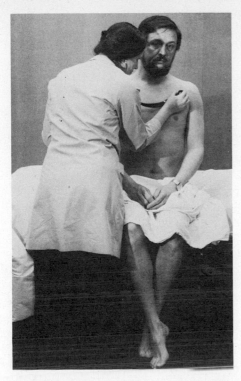

Fig. 26-3. Client seated (uncovered to waist), examiner facing client.

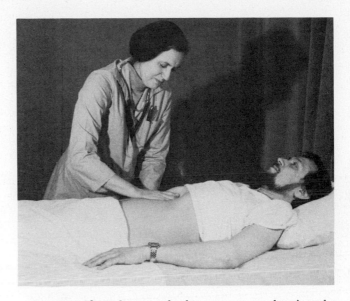

Fig. 26-4. Client lying on back, examiner at client's right side.

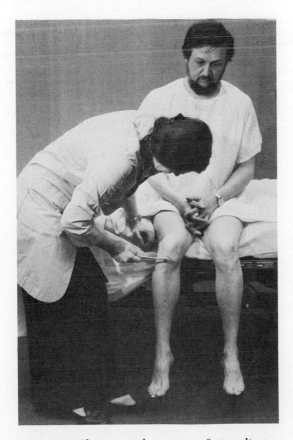

Fig. 26-5. Client seated, examiner facing client.

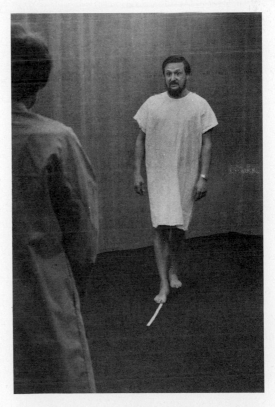

Fig. 26-6. Client standing, examiner standing.

1. Observe with client bending over.
2. Test for range of motion.
B. Assess neural system.
   1. Observe gait.
   2. Perform Romberg test.
   3. Observe heel and toe walks.
C. Test for inguinal and femoral hernias.
D. Examine male rectum: palpate rectum.

RECORDING THE PHYSICAL EXAMINATION

In recording the physical examination, the practitioner is continuously attempting to achieve a balance between conciseness and comprehensiveness. The record should describe what was seen, heard, palpated, and percussed. Whenever appropriate, the exact description is written; evaluations such as "normal," "good," or "poor" are avoided or used judiciously. Too frequently, a major system, such as the cardiovascular system, is described in one word, "normal." This description does not indicate what components of that system were assessed or the examiner's parameters of normal.

Conciseness is achieved through the use of outlines, phrases, and abbreviations. Grammar is sacrificed, and only essential words are written. Often it is helpful to use a form for recording the physical examination. A form provides an outline into which data can be entered. Forms serve as reminders for completeness; they save time; and, if they are used by all of the members of a health care system, they are useful as indices for rapid information identification. An example of a worksheet for recording a physical examination is included at the end of this chapter.

As recommended in the recording of the history (see Chapter 3 on the health history), the beginning practitioner should overrecord. The beginner should record all findings from the examination. With increased skill and discrimination regarding the significance of findings, the practitioner will be able to weed out the irrelevant information and consolidate the significant data.

Table 26-1 is a guideline that is designed to be of assistance to the beginning recorder. The first column indicates the body systems or regions that are examined. The second column contains a list of the areas of recording. These areas should be described for all clients. The third column is a partial list of areas to be recorded if abnormalities are identified in the examination of that system. The fourth column contains examples of recording for each body system or area. The examples of recording do not relate to one client; they should not be read as an example of the composite physical examination of one client.

Table 26-1. Areas and examples of recording for the physical examination

Area of examination	Descriptions usually recorded	Descriptions recorded in detail if abnormalities are present (partial listing only)	Examples of recording

Vital signs	Temperature: oral or rectal
	Pulse
	Respiration
	Blood pressure: both arms in at least two positions (lying and sitting recommended)
	Weight: indicate if client is clothed or unclothed
	Height: without shoes
		Blood pressure in standing position and in both thighs	T: 98.6° F (oral)
			P: 76/min—strong and regular; R: 16/min
			BP:
			  Lying: R, 110/70/60; L, 112/68/60
			  Sitting: R, 116/74/67; L, 120/76/65
			Wt: 130 lb unclothed
			Ht: 5 ft 3 in

General health	Appearance as relative to chronological age Apparent state of health Awareness Personal appearance Emotional status Nutritional status Affect Response Cooperation	Handshake Speech Respiratory difficulties Gross deformity Movements Unusual behavior	Slightly obese, alert, white male who looks younger than his stated age of 45. Moves without difficulty; no gross abnormalities apparent. Appears healthy and in no acute distress; is neatly dressed, responsive, and cooperative. Responds appropriately; smiles frequently.
Skin and mucous membranes	Color Edema Moisture Temperature Texture	Discharge Drainage Lesions: distribution, type, configuration Superficial vascularity	*Skin:* Uniformly brown in color; soft, warm, moist, elastic, of normal thickness. No edema or lesions. *Mucous membranes:* Pink, moist, slightly pale.

Table 26-1. Areas and examples of recording for the physical examination—cont'd

Area of examination	Descriptions usually recorded	Descriptions recorded in detail if abnormalities are present (partial listing only)	Examples of recording
	Turgor	Mobility Thickness	
Nails	Color of beds Texture	Lesions Abnormalities in size or shape Presence of clubbing	Nail beds pink, texture hard, no clubbing.
Hair and scalp	Quantity Distribution Color Texture	Lesions Parasites	*Hair:* Normal male distribution; thick, curly; black color with graying at temples. *Scalp:* Clean, no lesions.
Cranium	Contour Tenderness	Lesions	Normocephalic, no tenderness.
Face	Symmetry Movements Sinuses CN V CN VII	Tenderness Edema Lesions Parotid gland	Symmetrical at rest and with movement. Jaw muscles strong, no crepitations in temporomandibular joint. Sinus areas not tender. Sensory: pain and light touch intact.
Eyes	Visual acuity Visual fields Alignment of eyes Alignment of eyelids Movement of eyelids Conjunctiva Sclera Cornea Anterior chamber Iris Pupils: size, shape, symmetry, reflexes (PERRLA may be used for "Pupils, equally round, react to light and accommodation") Lens Lacrimal apparatus Ophthalmological examination (media, disc, vessels, retina, macular areas)	Eyebrows Tonometry Lesions Exophthalmia	Vision (with glasses): R, 20/40; L, 20/30; can read newspaper at 18 in. Visual fields full. Alignment: no deviation with cover test; light reflex equal; palpebral fissure normal. Extraocular movements: bilaterally intact; no nystagmus, ptosis, lid lag. Conjunctiva: clear, slightly injected around area of R inner canthus. Sclera: white. Cornea: clear, arcus senilis, R eye. Anterior chamber: not narrowed. Iris: blue, round. Pupils: PERRLA. Lens: clear. Funduscopic examination: normal veins and arteries; disc round, margins well defined, color yellowish pink; macular areas normal; no arteriolovenous nicking, hemorrhages, or exudates. Lacrimal system: no swelling or discharge. Corneal reflex: present.
Ears	Auricle Canal Otoscopic examination (color, presence of landmarks) Rinné and Weber tests	Discharge Pathological alterations, present on otoscopic examination Lesions Mastoid tenderness General tenderness	Auricle: no lesions, canal clean. Otoscopic examination: drum intact, color gray, landmarks present. Hearing: finger rub heard in both ears at 3 ft. Rinné and Weber tests: normal, AC 2× > BC.
Nose	Patency of each nostril Olfaction Turbinates and mucous membranes	External nose Vestibule Transillumination of sinuses	Nostrils patent, odors identified. Septum: slightly deviated to R. Turbinates and membranes: pink, moist, no discharge.

Continued.

Table 26-1. Areas and examples of recording for the physical examination—cont'd

Area of examination	Descriptions usually recorded	Descriptions recorded in detail if abnormalities are present (partial listing only)	Examples of recording
Oral cavity	Buccal mucosa Gums Teeth (decayed, missing, filled) Floor of mouth Hard and soft palate Tonsillar areas Posterior pharyngeal wall Taste Tongue	Breath Lips Lesions Laryngoscopic examination Palpation of mouth Parotid duct	Membrane: pink and moist, no lesions. Gums: no edema. Teeth: 3D, 1M, 10F (approximately). Palate: intact, moves symmetrically with phonation, gag reflex present. Tonsils: present, not enlarged. Pharynx: pink and clean. Tongue: strong, moves symmetrically. Taste: able to differentiate sweet and sour.
Neck	Movements: rotation and lateral bend Symmetry Thyroid gland Tracheal position Glands and nodes	Postural alignment Tenderness Tone of muscles Lesions Masses	Full ROM, strong symmetrically, thyroid not palpable, trachea midline, no enlargement of head and neck regional nodes.
Breasts	Axillary nodes Supraclavicular nodes Infraclavicular nodes Breasts: observation and palpation Nipples Discharge Masses	Retraction Dimpling	No nodes palpable—axillary, infraclavicular, or supraclavicular; no masses, retraction, or discharge; L breast slightly larger than R breast, otherwise symmetrical at rest and with movement.
Chest and respiratory system	Shape of thorax Symmetry of thorax Respiratory movements Respiratory excursion Palpation: tactile fremitus, tenderness, masses Percussion notes Diaphragmatic excursion and level Auscultation: breath sounds, adventitious sounds	Adventitious sounds Deformity Use of accessory muscles of respiration Vocal fremitus Egophony, bronchophony, whispered pectoriloquy	Thorax oval, AP diameter < lateral diameter; symmetrical at rest and with movements; excursion normal; tactile fremitus equal bilaterally; no masses or tenderness; percussion tones resonant, diaphragmatic excursion 5 cm bilaterally between T10 and T12; vesicular breath sounds bilaterally; no adventitious sounds.
Central cardio-vascular system	Position in which the heart was examined; lying, sitting, left lateral, recumbent Inspection: bulging depression, pulsation (precordial and juxtaprecordial) Palpation: thrusts, heaves, thrills, friction rubs Point of PMI Auscultation: rate and rhythm, character of S_1, character of S_2, comparison of S_1 in aortic and pulmonic areas, comparison of S_1 and S_2 in major auscultatory areas, presence or absence of extra sounds—if present, description	Murmur or extra sound: whether systolic or diastolic; intensity; pitch; quality; site of maximal transmission; effect of position, respiration, and exercise; radiation	Examined in sitting and lying positions; no abnormal pulsations or lifts observed; PMI in the 5th ICS, slightly medial to the LMCL; no abnormal pulsations palpated. Apical pulse: 72, regular; S_1 single sound; S_2 splits with inspiration; A_2 is louder than P_2, S_1 heard loudest at apex, S_2 heard loudest at base; no murmurs or other sounds.
Arterial pulses	Radial pulse: rate, rhythm; consistency and tenderness of arterial wall	Any abnormality: analysis of type	Radial pulse: bilaterally equal, regular, strong; no tenderness or thickening of vessels; 76/min.

Table 26-1. Areas and examples of recording for the physical examination—cont'd

Area of examination	Descriptions usually recorded	Descriptions recorded in detail if abnormalities are present (partial listing only)	Examples of recording
	Amplitude and character of peripheral pulses: superficial temporal, brachial, femoral, popliteal, posterior tibial, dorsal pedal Carotid pulses: equality, amplitude, thrills, bruits		Peripheral pulses: Temporal — Brachial — Femoral R as above — as above — as above L as above — as above — as above — Posterior Popliteal — tibial — Dorsal pedal R not felt — as above — as above L not felt — as above — as above Carotid pulses: equal, strong, no bruits.
Venous pulses and pressures	Jugular venous pulsations, presence of waves a, c, and v Venous pressure: distention present at 45 degrees	Hepatojugular reflex Analysis of jugular venous waves	Jugular venous pressure, 5 cm with client at 45 degrees; venous a and v waves present, a wave strongest.

Abdomen	Inspection: scars, size, shape, symmetry, muscular development, bulging, movements
	Auscultation: peristaltic sounds—present or absent; vascular bruits—present or absent
	Palpation
	  Masses
	  Tenderness (local, referred, rebound), tone of musculature
	  Liver: size, contour, character of edge, consistency, tenderness
	  Kidney (indicate if palpable or not)
	  Costovertebral area: tenderness
	Percussion: liver size at MCL, spleen, masses
		Diastasis
		Distention
		Mass or bulging: specific description
		Palpable spleen: indication of size, surface contour, splenic notch, consistency, tenderness, mobility
		Palpable kidney: indication of location, size, shape, consistency
		Distension of urinary bladder
		Fluid wave
		Flank dullness
		Shifting dullness
		Aorta
		Gallbladder
			Healed scar RLQ (appendectomy); slightly obese, protuberant; symmetrical, no bulging, normal bowel sounds, no bruits, no abnormal movements, symmetrical; no masses; no tenderness; liver 11 cm in RMCL; no CVA tenderness; no organs palpated; muscle tones lax.
			Area of midline diastasis: 6 cm × 2 cm inferior and superior to the umbilicus.

Neural system	Orientation
	Intellectual performance
	Emotional status
	Insight
	Memory
	Cranial nerves
	Coordination
	Sensory: touch, pain, position, vibration
	Babinski's sign
	Romberg's sign
		Thought content
		Speech
		Sensory: hot, cold, two-point discrimination
		Stereognosis
		Involuntary movements
		
			Alert, oriented ×3; mood appropriate and stable; remote and recent memory intact; several calculations by 6 accurate; insight normal; cranial nerves all intact, examined and recorded in head and neck regions; all movements coordinated; able to perform rapid coordinated movements with upper and lower extremities.
			
			Reflexes (0-4+)
			  0 = absent
			  + (or 1+) = decreased
			  ++ (or 2+) = normal
			  +++ (or 3+) = hyperactive
			  ++++ (or 4+) = clonus

Continued.

Table 26-1. Areas and examples of recording for the physical examination—cont'd

Area of examination	Descriptions usually recorded	Descriptions recorded in detail if abnormalities are present (partial listing only)	Examples of recording
Neural system—cont'd			Sensory: light touch, pain, and vibration to face, trunk, and extremities normal and symmetrical; walks with coordination, able to maintain standing position with eyes closed.
Extremities and musculoskeletal system	Both upper and lower extremities: general assessments—size, shape, mass, symmetry, hair distribution, color; temperature; edema; varicosities; tenderness; epitrochlear lymph nodes Bones and joints: range of motion, tenderness, gait Muscles: size, symmetry, strength, tone, tenderness, consistency Back: posture, tenderness; movement—extension, lateral bend, rotation	Lesions Deformities Color and temperature changes on elevation and dependency Homans' sign Redness Heat Swelling Deformity Crepitations Contractures Muscle spasms Tenderness Atrophy Hypertrophy	Muscular development and mass normal for age; arms and legs symmetrical; skin warm, soft, neither moist nor dry; normal male hair growth on arms, legs, and feet; no edema, varicosities, or tenderness; no nodes palpated; joints nontender, not swollen; normal ROM; muscle tone and strength normal bilaterally; back—full ROM; no tenderness or deformities.
Rectal area	Anal area Skin Hemorrhoids Sphincter tone Rectum Tumors Stool color Occult blood	Lesions Fissures Pilonidal sinus Condition of perineal body Tenderness Proctoscopic examination	Skin clean, no lesions; sphincter tone good; no hemorrhoids or masses noted; stools brown, guiac negative.
Inguinal area	Hernia: inguinal, femoral Nodes	Size, shape, consistency, tenderness, reducibility of hernia or nodes	Hernias not present; no enlargement of nodes noted.

Table 26-1. Areas and examples of recording for the physical examination—cont'd

Area of examination	Descriptions usually recorded	Descriptions recorded in detail if abnormalities are present (partial listing only)	Examples of recording
Male genitalia	Penis: condition of prepuce, skin Scrotum: size, skin, testes, epididymides, spermatic cords Prostate gland: size, shape, symmetry, consistency, tenderness Seminal vesicles: size, shape, consistency	Scars Lesions Structural alterations Masses Swelling Nodules	Penis: circumsized, clean, no lesions. Scrotum and contents: normal size, no masses or tumors noted. Prostate and inferior portions of seminal vesicles: palpated. Prostate: not enlarged, rubbery, not tender. Seminal vesicles: soft, not nodular.
Female genitalia	External: hair distribution; labia; Bartholin's glands, urethral meatus, Skene's glands (BUS); hymen; introitus Vaginal observation: presence or absence of rectocele, urethrocele, cystocele; tissue; discharge (smears or cultures taken); cervix Bimanual examination: cervix, uterus, adnexa Rectovaginal examination; uterus, cul-de-sac, septum	Lesions Tumors Prolapses	Normal female hair distribution; no lesions or masses. BUS: no tenderness, redness, or discharge. Hymen: present in caruncles. Labia: approximate, intact. Introital tone: good; no prolapses; no scars, perineum thick. Vagina: pink; discharge—small amount, thin, clean, nonodorous. Cervix: pink, nulliparous, firm, not tender, movable, midline. Uterus: pear-shaped, movable, normal size, firm, no masses. Tubes: not palpable. Ovaries: palpable, movable, not tender, approximately 2 × 3 × 2 cm; smooth surface, no lesions, firm consistency. Rectovaginal septum: thick and firm; no masses palpated in rectum or cul-de-sac.

WORKSHEET FOR RECORDING A PHYSICAL EXAMINATION

Vital signs

Temperature _____ Respiration _____ BP   (L)   Arm   (R)

  _____ Supine _____

  _____ Sitting _____

  _____ Standing _____

Height _____ Weight _____ (Stripped or clothed)

General

Skin, hair, nails, mucous membranes

Head

Scalp _____

Face _____

(CNs V, VII) _____

_____

Sinus areas _____

Nodes _____

Cranium _____

Eyes

Visual acuity _____

Visual fields _____

Ocular movements (CNs III, IV, VI) _____

Corneal light reflex _____

Lids, lacrimal organs _____

Conjunctiva, sclera _____

Cornea (CN V) _____

Lens and media _____

Pupils: Pupillary reflexes (CN III) _____

     Light, direct and consensual _____

     Near point _____

Fundi (CN II) _____

Intraocular pressure _____

Ears

External structures _____

Canal _____

Tympanic membranes _____

Hearing (CN VIII) _____

2

Nose

Septum _____

Mucous membranes _____

Patency _____

Olfactory sense (CN I) _____

Oral cavity

Lips _____

Mucous membranes _____

Gums _____

Teeth _____

Palates and uvula (CNs IX and X) _____

Tonsillar areas _____

Tongue (CN XII) _____

Floor _____

Voice _____

Breath _____

Neck

General structure _____

Trachea _____

Thyroid _____

Nodes _____

Muscles (CN XI) _____

Breasts and area nodes

_____

_____

_____

Chest, respiratory system

Chest shape _____

Type of respiration _____

Expansion _____

Fremitus _____

General palpation _____

Percussion _____

_____ Diaphragmatic excursion: (R) _____ cm (L) _____ cm

Breath sounds _____

_____

_____

_____

_____

Adventitious sounds _____

_____

Continued.

WORKSHEET FOR RECORDING A PHYSICAL EXAMINATION—cont'd

3

Cardiovascular system

      Rate and rhythm: Radial (palpation) _____

                        Apical (auscultation) _____

      Precordium: Inspection _____

                Palpation _____

                Auscultation _____

                  S_1 _____

                  S_2 _____

                  S_3 _____

                  S_4 _____

                Extra sounds _____

                Murmur(s): Systolic _____

                        Diastolic _____

      Carotids _____

      Jugular venus pulse and pressure _____

      _____

      Description of peripheral pulses

	Brachial	Radial	Femoral	Popliteal	Dorsal pedal	Post. tibial
R						
L						

Abdomen and inguinal areas

      Contour, tone _____

      Scars, marks _____

      Auscultation _____

      _____

      Liver _____ Span _____ cm at RMCL

      Spleen _____

      Kidneys _____ CVA tenderness _____

      Bladder _____

      Hernias _____

      Masses _____

      Palpation _____

      _____

      Percussion _____

Genitalia and area nodes

_____

_____

_____

_____

_____

Rectal examination

4

Musculoskeletal system

Gait _____

Deformities _____

Joint evaluation _____

_____

Muscle strength _____

_____

Muscle mass _____

Range of motion _____

Spine

Contour _____

Position _____

Motion _____

_____

Nervous system

Mental status _____

Language _____

Cranial nerves (summarize) _____

Motor: Coordination: Upper extremities _____

Lower extremities _____

Involuntary movements _____

Deep tendon reflexes:

Note: +s denote finger jerks, brachioradialis, biceps, triceps, reflexes, 4-quadrant abdominal scratch reflexes, patellar Achilles reflexes, and plantar reflexes. Abdominal reflexes are recorded as 0 or +. Scale: 0-4 (++++); normal = 2 (++).

Sensory

Light touch _____

Pain (pinprick) _____

Vibration _____

Position _____

27 Clinical laboratory procedures

The information obtained through the physical examination is augmented and in many cases verified through the judicious use of laboratory diagnostic procedures to provide a biochemical data base for use in the analysis of the client's state of health.

The tests most frequently included in a screening workup include a blood chemistry profile, hematology, a serological test for syphilis, urinalysis, a chest roentgenogram, the Papanicolaou (Pap) cytological examination for cancer diagnosis, hormonal evaluation of ovarian function in women from puberty onward, a proctoscopic examination, and an electrocardiogram (ECG) for all persons older than 40 years of age.

Blood chemistry profiles characteristically include determinations of sodium, potassium, chloride, calcium, phosphorus, glucose, bilirubin, blood urea nitrogen (BUN), uric acid, total proteins, albumin, cholesterol, serum glutamic-oxaloacetic transaminase (SGOT), lactic dehydrogenase (LDH), and alkaline phosphatase.

The hematology screening examination includes a study of the red blood cell (RBC) count, hematocrit, hemoglobin, mean corpuscular volume, and mean corpuscular hemoglobin concentration. In addition, the total white blood cell (WBC) count and a differential count based on morphological types are included.

Urinalysis is performed for analysis of specific gravity, pH, and the presence of glucose, protein, acetone, blood, and microscopic formed elements.

The procedure for the Pap smear is described in Chapter 20 on assessment of the female genitalia and procedures for smears and cultures.

The tables of normal ranges found in textbooks of clinical pathology are to be considered as relative guidelines. The values are often those of medical or nursing student volunteers and laboratory technicians and thus are not specific as to sex and age.

Furthermore, values vary from one clinical laboratory to another even though the same procedure may be used in each laboratory.

There may be real differences in values observed in geographically separated population groups; for example, generally higher cholesterol values are observed in sample populations in San Francisco. Seasonal changes may also play a role; for example, uric acid levels are observed to be greater in winter than in other seasons.

When abnormal values are observed in test results, the examiner should review the interview data to determine if any circumstances in the client's lifestyle, environment, drug use, or state of nutrition or hydration may have influenced the value. For instance, an elevated protein-bound iodine (PBI) level and low resin-uptake value (triiodothyronine [T_3]) may indicate that the client has been taking oral contraceptives.

Posture is known to affect laboratory values. Blood albumin, total protein, hemoglobin, cholesterol, and calcium values are known to be higher in the client who has been standing for a long period of time.

Diet and alcohol may also alter laboratory values. Bilirubin and SGOT values have been shown to be elevated during fasting. High fat content in the diet will produce hyperlipemia. High-protein meals may produce an increased BUN level. Most professionals are aware of the possibility of increased blood glucose values incurred as a result of a "carbohydrate binge." Alcohol consumption or alcoholic liver damage has been shown to result in increased levels of uric acid, glucose, calcium, phosphorus, LDH, SGOT, creatine phosphokinase (CPK), alkaline phosphatase, and triglycerides, accompanied by a low PBI level and albumin-globulin (A/G) ratio.

The blood specimens collected from a dehydrated individual will show the values to be consistent with the more concentrated fluid. These include increased levels of sodium, potassium, chloride, calcium, phosporus, glucose, BUN, uric acid, cholesterol, total protein, globulin, LDH, SGOT, and creatinine.

The overhydrated client might be expected to have decreased concentrations of sodium, potassium, chloride, calcium, phosphorus, BUN, uric acid, albumin, total proteins, and cholesterol in the blood.

Improper handling of specimens may also result in erroneous test results. Test tubes that have been washed with detergent and poorly rinsed may cause spuriously elevated calcium, sodium, and potassium levels.

Possible applications of results of laboratory procedures include:

1. Provision of health assessment parameters of both a morphological and biochemical nature that are unavailable through the health history and physical examination.
2. Confirmation of a biochemical state of health when physical examination findings are negative.
3. Provision of further information in the differential diagnosis of disease. For example, the client with easy fatigability, shortness of breath on exertion, dizziness on exercise, and pale buccal mucosa may have a diagnosis of anemia confirmed through the results of screening hematological studies.
4. Provision of a gauge of the severity of disease. The degree of anemia that is disclosed may determine the therapeutic regimen for the client. The milder form of iron deficiency anemia may well be ameliorated in time through diet and rest, allowing the client's blood-forming organs to make up the deficit. Medication may be necessary for more severe involvement, and blood replacement by transfusion may be necessary for marked reduction in hemoglobin and RBCs.
5. Provision of biochemical clues that will indicate appropriate dosages of medication. A serum iron determination may be made for the client who is suspected of having iron deficiency anemia to substantiate the physical examination findings. The serum iron levels may be used to monitor the efficiency of the treatment regimen.

BLOOD CHEMISTRY PROFILE

Automated machines are available in many pathology laboratories for the purpose of performing chemistry tests. These machines commonly perform 6 to 24 determinations, using a single small sample of blood. Two types of machines are utilized. The first type is a discrete sample analyzer (DSA), which separates the sample into as many chambers as there are tests to be performed. Translated into the language of technician-performed testing, this means the sample is separated into an individual test tube for each ordered test. The second type is a continuous flow analyzer (CFA), which separates the sample within a single tubing into discrete sections through

Table 27-1. Machines used in the performance of blood chemistry profiles

Instrument	Type	Size of sample required (ml)	Number of tests possible	Choice of test or machine runs all possible tests
SMA 12/60	CFA	1.0	12	All
SMA C	CFA	0.5	20	All
AcuChem	DSA	0.5	17	Choice
Coulter Chemistry	DSA	3.0	21	Choice
Hycel 17, Super 17	DSA	1.2	17	Choice

the use of bubbles. These sections pass through the tubing, stopping at specific sites for analysis. Some caution must be used with these machines to be certain that the tubing is thoroughly cleaned between samples.

Table 27-1 lists some of the machines used in the performance of blood chemistry profiles.

Most of these machines provide a printout sheet that records the client's data against a range of normal for the particular instrument. Graphs provided with the SMA 12/60 and SMA 6/60 are seen in Figs. 27-1 and 27-2.

Blood chemistry tests are performed on venous samples that are obtained following a period of fasting (usually at least 6 hours).

Some of these machines provide test results at a rate of greater than 3,000 per minute and thus provide significantly more data at less cost to the consumer.

In general, the machines are carefully self-calibrated and are more accurate than the results produced when humans do the testing.

One disadvantage to the practitioner and the client is that more data may be generated than is actually necessary to assess the client's health status.

Electrolytes

Some electrolytes that are routinely analyzed in a screening examination include sodium (Na^+), potassium (K^+), chloride (Cl^-), and carbon dioxide (CO_2) combining power.

Plasma is an aqueous solution (90% water) that contains approximately 1% electrolytes.

The distribution of electrolytes in the normal individual is represented by the following values:

Na^+ 136 to 142 mEq/L	Cl^- 95 to 103 mEq/L
K^+ 3.8 to 5 mEq/L	PO_4^{3-} 1.8 to 2.6 mEq/L
Ca^{2+} 4.5 to 5.3 mEq/L	SO_4^{2-} 0.2 to 1.3 mEq/L
Mg^{2+} 1.5 to 2.5 mEq/L	HCO_3^- 21 to 28 mEq/L

Protein $\cong$ 17 mEq/L

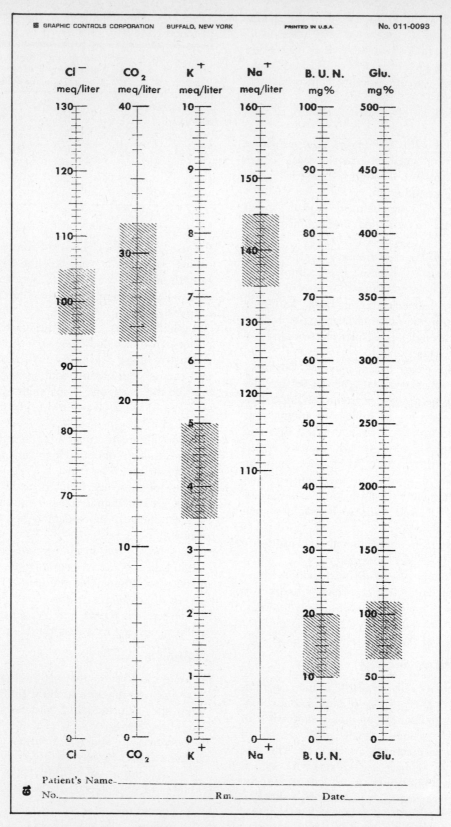

Fig. 27-1. SMA 6/60 graph sheet. Shaded areas in each column represent normal ranges. The machine draws a line representing the values of the specimen. Thus, deviation from the normal range is prominently displayed. (Courtesy Graphics Controls Corp., Buffalo, N.Y.)

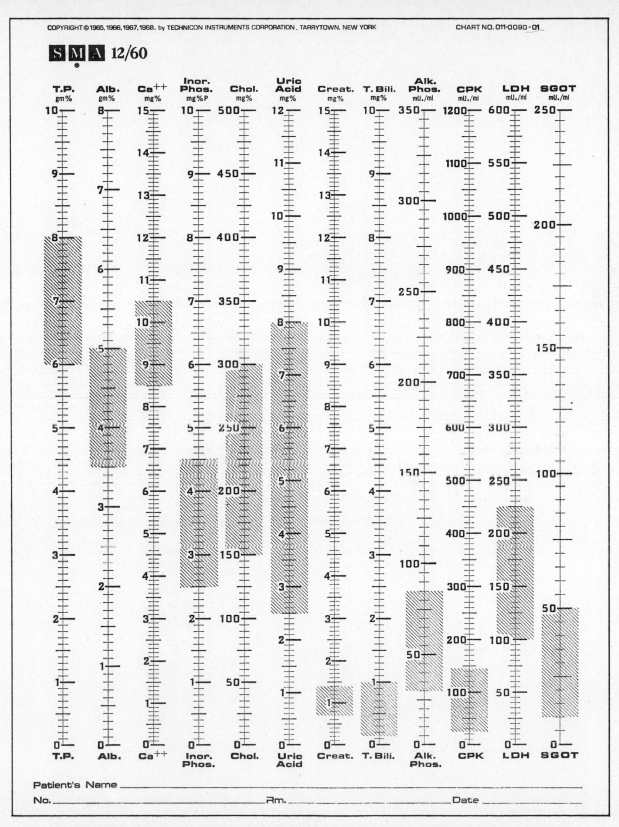

Fig. 27-2. Chart paper for Technicon™ SMA™ 12/60 multichannel analyzer. (Courtesy Technicon Instruments Corp., Tarrytown, N.Y.)

The distribution of these ions in the plasma is compared with those of the interstitial and cellular fluids in Fig. 27-3.

Electrolytes are carefully controlled through a variety of physical and chemical mechanisms, so that the range of normal for each of these compartments is quite narrow.

SODIUM

Sodium is the major cation of the body. It is the most abundant extracellular ion and as such plays a prominent role in the osmolality of the extracellular fluid. The ion is necessary to the resting potential of excitable cells. The intake of sodium in the average adult diet is 10 to 12 g, but the amount is variable.

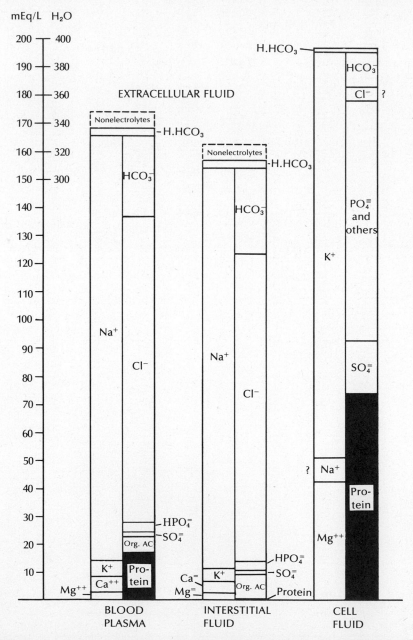

Fig. 27-3. Electrolyte distribution in the fluid compartment of the body. The column of figures on the left (200, 190, 180, and so on) indicates amounts of cations or anions; the figures on the right (400, 380, 360, and so on) indicate the sum of cations and anions. Note that chloride and sodium values in cell fluid are questioned. It is probable that at least muscle intracellular fluid contains some sodium but no chloride. (From Anthony, C. P., and Thibodeau, G. A.: Textbook of anatomy and physiology, ed. 10, St. Louis, 1979, The C. V. Mosby Co. Adapted from Mountcastle, V. B., editor: Medical physiology, vol. 2, ed. 14, St. Louis, 1980, The C. V. Mosby Co.; after Gamble, J. L.: Harvey Lect. **42:**247, 1946-1947.)

The kidney plays the principal role in homeostasis of sodium in the body fluids. Aldosterone is secreted by the adrenal cortex due to activation of the renin angiotensin system when the whole blood sodium concentration or blood volume are decreased or when the potassium concentration is increased. ACTH directly stimulates the cells of the adrenal cortex. Thus, aldosterone is also secreted in times of stress. Aldosterone facilitates the reabsorption of sodium in the distal tubule of the kidney.

The concentration of the ions is necessarily dependent on the water content of the blood. Although the whole blood sodium content might stay constant, the concentration of the sodium ions will be greater when water stores are less in quantity.

Osmotic diuretic agents, such as mannitol and glucose, are known to carry out sodium with them. In some cases of acidemia, the concentration of SO_4^{2-}, Cl^-, PO_4^{3-}, and organic acids overwhelms the kidney's capacity to secrete H^+ and NH_3 while exchanging Na^+. Thus, the ions are excreted in the urine with fixed base, which is sodium for the most part. In conditions where potassium is lost from the cellular compartment, sodium replaces the ion. This situation may occur in acidosis or when the sodium-potassium pump is malfunctioning.

SERUM SODIUM: NORMAL VALUES AND DEVIATIONS

Normal values: 136 to 142 mEq/L
Normal osmolality of the blood: 280 to 295 mOsm/L

Deviations	Etiology
Hyponatremia	Dehydration with loss of electrolytes
	Sweating
	Diarrhea
	Burns
	Nasogastric tube
	Addison's disease
	Diuretics
	Mercurial
	Chlorothiazide
	Chronic renal insufficiency
	Chronic glomerulonephritis
	Pyelonephritis
	Starvation
	Diabetic acidosis
	Water retention or dilution
	Cirrhosis
	Congestive heart failure
	Renal insufficiency
	Excessive ingestion of water
	Overhydration with intravenous therapy
Hypernatremia (uncommon)	Deficient water intake
	Excessive water loss—lack of antidiuretic hormone (ADH)
	Cushing's disease
	Primary hyperaldosteronism

POTASSIUM

Potassium is the most abundant intracellular cation; since the majority of potassium is found within the cells, the total body content of the ion cannot be measured readily. Furthermore, the relationship between intracellular potassium and serum potassium is a highly dynamic one. For instance, intracellular potassium readily leaves the cell in the event of serum potassium deficiency. Potassium ions compete with hydrogen ions for excretion by the kidney; potassium is excreted largely by this mechanism, though some may be lost in sweat and gastrointestinal secretions.

The importance of homeokinetic control of extracellular potassium ions relates to the function of potassium in neuromuscular excitability. The resting membrane potential of the cells of these tissues is directly related to the ratio of intracellular potassium concentrations.

SERUM POTASSIUM: NORMAL VALUES AND DEVIATIONS

Normal values: 3.8 to 5 mEq/L

Deviations	Etiology	Possible effects
Hyperkalemia	↓ Excretion of K^+	Changes in ECG; >8
	Kidney disease	mEq/L
	Intestinal	Widened P wave
	obstruction	Symmetrical peaking
	Addison's disease	of T wave
	Hypoaldosteronism	Widened QRS complex
	Iatrogenic K^+ replacement therapy	plex
	Trauma	Depressed ST segment; >11 mEq/L
	Burns	Ventricular fibrillation
	Diuretics such as	Heart block in diastole
	spironolactone that	Neuromuscular
	cause ↓ K^+ excretion	changes
	K^+ shift from tissues	Flaccidity
	Muscle crush	Muscle paralysis
	Acidosis	Numbness
		Tingling
Hypokalemia	↓ Ingestion of K^+	Changes in ECG
	↑ Excretion of K^+	Flattening and inversion of T wave
	Prolonged gastrointestinal suctioning	Prominent U wave
	Vomiting	Sagging of ST segment
	K^+ depleting diuretics	Muscle weakness
	Excessive administration of bicarbonate (K^+ enters the cells)	Malaise
	Cirrhosis	Apathy
	Cushing's disease	Nausea and vomiting
	Treatment with steroids	↓ Reflexes
	Aldosteronism	↓ Smooth muscle tone
	Excessive licorice intake	Distention
	Intravenous infusion of K^+ free fluids	Paralytic ileus
	Fasting, starvation	↓ Diastolic blood pressure
		Impairment of renal tubular function
		Polyuria

CHLORIDE

Chloride is the major anion of the body and in general is found to behave in concert with sodium. More precisely, the chloride passively follows sodium in its transport through membranes. Chloride plays a prominent role in acid-base balance. In acidemia, Cl^- concentration is increased, and thus more Cl^- is associated with sodium. In alkalemia, more bicarbonate (HCO_3^-) is associated with sodium. Chloride deficit leads to increased reabsorption of bicarbonate in the distal tubules of the kidney and thereby leads to alkalemia. Since chloride is necessary to the synthesis of hydrochloric acid in the stomach, excessive loss of gastric secretions leads to alkalemia. Chloride is also lost from the intestinal tract in diarrhea or as a result of intestinal fistula. Chloride is excreted in the urine with cations in diuresis.

SERUM CHLORIDE: NORMAL VALUES AND DEVIATIONS

Normal values: 95 to 103 mEq/L

Deviations	Etiology	Possible effects

Hypochloremia	Hypokalemic alkalosis
	Ingestion of potassium
	  compounds that do
	  not contain chloride
	Potassium-sparing
	  diuretics
	Excessive loss of
	  gastric secretions
	Vomiting
	Nasogastric tube
		Associated with
		↓ K^+ and ↑ CO_2
		combining power

Hyperchloremia (rare)	Diarrhea Iatrogenic Ammonium chloride ingestion	Fistulas

CALCIUM

Plasma calcium (Ca^{2+}) occurs in three forms. About half of the calcium is bound to protein. Calcium in this form does not diffuse through the capillary wall. A second, nonionized, nondiffusable group of calcium compounds makes up approximately 5% of the plasma calcium. Somewhat less than half (45%) of the plasma calcium is ionized. This third form of calcium diffuses through the capillary membrane and is physiologically active.

The effects of calcium on skeletal and cardiac muscle, nerve tissue, and bone are due to the ionized calcium. The ionized calcium of the plasma is maintained within a fairly narrow range (±5%) due to the influence of parathyroid hormone (PTH) and thyrocalcitonin (TCT). PTH increases plasma ionized calcium by increasing absorption of calcium from the intestinal tract and reabsorption of calcium from the renal tubules of the kidney and by absorbing calcium salts from the bones through its action of osteoclasts. TCT lowers serum ionized calcium by increasing depositions of calcium in the bones through its influence on the osteoblasts.

A metabolite of vitamin D increases the absorption of calcium from the intestine through the stimulation of a calcium-binding protein.

SERUM CALCIUM: NORMAL VALUES AND DEVIATIONS

Normal values
Adults:
Ionized: 4.2 to 5.2 mg/100 ml
      2.1 to 2.6 mEq/L
Total: 9 to 10.6 mg/100 ml
      4.5 to 5.3 mEq/L
Infants: 11 to 13 mg/100 ml

Deviations	Etiology	Possible effects

Hypercalcemia	↑ PTH ⎤ Hyperpara-
	↓ TCT ⎦ thyroidism
	   associated
	   with alkaline
	   phosphatase)
	↑ Vitamin D intake
	↑ Absorption of
	   Ca^{2+} in intestine
	↑ Reabsorption
	   of Ca^{2+} in
	   renal tubules
	Acidosis
	Paget's disease
	Destructive bone
	   lesions
	Osteoporosis
	Immobilization
	Hypothyroidism
	Malignancy (associated
	   with hypergamma-
	   globulinemia)
	↓ Urinary excretion
	Na^+ depletion
	Thiazide diuretics
		Polyuria; polydipsia
		↓ Neuromuscular
		   excitability
		Skeletal muscle
		   (↓ tone, weak-
		   ness, atrophy)
		Smooth muscle
		   (↓ tone, observed
		   in such signs as
		   nausea, vomiting,
		   and constipation)
		Heart muscle
		Shortening of Q-T
		   interval of the
		   ECG
		Arteriovenous block
		↓ Plasma phosphate
		Renal calculi due to
		   precipitation of
		   calcium phosphate
		   ($Ca_3[PO_4]_2$)
		Alkalosis
		Ataxia
		Hyperreflexia

Hypocalcemia	↑ TCT ⎤ Hypopara-
	↓ PTH ⎦ thyroidism
	↓ Absorption of Ca^{2+}
	   from the gastrointes-
	   tinal tract
	Steatorrhea
	Sprue
	Celiac disease
	Acute pancreatitis
	↓ Vitamin D (hypovita-
	   minosis)
	Hypoalbuminemia
	Pregnancy
	Diuretic ingestion
	Starvation
	↓ Magnesium
		↓ Neuromuscular
		   excitability (tetany)
		Prolongation of the
		   S-T segment of the
		   ECG
		Osteomalacia in
		   adults
		Rickets in children

PHOSPHORUS

The serum level of phosphate (PO_4^{3-}) generally bears a combination relationship with serum calcium concentration. Parathyroid hormone increases the amount of phosphate absorbed in the intestinal tract since phosphate is absorbed when calcium is absorbed. The excretion of phosphate is accomplished largely by the kidney and is determined by the fact that phosphate is a threshold substance. Thus, the kidney regulates the serum phosphate level by secreting phosphate when the serum level exceeds

1 mMol/L and retaining phosphate when the serum concentration is less.

SERUM PHOSPHORUS: NORMAL VALUES AND DEVIATIONS

Normal values

Adults: 3 to 4.5 mg/100 ml
1.8 to 2.6 mEq/L
Children: 4 to 7 mg/100 ml
2.3 to 4.1 mEq/L

Deviations	Etiology	Possible effects
Hyperphos-phatemia	↑ TCT ↑ Growth hormone ↑ Ingestion of PO_4^{3-} Chronic glomerulo-nephritis Sarcoidosis	Associated with ↓ BUN, creatinine Symptoms of hypocalcemia Associated with ↓ gamma globulin
Hypophos-phatemia	↑ PTH ↓ Ingestion of PO_4^{3-} Hyperinsulinism	↓ ATP Symptoms of hypercalcemia Associated with indications of hypoglycemia

MAGNESIUM

Magnesium (Mg^{2+}) influences muscular activity in much the same direction as does calcium. The ion appears to be necessary for the coenzyme activity in the metabolism of carbohydrate and protein.

SERUM MAGNESIUM: NORMAL VALUES AND DEVIATIONS

Normal values: 1.5 to 2.5 mEq/L
1.8 to 3 mg/100 ml

Deviations	Etiology	Possible effects
Hypermag-nesemia	↑ Ingestion of Mg^{2+} (milk of magnesia)	↓ Neuromuscular excitation ↓ Muscle tone
Hypomag-nesemia	Malabsorption syndrome Acute pancreatitis	↑ Neuromuscular excitation (tetany) Peripheral vasodilatation Arrhythmias

Gases and pH

The blood gases are not usually tested in the screening examination but may be indicated as necessary tests by clinical signs such as cyanosis or hyperventilation.

OXYGEN

Tests for blood oxygen analysis are generally performed on arterial blood. The blood may be tested for oxygen content, hemoglobin saturation, and the gas tension (Pa_{O_2}, arterial blood; Pv_{O_2}, venous blood). The oxygen content of the blood reflects the hemoglobin concentration. At standard temperature and pressure 1.34 ml of oxygen combines with 1 g of hemoglobin at full saturation. The oxygen saturation of hemoglobin is a comparison of the percentage of oxygen that is bound to hemoglobin with the total amount that it is possible for the hemoglobin to carry.

The erythrocyte carries 98.5% of the oxygen in the blood bound to hemoglobin. Since the normal hemoglobin content of the adult male is 15 g/100 ml, the oxygen-carrying capacity is approximately 20 ml/100 ml of blood, or 20 vol%.

BLOOD OXYGEN: NORMAL VALUES AND DEVIATIONS

Normal values

	Arterial blood	Mixed venous blood
Content:	15 to 23 vol%	
Saturation:	94% to 100%	70% to 75%
Tension:	95 to 100 mm Hg	35 to 40 mm Hg

Deviations	Etiology	Possible effects
Anoxic hypoxia	Inadequate environmental O_2 supply, such as occurs in high altitude (acute) Impaired respiratory exchange	Low Pa_{O_2} Inadequate saturation of the arterial blood with oxygen Cyanosis ↑ Respiratory rate
Chronic hypoxia	Living at high altitude	↑ O_2 carrying capacity as RBCs increase
Anemic hypoxia	↓ Hemoglobin Competition for hemoglobin-binding sites (carbon monoxide poisoning)	↓ Saturation of hemoglobin possible
Stagnant hypoxia	↓ Circulatory function (failure to deliver O_2 to tissues) Cardiac failure Shock Peripheral impairment of flow (embolism)	Blood O_2 values may be normal
Histotoxic hypoxia	↓ Ability of cells to take up or utilize O_2, such as in poisoning	
Hyperoxia	Pure O_2 delivered at 1 atmosphere (766 mm Hg)	Bronchitis in 12 to 24 hours Fall in vital capacity in 60 hours Retrolental fibroplasia

At standard conditions arterial blood contains 0.3 ml of oxygen dissolved in 100 ml of plasma; this exerts a pressure of 100 mm Hg. The amount of oxygen combined with hemoglobin is decreased with an increase in temperature, acidity, and carbon dioxide tension (Pa_{CO_2}, arterial blood; Pv_{CO_2}, venous blood).

CARBON DIOXIDE

Carbon dioxide in the blood occurs in three forms: as bicarbonate, combined with protein (carbamino), and in simple solution. Carbon dioxide in an aqueous solution is in potential equilibrium with carbonic acid. The enzyme carbonic anhydrase is necessary to the catalysis of the equilibrium:

$$CO_2 + H_2O \rightleftharpoons H_2CO_3$$

The only test for carbon dioxide that is generally performed as part of the screening battery is the carbon dioxide–combining power, which measures the buffering capacity of the blood. The sample is collected, and the serum is removed after clotting and centrifugation. The carbon dioxide tension of the serum is equilibrated to normal alveolar tensions of 40 mm Hg. The bicarbonate is converted to carbon dioxide by hydrolysis, and the gas that is given up is measured. Subtraction of the known amount of dissolved carbon dioxide in the blood gives a value that is essentially that of bicarbonate alone.

Normal Pa_{CO_2}: 35 to 45 mm Hg
Normal Pv_{CO_2}: 41 to 55 mm Hg
Normal arterial whole blood HCO_3^-: 22 to 26 mEq/L
Normal venous whole blood HCO_3^-: 22 to 26 mEq/L

The base excess (BE) is a measure of alkaline substances in the blood. This includes bicarbonate and other bases in the blood.

Normal arterial BE: -2 to $+2$
Normal venous BE: -2 to $+2$

pH

Hydrogen ion concentration of the blood is reflected in the pH value. The degree of alkalinity or acidity of the body is important in that many enzymes are active only within narrow pH ranges. Furthermore, many other physiological processes are pH dependent, notably respiration. Acidosis is the process whereby an individual develops acidemia, the accumulation of excess hydrogen ions in the blood—or decreased pH. The affected person is described as acidotic.

Alkalosis, on the other hand, is the process whereby alkalemia is incurred. Alkalemia may be defined as decreased hydrogen ion concentration in the blood—or increased pH—and the individual may be described as alkalotic.

The Henderson-Hasselbalch equation describes pH relationships:

$$pH = pK + \log \frac{base}{acid}$$

pK is the dissociation constant (the ability to release hydrogen ions of the acid described). In the human being the bicarbonate ion is the most important buffering system, since the ion is present in large quantities. Thus, the equation may be written:

$$pH = 6.1 + \log \frac{HCO_3^-}{H_2CO_3}$$

The ratio $\dfrac{HCO_3^-}{H_2CO_3} = \dfrac{20}{1}$ in the normal person.

The bicarbonate ion is controlled by the lungs through the expiration of carbon dioxide and the kidneys, which control excretion of bicarbonate and hydrogen ions.

WHOLE BLOOD pH: NORMAL VALUES AND DEVIATIONS

Normal values
 Arterial: 7.38 to 7.44 (7.40)
 Venous: 7.30 to 7.41 (7.36)
Deviations
 Acidemia (acidosis): <pH 7.35
 Alkalemia (alkalosis): >pH 7.45

Glucose

Sucrose, lactose, and starches make up the majority of the carbohydrates ingested by humans. Slight amounts of alcohol, lactic acid, pyruvic acid, pectins, and dextrins are also consumed. These carbohydrates are hydrolyzed in the intestinal tract and broken down to the monosaccharides: glucose (80%), fructose (10%), and galactose (10%), in which form they are absorbed into the bloodstream.

Glucose is the principal form of fuel for cellular function; the liver can convert fructose and galactose to glucose, so that all of the absorbed sugars can be used. Fats and proteins may also be converted to glucose during fasting states or in times of increased glucose use, as in exercise. Glucose in excess of energy needs is converted to storage forms. The body is capable of storing about 100 g of glucose as glycogen. The majority of the remainder of glucose is converted to fat, but some is converted to amino acids.

The pancreatic hormones, insulin and glucagon, play a prominent role in glucose metabolism, as well as in the metabolism of protein and lipid. Insulin is produced by the beta cells of the pancreas, and its secretion is primarily determined by the concentration of blood glucose. The secretion of insulin is increased by an increase from basal of blood glucose; it is decreased as the concentration of blood glucose becomes less than normal. Blood insulin values in excess of normal produce the following major changes in glucose metabolism: (1) the rate of glucose metabolism is increased by facilitating the transport of glucose into the cells via facilitated diffusion, (2) the process of glycogen storage is enhanced, (3) the process of glucose entry into fat cells is enhanced and fat sotrage increased, and (4) the process of glucose entry into muscle cells is enhanced.

On the other hand, a decrease of blood insulin is accompanied by (1) glycogenolysis, a breakdown of glycogen to glucose, and (2) glyconeogenesis, the manufacture of glucose by the liver from amino acids derived from protein stores and from glycerol derived from fat stores. These two processes are functions of glucagon.

Thus, blood glucose concentration in the fasting state is maintained within reasonably narrow limits. Blood glucose determination at any one time will provide data concerning the state of the body's metabolism for that specific point in the individual's daily cycle. However, the practitioner must bear in mind that the metabolic processes are determined by the state of nutrition and the energy expenditure. The normal individual, in dynamic equilibrium, will show remarkable variation throughout the day; the picture is even more complex in disease.

Care of specimens for blood glucose determination deserves special attention; glucose values for whole blood decrease 10 mg/100 ml per hour (at room temperature) unless a satisfactory preservative is employed. Fluoride is currently recognized as the most effective preservative.

Glucose analysis is accomplished by reducing and enzymatic methods. In both cases a protein-free filtrate of the blood sample is tested. The reducing methods include the Folin-Wu and Somogyi-Nelson tests, both of which consist of color changes that occur in copper solutions. The enzymatic (glucose oxidase) tests measure hydrogen peroxide that is released during the enzymatic conversion of glucose to gluconic acid.

Blood glucose values are 120 to 130 mg/100 ml in mild hyperglycemia, and greater than 500 mg/100 ml in marked hyperglycemia.

BLOOD GLUCOSE: NORMAL VALUES AND DEVIATIONS

Normal values
Serum or plasma: 70 to 110 mg/100 ml (Folin-Wu)
65 to 90 mg/100 ml (Somogyi-Nelson)
65 to 90 mg/100 ml (glucose oxidase)

Deviations	Etiology	Possible effects
Hyperglycemia	Diabetes mellitus (most common cause)	Ketoacidosis
	Pancreatic insufficiency	Diuresis if >160 to 180 mg/1
	Cushing's disease	bond
	Treatment with steroids	↓ CO$_2$ combining
	↑ Catecholamines	power >500
	Pheochromocytoma	mg/100 ml
	Pancreatic neoplasm	
	Hyperthyroidism (look for hypocholesterolemia)	
	Thiazide diuretics	
Hypoglycemia	Beta cell neoplasm (hyperinsulinism)	
	Addison's disease	
	Hypothyroidism	
	Hepatocellular disease	
	Starvation (late)	
	Glycogen storage diseases	

A rising blood glucose concentration stimulates excessive insulin secretion in some individuals. Some amino acids (leucine) may also stimulate excessive beta cell secretion. Thus, glucose levels may be depleted as the insulin effects are manifested.

Two-hour postprandial glucose test. The 2-hour postprandial glucose test consists of the serial collection of samples for blood glucose determination following a 100-g carbohydrate meal given to a client who has fasted for 12 hours. The following represent hyperglycemia results:

Time	Blood glucose determination
1 hour after meal	>170 mg/100 ml
2 hours after meal	>120 mg/100 ml

Glucose tolerance test. The glucose tolerance test is performed in the fasting individual following the ingestion of 100 g of glucose; the blood glucose level rises 30 to 60 mg/100 ml above the fasting level by 30 minutes. By the end of an hour the blood glucose level begins to decline (20 to 50 mg/100 ml), and after 2 to 3 hours returns to the fasting level. Urine specimens are collected. Glucose does not appear in the urine of the normal individual during the course of the glucose tolerance test. The glucose tolerance test shows elevated values in the period following myocardial infarction.

Bilirubin

Bilirubin is a pigment that is mainly derived from the breakdown of heme in the hemoglobin of RBCs in Kupffer's cells of the reticuloendothelial system. The pigment has a golden hue and is the major pigment found in bile. Plasma containing the pigment enters the hepatic parenchymal cells and is enzymatically conjugated with glucuronic acid in preparation for excretion. The conjugated bilirubin is soluble in an aqueous medium and is actively excreted into the bile. A small amount of the conjugated bilirubin is returned to the blood and accounts for the direct-reacting bilirubin found in the plasma of normal subjects. Because it passes through membranes, it may be detected in the urine.

Intestinal bacteria act on bilirubin to form urobilinogen. Since urobilinogen is highly soluble, it is readily reabsorbed through the intestinal mucosa into the blood and is for the most part recycled in the liver back to the intestine; some, however, is excreted in the urine.

Bilirubin is analyzed through its reaction (color change) with diazo reagents; this is the basis of van den Bergh's test. The conjugated form reacts expediently with the diazo reagents in aqueous solution and is called direct reacting. The unconjugated form must be treated with methyl alcohol for the reaction to occur and is called indirect reacting.

Bilirubin is called unconjugated, free, or indirect reacting before it is combined with glucuronic acid in the liver cell. It does not cross the membranes of the capillary or of the glomerular capsule. After combination with glucuronic acid in the hepatic cells, bilirubin is referred to as conjugated, glucuronide, or direct reacting. The routine test, however, gives only the total value.

The occurrence of jaundice (yellowish tint of the skin) represents the failure to remove or excrete the bilirubin. The skin may appear jaundiced when serum bilirubin levels are about three times the normal value. In most individuals pigmentation of the tissues is visible when serum bilirubin levels exceed 1.5 mg/100 ml.

SERUM BILIRUBIN: NORMAL VALUES AND DEVIATIONS

Normal values

Total: 0.1 to 1.2 mg/100 ml
Newborn total: 1 to 12 mg/100 ml

Deviations	Etiology	Possible effects
Hyperbili-rubinemia	Destruction of red cells Hemolytic diseases ($\downarrow$ hemoglobin) Hemorrhage Hematoma Hepatic dysfunction	Jaundice
$\uparrow$ Unconjugated bilirubin	Autoimmune disease Transfusion-initiated hemolysis Hemolytic diseases Sickle cell anemia Pernicious anemia Glucuronyl transferase deficiency (hemolytic disease of the newborn) Hemorrhage (bleeding into body cavities) Hematoma Impaired hepatic uptake of bile (infectious or toxic hepatitis)	Brain damage (22 mg/100 ml or more)
$\uparrow$ Conjugated bilirubin	Impaired glucuronide excretion Hepatocellular disease (infectious, toxic, or autoimmune hepatitis) Cirrhosis Obstruction of biliary ducts Calculi Tumor Extrinsic pressure Cholangiolitis	"Regurgitation" of conjugated bilirubin back into the blood

Blood urea nitrogen

Urea is the end product of protein metabolism and is formed through deamination of amino acids in the liver. Urea is excreted by the kidneys.

Ingestion of protein does not cause a significant change in the BUN level. However, in the interest of accuracy this test is done in the fasting individual.

The severity of uremia is an indicator of the seriousness of renal involvement.

BUN: NORMAL VALUES AND DEVIATIONS

Normal values

8 to 18 mg/100 ml
Normal values tend to be higher in male subjects that in female subjects.

Deviations	Etiology
Increased BUN level (uremia)	High protein intake Dehydration Protein catabolism Burns Intestinal obstruction Gastrointestinal hemorrhage Renal disease Glomerulonephritis Pyelonephritis Prostate hypertrophy
Decreased BUN level	$\downarrow$ Protein ingestion Starvation Liver dysfunction Cirrhosis (loss of 80% to 85% hepatic function)

Creatinine

The metabolism of creatinine phosphate, a high-energy compound produced in skeletal muscle, results in the production of creatinine. The serum creatinine level does not vary markedly with diet or exercise and may be regarded as an indicator of total muscle mass.

Creatinine clearance by the kidney has been used as a measure of renal function. In addition to the serum creatinine level being fairly constant, creatinine clearance as a measure offers another advantage to the client in that an intravenous injection of the substance used in the clearance study is not needed. Renal plasma clearance of creatinine (C) is equal to the rate of creatinine excretion (UV) divided by the plasma concentration of creatinine (P):

$$C = \frac{UV}{P}$$

Since endogenous creatinine is fully filtered in the glomerulus and not reabsorbed by the tubules, its clearance is a useful clinical tool for estimation of the glomerular filtration rate (GFR). Thus, the removal of creatinine from the blood is a measure of renal efficiency. As renal function declines, the creatinine level rises.

SERUM CREATININE: NORMAL VALUES AND DEVIATION

Normal values

0.6 to 1.2 mg/100 ml
Normal values for male subjects are slightly higher than for female subjects.

Deviation	Etiology	Possible effects
Hypercreatinemia	Renal disease (75% of nephrons are nonfunctional) Chronic glomerulonephritis Nephrosis Pyelonephritis Hyperthyroidism	Signs of renal failure

Uric acid

Uric acid production is the final step in purine metabolism. Uric acid is not in stable solution at a normal human blood pH of 7.4. Uric acid is continuously produced in the human being and is excreted by the kidney. The quantity of uric acid found in the urine is about 10% of that which is filtered. Thus, it is obvious that uric acid is reabsorbed in the proximal tubules. It has been further shown that uric acid is secreted in the proximal tubules.

However, reabsorption overrides this process, and the plasma uric acid represents the balance of uric acid production and excretion.

SERUM URIC ACID: NORMAL VALUES AND DEVIATION

Normal values
Females: 2 to 6.4 mg/100 ml
Males: 2.1 to 7.8 mg/100 ml

Deviation	Etiology	Possible effects
Hyperuricemia (gout)	↑ Destruction of nucleic acid and purine products	Monosodium urate precipitate in joints (tophi)
	Chronic lymphocytic and granulocytic leukemia	Often associated with hyperlipidemia, atheromatosis
	Multiple myeloma	
	Chronic renal failure	Impaired clearance of uric acid
	Fasting	
	↑ Ingestion of protein	
	↓ Excretion of uric acid	
	Gout	
	Fasting	
	Toxemia of pregnancy	
	Glomerulonephritis	
	Thiazide diuretics	
	Alpha-lipoprotein deficiency (Tangier disease)	
	Hypoparathyroidism	
	↑ Salicylate ingestion	
	Ethanol ingestion	

Monosodium urate deposits may occur in the presence of a normal serum uric acid value.

Hypouricemia is seldom observed unless the client is being treated with allopurinol, which depresses uric acid production.

Total proteins

Plasma proteins make up approximately 7% of the plasma volume. Albumin and globulin in the free state, as well as in combination with lipid and carbohydrate substances, are the major plasma proteins. Through the application of zone electrophoresis and ultracentrifugation, the plasma proteins have been defined as albumin, the globulins (alpha-1, alpha-2, beta-1, beta-2, and gamma), lipoproteins, and fibrinogen. Separation through centrifugation is possible because the sedimentation rate at high speeds is determined by molecular size and shape. Electrophoresis is the process of migration of charged particles in an electrolyte solution through which an electrical current is passed. The proteins move at various rates, depending on size, shape, and electrical charge.

Immunoelectrophoresis separates the immune globulin fractions through a combination of electrophoresis and immunodiffusion.

The plasma proteins are large molecules that do not readily diffuse through the capillary membrane. The small amount of protein that does pass through the capillary wall is taken up by the lymphatic system and returned to the blood. It has been demonstrated that the plasma protein concentration exceeds that of the interstitial space nearly four times. Since the plasma proteins are the only dissolved substances in the plasma that do not pass through the capillary membrane, they are responsible for plasma oncotic pressure. Thus, proteins help to regulate intravascular volume. The plasma proteins also serve as buffers in acid-base balance and as binding and transporting agents for lipids, triglycerides, hormones, vitamins, calcium, and copper. In addition, they participate in blood coagulation. Furthermore, in the event that body tissues become depleted of protein, plasma proteins may be used for replenishment. The liver synthesizes nearly all of the plasma albumin and fibrinogen and about one-half of the globulins.

The rate of synthesis is dependent on the availability of amino acids in the plasma.

Normal plasma protein values
Total: 6 to 7.8 g/100 ml
Albumin: 3.2 to 4.5 g/100 ml
Globulins: 2.3 to 3.5 g/100 ml
  Alpha-1 globulin   0.2 to 0.4 g/100 ml
  Alpha-2 globulin   0.5 to 0.9 g/100 ml
  Beta globulin   0.5 to 1.0 g/100 ml
  Gamma globulin   1.0 to 2.0 g/100 ml
Fibrinogen: 0.2 to 0.4 gm/100 ml

ALBUMIN

Normal plasma albumin, essentially all of which is synthesized in the liver, makes up 52% to 68% of the blood protein and is responsible for 80% of the oncotic pressure. Thyroxine, bilirubin, fatty acids, salicylates, barbiturates, and other drugs are bound and transported by albumin. Since the albumin molecule is small in comparison to other blood proteins, it is the plasma protein most frequently detected in the urine in the event of renal damage.

SERUM ALBUMIN: NORMAL VALUES AND DEVIATION

Normal values: 3.2 to 4.5 g/100 ml

Deviation	Etiology
Hypoalbuminemia (2.5 g or less)	Chronic liver disease
	Protein malnutrition
	Malabsorption syndrome, especially of protein
	Nephrotic syndrome
	Chronic infection
	Acute stress

Serum albumin elevation is seldom encountered.

The normal pregnant woman has decreased albumin levels that are progressive through delivery and do not return to normal until 8 weeks postpartum.

GLOBULINS

The five globulin fractions serve as transport media or antibodies. Approximately 50% of the globulins are manufactured by the liver; the remainder are synthesized in the lymphatic tissue and other reticuloendothelial cells.

Alpha-1 globulins are known to bind or act carriers for cortisol (transcortin), thyroxine (thyroxine-binding globulin), fats, lipids, and fat-soluble vitamins.

Alpha-2 globulins contain copper (ceruloplasmin), hemoglobin (haptoglobin), lipids, triglycerides, erythropoietin, glycoprotein, mucoprotein, prothrombin, angiotensinogen, enzymes such as cholinesterase, lactic acid dehydrogenase, and alkaline phosphatase.

Beta globulins bind and transport heme (hemopexin) and iron (transferrin) and include lipid-soluble vitamins, hormones, glycerides, phospholipids, lipoprotein, cholesterol, fibrinogen, profibrinolysin, and complement components.

The gamma globulin fraction includes the immunoglobulins, or antibodies, and the cryoglobulins, or cold agglutinins.

SERUM GLOBULIN: NORMAL VALUES AND DEVIATIONS

Normal values: 2.3 to 3.5 g/100 ml

Deviations	Etiology
Hyperglobulinemia	Hypergammaglobulinemia
	Hodgkin's disease
	Leukemia
	Myeloproliferative diseases (multiple myeloma)
	Chronic granulomatous infectious diseases (tuberculosis)
	Chronic hepatitis
	Collagen disease
	Sarcoidosis
Alteration in globulin fractions	
Absence of alpha-1 globulins	Alpha-1 (antitrypsin deficiency)
↓ Alpha-1 globulins	Nephrotic syndrome
↑ Alpha-2 globulins	Stress situations
	Infection
	Injury
	Surgery
	Tissue necrosis
	Myocardial infarction
	Nephrotic syndrome
↑ Beta globulins	Pregnancy (third trimester)
	Associated with serum cholesterol
	Hypothyroidism
	Biliary cirrhosis
	Nephrosis

↓ Gamma globulins	Obstructive jaundice
	Hepatitis
	Hypogammaglobulinemia
	Nephrotic syndrome
	Lymphosarcoma
	Lymphocytic leukemia
	Multiple myeloma
↑ Gamma globulins	Infections
	Collagen diseases
	Hypersensitivity diseases
	Hodgkin's disease
	Malignant lymphoma
	Chronic lymphocytic leukemia
	Multiple myeloma
	Liver disease
	Hepatitis
	Cirrhosis
	Obstructive jaundice

ALBUMIN-GLOBULIN RATIO

In the normal client, the albumin is about double that of globulin.

Normal A/G ratio: 1.5:2.5

An A/G ratio of 2.5:3 is strongly suggestive of chronic liver disease.

The levels of each of the globulins obtained from the electrophoretic zone patterns are more valuable data than the A/G ratio.

FIBRINOGEN

The bulk of fibrinogen is produced in the liver. Fibrinogen is the precursor of fibrin.

SERUM FIBRINOGEN: NORMAL VALUES AND DEVIATIONS

Normal values: 0.2 to 0.4 g/100 ml

Deviation	Etiology	Possible effects
Hypofibrinogenemia	Hepatic dysfunction	Disseminated intravascular coagulation

Lipids

Several lipid elements are present in the normal plasma: triglyceride, cholesterol, and phospholipid. They circulate as lipoproteins, which are macromolecular complexes of lipids and carrier proteins (apoproteins) that render them soluble in the aqueous media of the blood. The lipids that are transported in the blood are comprised of exogenous triglycerides (glycerol esterified with fatty acids from ingested foods), endogenous triglycerides (manufactured by the liver), cholesterol, and phospholipids. All of the serum lipoproteins contain these same substances and vary only in the amount of each substance and in the size of the molecule.

EXOGENOUS TRIGLYCERIDES

Exogenous triglycerides are the major constituent of chylomicrons, the largest lipids; these lipids contain a lesser quantity of cholesterol (10%), phospholipids (7%), and protein (24%). Chylomicrons transport exogenous triglyceride following absorption from the small intestine to sites for use or storage.

The high triglyceride content results in a density less than water. Thus, the chylomicrons may rise to the top of blood that is left standing. The large size of the molecule results in light scattering, resulting in a turbid appearance of the plasma. The disappearance of chylomicrons from the blood is dependent on the presence of the enzyme lipoprotein lipase. The chylomicrons should return to basal levels within 6 hours following a fat-containing test meal. Chylomicrons are absent during fasting.

Since the chylomicron (and thus, triglyceride) level varies with dietary intake of fats, the most valuable data concerning lipid levels are obtained from testing done in the fasting state.

ENDOGENOUS TRIGLYCERIDES

Endogenous triglycerides are manufactured by the liver. Hepatic triglyceride synthesis appears to be independent of the sudden increase in dietary intake of fats but shows a relationship to the total ingestion of foodstuffs, particularly in regard to caloric value.

Endogenous triglycerides are transported to sites for use or storage in molecules that are less dense than chylomicrons; these molecules are called very low-density (prebeta) lipoproteins (VLDLs). Endogenous triglycerides are the major constituent (55%) of these molecules; protein contributes a lesser amount (2% to 15%), and the remainder is made up of free and esterified cholesterol and phospholipids. Since chylomicrons are absent after a 6-hour fast, the majority of the circulating triglyceride is in the VLDL fraction.

Low-density lipoproteins (LDLs). Use and storage of triglyceride (exogenous and endogenous) is possible following release from the chylomicrons and VLDLs. The chylomicrons are cleared by the liver while the VLDL remnants become an intermediate density called low-density (beta) lipoproteins (LDLs).

High-density lipoproteins (HDLs). The enzyme lecithin-cholesterol acyltransferase and high-density (alpha) lipoproteins (HDLs) are responsible for the clearance of cholesterol from peripheral tissues. The HDLs transport cellular cholesterol from the periphery to the liver. It has been suggested that less than normal levels of HDL may be responsible for ineffective cholesterol clearance from the cells. Since the cholesterol remains in the cell, the entry of LDL cholesterol would be inhibited, resulting in increased plasma levels of LDL.

Epidemiological data as well as genetic and metabolic studies have served to associate LDL cholesterol directly to coronary artery disease, while an inverse relationship exists between HDL and coronary heart disease. Thus, HDL is the most positive indicator of the risk of coronary heart disease.

Lipoprotein phenotype	Cholesterol	Triglyceride	Lipoprotein
Type I		↑	Severe hyperchylomicronemia
Type IIa	↑		↑ LDL increase
Type IIb	↑	↑	↑ LDL and VLDL
Type III	↑	↑	↑ Remnants
Type IV		↑	↑ VLDL
Type V		↑	↑ Chylomicrons and VLDL

Lipoprotein phenotypes	Genetic classification	Plasma lipoprotein elevation
Type I	Familial lipoprotein lipase deficiency	Chylomicrons
Type IIa	Hypercholesterolemia (monogenic)	LDL
Type IIb	Hypercholesterolemia (polygenic)	LDL and VLDL
Type IIa, IIb, or IV	Familial hyperlipidemia (combined)	LDL and VLDL
Type III	Broad beta disease	Remnants
Type IV or V	Familial hypertriglyceridemia	VLDL

Familial lipoprotein lipase deficiency and familial hypertriglyceridemia have not been shown to be related to coronary artery disease. Monogenic hypercholesterolemia is the result of a defect in LDL uptake by peripheral cells. Affected individuals may have cutaneous xanthomas, xanthelasma, and retinal lipemia.

Laboratory tests of plasma lipids and lipoproteins include total cholesterol, total triglyceride, HDL, LDL, cholesterol/HDL ratio, phenotype determination, and centrifugation and separation.

Clinically significant hyperlipoproteinemia is said to exist with the following values:

Age of subject	Total plasma cholesterol	Plasma triglyceride
20 years	200 mg/100 ml	140 mg/100 ml
20 years	240 mg/100 ml	200 mg/100 ml

PHOSPHOLIPIDS

Lecithin and sphingomyelin are the major serum phospholipids. Phospholipids are constituents of both HDLs and LDLs.

Normal serum phospholipid values: 150 to 375 mg/100 ml

TOTAL SERUM LIPIDS: NORMAL VALUES AND DEVIATIONS

Normal values: 350 to 800 mg/100 ml (adult)

Deviations	Etiology	Predominant lipoprotein
Cholesterol: marked elevation; triglyceride: no change or elevation	↑ Ingestion of cholesterol	LDL (Type IIa)

Deviations	Etiology	Predominant lipoprotein

Cholesterol: elevation; triglyceride: no change or elevation	↑ Cholesterol manufacture by liver
	  Obesity
	  Hereditary
	↓ LDL catabolism
	  Hypothyroidism
	  Hereditary
		LDL (Type IIa) or LDL and VLDL (Type IIb)

	↓ Remnant removal
	  Hypothyroidism
	  Hereditary
		Remnants (Type III) or VLDL and chylomicrons (Type V)

Cholesterol: no change or elevation; triglyceride; elevation	↑ Triglyceride synthesis
	  Dietary intake (caloric)
	  Alcohol
	  Hyperinsulinism
	    Obesity
	    Corticosteroids
	  Estrogen
	  Hereditary
		VLDL (Type IV) or VLDL and chylomicrons (Type V)

	↓ Triglyceride clearance
	  Insulin (diabetes)
	  Hypothyroidism
	  Renal failure
	  Hereditary
		VLDL (Type IV) or VLDL and chylomicrons (Type V)

Deviations	Etiology	Possible effects
Hypercholesterolemia (marked: >400 mg/100 ml)	Liver disease Nephrotic stage of glomerulonephritis Familial hypercholesterolemia Hypothyroidism Pancreatic dysfunction Diabetes mellitus	Associated with ↑ alkaline phosphatase, ↑ bilirubin, ↑ BUN, ↑ creatinine
Hypocholesterolemia (significant: <150 mg/100 ml)	↓ Ingestion of cholesterol Malnutrition Fasting Liver disease Megaloblastic or hypochromic anemia ↑ Estrogen ↑ Thyroid hormone Hypermetabolic states Fever Exercise	

CHOLESTEROL

Exogenous cholesterol is absorbed from the small intestine into the lymph. Endogenous cholesterol is formed by all the cells of the body. Most of the endogenous cholesterol in the plasma is formed by the liver from acetate. It is the endogenous cholesterol that is measured in blood chemistry profiles. A control mechanism exists for these two processes, since endogenous cholesterol production is inhibited when cholesterol ingestion is increased. Cholesterol is present in the plasma primarily as LDLs. The LDL cholesterol is taken up by most peripheral tissues. This is a modified receptor process. In addition, most tissues are capable of cholesterol synthesis. Increased uptake of LDL inhibits cellular cholesterol production and decreased uptake results in increased cholesterol synthesis in the peripheral cells.

Cholesterol testing was the forerunner of serum lipid analysis and has served as a valuable but debatable tool for prediction of coronary artery disease due to atheromatous or arteriosclerotic artery disease.

Because the liver esterifies cholesterol, the ratio of esterified to unesterified cholesterol may be considered an indication of liver function. The normal serum esterified cholesterol value ranges from 20% to 30%.

Obstruction of the biliary ducts is typified by an increased cholesterol level with a decrease in the amount of esterified cholesterol.

SERUM CHOLESTEROL: NORMAL VALUES AND DEVIATIONS

Normal values: 150 to 250 mg/100 ml

Enzymes

Enzymes are individual molecules or aggregates of protein molecules occurring in globular form. Enzymes act as catalysts to biochemical reactions. In the event of cellular destruction of an organ or tissue, the cytoplasmic enzymes are released into the plasma from the diseased cells. Enzymes are categorized by their functional effect. These groupings are called isoenzymes. Isoenzymes are enzymes with the same functional effect but with variations in configuration and physical characteristics. The isoenzyme content of many tissues and structures has been determined. There is sufficient variation in the enzyme content of the various organs that changes in the enzyme concentration in the blood may serve as an indicator of the site of disease. Electrophoresis may be used to separate these proteins. Serum enzyme determination results are also used to assess tissue rejection following transplantation procedures.

SGOT, serum LDH, and serum alkaline phosphatase determinations are included in most screening laboratory examinations. Enzyme determinations currently and commonly encountered in clinical practice are described in this section.

SERUM GLUTAMIC-OXALOACETIC TRANSAMINASE (SGOT)

SGOT is found in many tissues. The transaminase enzymes catalyze the conversion of an amino acid to a keto acid while another keto acid is converted to an amino acid in the glycolytic cycle. This enzyme catalyzes conversions of glutamic and oxaloacetic acids. High tissue concentrations of SGOT have been demonstrated for the heart and liver, but appreciable amounts are found in RBCs, muscle, and kidney.

Colorimetric and spectrophotometric techniques are used in determining the serum concentration of these enzymes. Elevated levels of the enzyme may be identified 8 hours after tissue damage occurs. In the case of a single injury (such as myocardial infarction) that is not followed by further damage, the enzyme reaches a peak level in 24 to 36 hours and declines to basal levels in about 4 to 6 days.

The SGOT concentration is directly related to the degree of cellular damage.

SGOT: NORMAL VALUES AND DEVIATION

Normal values: 8 to 33 U/100 ml (Reitman-Frankel)
10 to 40 mU/ml (SMA 12/60)

Deviation	Etiology
Elevation of SGOT values	
Elevation greater than 1,000 U/ml (or more than 10 times normal)	Myocardial infarction
	Hepatocellular disease
	Infectious or toxic hepatitis
	Liver necrosis
Elevation to 40 to 100 U/ml	Tachyarrhythmias
	Congestive heart failure
	Myocarditis
	Pericarditis
	Pulmonary infarction
	Cirrhosis
	Cholangitis
	Pancreatitis
	Metastatic liver disease
	Generalized infection (infectious mononucleosis)
	Trauma
	Shock
	Muscle disease
	Muscular dystrophy
	Dermatomyositis
	Skeletal muscle damage
	Generalized infection

SERUM GLUTAMIC-PYRUVIC TRANSAMINASE (SGPT)

SGPT catalyzes conversions between glutamic and pyruvic acid in the glycolytic pathway. The liver contains the highest concentration of SGPT, but the enzyme is prominent in kidney, heart, and skeletal muscle. The pattern of release of SGPT is similar to SGOT in the face of cellular damage, though more damage than that necessary to produce an elevation of SGOT is generally present when SGPT levels are increased.

SERUM SGPT: NORMAL VALUES AND DEVIATION

Normal values: 5 to 35 U/ml (Reitman-Frankel)

Deviation	Etiology
Elevation of SGPT values	
Marked elevation	Infectious or toxic hepatitis
	Infectious mononucleosis
Moderate elevation	Obstructive jaundice
	Postnecrotic cirrhosis
Slight elevation	Cirrhosis
	Myocardial infarction

LACTIC DEHYDROGENASE (LDH)

The tissue concentrations of LDH mimic those of SGOT. Furthermore, elevations in serum LDH levels correlate with the same conditions underlying increases in SGOT concentrations. LDH catalyzes the conversions between pyruvate and lactate in the glycolytic cycle. Following myocardial infarction, serum LDH levels increase five to six times in the first 48 hours and may remain elevated for 6 to 10 days. LDH has been separated into five isoenzymes, making it a sharper diagnostic tool. These isoenzymes may be separated by electrophoresis.

A variety of colorimetric tests are available for assessment of this serum enzyme concentration.

A hemolyzed blood specimen may give spuriously high values for LDH concentration in the serum since the damaged RBCs give up LDH; this will be reflected in the concentration of the enzyme in the sample.

Since the 1970s particular emphasis has been placed on the use of the isoenzymes of LDH. There are five isoenzymes of LDH, designated LDH_1 to LDH_5. Normally LDH_2 is greater than LDH_1 in the serum. However, the myocardium has an abundant LDH_1 content, and following myocardial infarction, the serum value of LDH_1 may exceed LDH_2. Thus, the LDH_1/LDH_2 ratio becomes greater; this is referred to as a reversed or flipped ratio. Increases in LDH_1 also occur in hemolytic states, hyperthyroidism, megaloblastic anemia, renal disease, and gastric malignancy.

SERUM LDH: NORMAL VALUES AND DEVIATION

Normal values: 200 to 400 U/ml (Wroblewski)
100 to 225 mU/ml (SMA 12/60)

Deviation	Etiology
Evaluation of LDH values	
Elevation greater than 1,400 Wroblewski units	Hemolytic disorders (marked hemolysis)
	Pernicious anemia
	Myocardial infarction
Elevation of 500 to 700 Wroblewski units	Chronic viral hepatitis
	Malignant neoplasms
	Liver
	Kidney
	Brain
	Skeletal muscle
	Heart
	Destruction of lung tissue
	Pulmonary emboli
	Pneumonia
	Destruction of renal tissue
	Infarction
	Infection
	Generalized viral infection

ALKALINE PHOSPHATASE

Determinations of serum alkaline phosphatase levels are frequently used to determine the presence of liver and bone cell disease since the enzyme has its greatest content in these two tissues. However, it is also found in significant concentrations in intestine, kidney, and placenta. The enzyme is thought to catalyze reactions in the process of bone matrix formation, because increased serum alkaline phosphatase levels correlate with osteoblastic activity. The isoenzymes from the liver, bone, intestine, kidney, and placenta can be separated by electrophoresis; thus, the source of the enzyme can be determined. Synthesis of alkaline phosphatase is thought to be small in the normal hepatic cell. The serum alkaline phosphatase level reflects placental function and may be used to monitor the progress of pregnancy.

A low alkaline phosphatase level may be associated with hypophosphatemia, hypothyroidism, or vitamin C deficiency.

SERUM ALKALINE PHOSPHATASE: NORMAL VALUES AND DEVIATION

Normal values

Adults: 1.5 to 4.5 U/100 ml (Bodansky)
4 to 13 U/100 ml (King-Armstrong)
0.8 to 2.3 U/ml (Bessey-Lowry)
30 to 100 mU/ml (SMA 12/60)

Children: 5 to 14 U/100 ml (Bodansky)
3.4 to 9 U/ml (Bessey-Lowry)
15 to 30 U/100 ml (King-Armstrong)
(The level in children is about three times that of the adult.)

Deviation	Etiology
Elevation of alkaline phosphatase values	
Marked elevation (15 U/100 ml or more—Bodansky)	Liver disease
	Obstructive disease
	Neoplasm
	Bone disease
	Paget's disease
	Sarcoma
	Metastatic carcinoma
Slight to moderate elevation (8 to 10 U/100 ml—Bodansky)	Liver disease
	Cholangitis
	Cirrhosis
	Hyperparathyroidism
	Osteomalacia
	Renal infarction, tissue rejection

ACID PHOSPHATASE

Acid phosphatase occurs in greatest amount in prostatic tissue. In the normal individual the enzyme is excreted in prostatic fluids. However, in prostatic metastatic carcinoma, the serum acid phosphatase level rises and thus becomes a tool in differential diagnosis.

Normal serum acid phosphatase values: 1 to 4 U/100 ml (King-Armstrong)

CREATINE PHOSPHOKINASE (CPK)

CPK catalyzes the phosphorylation of creatine by adenosine triphosphate (ATP). The greatest tissue content of CPK is found in skeletal and cardiac muscle, although significant amounts occur in the brain. The serum CPK level may be elevated as a result of intramuscular injection or following surgery and returns to basal levels in 24 to 48 hours. Since CPK is not produced by the liver, elevated serum values of this enzyme may help eliminate liver disease in differential diagnosis.

Recent investigations have shown the usefulness of measuring the three isoenzymes of CPK, designated as M, B, and MB. The M isoenzyme is present in skeletal and cardiac muscle, the B isoenzyme is found in the brain, and the MB isoenzyme is found in relatively high concentrations in the cardiac muscle but is also present in the skeletal muscle. The MB fraction has specific predictability in relation to myocardial infarction; it is typically the first enzyme detectable in abnormal concentration in serum following myocardial damage. The isoenzyme is first detectable 3 to 5 hours after infarction and reaches its peak 12 to 24 hours, with a rapid decline to normal values in 24 to 48 hours.

CPK–MB is also elevated in individuals with muscle trauma, polymyositis, muscular dystrophy, neuromuscular disease, pulmonary embolism, tachyarrhythmias, and unstable angina.

SERUM CPK: NORMAL VALUES AND DEVIATION

Normal values: 0 to 200 units (Sigma)
Males: 5 to 50 mU/ml (Oliver-Rosalki)
Females: 5 to 30 mU/ml (Oliver-Rosalki)

Deviation	Etiology
Elevation of serum CPK values	Muscle disease
	Duchenne's muscular dystrophy (early)
	Dermatomyositis
	Polymyositis
	Trauma
	Myocardial infarction
	Encephalitis
	Bacterial meningitis
	Cerebrovascular accident
	Hepatic coma
	Uremic coma
	Strenuous exercise
	Ingestion of salicylates

ALDOLASE

Aldolase catalyzes the splitting of fructose 1,6-diphosphate into glyceraldehyde phosphate and dihydroxyacetone phosphate. Aldolase occurs in greatest concentration in skeletal and heart muscle, but the liver contains a moderate amount, and all tissues contain some of the enzyme.

SERUM ALDOLASE: NORMAL VALUES AND DEVIATION

Normal values: 3 to 8 U/100 ml (Sibley-Lehninger)

Deviation	Etiology
Elevation of serum aldolase values	Muscle disease
	Progressive muscular dystrophy

Elevation of serum aldolase
values—cont'd

    Dermatomyositis
    Trichinosis
    Myocardial infarction
    Viral hepatitis
    Hepatic cellular necrosis
    Granulocytic leukemia
    Carcinomatosis

AMYLASE

Pancreatic amylase is synthesized in the pancreatic cells and secreted into the pancreatic ducts for transport to the duodenum, where it catalyzes the hydrolysis of starch and glycogen. Elevated serum amylase levels may be used to monitor damage to pancreatic cells. Although the salivary glands produce amylase, diseases of these cells do not affect the serum lipase level.

SERUM AMYLASE: NORMAL VALUES AND DEVIATION

Normal values: 60 to 150 U/100 ml (Somogyi)

Deviation	Etiology
Elevation of serum amylase values	Acute pancreatitis

LIPASE

Lipase is synthesized by the pancreatic cells and secreted into the pancreatic ducts for transport to the duodenum, where it catalyzes the hydrolysis of triglycerides to fatty acids. Elevation of serum lipase concentrations indicates damage to pancreatic cells. Serum lipase levels remain elevated longer following acute pancreatitis than do amylase levels.

SERUM LIPASE: NORMAL VALUES AND DEVIATION

Normal values: 0 to 1.5 U/ml (Cherry-Crandall)

Deviation	Etiology
Elevation of serum lipase values (lipasemia)	Acute pancreatitis

CHOLINESTERASE

Cholinesterase (ChE) catalyzes the hydrolysis of acetylcholine and other cholinesters and has been classified as "true" cholinesterase or as pseudocholinesterase. True cholinesterase, or acetylcholinesterase, is more rapid in its action on acetylcholine and is found in greatest concentration in the brain and in RBCs. Pseudocholinesterase is found in plasma but not in the erythrocytes and is thought to be manufactured by the liver. Both of these enzymes are inactivated by organophosphates. Testing of acetylcholinesterase provides an indication of toxicity from insecticides containing these compounds.

    Normal ChE (RBC) values: 0.65 to 1.00 pH units
    Pseudocholinesterase (plasma): 0.5 to 1.3 pH units

SCREENING HEMATOLOGICAL EXAMINATIONS

The hemogram, or complete blood cell count (CBC), includes the following determinations: RBC count, hematocrit (HCT), hemoglobin (Hgb), white blood cell (WBC) count, and differential WBC count. Other commonly performed hematological examinations are determinations of the mean corpuscular volume (MCV), mean corpuscular hemoglobin (MCH), and mean corpuscular hemoglobin concentration (MCHC).

Red blood cells

RBC COUNT

Erythropoiesis, the manufacture of RBCs, occurs in the bone marrow. Erythropoietin, a hormone produced by the kidney exposed to hypoxia, plays a prominent role in the control of erythropoiesis.

Electronic counting devices (such as the Coulter device) are faster and produce more accurate blood cell determinations than those of a technician counting the smear under a microscope.

Both anemias and polycythemias are classified as relative if they result from changes in plasma volume.

RED BLOOD CELLS: NORMAL COUNTS AND DEVIATIONS

Normal counts
    Males: 4.6 to $6.2 \times 10^6/\mu l$
    Females: 4.2 to $5.4 \times 10^6/\mu l$

Deviations	Etiology	Possible effects
Elevated RBC count (polycythemia)	Bone marrow hyperplasia (polycythemia vera)	Hyperviscosity of blood Tendency toward thrombosis Sluggish blood flow to tissues (tissue hypoxia) Hypervolemia Headache Tinnitus Dizziness Ruddy cyanosis

Decreased RBC count (anemia)	RBC production deficiency states
	  Protein
	  Iron
	  Vitamin B_{12}
	  Folic acid
	Toxicity (depressed bone marrow)
	Metabolites (urea, creatinine)
	Drugs (chloramphenicol)
	Ionizing radiation
	Hypothyroidism
	Hereditary (thalassemia)
		Pallor
		Fatigue
		Rapid pulse
		Irritability
		Headache
		Dizziness
		Postural hypotension
		Menstrual irregularities
		Angina
		Shortness of breath

HEMATOCRIT

The hematocrit examination is used to determine the volume-packed (centrifuged) RBCs in 100 ml of blood.

Normal hematocrit values
Males: 40% to 54%
Females: 38% to 47%

HEMOGLOBIN

Hemoglobin consists of heme, a pigmented compound containing iron, and globin, a colorless protein. Hemoglobin binds with oxygen as well as with carbon dioxide. The hemoglobin molecule binds oxygen and transports it to the periphery; it binds carbon dioxide as it is transported to the lung.

Normal hemoglobin values
Males: 13.5 to 18 g/100 ml
Females: 12.0 to 16 g/100 ml

MEAN CORPUSCULAR VOLUME

The MCV test measures RBCs in terms of individual cell size. The value can be calculated through the use of the following formula:

$$MCV = \frac{HCT}{RBC}$$

The result is expressed in microcubic millimeters per blood cell.

Normal MCV: 80 to 94 μmm^3

This test is used to classify anemias as microcytic (RBC size smaller than normal), normocytic, or macrocytic (larger than normal).

Deviations	Etiology
Microcytic anemia	Hypochromic
	Iron deficiency
	Thalassemia
	Chronic infections
	Chronic renal disease
	Malignancy
Normocytic anemia	Hypochromic
	Lead poisoning
	Chronic infection
	Chronic renal disease
	Malignancy
	Normochromic
	Hemorrhage
	Hemolytic anemia
	Bone marrow hypoplasia
	Splenomegaly
Macrocytic anemia	Normochromic
	Pernicious anemia
	Folic acid deficiency
	Hypothyroidism
	Hepatocellular disease

MEAN CORPUSCULAR HEMOGLOBIN

The MCH examination measures the hemoglobin concentration of the individual RBCs. Expressed in picograms (micromicrograms), it can be calculated by dividing the hemoglobin in grams by the RBCs:

$$MCH = \frac{Hgb}{RBC}$$

The test allows the classification of anemia as hypochromic or normochromic.

Normal MCH values: 27 to 31 pg

MEAN CORPUSCULAR HEMOGLOBIN CONCENTRATION

The MCHC test measures the concentration of hemoglobin in grams per 100 ml of RBCs. Expressed in percentages, it can be calculated using the following formula:

$$MCHC = \frac{Hgb\ in\ grams}{HCT}$$

Normal mean cell hemoglobin concentration: 32% to 36%

An elevation of MCHC is seen only in hereditary spherocytosis.

SEDIMENTATION RATE

The erythrocyte sedimentation rate (ESR) is the speed with which RBCs settle in unclotted blood. The speed with which the RBCs settle is dependent on the concentration of the various plasma protein fractions and on the concentration of the RBCs. The cells settle out more rapidly when the plasma concentration is high and the RBC count is low. Increased concentration of fibrinogen or of the globulins speeds up the rate of sedimentation. The rate of settling is accelerated in many inflammatory conditions, in pregnancy, and in multiple myeloma. The sedimentation rate is decreased is sickle cell anemia; this may be caused by the abnormal shape and stickiness of the RBCs.

Normal ESR rate (Westergren)
Men under 50: <15 mm/hr
Men over 50: <20 mm/hr
Women under 50: <20 mm/hr
Women over 50: <30 mm/hr

MICROSCOPIC RBC EXAMINATION

A stained smear of whole blood is examined microscopically to assess the morphological characteristics of the RBCs.

Normal RBC: nonnucleated, biconcave disc, 7 μ to 8 μ in diameter; contains 95% hemoglobin (Fig. 27-4)

Nucleated RBCs may be observed in periods of marked erythropoiesis as a result of marrow stimulation. These immature cells are released from the marrow and are found in the circulating blood.

Reticulocytes. A reticulocyte is a precursor to the RBC, is larger than the normal RBC, and stains more with basic dye. The center does not appear pale, as does the normal RBC. In the normal individual 0.5% to 1.5% reticulocytes are present in the circulating blood. During periods of accelerated erythropoiesis the number of reticulocytes in the general circulation increases. The reticulocyte count is generally elevated as a result of hemorrhage or hemolysis.

Nuclear fragments. Structures that represent the degenerated nucleus of the erythroblast are seen as coarse dots, blue lines, and imperfect rings in the smear.

Basophilic stippling. The term basophilic stippling refers to the presence of hemogenous blue dots observed in RBCs treated with Wright's stain. This stippling may indicate thalassemia or toxic manifestations, resulting in abnormal hemoglobin production.

Siderotic granules. Granules of iron-containing substances in addition to hemoglobin may be seen in some cells of smears of RBCs treated with Prussian blue dye. The cells are termed siderocytes and are increased in number following splenectomy and during the course of hemolytic anemias.

Heinz bodies. The RBCs of the individual with glu-

cose-6-phosphate dehydrogenase deficiency may contain inclusion bodies containing denatured hemoglobin called Heinz bodies, for example, in thalassemias.

Poikilocytosis. A poikilocyte is an RBC of abnormal shape. Poikilocytosis refers to the presence of abnormally shaped RBCs in the blood. Leptocytes (target, or "Mexican hat," erythrocytes) are characterized by a central pigment bulls-eye area surrounded by a clear area, which is ringed by a hemoglobinated peripheral border. This type of erythrocyte is seen in the blood of individuals with hemoglobin C or A, or a combination of C and S. They are frequently seen in thalassemia. Liver disease has been shown to be present in some individuals with demonstrated poikilocytosis. The sickle cell disease is characterized by long, crescent-shaped cells.

Anisocytosis. Anisocytosis is the term used for blood that contains erythrocytes with excessive variations in size.

Platelets (thrombocytes). Platelets may be seen in the microscopic examination of whole blood smears. The platelets are granular fragments of cytoplasm of megakaryocytes in the bone marrow. The platelets are largely phospholipids and polysaccharides. They are carriers for a variety of enzymes as well as for clotting factors and serotonin. Thus, platelets play a major role in blood coagulation.

Thrombocytopathy refers to platelet cells of unusual size or shape.

PLATELETS: NORMAL COUNT AND DEVIATIONS

Normal count: 300,000/μl

Deviations	Etiology
Thrombocytopenia	Bone marrow depression
Thrombocytosis	Polycythemia
	Splenectomy

WHITE BLOOD CELLS: NORMAL COUNTS AND DEVIATIONS

Normal counts: 4,500 to 11,000/μl whole blood

Deviations	Etiology
Elevated WBC count (leukocytosis)	Leukemia
	Bacterial infection
	Polycythemia (resulting from bone marrow stimulation)
Decreased WBC count (leukopenia)	Bone marrow depression
	Ionizing radiation
	Chloramphenicol
	Phenothiazines
	Sulfonamides
	Phenylbutazone
	Agranulocytosis
	Acute viral infection
	Acute alcohol ingestion

White blood cells
WBC COUNT

The WBC count is the assessment of the number of WBCs (leukocytes) in 1 μl of whole blood. The

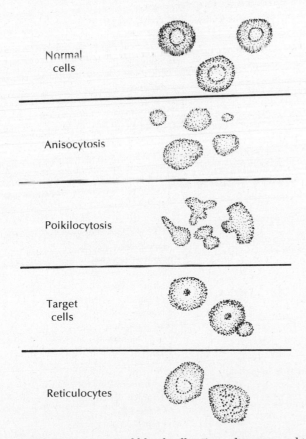

Fig. 27-4. The average red blood cell is 7μ in diameter and is slightly indented in the center. This produces a gradual lessening of color toward the center of the cell. In evaluation of shape, only cells that do not touch neighboring cells are considered. Irregularity in size is referred to as anisocytosis. Irregularity in shape is referred to as poikilocytosis. Increased basophilia is seen in younger cells, such as reticulocytes. (From Fowkes, W. C., Jr., and Hunn, V. K.: Clinical assessment for the nurse practitioner, ed. 1, St. Louis, 1973, The C. V. Mosby Co.)

WBCs function to protect the body against infectious disease. Neutrophils and monocytes destroy microorganisms by phagocytosis. Lymphocytes and plasma cells are thought to produce antibodies. Eosinophils play a role in allergy. Granulocytes, monocytes, and some lymphocytes are produced in the bone marrow; lymphocytes and plasma cells are produced in the lymph nodes and thymic tissue. Disease processes may result in changes within individual leukocyte groups, which may include morphological and functional changes as well as variations in total numbers. These alterations may provide valuable clues that can be used in differential diagnosis.

DIFFERENTIAL WBC COUNT

Six different types of WBCs have been identified in the blood: polymorphonuclear neutrophils (PMNs), polymorphonuclear eosinophils (PMEs), polymorphonuclear basophils (PMBs), monocytes, lymphocytes, and plasma cells. Platelets (thrombocytes) are particles of megakaryocytes.

Increased granulation of leukocytes may indicate toxicity reactions.

A shift to the left means that increased numbers of immature neutrophils are present in the specimen and that they are band forms rather than lobulations. Acute stress to the bone marrow and severe bacterial infection may cause the release of early granulocytes. Increased lobulation (3 to 6) or segmentation of neutrophils is often observed in association with vitamin B_{12} deficiency.

Mild to moderate leukocytosis associated with mild to moderate lymphocytosis is characteristic of chronic infections such as tuberculosis. In relative lymphocytosis the total number of circulating lymphocytes remains constant but the WBC count is low because of neutropenia. Relative lymphocytosis is normal between 4 months and 4 years of age.

Monocytosis may occur even with no increase in WBCs.

ABNORMAL WHITE BLOOD CELLS OF DIAGNOSTIC IMPORTANCE

Plasma cells. Plasma cells are not normally found in the circulating blood. The presence of plasma cells in the blood predicates the necessity to differentiate multiple myeloma, infectious mononucleosis, serum sickness, and rubella.

Downey cells. Downey cells are abnormal lymphocytes that differ from the normal cells in size, cytoplasmic structures (vacuolated, foamy), and immature chromatin pattern. These cells are observed in individuals with infectious mononucleosis, viral disease (hepatitis), and allergic states.

LE cell. The LE cell is a polymorphonuclear leukocyte, generally a neutrophil that contains an inclusion body. The inclusion body has been shown to be denatured nuclear protein that is being phagocytosed by the neutrophil. The LE cell, which can be induced in the laboratory in the presence of LE factor, is present in the blood of many individuals who have lupus erythematosis.

DIFFERENTIAL WBC COUNT: NORMAL PERCENTAGES AND DEVIATIONS

Normal differential count

Type of cell	Percentage of total WBC count	Range
Neutrophils (PMNs)	56%	50% to 70%
Eosinophils (PMEs)	2.7%	5% to 6%
Basophils (PMBs)	0.3%	0 to 1%
Lymphocytes	34%	20% to 40%
Monocytes		0 to 7%

Deviations	Etiology
Neutrophilic leukocytosis	Bacterial infections
	Pneumonia
	Systemic infections
	Inflammatory disease
	Rheumatic fever
	Rheumatoid arthritis
	Pancreatitis
	Thyroiditis
	Carcinoma
	Trauma (tissue destruction)
	Burns
	Crush injury
	Stress
	Cold
	Heat
	Exercise
	Electroshock therapy
	Panic, fear, anxiety
	Increased catecholamines
	Increased corticosteroids
	Cushing's disease
	Acute gout
	Diabetes mellitus
	Lead poisoning
	Acute hemorrhage
	Hemolytic anemia
Neutrophilopenia	Acute viral infections
	Bone marrow damage
	Nutritional deficiency
	Vitamin B_{12}
	Folic acid
Basophilic leukocytosis	Myeloproliferative diseases
	Myelofibrosis
	Polycythemia vera
Basophilopenia	Anaphylactic reaction
Eosinophilic leukocytosis	Allergic manifestations
	Asthma
	Hay fever
	Parasitic infestations
	Roundworm
	Flukes

Malignancy (Hodgkin's disease)
Colitis
Eosinophilic granulomatosis
Eosinophilic leukemia

Lymphocytosis — Leukemia (80% to 90% of total WBCs)
Infectious diseases
  Infectious mononucleosis
  Pertussis
Viral infections with exanthema
  Measles
  Rubella
  Roseola
  Chickenpox
Thyrotoxicosis
Cushing's disease

Monocytosis — Typhoid fever
Tuberculosis
Subacute bacterial endocarditis
Malaria

DETECTION OF SYPHILIS (LUES)

Syphilis is the disease caused by the spirochete *Treponema pallidum*. The disease is described in terms of its early or late manifestations or in terms of primary, secondary, and tertiary stages. It is transmitted by intimate mucous membrane contact or in utero. The destructiveness of the organism is attributed to its invasiveness and the elaboration of a weak endotoxin. Immunity is established by a single infection. One to 4 months after contraction of syphilis, two distinct antibodies appear in the serum. The complement fixation and flocculation diagnostic tests are based on one of these, syphilitic reagin, which combines with certain tissue lipids. *T. pallidum* is sensitive to penicillin. Thus, detection provides an opportunity for curative intervention.

Immunological tests for syphilis

The first serological test for syphilis (STS) was devised by Wassermann and, along with Kolmer's modification that superseded it, was a complement fixation test. Wassermann used extract from a syphilitic liver that had as its reactive ingredient cardiolipin, which is found in many tissues and is not actually specific for syphilis. Thus, it was fortuitous that the syphilitic reagin reacted with it. A lipoidal substance is found in spirochetes that is thought to be similar to the cardiolipin lipoprotein complex, which would explain the reaction.

The procedure for the complement fixation test involves first mixing the sample serum with cardiolipin reagent. The antigen-antibody reaction serves to bind the complement, removing it from the reaction. Sheep blood indicator is then added to the mixture. Hemolysis of the blood cells indicates the presence of free complement. If the cells do not hemolyze, complement is absent because of an earlier antigen-antibody reaction. False positive results may occur if the serum contains anticomplement activity.

The flocculation tests include the Venereal Disease Research Laboratory (VDRL), rapid plasma reagin (RPR), Kahn, Hinton, Kline, and Mazzini tests. These tests are performed by adding a suspension of cardiolipin antigen particles to the sample serum. If the syphilitic reagin (antibody) is present, it produces clumping, or flocculation. The reaction is quantitated by the degree of flocculation.

T. PALLIDUM IMMOBILIZATION (TPI) TEST

Nichols strain of pathogenic spirochetes can be cultured in rabbits. These spirochetes are incubated with the suspected serum for the TPI test. If the specific antibody is present, the spirochetes are immobilized. This reaction can be observed under the microscope. Other treponema spirochetes are known to give positive reactions to this test.

REITER PROTEIN COMPLEMENT FIXATION (RPCF) TEST

The nonpathological Reiter strain of spirochetes can be cultured in artificial media for the RPCF test. Antigen has been prepared from this strain and used in a complement fixation technique.

FLUORESCENT TREPONEMAL ANTIBODY ABSORPTION (FTA-ABS) TEST

In the FTA-ABS test, nonspecific cross-reacting antibodies are absorbed from the suspected serum through the use of the Reiter treponema antigen. The remaining serum is incubated on a smear of killed Nichols spirochetes. Following this, a solution containing fluorescent antibodies produced against human globulins is exposed to the sample.

ACCURACY OF TEST RESULTS

The STS tests are reported to produce as many as 25% to 45% biological false positive (BPF) results. That is, many positive tests have been reported for individuals who definitely have not been exposed to or do not have syphilis. Further investigation has shown these individuals to have acute viral or bacterial infections, hypersensitivity reactions, or a recent vaccination; in some cases such individuals have been found to have chronic systemic illness, such as collagen disease, malaria, or tuberculosis.

Positive test results obtained from nonspecific methods may be confirmed with the FTA-ABS test, which yield positive results midway through or at the end of the primary stage. Thus, in screening procedures a flocculation STS test is done initially and is followed up with the more specific FTA-ABS test.

All tests for syphilis give positive results in the secondary stage.

Antibiotic therapy may cause tests for syphilis to be negative.

Darkfield examination

Serous fluid exudate may be removed from a syphilitic lesion by pipet. *T. pallidum*, if present, may then be identified by darkfield microscopy. This provides positive identification of the spirochete and may be the earliest method of identification, since antibodies are not apparent until late in the primary stage.

URINALYSIS

The urine examined for screening purposes is generally a voided specimen collected without regard to circadian variation of the components; that is, it is voided at any time during the 24-hour period. More accuracy can be expected in electrolyte determination and less likelihood of bacterial contamination can be expected if a midstream or clean-catch specimen is employed. Ideally, the urine is collected on the client's arising, following a period of 12 hours in which no fluids were taken. The urine should be tested within 2 hours following its collection; spurious results may be obtained if urine is allowed to stand for long periods at room temperature; the urine pH is greater, bacteria multiply, and leukocytes and casts are known to deteriorate.

The standard urinalysis includes description of appearance, determination of specific gravity, pH, glucose, protein ketones, and microscopic examination of urinary sediment.

Appearance

The normal color of urine is pale golden yellow. Diluted urine is even more pale in hue. The color is only reported in the event of abnormality. Orange, red, and brown hues of the urine may be associated with porphyria, hemoglobinuria, urobilinuria, or bilirubinemia. Porphyria may be indicated by urine that becomes burgundy red on exposure to light.

Deviations	Etiology
Orange hue	Bile
	Ingestion of phenazopyridine (Pyridium)
Red hue	Blood
	Porphyria
	Urates
	Ingestion of dihydroxyanthraquinone (Dorbane)
Brown hue	Blood
	(melanin may turn black on standing)

Specific gravity

The specific gravity of the urine provides an indicator of the ability of the kidney to concentrate urine. The test is reported as the ratio of the weight of the urine tested to the weight of water.

Normal specific gravity of the urine
1.016 to 1.022 (in states of euhydration)
1.001 to 1.035 (range of normal without reference to hydration)

Low values suggest renal tubular dysfunction. Concentrated urine is observed in ADH deficiency.

pH

pH OF URINE: NORMAL pH AND DEVIATION

Normal pH: freshly voided urine is generally acidic, with a pH of 4.6 to 8

Deviation	Etiology
Alkaline urine	Metabolic alkalemia (except hypokalemic chloremia)
	Proteus infections
	Aged specimen

Glucose

The presence of glucose is not a normal finding for urine. Although glucose is freely filtered by the renal glomerulus, it is fully reabsorbed by the tubules. Only when the blood glucose levels reach the tubular maximum (T_m) of glucose (320 mg/min) or plasma threshold of 160 to 190 mg/100 ml is the kidney unable to completely reabsorb it. Glycosuria may indicate that the individual has a low renal threshold for glucose. The most common cause, however, is the presence of diabetes mellitus. Occasionally after high carbohydrate intake the blood glucose level may be high enough to allow spilling of glucose into the urine. Both reducing and enzymatic tests may be used to identify urinary glucose.

The practitioner may measure both blood and urinary glucose concentrations through the means of dipsticks, chemically treated papers that change color on exposure to glucose. Color charts provided with the testing materials allow standard comparison and subsequent identification of the degree of glucose concentration of the tested body fluid.

Deviation	Etiology
Glucosuria	Diabetes mellitus
	Increased intracranial pressure
	Cushing's disease
	Pheochromocytoma
	Pregnancy

Protein

Tests for the protein content in urine are dependent on the principle that protein precipitates in the presence of heat in acidic urine. Sulfosalicylic acid is the acid most frequently used for this purpose. An estimate of the protein content is made from the density of the precipitate as follows:

Precipitate description	Value	Percent protein
Faintly cloudy	1+	
Cloudy but transparent	2+	0.1
Opaque with clumping	3+	0.2 to 0.3
Dense, solid gel	4+	0.5

Normally, very small amounts of protein appear in urine that are not detectable by routine methods. Even trace quantities are an indication that follow-up should be done. A 24-hour quantitation of the protein excreted by the kidneys may be done. In addition, an electrophoretic determination of the type of protein in the urine may be done. Albumin is the most frequently encountered protein, since its molecular size is smaller than that of the globulins or fibrinogen.

The urine specimen of the female client may be contaminated with vaginal secretions. In many agencies it has become routine to use a clean-catch urine collection technique in order to obviate this protein contamination.

Bence Jones protein is an abnormal protein that appears in the urine of individuals with multiple myeloma.

URINARY PROTEIN: NORMAL EXCRETION AND DEVIATION

Normal excretion: 0.1 g/24 hr

Deivation	Etiology
Proteinuria	Pregnancy
	Strenuous physical exercise
	Orthostatism
	Fever
	Kidney disease
	Glomerulonephritis
	Nephrotic syndrome
	Neoplasm
	Infarction
	Postrenal infection

Acetone and diacetic acid (ketone bodies)

Ketones are products of fat metabolism and are increased in the blood during periods when increased fats are being used as fuel, such as in starvation, after glycogen stores have been depleted. In diabetes mellitus, the lack of insulin makes glucose relatively unavailable to the cells, so that fats are again metabolized in greater quantity. The blood ketones are increased more rapidly than they can be metabolized and are excreted in the urine. Acetone determinations are indicated whenever the urinary glucose test is positive or blood glucose is elevated.

The acetone level of urine may be tested with a chemically treated dipstick that changes color in the presence of ketone bodies. This is read against a standard scale provided with the test papers.

Microscopic examination of urinary sediment

The normal urinary sediment may contain one or two RBCs as well as WBCs and an occasional cast. All other substances are considered pathological.

Red blood cells. Since RBCs are too large to filter through the glomerulus, the presence of blood in the urine indicates bleeding within the genitourinary tract. Common causes are calculi, cystitis, neoplasm, tuberculosis, and glomerulonephritis.

White blood cells. WBCs may indicate infection in any part of the genitourinary tract. Glomerulonephritis is typified by the presence of WBCs, casts, and bacteria. As a rule, pyuria from the kidney is associated with proteinuria, whereas only very small amounts of protein are present in the urine of the individual with an infection of the lower urinary tract.

Casts. Gelled protein and cellular debris precipitated in the renal tubules and molded to the tubular lumen are called casts. Portions of these casts may break off and are found in the urine. The casts are hyaline, granular, or cellular in nature. Epithelial casts are made up of columnar renal epithelium or round cells. The hyaline casts are almost transparent and consist of homogeneous protein. The granular casts are dark colored and a degenerated form of the hyaline casts. The tubular shape of the casts has led to the use of the term cylindruria.

Casts consisting of WBCs are typical of pyelonephritis and the exudative stage of acute glomerulonephritis. Casts containing RBCs may appear clear or yellow.

The deposition of amyloid substance in urinary casts gives them a waxy appearance.

Urine that contains hyaline casts and protein may indicate a nephrotic syndrome.

Crystals. The acidity or alkalinity of the urine determines the type of crystals that may be identified in it. A urine with low pH is characterized by calcium oxalate, cystine, uric acid, and urate crystals. Alkaline urine is most frequently associated with carbonate crystals and amorphous phosphates.

EXAMINATION OF THE STOOL

In most cases a stool specimen is obtained by asking the individual to defecate, but digital removal of feces from the rectum can be done to facilitate collection when time constraints so dictate. Frequently a laxative is recommended to soften the stool, particularly if the individual has given a history of constipation. Because chemical analyses are calculated on the basis of daily output, the entire stool is sent to the laboratory. The feces are analyzed for size, shape, consistency, and color.

The normal individual excretes 100 to 200 g of feces daily. The volume is dependent on the fluid content of the bowel. About 500 to 1,000 ml of chyme (liquid stool) are delivered to the colon each day, but most of the water and electrolytes are reabsorbed, primarily in the proximal colon. Sodium is absorbed, and chloride follows passively. The gradient established results in absorption of water. In addition, bicarbonate ions are secreted by the colon, and an equal amount of chloride is absorbed. About one-fourth of the stool is solid material, which consists of the undigested residue of food, intestinal mucus and epithelium, bacteria, fat, and waste materials from the blood.

The rapid passage of stool through the colon in diarrhea results in larger stools (by volume) containing more liquid. Diarrhea is generally caused by inflammation of the colon but may also result from malabsorption syndromes.

A fecalith or stercolith is a dried, hardened fecal mass.

Color

The normal color of the stool is brown as a result of food pigments as well as the breakdown products of bilirubin. Bilirubin is converted to biliverdin (green bile) by intestinal bacteria and then to stercobilin (a brown substance). Increased motility of the stool in diarrhea may result in green stools because of the presence of biliverdin that was allowed insufficient time for bacterial conversion in the colon.

Melena is a black stool caused by gastrointestinal bleeding (more than 100 ml) high enough in the tract that it is partially digested. Bleeding of the lower gastrointestinal tract is observed as bright- to dark-red blood in the stool. The guiac test for occult blood is described in Chapter 15 on assessing the abdomen and rectosigmoid region.

Deviation	Etiology
Melena	Esophagitis
	Esophageal varices
	Hiatus hernia
	Gastritis
	Peptic ulcer
	Carcinoma
Presence of bright- to dark-red blood	Polyps of the colon
	Carcinoma of the colon
	Diverticulitis
	Colitis
	Hemorrhoids

Ingestion of iron or bismuth compounds may cause the stool to be green to black. Green vegetables ingested in excessive amounts may also turn the stool green. A dietary intake that contains a good deal of milk but is low in protein may result in a light-colored stool.

Odor

The odor of feces and flatus is the result of bacterial action and is dependent on the colonic bacterial flora and the type of food ingested.

The normal stool is 10% to 20% fat. Excessive amounts of fat in the stool is termed steatorrhea. The stool may appear grossly oily. Steatorrhea may be the result of pancreatic or small bowel malabsorption problems or liver disease. Sudan stain is an iodine compound that colors fat droplets, rendering them visible under the microscope. Excessive fat loss in the stool may also be associated with deficiency of the fat soluble, vitamin D.

Quantitative evaluation of fecal fat content is sometimes performed. In the performance of this test, the amount of dietary fat is usually controlled at 100 g of fat per day. A 3-day stool collection containing more than 5 g of fat for each day is considered pathological.

Microscopic examination

The stool may be examined under the microscope in order to identify ova and parasites. At least three separate specimens are examined, since one negative examination is not sufficient to rule out the infestation.

The presence of WBCs in the stool is indicative of an inflammation in the gastrointestinal tract.

BIBLIOGRAPHY

Bauer, J. D., Ackermann, P. G., and Toro, G.: Clinical laboratory methods, ed. 8, St. Louis, 1974, The C. V. Mosby Co.

Cromwell, L., and others: Medical instrumentation for health care, Englewood Cliffs, N.J., 1976, Prentice-Hall, Inc.

Eastham, R. D.: Clinical hematology, ed. 4, Baltimore, 1974, The Williams & Wilkins Co.

French, R. M.: Guide to diagnostic procedures, ed. 4, New York, 1975, McGraw Hill Book Co.

Henry, J. B.: Todd. Sanford. Davidsohn. Clinical diagnosis and management by laboratory methods, Philadelphia, 1979, W. B. Saunders Co.

Ravel, R.: Clinical laboratory medicine, ed. 2, Chicago, 1973, Year Book Medical Publishers, Inc.

Skydell, B., and Crowder, A. S.: Diagnostic procedures; a reference for health practitioners and a guide to patient counseling, Boston, 1975, Little, Brown and Co.

Tilkian, S. M., and Conover, M. H.: Clinical implication of laboratory tests, ed. 2, St. Louis, 1979, The C. V. Mosby Co.

Wallach, J.: Interpretation of diagnostic tests, a handbook synopsis of laboratory medicine, ed. 2, Boston, 1974, Little, Brown and Co.

Widmann, F. K.: Goodale's clinical interpretation of laboratory tests, ed. 7, Philadelphia, 1973, F. A. Davis Co.

Health hazards of the workplace*

BIOLOGIC AND INDUSTRIAL HAZARDS
Biologic hazards

Occupation	Disease or agent	Occupation	Disease or agent
Athletes	Dermatophytosis	Farmers—cont'd	Histoplasmosis
Bakers	Candidiasis		Sporotrichosis
Bartenders	Candidiasis		Chromoblastomycosis (southern U.S.)
Bulldozer operators	Coccidioidomycosis		
Butchers	Erysipeloid		Dermatophytosis
	Tularemia		Farmer's lung
Cattle breeders	Milkers' nodules		Chiggers (especially southern U.S.)
	Anthrax		
	Brucellosis		Mites
	Leptospirosis		Ticks
Construction workers	Rocky Mountain spotted fever	Fisherman (Gulf Coast)	Mycobacterial infections
	Coccidioidomycosis (southwestern U.S.)	Forestry workers	Rocky Mountain spotted fever
	Histoplasmosis		Tularemia
	Chiggers (especially southern U.S.)		Sporotrichosis (tree nursery workers)
Cooks	Tularemia		Ticks
	Candidiasis	Gardeners	Sporotrichosis
Cork workers	Farmer's lung		Creeping eruption
Cotton mill workers	Coccidioidomycosis		Hookworm disease
Dairy farmers	Milkers' nodules		Ascariasis
	Q fever		Mites
	Anthrax	Grain mill workers	Aspergillosis
	Leptospirosis		Mites
	Aspergillosis		Ticks
	Dermatophytosis	Health workers	Viral hepatitis
	Farmer's lung (especially handlers of hay in confined areas)		Tuberculosis (hospital employees)
			Mycobacterial infections
	Ticks		Candidiasis
Delivery personnel	Rabies	Hide workers	Q fever
Dishwashers	Candidiasis		Anthrax
Dockworkers	Swimmers' itch		Dermatophytosis
Farmers	Rabies	Laboratory workers	Cat-scratch disease
	Rocky Mountain spotted fever		Rocky Mountain spotted fever
	Tetanus		Ornithosis
	Plague (western U.S.)		Mycobacterial infections
	Tularemia		Tularemia
	Kerosene		Coccidioidomycosis
	Aspergillosis		Dermatophytosis
	Coccidioidomycosis (southwestern U.S.)		

Continued.

Biologic hazards—cont'd

Occupation	Disease or agent	Occupation	Disease or agent
Lifeguards	Dermatophytosis	Ranchers—cont'd	Brucellosis
	Swimmers' itch		Leptospirosis
	Creeping eruption		Plague (western U.S.)
	Hookworm disease		Dermatophytosis
	Ascariasis		Ticks
Linemen	Chiggers (especially southern U.S.)	Sawmill workers	Farmer's lung
		Sewer workers	Leptospirosis
Migrant workers	Coccidioidomycosis (southwestern U.S.)	Stockyard workers	Q fever
			Brucellosis
Military personnel	Leptospirosis		Leptospirosis
	Coccidioidomycosis (southwestern U.S.)	Sugarcane workers	Leptospirosis
			Farmer's lung
Miners	Leptospirosis	Surveyors	Chiggers (especially southern U.S.)
Packinghouse workers	Candidiasis		
Pet shop workers	Ornithosis	Taxidermists	Ornithosis
	Mycobacterial infections (tropical fish stores)	Textile workers	Farmer's lung
		Veterinarians	Rabies
	Aspergillosis (birds)		Cat-scratch disease
	Dermatophytosis		Milkers' nodules
Plumbers	Creeping eruption		Newcastle disease
	Hookworm disease		Brucellosis
	Ascariasis		Leptospirosis
Poultry handlers	Newcastle disease		Tularemia
	Ornithosis		Dermatophytosis
	Erysipeloid	Wool handlers	Q fever
	Candidiasis		Anthrax
	Aspergillosis		Dermatophytosis
	Histoplasmosis	Workers at risk of penetrating or crush-type trauma	Tetanus
	Mites		
Ranchers	Rabies		
	Rocky Mountain spotted fever	Zoo attendants	Ornithosis
	Q fever		Histoplasmosis
	Tetanus		Dermatophytosis
	Anthrax		

Industrial hazards

Occupation	Disease or agent	Occupation	Disease or agent
Adhesive workers	Isocyanates	Chemists	Carbon tetrachloride
	Benzene		Chloroform
	Styrene/ethyl benzene		Benzene
	Xylene hydrogen chloride		Toluene
	Sulfuric acid		Quinone
Agricultural workers	Calcium cyanamide		Benzidine salts
	Diphenyl		Picric acid
	Dinitro-o-cresol		Nickel and compounds
	Arsenic	Construction workers	Portland cement
	Nitrogen oxides	Cosmetic manufacturers	Paraffin
Automotive workers	Gasoline		Amyl alcohol
	Kerosene		Ethyl alcohol
	Ketones		Ethyl ether
	Trichloroethylene		Ketones
	Lead, inorganic		1, 2-Dichloroethane
	Nitrogen oxides		Ethyl chloride

Industrial hazards—cont'd

Occupation	Disease or agent	Occupation	Disease or agent
Cosmetic manufacturers—cont'd	Trichloroethylene	Dye makers—cont'd	Quinone
	Toluene		Benzyl chloride
	Quinone		Chlorodiphenyls and derivatives
	Benzyl chloride		Chlorinated benzenes
	Aniline		Aniline
	Dimethyl sulfate		Benzidine salts
	Zinc oxide		Dinitrobenzene
Detergent makers	Benzene		Dinitro-o-cresol
Drug manufacturers	Turpentine		Dinitrophenol
	Allyl alcohol		Dinitrotoluene
	Amyl alcohol		Picric acid
	Ethyl alcohol		n,n-dimethylformamide
	Ethylene chlorohydrin		Pyridine
	Ethyl ether		Carbon disulfide
	Acetic acid		Dimethyl sulfate
	Ketones		Bromine/hydrogen bromide
	Chloroform		Fluorides
	Ethyl chloride		Hydrogen chloride
	Methyl chloride		Arsenic
	Trichloroethylene		Magnesium and compounds
	Benzene		Thallium and compounds
	Benzyl chloride		Tin and compounds
	Aniline		Vanadium
	Picric acid		Zinc chloride
	n,n-dimethylformamide		Nitrogen oxides
	Pyridine		Phosgene
	Dimethyl sulfate	Electrical and electronic equipment makers	Chlorodiphenyls and derivatives
	Bromine/hydrogen bromide		Chlorinated naphthalenes
	Hydrogen chloride		Picric acid
	Arsenic		Beryllium
	Antimony		Lead, inorganic
	Cobalt and compounds		Magnesium and compounds
	Magnesium and compounds		Mercury, inorganic
	Manganese and compounds		Nickel and compounds
	Mercury, inorganic		Platinum and compounds
	Phosgene		Selenium and compounds
Dry cleaners	Naphtha		Graphite
	Dichloroethyl ether	Electroplaters	Hydrogen cyanide
	Carbon tetrachloride		Carbon disulfide
	1,2-Dichloroethane		Hydrogen chloride
	Propylene dichloride		Chromium and compounds
	Tetrachloroethane		Cobalt and compounds
	1,1,1-Trichloroethane		Germanium
	Trichloroethylene		Platinum and compounds
	Carbon disulfide		Zinc oxide
Dye makers	Ethyl alcohol	Enamel makers	Methyl alcohol
	Ethylene chlorohydrin		Cresol
	Methyl alcohol		Carbon disulfide
	Acetic acid		Arsenic
	Oxalic acid		Cobalt and compounds
	Ketones		Lead, inorganic
	1,2-Dichloroethane		Nickel and compounds
	Methyl and ethyl bromide	Epoxy resin makers	Epichlorohydrin
	Trichloroethylene		Ketones
	Benzene	Fat processors	n-hexane
	Naphthalene		Naphtha
	Cresol		Amyl alcohol

Continued.

Industrial hazards—cont'd

Occupation	Disease or agent	Occupation	Disease or agent
Fat processors— cont'd	Dichloroethyl ether	Laundry workers	Acetic acid
	Ethyl ether		Oxalic acid
	Ketones	Leather workers	Methyl alcohol
	Carbon tetrachloride		Ketones
	Ethyl chloride		Methylene chloride
	Methylene chloride		Aniline
	Propylene dichloride		Arsenic
	Tetrachloroethane		Sulfuric acid
	Trichloroethylene	Lithographers	Turpentine
	Carbon disulfide		Aniline
Food preservers	Acetic acid		Chromium and compounds
Food processors	Hydrogen chloride	Match and explosive manufacturers	Picric acid
	Sulfuric acid		Tetryl
Foundry workers	Methyl alcohol		Trinitrotoluene
	Cresol		Pyridine
	Chlorinated naphthalenes		Arsenic
	Fluorides		Antimony
	Arsenic		Lead, inorganic
	Beryllium		Magnesium and compounds
	Brass		Manganese and compounds
	Cadmium and compounds		Thallium and compounds
	Cobalt and compounds		Graphite
	Germanium		Sulfuric acid
	Lead, inorganic	Medical personnel	Nitrogen oxides
	Magnesium and compounds	Metal cleaners	Kerosene
	Manganese and compounds		Naphtha
	Nickel carbonyl		Ethylene chlorohydrin
	Thallium and compounds		Dichloroethyl ether
	Tin and compounds		Dioxane
	Zinc oxide		Ketones
	Graphite		Carbon tetrachloride
Grain workers	Carbon disulfide		1,2-Dichloroethane
	Sulfur dioxide		Propylene dichloride
Insecticide makers	1,-2-Dichloroethane		Tetrachloroethane
	Tetrachloroethane		1,1,1-Trichloroethane
	Trichloroethylene		Trichloroethylene
	Acrylonitrile		Fluorides
	Chlorinated benzenes		Sulfuric acid
	Chlorinated naphthalenes	Millinery workers	Methyl alcohol
	Fluorides	Oil processors	n-hexane
	Arsenic		Naphtha
	Cadmium and compounds		Dichloroethyl ether
	Lead, inorganic		Dioxane
	Selenium and compounds		Ethyl ether
	Phosgene		Ketones
Insulation workers	Isocyanates		Carbon tetrachloride
Lacquerers and makers	Epichlorohydrin		Methylene chloride
	Ketones		Propylene dichloride
	Carbon tetrachloride		Tetrachloroethane
	Chloroform		Trichloroethylene
	Tetrachloroethane		Carbon disulfide
	Styrene/ethyl benzene	Organic chemical synthesizers	Allyl alcohol
	Toluene		Ethyl alcohol
	Xylene		Ethylene chlorohydrin
	Chlorodiphenyls and derivatives		Methyl alcohol
	Chlorinated benzenes		Bis (chloromethyl) ether
	Zinc oxide		Epichlorohydrin

Industrial hazards—cont'd

Occupation	Disease or agent	Occupation	Disease or agent
Organic chemical synthesizers—cont'd	Phthalic anhydride	Photographic film developers	Quinone
	Methyl chloride		Hydrogen chloride
	Propylene dichloride	Pitch workers	Creosote
	Vinyl chloride	Plastics workers	Allyl alcohol
	Acrylonitrile		Amyl alcohol
	Calcium cyanamide		Ethyl alcohol
	Hydrogen cyanide		Methyl alcohol
	Isocyanates		Acetic acid
	Diphenyl		Phthalic anhydride
	Styrene/ethyl benzene		Ketones
	Creosote		Chloroform
	Quinone		1,2-Dichloroethane
	Aniline		Propylene dichloride
	Benzidine salts		Styrene/ethyl benzene
	Dinitrobenzene		Cresol
	Dinitrophenol		Benzyl chloride
	Dinitrotoluene		Chlorodiphenyls and derivatives
	n,n-dimethylformamide		Chlorinated naphthalenes
	Ethyleneimine		Aniline
	Pyridine		Benzidine salts
	Dimethyl sulfate		n,n-dimethylformamide
	Bromine/hydrogen bromide		Tricresyl phosphates
	Hydrogen chloride		Carbon disulfide
	Boron hydrides		Fluorides
	Magnesium and compounds		Hydrogen chloride
	Nickel carbonyl		Boron hydrides
	Selenium and compounds		Selenium and compounds
	Vanadium		Tin and compounds
	Ozone		Zinc oxide
Painters	Naphtha	Potato growers	Ethylene chlorohydrin
	Turpentine	Printers	Aniline
	Methyl alcohol		Arsenic
	Dioxane		Antimony
	Ketones		Paraffin
	Isocyanates	Refinery workers	N-heptane
	Arsenic		Kerosene
	Lead, inorganic		Naphtha
Paint manufacturers	Xylene		Amyl alcohol
	Chlorinated benzenes		Methyl chloride
	Pyridine		Benzene
	Carbon disulfide		Styrene/ethyl benzene
	Hydrogen chloride		Toluene
	Arsenic		Fluorides
	Antimony		Chlorinated naphthalenes
	Cadmium and compounds		n,n-dimethylformimide
	Lead, inorganic		Tricresyl phosphates
	Manganese and compounds		Bromine/hydrogen bromide
	Nickel and compounds		Boron hydrides
	Graphite		Lead, inorganic
Paper makers	Ethyleneimine		Nickel carbonyl
	Zinc chloride		Zinc chloride
	Ozone		Sulfur dioxide
	Sulfur dioxide	Refrigeration workers	Methyl chloride
	Sulfuric acid	Rubber manufacturers	Turpentine
Photoengravers	Methyl alcohol		Amyl alcohol
	Hydrogen chloride		Ethyl alcohol
	Chromium and compounds		Ethyl ether
	Nitrogen oxides		Acetic acid

Continued.

Industrial hazards—cont'd

Occupation	Disease or agent	Occupation	Disease or agent
Rubber manufac- turers—cont'd	Oxalic acid		Quinone
	Carbon tetrachloride		Ethyleneimine
	Methyl chloride		Arsenic
	Propylene dichloride		Antimony
	Vinyl chloride		Cadmium and compounds
	Isocyanates		Chromium and compounds
	Benzene		Magnesium and compounds
	Styrene/ethyl benzene		Mercury, inorganic
	Benzyl chloride		Nickel and compounds
	Chlorodiphenyls and derivatives		Selenium and compounds
	Chlorinated naphthalenes		Tin and compounds
	Aniline		Zinc chloride
	Benzidine salts	Upholsterers	Isocyanates
	Pyridine	Varnish makers	Paraffin
	Carbon disulfide		Turpentine
	Hydrogen chloride		Amyl alcohol
	Antimony		Dichloroethyl ether
	Boron hydrides		Epichlorohydrin
	Lead, inorganic		Ketones
	Selenium and compounds		Carbon tetrachloride
	Zinc chloride		1,2-Dichloroethane
	Zinc oxide		Tetrachloroethane
Steel workers	Calcium cyanamide		Trichloroethylene
	Hydrogen cyanide		Styrene/ethyl benzene
Tannery workers	Naphthalene		Xylene
	Quinone		Aniline
	Picric acid		Carbon disulfide
	Hydrogen chloride		Manganese and compounds
	Mercury, inorganic		Nickel and compounds
	Sulfur dioxide	Welders	Benzene
Textile workers	Amyl alcohol		Brass
	Ethylene chlorohydrin		Cadmium and compounds
	Methyl alcohol		Chromium and compounds
	Dioxane		Magnesium and compounds
	Acetic acid		Manganese and compounds
	Oxalic acid		Stibine
	Ketones		Zinc oxide
	Isocyanates		Nitrogen oxides
	Naphthalene		Ozone

DICTIONARY OF INDUSTRIAL CHEMICALS
Exposure route plus signs and symptoms of reactions to common agents

Acetic acid (INH)*

LOCAL: Vapor may irritate eyes, nose, throat, and lungs. Concentrated liquid may cause severe skin damage. Repeated exposure to liquid may cause dental erosion, chronic inflammation of nose, throat, and bronchi.

SYSTEMIC: Acute exposure may cause bronchopneumonia and pulmonary edema. Chronic exposure may cause pharyngitis or catarrhal bronchitis.

Acrylonitrile (INH, PA)*

LOCAL: Repeated exposure may cause skin irritation. When absorbed from leather or clothing, it may cause blisters after several hours of apparent harmlessness.

SYSTEMIC: Nausea, vomiting, headache, sneezing, weakness, light-headedness.

Allyl alcohol (INH, PA)*

LOCAL: Highly irritating to eyes and upper respiratory tract. Skin irritation and burns may follow contact with liquid. Onset may be delayed and symptoms prolonged.

SYSTEMIC: Local muscle spasms occur at absorption sites.

Amyl alcohol (INH, PA)*

LOCAL: Mild irritation of eyes, upper respiratory tract, and skin.

SYSTEMIC: Low concentration may cause nausea, vomiting, flushing, headache, diplopia, vertigo, and muscular weakness. Higher doses are narcotic.

Aniline (INH, PA)*

LOCAL: Liquid is mildly irritating to eyes and may cause corneal damage.

SYSTEMIC: Anoxia due to formation of methemoglobin. Initial cyanosis may be associated with headache, weakness, irritability, drowsiness, dyspnea, and unconsciousness as anoxia increases. If treatment not given promptly, death can occur.

Antimony (ING, INH, PA)*

LOCAL: Dust and fume irritate skin (though lesions rarely occur on the face), eyes, nose, and throat, with gingivitis and ulcerated nasal septum and larynx. Antimony trioxide may cause a dermatitis—"antimony spots"— with intense itching.

SYSTEMIC: Chronic accidental ingestion may cause chronically dry throat, nausea, sleep disturbance, anorexia, and dizziness.

Arsenic (INH, ING)*

LOCAL: Prolonged exposure causes local hyperemia and vesicular or pustular eruption.

SYSTEMIC: Toxic effects due to ingestion are rare in industry, but inhalation of inorganic compounds may cause chronic intoxication. Early findings are anorexia, nausea, vomiting, diarrhea. Conjunctivitis, coryza, hoarseness, and mild tracheobronchitis may follow continued exposure. Further exposure may involve symptoms of peripheral neuritis and depression of bone marrow. Arsenical compounds are lung and skin carcinogens. Acute poisoning causes death within 24 hours.

Benzene (INH)*

LOCAL: Irritates skin, eyes, and upper respiratory tract. Aspiration may cause pulmonary edema and hemorrhage. Defatting of skin causes erythema, vasiculation, and dry, scaly dermatitis.

SYSTEMIC: Acute exposure causes central nervous system depression, headache, dizziness, nausea, convulsions, coma, and death. Chronic exposure causes blood dyscrasias. Myelotoxic activity initially elevates, then decreases, erythrocyte, leukocyte, and thrombocyte counts, resulting in aplastic anemia, leukopenia, and thrombocytopenia. Strong evidence of leukemogenicity, especially for acute myelogenous leukemia and acute erythroleukemia.

Benzidine salts (INH, ING, PA)*

LOCAL: Contact dermatitis due to irritation or sensitization has been reported.

SYSTEMIC: A known urinary tract carcinogen; average latency period—16 years.

Benzyl chloride (INH)*

LOCAL: Severe irritation of eyes and respiratory tract. Liquid contact with eyes may injure the cornea.

SYSTEMIC: Pulmonary edema.

Beryllium (INH)*

LOCAL: Salts are skin sensitizers and irritants. Onset of contact dermatitis is delayed about two weeks following exposure.

SYSTEMIC: Acute exposure causes substernal pain, shortness of breath, and nonproductive cough. Chronic exposure causes respiratory distress, weakness, fatigue, and nonproductive cough. Symptoms can be delayed 5-10 years following exposure. Symptoms frequently are precipitated by illness, pregnancy, or surgery. Berylliosis is of long duration, with exacerbations and remissions.

Boron hydrides (INH, PA)*

LOCAL: Vapors irritate skin and mucous membranes.

SYSTEMIC: Many of these compounds are CNS depressants. Typical symptoms are excitability, muscular twitching, convulsions, dizziness, disorientation, and unconsciousness, which may be delayed 24 hours or more. Chronic exposure may lead to wheezing, dyspnea, dry cough, rales, and hyperventilation, which may persist for several years after cessation of exposure.

Brass (INH)*

LOCAL: Particulates may cause dermatitis via mechanical irritation.

SYSTEMIC: Metal fume fever, as a result of zinc oxide liberated in the foundry process (see zinc oxide). (The symptom is colloquially termed "brass founder's ague.") Similarly, brass foundries may liberate toxic amounts of lead (see lead, inorganic).

Bromine and hydrogen bromide (INH, PA)*

LOCAL: Both are highly irritating to eyes, skin, and mucous membranes of the upper respiratory tract.

---

*INH = inhalation; ING = ingestion; PA = percutaneous absorption.

SYSTEMIC: Spasm of the glottis, asthmatic bronchitis, and pulmonary edema may occur several hours after inhalation. Chronic exposure may cause cough, copious mucus secretion, nosebleeds, respiratory distress, vertigo, and headache. Bromine accumulates in tissue; hence, chronic exposure to low concentrations may cause symptoms after a latent period. Hydrogen bromide may cause similar, though less severe symptoms.

Cadmium and compounds (INH, ING)*

LOCAL: Prolonged exposure may cause anosmia, yellow-stained teeth. Once absorbed, cadmium remains in the kidney and liver.

SYSTEMIC: A few hours after acute exposure, usually via inhalation of fumes, slight upper respiratory tract irritation appears. A few hours after that, cough, chest pain, sweating, chills, appear. Up to 24 hours following initial exposure, severe pulmonary irritation develops, with coughing, chest pain, and edema. Mortality incidence is about 15 percent. Survivors may develop emphysema or cor pulmonale. Emphysema may follow chronic exposure. Chronic exposure may also cause kidney damage, with proteinuria, anemia, and elevated sed rate.

Calcium cyanamide (INH)*

LOCAL: Irritation of mucous membranes of eyes, skin, and respiratory tract. Inhalation may cause rhinitis, laryngitis, pharyngitis, or bronchitis.

SYSTEMIC: Erythema, nausea, fatigue, headache, dyspnea, vomiting, "oppression" in chest, shivering. Pneumonia or pulmonary edema may develop.

Carbon disulphide (INH, PA)*

LOCAL: Vapor irritates eyes, skin, mucous membranes. Liquid contact causes severe burns. Local absorption may damage peripheral nerves.

SYSTEMIC: Psychological, neurologic, and cardiovascular disorders. Irritability, anger, suicidal ideation, and manic depressive psychosis may follow repeated exposure. Chronic exposures may cause insomnia, nightmare, defective memory, and impotence. Polyneuritis, atherosclerosis, and coronary artery disease have been linked to chronic exposure. In women, chronic menstrual disorders may occur.

Carbon tetrachloride (INH)*

LOCAL: Defatting of the skin. Repeated contact may cause dry, scaly, fissure dermatitis.

SYSTEMIC: Psychological, neurologic, and cardiovascular; exposure may cause liver and kidney damage, toxic hepatitis. Hazard is increased by alcohol ingestion.

Chlorinated benzenes (INH, PA)*

LOCAL: Irritation of skin, conjunctiva, and upper respiratory tract.

SYSTEMIC: Acute exposure causes drowsiness, incoordination, and unconsciousness. Chronic exposure may cause liver, kidney, and lung damage.

Chlorinated naphthalenes (INH, PA)*

LOCAL: Chronic exposure may cause "chloracne," erythematous eruptions, pustules, papules, and comedones.

SYSTEMIC: Headache, fatigue, vertigo, and anorexia. Liver damage and jaundice may occur.

Chlorodiphenyls and derivatives (INH, PA)*

LOCAL: Prolonged contact with fumes or cold wax may cause comedones, sebaceous cysts, pustules ("chloracne").

SYSTEMIC: Acute and chronic exposure may cause liver damage, with edema, jaundice, vomiting, anorexia, abdominal pain, and fatigue. Causes stillbirth if exposure during pregnancy.

Chloroform (INH)*

LOCAL: Burns may follow long-term skin contact.

SYSTEMIC: General anesthesia at high concentration. Chronic exposure may cause hepatomegaly and kidney damage.

Chromium and compounds (INH, ING, PA)*

LOCAL: Compounds are allergenic and may cause pulmonary sensitization. Chromic acid is corrosive to skin and mucous membranes.

SYSTEMIC: Acute exposure may cause coughing, headache, dyspnea, pain on deep inspiration, fever, and weight loss. Chromate industrial workers have increased risk of lung cancer.

Cobalt (INH)*

LOCAL: Cobalt is an allergen; may cause sensitivity dermatitis even at very low concentration. Cross-sensitization occurs between cobalt and nickel, cobalt and chromium.

SYSTEMIC: Asthmalike disease, with cough and dyspnea, possibly progressing to interstitial pneumonia with marked fibrosis.

Creosote (PA)*

LOCAL: Liquid and vapors are strong irritants, causing local erythema, burning, itching, grey-to-bronze pigmentation, vesiculation, ulceration, and gangrene. May cause skin cancer.

SYSTEMIC: Salivation, vomiting, vertigo, headache, loss of pupillary reflex, hypothermia, cyanosis, convulsions, thready pulse, respiratory distress, and death in severe exposures.

Cresol (INH, PA)*

LOCAL: Extremely corrosive to all tissues. Low-level chronic exposure may cause skin rash, discoloration.

SYSTEMIC: Muscle weakness, headache, dizziness, dimmed vision, tinnitus, rapid breathing, mental confusion, loss of consciousness, and death may follow absorption. Chronic exposure may cause vomiting, difficulty in swallowing, salivation, diarrhea, anorexia, headache, fainting, dizziness, mental disturbance, and skin rash. Further exposure may cause fatal liver and kidney damage.

1,2-Dichloroethane (INH, PA)*

LOCAL: Repeated contact with liquid may cause dry, scaly, fissured dermatitis. Liquid and vapor may damage eyes.

SYSTEMIC: Inhalation of high concentrations may cause nausea, vomiting, mental confusion, dizziness, and pulmonary edema. Chronic exposure may cause liver and kidney damage.

---

*INH = inhalation; ING = ingestion; PA = percutaneous absorption.

Dichloroethyl ether (INH, PA)*

LOCAL: Irritation of conjunctiva, profuse lacrimation, and irritation of mucous membranes of upper respiratory tract may follow acute exposure.

SYSTEMIC: Chronic exposure to low levels may cause mild bronchitis.

Dimethyl sulfate (INH, PA)*

LOCAL: Liquid is highly irritating, causing skin vesiculation and analgesia. Analgesia may persist for several months. Skin irritation may be delayed.

SYSTEMIC: Acute exposure may cause pulmonary edema, bronchitis, or pneumonitis 6-24 hours later. Pulmonary effects may predispose to infection. CNS effects.

n,n-Dimethylformamide (INH, PA)*

LOCAL: Dermatitis.

SYSTEMIC: Inhalation may cause colicky abdominal pain. anorexia, nausea, vomiting, constipation, diarrhea, facial flushing, hypertension, hepatomegaly, and other signs of liver damage.

Dinitro-o-cresol (INH, PA)*

LOCAL: None.

SYSTEMIC: Rise in metabolic rate, temperature, with fatigue, sweating, thirst, and weight loss. May resemble thyroid crisis.

Dinitrobenzene (INH, PA)*

LOCAL: Yellowish discoloration of skin, eyes, and hair.

SYSTEMIC: Methemoglobin, with headache, irritability, dizziness, weakness, nausea, vomiting, dyspnea, drowsiness, and unconsciousness. May also cause a bitter almond taste in the mouth, dry throat, thirst, reduced vision, hearing loss, tinnitus, and liver damage.

Dinitrophenol (INH, PA)*

LOCAL: Yellow staining of exposed skin.

SYSTEMIC: Increased metabolism, oxygen consumption, and heat production. Acute onset entails sudden fatigue, thirst, sweating, feeling of oppression in chest, tachycardia, and fever. Less severe intoxication entails nausea, vomiting, anorexia, weakness, dizziness, vertigo, headache, and sweating. Chronic exposure may cause kidney and liver damage, cataracts.

Dinitrotoluene (INH, PA)*

LOCAL: None.

SYSTEMIC: Formation of methemoglobin causes anoxia, cyanosis, with headache, irritability, dizziness, weakness, nausea, vomiting, dyspnea, drowsiness, and unconsciousness. Symptom onset may be delayed several hours.

Dioxane (INH, PA)*

LOCAL: Liquid and vapor irritate eye, nose, and throat.

SYSTEMIC: Exposure to vapor may cause drowsiness, dizziness, loss of appetite, headache, nausea, vomiting, stomach pain, and liver and kidney damage.

Diphenyl (INH, PA)*

LOCAL: Irritation of skin or respiratory tract. Repeated exposure may cause sensitization dermatitis.

SYSTEMIC: Acute exposure may cause a CNS, peripheral nervous system, or hepatic toxic reaction, with headache, diffuse GI pain, nausea, indigestion, numbness and aching of limbs, and general fatigue. Liver function tests may be abnormal.

Epichlorohydrin (INH, PA)*

LOCAL: Severe irritation of eyes, skin, and respiratory tract. Blistering and deep-seated pain may be delayed.

SYSTEMIC: Earliest effects are nausea, vomiting, abdominal discomfort, followed by respiratory distress, dyspnea, and cyanosis. Onset of chemical pneumonitis may be delayed several hours after exposure.

Ethyl alcohol (INH, PA)*

LOCAL: Mild irritation of eyes and nose at high concentrations. Liquid may defat the skin, causing dry, fissured dermatitis.

SYSTEMIC: Prolonged inhalation of high concentration may cause headache, drowsiness, tremor, and fatigue. Bizarre symptoms may result from denaturants.

Ethyl chloride (INH, PA)*

LOCAL: Liquid is mildly irritating to eyes and skin. Frostbite may occur due to rapid evaporation.

SYSTEMIC: Headache, dizziness, incoordination, abdominal cramps, possible loss of consciousness.

Ethyl ether (INH)*

LOCAL: Mild irritation of eyes, nose, and throat. Liquid contact may cause dry, scaly, fissured dermatitis.

SYSTEMIC: Narcosis. Chronic exposure may cause anorexia, exhaustion, headache, drowsiness, dizziness, excitation, psychic disturbances, increased susceptibility to alcohol.

Ethylene chlorohydrin (INH, PA)*

LOCAL: High vapor concentrations can irritate eyes, nose, throat, and skin.

SYSTEMIC: Inhalation causes nausea, vomiting, dizziness, headache, thirst, delirium, low blood pressure, collapse. There is little safety margin between these symptoms and death due to lung and brain damage.

Ethyleneimine (INH, PA)*

LOCAL: Vapor and liquid exposure cause severe eye, nose, throat, skin, and upper respiratory tract irritation. Skin sensitization may occur.

SYSTEMIC: Acute exposure may cause nausea, vomiting, headache, dizziness, and pulmonary edema. Chronic effects have not been established in man.

Fluorides (INH, ING)*

LOCAL: Elemental fluorine and compounds are irritants of skin, eyes, mucous membranes, and lungs. Chemical burns may not become symptomatic for several hours following exposure. Burns (even as small as 3 percent of area) may cause systemic effects through absorption of the fluoride.

SYSTEMIC: Inhalation may cause bronchospasm, laryngospasm, and pulmonary edema. Ingestion of compounds causes GI symptoms associated with severe irritation. Prolonged absorption of compounds may cause osteosclerosis, first in lumbar spine and pelvis. Severe skeletal fluorosis may exist without other physical effects or general physical impairment.

Gasoline (INH, ING)*

LOCAL: Irritates conjunctiva, skin, and mucous membranes. May sensitize.

SYSTEMIC: Vapor is a CNS depressant. Low concentrations may cause facial flushing, staggering, slurred speech, and mental confusion. Acute exposure may cause pancreatic hemorrhage, fatty degeneration of the liver, fatty degeneration of the proximal convoluted tubules and glomeruli of the kidneys, and passive congestion of the spleen. Ingestion or aspiration may cause chemical pneumonitis, pulmonary edema, or hemorrhage.

Germanium (INH)*

LOCAL: Germanium oxide dust irritates eyes. Germanium tetrachloride irritates skin.

SYSTEMIC: Bronchitis and pneumonitis may follow exposure to germanium tetrachloride. Prolonged exposure may damage liver, kidney, and other organs. Germanium tetrahydride is a toxic hemolytic gas that can damage kidneys.

Graphite (INH)*

LOCAL: None.

SYSTEMIC: Chronic exposure may cause a progressive and disabling pneumoconiosis similar to anthracosilicosis, with headache, cough, depression, anorexia, dyspnea, and black sputum. Some patients may be symptom-free for years, then become suddenly disabled.

n-Heptane (INH)*

LOCAL: Dermatitis and mucous membrane irritation.

SYSTEMIC: Effects may arise without complaints relating to local irritation. These effects are vertigo, incoordination, hilarity, nausea, anorexia, and persistent gasoline taste.

n-Hexane (INH)*

LOCAL: Dermatitis and irritation of mucous membranes of upper respiratory tract.

SYSTEMIC: Acute exposure may cause narcosis, with nausea, headache, and dizziness. Peripheral neuropathy may be a long-term result.

Hydrogen chloride (INH)*

LOCAL: Highly corrosive to eyes, skin, and mucous membranes. Produces burns, ulceration, and scarring. Prolonged exposure to low concentrations causes dental discoloration and erosion.

SYSTEMIC: Laryngitis, glottal edema, bronchitis, pulmonary edema, and death.

Hydrogen cyanide (INH, PA)*

LOCAL: Mild irritation of upper respiratory tract.

SYSTEMIC: Extremely toxic in high concentration; lower concentration may cause weakness, headache, confusion, nausea, and vomiting. These symptoms may progress to unconsciousness and death if exposure continues.

Isocyanates (INH, PA)*

LOCAL: Toluene diisocyanate and methylene disphenylisocyanate irritate eyes, respiratory tract, and skin. Possible bronchitis, pulmonary edema, nausea, vomiting, and abdominal pain if the irritation is severe.

SYSTEMIC: Sensitization with wheezing, dyspnea, and cough may occur.

Kerosene (INH)*

LOCAL: Defatting, irritation of skin. Aspiration may cause extensive pulmonary injury, chemical pneumonitis.

SYSTEMIC: Inhalation may cause headache, nausea, con-

fusion, or drowsiness. Accidental ingestion may cause nausea, vomiting, or renal damage.

Ketones (INH, PA)*

LOCAL: Dry, scaly, fissured dermatitis after repeated exposure. Irritation of conjunctiva and mucous membranes of nose, eyes, and throat following exposure to high concentration of vapor.

SYSTEMIC: Narcosis, headache, nausea, vomiting, decreased motor coordination following exposure to high concentration of vapor.

Lead, inorganic (INH, ING)*

LOCAL: None.

SYSTEMIC: Early symptoms difficult to differentiate from seasonal flulike illness. Later findings include pallor, anemia, "leadline" on gums, decreased hand grip strength, abdominal pain, and severe constipation. Continued exposure causes peripheral nerve damage, especially the radial nerve, causing "wrist drop."

Magnesium and compounds (INH)*

LOCAL: Mild irritation of conjunctiva and nasal mucosa.

SYSTEMIC: "Metal fume fever"; symptoms similar to that of zinc oxide.

Manganese and compounds (INH, PA)*

LOCAL: Mild irritation of eyes and respiratory tract. Innocuous to intact skin.

SYSTEMIC: Deposition in body organs, especially liver, spleen, and parts of brain and spinal cord. Onset of intoxication is insidious, with apathy, anorexia, and asthenia. Psychosis, with inappropriate laughter, euphoria, impulsive acts, absentmindedness, confusion, aggression, and hallucinations. Late stage indistinguishable from parkinsonism.

Mercury-alkyl (INH, ING)*

LOCAL: Primary skin irritant and prolonged contact may cause second degree burns.

SYSTEMIC: Progressive central nervous system deterioration may follow chronic exposure.

Mercury, inorganic (INH, PA)*

LOCAL: Irritation of skin and mucous membranes. May sensitize skin.

SYSTEMIC: Acute poisoning causes interstitial pneumonitis, bronchitis, and bronchiolitis. Fatigue, anorexia, weight loss, insomnia, indigestion, diarrhea, metallic taste in mouth, inflammation of gums, black line on gums, loosened teeth, irritability, memory loss and tremors of tongue, fingers, eyelids, and lips. Continued exposure causes aggravation of symptoms plus anxiety, delirium, hallucinations, depression, or manic depressive psychosis.

Methyl alcohol (INH, PA)*

LOCAL: Contact with liquid may defat skin, produce a mild dermatitis.

SYSTEMIC: May cause optic nerve damage and blindness. Other CNS depressive symptoms include headache, nausea, giddiness, loss of consciousness.

Methyl chloride (PA)*

LOCAL: Liquid may damage eyes.

SYSTEMIC: Staggering gait, speech difficulty, nausea,

---

*INH = inhalation; ING = ingestion; PA = percutaneous absorption.

headache, dizziness, and blurred vision may follow acute exposure after a short latency period. Chronic exposure entails similar symptoms after a period of several hours.

Methylene chloride (INH, PA)*

LOCAL: Dry, fissured, scaly dermatitis from continued contact.

SYSTEMIC: A mild narcotic, methylene dichloride may cause headache, giddiness, stupor, numbness, and tingling sensation in limbs. Exposure may cause increased carboxyhemoglobin, which may be significant in smokers or patients with anemia or heart disease.

Methyl and ethyl bromide (INH, PA)*

LOCAL: Methyl bromide irritates skin, eyes, and mucous membrane of upper respiratory tract. May cause itching dermatitis. May be absorbed by leather, causing prolonged contact. Ethyl bromide may cause skin irritation on prolonged contact.

SYSTEMIC: High concentrations of either may cause pulmonary edema. Acute exposure to methyl bromide causes malaise, visual disturbances, headache, nausea, vomiting, somnolence, vertigo, and hand tremor. Onset may be delayed 30 minutes to 6 hours. Chronic poisoning entails CNS depression. Ethyl bromide has not been associated with chronic systemic effects.

Naphtha (INH)*

LOCAL: Irritation and "chapping" of skin and photosensitivity may follow repeated contact with liquid.

SYSTEMIC: High concentration may cause CNS depression.

Naphthalene (INH)*

LOCAL: Erythema and dermatitis on repeated contact. An allergen, it may cause sensitization dermatitis.

SYSTEMIC: Inhalation may cause intravascular hemolysis. Early symptoms include eye irritation, headache, confusion, excitement, malaise, profuse sweating, nausea, vomiting, abdominal pain, and bladder irritation. There may be progressive jaundice, hematuria, hemoglobinuria, renal tubular blockade, and acute renal shutdown. Hematologic effects include red cell fragmentation, anemia, with nucleated red cells, leukocytosis, and sharp decrease in hemoglobin, hematocrit, and red cell count.

Nickel and compounds (INH)*

LOCAL: Skin sensitization is common. May lead to chronic eczema, "nickel itch," with lichenification resembling atopic or neurodermatitis. Nickel and compounds irritate conjunctiva and mucous membranes of the upper respiratory tract.

SYSTEMIC: Elemental nickel and its salts are probably carcinogenic.

Nickel carbonyl (INH, PA)*

LOCAL: Nickel dermatitis (see nickel)

SYSTEMIC: Mild frontal headache, giddiness, nausea, limb weakness, sweating, cough, vomiting, clammy skin, dyspnea result from acute exposure. Even lethal exposure may entail symptoms so mild that they are ignored. Hours or days later, a chemical pneumonitis with adrenal cortical suppression develops. Nickel carbonyl is also carcinogenic.

Nitrogen oxides (INH)*

LOCAL: Irritation of eyes and mucous membranes by gases. Acids are extremely corrosive, may cause severe burns, ulcers, and necrosis.

SYSTEMIC: Exposure to high concentration may cause pulmonary irritation and methemoglobinemia. Nitrogen oxides may be formed by green silage in hazardous concentrations, causing bronchiolitis fibrosa obliterans ("Silo-filler's disease"). Victims may develop severe and progressive dyspnea, with fever and cyanosis. Symptoms may appear a few days or as long as six weeks after exposure. Chronic exposure may cause exertional dyspnea, decreased vital capacity, maximum breathing capacity, lung compliance, and increased residual volume. Signs include moist rales, wheezes, sporadic cough with mucopurulent, expectoration, decreased blood pH, serum proteins, and increased urinary hydroxyproline and acid mucopolysaccharides.

Oxalic acid (INH)*

LOCAL: Liquid causes ulceration of skin and mucous membranes.

SYSTEMIC: Chronic exposure to mist may cause chronic inflammation of the upper respiratory tract. Accidental ingestion is rare.

Ozone (INH)*

LOCAL: Irritation of eyes and mucous membranes. Severe exposure causes choking, coughing, substernal soreness and, hours after exposure, pulmonary edema.

SYSTEMIC: Chronic exposure may cause headache, malaise, drowsiness, shortness of breath, reduced ability to concentrate, slowed heart and respiration rate, visual impairment, and reduced desaturation of oxyhemoglobin in capillaries.

Paraffin (INH)*

LOCAL: Chronic exposure may cause chronic dermatitis, wax boils, folliculitis, comedones, melanoderma, papules, and hyperkeratoses.

SYSTEMIC: Carcinoma of the scrotum, latency period 10 years or more.

Phosgene (INH)*

LOCAL: Conjunctivitis, lacrimation, and upper respiratory tract irritation. Liquid contact may cause burns.

SYSTEMIC: Pulmonary edema between 5-12 hours following exposure, with dizziness, chills, thirst, tormenting cough, viscous sputum. Sputum may become thin and foamy. Tracheal rhonchi and grey-blue cyanosis may follow. Death may result from respiratory or cardiac failure. Chronic exposure may entail some tolerance to edemagenic effects but cause irreversible emphysema and fibrosis.

Phthalic anhydride (INH)*

LOCAL: Severe irritation of eyes, skin, and respiratory tract. Sensitization reactions are also possible.

SYSTEMIC: Repeated exposures may cause bronchitis, emphysema, allergic asthma, urticaria, and chronic eye irritation.

Picric acid (INH, ING, PA)*

LOCAL: Dust or solutions are potent skin sensitizers. Dust or fume may cause eye irritation and sensitization.

SYSTEMIC: Ingestion may cause headache, vertigo, nausea, vomiting, diarrhea, yellow pigmentation of skin, hematuria, or albuminuria. High dosage pigments all tissue, including aqueous humor, causing yellow vision; and it may cause destruction of erythrocytes, hemorrhagic nephritis, and hepatitis.

Platinum and compounds (INH)*

LOCAL: Salts (not elemental platinum) may sensitize skin, nasal mucosa, and bronchi.

SYSTEMIC: Bronchial irritation, respiratory distress may be delayed 2-6 months after exposure. Status asthmaticus may develop. After recovery most patients remain allergic to dust or mist bearing the compounds.

Portland cement (INH)*

LOCAL: Acute exposure may cause "cement dermatitis," which may be prolonged and involve covered parts of the body as well as exposed. Components of cement may cause allergic sensitivity.

SYSTEMIC: None.

Propylene dichloride (INH)*

LOCAL: Dermatitis due to defatting action.

SYSTEMIC: None known, though animal experiments show CNS narcosis and fatty degeneration of liver and kidneys following acute exposure.

Pyridine (INH, PA)*

LOCAL: Irritation of conjunctiva, cornea, and mucous membranes of upper respiratory tract and skin. May cause skin sensitization.

SYSTEMIC: Repeated or continued low-level exposure may cause CNS depression and GI complications, with headache, dizziness, insomnia, nervousness, anorexia, nausea, vomiting, and diarrhea.

Quinone (INH)*

LOCAL: Contact with the crystals causes ulceration. Prolonged contact with vapor causes severe eye irritation, with brownish conjunctival stains. These may be followed by corneal opacities and loss of visual acuity due to corneal dystrophy. Early staining is reversible. Corneal dystrophy tends to be progressive.

SYSTEMIC: None observed.

Selenium and compounds (INH, ING, PA)*

LOCAL: Some compounds are irritant to skin and may be allergenic. May cause excruciating pain if the oxide penetrates under the free edge of the nail.

SYSTEMIC: First signs of absorption is "garlic" odor of breath. Other effects are pallor, lassitude, irritability, vague GI complaints, and giddiness.

Stibine (INH)*

LOCAL: None reported.

SYSTEMIC: Stibine is a potent CNS toxin and hemolytic agent. Acute intoxication entails severe headache, nausea, weakness, abdominal and lumbar pain, slow breathing, and weak, irregular pulse. Chronic exposure has not been reported.

Styrene/ethyl benzene (INH, PA)*

LOCAL: Irritates eyes, nose, throat, and skin. May cause dry, scaly, fissured dermatitis.

SYSTEMIC: Acute exposure to high concentrations may cause irritation of the mucous membranes of the upper respiratory tract, followed by narcosis, cramps, and death due to respiratory center paralysis.

Sulfur dioxide (INH, PA)*

LOCAL: Gas is extremely irritating to upper respiratory tract. Chronic effects include rhinitis, dry throat, and cough.

SYSTEMIC: Acute exposure survivors may develop bronchopneumonia with bronchiolitis obliterans. Moderate exposure may cause bronchoconstriction with high-pitched rales. Chronic exposure may cause nasopharyngitis, fatigue, altered sense of smell, and chronic bronchitis.

Sulfuric acid (INH)*

LOCAL: Burning and charring of skin.

SYSTEMIC: Irritates upper respiratory tract epithelium. Low-level exposure causes reflex increase of respiratory rate, decrease of depth, bronchoconstriction. A single exposure may cause laryngeal, tracheobronchial, and pulmonary edema. Chronic exposure may cause conjunctivitis, frequent respiratory infections, emphysema, and digestive disturbances.

Tetrachloroethane (INH, PA)*

LOCAL: Scaly, fissured dermatitis from prolonged contact.

SYSTEMIC: Some evidence that CNS depression is associated with percutaneous absorption only. Early effects of inhalation include narcosis, with tremors, headache, numbness, and prickling sensation of limbs, loss of knee jerk, and profuse sweating. Blood changes include increased mononuclear leukocytes, progressive anemia, slight thrombocytosis. Continued exposure entails fatigue, headache, constipation, insomnia, irritability, anorexia, nausea. Liver dysfunction may follow, with abdominal pain, hematemesis, and purpuric rash.

Tetryl (INH, PA)*

LOCAL: Allergic dermatitis, with generalized edema requiring hospitalization in severe cases. Contact may stain skin and hair yellow or orange.

SYSTEMIC: Irritability, fatigability, malaise, headache, lassitude, insomnia, nausea, and vomiting. Anemia has been observed among exposed workers.

Thallium and compounds (INH, ING, PA)*

LOCAL: Rarely, skin irritation and sensitization.

SYSTEMIC: Prolonged exposure, when not fatal, entails fatigue, limb pain, metallic taste in mouth, loss of hair, followed by peripheral neuritis, proteinuria, and arthralgia. Thallium is extremely toxic and cumulative in man.

Tin and compounds (INH, ING, PA)*

LOCAL: Organic tin compounds may burn the skin. Clothing contaminated by vapors or liquids may produce diffuse erythematoid dermatitis on lower abdomen, thighs, and groin.

SYSTEMIC: Inorganic dust or fume causes a benign pneumoconiosis (stannosis). There are no progressive changes after removal from contact, and early X-ray

---

*INH = inhalation; ING = ingestion; PA = percutaneous absorption.

diagnosis is facilitated by radiopacity of the element. Many organic tin compounds are highly toxic when ingested.

Toluene (INH, PA)*

LOCAL: Irritation of eyes, respiratory tract, and skin. Repeated or prolonged contact may cause defatting of skin—a dry, fissured dermatitis.

SYSTEMIC: Acute exposure entails CNS depression, headache, dizziness, fatigue, drowsiness, muscular incoordination, staggering gait, skin paresthesia, collapse, and coma.

1,1,1-Trichloroethane (INH, PA)*

LOCAL: Irritation of eyes on contact. Dry, scaly, fissured dermatitis may follow repeated contact due to defatting action.

SYSTEMIC: Narcosis, CNS depression.

Trichloroethylene (INH, PA)*

LOCAL: Irritation of eyes, nose, and throat. Dermatitis may be caused by chronic exposure to liquid.

SYSTEMIC: Acute exposure involves CNS depression, headache, dizziness, vertigo, tremor, nausea, vomiting, irregular heartbeat, sleepiness, fatigue, blurred vision. May resemble alcohol intoxication.

Tricresyl phosphates (INH, ING, PA)*

SYSTEMIC: Major effects are on the spinal cord and peripheral nerves. GI symptoms of acute exposure (pain, diarrhea, nausea, vomiting, and abdominal pain) are followed in 3-30 days by progressive neurologic symptoms: numbness, muscle soreness, foot and wrist drop. In chronic poisoning, the GI symptoms are usually unnoticed, and flaccid paralysis of arm and leg muscles gradually develops.

Trinitrotoluene (INH, ING, PA)*

LOCAL: Irritation of eyes, nose, and throat, with sneezing, coughing, sore throat.

SYSTEMIC: Toxic hepatitis and aplastic anemia. Exposure may cause methemoglobinemia, with cyanosis, weakness, drowsiness, dyspnea, unconsciousness, muscular pain, cardiac arrhythmias, renal irritation, menstrual irregularity, and peripheral neuritis.

Turpentine (INH, PA)*

LOCAL: Highly irritating to skin, eyes, nose, and bronchi. Liquid may cause eczema.

SYSTEMIC: Acute exposure may cause CNS depression, with headache, anorexia, anxiety, excitement, mental confusion, and tinnitus. Vapor may cause kidney and bladder damage. Chronic nephritis with albuminuria and hematuria may follow repeated exposure.

Vanadium and compounds (INH)*

LOCAL: Irritation of eyes and skin. Skin may itch intensely. Possible general urticaria and greenish tongue.

SYSTEMIC: Serous or hemorrhagic rhinitis, sore throat, cough, tracheitis, bronchitis, expectoration, and chest pain may follow brief exposure. Pneumonia and pulmonary edema may follow. Patients who recover may have persistent bronchitis resembling asthma and episodes of dyspnea.

Vinyl chloride (INH)*

LOCAL: Severe skin irritation.

SYSTEMIC: Acute exposure may cause CNS depression, with symptoms resembling mild alcoholic intoxication. Chronic exposure entails the triad of acro-osteolysis, Raynaud's phenomenon, and sclerodermatous skin changes. Agent is also a carcinogen.

Xylene (INH, PA)*

LOCAL: Irritates eyes, nose, and throat.

SYSTEMIC: Acute exposure to vapor may cause CNS depression. High concentration may cause pulmonary edema, anorexia, nausea, vomiting, and abdominal pain.

Zinc chloride (INH, ING)*

LOCAL: Solid or aqueous solution is extremely corrosive. May produce eczemoid dermatitis due to sensitization. Accidental ingestion may cause pyloric stenosis in addition to effects of corrosive properties.

Zinc oxide (INH)*

LOCAL: Red, papular dermatitis, "oxide pox," itching.

SYSTEMIC: "Metal fume fever," begins 4-12 hours after exposure, heralded by metallic taste in the mouth. Cough, general malaise, and pains in muscles and joints occur. Fever up to 104° F then develops, with shaking and profuse sweating. Episode typically resolves in 24-48 hours.

B Tables of normal values*

ABBREVIATIONS USED IN TABLES

<	=	less than
>	=	greater than
dl	=	100 ml
gm	=	gram
IU	=	International Unit
kg	=	kilogram
mEq	=	milliequivalent
mg	=	milligram
ml	=	milliliter
mM	=	millimole
mm Hg	=	millimeters of mercury
mIU	=	milliInternational Unit
mOsm	=	milliosmole
$m\mu$	=	millimicron
ng	=	nanogram
pg	=	picogram
μEq	=	microequivalent
μg	=	microgram
μIU	=	microInternational Unit
μl	=	microliter
μU	=	microunit

*From Henry, J. B.: Todd-Sanford-Davidsohn clinical diagnosis and management by laboratory methods, ed. 16, Philadelphia, 1979, W. B. Saunders Co.

Table B-1. Whole blood, serum, and plasma chemistry

| Component | System | Typical reference intervals | | |
		In conventional units	Factor*	In SI units†
Acetoacetic acid:				
qualitative	Serum	Negative		Negative
quantitative	Serum	0.2-1.0 mg/dl	98	19.6-98.0 µmol/l
Acetone:				
qualitative	Serum	Negative		Negative
quantitative	Serum	0.3-2.0 mg/dl	172	51.6-344.0 µmol/l
Albumin:				
quantitative	Serum	3.2-4.5 g/dl (salt fractionation)	10	32-45 g/l
		3.2-5.6 g/dl (electrophoresis)	10	32-56 g/l
		3.8-5.0 g/dl (dye binding)	10	38-50 g/l
Alcohol, ethyl	Serum or whole blood	Negative—but presented as mg/dl	0.22	Negative—but presented as mmol/l
Aldolase	Serum:			
adults		3-8 Sibley-Lehninger U/dl at 37° C.	7.4	22-59 mU/l at 37° C.
children		Approximately 2 times adult levels		Approximately 2 times adult levels
newborn		Approximately 4 times adult levels		Approximately 4 times adult levels
Alpha-amino acid nitrogen	Serum	3.6-7.0 mg/dl	0.714	2.6-5.0 mmol/l
δ-Aminolevulinic acid	Serum	0.01-0.03 mg/dl	76.3	0.76-2.29 µmol/l
Ammonia	Plasma	20-120 µg/dl (diffusion)	0.554	22.2-44.3 µmol/l
		40-80 µg/dl (enzymatic method)	0.554	11.1-67.0 µmol/l
		12-48 µg/dl (resin method)	0.554	6.7-26.6 µmol/l
Amylase	Serum	60-160 Somogyi units/dl	1.85	111-296 U/l
Argininosuccinic lyase	Serum	0-4 U/dl	10	0-40 U/l
Arsenic‡	Whole blood	<7 µg/dl	0.13	<0.91 µmol/l
Ascorbic acid (vitamin C)	Plasma	0.6-1.6 mg/dl	56.8	34-91 µmol/l
	Whole blood	0.7-2.0 mg/dl	56.8	40-114 µmol/l
Barbiturates	Serum, plasma, or whole blood	Negative	—	Negative
Base excess	Whole blood:			
male		−3.3 to +1.2 mEq/l	1	−3.3 to +1.2 mmol/l
female		−2.4 to +2.3 mEq/l	1	−2.4 to +2.3 mmol/l
Base, total	Serum	145-160 mEq/l	1	145-160 mmol/l
Bicarbonate	Plasma	21-28 mM	1	21-28 mmol/l
Bile acids	Serum	0.3-3.0 mg/dl	10	3.0-30.0 mg/l
Bilirubin:	Serum			
direct (conjugated)		Up to 0.3 mg/dl	17.1	Up to 5.1 µmol/l
indirect (unconjugated)		0.1-1.0 mg/dl	17.1	1.7-17.1 µmol/l
total		0.1-1.2 mg/dl	17.1	1.7-20.5 µmol/l
newborns total		1-12 mg/dl	17.1	17.1-205.0 µmol/l
Blood gases:	Whole blood			
pH		7.38-7.44 (arterial)	1	7.38-7.44
		7.36-7.41 (venous)	1	7.36-7.41
P_{CO_2}	Whole blood	35-40 mm Hg (arterial)	0.133	4.66-5.32 kPa[a]
		40-45 mm Hg (venous)	0.133	5.32-5.99 kPa[a]
P_{O_2}	Whole blood	95-100 mm Hg (arterial)	0.133	12.64-13.30 kPa[a]
Bromide	Serum	0-5 mg/dl	0.125	0-0.63 mmol/l

*Factor = Number factor (note that units are not presented).   *Continued.*
†Value in SI units = Value in conventional units × factor.
‡Usually not measured in blood (preferred specimen is urine, hair, or nails except in acute cases where gastric contents are used).

Table B-1. Whole blood, serum, and plasma chemistry—cont'd

Component	System	Typical reference intervals		
		In conventional units	Factor*	In SI units†
BSP (Bromosulphalein) (5 mg/kg)	Serum	Less than 6% retention 45 min. after injection	0.01[b]	Less than 0.06 retention 45 min. after injection
Calcium:				
ionized	Serum	4-4.8 mg/dl	0.25	1.0-1.2 mmol/l
		2.0-2.4 mEq/l	0.5	
		30-58% of total	0.01[b]	0.30-0.58 of total
Total		9.2-11.0 mg/dl	0.25	2.3-2.8 mmol/l
		4.6-5.5 mEq/l	0.5	23-28 mmol/l
Carbon dioxide (CO_2 content)	Whole blood (arterial)	19-24 mM	1	19-24 mmol/l
	Plasma or serum (arterial)	21-28 mM	1	21-28 mmol/l
Carbon dioxide	Whole blood (venous)	22-26 mM	1	22-26 mmol/l
	Plasma or serum (venous)	24-30 mM	1	24-30 mmol/l
CO_2 combining power	Plasma or serum (venous)	24-30 mM	1	24-30 mmol/l
CO_2 partial pressure (P_{CO_2})	Whole blood (arterial)	35-40 mm Hg	0.133	4.66-5.32 kPa[a]
	Whole blood (venous)	40-45 mm Hg	0.133	5.32-5.99 kPa[a]
Carbonic acid (H_2CO_3)	Whole blood (arterial)	1.05-1.45 mM	1	1.05-1.45 mmol/l
	Whole blood (venous)	1.15-1.50 mM	1	1.15-1.50 mmol/l
	Plasma (venous)	1.02-1.38 mM	1	1.02-1.38 mmol/l
Carboxyhemoglobin (carbon monoxide hemoglobin)	Whole blood:			
	suburban non-smokers	<1.5% saturation of hemoglobin	0.01[b]	<0.015 saturation of hemoglobin
	smokers	1.5-5.0% saturation	0.01	0.015-0.050 saturation
	heavy smokers	5.0-9.0% saturation	0.01	0.050-0.090 saturation
Carotene, beta	Serum	40-200 μg/dl	0.0186	0.75-3.72 μmol/l
Ceruloplasmin	Serum	23-50 mg/dl	10	230-500 mg/l
Chloride	Serum	95-103 mEq/l	1	95-103 mmol/l
Cholesterol				
total	Serum	150-250 mg/dl (varies with diet, sex, and age)	0.026	3.90-6.50 mmol/l
esters	Serum	65-75% of total cholesterol	0.01[b]	0.65-0.75 of total cholesterol
Cholinesterase	Erythrocytes	0.65-1.3 pH units	1	0.65-1.3 units[e]
(Pseudocholinesterase)	Plasma	0.5-1.3 pH units	1	0.5-1.3 units
		8-18 IU/l at 37° C.	1	8-18 U/l at 37° C.
Citrate	Serum or plasma	1.7-3.0 mg/dl	52	88-156 μmol/l
Copper	Serum, plasma:			
	male	70-140 μg/dl	0.157	11.0-22.0 μmol/l
	female	80-155 μg/dl	0.157	12.6-24.3 μmol/l
Cortisol	Plasma:			
	8 a.m.-10 a.m.	5-23 μg/dl	27.6	138-635 nmol/l
	4 p.m.-6 p.m.	3-13 μg/dl	27.6	83-359 nmol/l
Creatine as creatinine	Serum or plasma:			
	male	.1-.4 mg/dl	76.3	7.6-30.5 μmol/l
	female	.2-.7 mg/dl	76.3	15.3-53.4 μmol/l

*Factor = Number factor (note that units are not presented).

†Value in SI units = Value in conventional units × factor.

‡Usually not measured in blood (preferred specimen is urine, hair, or nails except in acute cases where gastric contents are used).

Table B-1. Whole blood, serum, and plasma chemistry—cont'd

Component	System	Typical reference intervals		
		In conventional units	Factor*	In SI units†
Creatine kinase (CK)	Serum:			
	male	55-170 U/l at 37° C.	1	55-170 U/l at 37° C.
	female	30-135 U/l at 37° C.	1	30-135 U/l at 37° C.
Creatinine	Serum or plasma	0.6-1.2 mg/dl (adult)	88.4	53-106 μmol/l
		0.3-0.6 mg/dl (children <2 yr.)	88.4	27-54 μmol/l
Creatinine clearance (endogenous)	Serum or plasma and urine:			
	male	107-139 ml/min.	0.167	1.78-2.32 ml/s
	female	87-107 ml/min	0.0167	1.45-1.79 ml/s
Cryoglobulins	Serum	Negative	—	Negative
Electrophoresis, protein	Serum	Per cent:	0.01[b]	0.52-0.65 of total protein
Albumin		52-65% of total protein	0.01	0.025-0.05 of total protein
Alpha-1		2.5-5.0% of total protein	0.01	0.07-0.13 of total protein
Alpha-2		7.0-13.0% of total protein	0.01	0.08-0.14 of total protein
Beta		8.0-14.0% of total protein	0.01	0.12-0.22 of total protein
Gamma		12.0-22.0% of total protein		
	Serum	Concentration	10	32-56 g/l
Albumin		3.2-5.6 gm/dl		1-4 g/l
Alpha-1		0.1-0.4 gm/dl		4-12 g/l
Alpha-2		0.4-1.2 gm/dl		5-11 g/l
Beta		0.5-1.1 gm/dl		5-16 g/l
Gamma		0.5-1.6 gm/dl		
Fats, neutral (see Triglycerides)				
Fatty acids:				
total (free and esterified)	Serum	9-15 mM	1	9-15 mmol/l
free (non-esterified)	Plasma	300-480 μEq/l	1	300-480 μmol/l
Fibrinogen	Plasma	200-400 mg/dl	0.01	2.00-4.00 g/l
Fluoride	Whole blood	<0.05 mg/dl	0.53	<0.027 mmol/l
Folate	Serum	5-25 ng/ml (bioassay)	2.27	11-56 nmol/l
		>2.3 ng/ml (radioassay)	2.27	>5.2 nmol/l
	Erythrocytes	166-640 ng/ml (bioassay)	2.27	376-1452 nmol/l
		>140 ng/ml (radioassay)	2.27	>318 nmol/l
Galactose	Whole blood:			
	adults	None	0.055	None
	children	<20 mg/dl	0.055	<1.1 mmol/l
Gamma globulin	Serum	0.5-1.6 gm/dl	10	5-16 g/l
Globulins, total	Serum	2.3-3.5 gm/dl	10	23-35 g/l
Glucose, fasting	Serum or plasma	70-110 mg/dl	0.055	3.85-6.05 mmol/l
	Whole blood	60-100 mg/dl	0.055	3.30-5.50 mmol/l
Glucose tolerance	Serum or plasma:			
oral	fasting	70-110 mg/dl	0.055	3.85-6.05 mmol/l
	30 min.	30-60 mg/dl above fasting	0.055	1.65-3.30 mmol/l above fasting
	60 min.	20-50 mg/dl above fasting	0.055	1.10-2.75 mmol/l above fasting
	120 min.	5-15 mg/dl above fasting	0.055	0.28-0.83 mmol/l above fasting
	180 min.	Fasting level or below	0.055	Fasting level or below
	Serum or plasma:			
intravenous	fasting	70-110 mg/dl	0.055	3.85-6.05 mmol/l
	5 min.	Maximum of 250 mg/dl	0.055	Maximum of 13.75 mmol/l
	60 min.	Significant decrease	0.055	Significant decrease
	120 min.	Below 120 mg/dl	0.055	Below 6.60 mmol/l
	180 min.	Fasting level	0.055	Fasting level

Continued.

Table B-1. Whole blood, serum, and plasma chemistry—cont'd

Component	System	Typical reference intervals		
		In conventional units	Factor*	In SI units†
Glucose 6-phosphate dehydrogenase (G6PD)	Erythrocytes	250-500 units/10^6 cells	1	250-500 units/10^6 cells
		1200-2000 mIU/ml packed erythrocytes	1	1200-2000 U/l packed erythrocytes
γ-Glutamyl transferase	Serum	5-40 IU/l	1	5-40 U/l at 37° C.
Glutathione	Whole blood	24-37 mg/dl	0.032	0.77-1.18 mmol/l
Growth hormone	Serum	<10 ng/ml	1	<10 μg/l
Guanase	Serum	<3 nM/ml/min	1	<3 U/l at 37° C.
Haptoglobin	Serum	60-270 mg/dl	.01	0.6-2.7 g/l
Hemoglobin	Serum or plasma:			
	qualitative	Negative	10	Negative
	quantitative	0.5-5.0 mg/dl	10	5-50 mg/l
	Whole blood:			
	female	12.0-16.0 g/dl	10	1.86-2.48 mmol/l
	male	13.5-18.0 g/dl	10	2.09-2.79 mmol/l
α-Hydroxybutyrate dehydrogenase	Serum	140-350 U/ml	1	140-350 kU/l
17-Hydroxycorticosteroids	Plasma:			
	male	7-19 μg/dl	10	70-190 μg/l
	female	9-21 μg/dl	10	9-21 μg/l
	after 24 USP units of ACTH			
	I.M.	35-55 μg/dl	10	350-550 μg/l
Immunoglobulins:	Serum			
IgG		800-1801 mg/dl	0.01	8.0-18.0 g/l
IgA		113-563 mg/dl	0.01	1.1-5.6 g/l
IgM		54-222 mg/dl	0.01	0.54-2.2 g/l
IgD		0.5-3.0 mg/dl	10	5.0-30 mg/l
IgE		0.01-0.04 mg/dl	10	0.1-0.4 mg/l
Insulin	Plasma:			
	bioassay	11-240 μIU/ml[d]	0.0417	0.46-10.00 μg/l
	radioimmunoassay	4-24 μIU/ml	0.0417	0.17-1.00 μg/l
Insulin tolerance (0.1 unit/kg)	Serum:			
	fasting	Glucose of 70-110 mg/dl	0.055	Glucose of 3.85-6.05 mmol/l
	30 min.	Fall to 50% of fasting level	0.01[b]	Fall to 0.5 of fasting level
	90 min.	Fasting level		Fasting level
Iodine:				
Butanol-extraction (BEI)	Serum	3.5-6.5 μg/dl	0.079	0.28-0.51 μmol/l
Protein bound (PBI)	Serum	4.0-8.0 μg/dl		0.32-0.63 μmol/l
Iron, total	Serum	60-150 μg/dl	0.179	11-27 μmol/l
Iron binding capacity	Serum	300-360 μg/dl	0.179	54-64 μmol/l
Iron saturation	Serum	20-55%	0.01[b]	0.20-0.55 of total iron binding capacity
Isocitric dehydrogenase	Serum	50-240 units/ml at 25° C. (Wolfson-Williams Ashman units)	0.0167	0.83-4.18 U/l at 25° C.
Ketone bodies	Serum	Negative	—	Negative
17-Ketosteroids	Plasma	25-125 μg/dl	0.01	0.25-1.25 mg/l
Lactic acid (as lactate)	Whole blood:			
	venous	5-20 mg/dl	0.111	0.6-2.2 mmol/l
	arterial	3-7 mg/dl		0.3-0.8 mmol/l
Lactate dehydrogenase (LDH)	Serum	80-120 units at 30° C. (lactate → pyruvate)	0.48	38-62 U/l at 30° C. (lactate → pyruvate)

*Factor — Number factor (note that units are not presented).

†Value in SI units = Value in conventional units × factor.

‡Usually not measured in blood (preferred specimen is urine, hair, or nails except in acute cases where gastric contents are used).

Table B-1. Whole blood, serum, and plasma chemistry—cont'd

Component	System	Typical reference intervals		
		In conventional units	Factor*	In SI units†
		185-640 units at 30° C. (pyruvate → lactate)	0.48	90-310 U/l at 30° C. (pyruvate → lactate)
		100-190 U/l at 37° C. (lactate → pyruvate)	1	100-190 U/l at 37° C. (lactate → pyruvate)
Lactate dehydrogenase iso-enzymes:	Serum			
LDH₁ (anode)		17-27%	0.01[b]	0.17-0.27 of total LDH
LDH₂		27-37%		0.27-0.37 of total LDH
LDH₃		18-25%		0.18-0.25 of total LDH
LDH₄		3-8%		0.03-0.08 of total LDH
LDH₅ (cathode)		0.5%		0.00-0.05 of total LDH
Lactate dehydrogenase (heat stable)	Serum	30-60% of total	0.01[b]	0.3-0.6 of total LDH
Lactose tolerance	Serum	Serum glucose changes similar to glucose tolerance test	—	Serum glucose changes similar to glucose tolerance test
Lead	Whole blood	0-50 μg/dl	0.048	0-2.4 μmol/l
Leucine aminopeptidase (LAP)	Serum:			
	male	80-200 U/ml (Goldbarg-Rutenberg)	0.24	19.2-48.0 U/l
	female	75-185 U/ml (Goldbarg-Rutenberg)	0.24	18.0-44.4 U/l
Lipase	Serum	0-1.5 U/ml (Cherry-Crandall)	278	0-417 U/l
		14-280 mIU/ml	1	14-280 U/l
Lipids, total	Serum	400-800 mg/dl	0.01	4.00-8.00 g/l
Cholesterol		150-250 mg/dl	0.026	3.9-6.5 mmol/l
Triglycerides		10-190 mg/dl	0.109	1.09-20.71 mmol/l
Phospholipids		150-380 mg/dl	0.01	1.50-380 g/l
Fatty acids (free)		9.0-15.0 mM/l	1	9.0-15.0 mmol/l
		300-480 μEq/l	0.01	300-480 μmol/l
Phospholipid phosphorous		8.0-11.0 mg/dl	0.323	2.58-3.55 mmol/l
Lithium	Serum	Negative	—	Negative
therapeutic interval		0.5-1.4 mEq/l	1	0.5-1.4 mmol/l
Long-acting thyroid-stimulating hormone (LATS)	Serum	None	—	None
Lutenizing hormone (LH)	Serum:			
	male	6-30 mIU/ml	0.23	1.4-6.9 mg/l
	female	Mid cycle peak: 3 times baseline value	0.23	Mid cycle peak: 3 times baseline value
		Premenopausal <30 mIU/ml	0.23	Premenopausal <5 times baseline value
		Postmenopausal >35 mIU/ml		Postmenopausal >5 times baseline value
Macroglobulins, total	Serum	70-430 mg/dl	0.01	0.7-4.3 g/l
Magnesium	Serum	1.3-2.1 mEq/l	0.5	0.7-1.1 mmol/l
		1.8-3.0 mg/dl	0.41	0.7-1.1 mmol/l
Methemoglobin	Whole blood	0-0.24 g/dl	10	0.0-2.4 g/l
		<3% of total hemoglobin	0.01[b]	<.03 of total hemoglobin
Mucoprotein	Serum	80-200 mg/dl	0.01	0.8-2.0 g/l
Non-protein nitrogen (NPN)	Serum or plasma	20-35 mg/dl	0.714	14.3-25.0 mmol/l
	Whole blood	25-50 mg/dl	0.714	17.9-35.7 mmol/l
5'Nucleotidase	Serum	0-1.6 units at 37° C.	1	0-1.6 units at 37° C.
Ornithine carbamyl transferase	Serum	8-20 mIU/ml at 37° C.	1	8-20 U/l at 37° C.

Continued.

Table B-1. Whole blood, serum, and plasma chemistry—cont'd

Component	System	Typical reference intervals		
		In conventional units	Factor*	In SI units†
Osmolality	Serum	280-295 mOsm/kg	1	280-295 mOsm/l
Oxygen:				
pressure (Po₂)	Whole blood (arterial)	95-100 mm Hg	0.133	12.64-13.30 kPaᵃ
content	Whole blood (arterial)	15-23 volume %	0.01ᵇ	0.15-0.23 of volume
saturation	Whole blood (arterial)	94-100%	0.01ᵇ	0.94-1.00 of total
pH	Whole blood (arterial)	7.38-7.44	1	7.38-7.44
	Whole blood (venous)	7.36-7.41	1	7.36-7.41
	Serum or plasma (venous)	7.35-7.45	1	7.35-7.45
Phenylalanine	Serum:			
adults		<3.0 mg/dl	0.061	<0.18 mmol/l
newborns (term)		1.2-3.5 mg/dl	0.061	0.07-0.21 mmol/l
Phosphatase				
Acid phosphatase	Serum	0.13-0.63 U/l at 37° C. (paranitrophenyl phosphate)	16.67	2.2-10.5 U/l at 37° C. (*p*-nitrophenylphosphate)
Alkaline phosphatase	Serum	20-90 IU/l at 30° C. (paranitrophenylphosphate in AMP buffer)	1	20-90 U/l at 30° C. (*p*-nitrophenylphosphate) 25-97 U/l at 37° C. (*p*-nitrophenylphosphate)
Phospholipid phosphorus	Serum	8-11 mg/dl	0.323	2.6-3.6 mmol/l
Phospholipids	Serum	150-380 mg/dl	0.01	1.50-3.80 g/l
Phosphorus, inorganic	Serum:			
adults		2.3-4.7 mg/dl	0.323	0.78-1.52 mmol/l
children		4.0-7.0 mg/dl	0.323	1.29-2.26 mmol/l
Potassium	Plasma	3.8-5.0 mEq/l	1	3.8-5.0 mmol/l
Prolactin	Serum	1-25 ng/ml (females)	1	1-25 µg/l
		1-20 ng/ml (males)	1	1-20 µg/l
Proteins:	Serum			
total		6.0-7.8 g/dl	10	60-78 g/l
albumin		3.2-4.5 g/dl	10	32-45 g/l
globulin		2.3-3.5 g/dl	10	23-35 g/l
Protein fractionation		See electrophoresis		See electrophoresis
Protoporphyrin	Erythrocytes	15-50 µg/dl	0.018	0.27-0.90 µmol/l
Pyruvate	Whole blood	0.3-0.9 mg/dl	114	34-103 µmol/l
Salicylates	Serum	Negative	—	Negative
therapeutic interval		15-30 mg/dl	0.072	1.44-1.80 mmol/l
		150-300 µg/ml	0.0072	1.08-2.16 mmol/l
Sodium	Plasma	136-142 mEq/l	1	136-142 mmol/l
Sulfate, inorganic	Serum	0.2-1.3 mEq/l	0.5	0.10-0.65 mmol/l
		0.9-6.0 mg/dl as SO₄⁻⁻	0.104	0.09-0.62 mmol/l as SO₄⁻⁻
Sulfhemoglobin	Whole blood	Negative	—	Negative
Sulfonamides	Serum or whole blood	Negative	—	Negative
Testosterone	Serum or plasma:			
male		300-1200 ng/dl	0.035	10.0-42.0 nmol/l
female		30-95 ng/dl	0.035	1.1-3.3 nmol/l
Thiocyanate	Serum	Negative	—	Negative

*Factor = Number factor (note that units are not presented).

†Value in SI units = Value in conventional units × factor.

‡Usually not measured in blood (preferred specimen is urine, hair, or nails except in acute cases where gastric contents are used).

Table B-1. Whole blood, serum, and plasma chemistry—cont'd

Component	System	Typical reference intervals		
		In conventional units	Factor*	In SI units†
Thymol flocculation	Serum	0-5 units[f]	1	0-5 units
Thyroid hormone tests:	Serum			
a) Expressed as thyroxine:				
T_4 by column		5.0-11.0 μg/dl	13.0	65-143 nmol/l
T_4 by competitive binding—Murphy-Pattee		6.0-11.8 μg/dl	13.0	78-153 nmol/l
T_4 RIA		5.5-12.5 μg/dl	13.0	72-163 nmol/l
free T_4		0.9-2.3 ng/dl	13.0	12-30 pmol/l
b) Expressed as iodine:				
T_4 by column		3.2-7.2 μg/dl	79.0	253-569 nmol/l
T_4 by competitive binding—Murphy-Pattee		3.9-7.7 μg/dl	79.0	308-608 nmol/l
free T_4		0.6-1.5 ng/dl		47-119 pmol/l
T_3 resin uptake		25-38 relative % uptake	0.01[b]	0.25-0.38 relative uptake
Thyroxine-binding globulin (TBG)	Serum	10-26 μg/dl	10	100-260 μg/l
TSH	Serum	<10 μU/ml	1	<10^{-3} IU/l
Transferases				
Aspartate amino transferase (AST or SGOT)	Serum	10-40 U/ml (Karmen) at 25° C.	0.48	8-29 U/l at 30° C.
		16-60 U/ml (Karmen) at 30° C.		8-33 U/l at 37° C.
Alanine amino transferase (ALT or SGPT)	Serum	10-30 U/ml (Karmen) at 25° C.		
		8-50 U/ml (Karmen) at 30° C.	0.48	4-24 U/l at 30° C.
				4-36 U/l at 37° C.
Gamma glutamyl transferase (GGT)		5-40 IU/l at 37° C.	1	5-40 U/l at 37° C.
Triglycerides	Serum	10-190 mg/dl	0.011[e]	0.11-2.09 mmol/l
Urea nitrogen	Serum	8-23 mg/dl	0.357	2.9-8.2 mmol/l
Urea clearance:	Serum and urine			
maximum clearance		64-99 ml/min	0.0167	1.07-1.65 ml/s
standard clearance		41-65 ml/min, or more than 75% of normal clearance	0.0167	0.68-1.09 ml/s or more than 0.75 of normal clearance
Uric acid	Serum:			
male		4.0-8.5 mg/dl	0.059	0.24-0.5 mmol/l
female		2.7-7.3 mg/dl	0.059	0.16-0.43 mmol/l
Vitamin A	Serum	15-60 μg/dl	0.035	0.53-2.10 μmol/l
Vitamin A tolerance	Serum:			
fasting 3 hr. or 6 hr. after 5000 units vitamin A/kg		15-60 μg/dl	0.035	0.53-2.10 μmol/l
		200-600 μg/dl		7.00-21.00 μmol/l
24 hrs.		Fasting values or slightly above		Fasting values or slightly above
Vitamin B_{12}	Serum	160-950 pg/ml	0.74	118-703 pmol/l
Unsaturated vitamin B_{12} binding capacity	Serum	1000-2000 pg/ml	0.74	740-1480 pmol/l
Vitamin C	Plasma	0.6-1.6 mg/dl	56.8	34-91 μmol/l
Xylose absorption	Serum:			
normal		25-40 mg/dl between 1 and 2 hr.	0.067	1.68-2.68 mmol/l between 1 and 2 h
in malabsorption		Maximum approximately 10 mg/dl		Maximum approximately 0.67 mmol/l
Dose: adult		25 g D-xylose	0.067	0.167 mol D-xylose
children		0.5 g/kg D-xylose		3.33 mmol/kg D-xylose
Zinc	Serum	50-150 μg/dl	0.153	7.65-22.95 μmol/l

Table B-2. Urine

Component	Type of urine specimen	Typical reference intervals In conventional units	Factor	Typical reference intervals In SI units
Acetoacetic acid	Random	Negative	—	Negative
Acetone	Random	Negative	—	Negative
Addis count	12 hr. collection	WBC and epithelial cells:		
		1,800,000/12 hr.	1	$1.8 \times 10^6/12$ h
		RBC 500,000/12 hr.	1	$0.5 \times 10^6/12$ h
		Hyaline casts: 0-5000/12 hr.	1	$5.0 \times 10^3/12$ h
Albumin:				
qualitative	Random	Negative	—	Negative
quantitative	24 hr.	15-150 mg/24 hr.	1	0.015-0.150 g/24 h
Aldosterone	24 hr.	2-26 µg/24 hr.	2.77	5.5-72.0 nmol/24 h
Alkapton bodies	Random	Negative	—	Negative
Alpha-amino acid nitrogen	24 hr.	100-290 mg/24 hr.	0.0714	7.14-20.71 mmol/24 h
δ-Aminolevulinic acid	Random:			
	adult	0.1-0.6 mg/dl	76.3	7.6-45.8 µmol/l
	children	<0.5 mg/dl	76.3	<38.1 µmol/l
	24 hr.	1.5-7.5 mg/24 hr.	7.63	11.15-57.2 µmol/24 h
Ammonia nitrogen	24 hr.	20-70 mEq/24 hr.		
		500-1200 mg/24 hr.	0.071	35.5-85.2 mmol/24 h
Amylase	2 hr.	35-260 Somogyi units/hr.	0.185	6.5-48.1 U/h
Arsenic	24 hr.	<50 µg/l	0.013	<0.65 µmol/l
Ascorbic acid	Random	1-7 mg/dl	0.057	0.06-0.40 mmol/l
	24 hr.	>50 mg/24 hr.	0.0057	>0.29 mmol/24 h
Bence Jones protein	Random	Negative	—	Negative
Beryllium	24 hr.	<0.05 µg/24 hr.	111	<5.55 nmol/24 h
Bilirubin, qualitative	Random	Negative	—	Negative
Blood, occult	Random	Negative	—	Negative
Borate	24 hr.	<2 mg/l	16	<32 µmol/l
Calcium:				
qualitative (Sulkowitch)	Random	1+ turbidity	1	1+ tubidity
quantitative	24 hr.:			
	average diet	100-240 mg/24 hr.	0.025	2.50-6.25 mmol/24 h
	low calcium diet	<150 mg/24 hr.	0.025	<3.75 mmol/24 h
	high calcium diet	240-300 mg/24 hr.	0.025	6.25-7.50 mmol/24 h
Catecholamines	Random	0-14 µg/dl	0.059	0-0.83 µmol/l
	24 hr.	<100 µg/24 hr. (varies with activity)	0.0059	<0.59 µmol/24 h
Epinephrine		<10 ng/24 hr.	5.46	<55 nmol/24 h
Norepinephrine		<100 ng/24 hr.	5.91	<590 nmol/24 h
Total free catecholamines		4-126 mcg./24 hr.	5.91	24-745 nmol/24 h
Total metanephrines		0.1-1.6 mg./24 hr.	5.07	0.5-8.1 µmol/24 h
Chloride	24 hr.	140-250 mEq/24 hr.	1	140-250 mmol/24 h
Concentration test (Fishberg):	Random—after fluid restriction			
specific gravity		>1.025	1	>1.025
osmolality		>850 mOsm/l	1	>850 mOsm/l
Copper	24 hr.	0-30 µg/24 hr.	0.016	0-0.48 µmol/24 h
Coproporphyrin	Random:			
	adult	3-20 µg/dl	0.015	0.045-0.30 µmol/l
	24 hr.:			
	adult	50-160 µg/24 hr.	0.0015	0.075-0.24 µmol/24 h
	children	0-80 µg/24 hr.	0.0015	0.00-0.12 µmol/24 h
Creatine	24 hr.:			
	male	0-40 mg/24 hr.	0.0076	0-0.30 mmol/24 h
	female	0-100 mg/24 hr.	0.0076	0-0.76 mmol/24 h

Table B-2. Urine—cont'd

Component	Type of urine specimen	Typical reference intervals		
		In conventional units	Factor	In SI units
		Higher in children and during pregnancy	0.0076	Higher in children and during pregnancy
Creatinine	24 hr.:			
	male	20-26 mg/kg/24 hr.	0.0088	0.18-0.23 mmol/kg/24 h
		1.0-2.0 g/24 hr.	8.8	8.8-17.6 mmol/24 h
	female	14-22 mg/kg/24 hr.	0.0088	0.12-0.19 mmol/kg/24 h
		0.8-1.8 g/24 hr.	8.8	7.0-15.8 mmol/24 h
Cystine, qualitative	Random	Negative	—	Negative
Cystine and cysteine	24 hr.:	10-100 mg/24 hr.	.0083^g	0.08-0.83 mmol/24 h
Diacetic acid	Random	Negative	—	Negative
Epinephrine	24 hr.	0-20 μg/24 hr.	0.0055	0.00-0.11 μmol/24 h
Estrogens				
total	24 hr:			
	male	5-18 μg/24 hr.	1	5-18 μg/24 h
	female:			
	ovulation	28-100 μg/24 hr.	1	28-100 μg/24 h
	luteal peak	22-80 μg/24 hr.	1	22-80 μg/24 h
	at menses	4-25 μg/24 hr.	1	4-25 μg/24 h
	pregnancy	Up to 45,000 μg/24 hr.	1	Up to 45,000 μg/24 h
	postmeno-pausal	Up to 10 μg/24 hr.	1	Up to 10 μg/24 h
fractionated	24 hr., non-pregnant, midcycle			
Estrone (E^1)	—	2-25 μg/24 hr.	3.7	7-93 nmol/24 h
Estradiol (E^2)	—	0-10 μg/24 hr.	3.7	0-37 nmol/24 h
Estriol (E^3)	—	2-30 μg/24 hr.	3.5	7-105 nmol/24 h
Fat, qualitative	Random	Negative	—	Negative
FIGLU (N-formiminoglutamic acid)	24 hr.	<3 mg/24 hr.	5.7	<17.0 μmol/24 h
	after 15 g of L-histidine	4 mg/8 hr.	5.7	23.0 μmol/8 h
Fluoride	24 hr.	<1 mg/24 hr.	0.053	0.053 mmol/24 h
Follicle-stimulating hormone (FSH)	24 hr.:			
	adult	6-50 Mouse uterine units (MUU)/24 h	1	4-25 mIU/ml
	prepubertal	<10 MUU/24 h	1	4-30 mIU/ml
	postmenopausal	>50 MUU/24 h	1	40-50 mIU/ml
	midcycle	2+ baseline		
Fructose	24 hr.	30-65 mg/24 hr.	0.0056	0.17-0.36 mmol/24 h
Glucose:				
qualitative	Random	Negative	—	Negative
quantitative:	24 hr.			
copper-reducing substances		0.5-1.5 g/24 hr.	1	0.5-1.5 g/24 h
total sugars		average 250 mg/24 hr.	1	Average 250 mg/24 h
glucose		average 130 mg/24 hr.	0.0056	Average 0.73 mmol/24 h
Gonadotropins, pituitary (FSH and LH)	24 hr.	10-50 MUU/24 hr.	1	10-50 MUU/24 h
Hemoglobin	Random	Negative	—	Negative
Homogentisic acid	Random	Negative	—	Negative
Homovanillic acid (HVA)	24 hr.	<15 mg/24 hr.	5.5	<83.0 μmol/24 h
17-Hydroxycorticosteroids	24 hr.			
	male	5.5-14.5 mg/24 hr.	1	5.5-145 mg/24 h
	female	4.9-12.9 mg/24 hr.		4.9-12.9 mg/24 h

Continued.

Table B-2. Urine—cont'd

Component	Type of urine specimen	Typical reference intervals		
		In conventional units	Factor	In SI units
5-Hydroxyindoleacetic acid (5-HIAA)				
qualitative	Random	Negative	—	Negative
quantitative	24 hr.	<9 mg/24 hr.	5.2	<47 μmol/24 h
Ketone bodies	Random	Negative		Negative
17-Ketosteroids	24 hr.			
male		8-20 mg/24 hr.	1	8.0-20 mg/24 h
female		4-15 mg/24 hr.		4.0-15 mg/24 h
Androsterone	24 hr.			
male		2.0-5.0 mg/24 hr.	3.44	6.9-17.2 μmol/24 h
female		0.8-3.0 mg/24 hr.		2.8-10.3 μmol/24 h
Etiocholanolone	24 hr.:			
male		1.4-5.0 mg/24 hr.	3.44	4.8-17.2 μmol/24 h
female		0.8-4.0 mg/24 hr.	3.44	2.8-13.8 μmol/24 h
Dehydroepiandroste-rone	24 hr.:			
male		0.2-2.0 mg/24 hr.	3.46	0.7-6.9 μmol/24 h
female		0.2-1.8 mg/24 hr.	3.46	0.7-6.2 μmol/24 h
11-Ketoandrosterone	24 hr.:			
male		0.2-1.0 mg/24 hr.	3.28	0.7-3.3 μmol/24 h
female		0.2-0.8 mg/24 hr.	3.28	0.7-2.6 μmol/24 h
11-Ketoetiocholanolone	24 hr.:			
male		0.2-1.0 mg/24 hr.	3.28	0.7-3.3 μmol/24 h
female		0.2-0.8 mg/24 hr.	3.28	0.7-2.6 μmol/24 h
11-Hydroxyandosterone	24 hr.:			
male		0.1-0.8 mg/24 hr.	3.26	0.3-2.6 μmol/24 h
female		0.0-0.5 mg/24 hr.	3.26	0.0-1.6 μmol/24 h
11-Hydroxyetiocholano-lone	24 hr.:			
male		0.2-0.6 mg/24 hr.	3.26	0.7-2.0 μmol/24 h
female		0.1-1.1 mg/24 hr.	3.26	0.3-3.6 μmol/24 h
Lactose	24 hr.	14-40 mg/24 hr.	2.9	41-116 μmol/24 h
Lead	24 hr.	<100 μg/24 hr.	0.0048	<0.48 μmol/24 h
Magnesium	24 hr.	6.0-8.5 mEq/24 hr.	0.5	3.0-4.3 mmol/24 h
Melanin, qualitative	Random	Negative	—	Negative
3-Methoxy-4-hydroxyman-delic acid (VMA)	24 hr.:			
adults		1.5-7.5 mg/24 hr.	5.05	7.6-37.9 μmol/24 h
infants		83 μg/kg/24 hr.	0.0051	0.4 μmol/kg/24 h
Mucin	24 hr.	100-150 mg/24 hr.	1	100-150 mg/24 h
Myoglobin				
qualitative	Random	Negative	—	Negative
quantitative	24 hr.	<4 mg/l	1	<4 mg/l
Osmolality	Random	500-800 mOsm/kg water	1	500-800 mOsm/kg water
Pentoses	24 hr.	2-5 mg/kg/24 hr.	1	2-5 mg/kg/24 h
pH	Random	4.6-8.0	1	4.6-8.0
Phenosulfonphthalein (PSP)	Urine timed after 6 mg PSP IV			
15 min.		20-50% dye excreted	0.01[b]	0.2-0.5 dye excreted
30 min.		16-24% dye excreted	0.01	0.16-0.24 dye excreted
60 min.		9-17% dye excreted	0.01	0.09-0.17 dye excreted
120 min.		3-10% dye excreted	0.01	0.03-0.10 dye excreted

Table B-2. Urine—cont'd

Component	Type of urine specimen	Typical reference intervals		
		In conventional units	Factor	In SI units
Phenylpyruvic acid, qualitative	Random	Negative	—	Negative
Phosphorus	Random	0.9-1.3 g/24 hr.	32	29-42 mmol/24 h
Porphobilinogen:				
qualitative	Random	Negative	—	Negative
quantitative	24 hr.	0-1.0 mg/24 hr.	4.42	0-4.4 μmol/24 h
Potassium	24 hr.	40-80 mEq/24 hr.	1	40-80 mmol/24 h
Pregnancy tests	Concentrated morning specimen	Positive in normal pregnancies or with tumors producing chorionic gonadotropin	—	Positive in normal pregnancies or with tumors producing chorionic gonadotropin
Pregnanediol	24 hr.:			
male		0-1.5 mg/24 hr.	3.12	0-4.7 μmol/24 h
female		1-8 mg/24 hr.	3.12	3-25 μmol/24 h
peak		1 week after ovulation	3.12	1 week after ovulation
pregnancy		<50 mg/24 hr.	3.12	<156 μmol/24 h
children		Negative	—	Negative
Pregnanetriol	24 hr.:			
male		0.4-2.4 mg/24 hr.	2.97	1.2-7.1 μmol/24 h
female		0.5-2.0 mg/24 hr.	2.97	1.5-5.9 μmol/24 h
children		Up to 1 mg/24 hr.	2.97	Up to 3 μmol/24 h
Protein, qualitative	Random	Negative	—	Negative
	24 hr.	40-150 mg/24 hr.	1	40-150 mg/24 h
Reducing substances, total	24 hr.	0.5-1.5 mg/24 hr.	1	0.5-1.5 mg/24 h
Sodium	24 hr.	75-200 mEq/24 hr.	1	75-200 mmol/24 h
Solids, total	24 hr.	55-70 g/24 hr.	1	55-70 g/24 h
		Decreases with age to 30 gm/24 hr.	—	Decreases with age to 30 g/24 h
Specific gravity	Random	1.016-1.022 (normal fluid intake)	1	Relative density (U 20° C./ water 20° C.) 1.016-1.022 (normal fluid intake)
		1.001-1.035 (range)		1.001-1.034 (range)
Sugars (exluding glucose)	Random	Negative	—	Negative
Titratable acidity	24 hr.	20-50 mEq/24 hr.	1	20-50 mmol/24 h
Urea nitrogen	24 hr.	6-17 g/24 hr.	0.0357	0.21-0.60 mol/24 h
Uric acid	24 hr.	250-750 mg/24 hr.	0.0059	1.48-4.43 mmol/24 h
Urobilinogen	2 hr.	0.3-1.0 Ehrlich units	—	
	24 hr.	0.05-2.5 mg/24 hr. or	1.69	0.09-4.23 μmol/24 h
		0.5-4.0 Ehrlich units/24 hr.	—	
Uropepsin	Random	15-45 units/hr. (Anson)	7.37	111-332 U/h
	24 hr.	1500-5000 units/24 hr. (Anson)	7.37	11-37 kU/h
Uroporphyrins:				
qualitative	Random	Negative	—	Negative
quantitative	24 hr.	10-30 μg/24 hr.	0.0012	0.012-0.037 μmol/24 h
Vanillylmandelic acid (VMA)	24 hr.	1.5-7.5 mg/24 hr.	5.05	7.6-37.9 μmol/24 h
Volume, total	24 hr.	600-1600 ml/24 hr.	0.001	0.6-1.61/24 h
Zinc	24 hr.	0.15-1.2 mg/24 hr.	15.3	2.3-18.4 μmol/24 h

Table B-3. Synovial fluid

Component	Typical reference intervals		
	In conventional units	Factor	In SI units
Blood-serum-synovial fluid glucose difference	<10 mg/dl	0.055	<0.55 mmol/l
Differential cell count	Granulocytes <25% of nucleated cells	0.01[b]	Granulocytes <0.25 of nucleated cells
Fibrin clot	Absent	—	Absent
Mucin clot	Abundant	—	Abundant
Nucleated cell count	<200 cells/μl	10^6	<2 × 10^8 cells/l
Viscosity	High	—	High
Volume	<3.5 ml	0.001	<0.00351

Table B-4. Seminal fluid

Component	Typical reference intervals		
	In conventional units	Factor	In SI units
Liquefaction	Within 20 min.	1	Within 20 min
Sperm morphology	>70% normal, mature spermatozoa	0.01[b]	>0.7 normal, mature spermatozoa
Sperm motility	>60%	0.01[b]	>0.6
pH	>7.0 (average 7.7)	1	>7.0 (average 7.7)
Sperm count	60-150 million/ml	10^3	60-150 × 10^9/l
Volume	1.5-5.0 ml	0.001	0.0015-0.005/1

Table B-5. Gastric fluid

Component	Typical reference intervals		
	In conventional units	Factor	In SI units
Fasting residual volume	<50 ml	0.001	<.05/1
pH (stimulated specimen)	<2.0	1	<2.0
Basal acid output (BAO)	0-6 mEq/hr.	1	0-6 mmol/h
Maximum acid output (MAO) (after histamine stimulation)	5-40 mEq/hr.	1	5-40 mmol/h
BAO/MAO ratio	<0.4	1	<0.4

Table B-6. Hematology

Component	Typical reference intervals		
	In conventional units	Factor	In SI units
Red cell volume:			
male	25-35 ml/kg body weight	0.001	0.025-0.035 l/kg body weight
female	20-30 ml/kg body weight	—	0.020-0.030 l/kg body weight
Plasma volume:			
male	40-50 ml/kg body weight	0.001	0.040-0.050 l/kg body weight
female	40-50 ml/kg body weight	—	0.040-0.050 l/kg body weight
Coagulation tests:			
Bleeding time (Ivy)	1-6 minutes	1	1-6 min
Bleeding time (Duke)	1-3 minutes	1	1-3 min
Clot retraction	½ the original mass in 2 hr.	1	0.5 the original mass in 2 h
Dilute blood clot lysis time	Clot lysis between 6 and 10 hr at 37° C.	1	Clot lysis between 6 and 10 h at 37° C.
Euglobin clot lysis time	Clot lysis between 2 and 6 hr. at 37° C.	1	Clot lysis between 2 and 6 h at 37° C.
Partial thromboplastin time	60-70 seconds	1	60-70 s
Kaolin activated	35-50 seconds	1	35-50 s
Prothrombin time	12-14 seconds	1	12-14 s
Venous clotting time:			
3 tubes	5-15 minutes	1	5-15 min
2 tubes	5-18 minutes	—	5-8 min
Whole blood clot lysis time	None in 24 hr	—	None in 24 h
Complete blood count (CBC)			
Hematocrit:			
male	40-54%	0.01[b]	0.40-0.54
female	38-47%	—	0.38-0.47
Hemoglobin:			
male	13.5-18.0 g/dl	0.155	2.09-2.79 mmol/l
female	12.0-16.0 g/dl	—	1.86-2.48 mmol/l
Red cell count:			
male	$4.6\text{-}6.2 \times 10^6/\mu l$	0.155	$4.6\text{-}6.2 \times 10^{12}/l$
female	$4.2\text{-}5.4 \times 10^6/\mu l$	—	$4.2\text{-}5.4 \times 10^{12}/l$
White cell count	$4.5\text{-}11.0 \times 10^3/\mu l$	10^6	$4.5\text{-}11.0 \times 10^9/l$
Erythrocyte indices:			
Mean corpuscular volume (MCV)	80-96 cu. microns	1	80-96 fl
Mean corpuscular hemoglobin (MCH)	27-31 pg	1	27-31 pg
Mean corpuscular hemoglobin concentration (MCHC)	32-36%	0.01[b]	0.32-0.36

White blood cell differential (adult):	Mean per cent	Range of absolute counts		Mean fraction*	Range of absolute count
Segmented neutrophils	56%	1800-7000/μl	10^6	0.56	$1.8\text{-}7.0 \times 10^9/l$
Bands	3%	0-700/μl	10^6	0.03	$0\text{-}0.70 \times 10^9/l$
Eosinophils	2.7%	0-450/μl	10^6	0.027	$0\text{-}0.45 \times 10^9/l$
Basophils	0.3%	0-200/μl	10^6	0.003	$0\text{-}0.20 \times 10^9$-l
Lymphocytes	34%	1000-4800/μl	10^6	0.34	$1.0\text{-}4.8 \times 10^9/l$
Monocytes	4%	0-800/μl	10^6	0.04	$0\text{-}0.80 \times 10^9/l$

Component	In conventional units	Factor	In SI units
Hemoglobin A_2	1.5-3.5% of total hemoglobin	0.01[b]	0.015-0.035 of total hemoglobin
Hemoglobin F	<2%	0.01[b]	<0.02
Osmotic fragility	% NaCl % Lysis Fresh 24 hr. at 37° C.	% NaCl—171 % Lysis—0.01[b]	NaCl Fractional Lysis mmol/l Fresh 24 h at 37° C.

*All percentages are multiplied by 0.01[b] to give mean fraction.

Continued.

Table B-6. Hematology—cont'd

Component	Typical reference intervals					
	In conventional units			Factor	In SI units	
	0.2	—	95-100		34.2	—	0.95-1.00
	0.3	97-100	85-100		51.3	0.97-1.00	0.85-1.00
	0.35	90-99	75-100		59.8	0.90-0.99	0.75-1.00
	0.4	50-95	65-100		68.4	0.50-0.95	0.65-1.00
	0.45	5-45	55-95		77.0	0.05-0.45	0.55-0.95
	0.5	0-6	40-85		85.5	0-0.06	0.40-0.85
	0.55	0	15-70		94.1	0	0.15-0.70
	0.6	—	0-40		102.6	—	0-0.40
	0.65	—	0-10		111.2	—	0-0.10
	0.7	—	0-5		119.7	—	0-0.05
	0.75	—	0		128.3	—	0
Platelet count	150,000-400,000/μl			10^6	0.15-0.4 $\times$ 10^{12}/l	
Reticulocyte count	0.5-1.5%			0.01[b]	0.005-0.015	
	25,000-75,000 cells/μl			10^6	25-75 $\times$ 10^9/l	
Sedimentation rate (ESR) (Westergren)						
men under 50 yrs.	<15 mm/hr			1	<15 mm/h	
men over 50 yrs.	<20 mm/hr			1	<20 mm/h	
women under 50 yrs.	<20 mm/hr			1	<20 mm/h	
women over 50 yrs.	<30 mm/hr			1	<30 mm/h	
Viscosity	1.4-1.8 times water			1	1.4-1.8 times water	
Zeta sedimentation ratio	41-54%			0.01[b]	0.41-0.54	

Table B-7. Amniotic fluid

Component	Typical reference intervals		
	In conventional units	Factor	In SI units
Appearance:			
early gestation	Clear	—	Clear
term	Clear or slightly opalescent	—	Clear or slightly opalescent
Albumin:			
early gestation	0.39 g/dl	1	3.9 g/l
term	0.19 g/dl	1	1.9 g/l
Bilirubin:			
early gestation	<0.075 mg/dl	17.1	<1.28 μmol/l
term	<0.025 mg/dl	17.1	<0.43 μmol/l
Chloride:			
early gestation	Approximately equal to serum chloride	—	Approximately equal to serum chloride
term	Generally 1-3 mEq/l lower than serum chloride	1	Generally 1-3 mmol/l lower than serum chloride
Creatinine:			
early gestation	0.8-1.1 mg/dl	88.4	70.7-97.2 μmol/l
term	1.8-4.0 mg/dl (generally >2 mg/dl)	88.4	159.1-353.6 μmol/l (generally >176.8 μmol/l)
Estriol:			
early gestation	<10 μg/dl	0.035	<0.35 μmol/l
term	>60 μg/dl	0.035	>2.1 μmol/l
Lecithin/sphingomyelin			
early (immature)	<1:1	1	<1:1
term (mature)	>2:1	1	>2:1

Table B-8. Selected pediatric reference values*

S†-Acid phosphatase
Newborn: 7.4-19.4 U/l
2-13 yrs: 6.4-15.2 U/l

S-Aldolase
Newborn: to 4 × adult value
Child: to 2 × adult value

S-Alkaline phosphatase
Newborn: 40-300 U/l
Child: 60-270 U/l

S-Alpha fetoprotein:
Newborn: up to 100 mg/l
2 weeks: undetectable

S-Amylase
Newborn: little, if any, amylase activity
1 year: adult values

S-Aspartate aminotransferase
Newborn: 16-74 U/l
1-3 yrs: 6-30 U/l

S-Bilirubin
Newborn:

	Pre-term	**Full-term**
24 h	17.1-102.8 μmol/l (10-60 mg/l)	34.2-102.8 μmol/l (20-60 mg/l)
48 h	102.8-137.0 μmol/l (60-80 mg/l)	102.8-119.9 μmol/l (60-70 mg/l)
3-5 d	171.0-266.5 μmol/l (100-150 mg/l)	68.6-205.2 μmol/l (40-120 mg/l)

S-Calcium
Pre-term, first week: 1.5-2.5 mmol/l (60-100 mg/l)
Full-term, first week: 1.75-3.00 mmol/l (70-120 mg/l)
1-2 yrs: 2.5-3.0 mmol/l (100-120 mg/l)
2-16 yrs: 2.25-2.88 mmol/l (90-115 mg/l)

U†-Catecholamines

	Norepinephrine	**Epinephrine**
1 yr:	29.5-86.8 nmol/d (5.4-15.9 μg/d)	0.6-25.4 nmol/d (0.1-4.3 μg/d)
1-5 yrs:	44.2-168.1 nmol/d (8.1-30.8 μg/d)	4.7-53.8 nmol/d (0.8-9.1 μg/d)
6-15 yrs:	103.7-388.1 nmol/d (19.0-71.1 μg/d)	7.7-62.1 nmol/d (1.3-10.5 μg/d)
>15 yrs:	188.8-474.8 nmol/d (34.4-87.0 μg/d)	20.7-78.0 nmol/d (3.5-13.2 μg/d)

U-Chloride
Infant: 1.7-8.5 mmol/d (1.7-8.5 mEq/24 hr.)
Child: 17-34 mmol/d (17-34 mEq/24 hr.)

S-Cholesterol
Cord blood: 1.2-2.5 mmol/l (460-980 mg/l)
1-2 yrs: 1.8-4.9 mmol/l (700-1900 mg/l)
2-16 yrs: 3.5-6.5 mmol/l (1350-2500 mg/l)

U-Cortisol (free)
4 mos-10 yrs: 5.5-74.4 nmol/d (2-27 μg/d)
11-20 yrs: 1.9-151.7 nmol/d (0.7-55 μg/d)

S-Creatine kinase
Newborn: 3 × adult values
3 wks-3 mos: 1.5 × adult values
>1 yr: at adult values

S-Creatinine
Upper reference value:
Up to 5 yrs: 44 μmol/l (5.0 mg/l)
Up to 6 yrs: 53 μmol/l (6.0 mg/l)
Up to 7 yrs: 62 μmol/l (7.0 mg/l)
Up to 8 yrs: 70 μmol/l (8.0 mg/l)

---

*Information based on Meites, S., editor: Pediatric clinical chemistry, Washington, D.C., 1977, American Association for Clinical Chemistry.
†S = serum; U = urine

Continued.

Table B-8. Selected pediatric reference values—cont'd

Up to 9 yrs: 79 μmol/l (9.0 mg/l)
Up to 10 yrs: 88 μmol/l (10.0 mg/l)
>10 yrs: 106 μmol/l (12.0 mg/l)

S-Estradiol

0-2 yrs: 0-26 pmol/l (0-7 pg/ml)
2-4 yrs: 0.26 pmol/l (0-7 pg/ml)
4-6 yrs: 0-51 pmol/l (0-14 pg/ml)
6-8 yrs: 0-37 pmol/l (0-10 pg/ml)
8-10 yrs: 0-367 pmol/l (0-100 pg/ml)
10-12 yrs: 0-367 pmol/l (0-100 pg/ml)
12-14 yrs: 0.367 pmol/l (0-100 pg/ml)
14-16 yrs: 26-285 pmol/l (7-105 pg/ml)
16-25 yrs: 26-1175 pmol/1 (7-320 pg/ml)

Fecal Fat:

Pre-term newborn: up to 40% excreted
Full-term newborn: up to 20% excreted
3 mos-1 yr: up to 15% excreted
1 yr: up to 8.5% excreted

P-Nonesterified fatty acids

Newborn: 0-1845 mmol/l
4 mos-10 yrs: 300-1100 mmol/l

S-Glucose

Pre-term newborn: 1.2-3.6 mmol/l (200-656 mg/l)
Full-term newborn: 1.1-6.0 mmol/l (200-1100 mg/l)
Child: 3.3-5.8 mmol/l (600-1050 mg/l)

S-γ-Glutamyltransferase

Premature newborn: 56-233 U/l
Newborn-3 wks: 10-103 U/l
3 wks-3 mos: 4-111 U/l
1-5 yrs: 2-23 U/l
6-15 yrs: 2-23 U/l
16 yrs-adult: 2-35 U/l

S-Haptoglobin

Newborn: detectable haptoglobin in only 10-20%
1 yr and older: at adult values

S-Immunoglobulin IgG

0-5 wks: 7500-15,000 mg/l
6 mos: 1500-7000 mg/l
1 yr: 1400-10,300 mg/l
5 yrs: 3700-15,000 mg/l
10 yrs: 4400-15,500 mg/l

S-Immunoglobulin IgA

0-5 wks: none
6 mos: 200-1300 mg/l
1 yr: 200-1300 mg/l
5 yrs: 300-200 mg/l
10 yrs: 500-2300 mg/l

S-Immunoglobulin IgM

0-5 wks: less than 200 mg/l
6 mos: 300-600 mg/l
1 yr: 300-1600 mg/l
5 yrs: 200-2200 mg/l
10 yrs: 300-1700 mg/l

Table B-8. Selected pediatric reference values—cont'd

Inulin clearance

<1 mo: 29-88 ml/min per 1.73 m² of body surface
1-6 mos: 40-112 ml/min per 1.73 m² of body surface
6-12 mos: 62-121 ml/min per 1.73 m² of body surface
>1 yr: 78-164 ml/min per 1.73 m² of body surface

U-17-Ketosteroids

0-3 days: 0-0.5 mg/d
1-3 yrs: <2.0 mg/d
3-6 yrs: 0.5-3.0 mg/d
6-9 yrs: 0.8-4.0 mg/d
10-12 yrs: male: 0.7-6.0 mg/d
female: 0.7-5.0 mg/d
Adolescent: male: 3-15 mg/d
female: 3-12 mg/d

S-Lactate dehydrogenase

1-3 days: up to 2 × adult values

S-Phosphorus (inorganic)

	Pre-term	Full-term
Newborn:	1.8-2.6 mmol/l (56.0-80.0 mg/l)	1.6-2.5 mmol/l (50.0-78.0 mg/l)
6-10 days:	2.0-3.8 mmol/l (61-117 mg/l)	1.6-2.9 mmol/l (49-89 mg/l)
4 mos:	1.6-2.6 mmol/l (48-81 mg/l)	
1 yr:	1.25-2.1 mmol/l (39-60 mg/l)	
2-16 yrs:	0.9-1.5 mmol/l (26-50 mg/l)	

S-Potassium

Pre-term newborn: 4.5-7.2 mmol/l (4.5-7.2 mEq/l)
Full-term newborn: 5.0-7.7 mmol/l (5.0-7.7 mEq/l)
2 d-2 wks: 4.0-6.4 mmol/l (4.0-6.4 mEq/l)
2 wks-3 mos: 4.0-6.2 mmol/l (4.0-6.2 mEq/l)
3 mos-1 yr: 3.7-5.6 mmol/l (3.7-5.6 mEq/l)
1-16 yrs: 3.6-5.2 mmol/l (3.6-5.2 mEq/l)

S-Testosterone

Age	Male	Female
0-2 yrs:	0.1-1.3 nmol/l (40-370 ng/l)	0.2-0.6 nmol/l (70-180 ng/l)
2-4 yrs:	0.2-0.6 nmol/l (50-160 ng/l)	0.2-0.7 nmol/l (70-200 ng/l)
4-6 yrs:	0.3-1.4 nmol/l (80-400 ng/l)	0.3-0.7 nmol/l (100-200 ng/l)
6-8 yrs:	0.2-1.0 nmol/l (60-280 ng/l)	0.5-1.0 nmol/l (150-300 ng/l)
8-10 yrs:	0.3-1.7 nmol/l (90-500 ng/l)	0.7-1.4 nmol/l (200-400 ng/l)
10-12 yrs:	0.3-10.1 nmol/l (80-2900 ng/l)	0.7-1.7 nmol/l (200-500 ng/l)
12-14 yrs:	0.2-24.6 nmol/l (50-7600 ng/l)	1.0-2.4 nmol/l (300-700 ng/l)
14-16 yrs:	3.1-19.5 nmol/l (900-5600 ng/l)	1.2-3.3 nmol/l (350-950 ng/l)
16-18 yrs:	9.0-25.4 nmol/l (2600-7300 ng/l)	1.4-3.3 nmol/l (400-950 ng/l)
18-20 yrs:	13.9-25.0 nmol/l (4000-7200 ng/l)	1.4-3.3 nmol/l (400-950 ng/l)
20-25 yrs:	11.8-38.9 nmol/l (3400-11,200 ng/l)	1.4-3.3 nmol/l (400-950 ng/l)

S-Thyroxine

1-3 days: 142-296 nmol/l (11-23 µg/dl)
1 wk-1 mo: 116-232 nmol/l (9-18 µg/dl)
1-4 mos: 97-212 nmol/l (7.5-16.5 µg/dl)
4-12 mos: 71-187 nmol/l (5.5-14.5 µg/dl)
1-6 yrs: 71-174 nmol/l (5.5-13.5 µg/dl)
6-10 yrs: 64-161 nmol/l (5.0-12.5 µg/dl)

Glossary

abduction Movement away from the axial line (for a limb) or the median plane (for the digits).

abscess Localized collection of pus.

abulia Loss or deficiency in ability to make decisions or to act on decisions; may occur in depression (absence of will power).

achalasia Failure of smooth muscle of the gastrointestinal tract to relax; particularly significant for sphincters, such as the esophagogastric sphincters.

achondroplasia Disturbance in cartilage development.

acini Small, sacklike dilatations found in various glands.

acromegaly Chronic disease caused by hypersecretion of growth hormone; characterized by overgrowth of the small parts.

acrophobia Fear of heights.

acute Severe symptoms, usually of rapid onset and of short duration.

adduction Movement toward the axial line (for a limb) or the median plane (for the digits).

adenoid Resembling a gland; hypertrophy of the adenoid tissue situated in the pharynx; sometimes called pharyngeal tonsil.

adenoma Tumor consisting of glandular cells.

adiposis Excessive accumulation of adipose (lipoid) tissue; obesity or corpulence; fatty infiltration of an organ or tissue.

affect A mood or inner feeling; disturbances in affect are seen in most psychiatric illnesses.

afferent Carrying to the center from the periphery.

ageusia Loss of the sensation of taste or the ability to discriminate sweet, sour, salty, and bitter tastes.

agitation Restlessness; inability to concentrate or remain motionless.

agnosia Inability to discriminate sensory stimuli. *Acoustic or auditory agnosia:* impaired ability to recognize familiar sounds. *Tactile agnosia:* impaired ability to recognize familiar objects by touch or feel. *Visual agnosia:* impaired ability to recognize familiar objects by sight. *Autotopagnosia:* disturbance in recognition of body parts.

alienation Inability to identify with family, peer group, society, or culture; associated with schizophrenia.

amaurosis Blindness without perceptible disease of the visual structures.

amyotonia Lack of tone of the musculature of the body.

amyotrophy Wasting or atrophy of muscle tissue.

analgesia Loss of sensation; used particularly to denote relief of pain without loss of consciousness.

anarthria Loss of articulation.

anesthesia Loss of sensation.

aneurysm Dilatation of an artery.

angina pectoris Pain—substernal or radiating to the left arm, neck, or jaw; frequently correlated with myocardial ischemia.

anisocoria Unequal dilatation of the pupils.

anorexia Loss of appetite.

anosmia Inability to smell.

anosognosia Lack of insight or loss of ability to recognize one's disease.

antrum Cavity or chamber.

anuria Absence of excretion of urine.

anxiety Uncomfortable perception of apprehension, uncertainty, or fear associated with physiological changes, including sympathetic nervous system arousal.

apathy Lack of interest and blunting of affect in conditions that would normally stimulate interest or elicit feeling.

aphasia Dysfunction or loss of the ability to express thoughts by speech, writing, symbols, or signs. *Fluent aphasia:* ability to produce words but with frequent errors in the appropriate choice of words or in the creation of words. *Nonfluent aphasia:* inability to produce words, either in spoken or written form.

aphonia Inability to produce laryngeal voice sounds.

aplasia Failure of cellular formation or development of an organ or tissue or the cellular products from an organ or tissue, as an impairment in blood formation.

apraxia Impairment of the ability to carry out purposeful movement (although muscle and sensory apparatus are intact), as an inability to draw or construct forms of two or three dimensions.

aqueous humor Fluid secreted in the ciliary body and found in the anterior and posterior chambers of the eye.

arcus senilis Gray to white opaque ring surrounding the cornea, generally seen in individuals older than 50 years of age, caused by lipoid position.

arrhythmia Any deviation from the normal pace of the heart.

arteriosclerosis Hardening (sclerosis) and thickening of the walls of arterioles.

arthritis Inflammation of a joint.

arthropathy General term for disease in a joint.

ascites The accumulation of free fluid within the abdominal cavity.

asterixis Liver flap, flapping tremor, or wrist flapping as a result of a sudden relaxation of wrist extensors; appears in hepatic failure with the occurrence of metabolic encephalopathy.

asthenia Weakness; loss of strength or energy.

asthma Proxysmal dyspnea (wheezing) resulting from obstruction of the bronchi or spasm of smooth muscle.

ataxia Impairment of coordination of muscular activity.

atelectasis Incomplete expansion of a lung compromised since birth; collapse of the adult lung.

atherosclerosis Type of arteriosclerosis characterized by deposits (atheromas) of cholesterol, lipoid material, and lipophages in the walls of large arteries and arterioles.

athetosis Slow, sustained, involuntary large amplitude muscle movements that are sinous, writhing, or squirming in character.

atrophy Wasting; decrease in the size of a cell, tissue, organ, or body part.

aura Premonitory sensation, generally applied to sensations preceeding epileptiform convulsions.

auscultation Examination made by listening, usually through the stethoscope.

AV block Impairment of impulse conduction from the atria to the ventricles.

ballottement A palpation technique used to assess a floating object; fluid-filled tissue is pushed toward the examining hand so that the object will float against the examining fingers.

basophilia An abnormal increase in the basophilic leucocytosis.

Battle's sign Bluish discoloration along the course of the posterior auricular artery, with ecchymosis first appearing near the tip of the mastoid process; associated with basal skull fracture.

borborygmus Audible bowel sounds, generally caused by gas propulsion through the intestine.

bradycardia Slower than normal heart rate (<50 beats per minute).

bronchiectasis Chronic dilatation of one or more bronchi.

bronchitis Inflammation of one or more bronchi; condition may be chronic or acute.

bronchophony The sound of the voice as heard with abnormally increased clarity and intensity through the stethoscope over the lung parenchyma.

bruit Murmur (blowing sound) heard over peripheral vessels.

buccal Pertaining to the cheek.

bullous Characterized by vesicles (blisters) usually 2 cm or more in diameter.

bursa A sac or lined cavity filled with viscous fluid; located at anatomical sites at which tissues would otherwise create friction in rubbing over each other.

cachexia Marked malnutrition.

cataract Opacity of the lens of the eye.

chalazion Sebaceous cyst on the eyelid formed by distention of a meibomian gland with secretion.

cholesteatoma Cystlike mass common to the middle ear and mastoid region characterized by outer layer of stratified squamous epithelium filled with desquamating debris, including cholesterol; generally associated with chronic infection.

chorea Rapid, brief, involuntary, asymmetric movements worsened by emotional stress; improve or disappear during sleep.

chorionic Pertaining to the chorion, a fetal membrane composed of trophoblast that forms the fetal portion of the placenta.

chronic obstructive pulmonary disease (COPD) General term for disease involving airway obstruction, such as chronic bronchitis, emphysema, or asthma.

clonus Rhythmic alternation between contraction and relaxation of muscles, induced by stretching the muscle; may result in alternate flexion and extension.

clubbing Proliferation of soft tissue of terminal phalanges, generally associated with relative hypoxia of peripherial tissues, loss of the angle between the skin and nail base, and sponginess of the nail base.

coarctation A tightening or compression of the walls of a vessel, producing a narrowed lumen.

colic Acute abdominal pain associated with smooth muscle contraction of the gastrointestinal tract.

colitis Inflammation of the colon.

coma Deep unconsciousness from which the individual cannot be aroused, even by painful stimuli. *Comatose:* the condition of being affected by coma.

complex Emotionally charged attitudes and ideas that are unconscious and influence the behavior of the individual, such as an Oedipus complex.

compulsion behaviors Behaviors resulting from obsessions.

confabulation Psychiatric term for conversation by an individual in which the truth is little regarded; fabrication.

consensual Reflex reaction in one pupil mimicking that occurring in the other, which is being stimulated.

consolidation Process in which liquid or solid replacement of lung parenchyma as exudate from an inflammatory condition is amassed.

constipation Infrequent or difficult evacuation of feces; often associated with drying and hardening of the stool.

contralateral On the opposite side.

conversion Psychiatric term for the unconscious mechanism in which emotions are converted to an increase or decrease in motor activity or sensory change.

convulsion Series of involuntary muscle contractions.

Cooper's ligaments Suspensory ligaments of the breast.

corneal limbus The edge of the cornea where it meets the sclera.

cor pulmonale Disease of the heart secondary to pulmonary disease.

cramp Involuntary, painful skeletal muscle contraction.

crepitation, crepitus A dry, crackling sound in (1) the lung, when air passes through abnormally accumulated moisture; (2) the joints, when dry synovial surfaces rub together; and (3) the skin, when air is present subdermally.

cretinism Disease caused by congenital lack of thyroid hormone; characterized by retarded physical and mental development.

crisis Sudden change in the course of a disease.

cyanosis Dusky blue color imparted to skin when the hemoglobin saturation is less than 75% to 85% or Pa_{O_2} is less than 50 mm Hg.

cyst Collection of fluid surrounded by a membrane.

cystocele Herniation of the urinary bladder into the anterior vaginal wall.

decidua The endometrium during pregnancy that is shed in the postpartum period.

déjà vu A sensation of familiarity with a person, place, or activity during a first encounter; a feeling of "having been there before."

delusion A false belief, improbable in nature; not influenced by contrary experience nor related to the cultural and educational background of the client.

dementia Global impairment of intellectual functioning; may also include emotional and volitional deterioration.

depersonalization Loss of the sense of personal reality or identity; withdrawal and isolation result from disappointments or unbearable sufferings that make one a witness to personal experiences rather than a participant.

depigmentation Loss of pigment, usually of melanin.

depression Term used to define (1) a mood, (2) a syndrome, and (3) an illness. The mood of depression is described as dejection and lowering of functional activity; it is a normal experience that may be incurred in response to frustration and loss. The syndrome of depression includes a depressed mood in combination with one or more of the following symptoms: inability to concentrate, anorexia, weight loss, and suicidal ideas. The illness of depression is characterized by the syndrome of depression but lasts longer. Functional impairment may include inability to carry on daily activities, particularly work.

derealization Feeling that the world around one is not real; generally associated with depersonalization.

dermographia Abnormal skin sensitivity, so that firm stroking with a dull instrument or light scratching results in a wheal surrounded by a red flare; may be caused by allergy.

desquamation Scaling, shedding of epithelial tissue.

diarrhea Increased frequency and liquid content of fecal evacuation.

diastasis recti abdominis Separation of the rectus muscles of the abdominal wall; may occur in pregnancy.

dicrotic pulse Presence of two sphygmographic or polygraphic elevations to one beat of the pulse.

diopter Refractive power of a lens with a focal distance of 1 meter; a unit of measure of refractive power.

diplopia Double vision; perception of two images for a single object.

disease Cluster of symptoms or signs with a more or less predictable course.

disorientation Lack of awareness as to time, place, or person.

diverticulum Pouch or sac created by herniation of mucosal lining of a hollow organ (bladder or gastrointestinal tract) through a defect in the muscular wall.

dysarthria Difficulty in articulating single sounds or phonemes of speech. Individual letters: *f, r, g;* labials—sounds produced with the lips: *b, m, v* (cranial nerve [CN] VII); gutterals—sounds produced in the throat (CN X); linguals—sounds produced with the tongue: *l, t, n* (CN XII).

dyschezia Difficulty in passing stool; pain associated with defecation.

dyscoria Congenital abnormality in the shape of the pupil.

dysdiadochokinesia Impairment in the ability to stop a movement and to institute the opposite movement, such as pronation to supination.

dysesthesia Impairment of any sensation, particularly of touch.

dysgeusia Impairment or perversion of the sense of taste.

dyslexia Disturbance in understanding the written word; difficulty in reading.

dysmenorrhea Painful menstruation.

dyspareunia Difficult or painful sexual intercourse in women.

dyspepsia Impairment of the ability to digest food; especially, discomfort after eating a meal.

dysphagia Difficult or painful swallowing.

dysphasia Disturbance in speech evidenced by lack of coordination and failure to express words in proper order.

dysphonia puberum Difficulty in controlling laryngeal speech sounds that occurs as the larynx enlarges in puberty.

dysphoria Restlessness, agitation.

dysplasia Disorder in the size, shape, or organization of adult cells.

dyspnea Difficult or labored respiration. *Paroxysmal nocturnal dyspnea:* respiratory distress related to posture, especially noted when reclining at night.

dysprosody Difficulty in speech in which inflection, pronunciation, pitch, and rhythm are impaired.

dysuria Difficulty or painful urination.

ecchymosis A flat, round or irregular, blue or purplish lesion of the skin or mucous membranes resulting from intradermal or submucous hemorrhage.

echolalia Repetition by a client of words addressed to him; may also be the echo of his own thoughts; generally a sign of schizophrenia.

ectopic Abnormally located.

ectropion Eversion, or turning outward, of an edge, as of the eyelid.

eczema Superficial inflammatory process of the epidermis associated with redness, itching, weeping, and crusting; of multiple etiology.

edema Abnormal increase in the quantity of interstitial fluid.

efferent Carrying from the center to the periphery.

egophony Voice sound of a nasal (telephonelike or bleating) quality, heard through the stethoscope; often defined by asking the client to say "ee," which sounds like "ay."

elation Elevation of mood, emotional excitement; may be temporary response to fortuitous event in a normal individual. Elation is the characteristic mood of mania and also is observed in some schizophrenics.

embolism Sudden obstruction of an artery by a clot or other foreign substance.

emphysema Abnormal accumulation of air in tissues or organs, especially the lung.

encephalitis Inflammation of the brain.

enophthalmos Recession of the globe of the eye into the orbit.

enteritis Inflammation of the small intestine.

enterocele Herniation of intestinal contents.

entropion Inversion, or turning inward of an edge, as of the eyelid.

enuresis Involuntary urination during sleep.

epilepsy Paroxysmal disturbances in brain function characterized by loss of consciousness, motor or sensory impairment, and disturbance of emotions or thought processes.

epiphora Abnormal tearing of the eyes.

epispadias Congenital anomaly in which the urethra opens on the dorsum of the penis.

epistaxis Bleeding or hemorrhage from the nose.

epulis Tumor of the gingiva.

erectile tissue Tissue capable of becoming rigid and elevated.

eructation Act of belching or bring up gas (air) from the stomach.

erythema Enlargement of capillaries resulting in redness of the skin.

eversion A turning outward or inside out.

exanthem General eruption of the skin accompanied by fever.

exophthalmos (proptosis) Abnormal protrusion of the globe of the eye.

fasciculation Rapid, fine, twitching movements resulting from contraction of a fasciculus (bundle of muscle fibers) served by one anterior horn cell; usually does not cause movement of a joint.

festination Involuntary tendency to accelerate the speed of walking; occurs in paralysis agitans.

fever Pyrexia; elevation of the body temperature above normal for a given individual.

fiberoptics Transmission of an image along flexible bundles of coated glass or plastic fiber having special optical properties.

fibrillation Fine, continuous twitching caused by contraction of a single muscle or group of fibers.

flaccid Relaxed, without tone, flabby.

flatulence Excessive amount of gas in the gastrointestinal tract.

fremitus Palpable vibration.

friction rub A crackling, grating sound, heard through the stethoscope when two inflamed, roughened surfaces rub together.

fusiform Spindle or cigar shaped.

gallop rhythm Heart rate characterized by three sounds in the presence of tachycardia.

gastritis Inflammation of the stomach.

glomus jugulare Globus tympanicum tumor; tumor of the jugular bulb in the floor of the middle ear; may result in hearing loss, sense of fullness, and tinnitus; often seen as a bulging, reddish purple mass through the tympanic membrane.

goiter Increase in size of the thyroid gland.

gout Disease caused by deposition of crystals of monosodium urate; characterized by a disorder in purine metabolism and associated with exacerbations of arthritis of a single joint.

guilt Painful feeling caused by having transgressed personal or social ethical standards.

gumma Neoplasm composed of soft, gummy tissue resembling granulation tissue; may occur in tertiary syphilis or in tuberculosis.

gynecomastia Hypertrophy of breast tissue in a male subject.

hallucination Perception for which no external stimuli can be ascertained; an endogenous experience in an individual whose sensorium is clear. *Simple hallucination:* simple perception, such as seeing light. *Complex hallucination:* more detailed experience, such as seeing a figure or person.

hematemesis Vomiting of bright red or "coffee grounds" (partially digested) blood.

hematoma Localized collection of blood resulting from rupture of a blood vessel.

hematuria Presence of blood in the urine.

hemolytic Pertaining to the release of hemoglobin from red blood cells.

hemophilia Genetic predisposition to bleed more than normal because of a deficiency of the clotting factors.

hemoptysis Expectoration containing blood.

hernia Abnormal protrusion of an organ or tissue through an opening. *Incarcerated hernia:* protrusion of abdominal contents through a weakness in the abdominal wall, so that the contents cannot be returned to the abdominal cavity. *Inguinal hernia: direct*—protrusion of abdominal contents through a weakness in the abdominal musculature, region of Hesselbach's triangle; *indirect*—protrusion through an internal inguinal ring hernia descending beside the spermatic cord. *Scrotal hernia:* protrusion (generally indirect) of abdominal contents into the scrotal sac. *Strangulated hernia:* hernia in which the blood supply to the protruded tissue is obstructed.

herpes Virus disorder of the skin characterized by numerous small vesicles in clusters.

hordeolum Inflammation of a sebaceous gland of the eyelid; sty.

hyaline Glasslike, as of casts in the urine.

hydrocele Circumscribed collection of fluid, particularly in the scrotum.

hyperesthesia Abnormally increased sensitivity of the skin or another sense organ.

hyperpigmentation An excess of pigment in tissue.

hyperplasia Increase in the size of a tissue or organ caused by an increase in the number of cells.

hyperpnea Increased rate and depth of respiration.

hyperpyrexia Marked elevation of temperature, usually above 105.8° F (41° C).

hypertension Persistent elevation of blood pressure.

hypertrophy Increase in size of a tissue or organ.

hyphema Blood in the anterior chamber of the eye.

hypochondriasis Abnormal concern with one's state of health, frequently accompanied by symptoms that cannot be explained pathophysiologically.

hypochromic Abnormally decreased color; used to describe anemias in which the amount of hemoglobin in red blood cells is deficient.

hypoesthesia Abnormally decreased sensitivity of the skin or another sense organ.

hypoglossal Below the tongue.

hypopyon Purulent material in the anterior chamber of the eye.

hyposmia Partial loss of the sense of smell.

hypospadias A developmental anomaly in which the urethra opens on the under side of the penis.

icteric Jaundiced.

illusion Perception based on actual external stimulus with misinterpretation or distortion of the event.

infarction Obstruction of circulation followed by ischemic necrosis.

inflammation Localized protective condition associated with vascular dilatation, exudation of plasma, and leucocytes. Clinical signs include redness, swelling, pain, heat, and limitation of function.

ipsilateral On the same side.

iritis Inflammation of the iris.

joint An articulation or junction between two bones.

keratitis Inflammation of the cornea.

koilonychia Spoon-shaped nail surface, frequently associated with iron deficiency anemia.

kyphosis Increased posterior convexity of the spine (humpback).

lamella Small sheet or leaf.

leukopenia Abnormal diminution of leucocytes.

leukoplakia A disease appearing as white, thickened patches on mucous membranes.

linea nigra Pigmentation of the linea alba, the tendinous median line on the anterior abdominal wall, during pregnancy.

lordosis Anterior concavity of the lumbar spine (swayback, saddle back).

lymphadenopathy Disease of the lymph nodes.

lymphadenosis Hypertrophy or proliferation of lymphatic tissue.

lymphedema Edema caused by accumulation of lymph; may result from pathology of lymph ducts or nodes.

lymphoma Neoplastic disorder of lymphatic tissue.

lysis Gradual return to normal following a disease; generally refers to a fever.

macula Small spot on the skin that differs in color from the surrounding tissue and is not elevated.

malignant Tending to become progressively worse and life threatening, especially a disease or tumor.

malingering Simulation of illness.

mastitis Inflammation of breast tissue.

melanocyte A cell that produces melanin.

melena Dark-colored stools that may be black or tarry stained with partially digested blood.

menorrhagia Excessive menstruation.

metrorrhagia Irregular uterine bleeding.

microcephaly Head circumference measuring less than three standard deviations below the mean for age and sex.

migraine Paroxysmal headache, frequently unilateral.

miosis Abnormal contraction of the pupils.

Montgomery's glands Small, sebaceous glands located on the areola.

mumps Viral infection involving the parotid gland.

murmur Blowing sound caused by turbulence of blood flow, heard through the stethoscope over the heart or the great vessels.

mydriasis Extreme dilatation of the pupil resulting from paralysis of the oculomotor muscles or the effect of a drug.

myoclonus Jerking movement of one or more limbs or the trunk caused by muscle contractions.

myopathy Disease of the muscles.

nabothian follicles Cystlike formations on the mucosa of the uterine cervix resulting from an accumulation of retained secretion in occluded glands.

nausea Feeling that emesis is impending.

neologism Newly coined word; meaningless word often uttered by a psychotic patient.

neuralgia Pain associated with the course of a nerve.

neurosis Psychiatric term for an emotional problem thought to be related to unresolved conflict; differs from a psychosis in that hallucinations, delusions, and illusions generally do not occur.

nevus Well-demarcated malformation of the skin, such as an area of pigmentation or a mole.

nocturia Excessive urination at night.

nuchal Pertaining to the nape of the neck.

nystagmus Involuntary, rhythmic motion of the eye; may be horizontal, vertical, rotary, or mixed.

obsession Persistent, upsetting preoccupation with an idea that morbidly dominates the mind.

obstipation Severe constipation.

oliguria Abnormally decreased urine secretion (<400 ml/24 hours).

onychia Inflammation of the matrix of the nail.

opisthotonos Hyperextension of the neck and marked flexion of hips and legs.

orthopnea Dyspnea relieved by sitting upright.

orthostatic (postural) hypotension Lowering blood pressure that occurs on rising to an erect position.

otalgia Earache.

Paget's disease Condition characterized by excoriating or scaling lesion of the nipple, extending from an intraductal carcinoma of the breast.

palpate Examination conducted by feeling or touching the object to be evaluated.

palpebra Eyelid.

palpitation Subjective awareness of the pulsations of the heart and arteries.

papilledema Edema of the optic papilla.

paraesthesia Abnormal or perverted sensation; may include burning, itching, pain, or the feeling of electric shock.

paresis Slight or incomplete paralysis; weakness.

parosmia Perversion of the sense of smell; olfactory hallucinations.

percussion Examination conducted by listening to reverberation of tissue after striking the surface with short, sharp blows.

peristalsis Wave of contraction moving along a muscular tube, particularly the gastrointestinal tract.

petechiae Very small, flat, purple-to-red skin or mucous membrane lesions caused by submucous or intradermal hemorrhage.

phobia Persistent and exaggerated fear of a particular object or situation.

phoria Mild weakness of the extraocular muscle(s). *Esophoria:* inward deviation of the eye(s). *Exophoria:* outward deviation of the eye(s).

photophobia Abnormal visual intolerance to light.

-plegia Complete paralysis. *Diplegia:* paralysis of both upper or lower limbs. *Hemiplegia:* paralysis of one side of the body. *Paraplegia:* paralysis of both legs and the lower part of the body. *Quadraplegia:* paralysis of all four limbs.

plethora Pertaining to a red, florid complexion.

pleural effusion Fluid of any kind in the pleural cavity.

pleurisy Pain accompanying pleural inflammation.

polycythemia Abnormal increase in the number of red blood cells.

polydipsia Increased sensation of thirst.

polymenorrhea Abnormally frequent menstruation.

polyphagia Excessive ingestion of food.

polyuria Increased urinary excretion.

Poupart's ligament The inguinal ligament; the fibrous band which runs from the anterior superior iliac spine to the pubic spine.

prepuce Foreskin.

priapism Prolonged erection of the penis.

proctoscopy Examination of the rectum with a short cylindrical instrument called a proctoscope.

prognathism Protrusion of the jaw.

proprioceptive sensation Muscle and joint sensations of position in space.

pruritus Itching.

psoriasis Papulosquamous dermatosis; characteristic lesion is bright red macule, papule, or plaque covered with silver scales.

psychasthenia Neurosis characterized by depersonalization, delusions, fear, and feelings of inadequacy.

psychosis Psychiatric term for a mental disorder associated with thought disorders, pathological perception (delusions, hallucinations), or extremes of affect.

pterygium Abnormal triangular thickening of the bulbar conjunction on the cornea, with the apex toward the pupil.

ptosis Drooping of the eyelid.

pulse Palpable rhythmic expansion of the artery.

pyemia General septicemia marked by fever, chills, and abscesses.

pyorrhea Purulent inflammation of the gums.

pyrexia Fever; elevation of the body temperature above normal for a given individual.

pyrosis Heartburn.

pyuria Presence of pus in the urine.

rale Discrete, noncontinuous sound resembling fine crackling, radio static, or hairs being rubbed together, heard through the stethoscope; generally produced by air bubbling through an exudate.

rectocele Herniation of the rectum into the vagina.

regurgitation Reversal of the flow of a substance through a vessel, such as blood flow in the wrong direction or the return of food to the mouth without vomiting.

retraction Condition of being drawn back.

rhonchus Wheezing or snoring sound produced by airflow across a partially constricted air passage. *Sibilant rhonchus:* wheeze produced in a small air passage. *Sonorous rhonchus:* wheeze produced in a large air passage.

rigor Common term for shivering accompanying a chill or for muscle rigidity accompanying depletion of adenosine triphosphate, as in death (rigor mortis).

scoliosis Lateral deviation of the spine.

scotoma An islandlike blind gap in the visual field.

sebaceous Pertaining to or secreting sebum, an oily secretion composed of fat and epithelial debris.

sign Objective evidence of disease that is perceptible to the examiner.

somatic Pertaining to the body.

sordes Materia alba; undigested food bacteria encrusting the lips and teeth.

spasm Contraction of a single muscle or a group of muscles. *Clonic spasm:* rapid onset and brief duration; may cause movement of body part. *Tonic spasm:* prolonged or continuous; may cause movement or limitation of movement.

spastic Rigid; characterized by muscle spasm.

steatorrhea Abnormal increase of fat in the feces.

stereognosis Discrimination of objects by the sense of touch.

sthenic Sturdy or strong; active.

stomatitis Inflammation of the mouth.

strabismus Disparity in the anteroposterior axes of the eyes; the optic axes cannot be directed to the same object because of lack of muscular coordination.

stress incontinence Involuntary urination incurred on straining, coughing, or lifting.

striae gravidarum Atrophic, pinkish or purplish scarlike lesions observed on the breasts, thighs, abdomen, and buttocks during pregnancy; lesions later become silvery white.

stridor Harsh, high-pitched respiratory sound heard in respiratory obstruction.

stupor Decreased responsiveness; partial unconsciousness.

succussion Procedure involving shaking an individual to demonstrate fluid in a hollow cavity.

symptom Subjective perception of a client of an alteration of bodily or mental function from basal conditions; change perceived by the individual.

syncope Fainting; temporary unconsciousness.

syndrome Consistent group of symptoms and signs that are produced by a similar pathological change in different individuals.

tachycardia Rapid heart rate (>100 beats per minute). *Atrial flutter:* rapid, regular, uniform atrial contraction caused by AV block; ventricular rhythm varies with the degree of AV block. *Atrial tachycardia:* arrhythmia caused by the atria; rapid, regular beat of the entire heart. *Ventricular tachycardia:* arrhythmia caused by the ventricles; rapid, relatively regular heartbeat.

tachypnea Rapid respiratory rate.

telangiectasis Localized group of dilated capillaries.

tenesmus Uncomfortable straining; particularly, unsuccessful attempts at defecation or urination.

thrill Palpable murmur; vibration accompanying turbulence in the heart or the great vessels.

tic Sudden, short contractions of a muscle or group of muscles, always causing movement of affected part.

tinnitus Sensation of noise in the ear caused by abnormal stimulation of the auditory apparatus or its afferent pathways; may be described as ringing, buzzing, swishing, roaring, blowing, or whistling.

tophus Deposits of monosodium urate, seen in gout.

tremor Involuntary, somewhat rhythmic, oscillatory quivering of muscles, caused by alternate contraction of opposing groups of muscles. *Cerebellar tremor:* occurs during intentional movement, becoming more pronounced near end of the movement; associated with lesions of the dentate nucleus. *Coarse tremor:* slow rate and large amplitude movements. *Essential (familial) tremor:* begins usually around age 50 with fine tremors of the hands; aggravated by intentional movement; commonly affects head, jaws, lips, or voice. *Fine tremor:* rapid (10 to 20 oscillations per second) and low amplitude movements, usually in the fingers and hands. *Moderate tremor:* medium rate and medium amplitude movements. *Passive tremor:* present at rest, may improve during intentional movement; for example, pill-rolling tremor or Parkinson's disease. *Physiologic tremor:* experienced by healthy people in fatigue, cold and stress. *Toxic tremor:* caused by endogenous (thyrotoxicosis, uremia) or exogenous toxins (alcohol, drugs).

trimester A period of 13 weeks.

trophoblast The peripheral cells of the blastocyst that attach the fertilized ovum to the uterine wall and become the placenta and the membranes.

tropia Permanent deviation of the axis of an eye.

tympany Drumlike note produced by percussion, generally over a gas-filled region.

undulant Wavelike variations, particularly as in fever and diurnal circadian fluctuations.

urticaria Rash characterized by wheals.

valgus Angulation of an extremity toward the midline. *Genu valgum:* condition in which knees are abnormally close together; knock knee.

varicocele Distention of the veins of the spermatic cord.

varicose Dilated, particularly a vein.

varus Angulation of an extremity away from the midline. *Genu varum:* condition in which knees are abnormally separated; bowleg.

verbigeration (polyphasia) Repetition of meaningless words or phrases.

vertigo Illusion of movement, with imagined rotation of one's self (subjective vertigo) or of one's surroundings (objective vertigo).

vitiligo Skin affliction characterized by patches of depigmented skin caused by destruction of melanocytes.

whispered pectoriloquy Increased resonance of the whispered voice as heard through the stethoscope.

xerostomia Dryness of the mouth.

xiphisternum Xiphoid process of the sternum.

Index

A

a wave, 342
Abdomen
  assessment of, 348-375
    of aged client, 628-629
    in child, 600-603
    in pregnancy, 426-433
  changes of, in pregnancy, 419
  examination of, in pregnancy, 426
  masses of, palpation for, 367-368
  pain in, sites of, 373, 374-375
  reflexes of, 374
Abdominal aorta, 356
Abducens paralysis, 239
Abduction, 443, 444
Abductor strength, assessment of, 457
Abscesses of rectum, 383-384
Accidents in health history, 40
Acclimatization, 141
Achilles tendon reflex, 549-550, 552
Acid phosphatase, 662
Acidosis, 654
Acne, 192
Acoustic nerve, 524-527
Acoustical stethoscope, 18, 19
Acrochordons, 631
Acromegaly, 131
Active motion, 456
Acuity, auditory, loss of, 624
Adduction, 443, 444
Adductor strength, assessment of, 457
Adnexa, bimanual palpation of, 407
Adolescence
  development in, 74-77
  recommendations for, 9
Adulthood
  early, recommendations for, 10
  late, development in, 82-84
  middle
    development in, 78-82
    recommendations for, 12
  older, recommendations for, 13
  young
    development in, 78
    recommendations for, 11
    sleep patterns in, 118
Adventitious sounds, assessment of, 307-309
Affective disorders, 176
African pigmy, 130

Age
  assessment of, 132
  effect of, on temperature, 139
Age-related muscle weakness, 500
Ageusia, 524
Aging client
  assessment of, 623-631
  posture of, 132-134
  sleep patterns in, 119
Agnosia, 164-165, 555
Agraphia, 165
Agriculture Handbook No. 456, 97
Albumin, plasma, 657
Albumin-globulin ratio, 658
Alcoholism, 122-123
Aldolase, 662-663
Alkaline phosphatase, 661-662
Alkalosis, 654
Allergies in health, history, 40
Alopecia, 135, 184, 246
AMA; *see* American Medical Association
American Academy of Pediatrics, 61
American Cancer Society guidelines, 15
American Heart Association, 142-143, 156, 158
American Medical Association, 1
Amnesia, 171
Amniotic fluid, normal values for, 698
Amylase, 663
Amyotrophic lateral sclerosis, 521
Analysis, chemical, of food, 98
Anarthria, 136
Anatomical mapping, 348-351
Anemia, 663, 664
Aneroid sphygmomanometer, 155
Anesthesia, 537
Anisocoria, 241
Anisocytosis, 665
Ankle joint, 513, 516
  strength and range of motion of, testing for, 489-490
Anonychia, 185
Anorectal strictures, 377
Anorexia nervosa, 123
Anoscopy, 380
Anosmia, 519
Anterior axillary lines, 294
Anterior cervical chain, 260-265
Anterior chamber, 225
  examination of, 234-235
  pathology of, 240-241

Anthropometric parameters in children, 574-594
Anthropometry, 102-107
Anus
   assessment of, 376-384
   smear from, 415, 416
Anxiety, signs of, 26-27
Anxiety attacks, 119
Anxiety neurosis, 177
Aorta
   abdominal, 356
   coarctation of, 158
Aphasia, 136, 163, 164, 555
Aphonia, 136
Apical impulse, 337, 338
Apley's sign, 513, 514
Apnea, sleep, 124
Apocrine sweat glands, 180
Appearances
   effect of, on communication, 32
   physical, and behavior, 162-178
Appendicitis, 374
Apraxia, 165
Arcus senilis, 234, 241, 626
Areolae, 275
Areolar lymphatic drainage, 275
Argyll Robertson pupil, 241
Arm
   arteries of, 145
   reflexes, 548-549
Arteriovenous nicking, 243
Artery(ies)
   carotid, assessment of, 344-347
   insufficiency of, 151-153
   of lower extremities, 146
   temporal, 247, 248
   of upper extremities, 145
Arthritis, rheumatoid
   juvenile, 607
   and sleep disorders, 124
Articulation, assessment of, 162
Ascites
   demonstration of, by palpation, 366-367
   percussion of, 360-361
Ascorbic acid deficiency, 102
Asthenic body type, 130
"At risk" child, 61
Athletic injury, 607
Attention span, assessment of, 170
Auditory acuity, loss of, 624
Auditory canal, 205, 206, 208
Auricle, 205
Auscultation, 18
Axilla, examination of, 270, 283
Axillary fossa, lymph nodes of, 269
Axillary lines, 294
Axillary lymph nodes, 271, 283
Axillary tail of Spence, 277
Axillary temperature, 141
Axillary veins lymph center, 266

B

Babinski's reflex, 550, 553, 611, 620
Back, examination of, 374-375
Balding, 135
Ballottement, 366, 367
   of knee, 509, 512
Bárány chair rotation test, 525

Bárány's test, 524
Barlow's test, 606
Barrel chest, 298
Bartholin's glands, 399, 403
Basic Four food guide, 96-97
Basophilic stippling, 665
Basophilopenia, 666
Beau's lines, 185, 187
Behavior and physical appearance, 162-178
Bell's palsy, 523
Biceps reflex, 549
Biceps strength, assessment of, 454
Bigeminal pulse, 149
Bilirubin, blood, 655-656
Bimanual palpation, 364-365
   of breasts, 283
   of uterus and adnexa, 407
Bimanual rectovaginal examination, 408-414
Bimanual vaginal examination, 408-413
Biochemical appraisal of nutrients, 107-109
Biography, patient, in health history, 35-37
Biologic hazards of workplace, 671-672
Biological rhythms, 113-114
   and temperature, 139
Biopsy, muscle, 502
Bladder, urinary, 372
Blood bilirubin, 655-656
Blood chemistry, normal values for, 685-691
Blood chemistry profile, 647-653
Blood creatinine, 656
Blood flow cycles, 324
Blood gases, 653-654
Blood glucose, 654-655
Blood oxygen, 653
Blood pH, 654
Blood pressure, 153-159
   of child, 576-577
   examination of, in pregnancy, 425
Blood urea nitrogen, 656
Body movement, 30
Body types, 129-130
Bones
   examination of, 502
   of pelvis, 435
   of skull, 246-247
Bony pelvis, examination of, 434-442
Bowel segments, palpable, 368
Bowel sounds, 354, 355
Brachial pulse, 143, 146
Brachial veins lymph center, 266
Brachioradialis reflexes, 549, 550, 551
Bradycardia, 148, 150
Braxton-Hicks contractions, 419
Breast-feeding of infant, 561-562
Breasts
   assessment of, 275-288
      of aged client, 627
   changes of, in pregnancy, 419
   in health history, 43
   lymphatic drainage of, 270, 271
   palpation of, systematic, 259
Breath sounds, assessment of, 307
Bronchophony, 320
Brudzinski's sign, 556, 557
Bruits, auscultation for, 152
Bruxism, 123

Build and Blood Pressure Study, 103
Bulla, 197

C

Cacosmia, 520
Calcium, serum, 652
Calipers, skinfold, 103, 104
Cancer
  breast, 286-287
  metastatic, lymph nodes in, 274
  primary and lymph drainage, 260
Candida albicans, 416
Caput succedaneum, 595
Carbon dioxide, 653-654
Carcinoma of penis, 388
Cardiac cycle, 324-326
Cardiac examination, 336-340
Cardinal positions of gaze, six, 231, 232
Cardiovascular sounds, 326-327
Cardiovascular symptoms and sleep disorders, 124
Cardiovascular system
  of aged client, assessment of, 628
  changes of, in pregnancy, 420
  in health history, 43
Caring Infant Temperament Questionnaire, 66
Carotid arteries, assessment of, 344-347
Carotid pulse, 143, 144, 343
  arterial, 344
Carpal joint, 508
Carpal tunnel syndrome, 508
Casts, urinary, 669
Cataplexy, 121
Cataract, 241-242, 627
Cephalohematoma, 595
Cerumen
  evaluation of, 208
  removal of, 599
Cervical chain, anterior, 260-265
Cervix
  changes of, in pregnancy, 418-419
  examination of, 410-411
  normal, 404, 406
  smear from, 414
Chaddock's sign, 550
Chalazion, 240
Chemical(s), industrial, 677-683
Chemical analysis of food, 98
Chest; *see* Thorax
Childhood; *see also* Children; Pediatric client
  development during
    by age, 62-65
    early, 69-72
  health surveillance chart for, 612-620
  hypertension in, 159
  illnesses during, in health history, 40
  middle, 72-74
  recommendations for, 7-9
  sleep patterns in, 118-119
Children; *see also* Childhood
  assessment of, 559-622
  "at risk," 61
Chloride, serum, 651-652
Cholesterol, 660
Cholinesterase, 663
Chronemics, 32
Chvostek's sign, 500, 523
Circadian pattern of blood pressure, 157

Circadian rhythms, 113
  interference with, 114
  of nail growth, 184
Circumduction, 443, 445
Circumferences, body, measurement of, 105-107
Citizens Board of Inquiry into Hunger and Malnutrition, 91
Client
  contract with, 25-26
  participation by, in health care, 3-4
  pediatric; *see* Childhood; Children
  questioning of, 27-28
Clitoris, 398
Closed angle glaucoma, 244
Clubbing, finger, 188
Coarctation of aorta, 158
Cognition, assessment of, 171-172
Cognitive abilities, assessment of, 45
Cognitive development in middle childhood, 73-74
Colon, sigmoid, 376
Color
  inspection of, 137
  nail, 187, 189
  skin, 181-183
Coma, assessment of, 167-170
Commodity distribution program, 91
Communication
  development of, 60
  nonverbal, 25-26, 30-33
  process of, 26-32
Compulsional neurosis, 177
Computer-assisted histories, 46-47
Conduction, 138
  air and bone, 210
Condylomata, 388
Confabulation, 171
Conjugate, diagonal, 440
Conjunctiva, 223
  examination, 233-234
  pathology of, 240
Conscience, development of, in early childhood, 69, 71
Consciousness, assessment of, 165-169
Contractions, Braxton-Hicks, 419
Convection, 138
Cornea, 225
  examination of, 234
  pathology of, 241
Corneal light reflex, 231, 234
Cortex
  lesions of, 555
  map of, 545
Costal angle, 294
Cover-uncover test, 232, 233
CPK; *see* Creatine phosphokinase
Cramps, 500
  leg, in pregnancy, 426
Cranial nerve
  function of, 518-553
  relationship of, to eye structures, 229
Creatine phosphokinase, 662
Creatinine, blood, 656
Cremasteric reflex, 551
Crepitation, 503
  assessment of, 302
Crust, 198
Crystals, urinary, 669
Cullen's sign, 374
Curettement, 209

Current Pediatric Diagnosis and Treatment, 66
Curvature of nail, 185
Cushing's syndrome, 131-132
Cutaneous fields
    of head and neck, 521
    of peripheral nerves, 542-543
Cutaneous lymphatic drainage, 275
c-v waves, 342
Cyanosis, 181-183, 189
Cyst, pilonidal, 381
Cystocele, 404

D

Darkfield examination of *T. pallidum*, 668
DDST; *see* Denver Developmental Screening Test
Death, 83, 84
Decomposition of movement, 537
Deep cervical chain, 262
Deep lymphatic drainage, 275
Deep tendon reflex, 544-548
Defense mechanisms, 175
Deficiency, nutrient
    development of, 92, 93
    symptoms of, 101-102
Deformity, joint, 503
Delusion, 175
Denial, 175
Dental screening form, 221
Denver Articulation Screening Examination, 66
Denver Developmental Screening Test, 61, 66
Depersonalization, 175
Depression, 122
Deprivation, sleep, 119
Derealization, 175
Dermatitis, 191, 199
Dermatodes, spinal, 544
Dermis, 180
Developmental assessment, 58-90
Developmental data in health history, 46
Developmental stages, 66-89
Diaphragm, 295, 298
Diastasis recti abdominis, 348
Diastole, 325
Diastolic arterial blood pressure, 153
Diastolic murmurs, 335-336
Diastolic pressure, normal, 157
Diet
    clinical appraisal of, 99-102
    surveys of, 94-99
    vegetarian, 97
Differential WBC count, 666
Disc of retina
    examination of, 237
    pathology of, 242
Displacement, 175
Distances, proxemic, types of, 31-32
Distention of abdomen, 353-354
Doll's head maneuver, 520
Dorsal pedal pulse, 147
Downey cells, 666
Drainage pathways, lymphatic, 257
Dream anxiety attacks, 119
Drugs
    effect of, on temperature, 139
    psychotropic, 119
    use of; *see* Pharmaceutical history
Duodenal ulcer and sleep disorders, 124

Dwarfism, 130
Dysarthria, 136, 163
Dysdiadochokinesia, 537
Dysmetria, 537
Dysphonia, 136, 163
Dysprosody, 164

E

Ears
    assessment of, 205-213
        of aged client, 627
        of child, 598-599
    in health history, 42
    pathology of, lymph nodes involved in, 267
Ecchymoses, 631
Eccrine sweat glands, 180
Ectropion, 239
Edema, assessment of, 425-426
Education
    of client, 45
    health, 3
EEG; *see* Electroencephalograms
Effusion of knee, 511
Egophony, 320
Eidetic imagery, 175
Elasticity of arterial wall, 143
Elbow joint, 505, 507
    strength and range of motion of, testing for, 471-472
Elderly; *see* Aging client
Electroencephalograms, 115, 116
Electrolytes, 647-653
Electromyography, 502
Electronic stethoscope, 18, 21
Electronystagmography, 525
Elephantiasis, 274
Emotional status, assessment of, 173
Empathy, 32-33
Endocervical culture, 415-416
Endocervical smear, 414
Endocrine system in health history, 43
Endoscopy, 380-381
Energy intake, recommended, 97
Engagement, 430
Enterocele, 404
Entropion, 239
Enuresis, 123-124
Environment
    effect of, on temperature, 139
    physical, in health history, 45
    psychological, in health history, 45
Enzyme(s)
    muscle, levels of, 501
    serum, 660-663
Epidermis, 180
Epididymis, 389
Epispadias, 388
Epitrochlear lymph center, 266, 269
Eponychium, 184
Equipment
    for abdominal assessment, 348
    for eye examination, 228
    for health assessment, 24
    for musculoskeletal assessment, 443, 446
    for neurological assessment, 518
    for pelvic examination, 400-401
    for rectal examination, 377
    for respiratory assessment, 298

Erection, nocturnal, 123
Erosion, 198, 199
Esophoria, 239
Estrogen therapy, 629-630
Ethnic foods, 94, 97
Evaporation, 139
Eversion of upper eyelid, 234
Exercise testing, 152
Exophoria, 239
Exostosis, 222
Extension, 443, 444
External mammary lymph center, 266
External rotation, 443, 445
Extinction phenomenon, 529
Extraocular muscle function, 231-233
Extremities
    lower; see Leg
    measurement of, 450-451, 452
    upper; see Arm
Exudates of retinal background, 243
Eyes
    assessment of, 223
        of aged client, 626-627
        of child, 595-598
    in health history, 42
    muscles of, and posture, 132
    symptoms of, in nutrient deficiency, 101
    unilateral protrusion of, 520
Eyelashes, 223
    examination of, 233
    pathology of, 239-240
Eyelids, 223, 224
    examination of, 233
    infection of, 240
    pathology of, 239-240
    upper, eversion of, 234

F

Face
    assessment of, 247-249
    in health history, 42
Facial expression as kinesis, 30
Facial nerves, 247, 523-524
Failure to thrive, 130-131
Family dietary survey, 94
Family history in health history, 41
Fasciculations, 500-501
Fecal impaction, 382
Femoral hernias, 394
Femoral pulse, 145, 146-147
Fetal head diameters, 434
Fetal heart rate, 433-434
Fetal lie and presentation, 429
Fetal position and attitude, 430
Fetoscope, 433
Fever, 141-142, 575
Fibrinogen, serum, 658
Fibroadenoma, 288
Fibrocystic disease of breast, 288
Finger
    clubbing of, 188
    flexor reflex of, 549, 554
    strength of
        assessment of, 456
        and range of motion, testing for, 479-481
First heart sound, 327

Fissure, 198
    of lungs, 295
Fistula in ano, 382
Flexicon, 443, 444
Flocculation tests, 667
Fluorescent treponemal antibody absorption test, 667
Fontanels, 595, 596
Food
    chemical analysis of, 98
    composition tables for, 97-98
    effect of, on temperature, 139
    ethnic, 94, 97
    intake dietary survey of, individual, 94-95
    intake record of, 94-95
    list dietary survey of, 94
    record dietary survey of, 94
Food and Nutrition Board of National Research Council of National Academy of Sciences, 98
Foot
    deformation of, 605
    joints of, 513-516
    strength and range of motion of, testing for, 491
Forearm strength and range of motion, testing for, 472-473
Formula feeding of infant, 562-563
Fourth heart sound, 329-330
Fremitus, assessment of, 300-301
Friction rub, 309
    pericardial, 331
    peritoneal, 366-367
Friends of client, interviewing, 29-30
FTA-ABS test; see Fluorescent treponemal antibody absorption test
Fundus, uterine, 426, 427, 428, 431-432

G

Gait, 133-134
    assessment of, 502
Galeazzi's sign, 606
Gallbladder, assessment of, 368-369
Gallop, summation, 330
Gases, blood, 653-654
Gastric fluid, normal values for, 696
Gastrointestinal function of aged client, 629
Gastrointestinal system in health history, 43
Gaze, six cardinal positions of, 231, 232
Genital system in health history, 43
Genitalia
    female, 397-414, 603-604
    male, assessment of, 385-394, 603
Genitourinary system of aged client, assessment of, 629
Genu valgum, 606
Genu varum, 606
Gigantism, 131
Glands, symptoms of nutrient deficiency in, 102; see also specific gland
Glasgow coma scale, 167
Glaucoma, 238, 239, 241, 242, 244
Glaucomatous cupping, 242
Glenohumoral joint, 505, 506
Globulin-albumin ratio, 658
Globulins, plasma, 658
Glossopharyngeal nerve, 527
Glucose
    blood, 654-655
    urine, 668
Glucosuria, 668
Gluteal reflex, 551

Gluteal strength, assessment of, 457
Gonadal dysfunction, 131
Goniometers, 446, 455-456
Gonorrheal culture, 415-416
Gordon's reflex, 551
Grandparents, role of, 83
Graphesthesia, 542
Grasp reflex, 554, 609, 611
Graves speculum, 403
Great vessels, 323
Grooming, assessment of, 162
Group dietary survey, 94
Growth
    during adolescence, 76
    charts of, for children, 579-590
    definition of, 58
    in early childhood, 69
    of hair, in elderly, 630
    in infancy, 67
    in middle childhood, 72-73
    nail, 184
Growth hormone
    deficiency of, 130
    hypersecretion of, 131
Guaiac test, 380, 381
Gums, examination of, 219

H

Hair
    assessment of, 134-135, 180-204, 246-247
    changes in, in pregnancy, 419-420
    growth of, in elderly, 630
    in health history, 42
    symptoms of nutrient deficiency in, 102
Hallucinations, 175
    hypnagogic, 121
Hallux valgus, 415
Hammer toe, 514, 515
Hamstring strength, assessment of, 457
Hand grasp, assessment of, 456
Harvey stethoscope, 18
HCG; see Human chorionic gonadotropin
Head
    assessment of, 246
        of child, 595
    circumference of
        of child, 592-593
        measurement of, 106
    cutaneous fields of, 521
    diameters of, fetal, 434
    in health history, 42
    lymphatic drainage of, 260-261
Headaches, migraine, and sleep disorders, 125
Hearing; see also Auditory acuity
    loss of, 207
    testing of, 209-213
Heart, assessment of, 231-240
    of child, 600-601
Heart murmurs, 330-336
    in child, 600
Heart rate
    of child, 576
    fetal, 433-434
Heart sounds, 327-331
Heaves, 337
Hegar's sign, 424

Height
    of aged client, 626
    of children, 105, 591
Heinz bodies, 665
Hematocrit, 663-664
Hematology, normal values in, 697-698
Hematopoietic system in health history, 43
Hemianopia, 239
Hemiparesis, 523-524
Hemoglobin, 664
Hemophilus vaginalis, 416
Hemorrhages of retinal background, 243
Hemorrhoids, 382-383
Hepatomegaly, 368
Hernias
    assessment of, 393, 394-396
    umbilical, 372
Herpes zoster, 194, 523
Hip joint, 508, 509
    strength and range of motion of, testing for, 482-486
Hippocratic nails, 189
Hirsutism, 135, 136, 184
History
    of aging client, 623-626
    child's developmental, 61
    dietary, survey, 95, 96
    health, 35-37
        interview for, 33
        prenatal, 420-422
    pediatric, 559-565
    for sleep assessment, 125-126
Hobbies and leisure
    in late adulthood, 83
    in middle adulthood, 80, 81
Hodgkin's disease, lymph nodes in, 274
Homan's sign, 153
Hordeolum, 240
Hormonal changes of pregnancy, 418
Hormones
    effect of, on temperature, 139
    thyroid, alterations in, 122
Human chorionic gonadotropin test, 423
Hunger in America, 91
Hunger USA, 91
Hygiene, assessment of, 136
Hymen, 398
Hyperbilirubinemia, 656
Hypercalcemia, 652
Hyperchloremia, 652
Hypercreatinemia, 656
Hyperesthesia, 537
Hyperglobulinemia, 658
Hyperglycemia, 655
Hyperkalemia, 651
Hyperkeratosis, 631
Hypermagnesemia, 653
Hypernatremia, 651
Hyperphosphatemia, 653
Hypersensitivity, assessment of, 362, 363
Hypersomatotropism, 131
Hypersomnia, 120-121
Hypersthenic body type, 129
Hypertension, 153, 158-159, 346
    in children, 577
    in pregnancy, 425
Hyperthermia, 183
Hyperuricemia, 657

Hyphema, 241
Hypnagogic hallucinations, 121
Hypoalbuminemia, 657
Hypocalcemia, 652
Hypochloremia, 652
Hypoesthesia, 537
Hypoglossal nerve, 528, 532
Hypoglycemia, 655
Hypokalemia, 500, 651
Hypomagnesemia, 653
Hyponatremia, 651
Hyponychium, 184
Hypophosphatemia, 653
Hyposmia, 519
Hyposomatotropism, 130
Hypospadias, 388
Hyposthemic body type, 129-130
Hypotension, 159
Hypothyroidism, 131
Hypoxia, 653
Hysteria, 177

I

ICNND; *see* Interdepartmental Committee on Nutrition for National Defense
Iliopsoas muscle test, 372, 374
Illusion, 175
Impaction, fecal, 382
Incontinence, anal, 383
Industrial chemicals, 677-683
Industrial hazards of workplace, 672-676
Infancy; *see also* Pediatric client
    breast-feeding during, 561-562
    development in, 66-69
    recommendations for, 6
    sleep patterns, in, 118-119
Infection
    of eyelids, 240
    of lymph nodes, pyogenic, 273
    vaginal, 416
Infraclavicular lymph center, 266
Inguinal hernias, 394
Inguinal lymph center, superficial, 272-273
Injury, athletic, 607
Inner ear, 206
Insomnia, 120-121
Inspection, 15
Inspiration, 289
Intelligence of aged, 625
Intensity of sound, 17
Intercourse, phases of, in aged client, 629
Interdepartmental Committee on Nutrition for National Defense, 99, 108
Internal jugular chain, 263
Internal rotation, 443, 445
International survey, 99
Interspinous diameter, 440
Intertuberous diameter, 441
Interview, 25-34, 161
    of aging client, 623-626
    assessment of knowledge via, 172
    for dietary survey, 95-96
    form for, for nutritional assessment of child, 565-569
    for health history, 36
Intraocular pressure, 237-238
Iris, 225
    examination of, 235

Iris—cont'd
    pathology of, 241
Iritis, 241
Irrigation of ear, 209
Ischiorectal abscess, 383

J

Jaundice, 181-182
Jaw closure reflex, 548
Joints; *see also* specific joint
    deformity of, 503
    examination of, 502
    of foot, 513-516
    pain in, 502-503
    and posture, 132
    range of motion of; *see* Range of joint motion
    swelling of, 503
Jugular veins, 340-344
Jugular venous pressure, 343-344
Juvenile rheumatoid arthritis, 607

K

Kernig's sign, 556
Ketone bodies in urine, 669
Kidney
    assessment of, 370, 372
    relationship of, to twelfth rib, 360
    tenderness related to, 361
Kinesis, 25-26, 30-33
Kinesthetic sensation, 542
Knee joint, 509-514
    strength and range of motion of, testing for, 486-488
Knee-chest position, 360-361, 377
Koilonychia, 185, 186
Korotkoff sounds, 156, 157
Kyphosis, 450
    in elderly, 630

L

Labia majora, 398
Labia minora, 398
Laboratory procedures, 646-670
Lacrimal apparatus, 224, 225
    examination of, 235
    pathology of, 241
Lactic dehydrogenase, 661
Language
    using common, during interview, 28
    development of, 60
        by age, 62-65
        in early childhood, 72
Laron dwarfism, 130
Lateral palpation, 432
Lateral sclerosis, amyotrophic, 521
Lateroinferior lymph nodes, 271
LDH; *see* Lactic dehydrogenase
LE cell, 666
Leg
    arteries of, 146
    blood pressure of, 157
    cramps of, in pregnancy, 426
    lymphatic drainage of, 271-272
Leg-raising test, straight, 516
Leisure and hobbies
    in late adulthood, 83
    in middle adulthood, 80, 81

Lens, 225
  pathology of, 241-242
Lesions
  of breast, benign, 287-288
  cortical, 555
  primary, 196-197, 199
  secondary, 198-199
  skin, 189-204, 352
    configurations of, 195
    flat, 200-202
    raised, 203-204
Leukocytosis, 665, 666
Leukonychia, 187
Leukopenia, 665
LYMP; *see* Lifetime Health Monitoring Plan
Lid lag, 239
Life expectancy, 623
Life Experiences Survey, 84, 87-89
Life review, 83-84
Lifetime Health Monitoring Plan, 4-15
Lifts, 337
Light reflex, corneal, 231, 234
Light touch sensation, 537-539
Lipase, 663
Lipids, plasma, 658-660
Lips, examination of, 218, 219, 300
Lithotomy position, 377, 400
Liver, assessment of, 368
Liver span, assessment of, 357-359
Lordosis, 450, 451
Louis's angle, 289, 294
Lungs, 292
  borders of, 295
  conditions of, common, assessment of, 310-319
  fissures of, 295
Lymph, mechanical stasis, of, 258
Lymph centers, 260, 265, 266, 269, 271-273
Lymph nodes, 259
  assessment of, of child, 594-595
  axillary, 271, 283
  of axillary fossa, 269
  examination of, 259-260
  lateroinferior, 271
  pathology of, 273-274
Lymph node chains, examination of, 264-272
Lymphangitis, acute, 274
Lymphatic drainage, 271-272, 275, 276
Lymphatic drainage pathways, 257
Lymphatic system, assessment of, 256-274
Lymphedema, 258, 274
Lymphocytes, 257
Lymphocytosis, 667
Lymphography, 257-258

M

Macula, 227
  examination of, 237
Macule, 196
Magnesium, serum, 653
Magnetic stethoscope, 18, 20
Malnutrition
  development and nature of, 92
  drug-induced, 91
  in hospitalized clients, 91
Mammography, 286
Manometer, mercury, 154
Manubriosternal joint, 505

Manubriosternal junction, 289, 294
Marfan's syndrome, 130
Marriage, effect of, on development, 78
Masses
  abdominal, palpation for, 367-368
  of breast, 279, 282
Mastication, muscles of, 521
Mastoid lymph center, 260
Mazoplasia, 288
McMurray's sign, 513, 514
Mean corpuscular hemoglobin, 604
Mean corpuscular hemoglobin concentration, 664
Mean corpuscular volume, 664
Mediosuperior axillary lymph nodes, 271
Mee's lines, 187
Melanonychia, 189
Melena, 380
Memory, assessment of, 171
Men, examination of breast of, 287
Meningeal irritation, 555-556
Menopause
  breast changes during, 278
  role of, in development, 81
Mental status, assessment of, 137, 161-179
Mercury gravity manometer, 154
Metabolism
  of aged client, 626
  disorders of, and sleep disorders, 124
Metacarpal joint, 508
Metastatic cancer, lymph nodes in, 274
Metatarsus varus, 606
Microaneurysms of retinal background, 243
Midarm circumference, percentiles for, 105, 106
Midarm muscle circumference, percentiles for, 106, 107
Midaxillary lines, 294
Midclavicular lines, 294
Middle ear, 205
Midpelvis planes, 435
Midspinal line, 294
Midsternal line, 294
Migraine headaches and sleep, 125
Milk lines, 277
Minerals, daily intake of, 100
Miosis, 241
Mitral stenosis, 335
Moisture of skin, 183
Monocytosis, 667
Mood
  assessment of, 173
  changes of, 114
Moro reflex, 610, 611
Motor development, 60
  by age, 62-65
Motor neuron, upper and lower, involvement of, in muscle strength, 498
Mouth
  assessment of, 216-221
    of aged client, 627
    of child, 600
  in health history, 43
  lymph nodes of, 260
Mucous membranes, changes of, in pregnancy, 419-420
Murmurs
  auscultation for, 153
  heart, 330-336
    in child, 600
Murphy's sign, 369

Muscle
  biopsy of, 502
  cramps of, 500-501
  enzyme levels of, 501
  extraocular function of, 231, 233
  mass of, measurement of, 451, 452
  of mastication, 521
  of neck, 249-250
  palsy of, 499
  of pelvic floor, 399
  and posture, 132
  rectus abdominis, 349
  sounds of activity of, 357
  spasticity of, assessment of, 363
  strength of, testing for, 453-455
    by functional group, 458-495
  testing of, chart for, 496-498
  weakness of, 498-500
Musculoskeletal system
  assessment of, 443-517
    of aged client, 630
    of child, 604-607
  changes of, in pregnancy, 420
  in health history, 43-44
Myalgia, 501-502
Myasthenia gravis, 521
Mydriasis, 241
Myoclonus, nocturnal, 120

N

Nails
  assessment of, 136, 180-204
  examination of, 300
  in health history, 42
Narcolepsy, 121-122
National Center for Health Statistics, 103
  Task Force, 578
National High Blood Pressure Coordination Committee, 628
National Nutrition Survey, 91, 99, 101
NCHS; *see* National Center for Health Statistics
Neck
  assessment of, 249-255
    of child, 595
  cutaneous fields of, 521
  in health history, 43
  lymphatic drainage of, 260-266
  muscles of, 249-250
  musculature of, assessment of, 454
  strength and range of motion of, testing for, 458-460
  vessels in, assessment of, 340-347
Neonatal Behavioral Assessment Scale, 66
Nerves
  acoustic, 524-527
  cranial, relationship of, to eye structures, 229
  function of, 518, 553
  glossopharyngeal, 527
  optic, damage to, 238-239
  hypoglossal, 528, 532
  peripheral, cutaneous fields of, 542-543
  trigeminal and facial, 247, 523-524
Nervous system
  in health history, 43
  maturation of, 67
Neural system assessment in aged client, 631
Neuralgia, trigeminal, 523
Neuritis, 523
Neurofibromatosis, 182

Neurological adequacy, assessment of, 455
Neurological assessment, 518-559
  in child, 607-621
Neuromuscular aspects of vision, 227-228
Neuroses, 177
Neutrophilopenia, 666
Nevus, 182
Newborn reflexes, 68
Niacin deficiency, 101
Night terrors, 119
Nipples, 275
Nocturnal erection, 123
Nocturnal myoclonus, 120
Nodule, 196
  Sr. Mary Joseph's, 372
Nonverbal communication, 25-26, 30-33
Normal values, 684-701
Nose
  assessment of, 213-216
    of aged client, 627
    of child, 599-600
  in health history, 42
NREM sleep, 118
Nuchal rigidity, 556
Nuclear fragments, 665
Nursing bottle syndrome, 562
Nutrients
  bioavailability of, 93
  biochemical appraisal of, 107-109
  deficiency of
    development of, 92, 93
    symptoms of, 101-102
  intake of
    interpretation of, 101
    standards of evaluation of, 98
Nutritional assessment, 91-112
  of child, interview form for, 565-569
Nutritional data in health history, 46
Nutritional status, assessment of, 108
  form for, 110-111
Nylen-Bárány test, 524-525
Nystagmus, 233

O

Obesity, 103
  of child, 563-564
Object permanence, 68
Obsessional neurosis, 177
Obturator muscle test, 372, 374
Oculesics as kinesis, 30
Oculomotor paralysis, 239
Odor, body, assessment of, 136
Old age, recommendations for, 14
Olfactory area, 214
Olfactory nerve, 518-520
Onycholysis, 185, 186
Onychomadesis, 185
Open angle glaucoma, chronic, 244
Operations in health history, 40
Ophthalmoscope, 18, 22-23
  use of, 235-237
Oppenheim's reflex, 551, 553
Optic disk, 226
Optic nerve damage, 238-239
Oral cavity, symptoms of nutrient deficiency in, 102
Oral temperature, 141
Organic brain syndrome, 175-176

Orientation, assessment of, 170
Oropharynx
    assessment of, of child, 600
    culture from, 416
    orthopedic disorders involving, 605
Ortolani test, 606
Otosclerosis, 627
Otoscope, 23-24
    use of, 207-208
        with child, 599
Ovaries, 400
Oxygen, blood, 653

P

Paget's disease, 278
Pain
    abdominal, sites of, 373, 374-375
    joint, 502-503
    sensation of, 539
    and sleep disorders, 124
Pallor, 181-183
Palpation, 15
    bimanual, 364-365
        of adnexa and uterus, 407
        of breasts, 282, 285
    deep, 364
        pelvic, 432, 433
    fundal, 431-432
    lateral, 432
    light, 362-363
    moderate, 363-364
    Pawlick, 432-433
    of sinuses, 216
Palpitations, causes of, 150, 151
Palsy
    Bell's, 523
    muscle, 499
Pancreas, assessment of, 370
Papanicolaou smear, 414-415
Papilledema, 242
Papule, 196
Paralysis
    oculomotor and abducens, 239
    sleep, 122
Paranoid ideation, 175
Parasomnias, 123-124
Parenting in middle adulthood, 80-81
Paresthesia, 537
Parkinsonism, 498
Paronychia, 185-186
Parosmia, 520
Parotid gland, 216
Parotid lymph center, 260
Passive motion, 456
Patellar reflex, 549, 551
Patent urachus, 372
Pawlick palpation, 432-433
Peau d'orange breast, 278, 280
Pectoralis reflex, 548
Pectoriloquy, whispered, 320
Pectus carinatum, 298
Pectus excavatum, 298
Pederson speculum, 403
Pediatric client, assessment of, 559-622
Pediatric reference values, 699-701
Peers, effect of, in development, 73

Pelvis
    bones of, 435
    bony, examination of, 434-442
    inlet planes of, 435
    organs of, male, 386
    outlet of, 436
    palpation of, deep, 432, 433
    types of, 436, 437
Penis, 388-389
    circumcised, 386
Percussion, 15-18
    immediate, 302-303
    mediate, 304-305
Pericardial friction rub, 331
Pericardium, 323-324
Perihypersomnia, 121
Perionychium, 184
Peripheral nerves, cutaneous fields of, 542-543
Perirectal abscess, 383
Peristalsis, 354, 355
Peritoneal friction rub, 356-357
Personality development, 67
pH
    blood, 654
    urine, 668
Phalangeal joint, 508
Pharmaceutical agents, effect of, on sleep, 125
Pharmaceutical history of aged client, 625-626
Pharynx, 292
Phimosis, 389
Phobia, 177
Phoria, 239
Phospholipids, 659
Phosphorus, serum, 652-653
Physical examination, screening, 632-645
Physicians, control of health care by, 1
Pica, 419
Pigment band, 189
Pigmentation
    skin, 352
    variations in, 183
Pigmy, African, 130
Pilonidal cyst, 381
Piskacek's sign, 423-424
Pituitary hyposomatic dwarfism, 130
Plantar reflex, 550-551, 552
Plasma albumin, 657
Plasma cells, 666
Plasma globulins, 658
Plasma lipids, 658-660
Plasma proteins, 657-658
Platyonychia, 185
Play in toddler years, 71, 72
Pleural friction rub, 309
Pleximeter, 15, 16
Plexor, 15, 16
Poikilocytosis, 665
Polycythemia, 663
Polyps, rectal, 382
Popliteal lymph center, 271
Popliteal pulse, 147
Positions for rectal examination, 377
Postauricular lymph center, 260
Posterior axillary lines, 294
Posterior tibial pulse, 147-148
Postprandial glucose test, 655

Posture
  assessment of, 132-134
  and behavior, 162
  as kinesis, 30
Potassium, serum, 651
Preauricular lymph center, 260, 261
Precocious puberty, 132
Pregnancy
  assessment during, 418-442
  changes in breast during, 278
Pregnancy age group, recommendations for, 5
Prenatal client, health assessment of, 418-442
Presbycusis, 627
Preschool children, recommendation for, 7
Primary lesions, 196-197, 199
Proctoscopy, 380
Progeria, 132
Projection, 175
Prolapse
  rectal, 383
  uterine, 404
Proprioception, 532-537
  and posture, 132
Prostate gland, 380, 387, 388, 389-394
Proteins
  plasma, 657-658
  urine, 668-669
Proteinuria, 669
Protrusion of eyes, unilateral, 520
Proxemics, 31-32
Pruritus, 630
Pruritus ani, 381
Psoriasis, 187
Psychological system in health history, 45-46
Psychosocial development in middle childhood, 73-74
Psychotropic drugs, 119
Pterygium, 240, 241
Ptosis, 239
Puberty
  precocious, 132
  signs of, 76
Puddle sign, 360, 361
Pulsation, assessment of, 142-153
Pulse deficit, 148-149
Pulse pressure, 153
  assessment of, 158
Pulses
  of aged client, 628
  bigeminal, 149
  brachial, 143, 146
  carotid, 143, 144, 343
    arterial, 344
  of child, 575-576
  dorsal pedal, 147
  femoral, 145, 146-147
  jugular venous, 342-343
  popliteal, 147
  radial, 143, 145
  and temperature, 141
  tibial, posterior, 147-148
Pulsus alternans, 149-150
  assessment of, 158
Pulsus paradoxus, 150-151
  assessment of, 158
Pupils, 225
  Argyll Robertson, 241
  examination of, 235

Pupils—cont'd
  pathology of, 241
Pustule, 197
Pyogenic infection of lymph nodes, 273
Pyorrhea, advanced, 220
Pyridoxine deficiency, 102

Q

Quadriceps strength, assessment of, 457

R

Racket nails, 185
Radial pulse, 143, 145
Radiation, 139
Rales, 307-308
Range of joint motion
  assessment of, 455-457
  limitations of, 503
  testing for, by functional groups, 458-495
Rationalization, 175
Rebound tenderness, 365-366
Recent Life Changes Questionnaire, 84-87
Recommended Daily Allowances, 98-99
Rectocele, 404
Rectosigmoid region, assessment of, 376-384
Rectovaginal examination, bimanual, 408-414
Rectum, 376
  abscesses of, 383-384
  examination of, positions for, 377
  polyps of, 382
  prolapse of, 383
  temperature taken by, 141
Rectus abdominis muscles, 349
  diastasis of, 348
Red blood cells, 663-665
  urinary, 669
Red reflex, 237
Reflexes, 544-554
  abdominal, 374
  Babinski's, 550, 553, 611, 620
  corneal light, 231, 234
  grasp, 554, 609, 611
  Moro, 610-611
  newborn, 68
  red, 237
  rooting, 609-611
  tendon, deep, 544, 548
  tonic neck, 610, 620
Reiter protein complement fixation test, 667
Relatives of client, interviewing, 29-30
Relaxation techniques, 397
REM sleep, 117-118
Renal insufficiency, chronic, 122
Reproductive status of aged client, 629-630
Research, sleep, 115
Respiration, pattern of, 299
Respiratory alterations and sleep disorders, 124
Respiratory movement of abdomen, 354
Respiratory system
  assessment of, 289-320
    of aged client, 627-628
  changes of, in pregnancy, 420
  in health history, 43
Respiratory tract, upper, infections of, 498
Restless legs syndrome, 120
Reticulocytes, 664-665

Retina, 225-227
  disc of; *see* Disc of retina
Retinal background, 227
  pathology of, 243-244
Retinal vessels, 226-227
  examination of, 237
  pathology of, 242-243
Retirement, 623
Retropharyngeal lymph center, 260
Rheumatoid arthritis
  juvenile, 607
  and sleep disorders, 124
Rhythms
  biological, 113-114
    and temperature, 139
  circadian and seasonal, of nail growth, 184
Riboflavin deficiency, 101, 102
Ribs, inspection of, 299
Rinne test, 210, 211, 212
Risk factors, prenatal, 422
Ronchi, 308-309
Rooting reflex, 609, 611
Rotation, 443, 445
RPCF test; *see* Reiter protein complement fixation test

S

Sacrosciatic notch, 439
Salivary glands, 216
Salmon's law, 382
Scabies, 193
Scale, 198
Scapular line, 294
Scapular lymph center, 266
Scar(s), 198
  of abdomen, 352-353
Schäffer's reflex, 551
Schiøtz tonometer, 237
Schizophrenia, 122
Schizophrenic disorders, 176-177
School Breakfast Program, 91
School Lunch Program, 91
School-aged children, recommendations for, 8
Schools, effect of, in development, 73
Schwabach test, 213
Sclera, 223, 225
  examination of, 234
  pathology of, 240
Sclerosis, amyotrophic lateral, 521
Scoliosis, 447, 448, 607
Scotoma, 239
Scratch test, 356
Screening physical examination, 632-645
Screening tests, developmental, 61, 66
Scrotum, 385, 387, 389
  abnormalities of, 390-391
  palpation of, 603
Sebaceous glands, 180, 189
Second heart sound, 327-329
Secondary lesions, 198-199
Sedimentation rate, 664
Self-examination of breasts, 285
Seminal fluid, normal values for, 696
Seminal vesicles, 387, 388
Senile cataracts, 242
Senile telangiectasia, 631
Sensorimotor period, 67
Sensorium, assessment of, 165-175

Sensory function, 537-544
Sensory loss, 541, 542-544
  in aging, 624
Serum calcium, 652
Serum chloride, 651-652
Serum enzymes, 660-663
Serum fibrinogen, 658
Serum glutamic-oxaloacetic transaminase, 660-661
Serum glutamic-pyruvic transaminase, 661
Serum magnesium, 653
Serum phosphorus, 652-653
Serum potassium, 651
Serum sodium, 650-651
Serum uric acid, 657
Sexual identification in early childhood, 71
SGOT; *see* Serum glutamic-oxaloacetic transaminase
SGPT; *see* Serum glutamic-pyruvic transaminase
Shifting dullness, test for, 359, 360
Shingles, 523
Shoulder joint, 505, 506
  strength and range of motion of, testing for, 463-470
Siderotic granules, 665
Sigmoid colon, 376
Sigmoidoscopy, 380-381
Sims's position, 377
Sinuses
  development of, 597
  in health history, 42
  paranasal, 213-216
Sr. Mary Joseph's nodule, 372
Skene's glands, 398, 402
Skin
  assessment of, 180-204
    abdominal, 352-353
    in aged client, 630
    in child, 594
  changes of, in pregnancy, 419-420
  in health history, 42
  symptoms of nutrient deficiency in, 101-102
Skinfold thickness measurement, 103-106
Skull
  bones of, 246-247
  transillumination of, 595
Sleep, 117-118
Sleep apnea, 124
Sleep attacks, 121
Sleep research, 115
Sleeping pills, 119
Sleep-wakefulness patterns, assessment of, 113-127
Slow-wave sleep, 118
Smear procedures, 414-416
Smell, ability to, 519
Snellen chart, 229
Social-adaptive-personal development by age, 62-65
Social-personal behavior development, 60
Society of Actuaries, 103
Sociological system in health history, 44-45
Sociopath, 177-178
Sodium, serum, 650-651
"Soft" signs, 556-557
Somnambulism, 123
Soto's syndrome, 131
Sound(s)
  adventitious, assessment of, 307-309
  bowel, 354, 355
  breath, assessment of, 307
  cardiovascular, 326-327

Sound(s)—cont'd
  heart, 327-331
  percussion, 17
  properties of, 17-18
  vascular, of abdomen, 355-356
  voice, assessment of, 309, 320
Spasms, 500
Special Milk Program, 91
Specialization, effect of, 1-2
Specific gravity of, urine, 668
Speculums, 403, 404
  nasal, 214-215
Speech, assessment of, 136, 162-165
Spence, tail of, 277
Sphygmomanometer, 153-156
Sphygmomanometer cuff, 156-157
Spinal accessory nerve, 527
Spinal nerve, chain of, 263
Spleen, assessment of, 359, 368-370
Splitting of second heart sound, 328-329
Squatting position, 377
Standards of Child Health Care, 61
Stereognosis, 539, 540
Sternoclavicular joint, 504-505
Stethoscope
  development of, 18
  types of, 18-21
  use of, 339
Sthenic body type, 129
Stippling, basophilic, 665
Stomach, assessment of, 359
Stool, examination of, 380, 669-670
Stool cycle of infant, 564-565
Strabismus, 239
  testing child for, 598
Straight leg-raising test, 516
Strength, assessment of, 454, 457
Stretch reflex, 546
Striae of abdomen, 352
Strictures, anorectal, 377
Sty, 240
Subclavian lymph center, 266
Sublingual gland, 216
Submandibular gland, 216
Submandibular lymph center, 260, 265
Submental lymph center, 260, 265
Suboccipital lymph center, 260
Subpubic arch, 438
Suggested Guide to Interpretation of Nutrient Intake Data, 99
Summation gallop, 330
Superficial cervical chain, 260-261
Superficial inguinal lymph center, 272-273
Superficial temporal pulse, 143, 144
Supra–levator ani muscle abscess, 384
Suprasternal notch, 294
Surveys, dietary, 94-99
Sweat glands, 180
Swelling, joint, 503
Symphysis pubis, 438, 439
Symptom(s)
  description of, for health history, 33
  investigation of, 38-40
Synovial fluid, normal values for, 696
Syphilis, 667-668
  lymph nodes in, 274
Systole, 325
Systolic arterial blood pressure, 153

Systolic murmurs, 333-335
Systolic pressure, normal, 157

T

Tachycardia, 148, 150
Tactile discrimination, 539-541
Tail of Spence, 277
Talipes equinovarus, 605
Talocalcaneal joint, 514-515
Taste sensations, 524
Technicon SMA 12/60 multichannel analyzer, 648-649
Teeth
  of child, 600
  examination of, 218
Telangiectasia, senile, 631
Temperature
  assessment of, 138-141
  effect of age on, 139
  of children, 574-576
  sensation, 539
Temporal artery, 247, 248
Temporomandibular joint, 503-504
  palpation of, 218
Tendons and posture, 132
Tenesmus, rectal, 381-382
Tensilon test, 498
Ten-State Survey, 1968-1970, 91, 100, 101
Territoriality, 31-32
Tests
  Bárány's, 524, 525
  Barlow's, 606
  cover-uncover, 232, 233
  exercise, 152
  flocculation, 667
  fluorescent treponemal antibody absorption, 667
  glucose, postprandial, 655
  guaiac, 380, 381
  of hearing, 209-213
  human chorionic gonadotropin, 423
  iliopsoas muscle, 372, 374
  leg-raising, straight, 516
  Nylen-Bárány, 524-525
  obturator muscle, 372, 374
  Ortolani, 606
  of range of motion, 458-495
  Reiter protein complement fixation, 667
  Rinne, 210, 211, 212
  Schwabach, 213
  scratch, 356
  screening developmental, 61, 66
  Tensilon, 498
Tetanus, 523
Tetany, 500
Texture of skin, 183
Thayer-Martin culture, 415
Thermography, 286
Thermometry, 141
Third heart sound, 329
Thom's pelvimeter, 440
Thorax, 290, 291, 293, 294, 295, 296, 297
  barrel, 298
  cage of, 290, 291, 293, 294, 295, 296, 297
  of child
    assessment of, 600
    circumference of, 592-593
  expansion of, assessment of, 300-301
  inspection of configuration of, 298

Throat in health history, 43
Thrombocytes, 665
Thrombocytopenia, 665
Thrombocytosis, 665
Thumb strength and range of motion, testing for, 476-479
Thyroid gland, assessment of, 250-255
Thyroid hormone alterations, 122
Thyrolinguofacial chain, 262
Tibial pulse, posterior, 147-148
Tibial torsion, 606
Tic douloureux, 523
Tissue degeneration with aging, 626
Tissue thickness of child, 592-594
Toe
   hammer, 514, 515
   strength and range of motion of, testing for, 492-495
Tongue
   examination of, 218, 220
   pathology of, lymph nodes involved in, 267
   strength of, 528
Tonic neck reflex, 610, 620
Tonometer, Schiøtz, 237
Torticollis, 604
Touch as kinesis, 30
TPI test; *see Treponema pallidum* immobilization test
Trachea, 292, 298
   deviation of, assessment of, 301-302
Transient ischemic attacks, 499-500
Transillumination of skull, 595
Transverse cervical chain, 263
Tremor classification, 501
Treponema pallidum, 667
Treponema pallidum immobilization test, 667
Triceps reflex, 549, 550
Triceps strength, assessment of, 455
Trichomonads, 416
Trigeminal nerve, 247, 520-524
Trigeminal neuralgia, 523
Triglycerides, 658-659
Tropia, 239
Trousseau's sign, 500
Trunk strength and range of motion, testing for, 460-463
Tuberculosis, lymph nodes in, 274
Tuning fork, use of, 209-213
Turgor of skin, 184
Twenty-Four Hour Recall Dietary Survey, 95
Twitch, 500
Two-point discrimination, 539, 540
Tympanic membrane, 205, 207, 209

U

Ulcer, duodenal, and sleep disorders, 124
Ulnar pulse, 143, 145
Umbilicus, assessment of, 372-374
Uncover-cover test, 232, 233
Upper arm circumference, percentiles for, 105
Urachus, patent, 372
Urethral culture, 416
Urethral meatus, malposition of, 389
Uric acid, serum, 657
Urinalysis, 668-669
Urinary bladder, 372
Urinary casts, 669
Urinary crystals, 669
Urinary output of infant, 564
Urinary red blood cells, 669

Urinary system in health history, 43
Urine, normal values for, 692-695
Urine glucose, 668
Urine pH, 668
Urine proteins, 668-669
U.S. Census Bureau, 623
Uterus, 399
   bimanual palpation of, 407
   changes in, in pregnancy, 418-419
   enlargement of, in pregnancy, 423
   examination of, 411
   fundus of, 426, 427, 428, 431-432
   prolapse of, 404

V

Vagina, 399
   changes in, in pregnancy, 418-419
   examination of, bimanual, 408-413
   infections of, 416
   pool smear of, 415
Vagus nerve, 527
Valgus deformity, 447, 448
Valsalva's maneuver, 378
Valve
   alterations of, 331-333
   of heart, 321-323
Varus deformity, 447, 448
Vascular sounds of abdomen, 355-356
VDRL; *see* Venereal Disease Research Laboratory test
Vegetarian diets, 97
Veins, jugular, 340-344
Venereal Disease Research Laboratory test, 667
Venous engorgement, 374
Venous flow, direction of, 371
Venous hum, 335, 336, 355-356
Venous pressure, jugular, 343-344
Ventricles, hypertrophy of, 338-339
Vertebra prominens, 294
Vesicle, 196
Vessels
   great, 323
   of neck, assessment of, 340-347
   retinal, 226-227
      examination of, 237
      pathology of, 242-243
Vestibular division of acoustic nerve, 524
Vestibular oculogyric reflex, 520
Vestibular organs and posture, 132
Vibration sensation, 539
Vision
   development of, 70
      in middle childhood, 73
   loss of, 624
   neuromuscular aspects of, 227-228
   pathways and fields of, 227
Visual acuity, 229-230
   pathology of, 238
Visual fields, 230-231
   pathology of, 238-239
Vital signs, assessment of, 137-159
Vitamin A deficiency, 101
Vitamins, daily intake of, 100
Vitiligo, 182
Vocalics, 32
Voice sound assessment, 309, 320

W

Wakefulness-sleep patterns, assessment of, 113-127
Wartenberg's reflex, 551
Wassermann test, 667
Watch-glass nails, 189
Waves, pulse, abnormalities of, 342-343
Weber test, 210, 211, 212, 213
Weighing machines, 107
Weight
   of aged client, 626
   assessment of, 131-132
   of children, 105, 591-592
   desirable, 104
   gain of, in pregnancy, 425
   loss of, unexplained, 131
   smoothed average, 104
Wheal, 197
Whispered pectoriloquy, 320
White blood cell count, 665-666
White blood cells, urinary, 669
White House Conference on Aging, 1

White House Conference on Food, Nutrition, and Health, 91
WHO; *see* World Health Organization
Women in middle adulthood, 81
Workplace, hazards of, 671-676
Worksheet for recording physical examination, 642-645
World Health Organization, 3, 156, 158
Wrist joint, 507, 508
   strength of
      assessment of, 455
      and range of motion of, testing for, 474-475

X

x descent, 342
Xanthelasma, 240
Xerography, 286
Xerophthalmia, 101
Xerosis, 101

Y

y descent, 343
Young adults, sleep patterns in, 118